Ultrasound

A Practical Approach to Clinical Problems

Ultrasound

A Practical Approach to Clinical Problems

Editors

Edward I. Bluth, M.D.
Chairman, Department of Radiology
Ochsner Clinic
New Orleans, Louisiana

Peter H. Arger, M.D. F.A.C.R.
Professor of Radiology and Obstetrics and Gynecology
University of Pennsylvania Medical Center
Philadelphia, Pennsylvania

Carol B. Benson, M.D.
Associate Professor of Radiology
Harvard Medical School
Co-Director of High Risk Obstetrical Ultrasound
Brigham & Women's Hospital
Boston, Massachusetts

Philip W. Ralls, M.D.
Professor and Vice Chair
Department of Radiology
University of Southern California School of Medicine
Los Angeles, California

Marilyn J. Siegel, M.D.
Professor of Radiology and Pediatrics
Washington University School of Medicine
Mallinckrodt Institute of Radiology
St. Louis, Missouri

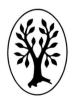

2000
Thieme
New York · Stuttgart

Thieme New York
333 Seventh Avenue
New York, NY 10001

Executive Editor: Jane Pennington
Editorial Director: Avé McCracken
Editorial Assistant: Todd Warnock
Developmental Manager: Kathleen P. Lyons
Director, Production & Manufacturing: Anne Vinnicombe
Production Editor: Gert A. Krueger
Marketing Director: Phyllis Gold
Sales Manager: Ross Lumpkin
Chief Financial Officer: Seth S. Fishman
President: Brian D. Scanlan
Cover Designer: Renate Stockinger
Compositor: primustype R. Hurler GmbH
Printer: G. Canale & C.

Library of Congress Cataloging-in-Publication Data

Ultrasound : a practical approach to clinical problems / editors,
Edward I. Bluth... [et al.].
  p. cm.
Includes bibliographical references and index.
ISBN 0-86577-895-7
1. Diagnosis, Ultrasonic. I. Bluth, Edward I.
[DNLM: 1. Ultrasonography. WN 208 U472 1999]
RC78.7.U4 U4462 1999
616.07'543 21–dc21   99-040816

Important Note: Medical knowledge is ever-changing. As new research and clinical experience broaden our knowledge, changes in treatment and drug therapy may be required. The authors and editors of the material herein have consulted sources believed to be reliable in their efforts to provide information that is complete and in accord with the standards accepted at the time of publication. However, in view of the possibility of human error by the authors, editors, or publisher of the work herein, or changes in medical knowledge, neither the authors, editors, publishers, nor any other party who has been involved in the preparation of this work, warrants that the information contained herein is in every respect accurate or complete, and they are not responsible for any errors or omissions or for the results obtained from use of such information. Readers are encouraged to confirm the information contained herein with other sources. For example, readers are advised to check the product information sheet included in the package of each drug they plan to administer to be certain that the information contained in the publication is accurate and that changes have not been made in the recommended dose or in the contraindications for administration. This recommendation is of particular importance in connection with new or infrequently used drugs.

Some material contained in this book was originally printed by the Radiological Society of North America in November 1996, as a syllabus to accompany a categorical course in ultrasound given at the 1996 Annual Meeting and Scientific Assembly. That material has been printed here with the approval of the RSNA. The editors would like to acknowledge the support of the RSNA in this project.

Some of the product names, patents, and registered designs referred to in this book are in fact registered trademarks or proprietary names even though specific reference to this fact is not always made in the text. Therefore, the appearance of a name without designation as propietary is not to be construed as a representation by the publisher that it is in the public domain.

Printed in Italy
5 4 3 2 1

TNY ISBN 0-86577-861-2
GTV ISBN 3-13-116831-5

Dedications

We dedicate this book to our families and friends who supported us in this project:

Ed Bluth to Elissa, Rachel, Jonathan, Marjorie, and Irene with gratitude and love.

Peter Arger to Afento and Harry, Donald and Anastasia, Eugenia and Nicholas, to whom he is immensely grateful as they have profoundly influenced his whole approach to life.

Carol Benson to her husband, Peter, and her children, Nicole and Benjamin.

Phil Ralls to Renee, Colin, and Whitney with love.

Marilyn Siegel to her husband, Barry.

Contents

Superficial Organs

Acknowledgement

The authors would like to thank Drs. Carol Stelling, Barbara Hertzberg and William Middleton for their help with the conceptual origins for this project.

List of Contributors

Ronald S. Adler, PhD, MD
Division of Ultrasound
The Hospital for Special Surgery
New York, NY
Professor of Radiology
Weill Medical College
Cornell University
Ithaca, NY

Peter H. Arger, MD
Professor of Radiology and OB/GYN
Department of Radiology
University of Pennsylvania Medical Center
Philadelphia, PA

Sam T. Auringer, MD
Associate Professor of Radiology and Pediatrics
Department of Radiology
Division of Radiological Sciences
Wake Forest University School of Medicine
Winston-Salem, NC

Catherine J. Babcook, MD, FRCP(C)
Associate Professor of Radiology and OB/GYN
Director of Women's Imaging
Department of Radiology
University of Utah Health Sciences Center
Salt Lake City, UT

Kurt Barnhart, MD, MSCE
Assistant Professor of Ob/GYN
Division for Reproductive Endocrinology and Infertility
University of Pennsylvania Medical Center
Philadelphia, PA

Thomas R. Beidle, MD, RVT
Associate Professor of Radiology
LSU School of Medicine
New Orleans, LA

Richard D. Bellah, MD
Associate Professor of Radiology and Pediatrics
University of Pennsylvania School of Medicine
Children's Hospital of Philadelphia
Philadelphia, PA

Beryl R. Benacerraf, MD
Director of Obstetrics and Ultrasound
Massachusetts General Hospital
Clinical Professor of OB/GYN and Radiology
Harvard Medical School
Boston, MA

Carol B. Benson, MD
Associate Professor of Radiology
Harvard Medical School
Codirector of High Risk Obstetrical Ultrasound
Department of Radiology
Brigham and Women's Hospital
Boston, MA

Edward I. Bluth, MD
Chairman
Department of Radiology
Ochsner Clinic
Clinical Professor
Tulane University School of Medicine
New Orleans, LA

Robert L. Bree, MD
Department of Radiology
University of Michigan Medical Center
Ann Arbor, MI

Gregory A. Broderick, MD, FACS
Department of Urology
Mayo Clinic
Jacksonville, FL

Douglas L. Brown
Associate Professor Radiology
Harvard Medical School
Department of Radiology
Brigham and Women's Hospital
Boston, MA

Peter W. Callen, MD
Professor of Radiology, OB-GYN, and Reproductive Sciences
Department of Radiology
University of California, School of Medicine
San Francisco, CA

Barbara A. Carroll, MD
Professor of Radiology
Department of Radiology
Duke University Medical Center
Durham, NC

Harris L. Cohen, MD
Professor of Radiology
Department of Radiology
Division of Ultrasound
SUNY Health Science Center at Brooklyn
Brooklyn, NY

Beverly G. Coleman, MD, FACR
Professor of Radiology
Director, Ultrasound Imaging
Department of Radiology
University of Pennsylvania Medical Center
Philadelphia, PA

Christos Coutifaris, MD
Assistant Professor and Interim Director
University of Pennsylvania Medical Center
Philadelphia, PA

T. David Cox, MD
Assistant Professor of Radiology and Pediatrics
Department of Radiology
Division of Radiological Sciences
Wake Forest University School of Medicine
Winston-Salem, NC

John T. Cronan, MD
Professor and Chairman
Department of Diagnostic Imaging
Brown University School of Medicine
Rhode Island Hospital
Providence, RI

Jeanne A. Cullinan, MD
Associate Professor, Chief of Service
Department of Radiological Sciences
City Avenue Hospital/Tenet Health System
Philadelphia, PA

Gerald D. Dodd, III, MD
Director of Abdominal Imaging
Professor- Department of Radiology
University of Texas Health Sciences Center
San Antonio, TX

Peter M. Doubleit, MD
Associate Professor of Radiology
Harvard Medical School

Vice Chairman
Depatment of Radiology
Brigham and Women's Hospital
Boston, MA

Arthur C. Fleischer, MD
Professor of Radiology and Radiological Sciences
Professor of OB/GYN
Chief, Diagnostic Sonography
Department of Radiology
Vanderbilt University Medical Center
Nashville, TN

W. Dennis Foley, MD
Professor of Radiology
Director, Section of Digital Imaging
Department of Radiology
Medical College of Wisconsin
Milwaukee, WI

Andrew M. Fried, MD
Professor of Radiology
Department of Diagnostic Radiology
University of Kentucky Medical Center
Lexington, KY

Ruth B. Goldstein, MD
Department of Radiology
University of California Medical Center
San Francisco, CA

Frank P. Hadlock, MD
Department of Radiology
Baylor College of Medicine
Houston, TX

Ulrike M. Hamper, MD
Associate Professor of Radiology & Urology
Director, Division of Ultrasound
John Hopkins Medical Institutions
Baltimore, MD

Barbara S. Hertzberg, MD
Professor of Radiology
Associate Professor of OB/GYN
Co-Director of Fetal Diagnostic Center
Department of Radiology
Duke University Medical Center
Durham, NC

R. Brooke Jeffrey Jr., MD
Professor of Radiology
Chief of Abdominal Imaging
Department of Radiology
Stanford University Medical Center
Stanford, CA

Robert A. Kane, MD, FACR
Associate Professor of Radiology
Harvard Medical School
Associate Chief for Administrative Affairs
Department of Radiology
Beth Israel Deaconess Medical Center
Boston, MA

Donna M. Kepple, RDMS
Vanderbilt University Medical Center
Nashville, TN

Mark A. Kliewer, MD
Associate Professor of Radiology
Department of Radiology
Duke University Medical Center
Durham, NC

Alfred B. Kurtz, MD
Professor and Vice Chair
Department of Radiology
Jefferson Medical College of
Thomas Jefferson University Hospital
Philadelphia, PA

Faye C. Laing, MD
Professor of Radiology
Director of Radiological Education & Training
Harvard Medical School
Department of Radiology
Brigham and Women's Hospital
Boston, MA

Debra M. Lau, MD
Department of Radiology
Stanford University School of Medicine
Sanford, CA

Doohi Lee, MD
Commonwealth Radiology
Richmond, VA

Janis Gissel Letourneau, MD, RVT
Professor of Radiology and Surgery
Louisiana State University Medical School
New Orleans, LA

Deborah Levine, MD
Department of Radiology
Beth Israel Deconess Hospital
Harvard Medical School
Boston, MA

Edward A. Lyons, MD, FRCP(C), FACR
Professor of Radiology and OB/GYN
Department of Radiology
University of Manitoba Health Sciences Center
Winnipeg, Manitoba

Jon McGrath, MD
Radiology Imaging Associates

Christopher R.B. Merritt, MD
Professor of Radiology
Jefferson Ultrasound Research and Education Institute
Thomas Jefferson University Hospital
Philadelphia, PA

William D. Middleton, MD
Professor of Radiology
Chief of Diagnostic Ultrasound
Washington University School of Medicine
Mallinckrodt Institute of Radiology
St. Louis, MO

Laurence Needleman, MD
Associate Professor of Radiology
Division of Ultrasound
Thomas Jefferson University Hospital
Philadelphia, PA

Harvey L. Nisenbaum, MD
Assistant Professor of Radiology
University of Pennsylvania Medical Center
Philadelphia, PA

Harriet J. Paltiel, MD
Assistant Professor of Radiology
Harvard Medical School
Department of Radiology
Children's Hospital
Boston, MA

John S. Pellerito, MD
Chief, Division of Ultrasound, CT & MRI
Department of Radiology
North Shore University Hospital
Assistant Professor of Radiology
New York University School of Medicine
Manhasset, NY

Joseph F. Polak, MPH
Department of Radiology
Harvard Medical School
Vascular Diagnostic Labratory
Brigham and Women's Hospital
Boston, MA

Philip W. Ralls, MD
Professor and Vice Chair
Department of Radiology
University of Southern California
School of Medicine
Los Angeles, CA

Cindy Rapp, RDMS
Radiology Imaging Associates

Carl L. Reading, MD
Professor of Diagnostic Radiology
Department of Radiology
Mayo Clinic
Rochester, MN

Michelle L. Robbin, MD
Chief of Ultrasound and
Assistant Professor of Radiology
Department of Radiology
University of Alabama Hospital at Birmingham
Birmingham, AL

Henrietta Kotlus Rosenberg, MD, FACR, FAAP
Chairman, Department of Radiology
Albert Einstein Medical Center
Professor of Diagnostic Imaging
Temple University School of Medicine
Philadelphia, PA

Marilyn J. Siegel, MD
Professor of Radiology and Pediatrics
Washington University School of Medicine
Mallinckrodt Institute of Radiology
St. Louis, MO

Carlos J. Sivit, MD
Professor of Radiology
Rainbow Babies and Children's Hospital
University Hospitals of Cleveland
Cleveland, OH

A. Thomas Stavros, MD, FACR
Medical Director of Ultrasound
and Nonvascular Imaging
Radiology Imaging Associates
Englewood, CO

Thomas E. Sumner, MD
Professor of Radiology and Pediatrics
Department of Radiology
Division of Radiological Sciences
Wake Forest University School of Medicine
Winston-Salem, NC

Sharlene A. Teefey, MD
Associate Professor of Radiology
Washington University School of Medicine
Mallinckodt Institute of Radiology
St. Louis, MO

Ronald R. Townsend, MD
Associate Professor of Radiology
University of Colorado Health Sciences Center
Denver, CO

Dirk J. van Leeuwen
Associate Professor of Medicine
Scientist UAB Cancer Center
Department of Gastroenterology
University of Alabama at Birmingham
Birmingham, AL

Geoffrey Wong, MD
Department of OB/GYN
Beth Israel Deaconess Medical Center
Harvard Medical School
Boston, MA

Ken Yamaguchi, MD
Department of Orthopedic Surgery
Washington University School of Medicine
St. Louis, MO

Harry L. Zinn, MD
Department of Radiology
Division of Ultrasound
SUNY-Health Science Center at Brooklyn
Brooklyn, NY

William J. Zwiebel, MD
Professor of Radiology
University of Utah School of Medicine
Chief, Radiology Service
Department of Radiology
VA Medical Center
Salt Lake City, UT

Preface

Ultrasonography has become accepted as a practical and accurate diagnostic procedure for the evaluation of pathologic processes in virtually every part of the body. The practice of ultrasonography continues to undergo remarkable changes related to improvements in instrumentation and development of new technology. These technologic advances have had a major impact on the evaluation of disease processes and present challenges for the clinician. They have stimulated a tremendous volume of literature that the practitioner should understand in order to maximize the clinical benefits of ultrasonography. In addition, these technologic improvements force the clinician to assess whether sonography or another imaging tool is the most appropriate for evaluating a clinical problem.

The role of the diagnostician is changing. Consultative responsibilities are much greater as managed care places greater demands on reduction of utilization. The choice of the most appropriate procedure becomes far more important to help minimize cost. It is the aim of this book to focus on clinical problems and help guide clinicians in choosing the most appropriate imaging examination.

The origins of this book can be traced to the 1996 Radiological Society of North America Annual Meeting at which Drs. Edward Bluth, Peter Arger, Barbara Hertzberg, and William Middleton directed a special course on ultrasound which attempted to begin to address this issue. This book expands greatly and updates that previous work.

It is the aim of this text to review the current state of sonography with regard to important clinical issues that clinicians are likely to face in their daily practice and to outline approaches for the effective use of sonography and other imaging methods. This volume is not a comprehensive textbook on ultrasonography, nor is it meant to be; rather the material included represents issues that the authors believe to be of current importance based on their daily experience. The Information in this text is intended primarily for practitioners who wish to understand the indications, limitations and clinical applications of sonography.

The book is divided into nine general areas: abdomen, female pelvis, obstetrics, vascular system, musculoskeletal system, male genital system, superficial organs, interventional and pediatrics. Practical sonographic techniques, basic sonographic anatomy, and the sonographic findings in a variety of important clinical problems are described and illustrated within each of these areas. For completeness, summary clinical information and differential diagnostic considerations of the various disorders are included in the discussion. Technical and interpretative errors that can occur with sonography are also described.

Because the clinician is often required to direct the imaging workup and select the best imaging examination for a given clinical indication, discussions of the relative values of sonography and other imaging studies are included within individual chapters. Each editor and author has an area of interest and expertise from which the current ideas and imaging approaches have been developed. We recognize that imaging approaches can vary based on personal experience and equipment. Nonetheless, we believe our recommendations and discussions on the optimal use of sonography in examining important clinical problems will serve to improve diagnostic evaluation of patients.

Edward I. Bluth, MD
Peter H. Arger, MD, FACR
Carol B. Benson, MD
Philip W. Ralls, MD
Marylin J. Siegel, MD

The Abdomen

1 Right Upper Quadrant Pain

William D. Middleton

Right upper quadrant (RUQ) pain is a common complaint that typically stimulates a work-up of the hepatobiliary system. In particular, evaluation of the gallbladder (GB) is important since cholelithiasis and its complications are a frequent cause of RUQ pain. For this reason, tests used in this condition must be capable of providing accurate information about the GB. This chapter will focus on the imaging evaluation of the patient with RUQ pain and illustrate why the use of ultrasound (US) is so important.

Differential Diagnosis

Gallstone disease is one of the most common causes of RUQ pain. Gallstones are present in approximately 10% of the population.[1] In North America, 75% of gallstones are cholesterol stones; the rest are pigment stones.[2] In women, factors that predispose to gallstones are increased weight, increased age, and increased parity. In men, increased age also predisposes to gallstones.[1]

Although gallstones are one of the most common causes of RUQ pain, the majority of patients with gallstones are asymptomatic.[2] Imaging studies performed for other reasons often discover patients with asymptomatic (silent) gallstones. Silent gallstones tend to become symptomatic at a rate of approximately 2% per year.[3,4] The overall risk after 20 years is 18%.[3] Patients with gallstones are unlikely to develop symptoms after 10—15 years of being asymptomatic. Those patients who ultimately do develop symptoms almost always have episodes of biliary colic first. It is very unusual for a patient to develop acute cholecystitis as the initial symptom of gallstone disease without previous incidents of colic. Based on these statistics and the known risk of cholecystectomy, it has been shown that performing prophylactic cholecystectomy in asymptomatic patients actually decreases their overall life expectancy and increases the cost of treatment.[5] For these reasons, asymptomatic gallstones are generally not treated surgically.

Approximately one-third of all patients with gallstones will develop symptoms. Patients with symptomatic gallstone disease generally first seek medical attention due to bouts of biliary colic. As mentioned above, patients that first present with acute cholecystitis generally will describe previous episodes consistent with biliary colic. Dyspeptic symptoms (pyrosis, flatulence, vague abdominal discomfort, and fatty food intolerance) may occur in patients with gallstones but it is hard to prove a cause-and-effect relationship because these symptoms are also very common in patients without gallstones.[2]

The symptom complex of biliary colic is produced when a stone obstructs the cystic duct. Classically, these patients experience acute RUQ or epigastric pain that increases in intensity over several seconds or minutes and then persists for several (usually 4 to 6) hours. The pain may begin in the RUQ and radiate to the epigastrium or vice versa. It may occasionally be most severe in the left upper quadrant, precordium, or even the lower abdomen.[2,6] Periodic exacerbations may occur during a given episode, but, in general, the pain is fairly steady (colic is a misnomer). In most cases, there is no obvious cause of biliary colic. In some patients, the pain is provoked by a meal. Tenderness to palpation is unusual.

Biliary colic may be relieved if the obstructing stone spontaneously disimpacts from the cystic duct. It may also be relieved if the stone passes through the cystic duct and into the bile duct. If the stone subsequently obstructs the common bile duct, a second episode of biliary colic may occur. The interval between attacks of biliary colic is very unpredictable and can vary from weeks to months to years.

Acute cholecystitis develops if there is persistent cystic duct obstruction. This diagnosis should be considered when the patient's symptoms persist beyond 6 hours. Acute cholecystitis is manifest as persistent RUQ pain that may radiate to the right shoulder, right scapula, or interscapular area. Nausea, vomiting, chills, fever, and RUQ tenderness and guarding are common. Leukocytosis and elevations of alkaline phosphatase, aminotransferase (transaminase), and amylase may occur. Mild hyperbilirubinemia is seen in as many as 20% of cases.[7] Bilirubin levels greater than 4 mg/100 ml may occur if there is common bile duct obstruction.

In addition to gallbladder disease, many other disease processes can potentially produce RUQ pain.[8] These are listed in **Table 1–1**. In particular, liver diseases should be strongly considered including diffuse hepatic parenchymal diseases such as hepatitis (viral, alcoholic, drug induced, or toxin induced) or passive hepatic congestion,

Table 1–1   Differential diagnosis of RUQ pain

1. Biliary colic
2. Acute cholecystitis
3. Acute pancreatitis
4. Acute appendicitis
5. Disorders of the liver
   A.   Acute hepatitis
        1. Alcoholic
        2. Viral
        3. Drug-related
        4. Toxins
   B.   Hepatic abscess
   C.   Hepatic tumors
        1. Metastases
        2. Hepatocellular cancer
        3. Hemangioma
        4. Focal nodular hyperplasia
        5. Hepatic adenoma
   D.   Hemorrhagic cyst
   E.   Hepatic congestion
        1. Budd-Chiari syndrome
        2. Acute hepatic congestion
6. Disorders of the bile ducts
   A.   Bile duct obstruction
   B.   Cholangitis
7. Disorders of the intestines
   A.   Peripyloric ulcers with or without perforation
   B.   Small bowel obstruction
   C.   Irritable bowel
   D.   Colitis
   E.   Ileitis
   F.   Intestinal tumors
8. Costochondritis of the lower right anterior chest
9. Perihepatitis due to gonococcal or chlamydial infection (Fitz-Hugh-Curtis syndrome)
10. Pleuroabdominal pain due to pneumonia or pulmonary infarction
11. Disorders of the right kidney
    A.   Acute pyelonephritis
    B.   Ureteral calculus
    C.   Renal or perirenal abscess
    D.   Renal infarction
    E.   Renal tumor
12. Unknown causes
13. *Herpes zoster*

Table 1–2   Causes of RUQ pain

Common	Uncommon	Rare
Biliary colic	Drug-related and toxic hepatitis	Budd-Chiari syndrome
Cholecystitis		Hepatic hemangioma
Acute pancreatitis	Hepatic abscess	Hepatic adenoma
Acute appendicitis	Hepatocellular carcinoma	Focal nodular hyperplasia
Alcoholic hepatitis	Ascending cholangitis	
Viral hepatitis	Acute pyelonephritis	Pneumonia/pleuritis
Hepatic metastases	Renal tumor	Renal abscess
Irritable bowel	Peptic ulcer disease	Perinephric abscess
Costochon- dritis		Renal infarction
Unknown causes		Perihepatitis (Fitz-Hugh-Curtis syndrome)

or focal hepatic diseases. Focal liver tumors can produce pain due to rapid growth, bleeding, or infarction. Hepatic abscesses, perihepatitis (Fitz-Hugh-Curtis syndrome), hematomas, and hemorrhagic cysts are also capable of producing RUQ pain.

The bile ducts can also be responsible for RUQ pain. Biliary colic from an obstructing common bile duct stone is probably the most frequent cause of bile duct-related RUQ pain. Cholangitis, choledochal cysts, and tumors are other possibilities.

Pancreatitis may also cause confusion because it can both simulate and coexist with GB disease. A transient episode of biliary colic may be followed by an episode of pancreatitis as the stone passes through the common duct and obstructs the pancreatic duct.

Gastrointestinal abnormalities should also be considered in the differential diagnosis. Appendicitis occasionally presents primarily as RUQ pain. Peptic ulcer disease, colitis, ileitis, intestinal obstruction, irritable bowel syndrome, and intestinal tumors are additional considerations.

The right kidney is another source of RUQ pain. Renal colic may present with atypical symptoms and be confused with GB disease. Pyelonephritis, renal abscess, hematoma, hemorrhagic cysts, tumors, and ischemia are other renal diseases that can cause RUQ pain.

Miscellaneous other processes to be considered in patients with RUQ pain are right lower-lobe pneumonia and pulmonary infarction, myocardial ischemia, local chest and abdominal wall lesions, local musculoskeletal lesions, right adrenal lesions and herpes zoster.

The relative prevalence of the different causes of RUQ pain varies from institute to institute. **Table 1–2** categorizes these causes by their approximate prevalence.

Diagnostic Evaluation

Nonimaging tests

In many patients with RUQ pain, a careful history and physical examination will help guide the work-up in the appropriate direction. However, the signs and symptoms of the many conditions potentially capable of causing RUQ pain overlap greatly. For this reason, there is a multitude of useful diagnostic tests. The most common tests are (1) liver function tests, (2) amylase levels, (3) urinalysis, (4) white blood cell counts, and (5) electrocardiograms (ECGs) .

Liver function tests (LFTs) are among the most useful initial laboratory tests because certain abnormalities strongly suggest hepatobiliary disease. In addition, the pattern of LFT abnormality on LFTs can point toward liver parenchymal processes or biliary processes. (Please see the chapter on evaluation of abnormal LFTs.) Renal, pancreatic, and cardiac abnormalities can be identified in many cases by obtaining a urinalysis, serum amylase level, and an ECG.

Imaging Tests Other than Ultrasound

The initial imaging tests in patients with RUQ pain should be radiographs of the chest and abdomen. These are rapid and inexpensive ways of evaluating the patient for pulmonary and intestinal sources of pain. In addition, abdominal radiographs can detect calcifications in the kidney, ureter, and pancreas. Gallstones that are sufficiently calcified to be radiopaque (10—15% of cases) can also be detected. Therefore, while abdominal radiographs may reveal gallstones, a negative study does not exclude the diagnosis.

If the patient presents with suspected biliary colic and the preliminary tests fail to suggest an alternative source of pain, then the GB should be evaluated to determine the presence or absence of gallstones. In addition to abdominal radiographs, there are a number of imaging tests that are capable of detecting gallstones. The sensitivity of these various tests is indicated in **Table 1–3**.

Table 1–3 Sensitivity of imaging tests for gallstones

Test	Sensitivity (%)
Radiography	15
CT	80
Oral cholecystography	65—90
Ultrasound	95

CT is much better at detecting small degrees of calcification than plain radiography and is therefore more sensitive at detecting gallstones. CT can also detect some cholesterol stones that are less dense than surrounding bile. In addition, unlike abdominal radiography, CT can determine the anatomic location of a calcification and confirm that it is in the gallbladder. Unfortunately, at least 20% of gallstones have the same attenuation as bile and are not detectable with CT.[9] For this reason, CT is useful when positive but not useful when negative.

Oral cholecystography (OCG) was the preferred means of diagnosing gallstones for many years. When the gallbladder is well opacified, OCG is similar to sonography in its ability to detect and exclude gallstones. Sensitivity decreases somewhat if opacification is faint on an OCG. In approximately 25% of OCGs, the gallbladder is not opacified. If nonvisualization of the gallbladder is considered a positive result, then the sensitivity of OCG for detecting stones is as high as 90—95%.[10,11] Unfortunately, there are many nonbiliary causes of nonvisualization. These include failure to take the contrast, vomiting, diarrhea, fasting, hiatal hernia, proximal intestinal obstruction, proximal intestinal diverticulum, malabsorption, and liver disease.[11] Therefore, nonvisualization of the gallbladder is less specific for gallstones than the typical finding of a mobile filling

defect in a well-opacified gallbladder. If a nonvisualized gallbladder is considered an inconclusive result, then the sensitivity of OCG is 65%.[10]

Ultrasound Imaging

Many investigations performed in the late 1970s and early 1980s analyzed the effectiveness of sonography in detecting gallstones. Despite using static scanners and first-generation real-time equipment, these studies almost all showed that sonography was highly accurate (> 90%) in detecting gallstones. Since then, sonography has essentially replaced the OCG for the detection of gallstones. Data from slightly more recent studies continues to support this approach. One blinded prospective comparison of these techniques showed a sonographic sensitivity of 93% and an OCG sensitivity of 65%.[10] In this same study, if a nonvisualized GB on OCG was considered positive for gallstones, then the sensitivity of OCG increased to 87%. Another study on patients who were morbidly obese showed a sonographic sensitivity of 91% and specificity of 100%. In this patient population which is not ideal for sonography, the negative predictive value was still very high at 97%.[12]

The typical sonographic appearance of a gallstone is a mobile, shadowing, echogenic structure in the lumen of the gallbladder (**Fig. 1–1**). The positive predictive value of this triad of findings is 100%. When shadowing is not detected, the differential includes gallstones and tumefactive sludge. Small, mobile nonshadowing intraluminal structures are generally gallstones (**Fig. 1–2**). On the other hand, tumefactive sludge generally forms larger mass-like aggregates (**Fig. 1–3**). There is some degree of overlap in the appearance of small gallstones and sludgeballs and, occasionally, a follow-up sonogram is helpful in distinguishing these two possibilities. Nonmobile, nonshadowing structures represent adherent sludge balls or polyps (**Fig. 1–4**).[13] Gallbladder cancer can appear as a polypoid mass and can potentially simulate a benign polyp or tumefactive sludge (**Fig. 1–5 A**). Detection of mobility and vascularity are important in distinguishing these possibilities (**Fig. 1–5 B & C**).

As indicated above, the documentation of acoustic shadowing is very important in the differential diagnosis of gallstones. To optimize the detection of acoustic shadowing, as high a frequency transducer as possible should be used and it should be focused at the depth of the gallstone. Changes in the patient's position may help by clumping multiple stones together and thereby increasing the collective attenuation. Changing the transducer position may alter the tissues displayed behind the GB and make shadowing easier to visualize.

Although sonography is very good at detecting gallstones, false-negative exams do occur. Approximately one out of 20 patients with gallstones will be missed by sonography. Therefore, if the clinical suspicion is ex-

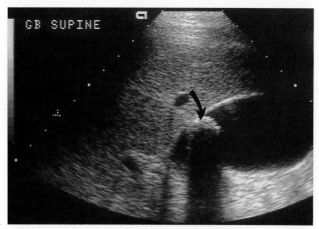

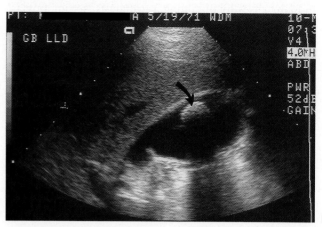

Figure 1–1 Typical gallstone. **A:** Longitudinal scan shows a shadowing echogenic structure (arrow) near the neck of the gall-bladder. **B:** Longitudinal scan with the patient in a left lateral decu-bitus position documents mobility of this stone (**arrow**) which is now seen in the body of the gallbladder.

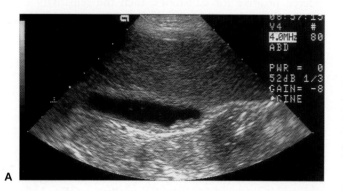

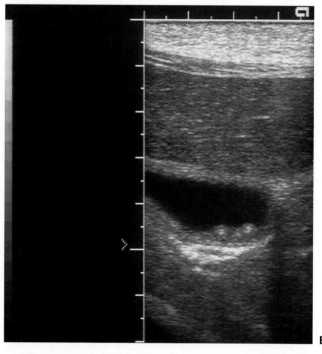

Figure 1–2 Small nonshadowing gallstones. **A:** Longitudinal scan using a 4-MHz transducer shows several small (2 mm) echogenic foci in the fundus of the gallbladder. No acoustic shadowing is ap-parent. **B:** Longitudinal scan using a 7-MHz linear array transducer shows similar findings. Although this sonographic appearance can, in general, be seen with sludge and stones, it is common to be un-able to detect shadowing in stones this small. It is very uncommon for sludge to aggregate into multiple, small, well-formed foci like this.

tremely high, it is reasonable to follow a negative US with an OCG or with a follow-up US. Reasons for a false-negative ultrasound exam include a contracted GB (**Fig. 1–6**), a GB in an anomalous or unusual location, small stones, stones impacted in the GB neck or cystic duct (**Fig. 1–7**), immobile patients, obese patients, or patients with extensive RUQ bowel gas.

Once gallstones are documented in a patient with RUQ pain, the next issue is whether the patient should undergo cholecystectomy. If the RUQ pain is clinically consistent with biliary colic, then approximately 40% of patients will have continued symptoms and 25% will have worsening symptoms. Because of this, surgery is ultimately necessary in approximately 45% of these patients.[4] The percentage of patients opting for surgery is likely to go up now that laparoscopic cholecystectomy is so widely available. Surgery is usually performed when the episodes of biliary colic are frequent or severe enough to seriously interfere with a patient's life-style or when there is a history of complications such as acute cholecystitis, pancreatitis, or cholangitis.

As with biliary colic, sonography is very valuable in patients presenting with suspected acute cholecystitis. Sonographic findings in acute cholecystitis are (1) gall-

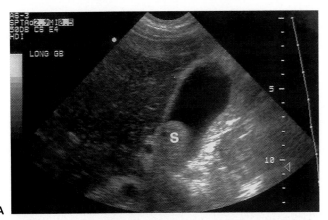

A

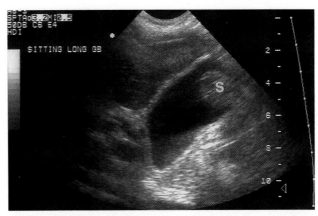

B

Figure 1–3 Tumefactive sludge. **A:** Longitudinal scan with the patient in a supine position demonstrates a nonshadowing mass-like structure (s) in the gallbladder neck. The differential diagnosis based on this single image is primarily that of a gallbladder tumor versus tumefactive sludge. **B:** Longitudinal scan with the patient sitting documents mobility of this mass (s) and confirms that it represents tumefactive sludge.

Figure 1–4 Gallbladder polyps. Longitudinal view demonstrates two small, round, nonshadowing lesions arising from the nondependent wall of the gallbladder (**arrows**). Views in multiple positions documented the lack of mobility of these lesions and the sonographic findings are typical of cholesterol polyps. (Reproduced with permission from **Ultrasound: The Requisites**, editors, A.B. Kurtz and W.D. Middleton. Mosby Yearbook, St. Louis, 1996.)

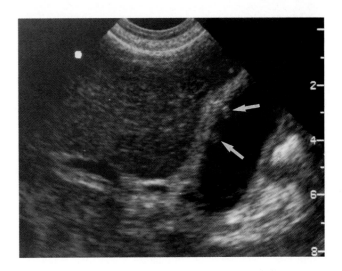

stones, (2) gallbladder wall thickening of greater than 3 mm, (3) gallbladder enlargement greater than 4 x 10 cm, (4) positive sonographic Murphy's sign, (5) pericholecystic fluid, and (6) impacted gallstones. The diagnostic value of several of the most important individual findings is shown in **Table 1–4**.[14, 15] The diagnostic value of different combinations of these findings is shown in **Table 1–5**.

Table 1–4 Analysis of single sonographic criteria for diagnosis of acute cholecystitis[a]

	Sensitivity (%)	Specificity (%)	PPV (%)	NPV (%)
Stones	83—98	52—77	86	96
Positive Murphy's sign	75—94	85—87	88	72
Thickened gallbladder wall	45—72	76—88	84	56

[a] Source: Reprinted with permission from Laing et al.[14] and Ralls et al.,[15] in which the prevalence of acute cholecystitis was 35 and 62%, respectively. PPV, positive predictive value; NPV, negative predictive value.

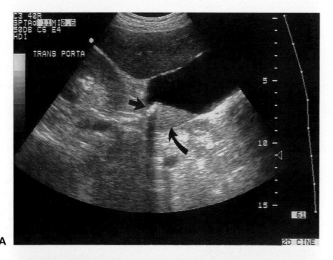

A

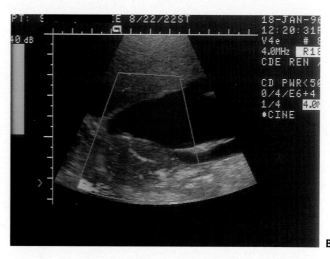

B

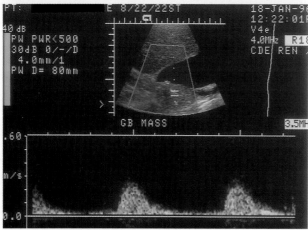

C

Figure 1–5 Gallbladder carcinoma. **A:** Longitudinal view of the gallbladder demonstrates shadowing stones (**straight arrow**) and nonshadowing echogenic material (**curved arrow**) in the dependent portion of the gallbladder. The straight border between this material and the lumen of the gallbladder simulates the appearance of layering sludge. **B:** Longitudinal power Doppler image documents the presence of internal vascularity within this echogenic material and confirms that this represents vascularized soft tissue rather than layering sludge. Its lack of mobility was demonstrated on upright views. **C:** Doppler waveform analysis documents arterial flow within the mass, which was histologically confirmed to represent gallbladder carcinoma.

Table 1–5 Predictive values of multiple sonographic criteria for diagnosis of acute cholecystitis[a]

Sonographic findings	Predictive value (%)
Positive	
Stones and positive Murphy's sign	90
Stones and thickened gallbladder wall	94
Stones, positive Murphy's sign, and thickened gallbladder wall	92
Negative	
No stones and negative Murphy's sign	97
No stones and normal gallbladder wall	98
No stones, negative Murphy's sign, and normal gallbladder wall	99

[a] Source: Reprinted with permission from Ralls et al.[15] Data were obtained from a patient population with a 62% prevalence of acute cholecystitis.

Approximately 95% of cases of acute cholecystitis are related to cystic duct obstruction due to gallstones. Therefore, detection of gallstones is very important in the sonographic diagnosis of acute cholecystitis. In most cases, freely mobile stones will be seen in the GB lumen, and the actual obstructing stone in the cystic duct will not be seen. When a stone is impacted in the GB neck, it is usually visible. Occasionally, small stones impacted in the cystic duct can also be detected. Acalculous cholecystitis may occur in extremely sick patients following major surgery, serious trauma, extensive burns, or prolonged parenteral nutrition. Therefore, in this patient population the absence of stones is not a reliable means of excluding the diagnosis and secondary sonographic signs of cholecystitis, described below, must be relied upon. Although some centers have reported good results in the sonographic diagnosis of acalculous cholecystitis,[16] it is often a difficult diagnosis to make or exclude by sonography or any other means.

GB wall thickening (defined as 3 mm or greater) occurs to some degree in the majority of cases of acute cholecystitis (**Fig. 1–8**). The positive predictive value of

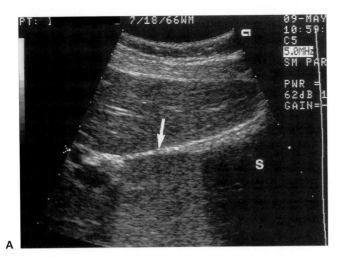

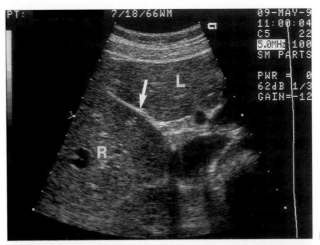

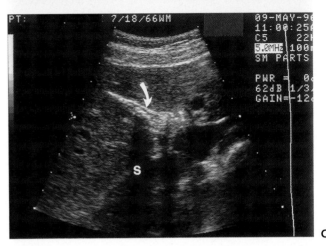

Figure 1–6 Contracted gallbladder filled with multiple small stones. **A:** Longitudinal view of the right upper quadrant demonstrates a region of clean shadowing (s) adjacent to the inferior edge of the liver. Note the echogenic linear structure (**arrow**) that extends from the shadowing focus to the region of the portal hepatis. This echogenic line represents the interlobar fissure. **B:** Transverse scan through the liver identifies the interlobar fissure (**arrow**) separating the left (L) and right (R) lobes of the liver. **C:** Transverse scan obtained immediately inferior to the level shown in **B** confirms that the echogenic shadowing structures (**curved arrow**) arise immediately inferior to the interlobar fissure. In addition, this image demonstrates the wall-echo-shadow complex that is typical of gallstones within a contracted gallbladder. Although stones are more difficult to diagnose in a completely contracted gallbladder, this case illustrates that careful scrutiny of the expected region of the gallbladder fossa can usually identify stones even in a very contracted gallbladder. s, shadow.

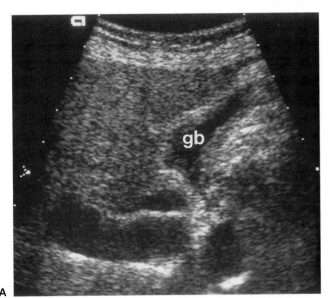

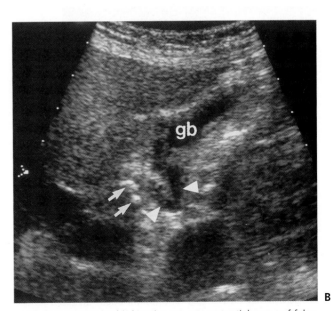

Figure 1–7 Cystic duct stones. **A:** Initial longitudinal view of the gallbladder demonstrates a contracted gallbladder (gb) but no evidence of gallstones. **B:** Repeat view of the gallbladder better demonstrates the gallbladder neck and cystic duct (**arrow heads**) and confirms the presence of two small gallstones (**arrows**) within the cystic duct. Stones in this location are one potential cause of false-negative sonograms. For this reason, careful attention to the gallbladder neck is very important during real time scanning. (Reproduced with permission from **Ultrasound: The Requisites**, editors, A.B. Kurtz and W.D. Middleton. Mosby Yearbook, St. Louis, 1996.)

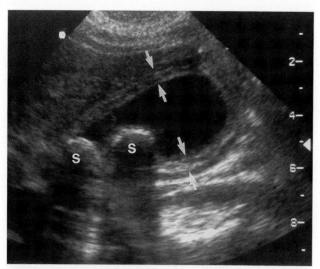

Figure 1–8 Acute cholecystitis with gallbladder wall thickening. Longitudinal view of the gallbladder demonstrates two stones (s) in the gallbladder. The gallbladder wall is diffusely thickened (**arrows**). This patient also demonstrated a positive sonographic Murphy sign and these findings are typical of acute cholecystitis. (Reproduced with permission from **Ultrasound: The Requisites**, editors, A.B. Kurtz and W.D. Middleton. Mosby Yearbook, St. Louis, 1996.)

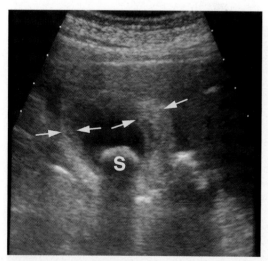

Figure 1–9 Gallbladder wall thickening not due to acute cholecystitis. Transverse view of the gallbladder demonstrates diffuse wall thickening (**arrows**) and a gallstone (s). This patient had congestive heart failure and diffuse right upper quadrant tenderness. The gallbladder wall thickening was felt to be related to either acute cholecystitis or congestive heart failure. Gallbladder scintigraphy was recommended for further evaluation. It demonstrated normal filling of the gallbladder thus excluding acute cholecystitis as the cause of this patient's thick gallbladder wall.

gallstones and wall thickening is as high as 94%. However, it is important to remember that asymptomatic gallstones are common and there are many causes of GB wall thickening besides cholecystitis (**Table 1–6**).

Table 1–6   Causes of gallbladder wall thickening

Biliary	Nonbiliary
Cholecystitis	Hepatitis
Adenomyomatosis	Pancreatitis
Cancer	Heart failure
AIDS cholangiopathy	Hypoproteinemia
Sclerosing cholangitis	Cirrhosis
	Portal hypertension
	Lymphatic obstruction

In patients with suspected acute cholecystitis and sonographic findings of gallstones and wall thickening, it is important to determine if there are possible nonbiliary causes for the thick GB wall. If there are other potential explanations for the wall thickening, assessment of the sonographic Murphy's sign is critical. Hepatobiliary scintigraphy is also an extremely valuable technique in this type of situation (**Fig. 1–9**).

Gallbladder enlargement is also commonly present in patients with cholecystitis (**Fig. 1–10 A**). The upper limits of normal for the size of the gallbladder is 8—10 cm in length and 4—5 cm in width. The width is clearly the more important dimension due to the normal variation in gallbladder length. In other words, a long, thin gallbladder is much less worrisome than a short, wide gallbladder.

Pericholecystic fluid is present in approximately 20% of patients with acute cholecystitis (**Fig. 1–11**). Recognizing this fluid is important since it implies a more advanced case of cholecystitis. It is usually seen as a focal collection adjacent to the GB wall. It should be distinguished from gallbladder wall edema, which is more concentric, and pericholecystic ascites, which is less mass-like and conforms to the shape of the GB and adjacent structures. In addition to sonography, CT is occasionally very helpful in determining the full extent of pericholecystic fluid collections. Although CT is rarely used as the initial imaging test in patients with suspected acute cholecystitis, it can provide useful information in cases of complicated cholecystitis that are difficult to fully sort out with sonography. CT can also be useful in distinguishing complicated cholecystitis from gallbladder carcinoma.

In addition to pericholecystic fluid, other signs of complicated cholecystitis include sloughed mucosal membranes (a rare finding), localized disruption of the mucosal layer of the GB wall (**Fig. 1–12**), striated intramural sonolucencies (**Fig. 1–13**), and intramural gas (**Fig. 1–14**). Patients with these findings of gangrenous cholecystitis have a higher morbidity and mortality than patients with uncomplicated cholecystitis and require

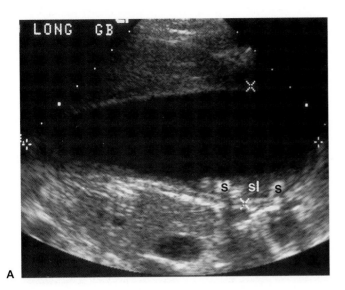

A

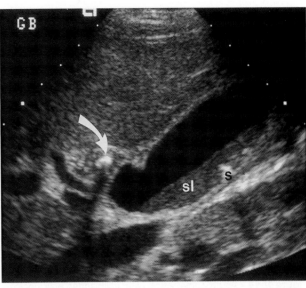

B

Figure 1–10 Acute cholecystitis with gallbladder enlargement. **A:** Longitudinal view of the gallbladder in a left lateral decubitus position demonstrates sludge (sl) and stones (s) in the gallbladder fundus as well as mild wall thickening. The gallbladder also is en-

larged measuring 5–12 cm in size. **B:** Longitudinal view of the gallbladder in an upright position demonstrates mobile sludge (sl) and stones (s) but also shows a stone impacted in the gallbladder neck/cystic duct (**curved arrow**).

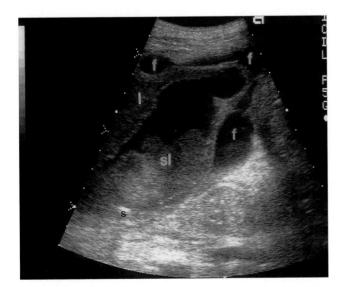

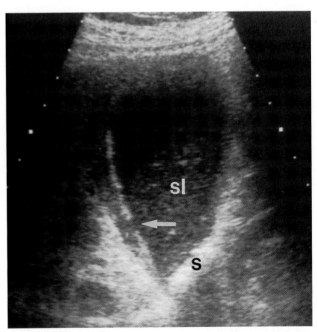

Figure 1–11 Cholecystitis with pericholecystic fluid. Longitudinal view of the gallbladder in a patient in the intensive care unit demonstrates sludge (sl) and a stone (s) in the gallbladder lumen. Also seen is loculated pericholecystic fluid (f) around the gallbladder fundus and over the anterior surface of the liver (l).

Figure 1–12 Cholecystitis with mucosal disruption. Longitudinal view of the gallbladder demonstrates intra-luminal sludge (sl) and stones (s). In addition, there is a region of mucosal disruption (**arrow**) along the superior wall of the gallbladder with fluid dissecting beneath the mucosa. This is a sign of complicated cholecystitis and indicates gallbladder wall necrosis. (Reproduced with permission from **Ultrasound: The Requisites**, editors, A.B. Kurtz and W.D. Middleton. Mosby Yearbook, St. Louis, 1996.)

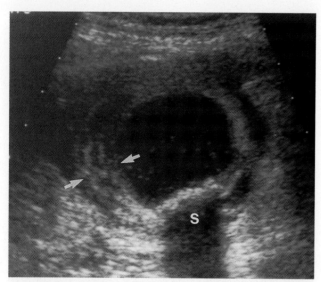

Figure 1–13 Acute cholecystitis with gallbladder wall necrosis. Transverse view of the gallbladder demonstrates stones (s) layering in the dependent portion of the gallbladder. Wall thickening with striated intramural sonolucencies (**arrows**) is detected along the lateral gallbladder wall. Although striated intramural sonolucencies are typically seen in patients with gallbladder wall thickening due to sources other than acute cholecystitis, in the setting of acute cholecystitis, this appearance suggests gallbladder wall necrosis. (Reproduced with permission from **Ultrasound: The Requisites,** editors, A.B. Kurtz and W.D. Middleton, Mosby Yearbook, St. Louis, 1996.)

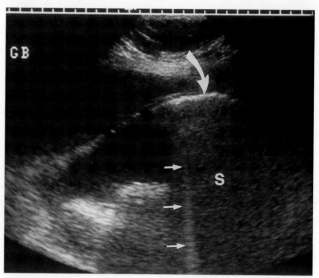

Figure 1–14 Emphysematous cholecystitis. Longitudinal view of the gallbladder demonstrates very bright reflectors (**curved arrow**) in the nondependent portion of the gallbladder wall. A dirty shadow (s) is seen deep to these bright reflectors. In addition, a ring down artifact (**straight arrows**) is identified. The ring down artifact is pathognomonic of gas and allows for a confident diagnosis of emphysematous cholecystitis.

more aggressive medical treatment and/or more urgent surgical treatment.

The sonographic Murphy's sign refers to localized tenderness directly over the GB. This sign is considered positive when pressure applied with the transducer elicits tenderness only over the GB or when maximum tenderness is located over the GB. A convincingly positive Murphy's sign is strong evidence of acute cholecystitis. The combination of gallstones and a positive sonographic Murphy's sign has a positive predictive value as high as 90%. A negative sonographic Murphy's sign is less helpful. Causes of a false-negative Murphy's sign include patient nonresponsiveness, pain medication, or inability to press directly on the GB (due to excessive ascites, a GB that is positioned very deep to the liver or a GB that is located deep to the ribs). Another important cause of a negative Murphy's sign is GB wall necrosis (**Fig. 1–15**). This occurs presumably due to damage to the GB innervation.[17] When the Murphy's sign is difficult to assess, scintigraphy can be helpful in determining the significance of morphologic changes seen on sonography.

The other major means of imaging patients with suspected acute cholecystitis is hepatobiliary scintigraphy. Scintigraphy is an excellent means of determining patency of the cystic duct and presence or absence of acute cholecystitis. Sensitivity of cholescintigraphy has been reported to range from 86 to 97% and specificity from 73 to 100%.[18–24] Sonographic sensitivity ranges from 81—100%, and specificity ranges from 60—100%.[14, 19—21, 24] The bulk of evidence indicates that sensitivity and specificity of sonography and scintigraphy are very similar. Therefore, the choice of initial imaging modalities is often made based on the preferences of the referring clinician and local expertise of the radiologist. Although either approach is acceptable, there are several good reasons to start the imaging evaluation with sonography.

1. Most patients with acute RUQ pain do not have acute cholecystitis. Sonography can rapidly exclude the diagnosis of cholecystitis by showing a stone free GB (**Fig. 1–16 and 1–17**).
2. Sonography is more likely to provide an alternative diagnosis[14, 19] than is scintigraphy (**Fig. 1–16 and 1–17**).
3. Sonography is more capable of establishing the presence of symptomatic gallstone disease in patients with biliary colic (**Fig. 1–18**) but without acute cholecystitis.[21] In fact, the positive predictive value of

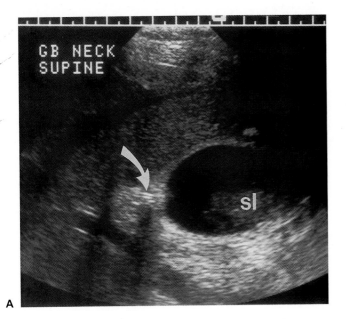
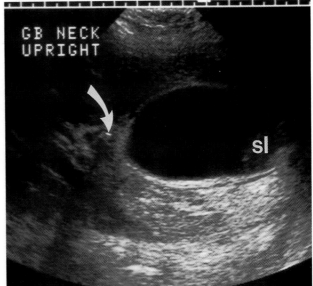

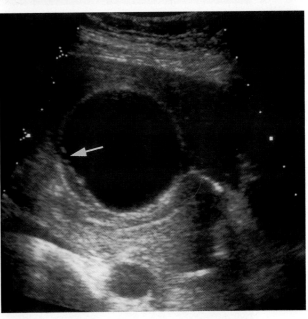

Figure 1–15 False-negative sonographic Murphy sign in the setting of gallbladder wall necrosis. **A:** Longitudinal view of the gallbladder with the patient supine demonstrates sludge (sl) in the lumen of the gallbladder. In addition, a gallstone is seen in the region of the gallbladder neck (**curved arrow**). **B:** Similar view with the patient standing upright demonstrates migration of the sludge (sl) into the gallbladder fundus but no motion of the stone (**curved arrow**) in the gallbladder neck. This suggests stone impaction in the gallbladder neck. Mild gallbladder wall thickening is also present. **C:** Transverse view of the gallbladder demonstrates an area of mucosal disruption (**arrow**) with a small amount of fluid dissecting beneath the mucosa. This patient presented as an outpatient with vague upper abdominal pain and a negative Murphy's sign. Although acute cholecystitis was not a major clinical consideration, the morphologic changes seen on sonography in conjunction with a negative Murphy's sign suggested acute cholecystitis with necrosis. Based on this, the patient was operated on later that day, and the sonographic findings were confirmed.

sonography for detecting patients who need a cholecystectomy is approximately 99%.[15] Occasionally, sonography may falsely classify patients with symptomatic gallstones as having acute cholecystitis, but the impact of this type of false-positive diagnosis is minimal because laparoscopic cholecystectomy is a well-accepted treatment for biliary colic and chronic cholecystitis.

4. Sonography can provide important preoperative information that is not readily available from scintigraphy (**Fig. 1–19**). This includes information about the size of the GB and the size of the largest stone, the appearance of the GB wall, the presence of peri-cholecystic fluid, the presence of common bile duct stones, and the status of adjacent organs (especially liver, right kidney, and pancreas). This information is more important in the current era of laparoscopic surgery since the surgeon is no longer able to carefully inspect and palpate the upper abdominal organs.

5. It is common to do sonography after either a negative hepatobiliary scan (see reason number 2 and 3 above) or a positive hepatobiliary scan (see reason number 4 above). On the other hand, positive and negative sonograms do not need to be followed by scintigraphy.

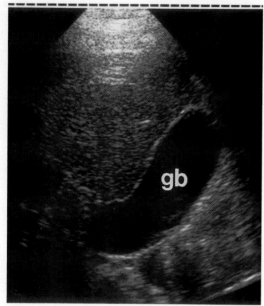

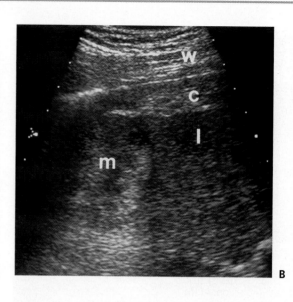

Figure 1–16   Ruptured hepatocellular carcinoma masquerading as acute cholecystitis. **A:** Longitudinal view of the right upper quadrant in a patient with resolving right upper quadrant pain demonstrates a normal gallbladder (gb) without evidence of stones or wall thickening. **B:** Longitudinal view of the superior aspect of the liver (l) demonstrates an inhomogenous mass (m) adjacent to the liver capsule. Echogenic blood clot (c) is seen between the liver and the abdominal wall (w). Echogenic ascites was also seen in the pelvis on other views. Based on the sonographic findings, a diagnosis of a ruptured hepatic mass with hemoperitoneum was made. The patient was then taken to the operating room where a ruptured hepatocellular carcinoma was confirmed.

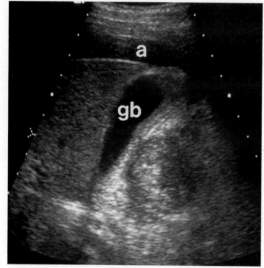

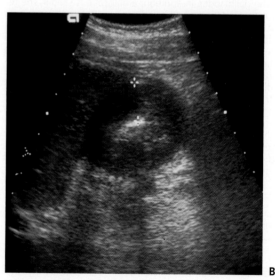

Figure 1–17   Ruptured duodenal ulcer simulating acute cholecystitis. **A:** Longitudinal view of the gallbladder (gb) demonstrates no evidence of gallstones. Ascites (a) is seen in the perihepatic region. **B:** Longitudinal scan in the peripyloric region demonstrates marked thickening of the bowel wall (**cursors**). This was interpreted as representing either neoplastic infiltration or inflammatory thickening due to ulcer disease. The patient was subsequently shown to have a perforated duodenal ulcer.

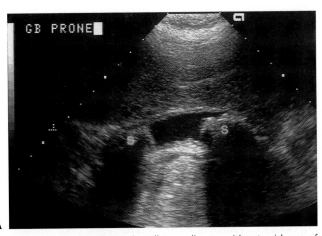

A

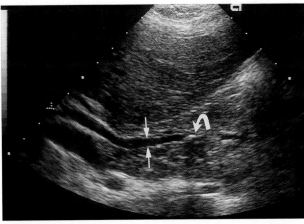

B

Figure 1–18 Symptomatic gallstone disease without evidence of acute cholecystitis. **A:** Longitudinal view of the gallbladder demonstrates multiple stones (s), mild gallbladder wall thickening and mild gallbladder contraction. At the time this patient was scanned, there was no localized tenderness over the gallbladder. However, she had previously experienced a severe episode of RUQ pain that lasted for three hours and was now resolving. **B:** Longitudinal view of the normal diameter distal bile duct (**arrows**) demonstrates a shadowing echogenic focus (**curved arrow**) consistent with a small distal common bile duct stone. This provides convincing evidence that the patient's recent pain was due to biliary colic as a stone passed through the cystic duct and into the common bile duct.

The ACR guidelines for imaging patients with suspected acute cholecystitis indicate that either sonography or scintigraphy are appropriate. However, sonography is given a higher score than scintigraphy for the reasons indicated above. Practice guidelines issued in 1988 by the American College of Physicians also recommended using sonography as the first imaging test for suspected acute cholecystitis.[25,26] Although both of these groups prefer to start with sonography in the evaluation of patients with suspected acute cholecystitis, scintigraphy should be recognized as a powerful problem solver when the sonogram is confusing or inconclusive. This may occur in up to 25% of patients with clinically suspected acute cholecystitis in whom ultrasound is done first. Therefore, cholescintigraphy continues to play an important role in the evaluation of acute cholecystitis.

Treatment for acute cholecystitis can initially be conservative with pain medication, IV hydration, and antibiotics. Approximately 75% of patients will respond to medical therapy. The rest will either be refractory to conservative treatment or will develop complications and require surgery. Of the patients that initially respond to medical treatment, recurrent cholecystitis will occur within one year in 25% and within 6 years in 60%. Therefore, the current approach is to perform cholecystectomy during or after the first episode of acute cholecystitis. The exact timing of the cholecystectomy is not uniformly agreed upon. It appears that early laparo-

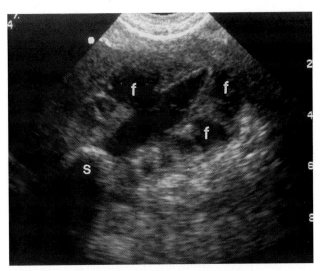

Figure 1–19 Acute cholecystitis with marked intramural fluid collections. Longitudinal view of the gallbladder demonstrates a stone (s) impacted in the gallbladder neck. Multiple fluid collections (f) are seen in the thickened gallbladder wall. Communication between the gallbladder lumen and the anterior intramural fluid collection is apparent. Identification of this severe gallbladder wall abnormality provides important preoperative information to the patient's surgeon. (Reproduced with permission from **Ultrasound: The Requisites**, editors, A.B. Kurtz and W.D. Middleton. Mosby Yearbook, St. Louis, 1996.)

scopic cholecystectomy is most effective if performed on patients presenting within 48 h of the onset of symptoms. Early cholecystectomy may also be necessary if the patient fails to respond to medical treatment. Delayed cholecystectomy is generally reserved for patients presenting after 48 h, for those patients at increased operative risk, or those patients in whom the diagnosis is unclear. Emergent cholecystectomy is reserved for patients that are clinically unstable or patients with complications identified clinically or on imaging studies.

Summary

Sonography is the primary imaging modality for evaluation of RUQ pain. It is more effective at diagnosing and evaluating gallstones than any other imaging test. Oral cholecystography has little role in the current evaluation RUQ pain. However, gallstones are well quantified by OCGs and if dissolution therapy or lithotripsy become more popular in the future, OCG may become more important. Sonography is similar in accuracy to scintigraphy in the evaluation of suspected acute cholecystitis and provides additional information that is not available on scintigraphy. Cholescintigraphy is a valuable test of gallbladder function that is very useful in the evaluation of suspected acute cholecystitis when ultrasound is confusing or indeterminate. CT is not a primary modality in the evaluation of RUQ pain but is very useful in further evaluating complicated cholecystitis and gallbladder neoplasm. CT may be useful in the diagnosis of acute acalculous cholecystitis.

References

1. Hopper K.D., Landis J.R., Meilstrup J.W., McCauslin M.A., Sechtin A.G. The prevalence of asymptomatic gallstones in the general population. *Invest Radiol* 1991;26:939—945.
2. Lee S.P., Kuver R. Gallstones. In: Yamada T., ed. *Textbook of Gastroenterology*, 2nd ed. Philadelphia, PA: J.B. Lippincott Co, 1995;2187—2212.
3. Gracie W.A. The natural history of silent gallstones. The innocent gallstone is not a myth. *N Engl J Med* 1982;307:798—800.
4. McSherry C.K., Ferstenberg H., Calhoun F., Lahman E., Virshup M. The natural history of diagnosed gallstone disease in symptomatic and asymptomatic patients. *Ann Surg* 1984;202:59—63.
5. Ransohoff D.F., Gracie W.A., Wolfenson L.B., Neuhauser D. Prophylactic cholecystectomy or expectant management for silent gallstones. *Ann Intern Med* 1983;99:199—204.
6. Way L.W., Sleisenger M.H. Cholelithiasis; chronic and acute cholecystitis. In: Sleisenger M.H., Fordtran J.S., eds. *Gastrointestinal Disease*, 4th ed. Philadelphia, PA: W.B. Saunders Co., 1989; p. 1691—1714.
7. Gadacz T.R. Cholelithiasis and cholecystitis. In: Zuidema G.D., ed. *Shackelford's Surgery of the Alimentary Tract*, 3rd ed. Philadelphia, PA: W.B. Saunders Co, 1991; p. 174—185.
8. Wiener S.L. Acute right hypochondriac pain. In: Wiener S.L., ed. *Differential Diagnosis of Acute Pain by Body Region*, 1st ed. New York, NY: McGraw Hill Inc. 1993; p. 217—226.
9. Barakos J.A., Ralls P.W., Lapin S.A., et al. Cholelithiasis: evaluation with CT. *Radiology* 1987;162:415—418.
10. Gelfand D.W., Wolfman N.T., Ott D.J., et al. Oral cholecystography vs gallbladder sonography: a prospective, blinded reappraisal. *AJR* 1986;151:69—72.
11. Berk R.N. Oral cholecystography. In: Berk R.N., Ferrucci J.T., Leopold G.R., eds. *Radiology of the Gallbladder and Bile Ducts: Diagnosis and Intervention*, 1st ed. Philadelphia PA: W.B. Saunders Co, 1983; p. 83—162.
12. Silidker M.S., Cronan J.J., Scola F.H., et al. Ultrasound evaluation of cholelithiasis in the morbidly obese. *Gastrointest Radiol* 1988;13:345—346.
13. Kurtz A.B., Middleton W.D., eds. *Ultrasound: The Requisites*. St. Louis, Mo: Mosby-Yearbook, 1996.
14. Laing F.C., Federle M.P., Jeffrey R.B., Brown T.W. Ultrasonic evaluation of patients with acute right upper quadrant pain. *Radiology* 1981;140:449—455.
15. Ralls P.W., Colletti P.M., Lapin S.A., et al. Real time sonography in suspected acute cholecystitis: Prospective evaluation of primary and secondary signs. *Radiology* 1985;155:767—771.
16. Mirvis S.E., Vainright J.R., Nelson A.W., et al. The diagnosis of acute acalculous cholecystitis: a comparison of sonography, scintigraphy, and CT. *AJR* 1986;147:1171—1175.
17. Simeone J.F., Brink J.A., Mueller P.R., et al. The sonographic diagnosis of acute gangrenous cholecystitis: Importance of the Murphy sign. *AJR* 1989;152:289—290.
18. Samuels B.I., Freitas J.E., Bree R.L., Schwab R.E., Heller S.T. A comparison of radionuclide hepatobiliary imaging and real-time ultrasound for the detection of acute cholecystitis. *Radiology* 1983;147:207—210.
19. Shuman W.P., Mack L.A., Rudd T.G., Rogers J.V., Gibbs P. Evaluation of acute right upper quadrant pain: sonography and 99mTcPIPIDA cholescintigraphy. *AJR* 1982;139:61—64.
20. Ralls P.W., Colletti P.M., Halls J.M., Siemsen J.K. Prospective evaluation of 99mTc-IDA cholescintigraphy and gray-scale ultrasound in the diagnosis of acute cholecystitis. *Radiology* 1982;144:369—371.
21. Worthen N.J., Uszler J.M., Funamura J.L. Cholecystitis: prospective evaluation of sonography and 99mTc-HIDA cholescintigraphy. *AJR* 1981;137:973—978.
22. Weissmann H.S., Frank M.S., Bernstein L.H., Freeman L.M. Rapid and accurate diagnosis of acute cholecystitis with 99mTc-HIDA cholescintigraphy. *AJR* 1979;132:523—528.
23. Weissmann H.S., Badia J., Sugarman L.A., et al. Spectrum of 99mTc-IDA cholescintigraphic patterns in acute cholecystitis. *Radiology* 1981;138:167—175.
24. Freitas J.E., Mirkes S., Fink-Bennett D.M., Bree R.L. Suspected acute cholecystitis—comparison of hepatobiliary scintigraphy and ultrasonography. *Clin Nuc Med* 1982;7:364—367.
25. Marton K.I., Doubilet P., et al. How to study the gallbladder. *Ann Intern Med* 1988;109:752—754.
26. Marton K.I., Doubilet P. How to image the gallbladder in suspected acute cholecystitis. *Ann Intern Med* 1988;109:722—729

2 Jaundice

Faye C. Laing

In most cases jaundice reflects the presence of cholestasis. It results from either hepatic parenchymal disease or biliary obstruction. It is usually manifest as an elevated serum alkaline phosphatase value and increased serum levels of substances such as bilirubin, bile acids, and cholesterol that are normally secreted in bile. Less commonly, jaundice results from increased bilirubin production or from a combination of bilirubin overproduction and defective bilirubin excretion. In these instances, hyperbilirubinemia is typically present as an isolated abnormality, unaccompanied by other clinical or laboratory evidence of hepatic or bilirubin dysfunction.

The workup for cholestasis has changed dramatically over the past two decades due to the development of newer radiologic and endoscopic techniques for visualizing the biliary tree. When a patient with cholestasis is examined, the overriding objective is to determine whether a potentially treatable cause of cholestasis is present without subjecting the patient to needless risk, discomfort, or expense. Clinical judgment is initially important to decide whether or not a patient is or is not likely to have biliary obstruction. If biliary obstruction is unlikely, then an aggressive, invasive workup is usually not indicated. Most patients with jaundice have hepatocellular injury as the cause for their cholestasis. In this case, the disease process is typically self-limiting and warrants only an expectant approach, with removal of any inciting agents and supportive therapy, as required.

Clinical Clues to the Presence of Obstruction

The possibility that cholestasis may be due to extrahepatic obstruction may initially be suggested by the patient's history, a physical examination, and laboratory studies. Abdominal pain, previous biliary surgery, prolonged or intermittent cholestasis, the absence of exposure to potential hepatotoxins (e.g., drugs), and the absence of hepatitis exposure or hepatitis-like symptoms suggest the presence of an obstruction.

Findings on physical examination that warrant additional imaging studies include a palpable gallbladder or abdominal mass, a high fever (characteristic of cholangitis), occult blood in the stool, absence of stigmata of chronic liver disease, and abdominal tenderness.

Laboratory test results suggestive of extrahepatic biliary obstruction include disproportionate elevation of the serum bilirubin and alkaline phosphatase relative to serum transaminase levels, complete normalization of a prolonged prothrombin time after administration of vitamin K, and negative serologic markers for viral hepatitis, chronic active hepatitis, or primary biliary cirrhosis.

Differential Diagnosis of Biliary Obstruction

Because biliary obstruction typically results in bile duct dilatation proximal to the level of obstruction, and because approximately 90% of obstructive processes develop at the level of the distal common bile duct, most patients develop diffuse dilatation of both the common and intrahepatic bile ducts.[1] Initial dilatation occurs just above the site of the pathologic condition, and in most cases it rather rapidly involves the more proximal bile ducts. In most obstructive conditions, therefore, the earliest change is dilatation of the extrahepatic duct, which may precede elevation of the serum bilirubuin level.[2] In general, a malignant and/or chronic obstruction results in relatively greater proximal dilatation than does an acutely obstructing process.

Extrahepatic Obstruction: Level & Causes

Intrapancreatic Obstruction

The three most common conditions that cause 90% of biliary obstructions occur at the level of the distal duct. These conditions include (1) choledocholithiasis, (2) chronic pancreatitis, and (3) pancreatic carcinoma (**Fig. 2–1**). In the United States, choledocholithiasis is the single most common cause for biliary obstruction. It occurs in approximately 15% of patients with cholelithiasis.[1]

With careful attention to the anatomic configuration and internal contents of the distal duct, and with technically adequate visualization of the pancreas, noninvasive imaging can often determine which of the three conditions is responsible for a distal obstruction.

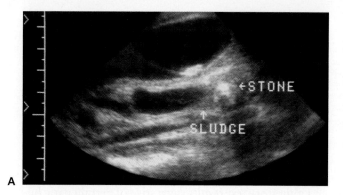

A

B

Figure 2–1 Extrahepatic bile duct obstruction. **A:** Sagittal US scan shows well-defined, echogenic, shadowing focus in the distal common bile duct due to a calculus. Small amount of echogenic, nonshadowing sludge is also present. **B:** Sagittal US scan shows pancreatic carcinoma as a heterogeneous mass in head of the pan-creas . The proximal interface of the mass has an irregular contour and produces an abrupt cutoff (**arrow**). Reprinted with permission from **Diagnostic Ultrasound** by F.C. Laing. Mosby, St. Louis, 1998. p. 175—223.

Suprapancreatic Obstruction

Suprapancreatic obstruction is defined as an obstruction that develops between the pancreas and porta hepatis. These obstructions occur in approximately 5% of patients, and are most often due to primary bile duct cancer (cholangiocarcinoma) or metastatic adenopathy (**Fig. 2–2**). Calculi and inflammatory strictures are uncommon at this level.

Portahepatis Obstruction

Obstruction at the porta hepatis occurs in approximately 5% of patients and is usually due to primary cholangiocarcinoma (Klatskin tumor), spread from an adjacent tumor (gallbladder or liver), or a surgical stricture (**Fig. 2–3**).

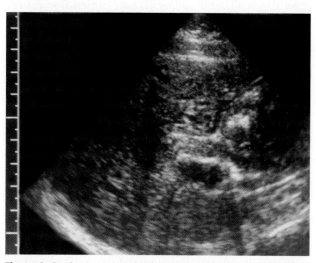

Figure 2–2 Suprapancreatic obstruction. Sagittal US scan shows abnormal echoes in dilated extrahepatic duct. This was due to a primary bile duct tumor. Reprinted with permission from **Diagnostic Ultrasound** by F.C. Laing. Mosby, St. Louis, 1998. p. 175—223.

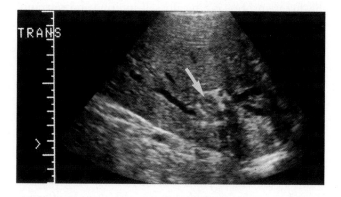

Figure 2–3 Portahepatis obstruction. Transverse US scan shows dilated right and left intrahepatic bile ducts. The was due to a poorly defined isoechic mass (**arrow**), pathologically confirmed to be a cholangiocarcinoma (Klatskin tumor). Reprinted with permission from **Diagnostic Ultrasound** by F.C. Laing. Mosby, St. Louis, 1998. p. 175—223

Unusual Causes for Obstruction

Relatively uncommon causes for extrahepatic bile duct obstruction include strictures, cholangitis, parasitic infestations, developmental abnormalities, hemobilia, and idiopathic narrowing.

Most benign strictures (95%) result from surgical injury, often after trauma associated with cholecystectomy.[3,4] Strictures typically occur in the common bile duct at the level of the hepatic hilus.[5] Postinflammatory strictures may also develop in association with pancreatitis, gallstones, infections, and duodenal ulcer disease.

A variety of unrelated cholangitides may cause biliary obstruction. These include recurrent pyogenic cholangitis (**Fig. 2–4** through **2–6**),[6] primary sclerosing cholangitis, and HIV infection related cholangiopathy (**Fig. 2–7**).

Recurrent pyogenic cholangitis is endemic to areas of Southeast Asia and is often associated with intrabiliary infestation by parasites (especially *Chlonorchis sinensis* and, to a lesser degree, *Ascaris lumbricoides*) and bacteria (*Escherichia coli*). In this condition, multiple strictures develop that result in massive dilatation of the common duct and, to a lesser degree, the intrahepatic ducts. Soft, mud-like calcium bilirubinate (pigment) calculi are frequently present in multiple ducts. In 25% of cases, these calculi are nonshadowing on ultrasound (US) imaging (**Fig. 2–4 B**).[7]

Primary sclerosing cholangitis, an uncommon disease of unknown cause, most often occurs in relatively young men with a preexisting condition, typically, ulcerative colitis or, to a lesser degree Crohn's disease.[8] The characteristic biliary appearance for primary sclerosing cholangitis is nonuniform, segmental, intrahepatic biliary dilatation, with beading and pruning of the ducts.[9] The extrahepatic bile duct is affected in a similar, but less severe manner, with involvement primarily involving the proximal duct.[9] An attempt should be made to distinguish the appearance of primary sclerosing cholangitis from cholangiocarcinoma, which develops in 6—9% of patients with primary sclerosing cholangitis.[10] Although the distinction may be difficult, if not impossible, findings that suggest a developing malignancy include marked ductal dilatation, progressive stricture or dilatation, and intraluminal polypoid masses.[11]

HIV cholangiopathy may involve the gallbladder and biliary tree in a focal or diffuse way. Characteristically, it causes mural thickening with a stricture of the distal common duct and relatively mild proximal dilatation (**Fig. 2–7**). Cytomegalovirus and cryptospiridium have been implicated as causes.

In addition to the development of recurrent pyogenic cholangitis in association with parasitic infestation, certain parasites that typically reside in the gastrointestinal tract may produce symptoms if they traverse the ampulla and enter the biliary tree. This most often occurs with *C. sinensis* and *A. lumbricoides*. *C. sinensis*, which is a liver fluke, does not typically cause radiographic abnormalities in and of itself. Occasionally, however, the flukes may be noted on cholangiograms or US images as small (10—15 mm) filling defects or as echogenic foci

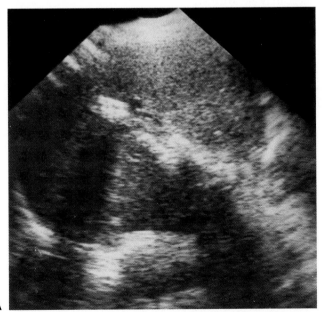

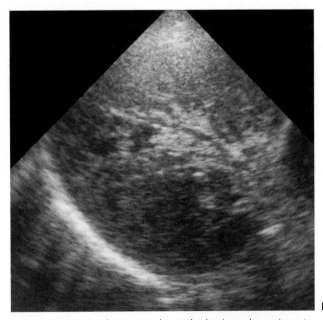

A

B

Figure 2–4   Recurrent pyogenic cholangiohepatitis. **A:** Transverse US scan reveals prominent echogenicity with acoustic shadowing in distribution of right intrahepatic bile duct. This appearance is due to multiple calcified intrahepatic biliary calculi. Reprinted with permission from Ultrasound diagnosis of choledocholithiasis by F.C. Laing. **Sem Ultrasound, CT and MR.** 1987;8:103—113. **B:** In another patient, transverse US scan reveals nonshadowing echogenic material in right intrahepatic bile duct, due to multiple noncalcified intrahepatic biliary calculi. Biliary sludge, pus, or hemobilia could have an identical appearance. Reprinted with permission from Ultrasound diagnosis of choledocholithiasis by F.C. Laing. **Sem Ultrasound, CT and MR.** 1987;8:103—113.

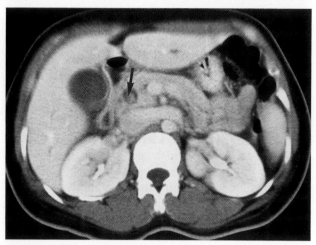

Figure 2–5 Choledocholithiasis due to recurrent pyogenic cholangiohepatitis. CT scan reveals a highly attenuating focus in the distal common duct (**arrow**).

Figure 2–6 Choledocholithiasis due to recurrent pyogenic ▷ cholangiohepatitis. Image from endoscopic retrograde cholangio-pancreatography (ERCP) shows multiple filling defects (**arrows**) in common duct, causing profound dilatation of both intra- and extrahepatic bile ducts.

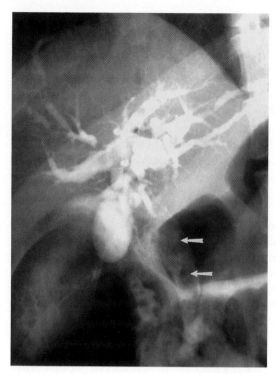

within the bile ducts. Mild intrahepatic dilatation has also been reported in patients with heavy infestation.[12, 13]

The adult ascaris worm is greater than 10 cm in length and 3—6 mm in diameter; therefore, it is readily visible by a variety of imaging modalities as a tubular structure, either straight or coiled (like spaghetti), in the extrahepatic duct (**Fig. 2–8**).[14–16] Not surprisingly, frank biliary obstruction by this parasite is relatively common.

In unusual cases, extrahepatic bile duct dilatation may be due to a congenital abnormality that results in a choledochal cyst. The pathogenesis for this condition is unknown, but it predominates among Asians and is

more common among women (approximate ratio of 3:1).[17] Various subtypes of these cysts result in either local cystic or aneurysmal dilatation of the extrahepatic bile duct.[18] Complications associated with a choledochal cyst include biliary obstruction, recurrent bacterial cholangitis, and biliary neoplasia. The latter typically involves the cyst, although the gallbladder and other bile ducts may be affected.[17]

Hemobilia or bleeding into the biliary tree has a variety of causes, but most often accompanies trauma, either iatrogenic or spontaneous. Patients with coagulopathy, either congenital (associated with hemophilia), or acquired (due to anticoagulation, severe liver disease, or multiple-organ failure) are at increased

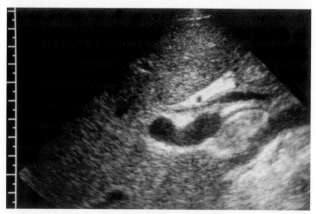

Figure 2–7 HIV cholangiopathy. US scan shows characteristic diffuse thickening of wall of common bile duct, without significant dilatation. Reprinted with permission from **Diagnostic Ultrasound** by F.C. Laing. Mosby, St. Louis, 1998. p. 175—223.

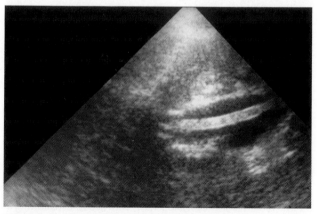

Figure 2–8 Ascariasis. US scan shows echogenic tubular structure due to an Ascaris worm in this markedly dilated common duct. Reprinted with permission from **Diagnostic Ultrasound: Text and Cases**. Yearbook, Chicago, IL, 1987, p. 142—153.

risk of developing hemobilia. With hemobilia, blood is present in the biliary tree, the gallbladder, or both. Its appearance will vary depending upon the imaging modality, the age of the blood, and its location.[19]

Intrahepatic Causes of Obstruction

Intrahepatic Neoplasms

Because it is distinctly unusual for primary bile duct carcinoma to originate within intrahepatic ducts, the most common primary intrahepatic biliary neoplasm is cystadenoma, and its malignant counterpart, cystadenocarcinoma. These uncommon tumors generally occur in middle-aged women and are usually quite large when they are discovered. Noninvasive imaging reveals a complex multiloculated cystic mass, with mural and septal nodules, as well as occasional calcifications within the soft tissue components of the tumor.[20, 21]

Mirizzi Syndrome

In this uncommon condition, the patient has intrahepatic bile duct dilatation with a common bile duct of normal size. The syndrome occurs when a large calculus in the neck of the gallbladder or cystic duct causes extrinsic mechanical compression on the common hepatic duct (**Fig. 2–9**).[22] Alternatively, a calculus may occasionally be lodged within the cystic duct remnant. In most cases, the insertion of the cystic duct into the common hepatic duct is relatively low. If the syndrome is not recognized preoperatively and correctly diagnosed, then major surgical complications can result, owing to inadvertent ligation and transection of the common duct. In suspicious cases, computed tomography (CT) and especially cholangiography should be considered for diagnostic confirmation.[23]

Caroli Disease

Caroli disease is a congenital abnormality that is most likely inherited in an autosomal recessive fashion. A recent review defines two distinct forms of this disease.[24] The originally described "pure" form can occur in a focal or diffuse pattern. It is characterized by saccular, communicating intrahepatic bile duct ectasia (**Fig. 2–10**). Complications include pyogenic cholangitis, hepatic abscess, intrahepatic biliary obstruction, calculi, and the development of cholangiocarcinoma (in 7% of cases). A variety of imaging modalities have been used to demonstrate and prove the existence of diverticulum-like sacculi of the intrahepatic biliary tree in the pure form of the disease.[24–27] To distinguish this condition from polycystic liver disease, it is important to show communication between the sacs and bile ducts.[27, 28]

The second form of Caroli disease appears in childhood, has relatively less bile duct dilatation, and is associated with hepatic fibrosis that results in portal hypertension and terminal liver failure. Associated condi-

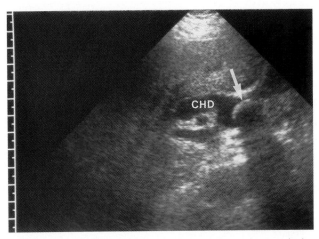

Figure 2–9 Mirizzi syndrome. US scan shows a large calculus (**arrow**) located in the cystic duct that is causing dilatation of proximal common hepatic duct (CHD). Reprinted with permission from **Diagnostic Ultrasound** by F.C. Laing. Mosby, St. Louis, 1998. p. 175—223.

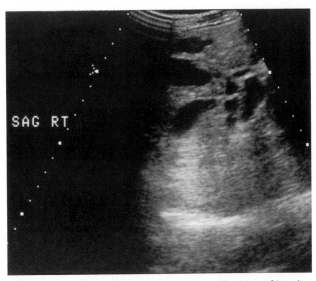

Figure 2–10 Caroli disease. US scan shows dilatation of intrahepatic bile ducts with cystic, diverticular out-pouchings (**arrows**). This appearance is highly suggestive of the pure form of Caroli disease.

tions include choledochal cyst, and infantile polycystic kidney disease. When Caroli disease is associated with hepatic fibrosis, noninvasive imaging studies reveal less pronounced biliary changes, with portal hypertension and cystic disease of the kidneys predominating.[29]

Miscellaneous Conditions

As discussed previously, various cholangidities (recurrent pyogenic cholangitis, primary sclerosing cholangitis, and HIV related) can affect the intra- and/or the extrahepatic biliary tree. Hemobilia can similarly occur in the intra- and/or the extrahepatic biliary tree.

Available Imaging Modalities (Other than US)

Because bile duct dilatation may precede the clinical onset of jaundice, the early diagnosis of biliary obstruction clearly depends on radiological imaging. Plain radiographs are seldom helpful and are usually not obtained in these patients. Currently, US imaging is used as the initial screening modality. The usefulness and the role of US imaging will be described in greater detail later in this chapter.

Noninvasive Modalities

Other noninvasive imaging modalities that can be used to evaluate the biliary tree include radionuclide imaging with technetium 99-m imino-diacetic acid (Tc-99 m IDA), CT imaging, and more recently magnetic resonance (MR) imaging.

Radionuclide imaging

With the advent of high-quality US imaging, Tc-99 m IDA hepatobiliary imaging has limited usefulness for the evaluation of patients with suspected biliary obstruction. Findings consistent with complete obstruction are lack of visualization of the biliary tree and good visualization of the liver. With incomplete obstruction, the tracer should be visible to the level of the obstruction. Occasionally, a filling defect may be identified at the site of the pathologic condition. Limitations of hepatobiliary imaging are that (1) it requires reasonably good hepatocyte function, and (2) the intrahepatic cholestasis produced by certain drugs can cause a pattern that cannot be distinguished from that of total extrahepatic obstruction.[30]

With unusual disease processes such as Caroli disease, Tc-99 m IDA hepatobilary imaging may play a pivotal role.[31] The diagnosis of Caroli disease can be especially challenging if the intrahepatic fluid collections are large and the US findings do not clearly indicate whether the patient has Caroli disease versus polycystic hepatic disease. In hepatobilary images obtained in patients with Caroli disease, persistent areas with focal accumulation of radiotracer will be evident.[26,27] In contrast, images obtained in patients with polycystic hepatic disease will show focal areas of decreased radiotracer, with normal liver washout and biliary excretion.

CT Imaging

Many CT examinations of the biliary tree are done to expand on or provide data complimentary to a previously performed US examination. Typically, CT examinations are performed to define a precise level and/or a cause for a dilated biliary system, obtain a more complete survey of the intrahepatic biliary tree, evaluate patients with intrabiliary air (US scans are technically limited in such cases), and measure the CT number of echogenic material within bile ducts to determine whether hemobilia is present.[32] It is particularly useful in the evaluation of jaundiced patients to detect and stage pancreatic carcinoma, detect choledocholithiasis, determine the extent of cholangiocarcinoma, and preoperatively assess patients undergoing laparoscopic cholecystectomy.[33]

The hallmark for the identification of biliary obstruction on CT scans is the presence of intra- and extrahepatic bile duct dilatation. Newer helical scanning technology has the advantage of volumetric data acquisition obtained during a single breath hold. This technique minimizes misregistration artifacts, allows overlapping axial reconstruction of slices, optimizes tissue contrast by obtaining images during the initial contrast bolus (rather than several minutes later as required by conventional equipment), and allows postprocessing of cholangiographically enhanced source images.[32,33] State of the art CT technology even allows occasional visualization of small, but normal diameter intrahepatic bile ducts.[34]

The key to defining the level and often the cause of biliary dilatation is careful evaluation of the transition zone at the level where the dilated duct narrows and often becomes invisible. An abrupt distal cutoff suggests a malignant process, whereas a tapered cutoff suggests a benign process.[35]

To optimize CT detection of a small, but distally obstructing pancreatic mass, overlapping thin sliced helical CT images are superior to conventional CT. Although the precise technique is still evolving, and varies somewhat from one institution to another, it is important to distend and fill adjacent bowel loops with contrast, and also inject intravenous contrast material. A single helical run is subsequently performed through the pancreas following a delay that is typically 70 s.[33] This results in vascular enhancement of the portal venous system, allowing more accurate evaluation of vascular encasement by tumors, and the detection of small metastatic deposits. In addition, pancreatic and biliary ductal anatomy is better defined when their walls are maximally enhanced by intravenous contrast material. Some authorities use a more rapid infusion of contrast material (5 mL/s), which permits biphasic scanning. The benefit of arterial phase imaging is that it can increase detection of small, noncontour deforming hypoattenuating tumors.[32]

Although highly specialized centers may be quite successful in using CT to detect choledocholithiasis, the detection of this condition may be quite challenging, especially if older equipment is used, and the staff is not familiar with newer CT imaging techniques. To a great degree, the appearance and detection rate of choledocholithiasis by CT imaging depends upon the calculus' chemical composition.[36] High-attenuation calculi (only about 20% of the total) are easily visible by CT examination due to their high calcium carbonate and phosphate content (**Fig. 2–5**). Approximately 50% of calculi are more difficult to diagnose confidently as their attenuation values are similar to soft tissue. These calculi may occasionally be detected because they create a "bull's eye" appearance, which is produced by a rim of bile surrounding the calculus. The remaining 30% of calculi may be extremely difficult, if not impossible to detect, because they are composed of cholesterol, which is isoechoic to bile.[32] A recent report emphasizes the importance of meticulous scanning in these patients, and suggests that helical axial CT, omitting both intravenous or oral contrast agents, but using thin-collimation scans with overlapping reconstructed images through the transition level can detect choledocholithiasis with a sensitivity of 88%, specificity of 97%, and an accuracy of 94%.[37]

A recently introduced CT technological advance that may be useful for evaluating patients with suspected biliary disease (both benign and malignant) is three-dimensional reconstruction of the biliary tree.[38, 39] If helical CT is performed after administering intravenous iodipamide meglumine, then the bile ducts will contain contrast medium, and a three-dimensional reconstruction can create a helical CT cholangiogram.[40, 41] Preliminary work suggests that, in selected patients with normal serum bilirubin levels, this noninvasive technique may be used in lieu of endoscopic retrograde cholangiography. Although the spatial resolution of a helical CT cholangiogram is less than endoscopic retrograde cholangiography, this noninvasive method can be used to detect choledocholithiasis. Because it is noninvasive, it can eliminate postprocedural hyperamylasemia, which occurs in one of four patients after endoscopic retrograde cholangiography.[42] It can be used to screen the biliary tree for anatomic variations, or choledocholithiasis prior to laparoscopic cholecystectomy, and it may in some patients obviate the need for laparoscopic interoperative cholangiography.[41, 43] It may also be useful to examine patients in whom endoscopic retrograde cholangiography is either technically not possible or unsuccessful.[41] A limitation of this technique is that it can be used for detection of diagnosis only, as it has no therapeutic options (unlike endoscopic retrograde cholangiography).

MRI Imaging

Without doubt, the most exciting new aspect of biliary MRI relates to MR cholangiopancreatography (**Fig. 2–11**).[44—47] Recent reports suggest the accuracy of MR cholangiopancreatography for identifying the cause of bile duct obstruction is comparable to endoscopic retrograde cholangiography.[48, 49] Calculi as small as 2 mm can be detected.[45] Published data report a sensitivity of 90—95% for biliary and pancreatic ductal dilatation and strictures,[45, 46, 50–53] and 72—95% for choledocholithiasis.[45, 48, 50, 52—54] Like helical CT cholangiography, the main advantage of MR cholangiopancreatography is that it can noninvasively provide a three-dimen-

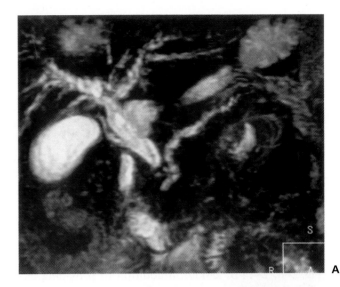

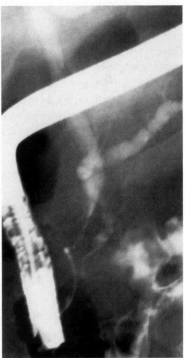

Figure 2–11 Pancreatic carcinoma. **A:** Image from MR cholangiopancreatography shows a double-duct sign, with dilatation of proximal bile ducts and distal pancreatic duct. **B:** ERCP image reveals identical findings.

sional overview of the biliary tree. Unlike CT imaging, however, three-dimensional biliary MR imaging does not require intravenous injection of contrast material.

MR imaging can also be used to evaluate jaundiced patients with malignant biliary obstruction, due to either bile duct involvement by hepatocellular carcinoma or cholangiocarcinoma.[55, 56] MR should also be considered as an alternative imaging method in patient's in whom ERCP (endoscopic retrograde cholangiopancreatography) is either unsuccessful or in whom there would be a risk of complications from ERCP such as acute pancreatitis.

The ultimate roles of helical CT cholangiography and MR cholangiopancreatography remain to be defined. In an environment of cost containment, economic considerations must obviously be considered. As compared to ERCP, the noninvasive nature of CT and MR imaging makes them attractive imaging modalities. Nonetheless, the ability of ERCP to combine diagnostic and therapeutic options continues to make this more invasive technique a necessity in many cases.

Invasive Modalities

Despite advances in noninvasive imaging that provide useful information about pathologic conditions of the biliary tract, direct cholangiography remains the single best way to optimally image the biliary tree (**Fig. 2–6, 2–11 B, 2–12**). In addition to providing exquisite anatomic detail and significant diagnostic information, direct cholangiographic techniques can also be used to obtain histologic material and provide therapeutic relief of biliary obstruction. On the other hand, direct cholangiography is more costly, invasive, and has associated procedure-related complications. As a result, direct cholangiography, is usually used as an adjunctive tool for biliary interventions, as it adds significant diagnostic information and facilitates treatment of a variety of biliary diseases.

Endoscopic Retrograde Cholangiography

In experienced hands, endoscopic retrograde cholangiography is relatively safe, with high success and accuracy rates (reported to be greater than 90%).[57] The diagnostic and therapeutic potential of endoscopic retrograde cholangiography is broader than that of percu-

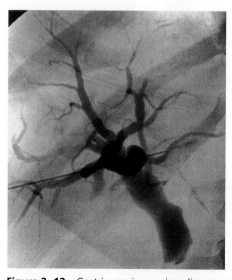

Figure 2–12 Gastric carcinoma invading common duct. Percutaneous transhepatic cholangiogram shows an abrupt and somewhat irregularly shaped cutoff in proximal common duct. This cholangiogram was done before placing a stent through the narrowed area.

taneous transhepatic cholangiography. Endoscopic retrograde cholangiography is used to diagnose and relieve obstructive jaundice that involves the distal duct (**Fig. 2–6, 2–11B**), to evaluate patients with postcholecystectomy syndrome and elucidate the cause of acute pancreatitis and cholangitis. Its limitations are that it is an invasive, technically challenging technique. ERCP is difficult to perform after a Billroth II anastomosis. It may by impossible with papillary obstruction; and it is relatively less effective in cases of proximal duct obstruction because of nonvisualization of the biliary tree above the site of obstruction. Complications occur in approximately 3% of patients, and result from pancreatitis, cholangitis, and sepsis.[58]

Percutaneous Transhepatic Cholangiography

Percutaneous transhepatic cholangiography may be used to delineate the biliary tree above an obstruction, but its primary uses are in conjunction with percutaneous biliary drainage procedures or to relieve biliary obstruction. In general, patients are selected for this approach (rather than endoscopic drainage) if the site of obstruction is proximal to the junction of the right and left hepatic ducts (**Fig. 2–12**).[59, 60] The reported success rate of this technique is 99% for dilated ducts and 85% for nondilated ducts.[61] When percutaneous transhepatic cholangiography is used to place an indwelling biliary stent, most authorities recommend it be done for relieving malignant, as opposed to benign obstructions.[62—64]

Significant complications of percutaneous transhepatic cholangiography occur in up to 1.5% of cases and include bile leakage, hemorrhage, and sepsis. The mortality rate is reported to be 0.07%.[65] Percutaneous transhepatic cholangiography is not used primarily for imaging because of its invasive nature; furthermore, similar visual information can usually be obtained using a variety of noninvasive imaging techniques.

Percutaneous Biliary Endoscopy and Endoscopic Ultrasound

These techniques are often complimentary to endoscopic retrograde cholangiography and percutaneous transhepatic cholangiography. Percutaneous biliary endoscopy is most often used as an adjunctive method to remove retained calculi in the common bile duct or gallbladder. It can also be used to determine the etiology of filling defects detected at cholangiography, guide biopsy of bile duct tumors, and help direct a guidewire across a tight biliary stricture.[66, 67] Complications of percutaneous biliary endoscopy are uncommon and include hemobilia, vagal reactions, laceration of the bile duct, and transient bacteremia.

Endoscopic ultrasound is another adjunctive technique that permits extremely high-resolution images (< 1 mm) to evaluate pancreaticobiliary and portal venous anatomy. This technique has a reported sensitivity that approaches 100% for detecting choledocholithiasis, and a reported accuracy of over 90% for detecting neoplasms in the head of the pancreas, common bile duct, and ampulla.[68] With a sensitivity of 95% and an accuracy of 93% for diagnosing portal vein invasion by pancreatobiliary neoplasms, it is superior to conventional ultrasound, CT, or angiography.[69] Limitations of endoscopic ultrasound include lack of therapeutic applications, difficulty evaluating obstructive lesions at the hilum or right hepatic duct, limited ability evaluating the distal bile duct/ampullary lesions in patients with significant pancreatic calcification or edema, and technical limitations if the endoscope cannot be positioned in the duodenum, or if there is air in the biliary tree.[68]

Use of US Imaging to Evaluate Jaundice

Despite the availability of newer imaging modalities, US remains the screening modality of choice for evaluating the biliary tree in most patients with jaundice or suspected biliary obstruction. The advantages of US imaging are well known and include the following: (1) it is a highly sensitive and accurate modality for determining whether intra- and/or extrahepatic bile duct dilatation is present; (2) it lacks ionizing radiation; (3) injection of contrast material is unnecessary; (4) it is speedy, flexible, portable, and safe; (5) it can successfully image patients independent of gastrointestinal, hepatic, biliary, and renal function; and (6) it can be used to examine multiple organs.

Accuracy of US Imaging

As a screening modality, the primary role of US imaging is to determine if biliary dilatation is present. Because US imaging is operator dependent, considerable variation exists in its ability to depict biliary obstruction. Reported sensitivities range from 68% to 99%, with reported specificities of 75—100%.[70]

The secondary role of US imaging is to determine the specific level and cause for an obstruction. Because bile ducts expand centrifugally from the site of obstruction, extrahepatic dilatation typically precedes intrahepatic dilatation.[71] It is important to identify the anatomic site and cause of an obstruction because this information may determine what other imaging examinations may be required for diagnostic evaluation. This information may also be used to suggest appropriate interventions, such as surgery, percutaneous biopsy, or endoscopic or percutaneous drainage. With real-time equipment and optimal scanning techniques, US imaging can define the level of obstruction in up to 92% of cases and can suggest the correct cause in up to 71% of cases.[72]

Limitations of US Imaging

Intrahepatic Duct Dilatation

Although intrahepatic duct dilatation is a highly specific finding for active biliary obstruction, it is a relatively insensitive finding, with a false-negative result rate of approximately 23%.[73] False-negative results typically occur in cases of acute extrahepatic obstruction or in cases where liver diseases (especially cirrhosis or diffuse neoplasm) limit the distensability of the intrahepatic ducts. Other causes for false-negative results include segmental obstruction, hemobilia, pneumobilia, and sclerosing cholangitis. In patients with hemobilia, the echogenicity of blood may be isoechoic with hepatic parenchyma. This may make the dilatation very subtle and difficult to detect.[74] Shadowing associated with pneumobilia can also make it impossible to determine either the diameter or internal contents of the duct (**Fig. 2–13**).[75] In patients with sclerosing cholangitis, fibrosis surrounding the intrahepatic ducts frequently prevents these duct dilatation.[76]

Although false-negative diagnoses are relatively common, a false-positive diagnosis of intrahepatic bile duct dilatation is quite unusual. It is important not to mistake a normally visible intrahepatic bile duct for mild dilatation. Revised criteria suggest that a pathologically dilated intrahepatic bile duct is greater than 2 mm in diameter and/or more than 40% of the diameter of the adjacent portal vein.[77] A pseudodilated intrahepatic duct can occur if an abnormally large hepatic artery mimics a dilated intrahepatic bile duct (**Fig. 2–14**).[78] Hepatic artery enlargement can occur with any condition that results in increased hepatic arterial flow, including

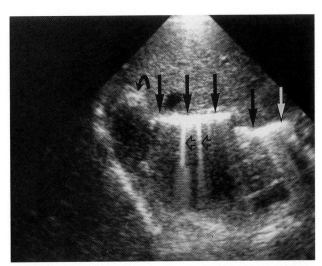

Figure 2–13 Pneumobilia. US scan of patient with surgically created biliary enteric anastomosis shows prominent linear areas of echogenicity (**straight solid arrows**) with comet tail artifacts (**open arrows**). These areas are due to pneumobilia. In this region, the biliary tree cannot be adequately evaluated with US imaging. Note also intrahepatic biliary calculus (**curved arrow**). Reprinted with permission from **Diagnostic Ultrasound** by F.C. Laing. Mosby, St. Louis, 1998. p. 175—223.

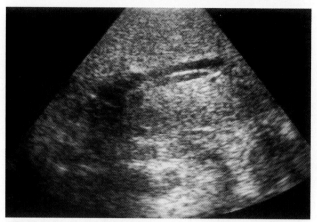

A

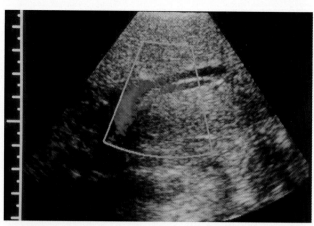

B

Figure 2–14   Pseudodilated intrahepatic bile ducts. **A:** Transverse US scans through left lobe of liver demonstrates two parallel tubular structures whose appearance suggests intrahepatic biliary dilatation. Reprinted with permission from **Diagnostic Ultrasound** by F.C. Laing. Mosby, St. Louis, 1998. p. 175—223. **B:** Color Doppler flow image reveals flowing blood within both of these tubular structures. Reprinted with permission from **Diagnostic Ultrasound** by F.C. Laing. Mosby, St. Louis, 1998. p. 175—223.

severe cirrhosis, portal hypertension, and hepatic neoplasms. The simplest way to detect a pseudodilated intrahepatic bile duct (due to an enlarged hepatic artery) from a truly dilated bile duct is to use color Doppler flow imaging to demonstrate blood flow within two parallel tubular structures—the portal vein and adjacent hepatic artery.[78]

Extrahepatic Duct Dilatation

Evaluation of the size of the extrahepatic duct is the most sensitive method of differentiating medical from surgical jaundice. Unfortunately, no single number determines if the extrahepatic duct is normal or dilated.

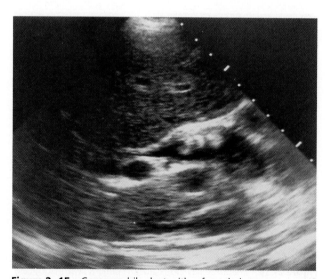

Figure 2–15   Common bile duct with a funneled appearance. US scan shows that the diameter of the distal duct is considerably more dilated than that of the proximal duct. If duct diameter is only measured in the porta hepatis, a falsely normal diameter would be obtained. This patient had acute obstruction due to choledocholithiasis. Reprinted with permission from **Diagnostic Ultrasound** by F.C. Laing. Mosby, St. Louis, 1998. p. 175—223.

Anteroposterior measurements as small as 4 mm or as large as 8 mm have been reported.[79, 80] A useful rule is that, after the patient reaches the fourth decade, the duct diameter is 10% of the patient's age. For example, in a 50-year-old patient, the maximum duct diameter is 5 mm, while in a 70-year-old patient, the maximum duct diameter is 7 mm. Although somewhat controversial, a recent study suggests that the diameter of the extrahepatic duct dilates slightly (about 2 mm) postcholecystectomy, and has a mean diameter of 6.1 mm.[81]

With the patient supine or in an oblique position, the duct diameter is typically measured in an anteroposterior direction. A recently reported study emphasizes that because the cross-sectional shape of the common bile duct is oval, the transverse diameter usually exceeds the anteroposterior diameter. Because transverse measurements correlate more closely with the measured diameter at endoscopic retrograde cholangiography, these investigators suggest measuring the transverse duct diameter to confirm or exclude biliary dilatation in patients with a larger than normal anteroposterior diameter.[82]

In most normal people, the diameter of the distal common bile duct is slightly greater than that of the proximal duct. This discrepancy in size is normally barely perceptible, unless the duct becomes abnormally funneled in configuration, with the distal duct diameter becoming several millimeters greater than the proximal diameter (**Fig. 2–15**). A funneled duct can be seen (1) in patients with early extrahepatic bile duct obstruction, (2) in patients whose extrahepatic obstruction has been relieved, or (3) in patients with an obstructed biliary tree and diffuse liver disease (particularly cirrhosis), in whom intrahepatic dilatation cannot readily occur. If, under these circumstances, the duct is measured only in the porta hepatis, then it may be falsely considered to be normal. More distal measurements will reveal borderline or frank dilatation.

Occasionally, anicteric dilation of the extrahepatic bile duct may occur (false-positive duct dilatation). This finding has been reported in patients with partial or incomplete biliary obstruction, in patients after cholecystectomy, and in patients whose prior obstruction has been relieved.

Alternatively, obstructive jaundice may occur without dilatation of either the intrahepatic or the extrahepatic bile ducts (false-negative duct dilatation).[83, 84] Underlying conditions usually responsible for these cases include cholangitis, partial obstruction, and intermittent obstruction from choledocholithiasis.

In questionable cases, biliary dynamics can be evaluated by repeating the US scan after the patient consumes a fatty meal. The fatty meal increases bile production, promotes gallbladder contraction, and relaxes the distal sphincter. In patients without biliary obstruction (true-negative cases), an initially normal-sized duct should remain unchanged or decrease in size after the meal, while an initially enlarged duct should decrease in caliber. In patients with biliary obstruction (true-positive cases), an initially normal or slightly dilated duct should increase in size after the meal.[85-87] This provocative test has been especially useful for detecting partial obstruction of the common bile duct. It has a reported sensitivity of 74% and specificity of 100%.[87]

Relation of US Imaging to Other Imaging Modalities

As the number of available imaging modalities used to evaluate jaundice continues to expand, clinical and imaging guidelines are becoming increasingly important (**Fig. 2–16**). In general, US imaging has been and continues to be the initial imaging modality of choice for evaluating a jaundiced patient. If the ducts are not dilated, then the patient is usually treated expectantly. Under exceptional circumstances, other imaging may be desirable or a liver biopsy may be performed.

If ductal dilatation is present, and the ultrasound examination can determine the level and the cause of the obstruction, then biopsy or therapy can often be performed directly. If the US examination is not successful in identifying the cause of the dilatation, additional problem-solving imaging studies (CT or MR imaging) are usually indicated. If a malignant obstruction is considered likely, either CT or MR imaging should be done to detect the precise location of the tumor and spread of disease, and guide a percutaneous biopsy. If a strong suspicion of calculus disease exists, then cholangiographic imaging may be desired. Although MR cholangiography appears to an excellent, noninvasive diagnostic cholangiographic examination, the therapeutic benefits of endoscopic retrograde cholangiography continue to make this more invasive technique attractive.

Curative or palliative surgical intervention is often indicated after the precise cause of the biliary obstruction has been determined. Techniques for radiologic intervention, however, continue to expand, and endoscopic retrograde cholangiography and percutaneous transhepatic cholangiography are frequently used to provide temporary or palliative therapeutic relief of biliary obstruction. In general, endoscopic retrograde cholangiography is used to treat distal obstruction, while percutaneous transhepatic cholangiography is used to treat proximal obstruction.[59, 60]

Other factors that must be considered in the selection of a particular imaging modality relate to a patient's body habitus, ability to cooperate, allergy history and renal function. Finally, when triage is considered, it is critical to evaluate the expertise of available radiologists as well as the availability of equipment.

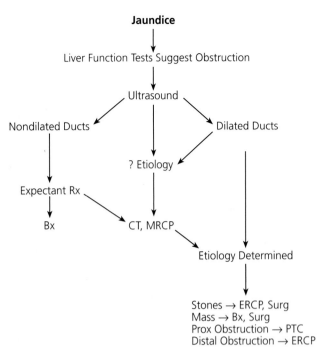

Figure 2–16 Algorithm for work-up of jaundice.

Summary

Jaundice continues to be a common and challenging indication for radiological imaging studies. Ultrasound remains the accepted imaging modality to be initially used in jaundiced patients. In the hands of a well-trained sonologist, this modality has reasonably acceptable sensitivity, specificity, and accuracy. Depending upon the ultrasound findings, additional imaging may be required. Most often this is CT, but as MRI evolves, it is playing a greater role for imaging the jaundiced patient. Despite the great ability of these more expensive noninvasive examinations to evaluate the biliary tree, interventional modalities such as ERC and PTC are often called upon to provide therapeutic relief of biliary obstruction.

References

1. Laing F.C. The gallbladder and bile ducts. In: Rumack C.M., Wilson S.R., Charboneau J.W., eds. *Diagnostic Ultrasound.* 2 nd ed. St Louis, Mo: Mosby, 1998; p. 175—223.

2. Zeman R.K., Taylor K.J.W., Rosenfield A.T., Schwartz A., Gold J.A. Acute experimental biliary obstruction in the dog. Sonographic findings and clinical implications. *AJR* 1981;136:965—967.

3. Standfield N.J., Salisbury J.R., Howard E.R. Benign non-traumatic inflammatory strictures of the extrahepatic biliary system. *Br J Surg* 1989;76:849—852.

4. Way L.W., Bernhoft R.A., Tomas M.J. Biliary stricture. *Surg Clin North Am* 1981;61:963—972.

5. Bismuth H. Postoperative strictures of the bile duct. In: Blumgart L.H., ed. *The Biliary Tract: Clinical Surgery International Series* (Vol. 5). Edinburgh: Churchill Livingstone 1982; p. 209—218.

6. Laing F.C: Ultrasound diagnosis of choledocholithiasis. *Sem Ultrasound, CT and MR* 1987;8:103—113.

7. Lim J.H., Ko Y.T., Lee D.H., et al. Oriental cholangiohepatitis. Sonographic findings in 48 cases. *AJR* 1990;155:511—514.

8. LaRusso N.F., Wiesner R.H., Ludwig J., et al. Primary sclerosing cholangitis. *N Engl J Med* 1984;310:899—903.

9. MacCarty R.L., LaRusso N.F., Wiesner R.H., et al. Primary sclerosing cholangitis; findings on cholangiography and pancreatography. *Radiology* 1983;149:39—44.

10. Farrant J.M., Hayllar K.M., Wilkinson M.L., et al. Natural history and prognostic variables in primary sclerosing cholangitis. *Gastroenterology* 1991;100:1710—1717.

11. MacCarty R.L., LaRusso N.F., May G.R., et al. Cholangiocarcinoma complicating primary sclerosing cholangitis: cholangiographic appearances. *Radiology* 1985;156:43—46.

12. Choi T.K., Wong K.P., Wong J. Cholangiographic appearance in clonorchiasis. *Br J Radiol* 1984;57:681—684.

13. Choi B.O., Kim H.J., Han M.C., et al. CT findings of clonorchiasis. *AJR* 1989;152:281—284.

14. Laing F.C: Ultrasonography of the gallbladder and biliary tree. In: Sarti D.A., ed. *Diagnostic Ultrasound: Text and Cases,* 2 nd ed. Chicago, IL: Yearbook, 1987; p. 142—153.

15. de Souza Rocha M. CT identification of ascaris in the biliary tract. *Abdom Imag* 1995;20:317—319.

16. Mehta P., Sharma A.K., Saluja S., et al. Biliary ascariasis: ultrasound diagnosis. *J Clin Ultrasound* 1995;23:500—501.

17. Yamaguchi M. Congential choledochal cyst analysis of 1,433 patients in the Japanese literature. *Am J Surg* 1980;140:653—657.

18. Kim O.H., Chung H.J., Choi B.G. Imaging of the choledochal cyst. *Radiographics* 1995;15:69—88.

19. Laing F.C., Frates M.C., Feldstein V., Goldstein R., Mondro S: Hemobilia: sonographic appearances in the GB and biliary tree with emphasis on intracholecystic blood. *JUM* 1997;16:537—544.

20. Choi B.I., Lim J.H., Han M.C., et al. Biliary cystadenoma and cystadenocarcinoma: CT and sonographic findings. *Radiology* 1989;171:57—61.

21. Korobkin M., Stephens D.H., Lee J.K.T., et al. Biliary cystadenoma and cystadenocarcinoma: CT and sonographic findings. *AJR* 1989;153:507—511.

22. Jackson V.P., Lappas J.C. Sonography of the Mirizzi syndrome. *J Ultrasound Med* 1984;3:281—283.

23. Becker C.D., Hassler H., Terrier F. Preoperative diagnosis of the Mirizzi syndrome. Limitations of sonography and computed tomography. *AJR* 1984;143:591—596.

24. Miller W.J., Sechtin A.G., Campbell W.L., Pieters P.C. Imaging findings in Caroli's disease. *AJR* 1995;165 333—337.

25. Sood G.K., Mahapatra J.R., Khurana A., et al. Caroli's disease: computed tomographic diagnosis. *Gastrointest Radiol* 1991;16:243—244.

26. Pavone P., Laghi A., Catalano C., et al. Caroli's disease: evaluation with MR cholangiopancreatography (MRCP). *Abdom Imag* 1996;21:117—117.

27. Desroches J., Spahr L., Leduc, et al. Noninvasive diagnosis of Caroli syndrome associated with congenital hepatic fibrosis using hepatobiliary scintigraphy. *Clin Nuc Med* 1995;20:512—514.

28. Sty J.R., Sullivan P., Wanger R., et al. Hepatic scinigraphy in Caroli's disease. *Radiology* 1978;127:732—■■.

29. Waters K., Howman-Giles R., Rossleigh M., et al. Intrahepatic bile duct dilatation and cholestasis in autosomal recessive polycystic kidney disease demonstration with hepatobiliary scintigraphy. *Clin Nuc Med* 1995;20:892—895.

30. Mettler F.A., Guiberteau M.J. Gastrointestinal tract. In:Mettler F.A., Guiberteau M.J., eds. *Essentials of Nuclear Medicine Imaging,* 3 rd ed. Philadelphia, Pa: WB Saunders Company, 1991; p. 201.

31. Pinos T., Xiol X., Herranz R., Figueras C., Catala I. Caroli's disease versus polycystic hepatic disease. Differential diagnosis with Tc-99 m DISIDA scintigraphy. *Clin Nuc Med* 1993;18:664—667.

32. Baron R.L. Computed tomography of the bile ducts. *Sem Roent* 1997;32:172—187.

33. Zeman R.K., Silverman P.M., Ascher S.M., et al. Helical (spiral) CT of the pancreas and biliary tract. *RCNA* 1995;33:887—902.

34. Liddell R.M., Baron R.L., Teefy S.A., et al. Normal intrahepatic bile ducts: CT depiction. *Radiology* 1990;176:633—655.

35. Baron R.L., Stanley R.J., Lee J.K.T., et al. Computed tomographic features of biliary obstruction. *AJR* 1983;140:1173—1178.

36. Brink J.A., Kammer B., Mueller P.R., et al. Prediction of gallstone composition: synthesis of CT and radiographic features in vitro. *Radiology* 1994;190:69—75.

37. Neitlich J.D., Topazian M., Smith R.C., et al. Detection of choledocholithiasis: comparison of unenhanced helical CT and endoscopic retrograde cholangiopancreatography. *Radiology* 1997;203:753—757.

38. Gilliams A., Gardener J., Richards R., Tan A.C., Linney A., et al. Three dimensional computed tomography cholangiography. A new technique for biliary tract imaging. *Br J Radiol* 1994;67:445—448.

39. Zeman R.K., Berman P.M., Silverman P.M., et al. Biliary tract. Three dimensional helical CT without cholangiographic contrast material. *Radiology* 1995;196:865—867.

40. Fleichmann D., Ringl H., Schofl R., et al. Three dimensional spiral CT cholangiography in patients with suspected biliary obstructive biliary disease. Comparison with endoscopic retrograde cholangiography. *Radiology* 1996;198:861—868.

41. Stockberger S.M., Wass J.L., Sherman S., Lehman G.A., Kopecky K.K. Intravenous cholangiography with helical CT. Comparison with endoscopic retrograde cholangiography. *Radiology* 1994;192:675—680.

42. Sherman S., Lehman G. ERCP and endoscopic sphincterotomy-induced pancreatitis. *Pancreas* 1991;3:350—367.

43. Van Beers B.E., Lacrosse M., Trigaux J.P., et al. Noninvasive imaging of the biliary tree before or after laparoscopic cholecystectomy: use of three dimensional spiral CT cholangiography. *AJR* 1994;162:1131—1135.

44. Soto J.A., Yucel E.K., Barish M.A., Chuttani R., Ferrucci J.T. MR cholangiopancreatography after unsuccessful or incomplete ERCP. *Radiology* 1996;199:91—98.

45. Guibaud L., Bret P.M., Reinhold C., Atri M., Barkun A.N. Bile duct obstruction and choledocholithiasis: diagnosis with MR cholangiography. *Radiology* 1995;197:109—115.

46. Hall-Craggs M.A., Allen C.M., Owens C.M., et al. MR cholangiography: clinical evaluation in 40 cases. *Radiology* 1993;189:423—427.

47. Reuther G., Kiefer B., Tuchmann A. Cholangiography before biliary surgery. Single-shot MR cholangiography versus intravenous cholangiography. *Radiology* 1996;198:561—566.

48. Chan Y., Chan A.C.W., Lam W.W.M., et al. Choledocholithiasis: comparison of MR cholangiography and endoscopic retrograde cholangiography. *Radiology* 1996;200:85—89.

49. Lee M.G., Lee H.J., Kim M.H., et al. Extrahepatic biliary diseases: 3 D MR cholangiopancreatography compared with endoscopic retrograde cholangiopancreatography. *Radiology* 1997;202:663—669.

50. Becker C.D., Grossholz M., Becker M., et al. Choledocholithiasis and bile duct stenosis: diagnostic accuracy of MR cholangiopancreatography. *AJR* 1996;167:1441—1445.

51. Ishizaki Y., Wakayama T., Okada Y., Kobayashi T. Magnetic resonance cholangiography for evaluation of obstructive jaundice. *Am J Gastroenterol* 1993;12:2072—2077.

52. Macaulay S.E., Shulte S.J., Sekijima J.H., et al. Evaluation of a non-breath-hold MR cholangiography technique. *Radiology* 1995;196:227—232.

53. Barish M.A., Yucel E.K., Soto J.A., Chuttani R., Ferrucci J.T. MR cholangiopancreatography: efficacy of three-dimensional turbo spin-echo technique. *AJR* 1995;165:295—300.

54. Regan F., Fradin J., Khazan R., et al. Choledocholithiasis: evaluation with MR cholangiography.

55. Soyer P., Laissy J.P., Bluemke D.A., et al. Dile duct involvement in hepatocellular carcinoma: MR demonstration. *Abdom Imag* 1995;20:114—121.

56. Murakami T., Nakamura H., Tsuda K., et al. Contrast-enhanced MR imaging of intrahepatic cholangiocarcinoma: pathologic correlation study. *JMRI* 1995;5:165—170.

57. Tobin R.S., Vogelzang R.L., Gore R.M., et al. A comparative study of computed tomography and ERCP in pancreaticobiliary disease. *JCAT* 1987;11:261—266.

58. Zeman R.K. Anatomy and techniques of examination of biliary tract and gallbladder (Oral cholecystography, computed tomography, cholescintigraphy, magnetic resonance imaging and cholangiography). In: Freeny P.C., Stevenson G.W., eds. *Margulis and Burhenne's Alimentary Tract Radiology*, 5 th ed. St. Louis MO: Mosby, 1995;1243.

59. Nelson K.M., Kastan D.J., Shetty P.C., et al. Utilization pattern and efficacy of nonsurgical techniques to establish drainage for high biliary obstruction. *JVIR* 1996,7;751—756.

60. England R.E., Martin D.F. Endoscopic and percutaneous intervention in malignant obstructive jaundice. *Cardiovasc Interv Radiol* 1996,19;381—387.

61. Ariyama J. Percutaneous transhepatic cholangiography. In: Margulis A.R., Burhenne H.J., eds. *Alimentary Tract Radiology*, 4 th ed. St. Louis MO: The CV Mosby Company, 1989;1995—2004.

62. Lammer J., Hausegger K.A., Flückiger F., et al. Common bile duct obstruction due to malignancy: treatment wih plastic versus metallic stents. *Radiology* 1996;201:167—172.

63. Lee B.H., Choe D.H., Lee J.H., et al. Metallic stents in malignant biliary obstruction: prospective long term clinical results. *AJR* 1997;168:741—745.

64. Hausegger K.A., Kugler C., Uggowitzer M., et al. Benign biliary obstruction: is treatment with the wallstent advisable? *Radiology* 1996;200:437—441.

65. Harbin W.P., Mueller P.R., Ferrucci J.T., Jr. Transhepatic cholangiography: complications and use patterns of the fine-needle technique: a multi-institutional survey. *Radiology* 1980;135:15—22.

66. Picus D. Percutaneous biliary endoscopy. *JVIR* 1995,6;303—310.

67. Rossi P., Bezzi M., Fiocca F., et al. Percutaneous cholangioscopy. *Semin Intervent Radiol* 1996,13;185—193.

68. Palazzo L., Levy P., Bernades P. Usefulness of endoscopic ultrasonography in the diagnosis of choledocholithiasis. *Abdom Imag* 1996,21;93—97.

69. Sugiyama M., Hagi H., Atomi Y., et al. Diagnosis of portal venous invasion be pancreatobiliary carcinoma: value of endoscopic ultrasonography. *Abdom Imag* 1997,22;434—438.

70. Zeman R.K., Burrell M.L. Biliary Obstruction—General Principles. In: Zeman R.K., Burrell M.L., eds. *Gallbladder and Bile Duct Imaging: A Clinical Radiologic Approach*. New York, NY: Churchill Livingstone, 1987; p. 403.

71. Shawker T.H., Jones B.L., Girton M.E: Distal common bile duct obstruction: an experimental study in monkeys. *J Clin Ultrasound* 1981;9:77—82.

72. Laing F.C., Jeffrey R.B., Jr., Wing V.W. Biliary dilatation. Defining the level and cause by real time US. *Radiology* 1986;160:9—42.

73. Sample W.F., Sarti D.A., Goldstein L.I., et al. Gray scale ultrasonography of the jaundiced patient. *Radiology* 1978;128:719—725.

74. Laffey P.A., Teplick S.K., Haskin P.H. Hemobilia: a cause of falsenegative ductal dilatation. *J Clin Ultrasound* 1986;14:636—638.

75. Lewandowski B.J., Withers C., Winsberg F. The airfilled left hepatic duct: the saber sign as an aid to the radiographic diagnosis of pneumobilia. *Radiology* 1984;153:329332.

76. Majoie C.B.L.M., Smits N.J., Phoa S.S.K.S., et al. Primary sclerosing cholangitis: sonographic findings. *Abdom Imaging* 1995;20:109—112.

77. Bressler E.L., Rubin J.M., McCracken S. Sonographic parallel channel sign. a reappraisal. *Radiology* 1987;151:343—346.

78. Wing V.W., Laing F.C., Jeffrey R.B. Sonographic differentiation of enlarged hepatic arteries from dilated intrahepatic bile ducts. *AJR* 1985;145:57—61.

79. Niederau C., Muller J., Sonnenberg A., et al. Extrahepatic bile ducts in healthy subjects, in patients with cholelithiasis, and in postcholecystectomy patients. A prospective ultrasonic study. *J Clin Ultrasound* 1983;11:23—27.

80. Behan M., Kazam E. Sonography of the common bile duct. Value of the right anterior oblique view. *AJR* 1978;130:701—709.

81. Feng B., Song Q. Does the common bile duct dilate after cholecystectomy? Sonographiuc evaluation in 234 patients. *AJR* 1995;165:859—861.

82. Wachsberg R.H., Kim K.H., Sundaram K. Sonographic versus endoscopic retrograde cholangiographic measurements of thebile duct revisited: importance of the transverse diameter. *AJR* 1998;170:669—674.

83. Weinstein B.J., Weinstein D.P. Biliary tract dilatation in the nonjaundiced patient. *AJR* 1980;134:899—906.

84. Zemen R., Taylor K.J.W., Burrell M.I., et al. Ultrasound demonstraton of anicteric dilatation of the biliary tree. *Radiology* 1980;134:689—692.

85. Simeone J.F., Butch R.J., Mueler P.R., et al. The bile ducts after a fatty meal. Further sonographic observations. *Radiology* 1986;160:29—31.

86. Willson S.A., Gosink B.B., vanSonnenberg E. Unchanged size of a dilated common bile duct after a fatty meal. Results and Significance. *Radiology* 1986;160:29—31.

87. Darweesh R.M., Dodds W.J., Hogan W.J. Fatty meal sonography for evaluating patients with suspected partial common duct obstruction. *AJR* 1988;151:63—68.

3

Sonography in the Evaluation of Abnormal Liver Tests

Michelle L. Robbin and Dirk J. van Leeuwen

An abdominal ultrasound (US) examination is frequently requested because a patient's liver tests are abnormal. This chapter is intended to provide the practicing radiologist with a framework for interpreting the results of liver tests. In conjunction with a patient's clinical history and the physical examination results, a differential diagnosis can be formulated for a specific patient. Then, imaging can be performed in a custom-tailored manner for that particular individual.

This review is intended to help the radiologist act as a consultant to the referring clinician and select the appropriate hepatobiliary imaging modality for a timely, cost-efficient workup. The goal is to become more comfortable with the clinical data and enhance a rational problem-solving approach.

The clinical data include the patient's history, physical findings, and laboratory tests. Possible diagnoses will be divided into two major categories—cholestasis and hepatocellular disease. An algorithmic approach to the patient will be outlined, with an emphasis on the role of ultrasound. Lastly, in the Addendum, the most commonly used liver tests are reviewed.

Clinical Questions

The clinician who refers a patient for an abdominal ultrasound examination may have a number of different questions to be answered, depending on the patient's initial history, physical examination, and laboratory work. The physician may consider a wide range of possible causes when minor liver test abnormalities are found.

When major liver test abnormalities are found, indications for an ultrasound examination include the initial evaluation of jaundice (the differentiation between parenchymal liver disease and biliary tract obstruction) and a more detailed study of already known chronic liver disease. This study should include a search for specific complications including ascites. One should keep in mind that liver disease may be asymptomatic, and an ultrasound examination may be the first indication of advanced liver disease. The following questions need to be addressed on every abdominal ultrasound examination. Although not usually stated, they are implicit when the clinician is concerned about possible hepatobiliary abnormalities:

1. Is there biliary tract dilatation? If so, what is the level of obstruction? Can the cause be identified?
2. Are the findings consistent with advanced liver disease, that is, cirrhosis?
3. Do any space-occupying lesions exist?
4. If no abnormalities are seen, what is the diagnostic certainty that none are present? Should a corroborating study such as computed tomography (CT), magnetic resonance imaging (MRI), or endoscopic retrograde cholangiopancreatography (ERCP) be performed?

Depending on the specific disease suggested by the clinical data or the ultrasound findings, a more focused examination may also be required. For example, in cases of suspected cirrhosis, the ultrasound examination must assess liver morphology and attempt to identify any signs of portal hypertension (discussed later).

Algorithmic Approach to Diagnosis

Fig. 3–1 shows an algorithm that is useful in thinking about liver disease. As already discussed, sonography is the imaging test of choice when the results of liver tests are abnormal. A low-cost, noninvasive screening modality, its primary initial role is to differentiate between dilated and nondilated ducts.

An elevated alkaline phosphatase (AP) and γ-glutamyl transpeptidase (GGT), with or without an elevation in bilirubin, is usually found in patients with obstruction of the biliary tree. The sonographic hallmark of biliary obstruction is bile duct dilatation, although sonographically normal ducts do not always exclude obstruction. When the ducts are dilated, the goal of sonography is to determine the level and cause of the obstruction. Sonographic findings can narrow the differential diagnosis and either suggest appropriate treatment, or, when required, point the way to the next appropriate diagnostic test. This limb of the algorithm will be further expanded in the section on cholestasis.

Elevations in transaminases, such as aspartate aminotransferase (AST) [serum glutamic oxaloacetic transaminase (SGOT)] and alanine aminotransferase (ALT) [serum glutamic pyruvic transaminase (SGPT)] are commonly found in parenchymal disease. Uncommonly, acute obstruction of the common bile duct by gallstones can cause very elevated levels of transaminases, mimicking acute hepatitis.[1]

When a negative sonogram makes biliary obstruction unlikely, many parenchymal liver diseases must still be considered in the differential diagnosis. Essentially, ultrasound imaging can confidently detect cirrhosis and can suggest fatty infiltration and hepatitis, but normal images do not exclude parenchymal disease. Likewise, the suggestion of fatty infiltration does not exclude the presence of more significant parenchymal disease. This topic will be discussed at greater length in the section on parenchymal disease.

A mixed pattern of elevated levels of alkaline phosphatase, γ-glutamyl transpeptidase (GGT), ALT, and AST can be confusing to the clinician because neither a typical cholestatic or parenchymal pattern is suggested by the laboratory tests. In this setting, ultrasound imaging is particularly valuable in sorting through the diagnostic pathways.

Cholestasis

Ultrasound imaging is usually the diagnostic test of choice in cases of suspected biliary tract obstruction. In certain cases, such as morbid obesity or a very fatty liver, ultrasound may not optimally image the biliary system, and CT can be a helpful alternative. CT imaging, and not ultrasound, is the usual staging modality for pancreatic malignancy in the United States. Thus, if a strong clinical suspicion exists that the patient has a pancreatic malignancy, institutional preference may favor CT as the initial exam.

An ultrasound examination is the primary screening test used to differentiate between dilated intrahepatic and extrahepatic ducts (so called "surgical jaundice") and nondilated ducts ("medical jaundice") and is accurate in more than 90% of cases.[2] It is important to realize that detecting the presence of dilated ducts does not always mean that biliary obstruction is present. Conversely, biliary obstruction may be present in the absence of dilatation, although this is uncommon.

When dilated ducts are detected, the level and cause of the biliary obstruction must be ascertained. Laing et al.[3] found that ultrasound imaging correctly determined the level of obstruction in 92% of the cases, almost all of which were at the intrapancreatic level. The ultrasound based interpretation was correct 71% of the time, with an accuracy of 81% in diagnosing choledocholithiasis, 83% accuracy in diagnosing pancreatitis (with clinical correlation), and 91% accuracy in the detection of primary and metastatic neoplasms as a cause of obstruction.[3]

Awareness of the most likely causes for obstruction at each level of the biliary tree helps in tailoring the ultrasound examination. At all levels, gallstones are the most

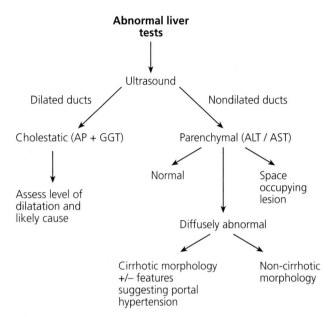

Figure 3–1 Algorithm for patient with abnormal liver tests. It is noteworthy that parenchymal liver disease may be very cholestatic (hepatitis A, drugs, primary biliary cirrhosis, and primary sclerosing cholangitis). Cholestasis of any cause may be responsible for significant weight loss and does not necessarily implicate malignancy. ALT, alanine aminotransferase; AP, alkaline phosphatase; AST, aspartate aminotransferase; GGT, γ-glutamyl transpeptidase.

common cause of obstructive jaundice. Detecting multiple bile duct stones, particularly in the elderly, does not exclude a coincident malignant cause of obstruction, such as cholangiocarcinoma. Also, when strictures (from cholangiocarcinoma or primary sclerosing cholangitis) are present, sludge and stones may develop. van den Hazel found that greater than 24% of initial diagnoses by CT or US were changed by ERCP in a study of 542 patients with presumed bile duct stones or a distal common bile duct stricture prior to ERCP (van den Hazel S.J., de Vries X.H., Speelman P., Huibregtse K., Tytgat G.N.J., van Leeuwen D.J., unpublished material).

Less common causes of intrahepatic biliary obstruction include primary sclerosing cholangitis (particularly in patients with ulcerative colitis), cholangiocarcinoma, and neoplasms (primary or metastatic).

The differential diagnosis of biliary obstruction in the porta hepatis includes cholangiocarcinoma, sclerosing cholangitis, gallbladder cancer, hepatocellular carcinoma, and metastatic disease (typically affecting the porta hepatis nodes in the hepatoduodenal ligament).[4] Benign inflammatory changes and reactive lymphadenopathy may occur in up to 13% of cases with "malignant" disease diagnosed by imaging.[5]

Supra- and intrapancreatic causes of biliary obstruction include choledocholithiasis, chronic pancreatitis, pancreatic or duodenal carcinoma, cholangiocarcinoma, and metastatic disease.[6] **Fig. 3–2** shows marked intra- and extrahepatic biliary ductal dilatation from a pancreatic neoplasm.

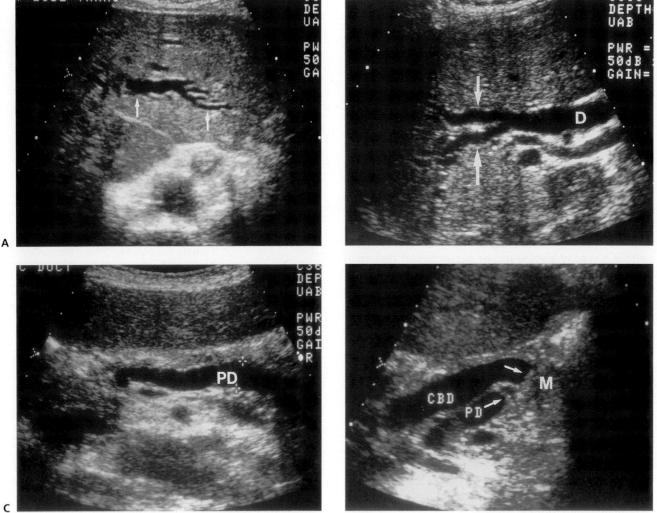

Figure 3–2   Ultrasound scans of dilated intra- and extrahepatic ducts from pancreatic carcinoma. (**A**) Transverse scan shows marked left-sided intrahepatic biliary ductal dilatation (**arrows**). (**B**) Long scan shows marked intrahepatic ductal dilatation (**arrows**) in right lobe of liver. Enlarged 1.3-cm common bile duct (D) is also shown. (**C**) Transverse scan shows marked pancreatic duct dilatation (PD). (**D**) Long scan shows common bile duct (CBD) and pancreatic ductal dilatation. Note abrupt shelflike termination of common bile duct and pancreatic duct (PD) (**arrows**) by pancreatic mass (M).

Parenchymal Liver Disease

The sonologist can observe several major morphologic patterns of hepatic disease caused by various types of diffuse hepatocellular injury. The liver may enlarge due to inflammation, fatty infiltration, or storage products. The liver may shrink due to acute liver failure with parenchymal collapse. The liver may have a cirrhotic appearance or findings strongly suggestive of cirrhosis. Characteristic morphologic features of cirrhosis include a nodular surface, a shrunken right lobe, and an enlarged left lobe and caudate lobe. It is important to realize that an enlarged cirrhotic liver may not have these typical morphologic features of cirrhosis. Thus, the absence of morphologic features of cirrhosis does not exclude that diagnosis, while the presence of a shrunken right lobe with enlarged left and caudate lobes is a reliable indicator of cirrhosis.

Parenchymal disease can be divided into two clinical situations—disease in relatively healthy individuals and disease in individuals who are ill and show clinical stigmata of chronic liver disease. Common diagnoses in apparently healthy people are chronic hepatitis B or C infection, and nonalcoholic steatohepatitis. Patients who appear to have a more serious problem may be diagnosed as having acute hepatitis, cirrhosis, or metastasis.

Chronic Hepatitis B or C

The number of people in the United States infected with chronic hepatitis B is around 1.9 million. Worldwide, over 400 million people suffer from hepatitis B. Although many of these patients have symptomatic liver disease, the majority are identified during routine screening procedures or when donating blood. Patients often have only minimal inflammatory changes and, therefore, a normal liver on ultrasound examination. The same statement applies to the over 200 million patients infected with hepatitis C, including 3.8 million in the United States. Both conditions are significant risk factors not only for cirrhosis but also for hepatocellular carcinoma. Hepatocellular carcinoma is a leading cause of death in Southeast Asia and South Africa.

Nonalcoholic Steatohepatitis

Patients who have a suggestion of a "fatty" liver on imaging studies such as CT or ultrasound and normal liver tests may only have fat accumulation in the liver. However, if patients have abnormal liver tests (a mixed cholestatic and a parenchymal pattern with mild elevations of alkaline phosphatase, GGT, AST, and ALT), it is more likely that they have steatohepatitis.[7] Steatohepatitis is a combination of both fat accumulation and inflammation which is pathologically identical to the features of alcoholic hepatitis and hepatitis seen after jejunoileal bypass surgery. Steatohepatitis is typically associated with obesity, diabetes, and middle-aged women, but it may be found in many other circumstances. The disease is very common and tends to have a relatively benign course. However, it may cause cirrhosis, which may require liver transplantation.[8]

In nonalcoholic patients, obesity is the most common condition associated with a fatty liver. Other frequently associated conditions are diabetes, especially in those who are poorly controlled and those who have an abnormal lipid profile. Various drugs have been implicated, including amiodarone. A fatty liver is also associated with chronic illnesses, such as heart failure and chronic pancreatitis, and with hyperalimentation. If the patient is asymptomatic and the abnormalities are mild, the patient should probably be followed up with periodic liver tests instead of further imaging examinations or a biopsy.

Typical sonographic findings of fatty liver are a diffusely echogenic liver and attenuation of the ultrasound beam,[9] as shown in **Fig. 3–3**. These findings are different from those of hepatic fibrosis, which usually does not cause an increase in attenuation of the liver parenchyma.[10—13]

The typical pattern of a fatty liver may be seen in patients with a combination of fatty liver and fibrosis. Thus, both the radiologist and the referring physician must not assume that an echogenic liver is solely due to "benign" fatty infiltration and overlook potential causes of coexistent fibrosis or inflammation. When significant attenuation of the ultrasound beam is present, focal lesions may be missed sonographically. If a mass is a clinical consideration, CT or MR imaging may be useful for further evaluation in these patients.

Areas of relatively decreased echogenicity are commonly seen in livers that have an overall increase in

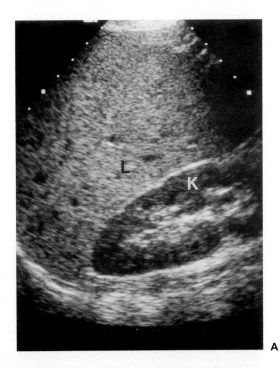

A

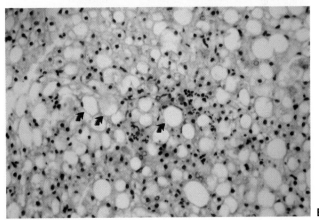

B

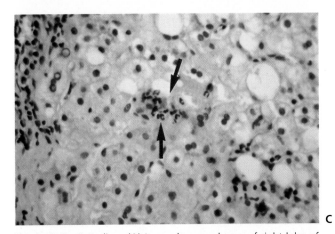

C

Figure 3–3 Fatty liver. (**A**) Long ultrasound scan of right lobe of liver (L) shows significantly increased echogenicity of liver as compared with that of renal cortex (K). Attenuation of the ultrasound beam causes loss of vessel wall definition in the posterior aspects of the liver. (**B**) Typical liver biopsy of steatohepatitis. There are abundant liver cells filled with large fat vacuoles (**arrows**). (**C**) The inset shows a neutrophilic infiltrate (**arrow**) as characteristically seen in steatohepatitis.

echogenicity consistent with infiltration of fat. These areas of decreased echogenicity usually represent focal sparing of the liver. The most common location for focal sparing is adjacent to the gallbladder fossa or in the periportal area, within the medial segment of the left lobe of the liver. These regions are usually ovoid, with sharply defined margins. Focal sparing does not produce a mass effect, and normal vessels are seen to course within it.[14] **Fig. 3–4** shows a typical fatty liver with an area of focal sparing adjacent to the gallbladder.

Focal fatty infiltration has similar findings and is found in the same locations. It appears as an echogenic area with geometric margins superimposed on a normal liver (**Fig. 3–5**). Occasionally, the diagnosis of fatty infiltration can be difficult if the borders are more irregular or multiple areas of involvement exist. In these cases, CT imaging can provide additional information, although a small percentage of cases may require MR imaging or biopsy.[15] An unusual case of innumerable echogenic lesions proven to be focal fat by biopsy is shown in **Fig. 3–6**.

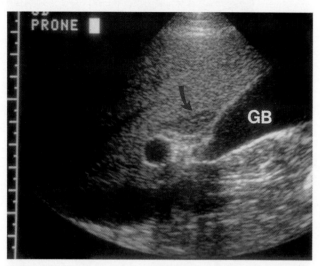

Figure 3–4 Region of focal sparing in a fatty liver. Long ultrasound scan shows focal, well-defined area of decreased echogenicity (**arrow**) adjacent to the gallbladder (GB), against the background of an echogenic liver.

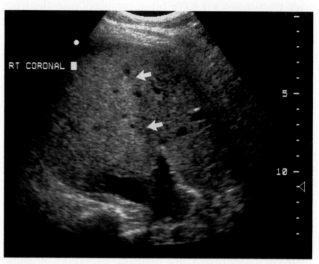

Figure 3–5 Focal fatty infiltration. Transverse image of the liver shows a well-defined, sharply marginated area of increased echogenicity in the anterior segment of the right lobe of the liver without mass effect (**arrows**). Vessels course smoothly through this area. These findings are characteristic of focal fat, and no further imaging studies are necessary.

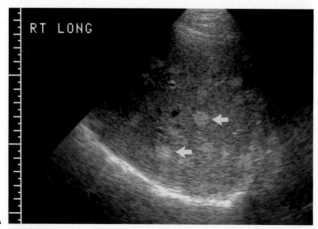

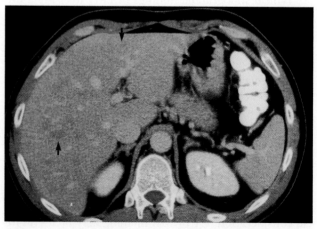

Figure 3–6 Unusual case of focal fatty infiltration. (**A**) Long ultrasound shows innumerable rounded echogenic foci of varying size (**arrows**) in this patient with a testicular tumor, initially thought to be metastatic disease. (**B**) Contrast-enhanced CT scan shows multiple low-attenuation areas corresponding to the areas of increased echogenicity on the ultrasound (**arrows**). Biopsy of the lesions demonstrated focal fat, without evidence of metastases.

Acute Hepatitis

Acute hepatitis results in variable degrees of liver cell damage. Large amounts of necrosis cause markedly elevated levels of ALT and AST, which often precede increases in bilirubin. Severe inflammation decreases the ability of the liver to excrete bilirubin, causing increases in serum-conjugated bilirubin and subsequent jaundice. Serologic tests are helpful in the diagnosis of viral hepatitis A, B, C, D, and E. **Table 3–1**[16] summarizes the most common viral markers used for diagnosis. Chronic hepatitis C infection often has normal or minimal increases in transaminases, but may have increases up to four or five times the upper limits of normal.

In most circumstances, imaging is unnecessary in patients with acute hepatitis A, as the diagnosis is obvious clinically. In acute hepatitis, the liver may have a diffusely decreased echogenicity, with prominence of the portal triads (**Fig. 3–7**).[17]A patient with acute alcoholic hepatitis is shown in **Fig. 3–8**, with areas of increased and decreased echogenicity without a focal mass. Interestingly, the CT image appeared relatively unremarkable in this very ill patient. Chronic hepatitis shows non-

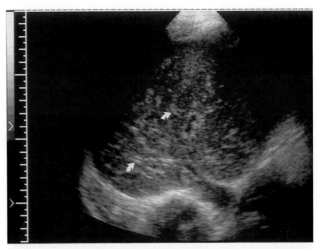

Figure 3–7 Acute hepatitis. Oblique ultrasound through the liver shows an overall decreased hepatic parenchymal echogenicity and increased prominence of the portal triads (**curved arrows**), a pattern that may be seen in acute hepatitis.

Table 3–1 Viral markers of hepatitis and their interpretation

Virus	Tests	Interpretation	Comments
HAV	Anti-HAV IgM	Acute hepatitis	Can remain positive for >1 yr
	Anti-HAV IgG	Past hepatitis, immunity	Is lifelong
HBV	HBsAG	Acute or chronic disease	
	Anti-HBc IgM	Acute infection (if high titer); chronic infection (if low titer)	
	Anti-HBc IgG	Past or recent HBV contact	Can be only serum indicator of past infection
	HBe	Active viral replication	Is becoming obsolete; has played major role in diagnosing replication
	Anti-HBe	Low or absent replicative state	Is typically present in long-standing HBV carriers
	Anti-HBs	Immunity	Shows immunity, after vaccination
	HBV-DNA	Active viral replication	Is expensive; may replace HBeAg if price declines
HCV	Anti-HCV	Past or current infection	Is not a neutralizing antibody
	RIBA	Test for various viral components	Is expensive; limited indications
	HCV-RNA	Active viral replication	Is expensive; limited indications (treatment)
HDV	Anti-HDV IgM	Acute or chronic infection	Consider only if HBsAg positive
	Anti-HDV IgG	Chronic infection (if high titer and IgM positive) Past infection (if low titer and IgM negative)	
	HDV-RNA	Replication of Δ	
HEV	Anti-HEV IgM	Acute hepatitis	Is not commercially available in United States
	Anti-HEV IgG	Past hepatitis	CDC may test in selected cases
	HEV-RNA	Viral replication	

Source: Reprinted with permission from Focal hepatic fatty infiltration as a cause of pseudotumors: ultrasonographic patterns and clinical differentiation by Wang, et al. J Clin Ultrasound 1990:18:401—409.
HAV, hepatitis A virus; HBV, hepatitis B virus; HCV, hepatitis C virus; HDV, hepatitis D virus; HEV, hepatitis E virus; anti-HAV, antibody to hepatitis A virus; anti-HBc, antibody to hepatitis B core antigen; anti-HBe, antibody to hepatitis B e antigen; anti-HBs, antibody to hepatitis B surface antigen; HBe, hepatitis B e antigen; HBs, hepatitis B surface antigen; IgG, immunoglobulin G; anti-HCV, antibody to hepatitis C virus; IgM, immunoglobulin M; RIBA, recombinant immunoblot assay. CDC, Centers for Disease Control

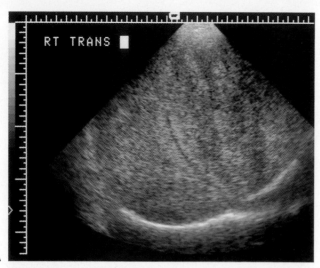

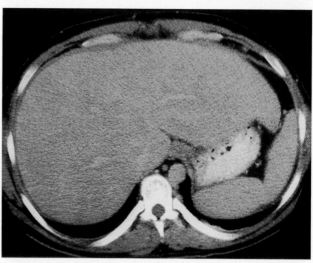

Figure 3–8   Acute alcoholic hepatitis. (**A**) Transverse ultrasound scan shows markedly heterogeneous liver, with multiple areas of adjacent increased and decreased echogenicity. No definite focal mass was identified. (**B**) Contrast-enhanced CT scan shows the liver, which was only minimally heterogeneous in this very ill patient.

specific coarsening of the echotexture at ultrasound imaging and, in the acute phase, a decrease in the bright portal vein walls.[17]

The sonographic findings of acute hepatitis may help to confirm (but never to exclude) the clinical diagnosis. In a patient with acute hepatitis, a decrease in liver size and an increase in ascites may be ominous and indicate impending liver failure due to parenchymal collapse. After a patient with cirrhosis develops ascites, measures to prevent spontaneous bacterial peritonitis will usually be taken by the clinician.

Edematous thickening of the gallbladder wall is often seen in patients with acute or chronic liver disease, and patients with low albumin levels, and does not necessarily indicate cholecystitis. Recognition of this association is very important, and may prevent confusion with cholecystitis and unnecessary surgery.[18]

Cirrhosis

Cirrhosis is caused by hepatic cell death and subsequent fibrosis and regeneration. The regeneration can be micronodular (< 1 cm) or macronodular.[19] Cirrhosis can be an insidious condition, with few symptoms and minor liver test abnormalities until late in the disease. Ultrasound findings of cirrhosis include morphologic signs of cirrhosis and evidence of portal hypertension. Echogenicity may be increased or normal, depending on the amount of fatty infiltration, inflammation, and fibrosis present. Only fatty infiltration causes increased echogenicity in the liver, as previously discussed. A nodular pattern may be seen. Morphologic changes, such as a nodular liver surface, are sensitive in the detection of cirrhosis (sensitivity 88%, specificity 82—95%).[20—22] The major differential diagnosis to be considered in a diffusely nodular liver is widespread metastatic disease.[23] It is usually easy to distinguish cirrhosis from metastatic disease clinically or from the imaging findings. In some but not all patients with cirrhosis, the right lobe decreases in size while the caudate and left lobes enlarge. When the ratio of the width of the caudate lobe to the width of the right lobe is greater than 0.65, cirrhosis is likely present. This ratio is a specific, but insensitive indicator of cirrhosis—specificity = 100%, sensitivity range 43—84% (**Fig. 3–9**). [24, 25] Typical ultrasound findings of cirrhosis are illustrated in **Fig. 3–10**.

After a cirrhotic morphology has been identified (particularly in a patient with decompensated liver disease), the following key questions must be answered by the ultrasound examination: (1) Are there signs of portal hypertension? (2) Is the portal venous system patent? (3) Are there focal liver masses?

Signs of portal hypertension include an enlarged spleen, ascites, biphasic or reversed flow in the left, right or main portal vein, and portosystemic collaterals.[26] The portosystemic collaterals most commonly visualized sonographically are an enlarged paraumbilical vein, splenic varices, splenorenal and splenoretroperitoneal collaterals, and enlarged coronary (left gastric) veins in the lesser omentum (gastrohepatic ligament). The portal vein may be enlarged, normal, or small. When the portal vein is small (< 7 mm), care should be taken not to mistake a venous collateral in the porta hepatis (found in cases of portal vein thrombosis) for the normal portal vein. Cavernous transformation of the portal vein is a potential vascular problem in patients who are candidates for a liver transplant. The superior mesenteric and splenic veins must then be imaged to insure that there is a vein sufficiently large to provide adequate venous inflow for the transplanted liver.

With color Doppler flow or spectral Doppler imaging, the absence of detectable flow in the portal vein can be problematic. The absence of flow in the portal vein is usually indicative of thrombus. However, approximately once a year we see no sonographic portal vein flow in a vein later proven (by another modality) to be widely patent, consistent with stagnant flow. When the portal vein is enlarged, filled with low-level echoes, and no flow is visualized despite optimal technique, we feel confident in identifying a portal vein thrombus (**Fig. 3–11**). Optimal sonographic technique includes high-sensitivity Doppler settings (low wall filter and pulse repetition frequency, high gain and power), good acoustic access, a low-scan angle, and visible flow in other vessels within the same field of view.[27, 28]

It is important to note that while spectral Doppler may be more sensitive than color or power Doppler in the detection of flow, it cannot differentiate partial thrombosis from occlusion. Presence of a venous flow signal in the region of the portal vein does not reliably distinguish a collateral vessel adjacent to a thrombosed vein from a totally or partially patent portal vein.

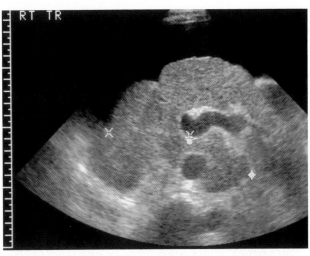

Figure 3–9 Enlarged caudate to right lobe ratio. Transverse ultrasound shows a nodular, cirrhotic liver outlined by ascites. The caudate to right lobe ratio is greater than 0.65, a finding specific for cirrhosis. Caudate length delimited by solid circles. Right lobe length delimited by asterisks.

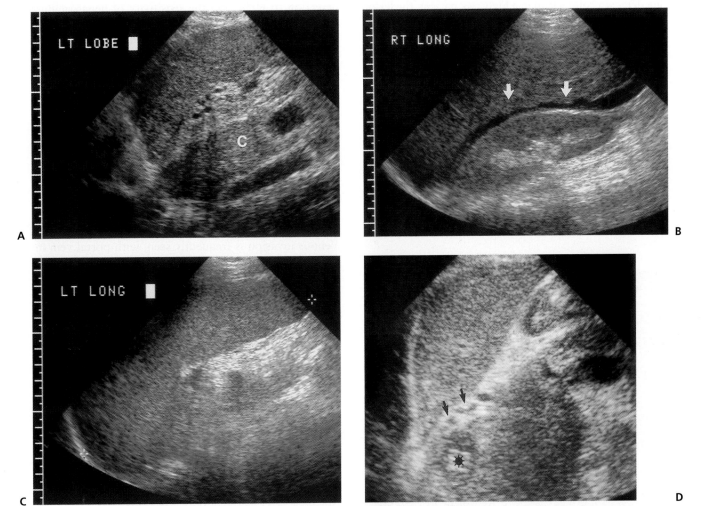

Figure 3–10 Cirrhosis. (**A**) Long ultrasound scan shows typical heterogeneous, nodular liver as seen in cirrhosis. Focal masses cannot be excluded sonographically in this liver. Note the caudate lobe enlargement (C). (**B**) Long ultrasound scan shows a markedly nodular contour of the inferior right liver border (**arrows**), outlined by ascites. (**C**) Long ultrasound scan shows markedly enlarged spleen (18 cm, X's), suggestive of portal hypertension. (**D**) Long ultrasound scan through left lobe of liver shows varices (arrows) around gastroesophageal junction (*).

If sonography cannot be definitive in the diagnosis of portal vein patency, local preference dictates whether angiography, MRI, or CT is used for further flow evaluation. The few patients in whom we are not able to definitively diagnose either portal vein patency or thrombosis are usually pre-TIPS (transjugular intrahepatic portosystemic shunt), and the differentiation between thrombosis and stagnant flow is made angiographically at the time of the TIPS procedure. Intra-arterial injection with drugs such as Tolazoline increase the contrast visualization of the portal venous system during angiography[29, 30], lessening the potential difficulty with visualization of the portal vein in patients with significantly altered portal hemodynamics (flow reversal, large collaterals, shunts, etc).

In a patient with known cirrhosis, new onset of clinical symptoms of weight loss, pain, and a significant increase in the amount of ascites should suggest the possibility of hepatocellular carcinoma. In this clinical setting, an ultrasound examination and α-fetoprotein (AFP) screening should be performed. When sonography detects a solid lesion in a high-risk patient, the lesion should be considered a hepatocellular carcinoma until proven otherwise.

Focal Liver Lesions

Hepatocellular Carcinoma

The most significant lesion found in patients with long-standing hepatitis and/or cirrhosis is hepatocellular carcinoma. The relative risk for hepatocellular carcinoma in patients who have had the hepatitis B virus for over 30 years is 100-fold that of the normal population.[31] The risk increases a further 10-fold in the presence of cirrhosis. In this high-risk population, AFP

screening is thought to be warranted.[32] Patients who are positive for hepatitis B surface antigen and who have chronic active hepatitis or cirrhosis should undergo measurement of AFP and an initial ultrasound examination,[31] and follow-up ultrasound considered.[33] The National Institutes of Health Consensus Conference in 1986 recommended an AFP screen every 3—4 months and an ultrasound examination every 4—6 months[32] for patients in this high-risk group.

The reported sensitivity and specificity of ultrasound imaging as compared to CT imaging in the detection of hepatocellular carcinoma is quite variable. Sensitivities range from 50—92% for ultrasound imaging and 73—94% for CT imaging.[34—36] Both CT and ultrasound imaging may not accurately assess the number and size of hepatocellular carcinomas.[37] In a retrospective analysis by Shapiro et al., hepatocellular carcinomas were identified by ultrasound in 67% of patients, and CT in only 57% of patients. Ultrasound detected 53% of individual tumors, while CT detected 45%. A combination of the two modalities increased the sensitivity of overall tumor detection to 60%, and the sensitivity of hepatocellular carcinoma detection to 80%.[38] Therefore, in end-stage cirrhotic livers and in heterogeneous livers, it is prudent to regard ultrasound, CT, and MR imaging as complementary tests that together can increase the sensitivity and specificity of hepatocellular carcinoma detection.

At sonography, hepatocellular carcinomas may be iso-, hypo-, or hyperechoic. Small tumors (< 5 cm) tend to be hypoechoic,[39] but can be very echogenic, mimicking cavernous hemangiomas and other tumors. **Fig. 3–12** shows a 3-cm hepatocellular carcinoma (AFP negative) with central arterial flow. Hepatocellular carcinomas can be single, multiple, or diffuse.[40] A high index of suspicion of tumor is required to differentiate some large diffuse tumors from a very nodular cirrhotic liver. Venous invasion is frequently seen, with portal vein invasion occurring more frequently than invasion of the hepatic vein.[41] Venous invasion may be the first or only definitive evidence that an hepatocellular carcinoma is present.

Metastases

Metastatic lesions are not infrequently found in patients with relatively new liver function test abnormalities and a history of a primary tumor. An isolated elevated alkaline phosphatase in a patient with a known malignancy is suspicious for liver metastasis, and may prompt a careful search for metastases. Metastatic disease of the liver is highly variable in its presentation on ultrasound imaging. Sonographic patterns of metastatic lesions include those with increased or decreased echogenicity, target, calcified, cystic, and diffuse.[42—44] Well-circumscribed lesions different from the background liver echogenicity are typically not difficult to diagnose with ultrasound (**Fig. 3–13**). This is distinct from diffuse

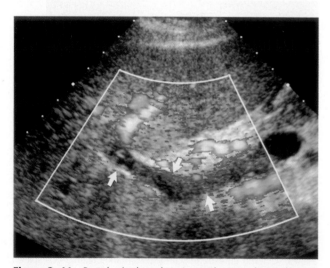

Figure 3–11 Portal vein thrombus. Long ultrasound scan through the main portal vein (**arrows**) shows no flow even with power Doppler. Note the low-level echoes filling the main portal vein, consistent with thrombus.

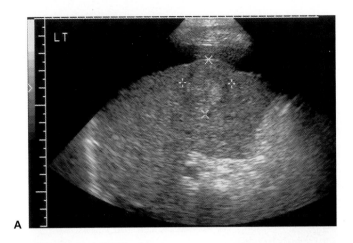

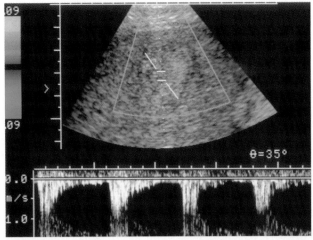

Figure 3–12 Hepatocellular carcinoma. (**A**) Long ultrasound scan through the liver demonstrates a 3-cm heterogeneous hepatocellular carcinoma (**cursors**). This tumor was AFP-negative in this patient with hepatitis B. (**B**) Color and spectral Doppler image shows central arterial flow in the tumor.

metastatic disease, typically from breast cancer, lung cancer, and malignant melanoma, which tend to be the most difficult tumor to detect on ultrasound scans.[40]

When the liver is absolutely normal in echotexture and appearance on ultrasound examination, and the patient's alkaline phosphatase, bilirubin, AST, and ALT are normal, we feel comfortable in excluding a diagnosis of metastatic disease. However, if ultrasound imaging shows heterogeneity or possible masses in the liver, a CT or MRI examination should be obtained to exclude diffuse disease. If a high clinical suspicion of metastatic disease exists, a CT examination may be a more useful initial test, because of its superiority as a screening test. In addition, it is often easier to perform serial, bidimensional measurements of multiple tumors on CT scans.

Benign Tumors

Benign liver tumors are typically incidental findings during an ultrasound examination and rarely cause liver function test abnormalities. Currently, the diagnosis of these tumors cannot be made solely on sonographic gray scale, color, and spectral Doppler criteria alone. Small hemangiomas are characteristically very echogenic, well-circumscribed masses <3 cm in diameter.[45] However, hepatocellular carcinomas, particularly small ones, can also be echogenic. It is therefore important to obtain a corroborating study such as a CT, MRI, or red blood cell scintigraphy for definite diagnosis of these echogenic lesions, particularly in the patient with hepatitis and or cirrhosis.[46]

Focal nodular hyperplasia[47,48] and adenomas likewise typically require additional imaging or biopsy to confirm a diagnosis. Occasionally, the characteristic central scar found in focal nodular hyperplasia tumors can be demonstrated at sonography (**Fig. 3–14**).[49]

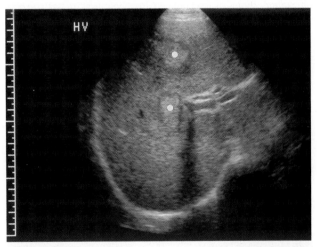

Figure 3–13 Lung cancer metastases to liver. Transverse ultrasound scan shows several echogenic irregular masses (solid circles) with a decreased echogenicity rim, consistent with metastases in this patient with a known lung tumor and abnormal (liver tests).

Vascular Abnormalities

Vascular abnormalities of the liver that are not related to cirrhosis are relatively uncommon. Ultrasound imaging, however, can play a crucial role in the noninvasive detection of conditions such as portal vein thrombosis,[50] pylephlebitis and Budd-Chiari syndrome.[51] Ultrasound findings in a patient with Budd-Chiari syndrome (partial or complete obstruction of one or more hepatic veins or the IVC), including absence of flow in the hepatic veins and a nonocclusive portal vein thrombus, are shown in **Fig. 3–15**. The portal vein thrombus is likely secondary to venous stasis from poor hepatic vein outflow.

Cardiac cirrhosis should be suspected when an enlarged liver and large hepatic veins are seen on ultra-

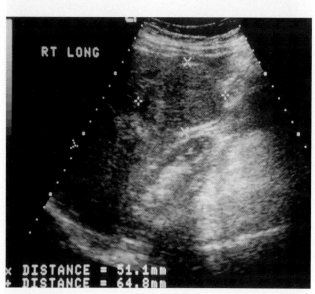

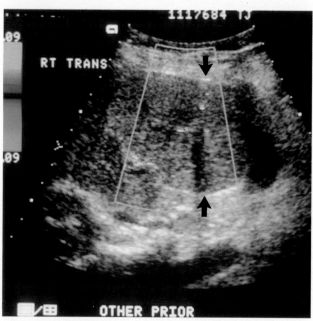

Figure 3–14 Biopsy proved focal nodular hyperplasia. (**A**) Long ultrasound shows a well-defined isoechoic liver mass (cursors).

(**B**) Transverse ultrasound scan shows central flow in a spokewheel pattern (**arrows**) in the region of the central scar.

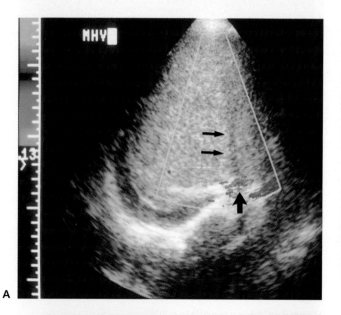

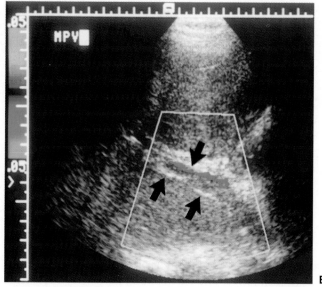

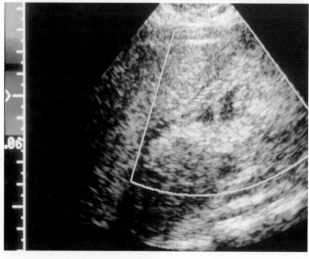

Figure 3–15 Budd-Chiari syndrome. (**A**) Transverse ultrasound scan shows absence of flow in middle hepatic vein. **Small arrows** indicate expected location of middle hepatic vein; **large arrow** = inferior vena cava. (**B**) Long color Doppler flow image of main portal vein (**arrows**) shows partial thrombosis. Color flow is seen in residual lumen. (**C**) Long color Doppler flow image shows color flow in paraumbilical vein.

sound. Some patients have prominent but normal hepatic veins. The presence of right ventricular failure or tricuspid regurgitation as a cause for the dilatation can be suspected if spectral flow in the inferior vena cava is not mostly toward the heart or if flow in the main portal vein has an accentuated pulsatile pattern[52–54] (**Fig. 3–16**).

Miscellaneous

Lymphoma and granulomatous diseases such as sarcoidosis may produce abnormal elevation in alkaline phosphatase, ALT, and AST. Various levels of difficulty have been reported with abscess detection sonographically, (**Fig. 3–17**) with recent excellent results.[55–57] However, if a strong clinical suspicion of abscess exists and the ultrasound scan is equivocal, a CT examination should be performed.

Summary

Ultrasound is the diagnostic imaging procedure of choice when a patient's liver tests are abnormal. The ability to correctly interpret liver tests in the context of a patient's physical examination and clinical history is useful in generating a clinical differential diagnosis.[58] These data are extremely valuable and allow a focused ultrasound examination that can provide maximum clinically relevant information and guide any future workup.

Addendum

Liver Tests

Liver tests can be divided into nonspecific and specific tests.

Nonspecific liver tests reflect liver damage and impaired function. Examples of nonspecific tests include transaminases, alkaline phosphatase, bilirubin, albumin, prothrombin time, glucose, and ammonia.[59–63]

Examples of specific tests include markers for (1) viral hepatitis (A through E), (2) metabolic diseases such as Wilson's disease (ceruloplasmin, alpha 1-antitrypsin and markers of iron overload), and (3) markers for autoimmune disease such as primary biliary cirrhosis (antimitochondrial antibodies), and classical autoimmune hepatitis (antinuclear antibody, anti-smooth-muscle antibodies, immunoglobulin G). Such tests help provide a specific diagnosis. Certain tumor markers may reflect a primary (AFP) or secondary (carcinoembryonic antigen) liver malignancy. Ca 19.9 may help in the diagnosis of cholangiocarcinoma.[64]

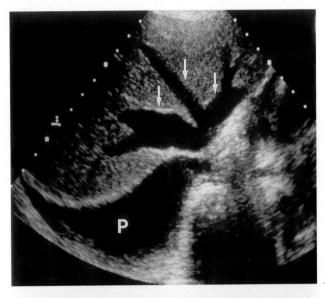

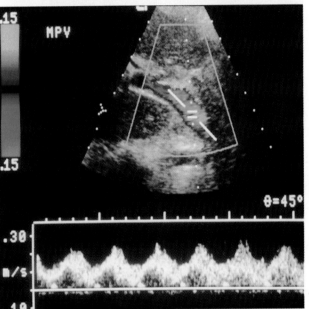

Figure 3–16 Pulsatile portal vein flow. (**A**) Transverse ultrasound scan shows dilated hepatic veins (**arrows**) and a right pleural effusion (P) in this patient with congestive heart failure. (**B**) Spectral and color Doppler shows pulsatile flow (minimum velocity is less than 60% of the peak velocity).

Liver Test Interpretation

Alkaline Phosphatase

Alkaline phosphatase is an enzyme that comes from bone, liver, intestine, and the placenta.[62] It rises in cholestasis and tends to be less elevated in parenchymal liver disease. When it is elevated, one should confirm its hepatic origin. Although fractionation of the alkaline phosphatase can be done, a corresponding rise in γ-glutamyl transpeptidase (GGT) serum levels is the simplest way to confirm liver disease as the cause.

Normal values of alkaline phosphatase usually exclude the diagnosis of a biliary tract problem. High values are classically found in extrahepatic biliary ob-

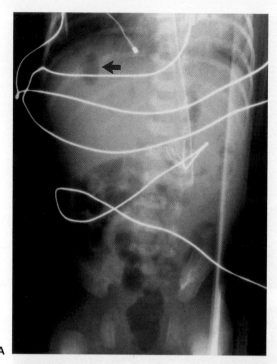

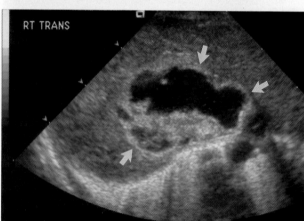

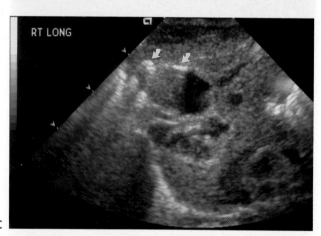

Figure 3–17   Liver abscess in septic premature infant born at 25 weeks gestation. (**A**) Left lateral decubitus abdominal radiograph shows an air collection with an air fluid level projecting over the liver (**arrow**). (**B**) Transverse ultrasound scan shows a lobular complex predominantly cystic collection (**arrows**) in the liver dome. (**C**) Long ultrasound scan shows multiple air bubbles (**arrows**) with shadowing.

struction. Gallstones are the most frequent cause. Bile duct and pancreatic malignancies and metastatic disease may cause obstruction at any level of the biliary system. However, a number of other conditions may cause marked elevations in alkaline phosphatase. These include drugs (macrolide antibiotics such as erythromycin; chlorpromazine, estrogens, methyltestosterone[58] and phenytoin,[61] granulomatous diseases (such as sarcoidosis), primary biliary cirrhosis and drug-induced hepatic injury. Primary and secondary malignancies of the liver may also produce alkaline phosphatase. Therefore, a rise in alkaline phosphatase levels may not necessarily indicate the presence of a large bile duct obstruction. Mild elevations can be seen in all forms of liver disease and other diseases that affect the liver indirectly, such as heart failure.

γ-Glutamyl transpeptidase (GGT)

Serum levels of GGT may rise in almost all forms of liver disease. Thus, GGT is very sensitive for the presence of hepatobiliary disease. However, its specificity is limited, as many systemic diseases incidentally involve the liver. The major utility of GGT is in confirming the hepatic source of an elevated alkaline phosphatase. This test may be useful in alcoholic patients, as it may indicate significant alcohol use, even without liver damage. However, its reported sensitivity is variable and elevated levels are nonspecific.

Transaminases

Levels of aspartate aminotransferase (AST) [serum glutamic oxaloacetic transaminase (SGOT)] and alanine aminotransferase (ALT) [serum glutamic pyruvic transaminase (SGPT)] are commonly used to diagnose hepatocellular damage and to monitor progress of disease. Their usefulness is limited to sorting among differential diagnostic possibilities.

AST is found in liver, muscle (skeletal and cardiac), kidney, pancreas, and red blood cells. ALT is found primarily in the liver, so it is more specific and often has more elevated levels than AST. The highest levels of AST and ALT are found in significant hepatic necrosis. Levels that are 20 times greater than normal suggest a diagnosis of acute hepatitis, viral or toxin-induced disease. Prolonged hypotension can cause very significant but usually very transient elevation of these transaminases. These diagnoses can usually be differentiated on clinical grounds.

Bilirubin (Total, Direct, Indirect)

Bilirubin values are used to diagnose and help differentiate among various causes of jaundice. Unconjugated bilirubin is formed from the breakdown of senescent red blood cells. Tightly bound to albumin in the blood, bilirubin is actively taken up by the liver and cannot be excreted by the kidneys. Unconjugated bilirubin is not soluble in water and must be converted to a water-soluble derivative to be excreted by the liver cells into bile. This conversion is accomplished by conjugation. Conjugated bilirubin is not reabsorbed by the intestinal mucosa and is excreted in the feces.

When an extrahepatic biliary obstruction is present, conjugated bilirubin cannot be secreted into the intestinal tract. As a small fraction of serum-conjugated bilirubin can be filtered by the glomerulus (unconjugated bilirubin cannot be filtered), an excess of conjugated bilirubin will be present in the urine. This excess will produce the classic symptoms of jaundice from biliary obstruction—namely, light-colored stools, dark urine, yellow skin, and sclera. The presence of bilirubin in the urine is consistent with liver damage and is present only with an excess of conjugated (direct) bilirubin. However, urinary bilirubin is no longer routinely measured, as bilirubin can be fractionated and the conjugated bilirubin directly measured. Imaging now helps in the differentiation of mechanical obstruction (of the larger bile duct) from parenchymal liver disease.

Normal values of bilirubin make a diagnosis of serious biliary tract disease somewhat less likely, but certainly do not exclude the possibility of parenchymal liver disease. Causes of elevated levels of bilirubin can be divided into four major categories: (1) overproduction (hemolytic anemia, resorption of hematoma, or multiple transfusions); (2) decreased hepatic uptake (drugs or sepsis); (3) decreased bilirubin conjugation (Gilbert syndrome[65], neonatal jaundice, hepatitis, cirrhosis, or sepsis); and (4) decreased excretion of bilirubin into bile (hepatitis, cirrhosis, drug-induced cholestasis, sepsis, or extrahepatic biliary obstruction).

Lactic dehydrogenase (LDH)

This enzyme is not helpful in the evaluation of liver disease due to its nonspecificity. However, marked increases are typically seen in primary or metastatic involvement of the liver.[63]

Albumin and Prothrombin

As these proteins are produced solely by the liver, decreased levels are indicators of decreased hepatic synthetic function. As such, these are true "liver function tests." A substantial decrease in these proteins often means significant impairment of liver function. Decreases in albumin and clotting factor levels may reflect very advanced liver disease, but are rarely helpful in distinguishing among causes of liver dysfunction. In addition, abnormalities occur in conditions that are not hepatic in origin. Low values of albumin may be found in patients with chronic diseases, inflammation, poor caloric intake, nephrotic syndrome, and protein-losing enteropathies. Vitamin K deficiency, which causes a prolonged prothrombin time, can result from dietary deficiency, antibiotic and anticoagulant use, and steatorrhea.

α-fetoprotein (AFP)

AFP is a fetal globulin expressed by many hepatocellular carcinomas. It is also expressed during liver cell regeneration. Early enthusiasm for AFP as a sensitive tumor marker for hepatocellular carcinoma has been tempered by a decrease in the overall percentage of AFP-positive hepatocellular carcinomas. This decrease has been found both in patients with alcoholic liver disease and those with hepatitis B or C.[66–70] Currently > 50% of patients with hepatocellular carcinomas have a negative AFP.[71] This is in part due to more aggressive ultrasound screening in at-risk patients, thereby finding smaller hepatocellular carcinomas (smaller tumors tend to have lower AFP levels). However, even large tumors may not be associated with elevated levels of AFP. In addition, liver metastases, especially those of gastrointestinal origin, may result in high levels of AFP.

It is important to remember that a normal value of this globulin does not exclude a diagnosis of hepatocellular carcinoma. Small (curable) tumors may be accompanied by normal or minimally elevated levels, and large hepatocellular carcinomas may not be accompanied by any elevation. AFP tends to be negative more often in small tumors (< 3 cm). When a focal mass is found in a cirrhotic liver, a level of AFP over 400 ng/mL strongly suggests the presence of hepatocellular carcinoma, and a biopsy is rarely necessary for diagnosis.[72] See **Table 3–2**[73] for a discussion of the implications of specific levels of AFP. Interestingly, it appears that patients with elevated levels of AFP who also have chronic hepatitis and cirrhosis have a high risk of liver-related death or development of hepatocellular carcinoma.[74] All these data make it clear that interpretation in the specific context is mandatory.

Table 3-2   Serum AFP determination in liver disease

AFP (ng/mL)	Interpretation
>400—500	HCC very likely if accompanied by space-occupying solid lesion(s) in cirrhotic liver or if levels are rapidly increasing
	Diffusely growing HCC may be difficult to detect on imaging
	Occasionally patients with active liver disease (particularly HBV or HVC infection) may have values in 5,000—10,000 range, reflecting inflammation/regeneration; levels tend to fluctuate over time
Normal value <400	Often from regeneration or inflammation (usually patient has elevated transaminases)
	If space-occupying lesion is present and transaminases are normal, then consider diagnosis of HCC
Normal value <10	Does not exclude HCC (cirrhotic and noncirrhotic liver)

Note: Very elevated AFP may exist in infants with liver tumors (hepatoblastoma may have values up to 50,000—100,000 ng/mL) and in young men with germ cell tumors. If a germ cell tumor is suspected, then the testes should be examined. The metastatic pattern of testicular tumor includes retroperitoneal spread and pulmonary lesions, while liver metastases, if any, appear late. Differentiation from hepatocellular carcinoma is based on clinical and imaging findings, so it is rarely a problem.
HCC, hepatocellular carcinoma.

Ceruloplasmin

Ceruloplasmin is a serum copper transport protein. Measurement of this protein is helpful if a diagnosis of Wilson disease is being considered. Low levels of ceruloplasmin are found in 90% of those homozygous for Wilson disease and 10% of heterozygotes.[63] Ceruloplasmin is an acute-phase reactant protein (a protein that increases secondary to inflammation). The levels may be high in inflammatory conditions, including inflammation of the liver itself. This explains why patients with active Wilson disease may have low normal levels (the usually low levels become elevated in cases with acute inflammation).

Iron

Serum ferritin levels and the percent of transferrin saturation provide an estimate of body iron stores and are an excellent screening test for the presence of hemochromatosis. If results of either of these tests are abnormal, a liver biopsy is nearly always mandatory for a definitive diagnosis of hemochromatosis. Quantitative iron levels obtained from the biopsy specimen are the most useful test in patients with suspected hemochromatosis and secondary iron overload due to hemolytic diseases and multiple transfusions. Hemochromatosis is a heritable disease, with major implications for the patient and family. If biopsy is considered too high risk, MR imaging may be helpful. Iron deposition in the liver shortens T1 greatly, leading to a "black liver" on most MRI sequences.

References

1. Isogai M., Hachisuka K., Yamaguchi A. Etiology and pathogenesis of marked elevation of serum transaminase in patients with acute gallstone disease. *HPB Surgery* 1991;4:95—107.
2. Taylor K.J.W, Rosenfield A.T., Spiro H.M. Diagnostic accuracy of gray scale ultrasonography for the jaundiced patient. *Arch Intern Med* 1979;139:60—63.
3. Laing F.C., Jeffrey R.B., Jr, Wing V.W., Nyberg D.A. Biliary dilatation: defining the level and cause by real-time US. *Radiology* 1986;160:39—42.
4. van Leeuwen D.J., Huibregtse K., Tytgat G.N.J. Carcinoma of the hepatic confluence 25 years after Klatskin's description: diagnosis and endoscopic management. *Sem Liver Disease* 1990;10:102—113.
5. Verbeek P.C.M, van Leeuwen D.J., de Wit L.T., et al. Benign fibrosing disease at the hepatic confluence mimicking Klatskin tumors. *Surgery* 1992;112:866—871.
6. Okuda K., Oshibuchi M. Imaging diagnosis of obstructive jaundice. *Hepatogastroenterol* 1989;36:398—405.
7. Bacon B.R., Farrahvash M.J., Janney C.G., Neuschwander-Tetri B.A. Nonalcoholic steatohepatitis: an expanded clinical entity. *Gastroenterology* 1994;107:1103—1109.
8. Neuschwander-Tetri B.A., Bacon B.R. Nonalcoholic steatohepatitis. *Med Clin North Am* 1996;50:1147—1166.
9. Scatarige J.C., Scott W.W., Donovan P.J., Siegelman S.S., Sanders R.C. Fatty infiltration of the liver: ultrasonographic and computed tomographic correlation. *J Ultrasound Med* 1984;3:9—14.
10. Garra B.S., Insana M.F., Shawker T.H., Russell M.A. Quantitative estimation of liver attenuation and echogenicity: normal state versus diffuse liver disease. *Radiology* 1987;162:61—67.
11. Joseph A.E., Saverymuttu S.H. US in the assessment of diffuse parenchymal liver disease. *Clin Radiol* 1991;44:219—221.
12. Saverymuttu S.H., Joseph A.E.A., Maxwell J.D. Ultrasound scanning in the detection of hepatic fibrosis and steatosis. *Brit Med J* 1986;292:13—15.
13. Joseph A.E., Saverymuttu S.H., Al-Sam A., Cook M.G., Maxwell J.D. Comparison of liver histology with ultrasonography in assessing diffuse parenchymal liver disease. *Clin Radiol* 1991;43:26—31.
14. White E.M., Simeone J.F., Mueller P.R., et al. Focal periportal sparing in hepatic fatty infiltration: a cause of hepatic pseudomass on US. *Radiology* 1987;162:57—59.
15. Wang S.S., Chiang J.H., Tsai Y.T., et al. Focal hepatic fatty infiltration as a cause of pseudotumors: ultrasonographic patterns and clinical differentiation. *J Clin Ultrasound* 1990;18:401—409.
16. van Leeuwen D.J., Dadrat A. *Infectious Diseases: Women's Medicine.* In: R.E. Blackwell, ed. Binghamton: Maple-Vail, 1996; p. 324—328.
17. Kurtz A.B., Rubin C.S., Cooper H.S., et al. Ultrasound findings in hepatitis. *Radiology* 1980;136:717—723.
18. Brogna A., Bucceri A.M., Catalano F., Ferrara R., Leocata V. Ultrasound demonstration of gallbladder wall thickening as a method to differentiate cirrhotic ascites from other ascites. *Invest Radiol* 1996;31:80—83.
19. Crawford J.M. *Robbins Pathologic Basis of Disease.* In: R.S. Cotran, S.L. Robbins, V. Kumar, eds. Philadelphia: WB Saunders Company, 1994; p. 831—883.
20. Di Lelio A.D., Cestari C., Lomazzi A., Beretta L. Cirrhosis: diagnosis with sonographic study of the liver surface. *Radiology* 1989;172:389—392.
21. Ferral H., Male R., Cardiel M., Munoz L., Ferrari F.Q. Cirrhosis: diagnosis by liver surface analysis with high-frequency US. *Gastrointest Radiol* 1992;17:74—78.
22. Gaiani S., Gramantieri L., Venturoli N., et al. What is the criterion for differentiating chronic hepatitis from compensated cirrhosis? A prospective study comparing ultrasonography and percutaneous liver biopsy. *J Hepatology* 1997;27:979—985.
23. Ladinheim J.A., Luba D.G., Yao F., et al. Limitations of liver surface US in the diagnosis of cirrhosis. *Radiology* 1992;185:21—24.
24. Goyal A.K., Pokharna D.S., Sharma S.K. Ultrasonic diagnosis of cirrhosis: reference to quantitative measurement of hepatic dimensions. *Gastrointest Radiol* 1990;15:32—34.
25. Giorgio A., Amoroso P., Lettieri G., et al. Cirrhosis: value of caudate to right lobe ratio in diagnosis with US. *Radiology* 1986;161:443—445.
26. van Leeuwen D.J. Assessment of portal hypertension: understanding will improve treatment. *Digest Dis* 1991;9:92—105.
27. Ralls P.W. Color Doppler sonography of the hepatic artery and portal venous system. *Am J Roentgenol* 1990;155:517—525.
28. Tessler F.N. Diagnosis of portal vein thrombosis: value of color Doppler imaging. *Am J Roentgenol* 1991;157(2):293—296.
29. Bron K.M., Baum R.A. *Abrams' Angiography—Vascular and Interventional Radiology.* M. Stanley Baum, ed. Little, Brown and Company, 1997; p. 1530—1531.
30. Redd D. *Abrams' Angiography—Vascular and Interventional Radiology.* M. Stanley Baum, ed. Little, Brown and Company, 1997; p. 57—58.
31. Smith C.S., Paauw D.S. Hepatocellular carcinoma: identifying and screening populations at increased risk. *Postgrad Med* 1993;94:71—74.

32. Bates S.E. Clinical applications of serum tumor markers. *Ann Intern Med* 1991;115:623—638.

33. Solmi L., Primerano A.M., Gandolfi L. Ultrasound follow-up of patients at risk for hepatocellular carcinoma; results of a prospective study on 360 cases. *Am J Gastroenterol* 1996;91:1189—1194.

34. Dodd G.D., III, Miller W.J., Baron R.L., Skolnick M.L., Campbell W.L. Detection of malignant tumors in end-stage cirrhotic livers: efficacy of sonography as a screening technique. *AJR* 1992;1992:727—733.

35. Tobe T. Primary liver cancer in Japan. *Cancer* 1987;60:1400—1411.

36. Shinagawa T., Ohto M., Kimura K., et al. Diagnosis and clinical features of small hepatocellular carcinoma with emphasis on the utility of real-time ultrasonography. *Gastroenterology* 1984;86:495—502.

37. Miller W.J., Federle M.P., Campbell W.L. Diagnosis and staging of hepatocellular carcinoma: comparison of CT and sonography in 36 liver transplantation patients. *AJR* 1991;157:303—306.

38. Shapiro R.S., Katz R., Mendelson D.S., et al. Detection of hepatocellular carcinoma in cirrhotic patients: sensitivity of CT and ultrasonography. *J Ultrasound Med* 1996;15:497—502.

39. Sheu J.C., Chen D.S., Sung J.L., et al. Hepatocellular carcinoma: US evolution in the early stage. *AJR* 1985;155:463—467.

40. Withers C.E., Wilson S.R. *Diagnostic Ultrasound*. In C.M. Rumack, S.R. Wilson, J.W. Charboneau, eds. St. Louis: Mosby Year Book, 1998; p. 131—134.

41. Subramanyam B.R., Balthazar E.J,. Hilton S., et al. Hepatocellular carcinoma with venous invasion. *Radiology* 1984;150:793—796.

42. Green B., Bree R.L., Goldstein H.M., Stanley C. Gray scale ultrasound evaluation of hepatic neoplasms: patterns and correlations. *Radiology* 1977;124:203—208.

43. Viscomi G.N., Gonzalez R., Taylor K.J. Histopathological correlation of ultrasound appearances of liver metastases. *J Clin Gastroenterol* 1981;3:395—400.

44. Scheible W., Skram C., Leopold G. High resolution real-time sonography of hemodialysis vascular access complications. *AJR* 1980;134:1173—1176.

45. Bree R.L., Schwab R.E., Neiman H.L. Solitary echogenic spot in the liver: is it diagnostic of a hemangioma? *AJR* 1983;140:41—45.

46. Withers C.E., Wilson S.R. *Diagnostic Ultrasound*. In C.M. Rumack, S.R. Wilson, J.W. Charboneau, eds. St. Louis: Mosby Year Book, 1998; p. 123—127.

47. Wang L.Y., Wand J.H., Lin Z.Y., et al. Hepatic focal nodular hyperplasia: findings on color Doppler ultrasound. *Abdom Imaging* 1997;22:178—181.

48. Di Staci M., Caturelli E., De Sio I., Natural history of focal nodular hyperplasia of the liver: an ultrasound study. *J Clin Ultrasound* 1996;24:345—350.

49. Withers C.E., Wilson S.R. *Diagnostic Ultrasound*. In C.M. Rumack, S.R. wilson, J.W. Charboneau, eds. St. Louis: Mosby Year Book, 1998; p. 127—128.

50. Pieters P.C., Miller W., DeMeo J. Evaluation of the portal venous system: complementary roles of invasive and noninvasive imaging strategies. *Radiographics* 1997;17:879—895.

51. Ralls P.W., Johnson M.B., Radin D.R., et al. Budd-Chiari Syndrome: detection with color Doppler sonography. *AJR* 1992;159:113—116.

52. Duerinckx A.J., Grant E.G., Perrella R.R., et al. The pulsatile portal vein in cases of congestive heart failure: correlation of duplex Doppler findings with right atrial pressures. *Radiology* 1990;176:655—658.

53. Abu-Yousef M.M., Milam S.G., Farner R.M. Pulsatile portal vein flow: a sign of tricuspid regurgitation on duplex Doppler sonography. *AJR* 1990;155:785—788.

54. Hosoki T., Arisawa J., Marikawa T., et al. Portal blood flow in congestive heart failure: pulsed duplex sonographic findings. *Radiology* 1990;174:733—736.

55. Halvorsen R.A., Foster W.L., Wilkinson R.H., Silverman P.M., Thompson W.M. Hepatic abscess: sensitivity of imaging tests and clinical findings. *Gastrointest Radiol* 1988;13:135—141.

56. Barnes P.F., DeCock K.M., Reynolds T.N., Ralls P.W. A comparison of amebic and pyogenic abscess of the liver. *Medicine* 1987;66:472—483.

57. Ralls P.W. Focal inflammatory disease of the liver. *Rad Clin North Am* 1998;36:377—389.

58. Kamath P.S. Clinical approach to the patient with abnormal liver test results. *Mayo Clin Proc* 1996;71:1089—1095.

59. Moseley R.H. *Textbook of Gastroenterology*. T. Yamada, ed. Philadelphia: Lippincott, 1991; p. 829—845.

60. Mendelson R.M., Kelsey P.J. Ultrasound and Liver Disease. *Australian Fam Physic* 1995;24:360—363.

61. McIntyre N., Rosalki S. *Bockus Gastroenterology*. W.S. Haubrich, F. Schaffner, J.E. Berk, eds. Philadelphia: WB Saunders, 1994; p. 293—309.

62. Podolsky D.K., Isselbacher K.J. *Principles of Internal Medicine* J.D. Wilson, et al, eds. New York: McGraw-Hill, 1991; p. 1308—1317.

63. Sherlock S., Dooley J. *Diseases of the liver and biliary system*. Edinburgh, Scotland: Blackwell, 1993; p. 17—32.

64. Ramage J.K., Donaghy A., Farrant J.M., Iorns R., Williams R. Serum tumor markers for the diagnosis of cholangiocarcinoma in primary sclerosing cholangitis. *Gastroenterology* 1995;108:865—869.

65. Bosma P.J., Chowdhury Jr., Bakker C., et al. The genetic basis of the reduced expression of bilirubin UDP-glucuronosyltransferase I in Gilbert's Syndrome. *N Engl J Med* 1995;333:1171—1175.

66. Lee H.S., Chung Y.H., Kim C.Y. Specificities of serum alphfetoprotein in HBsAg-positive and HBcAg-negative in the diagnosis of hepatocellular carcinoma. *Hepatology* 1991;14:68—72.

67. Wong C.B., Attar B.M., Shimoda S.S. Marked episodic elevations of alpha-fetoprotein without hepatocellular carcinoma in a patient with hepatitis B. *Am J Gastroenterol* 1995;1015—1016.

68. Taketa K. a-Fetoprotein: reevaluation in hepatology. *Hepatology* 1990;12:1420—1432.

69. Nomura F., Ohnishi K., Tanbe Y. Clinical features and prognosis of hepatocellular carcinoma with reference to serum alpha-fetoprotein levels. *Cancer* 1989;64:1700—1707.

70. The Liver Cancer Study Group. Primary liver cancer in Japan. *Cancer* 1987;60:1400—1411.

71. Pateron D., Ganne N., Trinchet J.C., et al. Prospective study of screening for hepatocellular carcinoma in caucasian patients with cirrhosis. *J Hepatology* 1994;20:65—71.

72. van Leeuwen D.J., Wilson L., Crowe D.R. Liver biopsy in the mid-1990s: questions and answers. *Sem Liver Dis* 1995;15:340—359.

73. van Leeuwen D.J., Shumate C.R. *Imaging in Hepatobiliary and Pancreatic Disease*. In: D.J. van Leeuwen, J.W. Reeders, J. Ariyama, eds. Philadelphia: W. B. Saunders, 1998.

74. di Bisceglie A., Hoofnagle J.H. Elevations in serum alpha-fetoprotein levels in patients with chronic hepatitis B. *Cancer* 1989;64:2117—2120.

4 Palpable Abdominal Mass

Ronald R. Townsend

Identification of an abdominal mass, incidentally by a patient or patient's family, or upon examination by a health care practitioner, is frequently ominous. Fear of a potentially life-threatening process, especially malignancy, is evoked. However, many "masses" noticed by patients or palpated by physicians are either not true masses or not clinically significant. Physical characteristics of a palpable mass, accompanying symptoms and signs, and patient history/demographic factors may lead to the likely diagnosis. In such cases, imaging is commonly requested to confirm that diagnosis. In other situations, the clinical differential diagnosis is long, and we are asked to facilitate patient management by providing as specific an imaging diagnosis as possible.

Differential Diagnosis

The differential diagnosis of palpable abdominal masses is extensive. Regional classification is useful, albeit imperfect. Clearly, a mass, especially when large, may be palpable outside of the usual location of the organ of origin. Common masses identified by location are listed in **Table 4–1**.

Right upper quadrant masses most commonly are hepatic in origin.

Liver metastases, hepatocellular carcinoma, hemangioma, adenoma, and focal nodular hyperplasia are common. In a young child, hepatoblastoma should be considered. Fluid-containing masses include abscesses (amebic, bacterial), hematomas, simple cysts and infectious (echinococcal) cysts. Multiple hepatic cysts in patients with autosomal dominant polycystic kidney disease may result in gross hepatic enlargement.

Nonhepatic causes of right upper quadrant palpable mass are less common. A distended gallbladder or a choledochal cyst (especially in an infant) may occur. A pseudomass in the right upper quadrant may be palpated when the liver edge is displaced inferiorly as a result of chronic obstructive pulmonary disease.

Palpable left upper quadrant masses are much less common than those on the right. Diffuse splenomegaly is common, with a long list of causes. Focal splenic masses are relatively uncommon. Causes of splenic mass include lymphoma, leukemia, cyst, abscess, hemangioma, angiosarcoma, and hematoma.

Other left upper quadrant masses include distended stomach due to gastric outlet obstruction (evident as a fluid-filled mass medial to the spleen) or solid gastric mass (adenocarcinoma, lymphoma). Less common left upper quadrant masses include those of colonic origin (neoplasm, abscess) or subphrenic abscess.

Epigastric masses are often caused by the same lesions as right and left upper quadrant masses. Gastric or colonic masses are often epigastric. The palpable mass ("olive") associated with pyloric stenosis in an infant is commonly epigastric/to the right midline. Pancreatic masses are typically close to the midline—adenocarcinoma, pseudocysts, pseudoaneurysm, cystic neoplasm, and inflammatory mass from acute pancreatitis.

Flank masses commonly arise from the kidney or adrenal gland. Renal cysts and renal cell carcinomas may be palpable. Less common causes of palpable mass in the kidney include angiomyolipoma, abscess, xanthogranulomatous pyelonephritis, and hematoma. In a child, Wilms tumor (nephroblastoma) may cause a solid palpable renal mass.

Hydronephrotic kidneys may be enlarged and palpable. Enlarged kidneys may be due to diffuse inflammatory processes (e.g., glomerulonephritis). Bilateral flank masses may also be present in conditions that result in renal enlargement due to multiple masses. These include autosomal dominant polycystic kidney disease (multiple cysts), tuberous sclerosis (cysts and angiomyolipomas), and autosomal recessive polycystic kidney disease.

Adrenal lesions occasionally large enough to palpate, include adrenocortical carcinoma, metastatic disease, myelolipoma, cyst, and neuroblastoma in children. Hormone-secreting adrenal adenomas are usually detected before they are large enough to palpate.

A palpable fullness in the mid-abdomen may relate to generalized abdominal distension, which may be caused by ascites, dilated GI tract (obstruction, adynamic ileus), or one or more masses. A pulsatile mass in the mid-abdomen in an adult must be considered an abdominal aortic aneurysm until proven otherwise. Pancreatic pseudocyst, lymphoma, liver masses, low-lying livers, etc, can cause mid-abdominal masses. Cystic masses associated with the mesentery (mesenteric cysts, gut duplication cysts) may be palpable. Palpable masses may be due to malignant or infectious mesenteric adenopathy,

Table 4-1   Common abdominal/pelvic masses

Right Upper Quadrant
  Hepatomegaly
  Hepatic Mass(es)
    Solid: Hepatocellular carcinoma
         Metastatic disease
         Hemangioma
         Adenoma
         Focal nodular hyperplasia
    Fluid: Cyst (solitary, multiple)
         Abscess (amoebic, bacterial)
         Hematoma
  Gallbladder — distended due to biliary obstruction
  Choledochal cyst (especially in children)
Epigastric
  Pancreatic carcinoma
       Pseudocyst
       Pseudoaneurysm
  Adenopathy
       Lymphoma/Metastasis-infectious
  Gastric/colonic
       Mass (neoplasm)
       Distension
  Pyloric stenosis (infant)

Flank:
  Kidney
    Nephromegaly
    Hydronephrosis (especially UPJ obstruction)
    ADPKD
    ARPKD (child)
    Multicystic dysplastic kidney (child)
    Focal mass, solid
       Renal cell carcinoma
       Wilms tumor (child)
       Angiomyolipoma
       Xanthogranulomatous pyelonephritis
    Focal mass, fluid
       Cyst
       Abscess
       Hematoma
  Adrenal
       Neuroblastoma (child)
       Cortical carcinoma
       Metastasis
       Myelolipoma
       Cyst/hematoma
Left upper quadrant:
  Splenomegaly
  Splenic mass(es):
    Solid: Lymphoma
         Leukemia
           Metastasis
    Cyst
  Gastric distension/mass
  Subphrenic abscess

Mid abdominal/general abdominal:
  Ascites
  Aortic aneurysm
  Adenopathy
  Bowel:
       Neoplasm
       Obstruction
       Adynamic ileus
       Intussusception (child)
  Abdominal wall:
       Hernia
       Lipoma
       Hematoma
  Mesentery
       Cyst, Neoplasm
Lateral pelvis:
  Ovary:
    Enlarged
       Infection
       Torsion
       Polycystic ovarian syndrome
    Mass: Functional cyst
         Cystadenoma/cystadenocarcinoma
         Teratoma
         Fibroma
  Endometrioma
  Hydro/pyosalpinx
  Paraovarian cyst
  Pedunculated leiomyoma
  Fluid Collections:
    Lymphocele
    Abscess
    Hematoma
    Urinoma
  Hernia
  GI tract:
  Appendiceal abscess/phlegmon/mucocele (right sided)
  Diverticular abscess (left more than right)
  Obstruction
  Colon carcinoma
Midline Pelvis:
  Uterus:
    Leiomyomata
    Adenomyosis
    Endometrial carcinoma
    Hemato/hydro metros
    Cervical carcinoma
  Urinary bladder:
    Outlet obstruction
    Carcinoma
  Prostate:
    BPH
    Malignancy
  GI tract:
    Obstruction
    Colon carcinoma
    Diverticulitis
Pseudomass:
  Stool-filled colon
  Edge of a normal organ in ectopic position
  Normal aorta in young, thin patient (especially female)
  Reidel lobe of liver

sarcoma, GI tract malignancies or intussusception (especially in young children). The possibility that a palpable abnormality is in the abdominal wall, rather than caused by intra or retroperitoneal pathology should be considered in all locations, but especially in the mid-abdomen. Abdominal wall masses include hernias, lipomas, desmoid tumors, and masses in abdominal wall muscles (rectus hematomas, etc).

Palpable pelvic masses may be grouped into those arising from structures at the midline and those originating laterally in the pelvis (**Table 4-1**). In an adult woman, masses of uterine and ovarian origin are very common. When large, these masses may be palpated abdominally, but when smaller may be detected only on bimanual pelvic examination. Masses include uterine leiomyomata, adenomyosis, endometrial carcinoma, hemato/hydrometros, advanced cervical carcinoma, colon adenocarcinoma, or diverticulitis with abscess. Lateral pelvic masses include masses of appendiceal and colonic origin (carcinoma, diverticular abscess) and ovarian masses. In a female of any age, ovarian pathology must be considered highly in the differential diagnosis for a pelvic mass lateral to midline. There is a long differential diagnosis for ovarian masses that can reach palpable size, including cystadenoma, functional (follicular, corpus luteum) cyst, teratoma, fibroma, polycystic ovaries, tubal and/or ovarian inflammatory mass/abscess, endometrioma, Paraovarian cysts, lymphocele, abscess, hematoma, and urinoma also occur.

Diagnostic Work Up

Historically, abdominal radiographs have been obtained as the initial imaging evaluation for almost any abdominal symptom or sign, including presence of a mass. However, radiographs are neither sensitive nor specific enough in characterizing abdominal masses to be routinely recommended. There remain occasional clinical situations in which radiographs can accurately confirm the nature of a palpable abnormality and effectively guide management. This is generally the case when there is a high clinical suspicion that the palpable abnormality is a dilated segment of the gastrointestinal tract. A stool-filled dilated colon may be palpable as a "mass" and, when this is clinically suspected, confirmed at radiography. Radiographs may confirm masses due to dilated colon with volvulus or other obstructing pathology. A dilated stomach, as with gastric outlet obstruction, can be confirmed radiographically when clinically suspected as the cause of an upper abdominal mass.

Cross-sectional imaging is required to accurately evaluate a palpable abdominal mass in most situations, however. Ultrasound and computed tomography have each been used successfully in evaluating patients with palpable masses.[1—10] While either modality may be appropriate in many situations, advantages of one over the other for specific types of masses will be addressed below. In general terms, ultrasound has the advantage of being less costly and is preferred by some as the initial imaging exam for that reason. It is also more widely available, especially in geographic areas with more limited resources or less dense populations. The ability to infinitely manipulate the imaging plane during the ultrasound exam offers an advantage in evaluating the organ of origin of a mass, but helical CT with multiplanar reconstruction makes this less of an issue than that in the past. Ultrasound remains more operator dependent than CT, requiring local expertise to optimally exploit its abilities. Relatively thin patients (including many pediatric patients) may be better evaluated with ultrasound. Obese patients frequently have pathology better resolved with CT. The inability of ultrasound to image through bowel gas may be a significant limitation relative to CT for some abdominal masses. Lack of ionizing radiation remains an advantage for ultrasound over CT in general terms, but this is obviously most important when dealing with pregnant or potentially pregnant patients.

Ultrasound Imaging

As one approaches the sonographic evaluation of the patient with a mass, clinical/demographic factors that may affect the likely diagnosis should be kept in mind. For example, a 5-cm solid soft tissue echogenicity renal mass in a 60-year-old would result in a likely diagnosis of renal cell carcinoma, while the same mass in a 3-year-old would likely be a Wilms tumor. Knowledge of the patient's symptoms, medical history, and physical findings, previous imaging/laboratory evaluation, and any known risk factors for specific pathology (family history, etc), will allow the sonographer/sonologist to make more clinically likely diagnoses/differential diagnoses.

For most adult patients, sonographers/sonologists begin their evaluation of the abdomen or pelvis with a 3—3.5 MHz sector or curved linear transducer. However, the optimal evaluation of a palpable mass may require creative use of other/additional equipment. The findings on physical exam, as confirmed by the sonographer, can guide this choice. If the mass feels superficial, possibly within the abdominal wall, then evaluation with a high-frequency linear or curved linear transducer is likely to be most useful. If the mass is deep, especially if the patient is obese, then a 2—2.5 MHz transducer may be necessary. Spectral/color/power Doppler evaluation may help characterize the vascular nature of a mass and/or help in the discrimination of inflammatory or neoplastic masses from others. Careful attention to echogenic interfaces demarcating tissue planes may help distinguish the organ/anatomic location of origin of a mass. Observation of the motion of a mass relative to adjacent structures, during respiration or with manual compression, may similarly help identify the site of origin of a mass.

The location of a palpable abnormality has obvious impact on its likely cause. For this reason, the sonographic approach to masses is discussed in terms of the location of the mass within the abdomen or pelvis. Masses may be localized as follows: right upper quadrant (RUQ), left upper quadrant (LUQ), epigastric, midabdominal, flank (left or right), right lower quadrant /right pelvis (RLQ), left lower quadrant/left pelvis (LLQ), and midline pelvis. These distinctions are somewhat artificial and clearly the edge of a mass, especially when large, may be palpable outside of the usual location of the organ of origin of the mass. Common masses identified by location are listed in **Table 4–1**. While common pediatric masses are included in this discussion, a more complete analysis of sonography of pediatric masses can be found elsewhere.[11—13]

Right Upper Quadrant Mass

A palpable mass in the right upper quadrant most commonly is due to hepatomegaly or focal hepatic mass. Accurate measurement of the liver to detect subtle hepatomegaly is problematic with ultrasound, because a normal-sized adult liver can exceed the size of the field of view of many transducers. However, hepatic enlargement sufficient to be palpable is readily evident at sonography (**Fig. 4–1**). The differential diagnosis of hepatomegaly without focal abnormality is long. If clinical/laboratory parameters do not lead to a specific diagnosis, biopsy (with ultrasound guidance as necessary) may be diagnostic. If an enlarged liver is diffusely increased in echogenicity with poor through transmission of sound, fatty infiltration can be suggested (**Fig. 4–2**).

Multiple solid hepatic masses may result in a palpably enlarged liver, frequently with a lobular surface, usually due to metastatic disease (**Fig. 4–3**). While technically optimal contrast-enhanced computed tomography may be more sensitive than sonography overall in detection of liver metastases, the diagnosis of metastatic disease as a cause of a palpable mass is generally not difficult. Ultrasound-guided biopsy may be useful to confirm the diagnosis.

Many different conditions may cause a solitary palpable hepatic mass, and ultrasound may help differentiate these lesions. Common solid hepatic masses in adults include hepatocellular carcinoma, hemangioma, adenoma, focal nodular hyperplasia, and metastasis (un-

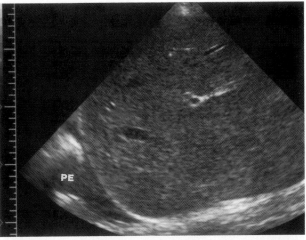

Figure 4–1 Hepatomegaly. Longitudinal image of a palpable right upper quadrant mass thought clinically to be enlarged liver. Liver is grossly enlarged (A-P dimension 19 cm) due to Hepatitis C. Incidentally noted is right pleural effusion (PE).

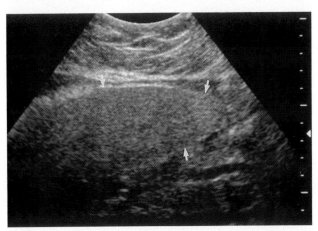

Figure 4–2 Hepatomegaly-left lobe. Longitudinal image of left lobe of liver (margins indicated with **white arrows**). The left lobe is enlarged and increased in echogenicity due to fatty infiltration associated with alcohol abuse.

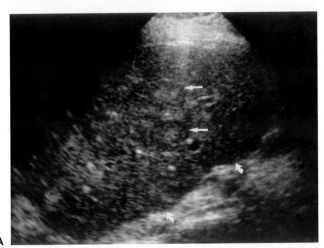

A

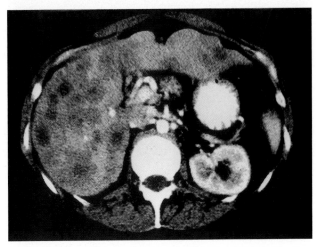

B

Figure 4–3 Hepatic metastatic disease. **A:** Longitudinal sonogram of right lobe of liver demonstrates masses (**straight arrows**) and lobular surface (**curved arrows**) in a patient with diffusely metastatic adenocarcinoma. **B:** Axial CT image through the liver confirms the diffuse metastatic disease.

usual to be solitary). In a young child, hepatoblastoma should be considered. Fluid-containing masses include abscesses (amoebic, bacterial), hematomas, simple cysts and infectious (echinococcal) cysts. Multiple hepatic cysts in patients with autosomal dominant polycystic kidney disease may result in gross hepatic enlargement (**Fig. 4–4**).

Nonhepatic causes of right upper quadrant palpable mass are less common. A palpably distended nontender gallbladder may be evident clinically and sonographically with common bile duct obstruction, as seen with pancreatic carcinoma. Patients with cystic duct obstruction/acute cholecystitis may also have a clinically evident mass that can be confirmed sonographically (**Fig. 4–5**).

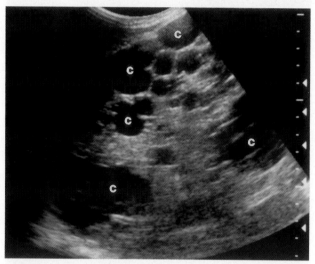

Figure 4–4   Multiple hepatic cysts with Autosomal Dominant Polycystic Kidney Disease (ADPKD). Transverse sonogram of left lobe of the liver shows it to be grossly enlarged with innumerable cysts (C). Patient had known ADPKD with upper abdominal mass thought to be enlarged liver with masses. Sonography confirmed hepatic cystic disease.

Other biliary causes of palpable mass include choledochal cyst, especially in an infant.

A pseudomass in the right upper quadrant may be palpated when the liver edge is displaced inferiorly as a result of chronic obstructive pulmonary disease or other lung abnormality displacing the diaphragm, and, therefore, the liver, inferiorly. Sonography fails to show any mass or hepatomegaly.

Left Upper Quadrant Mass

Palpable left upper quadrant masses are much less common than those on the right. A left upper quadrant mass may be easy to diagnose clinically as splenomegaly, and ultrasound may be used to confirm that diagnosis (**Fig. 4–6**). In other cases, it may be difficult to determine if a palpable finding is of splenic, gastric, or other origin. Splenomegaly without focal lesion is common, with a long list of causes. Focal splenic lesions as a cause of palpable abnormality or identified by sonography are relatively uncommon. Causes of splenic mass include lymphoma, leukemia, cyst, abscess, hemangioma, angiosarcoma, and hematoma.

Other left upper quadrant masses include distended stomach due to gastric outlet obstruction (evident as fluid-filled mass medial to the spleen) or solid gastric mass (adenocarcinoma, lymphoma). That a fluid mass is indeed the stomach may be confirmed by visualizing a nasogastric tube within, confirming gastric mucosa around the fluid, and/or confirming entry of fluid from the esophagus into the mass. In questionable cases, diagnosis can be confirmed with radiography or computed tomography. Less common left upper quadrant masses include those of colonic origin (neoplasm, abscess) or subphrenic abscess.

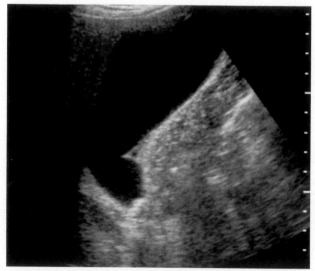

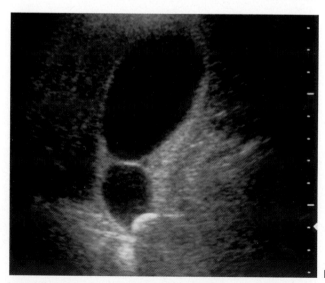

A

B

Figure 4–5   Palpable gallbladder. Patient with right upper quadrant pain and palpable mass, clinically thought to be gallbladder. Images of the gallbladder with the patient supine (**A**) and in the left lateral decubitus position (**B**) confirm a distended gallbladder with stone impacted in the neck. Acute cholecystitis was confirmed at surgery.

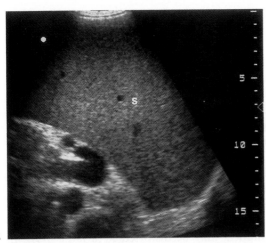

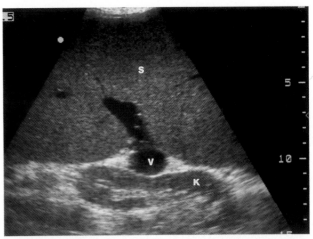

Figure 4–6 Splenomegaly. Grossly enlarged spleen (S) due to portal hypertension is confirmed as the cause of left upper quadrant mass on transverse (**A**) and longitudinal (**B**) images. Left kidney (K) is compressed by the enlarged spleen and dilated venous collaterals (V).

Epigastric Mass

Masses described under the headings right upper quadrant, left upper quadrant, and mid abdominal may appear to be localized to the epigastric (subxyphoid) area on physical exam in many cases. These include masses of gastric or colonic origin. The palpable mass ("olive") associated with pyloric stenosis in an infant is commonly epigastric/to the right midline.

Pancreatic masses are typically closed to the midline. These include solid masses (adenocarcinoma) and fluid-containing masses (pseudocysts, pseudoaneurysm, and cystic neoplasm). Hematoma within a pseudocyst or pseudoaneurysm may mimic solid neoplasm. In the clinical setting of pancreatitis, evaluation of any fluid collection identified in the upper abdomen with Doppler ultrasound is recommended because of the possibility of pseudoaneurysm.

Flank Mass

Flank masses commonly arise from the kidney or adrenal gland. Renal cysts are very common in older adults and occasionally reach palpable size (**Fig. 4–7**). Renal cell carcinomas are frequently palpable and are by far the most common solid renal mass in adults (**Fig. 4–8**). In a child, Wilms tumor (nephroblastoma) may cause a solid palpable renal mass. Less common causes of palpable mass in the kidney include angiomyolipoma, abscess, xanthogranulomatous pyelonephritis, and hematoma.

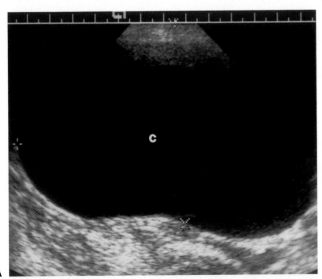

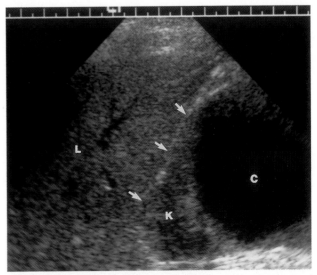

Figure 4–7 Palpable renal cyst. A 77-year-old woman with right flank mass found on physical exam. (**A**) Transverse image from the right flank shows a large anechoic fluid collection (C), which measured approximately 12 cm in greatest dimension. (**B**) Longitudinal image shows that the cyst (C) is of renal origin. There is renal cortex (K) cephalad to the cyst. An echogenic tissue plane (**arrows**) separates the kidney and cyst from the liver (L).

A hydronephrotic kidney, especially with congenital ureteropelvic junction obstruction, may be enlarged and palpable and is readily diagnosed with ultrasound. Enlarged kidneys due to diffuse inflammatory process (glomerulonephritis) or other processes can be confirmed as the cause of bilateral palpable flank masses with ultrasound. Bilateral palpable masses in the flank may also be evident with conditions that result in renal enlargement due to multiple masses. These include autosomal dominant polycystic kidney disease (multiple cysts) and tuberous sclerosis (cysts and angiomyolipomas) (**Fig. 4–9**). Autosomal recessive polycystic kidney disease may also result in palpably enlarged kidneys bilaterally, but the kidneys are large and echogenic, and cysts are frequently not resolved with sonography.

Adrenal lesions that may be large enough to palpate include neuroblastoma in children, adrenocortical carcinoma, myelolipoma, cyst, and metastatic disease. Hormone-secreting adrenal adenomas usually do not become large enough to palpate.

When flank masses are large, they can be difficult to localize in terms of their organ of origin. At times it is very difficult to distinguish a mass of renal or adrenal origin from one of hepatic origin.[14, 15] The echogenic plane, which can generally be visualized separating the intraperitoneal from the retroperitoneal structures in the upper abdomen, may be distorted by a large mass. In general, that plane is displaced anteriorly by retroperitoneal (especially renal/adrenal) lesions and displaced posteriorly by intraperitoneal (especially hepatic) lesions. The motion of the mass relative to these organs is also useful in terms of defining organ of origin. A mass that moves with the kidney and distinct from the liver is likely renal in origin and vice versa.[15]

Mid-abdominal Mass

A palpable fullness in the mid-abdomen may relate to generalized abdominal distension, which may be caused by ascites, dilated GI tract (obstruction, adynamic ileus), or one or more masses. Ascites is readily diagnosed as a cause of distension (**Fig. 4–10**), but the finding of ascites should lead to more complete sonographic examination of the abdomen and pelvis if the cause is unknown.

Focal palpable masses in the mid abdomen have many causes, which ultrasound can frequently differentiate. A pulsatile mass in the mid abdomen in an adult must be considered an abdominal aortic aneurysm until

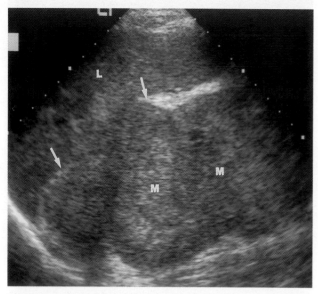

Figure 4–8 Palpable renal cell carcinoma. A 56-year-old man with palpable right flank mass and hematuria. Longitudinal image shows a lobulated mass (M) which replaces the kidney. An echogenic plane separating the mass from the liver (L) is evident in some areas (**arrows**) but not others.

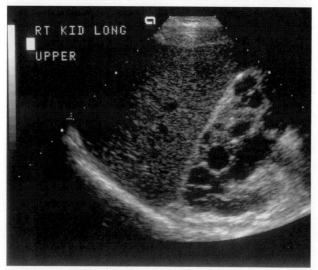

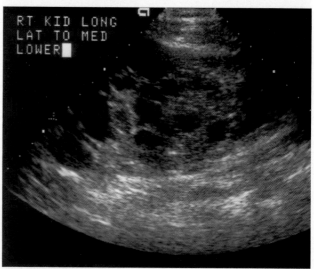

Figure 4–9 Autosomal Dominant Polycystic Kidney Disease with palpable kidneys bilaterally. Longitudinal images of the upper (**A**) and lower (**B**) parts of the right kidney show multiple cysts in a kidney which had a total length of 24 cm.

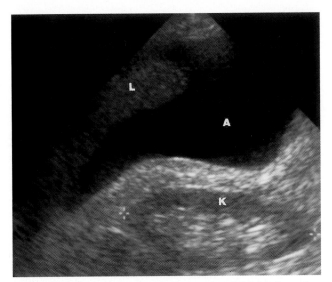

Figure 4–10 Ascites causing generalized abdominal distension. Longitudinal image from the right mid-abdomen angled laterally shows a large amount of ascites (A). L, liver; K, right kidney.

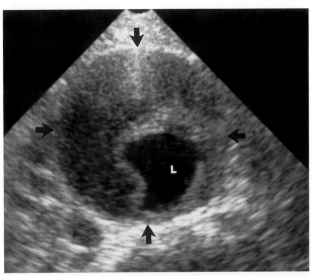

Figure 4–11 Abdominal aortic aneurysm presenting as a pulsatile mass. Transverse image of distal aorta shows an aneurysm (margins marked by **arrows**). Residual aortic lumen is marked L.

proven otherwise (**Fig. 4–11**). Ultrasound can readily diagnose an aneurysm in this situation in most cases. If there is so much bowel gas that the aorta is obscured, then computed tomography may be required. Because many other masses may mimic an abdominal aortic aneurysm clinically, a complete sonographic examination of the abdomen is necessary if the aorta appears normal.[16] Pancreatic pseudocyst, lymphoma, liver masses, low lying livers, etc, can cause pulsatile masses.[16] A normal aorta in a relatively thin patient (especially in young women) may result in prominant pulsations causing a false clinical impression of a pulsatile mass—easily proven with ultrasound.

Nonpulsatile masses in the mid-abdomen may be palpable as extensions of masses from structures in adjacent regions of the abdomen. Cystic masses associated with the mesentery (mesenteric cysts, gut duplication cysts) may be palpable. Solid masses may be due to malignant or infectious mesenteric adenopathy (**Fig. 4–12**) or a rare sarcoma of the mesentery. GI tract malignancies or intussusception (especially in young children) may cause palpable mass. While bowel gas may obscure pathology in the mid-abdomen, fluid-filled bowel may facilitate evaluation, and ultrasound may be successful in characterizing many GI tract abnormalities, particularly in children.[17]

The possibility that a palpable abnormality is due to abdominal wall, rather than intra- or retroperitoneal pathology, should be considered in all locations, but especially in the mid-abdomen. While a large abdominal wall mass may be obvious with any transducer, frequently a high-resolution linear or curved linear 5—12 MHz transducer will optimally delineate abdominal wall pathology. Definition of the plane of the anterior

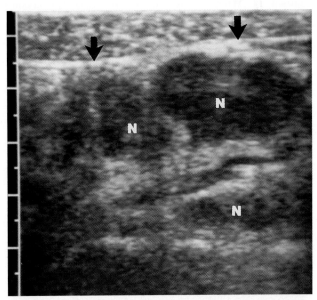

Figure 4–12 Mesenteric adenopathy due to mycobacterial infection causing palpable abdominal mass in a young man with AIDS. Transverse sonogram in the mid-abdomen shows multiple enlarged lymph nodes (N). Anterior parietal peritoneum indicated with **arrows**.

parietal peritoneum, separating abdominal wall from deeper structures, allows accurate localization of pathology. Optimal delineation of a hernia may require imaging with the patient upright or with whatever stress causes the palpable abnormality to appear (**Fig. 4–13**). Umbilical hernias, ventral hernias (commonly at previous surgical sites), and Spigelian hernias (lateral to the rectus muscle) may be be seen in this way. Lipomas and masses in abdominal wall muscles (rectus hematomas, etc.) may similarly be resolved.

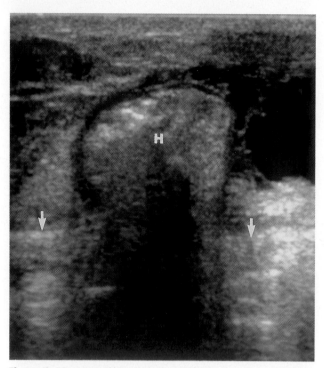

Figure 4–13 Ventral hernia. Patient complained of lower abdominal mass which would appear and disappear. A bowel containing hernia (H) is present, with anterior parietal peritoneum marked with **arrows**. The bowel herniated through the peritoneal defect when the patient laughed or strained, especially in the upright position, but reduced at rest, especially supine.

Midline Pelvic Mass

Palpable pelvic masses may be grouped into those arising from structures at the midline and those originating laterally in the pelvis (**Table 4–1**). In many situations this distinction will be uncertain clinically, and imaging findings will help in limiting the differential diagnosis.

A large smooth midline pelvic mass may be palpable when the urinary bladder is grossly distended (**Fig. 4–14**). The bladder may be distended as a result of outlet obstruction (posterior urethral valves in a male infant, benign prostatic hypertrophy, bladder, or urethral mass). Postvoid imaging will confirm the presence or absence of fixed obstruction. Continuity of the mass with the bladder neck should be confirmed while imaging to avoid dismissing other cystic pelvic mass (especially ovarian mass) as a distended bladder.

In an adult woman, masses of uterine origin are very common. When large, these masses may be palpated abdominally, but when smaller may be detected only on bimanual pelvic examination. Multiple uterine leiomyomata result in an enlarged uterus, with or without focal palpable masses (**Fig. 4–15**). When large and/or pedunculated myomata extend into the adnexal area, it may be impossible to determine clinically if these masses are uterine or ovarian in origin. This distinction is usually straightforward with ultrasound, with myomas evident as solid masses contiguous with the uterus. However, occasionally ultrasound can be misleading in this situation, with necrotic pedunculated myomata mimicking cystic ovarian masses or solid ovarian fibromas mimicking leiomyomata. Other causes of uterine enlargement, including adenomyosis, endometrial carcinoma, hemato/ hydrometros may cause a palpable mass and are detectable sonographically. Advanced cervical carcinoma may also present as a pelvic mass.

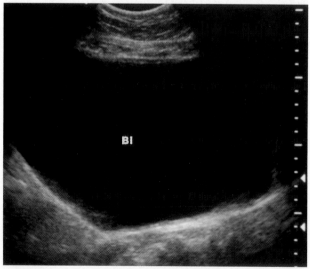

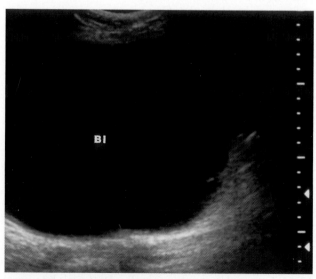

Figure 4–14 Distended urinary bladder causing palpable midline pelvic mass. Longitudinal (**A**) and Transverse (**B**) images demonstrate a grossly distended bladder (Bl). Patient was unable to void due to outlet obstruction caused by benign prostatic hypertrophy.

Colonic processes, including adenocarcinoma or diverticulitis with abscess, may present as a midline or lateral pelvic mass. While ultrasound may be able to suggest these diagnoses, further evaluation with computed tomography, barium enema, and/or endoscopy is commonly necessary. Masses of prostatic origin (BPH, malignancy) are not usually palpable abdominally, but are evident on rectal examination. When large, however, such masses may be detected sonographically through a urine-filled bladder.

Right or Left Lower Quadrant/Lateral Pelvic Mass

The differential diagnosis for masses laterally in the pelvis is largely the same for those to the right or left of midline (**Table 4–1**). Exceptions to this include masses of appendiceal origin in the right lower quadrant/right pelvis, including appendiceal abscess, phlegmon, and mucocele. Colonic masses (carcinoma, diverticulitis with abscess) may be palpated more frequently on the left.

In a female of any age, ovarian pathology must be considered highly in the differential diagnosis for a pelvic mass lateral to midline. Such masses may be either grossly obvious at abdominal palpation or evident only by bimanual pelvic examination. In adults, complex cystic/solid adnexal masses must be considered suspicious for ovarian carcinoma until proven otherwise (**Fig. 4–16**). There is a long differential diagnosis for ovarian masses that can reach palpable size, including cystadenoma, functional (follicular, corpus luteum) cyst, teratoma, fibroma, etc. A diffusely enlarged ovary without focal mass may be seen in polycystic ovarian syndrome (bilateral ovarian enlargement), with infection, or torsion. In the setting of infection, tubal and/or ovarian inflammatory mass/abscess must be suspected (**Fig. 4–17**). An endometrioma may be palpable and detected sonographically as a complex adnexal fluid collection within or outside the ovary. Paraovarian cysts may also become large and palpable.

In men or women, complex pelvic fluid collections may cause palpable masses, especially with previous pelvic surgery or other trauma. Lymphocele, abscess, hematoma, and urinoma may be included in the differential diagnosis, with clinical parameters effecting the likelihood of each. Ultrasound-guided aspiration may facilitate diagnosis.

In the pelvis, as higher in the abdomen, abdominal wall pathology should be considered in the differential diagnosis of palpable findings. Depending on the location of the mass, inguinal, femoral, ventral, or Spigelian hernia may be likely.

Sarcomas and lymphomas may arise in tissues between organs and result in masses anywhere in the abdomen or pelvis. A large soft tissue mass, not clearly related to any organ, should raise a suspicion of such a malignancy (**Fig. 4–18**).

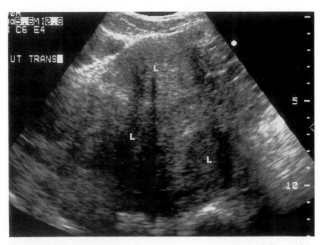

Figure 4–15 Multiple uterine leiomyomata causing midline pelvic mass in a 40-year-old woman. Transverse sonogram through the uterus shows multiple leiomyomata (L) resulting in a uterus measuring approximately 10 cm AP by 10 cm transverse.

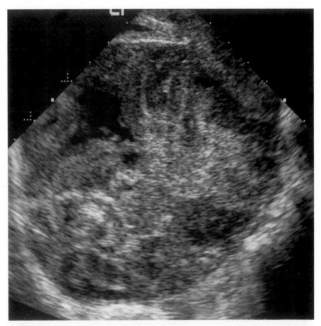

Figure 4–16 Palpable right adnexal mass due to ovarian mucinous cystadenocarcinoma in a 38-year-old woman. Longitudinal sonogram shows complex, predominantly solid, mass.

Benefits of Ultrasound

Ultrasound was employed in the evaluation of abdominal masses as soon as the technique was clinically available. In the 1970s, with extremely limited resolution, a role for ultrasound was recognized.[2,3] However, some authors reported a limited accuracy in the diagnosis of abdominal masses, with only 57% agreement with surgical findings in one report.[1]

With additional experience and improved equipment, reported accuracies of ultrasound examination of the patient with a palpable mass have improved substantially. Barker and Lindsell reported a 99% positive pre-

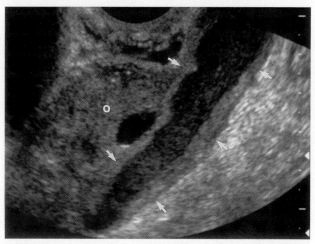

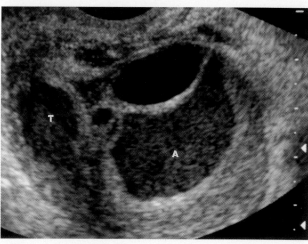

Figure 4–17   Palpable left adnexal mass due to pyosalpinx with ovarian abscess. (**A**) Longitudinal endovaginal sonogram shows thick walled tube (**arrows** at margins) with complex fluid within (pus at surgery). Ovary (O) is noted adjacent to pyosalpinx. (**B**) Transverse endovaginal sonogram shows thick walled tube in cross-section (T) with adjacent abscess (A) in ovary.

dictive value and 97% negative predictive value for ultrasound determination of the presence or absence of an abdominal mass in 104 patients referred with a palpable abdominal mass.[7] These figures match those of Williams et al., using computed tomography to evaluate a similar population (99% positive predictive value, 97% negative predictive value). In one study, analyzing findings at abdominal sonography for patients referred for all in-dications, the likelihood of a positive finding increased significantly when a palpable abnormality was present.[8]

Ultrasound is less accurate in giving a precise diagnosis than in determining the presence or abscess of a mass. In the study by Aspelin et al., ultrasound was 96% sensitive in mass detection, identified the correct organ/tissue of origin of the mass in 91%, and correctly diagnosed the exact nature of the pathology in 71%.[5] In another study, the correct pathological diagnosis was identified sonographically in 77% of cases.[7] In Williams et al., CT study,[9] the correct organ of origin was identified 93% of the time and the likely pathologic diagnosis was correctly given in 88%. Either technique is substantially more accurate than physical examination in making the diagnosis or excluding the presence of a mass.[5–7,9] Because there has been continued improvement in both sonographic and computed tomographic technology, the potential that current statistics for both exams exceed these levels exists. Some authors have emphasized the complimentary nature of the two techniques, with the second exam beneficial in cases where the first is equivo-cal.[4]

Summary

Ultrasound is an effective means to evaluate the patient with a clinically palpable abdominal or pelvic mass. Many masses can be completely characterized by ultrasound, facilitating treatment planning. In other situations, further workup (biopsy, endoscopy, radiographic contrast study, computed tomography, etc.) may be guided by the sonographic findings, leading to correct diagnosis.

Figure 4–18   Sarcoma as cause of lateral pelvic mass. A large pelvic soft tissue mass (**straight arrows** at margins) replaces the iliacus muscle ventral to the right iliac bone (**curved arrows**) and fills the right pelvis.

References

1. Richardson R., Norton L.W., Eule J., et al. Accuracy of ultrasound in diagnosing abdominal masses. *Arch Surg* 1975;110:933—939.
2. Cooperberg P.L., Cohen M.M. Grey-Scale ultrasound in the diagnosis of abdominal mass lesions. *Can Jour Surg* 1977;20:361—365.
3. Bryan P., Dinn W.M. Isodense masses on CT: differentiation by gray scale ultrasonography. *Am J Roentgenol* 1977;129:989—992.
4. Brasch R.C., Abols I.B., Gooding C.A., et al. Abdominal disease in children: a comparison of computed tomography and ultrasound. *Am J Roentgenol* 1980;134:153—158.
5. Aspelin P., Hildell J., Karlsson S., et al. Ultrasonic evaluation of palpable abdominal masses. *Acta Chir Scand* 1980;146:501—505.
6. Holm H.H., Gammelgaard J., Jensen F., et al. Ultrasound in the diagnosis of a palpable abdominal mass. *Gastrointest Radiol* 1982;7:149—151.
7. Barker C.S., Lindsell D.R.M. Ultrasound of the palpable abdominal mass. *Clin Radiol* 1990;41:98—99.
8. Colquhoun I.R., Saywell W.R., Dewbury K.C. An analysis of referrals for primary diagnostic abdominal ultrasound to a general X-ray department. *Br J Radiol* 1988;61:297—300.
9. Williams M.P., Scott I.H.K., Dixon A.K. Computed tomography in 101 patients with a palpable abdominal mass. *Clin Radiol* 1984;35:293—296.
10. Dixon A.K., Kingham J.G.C., Fry I.K., et al. Computed tomography in patients with an abdominal mass: effective and efficient? A controlled trial. *Lancet* 1981;5/30:1199—1201.
11. Wilson D.A. Ultrasound screening for abdominal masses in the neonatal period. *Am J Dis Child* 1982;136:147—151.
12. Wootton S.L. The child with an abdominal mass. In: Practical pediatric radiology. S.V.W. Hilton, D.K. Edwards, eds. Philadelphia: W.B. Saunders, 1994, p. 357—388.
13. Rumack C.M. Pediatric abdominal masses. Fr. Syllabus: A special course in ultrasound (E.I. Bluth et al. edSG). Oak Brook, IL. RSNA Publicating, 1996;8:81—90.
14. Graif M., Manor A., Itzchak Y. Sonographic differentiation of extra- and intrahepatic masses. *Am J Roentgenol* 1983;141:553—556.
15. Lim J.H., Ko Y.T., Lee D.H. Sonographic sliding sign in localization of right upper quadrant mass. *J Ultrasound Med* 1990;9:455—459.
16. Shawker T.H., Steinfeld A.D. Ultrasonic evaluation of pulsatile abdominal masses. *JAMA* 1978;239:419—422.
17. Seibert J.J., Williamson S.L., Gollady E.S., et al. The distended gasless abdomen: a fertile field for ultrasound. *J Ultrasound Med* 1986;5:301—308.

5

Periampullary Tumor: Is It Resectable?

Philip W. Ralls

Introduction

The prognosis for pancreatic carcinoma and other periampulary neoplasms is grim. Some have estimated that the overall cure rate for pancreatic ductal adenocarcinomas is less than 1%.[1] Despite this, surgical resection is popular, as it represents the only hope for cure. In a recent series, resection for cure has been possible in 15—20% of unselected patients[2–5] and 29—34% of patients screened as suitable candidates for curative resection.[6,7] Representative recent studies have reported five-year survival rates for pancreatic cancer of 6.8%, 9%, 17%, and 25%.[8–11] In pancreatic tumors other than ductal adenocarcinoma, five-year survival is higher, for example, 9% versus 36% in Wade, et al.'s study.[9] In the last decade, operative morbidity and mortality after Whipple pancreaticoduodenectomy resection have decreased. Several decades ago mortality ranged from 15—25%. More recently, mortality rates varying from 0%[11,12] to 8%[9] have been reported. Surgical mortality seems to be age-related; it is higher in elderly patients.[7,9] These facts have heightened interest in imaging as a means of selecting patients with pancreatic tumors for appropriate management: Whipple pancreaticoduodenectomy, palliative bypass surgery, or even nonsurgical management. High-resolution CT and magnetic resonance imaging[2,13] have been used to assess these patients. Sonography is often the first modality used to image patients with pancreatic carcinoma, as these patients usually present with jaundice or abdominal pain.[10] Despite this, relatively little work has been done to assess the usefulness of sonography in evaluating the resectability of pancreatic neoplasms.[14] In most recent discussions of imaging in pancreatic neoplasms, transabdominal sonography has been almost totally ignored.[2,5,16]

During the past several years, we have developed a technique to assess the resectability of pancreatic tumors using color flow sonography.[17] In a retrospective analysis of 45 patients referred for color flow sonographic evaluation of resectability of pancreatic neoplasm, a color Doppler scoring system was successful in identifying neoplasms as unresectable. Vessels that were touched or occluded by tumor were categorized according to a Pancreatic Color Doppler Score (**Table 5–1**). Others have been interested in the use of color Doppler sonography for this application as well.[18–20]

Table 5–1 Pancreatic Color Doppler Score

PCDS 0	Tumor *did not touch* a vessel.
PCDS 1	Tumor touched, *1—24%* around the vessel circumference
PCDS 2	Tumor touched, *25—49%* around the vessel circumference
PCDS 3	Tumor touched, *50—99%* around the vessel circumference
PCDS 4	Tumor touched, *100% around the vessel circumference*. "Encasement"
PCDS 5	*Occluded vessel*

Differential Diagnosis

Sonography is the primary imaging method to screen patients with jaundice and is often used to evaluate patients with abdominal pain. The differential diagnosis of jaundice is covered in another chapter. Sonography may reveal a pancreatic mass in both of these circumstances. Pancreatic masses may be benign or malignant, neoplastic or nonneoplastic.

Pancreatic Ductal Adenocarcinoma

Pancreatic ductal adenocarcinoma is by far the most common primary pancreatic neoplasm, comprising approximately 80% of all pancreatic tumors. Pancreatic carcinoma is one of the most common causes of cancer death in the United States. Pancreatic ductal adenocarcinoma is one of the most lethal malignancies. Overall five-year survival is poor—2% or less.

Nonneoplastic Masses

Focal pancreatic enlargement occurs in approximately 30% of patients with chronic pancreatitis. Carcinoma and pancreatitis-related masses can usually be differentiated clinically. In addition, the presence of calcification within a mass makes the diagnosis of pancreatitis almost certain. Hyperechoic masses, even without discrete calcifications, are usually related to chronic pancreatitis. An uncalcified iso- or hypoechoic mass is nonspecific (**Fig. 5–1**). In this instance, biopsy or ERCP is indicated to differentiate carcinoma from chronic pancreatitis. Carcinoma and pancreatitis may both cause obstruction of the pancreatic duct or extrahepatic bile duct. Obstruction of both ducts, the "double duct sign," is nonspecific, occurring in both pancreatitis and pancreatic carcinoma. Pseudocysts, while more frequent in pancreatitis, occur in both conditions.

Benign pancreatic cysts are fairly common as sporadic, incidental findings. Surprisingly, imageable pancreatic cysts are decidedly rare in polycystic disease (**Fig. 5–2**). Multiple pancreatic cysts should suggest the diagnosis of von Hippel Lindau disease, not polycystic disease.

Cystic Pancreatic Tumors

Cystic pancreatic tumors are relatively uncommon, comprising fewer than 15% of pancreatic cystic lesions and only a few percent of pancreatic tumors. Cystic pancreatic neoplasms include serous cystic neoplasms (microcystic adenoma) and mucinous cystic neoplasms (formerly called *cystadenoma/carcinoma*).[21,22] Serous cystic neoplasm (microcystic adenoma) are almost universally benign. When image findings typical for microcystic adenoma are present, asymptomatic or poor-risk patients need not undergo surgery. Serous cystic neoplasm is slightly more common in females and tends to occur in older individuals.

Morphologically, serous microcystic neoplasms comprise many tiny cysts, most smaller than 2 cm. Occasionally, a few larger cysts are present (**Fig. 5–3**). A distinctive, but inconsistent feature is a central stellate fibrotic scar that frequently calcifies (about one-half of tumors). Sonographically, microcystic adenomas are echogenic in regions of the tumor where there are many tiny cysts.

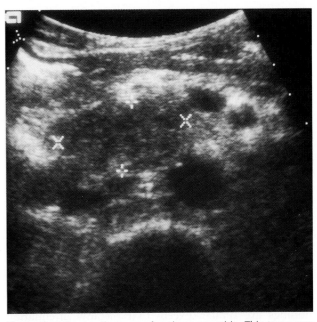

Figure 5–1 Pancreatic mass, chronic pancreatitis. This transverse sonogram demonstrates a 4-cm hypoechoic, uncalcified mass in the head and uncinate process of the pancreas. If typical features of chronic pancreatitis are lacking (calcification, focally dilated ducts), as in this patient, it may be difficult to distinguish masses such as this one from ductal adenocarcinoma.

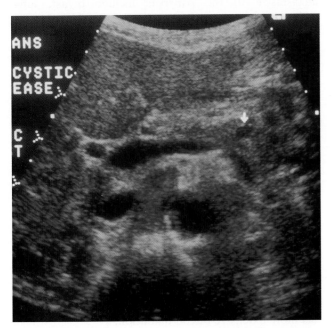

Figure 5–2 Small pancreatic cyst, polycystic disease. This transverse sonogram demonstrates a small pancreatic cyst. Imageable cysts are truly rare in polycystic disease. This is one of two examples seen by the author in 20 years of active practice in body imaging. Such cysts may be sporadic simple cysts, rather that one associated with polycystic disease. Imageable cysts in the pancreas should suggest von Hippel Lindau syndrome, not polycystic disease.

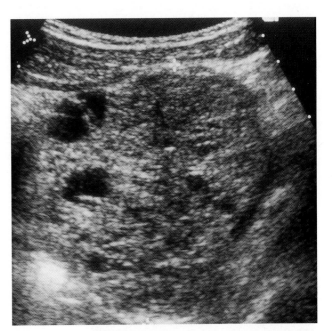

Figure 5–3 Serous cystic neoplasm (microcystic adenoma). This transverse sonogram reveals an 8-cm mass in the pancreatic head. On scanning, it was readily deformed by the pressure of the transducer. It is largely echogenic, owing to the many interfaces created by the very small cysts that make up the bulk of the tumor. Several larger cysts are noted in the periphery, a common finding in this neoplasm. This mass lacks the central calcification that is sometimes seen. This tumor is virtually always benign.

Transmission of sound is frequent. A central stellate scar and calcification may be identified, suggesting the diagnosis.

Mucinous cystic neoplasms consist of larger cysts, easily imaged with CT or sonography. Most tumors are located in the tail or body of the pancreas and are much more common in females, approaching 10:1 predominance. Because differentiation between benign and malignant, mucinous cystic neoplasms is often impossible even pathologically, all tumors are considered malignant and surgical removal is indicated. Calcifications occur in approximately 20% of these neoplasms (compared to about one-half of serous/microcystic neoplasms).

Sonography reveals cystic masses, comprised of septated cysts of variable size (**Fig. 5–4**). Unilocular lesions may occur. The septations may be few or many, quite thin or thick and polypoid. The internal architecture is shown to better advantage by sonography than CT. CT findings are similar, except that the low attenuation masses are more internally featureless and calcification is more frequently identified. These lesions may be confused with rarer cystic neoplasms such as papillary cystic tumor, cystic islet cell tumor, and cystic metastases, or nonneoplastic lesions such as pseudocyst, abscess, and echinococcal disease.

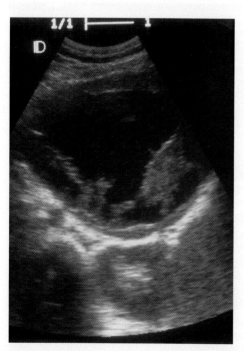

Figure 5–4 Mucinous cystic neoplasm. Transverse sonogram of the left upper abdomen shows a cystic mass with thick internal septations in the pancreatic tail. While not specific, a mass such as this is likely to be a mucinous cystic neoplasm. Differential diagnosis includes pancreatic pseudocyst and rare cystic neoplasms.

Neuroendocrine Tumors of the Pancreas

Neuroendocrine tumors, formerly called *islet cell tumors*, are a small but important group of pancreatic neoplasms that generally originate in pancreatic islet cells.[23] Insulinomas and gastrinomas are the commonest neuroendocrine tumors. Other tumors are glucagonoma, somatostatinoma, VIPoma, carcinoid tumors, pheochromocytoma, and combined histology tumors. These tumors tend to be small and, with the exception of insulinoma, malignant. It is difficult to image neuroendocrine tumors; they are usually small when the patient presents with hormonal abnormalities. Insulinomas and gastrinomas are frequently less than 2 cm in diameter. Thin-section dynamic incremental CECT or angiography sometimes reveal these lesions. Intraoperative sonography is useful in localizing occult neoplasms.

Sonographically, neuroendocrine tumors are usually well defined and round or oval in shape. They generally appear hypoechoic compared to the normal parenchyma.[24, 25] On occasion, the only detectable abnormality may be an alteration of the pancreatic contour. Increased echogenicity from calcification has been reported. Published success rates for the detection of insulinomas vary from 25—60% The results for gastrinomas are worse; approximately 20% are detected.

Unusual and Rare Pancreatic Neoplasms

In autopsy series, metastasis is the most common pancreatic neoplasm. Primary tumors that commonly metastasize to the pancreas include breast, lung, melanoma, colon, and stomach. Pancreatic metastases are rarely clinically significant, as they generally occur late in patients with widespread metastatic disease.

Many uncommon histologic variants of pancreatic ductal adenocarcinoma are indistinguishable on images from tumors with the usual histologic features.[23, 26] These include adenosquamous cell carcinoma, anaplastic carcinoma, and pleomorphic giant cell carcinoma. Acinar center cell carcinoma and pleomorphic giant cell carcinoma, though often indistinguishable from ductal adenocarcinoma, may be larger and exhibit central necrosis. Ductectatic carcinoma and mucin-hypersecreting carcinoma are variants of ductal adenocarcinoma. These lesions are characterized by cystically dilated mucin-filled pancreatic branch ducts, usually in the uncinate process and pancreatic head. Sonographically, ductectatic carcinomas show multiple sonolucent dilated ducts within the uncinate process. A discrete mass may not be evident. Mucin hypersecreting carcinoma usually has more extensive ductal dilatation.

Solid and papillary epithelial neoplasm is found most frequently in young females, often of African American descent. It is a low-grade malignancy, often curable by resection. The tumor tends to be large and well encapsulated. Tumors can be mostly solid, mixed cystic and solid, or almost entirely cystic. Images reveal a well-defined, round or oval mass with thick irregular walls. Varying areas of echogenic mass and cystic areas are seen depending on the morphology of the individual tumor. Hemorrhage and necrosis may be present.

Sarcomas of the pancreas, for which no specific sonographic findings have been reported, are prohibitively rare, accounting for less than 1% of all pancreatic neoplasms

Diagnostic Evaluation

Nonimaging tests

Nonimaging tests play little role in determining whether a neoplasm is resectable or unresectable. Clinical and laboratory information may suggest that a patient is not able to tolerate major surgery, but the actual determination of unresectability is generally made with imaging, laparoscopy, or laparotomy.

Imaging Tests Other than Sonography

The main contribution of imaging tests in patients with periampullary neoplasm has been the ability to quickly and safely identify patients with unresectable tumors. These individuals can then be managed in the most appropriate palliative fashion -- further, more invasive studies and diagnostic procedures are not necessary. Furthermore, the five-year survival of patients undergoing attempted curative resection is only 5—8%, although more recent studies have reported survival in the 10—20% range.

Because surgery is the only chance for cure of a periampullary carcinoma, surgeons are very interested in imaging as a means of selecting patients for Whipple pancreaticoduodenectomy, palliative bypass surgery, or even nonsurgical management. Preliminary imaging (10-mm thick section contrast-enhanced CT, routine sonography) often reveals evidence of metastasis or other signs of unresectability. If no evidence of unresectability is noted on the initial imaging study, more sophisticated evaluation is appropriate. High-resolution computed tomography (CT), magnetic resonance imaging (MRI) and, as we shall see, color flow sonography can often provide this information. High-resolution CT[2] and, to a lesser degree, magnetic resonance imaging[13] are the modalities used to assess these patients. Despite the fact that sonography is often the first modality used to image patients with pancreatic carcinoma, little work has been done to assess the usefulness of sonography in evaluating the resectability of pancreatic neoplasms.[14,27] In most recent discussions of imaging in pancreatic neoplasms, transabdominal sonography has been almost totally ignored.

Image findings of unresectability are reliable; only rarely can such a tumor be resected at the time of surgery.[28—30] The following findings correlate with unresectability: tumor larger than 2 cm, extracapsular extension, vascular invasion (venous or arterial), lymphadenopathy, or metastatic disease. High-resolution CT, performed in the arterial and venous phase, is good at showing extrapancreatic invasion and metastasis. It is also accurate in assessing whether there is vascular involvement—the most frequent local abnormality that makes a periampullary neoplasm unresectable. As the mortality of Whipple procedure declines, some surgeons have become more aggressive. Some surgeons now feel that pancreatic head lesions are unresectable only when the superior mesenteric artery is involved or when metastatic disease is present. New trials are needed to see if this more aggressive surgical approach will result in improved survival.

While findings of unresectability are reliable, many tumors believed resectable because of their image appearance on CT or sonography cannot be resected for cure at surgery. The recent CT studies by Meigibow et al., Fuhrman et al., and Freeny et al., yielded correct predictions of resectability in 28%, 88%, and 72% of patients, respectively.

Ultrasound Imaging

Sonographically, pancreatic carcinoma is typically (about 60%) a hypoechoic mass that deforms the gland's morphology. Homogeneous masses are slightly more common than heterogeneous masses. In our recent series, about 10% caused no glandular contour abnormality and were visualized only because tumor echogenicity differed from the normal pancreas.[31] Occasionally, pancreatic carcinoma is hyperechoic. Masses with increased echogenicity are common in chronic pancreatitis, rare in carcinoma. Slightly more than 60% occur in the pancreatic head; about 5% are diffuse, and the remaining one-third are found in the body or tail. Calcification occurs in about 5% of masses and is usually focal (**Fig. 5–5**) or scattered, unlike typical chronic pancreatitis calcifications. Small intralesional cysts occur in about 15% of patients. Pseudocysts, related to obstruction of a pancreatic duct, occur in about 5—10% of patients. Glandular atrophy may occur from obstruction caused by a tumor.

During the past several years, we have developed a technique to assess the resectability of pancreatic tumors using color flow sonography.[17] We performed a retrospective analysis of 45 patients with periampullary neoplasm referred for color flow sonographic evaluation of resectability. Vessels that were touched or occluded by tumor were categorized according to a Pancreatic Color Doppler Score (**Table 5–1**). Other factors affecting resectability (metastasis, enlarged nodes) were recorded. Findings were correlated to surgical and pathologic findings of resectability and unresectability. Patients were given a score corresponding to the most significantly affected vessel.

All 18 patients with circumferential tumor or vascular occlusion (PCDS 4 & 5) could not be resected (**Fig. 5–6** through **5–10**) . All 10 patients in whom tumor did not touch (PCDS 0) (**Fig. 5–11**) had negative margins. Patients with tumors that touched from 25 to 49% (PCDS 2) (**Fig. 5–12** through **5–13**) and from 50 to 99%

(PCDS 3) (**Fig. 5–14**) were sometimes resected surgically, but all had positive vascular margins. This correlates with a very poor prognosis. Of 6 patients with PCDS 1 (1—24% contiguity) (**Fig. 5–15**), all were resected. Two had positive vascular margins and 4 had surgically negative margins.

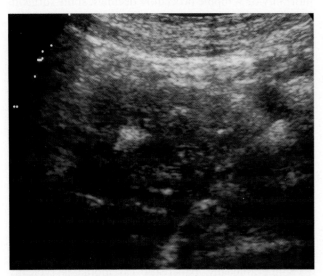

Figure 5–5 Calcification in pancreatic adenocarcinoma. This transverse sonogram of the pancreatic head reveals a single calcification in the mass caused by a ductal adenocarcinoma. The presence of calcification in about 5% of pancreatic carcinomas and the lack of calcifications in some chronic pancreatitis-related masses can occasionally lead to incorrect diagnosis.

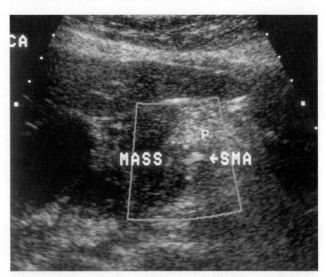

Figure 5–6 Hypoechoic pancreatic carcinoma obstructs the SMV—PCDS 5. This sonogram shows a mass that deforms the glands morphology and obliterates the superior mesenteric vein. This is a pancreatic color Doppler score of 5 (PCDS 5). The superior mesenteric artery (SMA) is encased. P, normal pancreas.

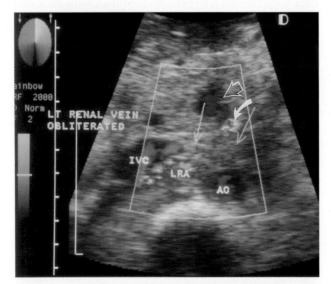

Figure 5–7 Pancreatic carcinoma obstructing the left renal vein (PCDS 5). This transverse color Doppler sonogram shows a pancreatic carcinoma that obliterates the left renal vein (**arrows**). The mass is also contiguous with the aorta (AO), inferior vena cava (IVC), left renal artery, superior mesenteric artery (**curved arrow**), and superior mesenteric vein (**open arrow**). This patient, as with all PCDS 4 or 5 patients, could not be resected.

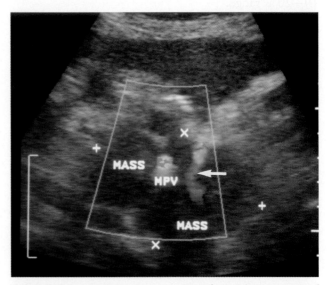

Figure 5–8 Pancreatic carcinoma – circumferential encasement of the portal vein. PCDS 4. A transverse color Doppler sonogram through the lower hepatoduodenal ligament reveals complete circumferential encasement of the main portal vein (MPV) by the irregular pancreatic carcinoma (MASS), outlined by calipers. The adjacent celiac axis (**arrow**) is approximately 80% circumferentially involved. Tumor did not completely encompass the cephalad aspect of the celiac axis (not shown). Tumors were graded according to the highest PCDS, in this case 4 (circumferential tumor).

Figure 5–9 Pancreatic cancer circumferentially surrounds the main ▷ portal vein, celiac axis, and common hepatic artery (PCDS 4). A transverse color Doppler sonogram reveals hypoechoic tumor (**arrows**) that is contiguous to the inferior vena cava and aorta and circumferentially surrounds the celiac axis from its origin. Also circumferentially involved are the main portal vein ("ENCASED main PV") and the common hepatic artery (CHA). The obstructed bile duct is seen ventral to the mass (CBD). The pancreatic color Doppler score is 4, circumferential contiguity. As with all other patients with PCDS of 4 or 5, this patient was unresectable at surgery.

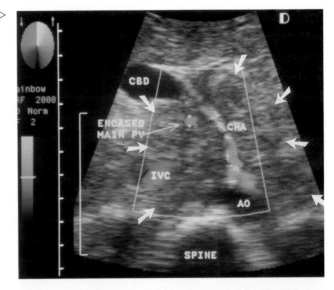

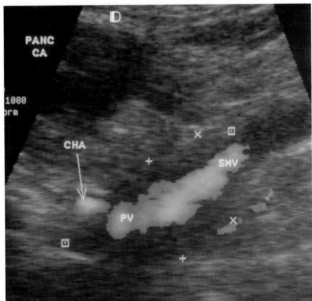

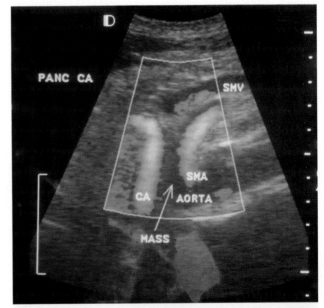

△
Figure 5–10 Pancreatic carcinoma circumferentially encircles the superior mesenteric vein (PCDS 4). The longitudinal power Doppler sonogram (**A**) of the superior mesenteric vein (SMV) reveals hypoechoic tumor circumferentially surrounding the vessel (outlined by calipers). Tumor is contiguous to the common hepatic artery (CHA), but it does not circumferentially surround it. Main Portal Vein—PV. The longitudinal color Doppler sonogram (**B**) shows the pancreatic tumor (mass) touching the aorta. The tumor is contiguous to both the celiac axis (CA) and the origin of the superior mesenteric artery (SMA). Superior mesenteric vein, SMV. All patients with completely circumferential tumor (PCDS 4) could not be resected.

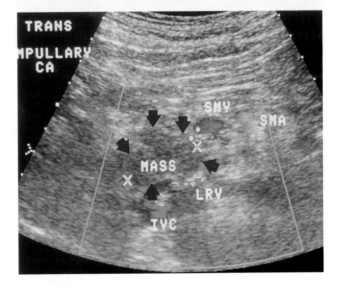

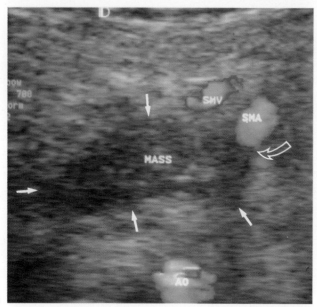

A

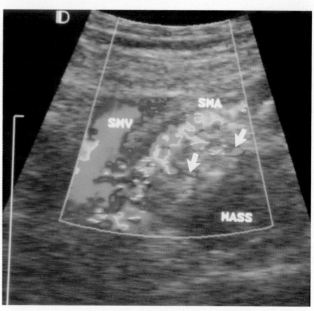

B

Figure 5–12 Pancreatic carcinoma touches the SMA (25—49% circumferential – PCDS 2). A transverse color Doppler sonogram through the region of the head of the pancreas (**A**) reveals a mass (mass, **arrows**) that touches, but does not completely encircle the superior mesenteric artery (**open curved arrow**). The tumor comes close to, but does not touch, the superior mesenteric vein (SMV). All PCDS 2 patients had positive surgical margins. A longitudinal color

Doppler sonogram (**B**) along the proximal superior mesenteric artery shows branches from the superior mesenteric artery (**arrows**) feeding the pancreatic cancer (mass). One of these feeding vessels (coded blue) is noted dorsal (posterior) to the superior mesenteric artery in Fig. 5–5 A. SMA, superior mesenteric artery; SMV, superior mesenteric vein.

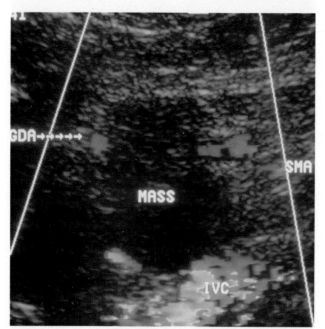

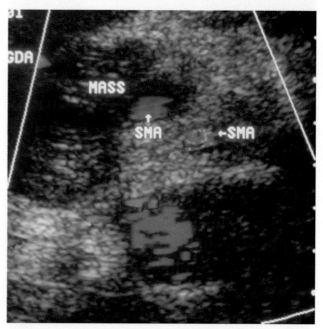

Figure 5–13 Pancreatic Carcinoma – PCDS 2. This transverse color Doppler sonogram through the head of the pancreas shows a mass that touches the superior mesenteric vein around slightly less than 50% of its circumference. This is classifed as a pancreatic color Doppler score of 2. The superior mesenteric artery (SMA) is free of tumor. GDA, gastroduodenal artery.

Figure 5–14 Pancreatic carcinoma—PCDS 3. This transverse color Doppler sonogram through the head of the pancreas shows a mass that touches the superior mesenteric vein (mislabeled SMA) around more than 50% of its circumference. This is classifed as a pancreatic color Doppler score of 3. Note the hypoechoic tongue of tumor that touches the superior mesenteric artery (SMA) medially. The pancreatic color Doppler score is assigned according to the vessel most affected by the tumor, in this case the superior mesenteric vein. GDA, gastroduodenal artery.

All 30 patients considered unresectable sonographically were also unresectable for cure based on surgical and pathological information. Six of 15 (40%) considered resectable sonographically were actually unresectable for cure. Color flow sonography influenced therapy in 10 of 45 patients (22% overall).

In the important area of determining definitively that a patient cannot be cured by surgical resection, our data showed a positive predictive value of 100%. That is, color flow sonography unresectability correlated with all 30 patients who were unresectable for cure. In this circumstance (at least 80% of all patients presenting with pancreatic carcinoma), no further evaluation is required; palliative management is appropriate.

Prediction of unresectability with CT is reliable. Our data suggest that color flow sonography likewise may be reliable. Identifying patients who are potentially resectable with a high probability for cure is more difficult. Sonographically 15 patients were classified as resectable. Only 9 of 15 (60%) were resectable with a significant probability of cure. This is comparable to the recent CT studies by Megibow et al., Fuhrman et al., and Freeny et al., which yielded correct predictions of resectability in 28%, 88%, and 72% of patients, respectively. On the other hand, when tumor did not touch on color flow sonography, tumor-free margins were achieved at resection in 10 of 10 patients.

One potential problem in using color flow sonography to assess resectability of pancreatic tumors is that the examiner must have significant experience in abdominal color flow imaging. We have learned, nevertheless, that color flow evaluation of patients with pancreatic masses is actually simpler than evaluation of patients with a normal pancreas. Pancreatic neoplasms tend to be noncompressible and are often immobile. Thus, compression with a large footprint-curved linear array transducer allows visualization of the mass and its relationship to any vessels. In this study we visualized 643 of 647 possible vessels (99.4% visualization rate) and achieved complete technical success in 49 of 51 patients (96%). It should also be remembered that the great majority of pancreatic neoplasms occur in the head and body, the easiest regions to visualize sonographically.

Benefits of Ultrasound

Can color flow sonography decrease the need for CT to assess resectability in pancreatic neoplasms? The role of color flow sonography in the evaluation of pancreatic tumors awaits the results of prospective trials. Our data, however, suggest that color flow sonography is promising. It was reliable in detecting unresectable lesions in our series, detecting all 30 patients who were unresectable for cure. Color flow sonography, a comfortable, noninvasive, and relatively inexpensive examination, may be an effective screening tool to evaluate resectabil-

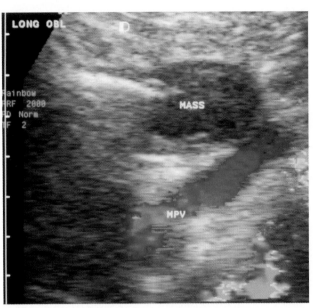

Figure 5–15 Ampullary carcinoma touching the main portal vein (PCDS 1—less than 25% circumferential). An oblique longitudinal color Doppler sonogram of the mass shows contiguity with the main portal vein (MPV) just above the confluence. Transverse color Doppler images (not shown) confirmed that less than 25% of the circumference was touched by tumor (PCDS 1). It was determined after resection that the surgical margins were clear by 0.5 mm. Two of six resected PCDS 1 patients had positive pathologic margins. A PCDS of 1 did not correlate well with either positive or negative surgical margins. Two-thirds (4 of 6 patients) of PCDS 1 patients were resected with negative margins.

ity. If color flow sonography can correctly predict unresectability, 80% of pancreatic carcinoma patients would require no further expensive and invasive imaging evaluation. Palliative management could proceed. Only 20% of patients would require further evaluation—CT, ERCP, laparoscopy, etc.

Summary

Sonography has been almost totally ignored in most of the recent discussions of imaging in pancreatic and periampullary neoplasms.[28–30] It seems clear from our data that color flow sonography can be very useful in evaluating the resectability of pancreatic neoplasms. Like high-resolution CT, color Doppler sonography is reliable in assessing resectability of periampullary neoplasm. Any future evaluation of imaging and management of pancreatic tumors should include color flow sonography.

References

1. Gudjonsson B. Carcinoma of the pancreas: critical analysis of costs, results of resections, and the need for standardized reporting. *J Am Coll Surgeons* 1995;181:483—503.
2. Warshaw A.L., Gu Z., Wittenberg J., Waltman A.C. Preoperative staging and assessment of resectability of pancreatic cancer. *Arch Surg* 1990;125:230—233.
3. Wade T.P., Radford D.M., Virgo K.S., Johnson F.E. Complications and outcomes in the treatment of pancreatic adenocarcinoma in the United States veteran. *J Am Coll Surgeons* 1994;179:38—48.
4. Geer R.J., Brennan M.F. Prognostic indicators for survival after resection of pancreatic adenocarcinoma. *Am J Surg* 1993;165:68—734.
5. Alvarez C., Livingston E.H., Ashley S.W., Schwarz M., Reber H.A. Cost-benefit analysis of the work-up for pancreatic cancer. *Am J Surg* 1993;165:53—60.
6. Fuhrman G.M., Charnsangavej C., Abbruzzese J.L., et al. Thin-section contrast-enhanced computed tomography accurately predicts the resectability of malignant pancreatic neoplasms. *Am J Surg* 1994;167:104—113.
7. Klinkenbijil, J.H.G., Jeekel J., Schmitz P.I.M., et al. Carcinoma of the pancreas and periampullary region: palliation versus cure. *Br J Surg* 1993;80;1575—1578.
8. Nitecki S.S., Sarr M.G., Colby T.V., vanHeerden J.A. Long-term survival after resection for ductal adenocarcinoma of the pancreas. Is it really improving? *Ann Surg* 1995;221:59—66.
9. Wade T.P., El-Ghazzawy A.G., Virgo K.S., Johnson F.E. The Whipple ressection for cancer in U.S. department of veterans affairs hospitals. *Ann Surg* 1995;221(3):241—248.
10. Warshaw A.L., Fernandez-del Castillo C. Pancreatic carcinoma. *N Engl J Med* 1992;326:455—465.
11. Trede M., Schwall G., Saeger H.D. Survival after pancreatoduodenectomy. *Ann Surg* 1990;211:447—458.
12. Cameron J.L., Pitt H.A., Yeo C.J., et al. One hundred and forty-five consecutive pancreaticoduodenectomies without mortality. *Ann Surg* 1993;217(5):430—438.
13. Vellet A.D., Romano W., Bach D.B., et al. Adenocarcinoma of the pancreatic ducts: comparative evaluation with CT and MR imaging at 1.5 T. *Radiology* 1992;183:87—95.
14. Campbell J.P., Wilson S.R. Pancreatic neoplasms: how useful is evaluation with US? *Radiology* 1988;167:341—344.
15. Megibow A.J. Pancreatic adenocarcinoma: designing the examination to evaluate the clinical questions. *Radiology* 1982;183:297—303.
16. Nghiem H.V., Freeny P.C. Radiologic staging of pancreatic adenocarcinoma. *Radiol Clin North Am* 1994;32(1):71—79.
17. Ralls P.W., Wren S.M., Radin D.R., et al. Color flow sonography in evaluating the resectability of periampullary and pancreatic tumors. *J Ultrasound Med* 1997;16:131—140.
18. Wren S.M., Ralls P.W., Stain S.C., et al. Assessment of resectability of pancreatic head and periampullary tumors by color flow Doppler sonography. *Arch Surg* 1996;131:812—818.
19. Tomiyama T., Ueno N., Tano S., et al. Assessment of arterial invasion in pancreatic cancer using color Doppler ultrasonography. *Am J Gastroenterol* 1996;91:1410—1416.
20. Angeli E., Venturini M., Vanzulli A., et al. Color Doppler imaging in the assessment of vascular involvement of pancreatic carcinoma. *AJR* 1997;168:193—197.
21. Johnson C.D., Stephens D.H., Charboneau J.W., Carpenter H.A., Welch T.J. Cystic pancreatic tumors: CT and sonographic assessment. *AJR* 1988;151:1133—1138.
22. Mathieu D., Guigui B., Valette P.J., et al. Pancreatic cystic neoplasms. *Radiol Clin North Am* 1898;27(1):163—176.
23. Cubilla A.L., Fitzgerald P.J. *Tumors of the Exocrine Pancreas, Atlas of Tumor Pathology*, 2nd series, Fascicle 19, Armed Forces Institute of Pathology, 1984.
24. Galiber A.K., Reading C.C., Charboneau J.W., et al. Localization of pancreatic insulinoma: comparison of pre-and intraoperative US with CT and angiography. *Radiology* 1988;166:405—408.
25. Rossi P., Allison D.J., Bezzi M., et al. Endocrine tumors of the pancreas. *Radiol Clin North Am* 1989;28(1):129—161.
26. Friedman A.C., Edmonds P.R. Rare pancreatic malignancies. *Radiol Clin North Am* 1989;27(1):177—190.
27. Campbell J.P., Wilson S.R. Pancreatic neoplasms: how useful is evaluation with US? *Radiology* 1988;167:341—344.
28. Megibow A.J., Zhou X.H., Rotterdam H., et al. Pancreatic adenocarcinoma: CT versus MR imaging in the evaluation of resectability-report of the radiology diagnostic oncology group. *Radiology* 1995;195:327—332.
29. Fuhrman G.M., Charnsangavej C., Abbruzzese J.L., et al. Thin-section contrast-enhanced computed tomography accurately predicts the resectability of malignant pancreatic neoplasms. *Am J Surg* 1994;167:104—113.
30. Freeny P.C., Traverso L.W., Ryan J.A. Diagnosis and staging of pancreatic adenocarcinoma with dynamic computed tomography. *Am J Surg* 1993;165:600—606.
31. Yassa N.A., Yang J., Stein S., Johnson M., Ralls P.W. Grayscale and color flow sonography of pancreatic ductal adenocarcinoma. *J Clin Ultrasound* 1997;25(9):473—480.

6 Hyperamylasemia

Philip W. Ralls

Introduction

Despite its many causes, hyperamylasemia is most often associated clinically with acute pancreatitis. Simultaneous elevation of serum lipase strongly suggests that hyperamylasemia is pancreatitis related. Acute pancreatitis is the clinical situation in which imaging is most often requested in hyperamylasemic patients. Our focus will be on these patients.

The clinical spectrum of acute pancreatitis ranges from a benign, self-limited disorder (about 75% of patients) to severe pancreatitis that may be fulminant and quickly cause death from multiorgan failure. Mild acute pancreatitis is generally a self-limited disease that resolves spontaneously with no special therapy other than supportive management. Acute interstitial/edematous pancreatitis results in an enlarged and congested gland without appreciable necrosis or hemorrhage. Although the clinical course in these patients is generally benign, progression to more severe pancreatitis and death may occur. Mortality in mild acute pancreatitis is generally only 1—2% — about 10—20% of all acute pancreatitis-associated deaths.[1]

Clinically and pathologically, necrotizing pancreatitis is a far more severe disease than acute edematous/interstitial pancreatitis. The most striking and significant histologic feature is pancreatic necrosis, often accompanied by intrapancreatic and peripancreatic hemorrhage and infection. This group comprises approximately 20—25% of all patients with acute pancreatitis, but is responsible for about 80% of acute pancreatitis-associated deaths. About one-third of all patients with severe acute pancreatitis die.[2]

Infection accounts for 80% of acute pancreatitis-related mortality. Inconsistent and sometimes confusing terminology has made evaluating studies that assess the therapy and diagnosis of patients with infected acute pancreatitis difficult. Using the definitions proposed by the Atlanta International Symposium on Acute Pancreatitis (see **Table 6–1**), there are two major infectious complications: pancreatic necrosis and pancreatic abscess. Pancreatic abscess is a circumscribed collection of pus that contains little or no necrosis. Infected pancreatic necrosis is a region of infected, nonviable pancreatic parenchyma. Infected pancreatic necrosis and pancreatic abscesses each occur in about 1—10% of all acute pancreatitis patients. Pancreatic abscess is associated with a lower mortality (7–33%) than is infected pancreatic necrosis (about 40%).[3]

Differential Diagnosis

Clinically significant hyperamylasemia is most often caused by acute pancreatitis. Increased serum amylase occurs in many conditions, however, ranging from ruptured ectopic pregnancy to mumps. Gastrointestinal conditions including appendicitis, perforation (from trauma, ulcers, and other causes), mesenteric ischemia or infarction, and portal thrombosis often result in hyperamylasemia. Other conditions, including salivary gland disorders, acute cholecystitis, dissecting abdominal aortic aneurysm, and neoplasms may also cause hyperamylasemia. The clinical presentation, as well as secondary laboratory tests and radiologic imaging, suffice to distinguish among the many causes of hyperamylasemia.

Diagnostic Evaluation

Nonimaging Tests

Clinical examination and laboratory data provide the most useful information in distinguishing among the many causes of hyperamylasemia. History and physical examination should guide further work-up and the imaging evaluation in patients with hyperamylasemia unrelated to acute pancreatitis.

Abdominal pain is by far the most common symptom in patients with acute pancreatitis. The onset of pain is usually sudden, peaking after a few hours and resolving in 2—3 days. Severe epigastric pain, often radiating to the back and making the patient lean forward, is common. Radiation of the pain to the back occurs in about half of all patients. On occasion, abdominal pain may be in the lower abdomen, rather than the epigastrium. Pancreatitis may be painless, even in severe cases.[4—6] Nausea and vomiting are almost always present.

While acute pancreatitis is usually obvious clinically, very mild cases may be missed. Rarely, the diagnosis may be missed in severe pancreatitis because pain is absent or

Table 6–1   The 1992 Atlanta International Symposium, Definition

Diagnosis	Definition
Acute pancreatitis	Acute pancreatitis is an acute inflammatory process of the pancreas with variable involvement of other regional tissues or remote organ systems.
Severe acute pancreatitis	Severe acute pancreatitis is associated with organ failure and/or local complications such as necrosis, abscess, or pseudocyst and may be characterized by either three or more Ranson criteria or eight or more APACHE II points. Organ failure is defined as shock (systolic BP less than 90 mm Hg), pulmonary insufficiency (P_aO_2 less than or equal to 60 mm Hg), renal failure (creatinine >2 mg % after rehydration), or GI bleeding (greater than 500 cc/24 hours). Systemic complications (e.g., disseminated intravascular coagulation, hypocalcemia) may occur. The hallmark of severe acute pancreatitis is pancreatic necrosis.
Mild acute pancreatitis	Mild acute pancreatitis is associated with little or no organ dysfunction and uneventful recovery. It lacks the features of severe acute pancreatitis.
Acute fluid collections	These occur early in the course of acute pancreatitis, in or near the pancreas. They lack a discernible wall of granulation or fibrous tissue. The crucial distinction between an acute fluid collection and a pseudocyst or abscess is the lack of a defined wall on imaging studies (CT or ultrasound).
Pancreatic necrosis	Pancreatic necrosis is a diffuse of focal area of nonviable pancreatic tissue, and is typically associated with peripancreatic fat necrosis. Dynamic contrast CT is the gold standard for the clinical diagnosis of pancreatic necrosis. Well marginated zones of nonenhanced pancreatic parenchyma greater than 3 cm in size or greater than 30% of the area of the pancreas are requisite for a CT diagnosis of pancreatic necrosis. Contrast attenuation fails to exceed 50 Hounsfield units after bolus injection of intravenous contrast. It is considered that the accuracy of dynamic CT is 80 to 90%. Biochemical markers for pancreatic necrosis, such as C-reactive protein and others are of limited usefulness. The clinical distinction between sterile necrosis and infected pancreatic necrosis is critical as infection of necrotic tissues triples the risk of mortality. Patients with sterile pancreatic necrosis can often be managed without surgical intervention, but infected necrosis is almost always fatal without surgical drainage. CT-guided aspiration is required to differentiate between these two conditions.
Acute pseudocyst	A pseudocyst is a collection of pancreatic juice enclosed by a defined wall. They are most often discovered by imaging. Formation of a pseudocyst requires 4 or more weeks from the onset of acute pancreatitis. Fluid collections less than 4 weeks of age or lacking a defined wall are more properly termed acute fluid collections. Bacterial contamination of a pseudocyst is often of no clinical significance. Pus means that the lesion should be more correctly termed a pancreatic abscess.
Pancreatic abscess	A pancreatic abscess is a circumscribed collection of pus usually near the pancreas that contains little or no pancreatic necrosis. A key distinction is that pancreatic abscesses likely arise as a consequence of limited necrosis as opposed to infected necrosis, which is a more broad-based less well-defined process. Pancreatic abscess and infected necrosis differ in clinical expression and the extent of the associated necrosis. The mortality for infected necrosis is double that for pancreatic abscess. Specific therapy may be markedly different. Abscesses that arise after pancreatic surgery are not properly termed pancreatic abscesses, but are more accurately classified as postoperative abscesses.
Obsolete terminology in pancreatitis	The symposium members suggested that the following terms are no longer useful clinically: phlegmon, infected pseudocyst, hermorrhagic pancreatitis, and persistent acute pancreatitis.

masked by other, more severe, symptoms.[4,5] In a series analyzing fatal pancreatitis reported in the 1980s and 1990s, 33% of cases were not diagnosed until autopsy.[5]

No single serologic abnormality is pathognomonic for acute pancreatitis. In mild cases, the patient may present after transient hyperamylasemia and elevated lipase levels have resolved; thus, no serologic indicators of pancreatitis may be present. In this instance, the diagnosis of mild acute pancreatitis is entirely clinical.[7,8] Rarely, serum amylase is normal in evere acute pancreatitis. Patients with gallstone-related pancreatitis tend to have higher serum amylase levels than alcoholics and other patients with acute pancreatitis.[9] Elevated serum amylase is nonspecific. Thus, pancreatic lipase is generally a more specific enzymatic indicator of pancreatitis.

Imaging Tests Other than Sonography

Computed Tomography

Both computed tomography (CT) and sonography are useful in imaging of patients with acute pancreatitis. CT may be used to confirm the diagnosis and assess potential complications of pancreatitis. CT is also useful in the early stages of severe acute pancreatitis as a guide to management.

Contrast CT is indicated early in the clinical course of severe pancreatitis if the diagnosis is uncertain or if complications such as abscess, hemorrhage, or necrosis are suspected. A preliminary noncontrast CT can detect high-attenuation pancreatic hemorrhage. CT may be useful to detect pseudoaneurysms or venous thrombus as a cause of bleeding. Angiography and color flow sonography are also effective techniques in diagnosing vascular abnormalities. Dynamic bolus contrast CT or, better, helical CT, can identify areas of focal pancreatic necrosis as relatively avascular nonenhancing regions. Contrast CT is the most reliable means of diagnosing pancreatic necrosis. When necrosis is detected and infection or sepsis is suspected, CT-guided aspiration of unenhancing regions of the pancreas is mandatory. Early diagnosis of pancreatic abscess is a prerequisite for cure. As the CT and sonographic features of pancreatic abscess are nonspecific, early and aggressive image-guided needle aspiration of suspicious fluid collections is critical for early diagnosis.

Magnetic Resonance Imaging

In some series, intravenous gadolinium-enhanced magnetic resonance imaging (MRI) has been able to image pancreatitis-related changes with success comparable to CT.[10, 11] MRI is not a primary modality to evaluate patients with pancreatitis because of its expense, inferior spatial resolution, poor tolerance to patient motion, difficulties in monitoring patients requiring life support, and its relative inability to guide interventional procedures. MRI may be potentially useful in patients with allergies to iodinated contrast, patients with renal failure, or in pregnant patients.

Angiography

Angiography was previously used to assess patients with vascular and hemorrhagic complications of acute pancreatitis. Venous thrombus and, less commonly, pseudoaneurysms, are causes of pancreatitis-associated gastrointestinal bleeding. Noninvasive techniques, mainly dynamic or helical CT or color Doppler sonography have now largely assumed this diagnostic role. While, angiography is still used diagnostically in cases that remain unclear after noninvasive imaging, its major use is therapeutic. Interventional angiography can be useful in many circumstances — from embolizing pseudoaneurysms to TIPS procedures.

Imaging in Acute Pancreatitis

Role of Ultrasound

— Detect gallstones as a cause of acute pancreatitis
— Follow known fluid collections
— Guide aspiration and drainage

Role of CT

— Confirm uncertain diagnosis of acute pancreatitis
— Detect complications of acute pancreatitis
— Detect pancreatic necrosis
— Guide aspiration and drainage

Ultrasound Imaging

Evaluation of the gallbladder and bile ducts is the focus of most sonographic examinations performed in patients with acute pancreatitis. After a careful search of the gallbladder for stones, the bile duct should be evaluated for choledocholithiasis (**Fig. 6–1**) and obstruction. The distal, intrapancreatic portion of the bile duct is often best imaged on transverse images with special scanning techniques. Compression scanning with a large footprint curved linear transducer often shows the pancreatic head and bile duct well. Another useful approach is to give the patient water orally, then scan the patient in an erect or semierect position. With careful technique, common duct stones can be identified in as many as 75% of patients.[12] The water-filled stomach may also reveal the pancreatic tail (**Fig. 6–2**), the most difficult portion of the pancreas to visualize sonographically. It may also be useful to obtain images coronally through the spleen and left kidney while the patient lies in a right lateral decubitus position. This scan plane, while usually

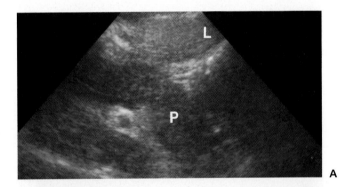
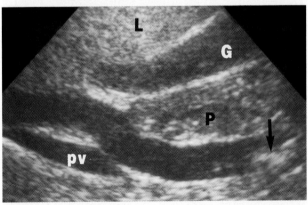

Figure 6–1 Acute pancreatitis, stone obstructing common bile duct. **A:** Transverse sonogram of the region of the body and tail of the pancreas reveals decreased echogenicity of the pancreas (P) compared to the liver (L). Most often, mild pancreatitis results in no alteration of the pancreatic echogenicity. A relatively hypoechoic pancreas, as noted in this case, is somewhat unusual. This patient's pancreatitis was caused by calculous obstruction of the common bile duct. **B:** The longitudinal image of the bile duct reveals extrahepatic bile duct dilatation and a distal stone (**arrow**). L, liver; G, gallbladder; PV, portal vein. Reprinted with permission from **Sonography of the Abdomen** by R. Brooke Jeffrey, Jr. and Philip W. Ralls. Raven Press, New York, 1995.

not revealing the normal pancreatic tail itself, may show abnormalities in the region of the tail of the pancreas (pseudocysts, masses, etc.) that are invisible on other views.

After scanning the pancreas, peripancreatic pathology should be sought in the lesser sac, anterior pararenal spaces, and the transverse mesocolon. An attempt should be made to visualize the lesser sac in both transverse and longitudinal planes. Sonographic landmarks identifying the inferior recess of the lesser sac include the body of the pancreas, spleen, and gastric an-

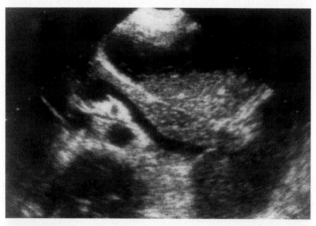

Figure 6–2 Normal pancreatic tail. The pancreatic tail is the most difficult part of the gland to image sonographically. An Rao position with water in the stomach may allow visualization of this region, as in this patient.

trum. Acute fluid collections that extend to the superior recess of the lesser sac are often best appreciated in the sagittal plane, as the superior recess reflects cranially over the pancreas. In the transverse plane, fluid in the superior recess of the lesser sac extends cranially next to the caudate lobe, to the left of the fissure for the ligamentum venosum. Fluid in the superior recess may sometimes insinuate itself to the right, posterior (dorsal) to the fissure for the ligamentum venosum, and anterior (ventral) to the caudate lobe.

The anterior pararenal spaces are best seen through a coronal flank approach. The patient is scanned while in a decubitus position with the transducer angled to achieve a sagittal scan plane through the flank. Areas of inflammation within the anterior pararenal space are often seen immediately adjacent to the echogenic fat within the perirenal space (**Fig. 6–3**). Acute pancreatic inflammation collections within the anterior pararenal space occasionally outline Gerota's fascia, but this is an inconsistent finding.

The transverse mesocolon is the most difficult of all peripancreatic compartments to directly visualize with sonography.[13] Gas in the transverse colon often precludes optimal sonographic imaging. The landmarks identifying the transverse mesocolon are the superior mesenteric artery and vein near the uncinate process of the pancreatic head. In the transverse plane, the transverse mesocolon lies directly ventral (anterior) to the

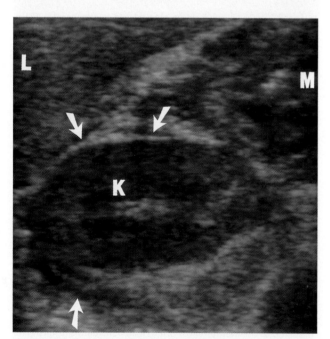

Figure 6–3 Perirenal inflammatory change, acute pancreatitis. Transverse sonogram through the region of the right kidney (K). Pancreatic inflammation often crosses multiple tissue planes. Note the decreased perirenal echogenicity caused by perirenal inflammation (**arrows**). A large predominantly hypoechoic mixed echogenicity mass (M) is seen ventromedial to the right kidney. L, liver. Reprinted with permission from **Sonography of the Abdomen** by R. Brooke Jeffrey, Jr. and Philip W. Ralls. Raven Press, New York, 1995.

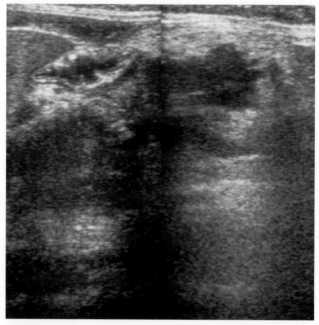

Figure 6–4 Inflammation in the transverse mesocolon. This longitudinal composite sonogram shows inflammation in the transverse mesocolon, caudal to the pancreas and stomach. This scan plane is best to identify transverse mesocolon inflammation. As in this patient, is it often much harder to identify the colon than the stomach.

head and uncinate process of the pancreas. The simplest way to identify inflammation in the transverse mesocolon is to scan longitudinally in the midline. Inflammation is seen extending caudally between the stomach and pancreatic body, toward the region of the transverse colon (**Fig. 6–4**).

Color and spectral Doppler sonography may be useful in detecting pancreatitis-associated pseudoaneurysms, demonstrating arterial flow in what appears to be a "cystic mass" on gray scale images (**Fig. 6–5**). All discrete cystic areas should be investigated with Doppler, as pseudoaneurysms may otherwise be misdiagnosed as a pseudocyst or other fluid collection. Venous thrombosis can be diagnosed with color flow sonography.

Sonographic Findings in Acute Pancreatitis

Normally, pancreatic echogenicity is equal to or slightly greater than the echogenicity of the liver. In alcoholic patients with increased liver echogenicity from fatty infiltration or cirrhosis, it may be more difficult to use this comparison (**Fig. 6–6**).

The reported prevalence of sonographic abnormality in acute pancreatitis varies widely — ranging from 33% to 90% of patients.[14, 15] Our recent retrospective evaluation using modern sonographic systems found abnormalities in 94% of patients with acute pancreatitis.[16] Pancreatic echogenicity typically decreases in acute pancreatitis because of interstitial edema (**Fig. 6–1 and 6–7**). In some patients, echogenicity is normal. Rarely, echogenicity may actually increase, possibly because of hemorrhage, necrosis, or fat saponification. Cotton et al.

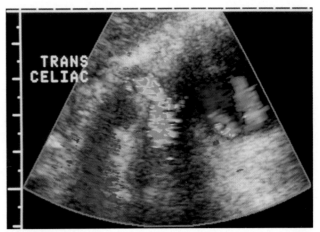

Figure 6–5 Psuedoaneurysm of the splenic artery from acute pancreatitis. This transverse color Doppler sonogram shows a splenic artery pseudoaneurysm, with bidirectional swirling flow. Note the aliased flow in the celiac axis, adjacent to the pseudoaneurysm. The splenic artery is the most frequent site of pancreatitis-associated pseudoaneurysms.

noted that, compared with the liver, the pancreatic echogenicity was increased in 16% of those normal patients and 32% of patients with acute pancreatitis.[17] Our recent study did not reveal any patients with globally increased echogenicity, although focal areas of increased echogenicity were observed.[16] With newer sonographic systems, inhomogenity of the parenchyma is often evident in acute pancreatitis (**Fig. 6–8**).

The pancreas may be diffusely enlarged, focally enlarged, or normal. Enlargement of the pancreas in acute pancreatitis is probably almost universal. Unfortunately,

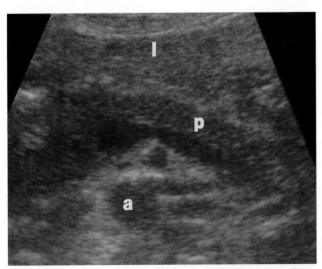

Figure 6–6 Pseudopancreatitis. Transverse sonogram at the level of the body and tail of the pancreas. When there is increased liver echogenicity, the normal pancreas may be relatively hypoechoic, simulating the findings sometimes associated with edematous acute pancreatitis. l, liver; p, pancreas; a, aorta. Reprinted with permission from **Sonography of the Abdomen** by R. Brooke Jeffrey, Jr. and Philip W. Ralls. Raven Press, New York, 1995.

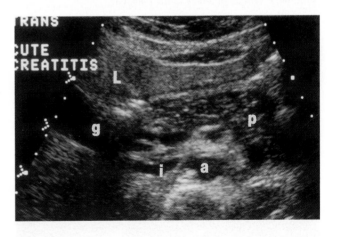

Figure 6–7 Acute pancreatitis with decreased pancreatic echogenicity. Transverse sonogram at the level of the upper head and body of the pancreas. Although the pancreas is often normal in acute pancreatitis, glandular echogenicity may be diffusely decreased. Echogenicity is usually judged by comparing the echogenicity of the liver (L) to that of the pancreas (p). a, aorta; i, inferior vena cava; g, gallbladder. Reprinted with permission from **Sonography of the Abdomen** by R. Brooke Jeffrey, Jr. and Philip W. Ralls. Raven Press, New York, 1995.

enlargement may be difficult to judge, as pancreatic size before the onset of pancreatitis is usually unknown and varies widely from individual to individual. A recently published measurement for the thickness of the body of the normal pancreas in 261 adults was 10.1 ± 3.8 mm with a range of 4—23 mm.[18] In our recent study, the mean anteroposterior measurement of the pancreatic body at the level of the superior mesenteric artery was 21.1 ± 6.4 mm. The range was 12—45 mm. It seems reasonable, then, to use 22 mm (mean plus 3 standard deviations) as the upper limit of normal.

It is not unusual to detect extrapancreatic inflammatory changes even when the pancreatic contour is normal and the pancreas is not obviously enlarged (**Fig. 6–9**). For this reason, extrapancreatic abnormalities are often the most important sonographic findings suggesting the diagnosis of acute pancreatitis (**Figs. 6–3** and **6–9** through **6–11**). Pancreatic inflammation, previously called *phlegmon*, is typically hypoechoic or anechoic and conforms to a known retroperitoneal space or peritoneal reflection. In addition to inflammation in the prepancreatic retroperitoneum, anterior pararenal spaces, and elsewhere, spread of inflammatory exudate along perivascular spaces is quite characteristic of acute pancreatitis (**Fig. 6–12**).[13]

Acute pancreatitis-associated fluid collections, present in 10 of 48 patients (21%) in our study, were seen only in patients who had evidence of extrapancreatic inflammation.[16] Fluid collections (**Fig. 6–13**) and abscesses may arise in these regions affected by inflammation. It may be difficult to distinguish fluid collections from hypo or anechoic inflammation. Fluid collections often have biconvex margins and sometimes, but not always, through transmission of sound. Fluid collections that persist for 6 weeks are called *pseudocysts*. The natural history of acute pancreatitis-associated fluid collections is that they are evanescent; more than half resolve spontaneously.

Often, the splenic or superior mesenteric veins are surrounded by hypoechoic inflammation, a phenomenon called *perivascular cloaking* (**Fig. 6–12**). This may lead to thrombosis of any or all of the portal veins (**Fig. 6–14**). While pancreatic abscesses may be detected with sonography, CT is preferred. CT is more able to comprehensively survey these patients. Optimal sensitivity is crucial, as the consequence of missing a pancreatic abscess is often the patient's death.

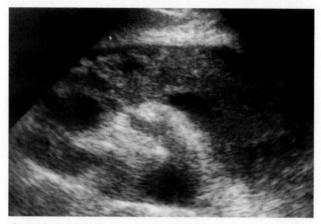

Figure 6–8 Inhomogeneous pancreas, acute pancreatitis. Pancreatic inhomogeneity is a common finding in acute pancreatitis. This patient also has a rim of hypoechoic inflammation in the retroperitoneum ventral (anterior) to the pancreas.

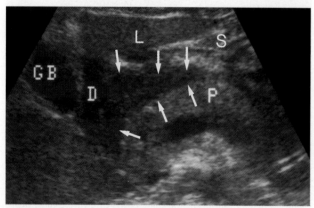

A

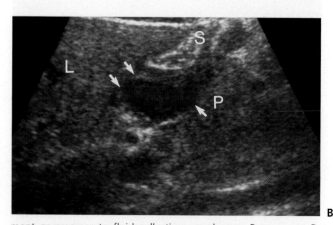

B

Figure 6–9 Peripancreatic inflammatory change. Peripancreatic abnormality is noted on both the transverse (**A**) and the longitudinal (**B**) sonograms. Hypoechoic enlargement of the peripancreatic tissue planes is a sign of inflammation (**arrows**). Abnormalities such as this may resolve spontaneously with conservative manage- ment or progress to fluid collections or abscess. P, pancreas; D, duodenum; GB, gallbladder; L, liver; S, stomach. Reprinted with permission from **Sonography of the Abdomen** by R. Brooke Jeffrey, Jr. and Philip W. Ralls. Raven Press, New York, 1995.

Figure 6–10 Intra- and peripancreatic inflammatory changes, ▷ acute pancreatitis. A transverse sonogram reveals both intrapancreatic (**open arrows**) and peripancreatic (**arrows**) abnormalities. In severe cases, definition of the pancreas itself may be lost. s, stomach; g, gallbladder; k, right kidney; a, aorta; l, liver. Reprinted with permission from **Sonography of the Abdomen** by R. Brooke Jeffrey, Jr. and Philip W. Ralls. Raven Press, New York, 1995.

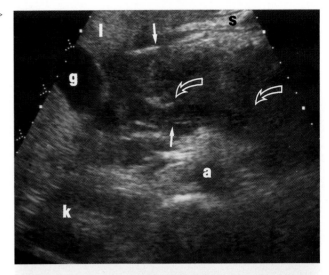

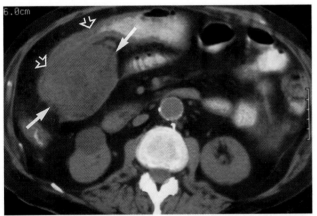

A

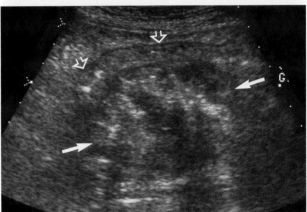

B

Figure 6–11 Inflammatory mass from pancreatitis adjacent to stomach and duodenum. **A**: Transverse sonogram in the region of the pancreatic head. **B**: CT scan in the same location. Inflammatory change related to acute pancreatitis may have a mixed echogenicity pattern, as noted in this case (**arrows**). The inflammatory mass (formerly called phlegmon) displaces the stomach and duodenum (**open arrows**). Reprinted with permission from **Sonography of the Abdomen** by R. Brooke Jeffrey, Jr. and Philip W. Ralls. Raven Press, New York, 1995.

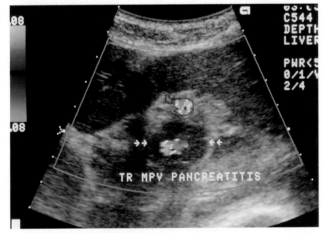

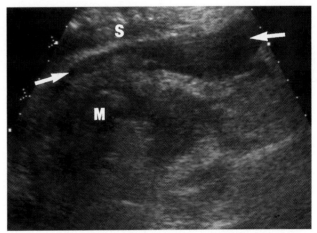

Figure 6–12 Acute pancreatitis, perivascular cloaking. Transverse color flow sonogram of the main portal vein (MPV). Pancreatic inflammation may surround blood vessels, resulting in hypoechoic areas that tracks along the vessels (**arrows**) near and around the pancreas. This perivascular inflammation is called **perivascular cloaking**. Reprinted with permission from **Sonography of the Abdomen** by R. Brooke Jeffrey, Jr. and Philip W. Ralls. Raven Press, New York, 1995.

Figure 6–13 Acute pancreatitis-related fluid collection. Transverse sonogram of region of the pancreatic body. Acute pancreatitis-associated fluid collections (**arrows**) generally conform to the tissue planes. Only a minority of these acute fluid collections persist to become well-defined pseudocysts. Most resolve spontaneously. An nonhomogeneous inflammatory mass (M) is seen dorsal to the fluid collection. S, stomach. Reprinted with permission from **Sonography of the Abdomen** by R. Brooke Jeffrey, Jr. and Philip W. Ralls. Raven Press, New York, 1995.

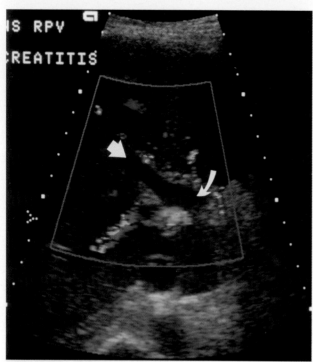

Figure 6–14 Thrombosis, right portal vein. Transverse color Flow sonogram of the right portal vein. Pancreatitis may lead to partial or complete thrombosis of the portal venous system. This patient developed complete venous thrombosis of the anterior segmental branch of the right portal vein (**arrow**), with partial clot of the main right portal vein (**curved arrow**). This is demonstrated on both color flow sonography and contrast-enhanced CT. This patient developed septic portal venous thrombosis (pylephlebitis) that led to a hepatic abscess (**open arrow**), visible on the CT scan. Reprinted with permission from **Sonography of the Abdomen** by R. Brooke Jeffrey, Jr. and Philip W. Ralls. Raven Press, New York, 1995.

Benefits of Ultrasound

Sonography's main use is to evaluate the biliary tract. Are gallstones the cause of acute pancreatitis? Are the bile ducts dilated? Sonography should be used to detect gallstones in all patients who present for the first time with acute pancreatitis. It is important to know if gallstones are a potential cause of acute pancreatitis, even in alcoholic patients.

When biliary dilatation or choledocholithiasis is present sonographically, a stone may be impacted in the distal common duct. Conventional wisdom suggests that urgent intervention to relieve obstruction is necessary in these patients.[19, 20] There is conflicting evidence, however, whether patients benefit from intervention in the acute setting. Neoptolemos et al. showed that early endoscopic sphincterotomy was beneficial in patients with biliary pancreatitis, regardless of the presence or absence of common duct stones at the time of endoscopic retrograde cholangiography (ERC).[21] Kelly et al., on the other hand, showed that early surgical removal of impacted common duct stones did not ameliorate or affect the progression of pancreatitis.[22]

Sonography may be used to serially follow masses and fluid collections that CT or sonography have already detected. Sonography can guide aspiration or drainage of known fluid collections. Color flow sonography should be used to ensure that well-defined anechoic pancreatic or peripancreatic "cystic masses" are not pseudoaneurysms.

Summary

All patients, even alcoholics, who have acute pancreatitis, should undergo biliary sonography, both to detect gallstones and determine if biliary obstruction is present. Sonography of the pancreas and the peripancreatic compartments may provide additional useful information. Sonography can guide intervention and noninvasively follow known lesions (e.g., pseudocysts, acute pancreatitis associated fluid collections). When CT is technically suboptimal or equivocal, sonography can provide additional information regarding the gallbladder and bile ducts, particularly in patients with suspected cholangitis and biliary sepsis.

References

1. DiMagno E.P. Treatment of mild acute pancreatitis. In E.L. Bradley III, ed. *Acute Pancreatitis: Diagnosis and Therapy*. New York: Raven Press, 1994.
2. Bradley EL III. The necessity for clinical classification of acute pancreatitis: the Atlanta System. In: E.L. Bradley III, ed. *Acute Pancreatitis: Diagnosis and Therapy*. New York: Raven Press, 1994.
3. Glazer G. Epidemiology and pathology of pancreatic abscess. In: E.L. Bradley III, ed. *Acute Pancreatitis: Diagnosis and Therapy*. New York: Raven Press, 1994.
4. Malfertheiner P., Buchler M. Clinical symptoms and signs and diagnostic requirement in acute pancreatitis. In: H.C. Beger, M. Buchler, eds. *Acute Pancreatitis*. Berlin: Springer Verlag, 1987, p. 104.
5. Lankisch P.G., Schirren C.A., Kunze E. Undetected fatal acute pancreatitis: why is the disease so frequently overlooked? *Am J Gastroenterol* 1991;86:322.
6. Read G., Braganza J.M., Howat H.T. Pancreatitis—a retrospective study. *Gut* 1976;17:945—952.
7. Sarner M. Clinical diagnosis of interstitial (edematous) pancreatitis. In: E.L. Bradley, III, ed. *Acute Pancreatitis: Diagnosis and Therapy*. New York: Raven Press, 1994.
8. Tietz N.W., Juang W.Y., Rauh D.F., Shuey D.F. Laboratory tests in the differential diagnoses of hyperamylasemia. *Clin Chem* 1986;32:301—307.
9. Marshall J.B. Acute pancreatitis. A review with an emphasis on new developments. *Arch Intern Med* 1993;153:1185—1198.
10. Semelka R.C., Kroeker M.A., Shoenut J.P., et al. Pancreatic disease: prospective comparison of CT, ERCP, and 1.5-T MR imaging with dynamic gadolinium enhancement. *Radiology* 1991;181:785—791.
11. Saifuddin A., Ridgway J.W., Chalmers A.G. Comparison of MR and CT scanning in severe acute pancreatitis: initial experiences. *Clin Radiol* 1993;48:111—116.

12. Laing F.C., Jeffrey R.B., Wing V.W. Improved visualization of choledocholithiasis by sonography. *AJR* 1984;143:949—952.

13. Jeffrey R.B., Laing F.C., Wing V.W. Extrapancreatic spread of acute pancreatitis: new observations with real-time US. *Radiology* 1986;159:707—711.

14. Freise J. Evaluation of sonography in the diagnosis of acute pancreatitis. In: H.G. Beger, M. Buchler, eds. *Acute Pancreatitis*. Berlin: Springer-Verlag, 1987, p. 118—131.

15. Jeffrey R.B. Jr. Sonography in acute pancreatitis. *Radiol Clin North Am* 1989;27:5—17.

16. Finstad T.A., Ralls P.W. Sonographic findings in acute pancreatitis. (Submitted for publication).

17. Cotton P.B., Lees W.R., Vallon A.G., et al. Gray scale ultrasonography and endoscopic pancreatography in pancreatitis diagnosis. *Radiology* 1980;134:453—459.

18. Guerra M., Gutierrez L., Carrasco R., Arroyo A. Size and echogenicity of the pancreas in Chilean adults: echotomography study in 261 patients. *Rev Med Chile* 1995;123(6):720—726.

19. Acosta J.M., Rossi R., Galli D.M. Early surgery for gallstone pancreatitis: evaluation of a systemic approach. *Surgery* 1978;83:367—371.

20. Stone H.H., Fabian T.C., Dunlop W.E. Gallstone pancreatitis, biliary tract pathology in relation to time of operation. *Ann Surg* 1981;194:305—312.

21. Neoptolemos J.P., London N.J., James D., et al. Controlled trial of urgent endoscopic retrograde cholangiopancreatography and endoscopic sphincterotomy versus conservative treatment for acute pancreatitis due to gallstones. *Lancet* 1988;2:979—983.

22. Kelly T.R. and Wagner D.S. Gallstone pancreatitis: a prospective randomized trial of the timing of surgery. *Surgery* 1988;104(4):600—605.

7 Flank Pain

Sharlene A. Teefey

Flank pain is a common complaint and most often, the primary symptom of ureteric stone disease. However, the differential diagnosis of flank pain is extensive and includes not only many different renal etiologies but nonrenal etiologies as well. The approach to the patient with flank pain begins with a thorough history and physical examination followed by appropriate laboratory studies. This information will help the clinician in consultation with the radiologist to determine which radiologic procedures are indicated. A list of the renal and nonrenal causes of acute flank pain is shown in **Table 7–1**.[1,2] Many of the disease processes listed in this table occur commonly, including renal calculus disease, acute pyelonephritis, and fibrositis (**Table 7–2**).[1,2] While many of the intraabdominal disease processes listed are also common, flank pain is an unusual manifestation. A brief summary of the important diagnostic features of these disease processes will be presented.

Differential Diagnosis of Flank Pain

An abrupt increase in intraluminal pressure in the collecting system is the primary cause of pain from calculus disease. The severity of the pain is directly related to the rapidity with which the obstructing stone raises intraluminal pressure.[3] The pain frequently radiates from the flank laterally into the abdomen and may be intermittent (renal colic) or steady. When the ureter is initially obstructed, there is an increase in the frequency of ureteral contractions causing colicky pain. Within a short time, ureteral contractions cease and while the intraluminal pressure remains elevated, the pain takes on a more steady character.[3] Nevertheless, the patient typically paces or writhes in bed, unable to find a comfortable position. The location of pain originating from the urinary tract has been carefully mapped out by McClellan and Goodell.[3] The authors distended various parts of the renal pelvis and ureter with small balloon catheters and observed that distention of the renal pelvis

Table 7–1 Renal and Nonrenal Etiologies of Flank Pain

Retroperitoneal	Renal	Calculus disease
		Pyelonephritis/abscess
		Xanthogranulomatous pyelonephritis
		Neoplasm/cyst
		Vascular compromise
	Nonrenal	Abdominal aortic aneurysm rupture
		Retroperitoneal fibrosis
		Retroperitoneal abscess
		Retroperitoneal adenopathy
		Retroperitoneal hemorrhage
		Retroperitoneal neoplasm
		Adrenal neoplasm with hemorrhage
Intraabdominal		Diverticulitis
		Perforated colon carcinoma
		Pancreatitis
		Cholecystitis
		Appendicitis
		Duodenal ulcer
		Splenic infarction/abscess
Musculoskeletal		Fibrositis
		Iliac/spine osteomyelitis
		Disk disease
		Spinal metastases
Miscellaneous		Münchhausen syndrome
		Narcotic abuse

Table 7–2 Disease Incidence [Incidence per 100,000 (approximate)]

Common (> 100)	Uncommon (> 5—100)	Rare (> 0—5)
Renal colic	Renal corticomedullary abscess	Renal cortical abscess
Acute pyelonephritis		Perinephric abscess
Fibrositis	Carcinoma of the kidney	Renal infarction
	Diverticulitis	Renal vein thrombosis
	Carcinoma of the colon with perforation	Adrenal neoplasm with hemorrhage
	Duodenal ulcer	Iliac osteomyelitis
	Acute cholecystitis	Retrocecal appendicitis
	Abdominal aortic aneurysm rupture	Splenic infarction
		Splenic abscess

produced costovertebral angle pain. When the upper, middle, or lower ureter was distended, pain occurred in the flank, middle inguinal canal or suprapubic region, respectively. Pain may also be referred from the upper or lower obstructed ureter to the ipsilateral scrotum in men or labia majora in women.[3] Symptoms of bladder irritation may occur. Because of the autonomic innervation of the kidney and stomach by the celiac ganglion, it is not unusual for patients to experience nausea, vomiting, and abdominal distention due to ileus. Diaphoresis and tachycardia may also occur in response to the pain, however, fever is not usually present unless there is a superimposed infection and pyonephrosis. Urinalysis usually reveals microscopic hematuria, however, 10% of patients may have gross hematuria. If ureteral obstruction is complete, then hematuria may be absent.[4]

Acute pyelonephritis is characterized by the abrupt onset of chills and fever, usually > 100 °F, in association with constant, dull flank pain and/or symptoms of cystitis, that is, dysuria, frequency, and urgency. In some cases, only irritative bladder symptoms are present, and it is difficult to differentiate pyelonephritis from cystitis.[5] The flank pain is usually less severe than that caused by stone disease. It may be associated with muscle spasm and tenderness that intensifies with movement. Nausea, vomiting, diarrhea, and abdominal pain may also occur. Laboratory findings show a leukocytosis with a neutrophil predominance. Urinalysis reveals numerous white blood cells and bacteria. Leukocyte casts and a specific type of cast characterized by the predominance of bacteria within the cast matrix are also frequently present in the urine.[5] Urine cultures usually grow *Escherichia coli*. When pyelonephritis occurs in the setting of stasis, calculi, pregnancy, diabetes mellitus or a neurogenic bladder, patients are predisposed to abscess formation.[5] If renal abscess develops from a hematogenous source, then urine cultures will frequently be negative.

An uncommon infectious process of the kidney, xanthogranulomatous pyelonephritis, predominantly affects women between the fifth and seventh decades of life. Patients frequently present with nonspecific constitutional symptoms such as malaise, low-grade fever, and flank pain which have usually been present for months to years.[6] On physical examination, there is costovertebral angle tenderness and frequently a palpable flank or abdominal mass. Laboratory findings reveal an elevated erythrocyte sedimentation rate, anemia and leukocytosis. Urinalysis shows pyuria, proteinuria, and occasionally hematuria. *Escherichia coli* and *proteus mirabilis* are often cultured from the urine, although urine cultures may be negative in up to one-third of patients if there is complete obstruction of the kidney.[6] An interesting syndrome of reversible hepatic dysfunction has been associated with xanthogranulomatous pyelonephritis in which abnormal liver function tests with or without hepatomegaly return to normal after nephrectomy.[6]

Renal neoplasms and cysts may also cause flank pain. The earlier literature stressed the importance of the triad of flank pain, a palpable mass, and hematuria as being characteristic of renal cell carcinoma.[7] However, fewer than 10% of patients present with this triad. The finding of a palpable mass and flank pain are late symptoms. Usually, patients with renal cell carcinoma present with painless hematuria.[7] Large renal cysts and complications such as infection or hemorrhage into the cyst may also cause acute flank pain.

Renal vascular compromise, in particular, when acute, may cause noncolicky flank pain. Etiologies include renal artery embolus, dissection of the renal artery, rupture of a renal artery aneurysm, and renal vein thrombosis. Renal artery emboli usually originate from the left atrium or ventricle in patients with myocardial infarction, rheumatic heart disease, arrhythmias, or subacute bacterial endocarditis.[8] Atherosclerotic plaque may also embolize to the renal arteries. Sudden interruption of the renal artery blood supply causes severe, sharp, constant flank pain that may radiate to the upper or mid-abdomen.[9] Nausea and vomiting may also occur. Urinalysis shows microscopic hematuria and proteinuria. Renal vein thrombosis, when acute, may also cause flank pain. Etiologies are many and include malignant neoplasm, a hypercoagulable state, or an underlying renal disease such as nephrotic syndrome, membranous glomerulonephritis, systemic lupus erythematosus, and amyloidosis. Other predisposing conditions include abdominal trauma, abdominal surgery, or pregnancy (ovarian vein thrombosis with inferior vena cava extension).[10] Patients typically present with flank or upper abdominal pain, nausea and vomiting, or costovertebral angle tenderness. Laboratory findings include hematuria, proteinuria, and azotemia.[1] Other much less common conditions may compromise renal blood flow and cause flank pain such as dissection of the renal artery and/or rupture of a renal artery aneurysm.

Several nonrenal retroperitoneal processes may also cause acute flank pain including abdominal aortic aneurysm rupture and retroperitoneal fibrosis, abscess, adenopathy, hemorrhage, or neoplasm. Patients with a ruptured abdominal aortic aneurysm most commonly present with abdominal, back and/or flank pain and syncope or loss of consciousness.[11] However, in one recent study,[12] abdominal and back pain were present in only 42% of patients, and the classic triad of abdominal pain, back pain, and a pulsatile mass was present in only 26%. Because an aneurysm frequently ruptures to the left of the root of the mesentery, the hematoma may extend inferiorly causing left groin or testicular pain that may be misinterpreted as renal colic. In fact, in the above study of 152 cases of ruptured abdominal aortic aneurysm, the leading misdiagnosis was renal colic followed by diverticulitis and gastrointestinal hemorrhage.[12]

Other retroperitoneal processes such as retroperitoneal fibrosis, abscess, adenopathy, hemorrhage, and neoplasm may also cause flank pain. Accompanying symptoms vary with the location of the process and which organs are encroached upon. Retroperitoneal fibrosis may cause colicky flank pain and tenderness due to entrapment and compression of the ureters.[13] A retroperitoneal abscess may cause abdominal or flank pain, tenderness, and fever.[14] Hemorrhage into an adrenal tumor has also been reported to cause acute flank and mid-back pain.[2]

There are multiple intraabdominal causes of flank pain including diverticulitis, perforated colon carcinoma, pancreatitis, cholecystitis, appendicitis, duodenal ulcer, and splenic infarction or abscess. The pain that is felt in the back or flank region is often referred to the posterior portion of the spinal segment that innervates that organ.[15] Patients with diverticulitis frequently present with acute left lower quadrant pain that may radiate into the left lumbar and flank region. Urinary tract symptoms may occur if the inflammatory process is adjacent to the bladder.[16] Perforation of a colon carcinoma may produce an identical clinical picture.[2]

Pancreatitis causes a constant, boring pain that radiates from the epigastrium into the lower abdomen as well as the back and flanks. The pain is usually more intense in the supine position; relief is often obtained by sitting. Physical examination reveals epigastric tenderness, however, signs of peritoneal irritation are initially absent due to the retroperitoneal location of the pancreas.[17]

While acute cholecystitis classically begins with acute right upper quadrant pain and localized tenderness, less typical presentations may also occur. The pain may be pleuritic and localized to the right lower posterior chest and flank.[2] Likewise, while the classic description of the pain from appendicitis is periumbilical with a shift to the right lower quadrant, an inflamed retrocecal appendix may cause right flank pain and tenderness. Local abdominal tenderness may not be present because the appendix is posterior to the cecum and deep to the parietal peritoneum.[2,18] Mid-epigastric pain and localized tenderness are the most common symptoms of duodenal ulcer. However, a duodenal ulcer may also cause right lower posterolateral chest and flank pain.[2] Finally, acute left upper abdominal and flank pain and tenderness may occur from acute splenic infarction or abscess. Respiration may intensify the pain in both conditions. In the latter disease process, fever and chills are invariably present.[2]

Musculoskeletal pain from various causes such as fibrositis, iliac/spine osteomyelitis, spinal metastases, and even disk disease may produce flank pain. The pain of fibrositis is usually of a dull, aching, continuous nature and is intensified by bending or lifting.[2,15] Osteomyelitis and spinal metastases can also cause flank pain and tenderness with guarding.

Finally, it is important to remember the Münchausen syndrome and narcotic abuse patients who present with fictitious hematuria, are well versed with the signs and symptoms of renal colic, and often give a history of contrast allergy to avoid imaging studies.[1]

Diagnostic Workup of the Patient with Flank Pain

Given the many different pathologic processes that can produce flank pain, the clinician must obtain a thorough history and perform a careful physical examination. Important historical points include the nature, quality, and severity of the pain; associated signs and symptoms; current medications; predisposing conditions such as previous renal disease, diabetes, or recent surgery; and any underlining history of neoplasm or metabolic, cardiovascular, or collagen vascular disease or family history of abdominal aortic aneurysm.[1] Findings at physical examination will assist in localizing the process to the retroperitoneum, abdominal cavity, or musculoskeletal system. Laboratory tests such as urinalysis, complete blood cell count, erythrocyte sedimentation rate, and amylase and/or lipase will further help to narrow the differential diagnosis.[1] At this point, the role of the radiologist as consultant becomes important.

While the intravenous urogram (IVU) has been the cornerstone in the evaluation of patients with suspected urinary tract obstruction, sonography and computed tomography have gained increasing acceptance as primary imaging studies. Nearly 20 years ago, Ellenbogen et al. reported that gray scale sonography can reliably exclude urinary tract obstruction with a sensitivity of 98%, which is important for a screening test.[19] However, their specificity was only 74%. False-positive results are often due to normal collecting system variants, high urine flow rate, postobstructive dilatation, blunted calyces (vesicoureteral reflux, papillary necrosis or congenital megacalyces), and renal sinus structures (blood vessels and parapelvic cysts).[19,20] While a higher false-positive rate is acceptable for a screening test, a high false-negative rate is not. Subsequent to Ellenbogen's study, reports of cases of nondilated or minimally dilated obstructive nephropathy began to appear in the literature[21-24] as did two other studies[25,26] which prospectively compared sonography with IVU in patients with acute flank pain due to suspected stone disease. Both of these latter studies found that gray scale sonography was only 65—69% accurate in diagnosing urinary tract obstruction.[25,26]

In an effort to overcome this serious limitation of gray scale sonography, intrarenal Doppler analysis [resistive index (RI)] has been advocated to distinguish obstructive from nonobstructive dilatation. In their original work involving a population of patients with acute and chronic obstruction, Platt et al. showed that the RI was significantly increased in obstructive pyelocalectasis in comparison to nonobstructive pyelocaliectasis and found that an RI of 0.70 was a reasonable upper limit of normal with a sensitivity of 92%, specificity of 88%, and overall accuracy of 90%.[27] In a later study of patients with acute obstruction (< 36 h), the same authors reported an elevated RI (0.70) in 87% of kidneys.[28] However, other authors have disagreed with Platt's findings. Deyoe et al. reported an elevated or asymmetric RI in only 30% of patients with acute complete obstruction[29] and Tublin et al. in only 47% of patients with acute high-grade obstruction,[30] although both found an elevated RI to be very specific when ureteral obstruction was suspected (**Fig. 7–1**).

There are several potential reasons why the RI may be falsely negative in the setting of acute renal obstruction. If the obstruction (whether complete or not) has been present for less than and six hours is partial or mild, then certain mediators that cause renal vasoconstriction and increased vascular resistance may not have been released.[31] In addition, spontaneous decompression of a dilated, obstructed collecting system (i.e., forniceal rupture) may normalize an elevated RI[28, 31] and medications such as nonsteroidal antiinflammatory drugs, which may be administered in the initial management of the patient with acute flank pain, may decrease the RI.[30] On the other hand, if RI values are increased due to renal medical disease, they are of little use unless the collecting system dilatation is unilateral in which case inter renal differences may help to distinguish obstructive from nonobstructive dilatation.[31] Still other considerations include the reported normal increase in the threshold value of RI with age,[32] and the variability in RI measurements.[33] Thus, while an elevated RI is very specific for ureteral obstruction in the proper clinical setting,[27, 29-31] it has been suggested that its low sensitivity limits its usefulness as a diagnostic test in the patient with acute flank pain.[29, 30]

Other strategies using sonography have emerged in an attempt to more accurately diagnose acute urinary tract obstruction. Haddad et al. combined gray scale sonography with KUB radiography and reported a sensitivity of up to 97% and specificity of 90% for diagnosing acute urinary tract obstruction.[34] Mallek et al. showed that the administration of furosemide before duplex sonography resulted in an accuracy rate of 95% in differentiating obstructive from nonobstructive pyelocaliectasis.[35] Laing used transvaginal sonography to detect 13 of 13 distal ureteral calculi.[36]

Another new technique has employed color Doppler sonography to search for ureteral jets. Ureteral jets are visualized with color Doppler sonography when density differences exist between bladder and ureteral urine.[37, 38] Before beginning ureteral jet analysis, patient hydration has been advocated to increase jet frequency and enhance the asymmetry between the normal and abnormal sides. However, if the patient voids and refills his bladder before jet analysis, jets may not be detected due to the loss of the density difference between the bladder and ureteral urine.[37] Two recent studies have shown that the absence of a ureteral jet is highly significant for complete obstruction[29, 38] (**Fig. 7–2**). Deyoe et al. demonstrated that the absence of a ureteral jet had a sensitivity of 100% and specificity of 91% for complete ureteral obstruction.[29] Burge et al. reported similar results.[38] However, ureteral jets may be normal in patients with partial or low-grade obstruction or nonobstructing stones.[38] Furthermore, it has been suggested that normal asymmetry in jet frequency may require a longer observation period to rule out obstruction than has been recommended.[39]

Recently, two studies have shown that unenhanced CT is a very valuable method for evaluating patients with acute flank pain because it can not only accurately detect ureteral stones, but determine other extraurinary causes of acute flank pain.[40, 41] In one of these studies using helical CT, the entire examination was completed in five min.[41] These same authors reported a sensitivity of 97%, a specificity of 96%, and an accuracy of 97%

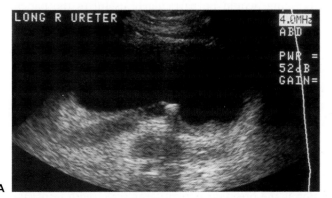

A

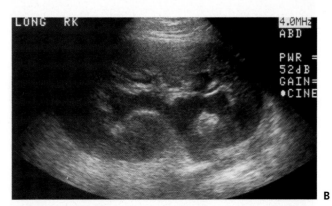

B

Figure 7–1 A sixty-one-year-old woman being treated with antibiotics for a urinary tract infection. After five days, fever recurred and the patient developed acute right abdominal pain. Sonography shows moderate right hydronephrosis with a uretero-vesical junction calculus (**A,B**).

Figure 7–1 C–E ▷

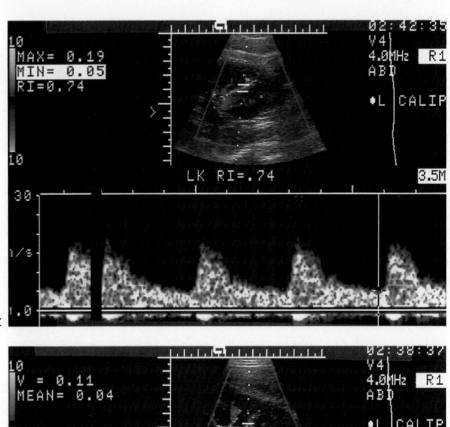

C

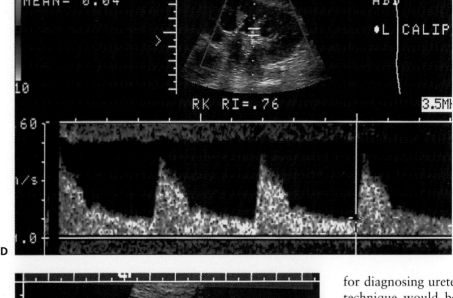

D

Figure 7–1 C, D Resistive indices are mildly elevated but symmetric, measuring 0.76 in the right kidney and 0.74 in the left kidney. Ureteral jet analysis shows a normal left ureteral jet but no right ureteral jet is visualized (**E**) indicating a high-grade ureteral obstruction.

E

for diagnosing ureteral calculus disease.[41] This imaging technique would be particularly useful in the patient with an elevated creatinine or contrast allergy.

What then is the role of sonography in the patient with acute flank pain due to suspected stone disease? The best answer depends upon the question being asked. If the question is the anatomic cause rather than the physiologic significance of the obstructing process, then an IVU or noncontrast helical computed tomography (CT) is the procedure of choice. If physiologic information is sought regarding the functional significance of the obstruction, then intrarenal Doppler analysis and analysis of ureteral jets may be more appropriate. An exception is the pregnant patient; gray scale (with transvaginal), duplex, and color Doppler sonography of ureteral jets should be used to obtain as much information as

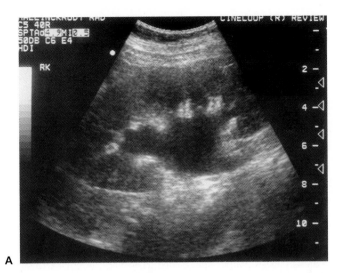

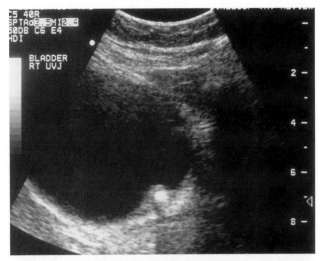

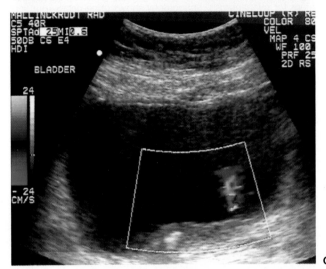

Figure 7–2 A sixty-seven-year old woman with a 10-day history of right flank pain. Sonography shows moderate right hydronephrosis with a uretero-vesical junction calculus (**A,B**). Resistive indices are normal and symmetric. Ureteral jet analysis demonstrates a normal left ureteral jet but no right ureteral jet is visualized indicating complete ureteral obstruction (**C**).

possible. Few studies have examined the role of sonography in the pregnant patient with suspected urinary tract obstruction. In one study, Hertzberg et al. showed that RI values are not elevated in normal pregnancy even in the presence of moderate physiologic pelvicaliectasis.[42] However, the authors also stated that the effects of other pathologic processes such as preeclampsia and pyelonephritis on RI values are as yet unknown and require further study.[42]

Most patients with uncomplicated acute pyelonephritis do not require an imaging study. The diagnosis is usually established based on clinical presentation and laboratory findings. An imaging study is indicated, however, when it is important to rule out obstruction or detect a complication such as a nephric or perinephric abscess. Patients who fail to respond to antibiotic therapy within 48—72 hours, or in whom the clinical diagnosis is uncertain should be imaged, as should patients with diabetes mellitus, recurrent pyelonephritis, or a history of stone disease.[43] Sonography or computed tomography are frequently used to evaluate such patients. Sonography is also very specific (100%) for diagnosing

pyonephrosis, a serious complication of ureteral obstruction[44] (**Fig. 7–3**). However, in this same study, Jeffrey et al. reported a sensitivity of only 62% and recommended percutaneous aspiration of potentially infected urine in cases of suspected pyonephrosis.[44] Sonography is less sensitive in detecting parenchymal inflammation or small nephric or perinephric abscesses compared to CT.[45—47] In fact, most kidneys appear normal on sonography despite obvious signs of parenchymal inflammation on contrast-enhanced CT.[45] While early sonographic reports described a variety of sonographic findings suggestive of pyelonephritis,[48—50] many of these features, such as an ill-defined hypoechoic mass (**Fig. 7–4**), are nonspecific and overlap with other disease processes. Thickening of the urothelium in native kidneys may be a fairly reliable indication of infection (**Fig. 7–5**) but has also been reported in patients with hydronephrosis and vesicoureteral reflux.[51, 52]

Recently, Morehouse et al.[53] evaluated 23 patients with pyelonephritis and found that a focal area of abnormal echogenicity had a sensitivity of only 30% and an RI > 0.70, a sensitivity of only 43% for diagnosing renal in-

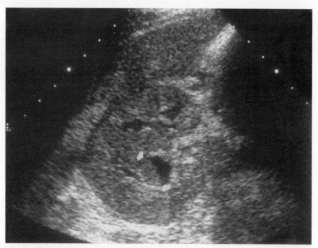

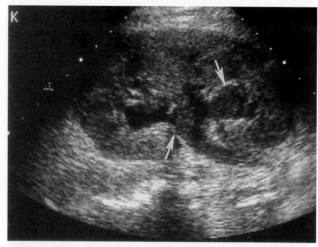

Figure 7–3 An elderly male with right nephrostomy stent placement for pyonephrosis. Sonography shows urine-debris (purulent material) levels within the dilated collecting system (**arrows**) (**A,B**).

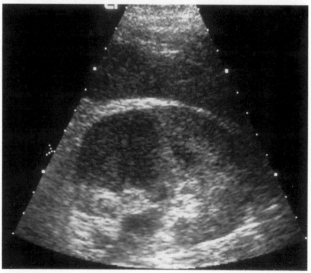

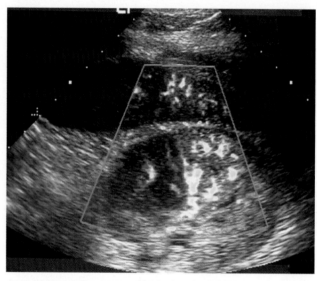

Figure 7–4 A thirty-eight-year-old woman with focal pyelonephritis. Sonography shows a hypoechoic region in the mid-left kidney on this transverse image (**A**). The power Doppler image shows a decrease in color flow due to intense vasoconstriction (**B**).

fection. These findings were reiterated by Keogan et al. They reported that while the mean RI in pregnant patients with pyelonephritis was significantly higher than in controls, the magnitude of the difference was too small and the overlap too great between the two groups for this index to be of clinical value.[54] Likewise, while sonography may demonstrate collecting system obstruction and a central calculus in patients with xanthogranulomatous pyelonephritis, CT will more precisely demonstrate extrarenal extension into the perirenal and pararenal spaces and soft tissues of the flank.[6]

Acute renal infarction can accurately be diagnosed in most cases with CT.[55–57] Little has been written about the role of sonography in evaluating acute native renal infarction. Theoretically, absence of parenchymal flow at color Doppler sonography should suggest complete occlusion of the main renal artery whereas patchy areas of absent parenchymal flow may indicate segmental arterial occlusion in the proper clinical setting. Nevertheless, angiography or scintigraphy may be required for a definitive diagnosis. Renal vein thrombosis, on the other hand, can be confidently diagnosed with color Doppler sonography which shows absence of flow in the renal vein (**Fig. 7–6**). Of interest, a recent study by Platt et al. showed that intrarenal Doppler analysis (RI) was neither sensitive nor specific in diagnosing renal vein thrombosis in native kidneys due to the early development of venous collaterals and subsequent decrease in renal vascular resistance.[58] CT is also capable of diagnosing renal vein thrombosis, however, optimal visualization of the renal veins is dependent on thin sections and an adequate intravenous contrast bolus with the proper scan delay. Recently, magnetic resonance (MR) angiography has been shown to be a valuable technique for evaluating the renal vessels. A larger prospective study comparing duplex and color Doppler sonography to MR angiography or CT is necessary to determine which technique is most accurate yet cost-effective.

While sonography is well established as a technique for following the asymptomatic patient with an abdominal aortic aneurysm, its sensitivity for detecting rupture (extraluminal blood) has been reported at only 4%.[59] Nevertheless, sonography is valuable in demonstrating the presence of an aneurysm in the hemodynamically unstable patient with abdominal pain. Sonography provided the correct diagnosis in 95% of such cases in which emergent surgery was performed.[59] Given the very low sensitivity of sonography in detecting rupture, in the hemodynamically stable patient, CT is the imaging study of choice.[59]

While sonography may demonstrate the presence of retroperitoneal pathology, the characteristics are often nonspecific. Usually biopsy and/or aspiration are necessary to obtain a specific diagnosis. CT and/or MRI are important in determining the location, size, extent, and characteristics of the retroperitoneal process as well as its encroachment on adjacent viscera.[60,61] If the suspicion for neoplasm is high and it is visible with sonography, a sonographically guided biopsy may expedite the patient's workup.

As discussed earlier, many intraabdominal processes such as diverticulitis, perforated colon carcinoma, pancreatitis, cholecystitis, appendicitis, duodenal ulcer and splenic infarction and/or abscess can cause acute flank pain. While flank pain is not a common presentation in most of these disease processes, in the proper clinical setting, these diagnoses should be considered.

Finally, of the musculoskeletal etiologies of flank pain, fibrositis is usually a clinical diagnosis requiring no imaging evaluation. Osteomyelitis, disk disease, and spinal metastases are best diagnosed using radionuclide imaging, MR imaging, and/or CT. The Münchhausen syndrome/narcotic abuse can only be diagnosed if a high level of suspicion is maintained by the clinician.

From the above discussion, it is evident that while the differential diagnosis of flank pain is extensive, the initial workup of the patient by the clinician should narrow the differential diagnosis sufficiently to allow the radiologist to recommend the appropriate imaging studies. While noncontrast helical CT may supplant the IVU as the study of choice in patients with suspected urinary tract obstruction, particularly, in those with a severe contrast allergy or elevated creatinine, sonography should remain as the initial test in the pregnant patient. It should also be used to rule out obstruction or a moderate to large abscess in the setting of pyelonephritis. Duplex and color Doppler sonography may also be useful in the patient with a question of renal infarction or renal

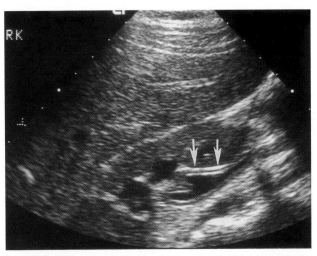

Figure 7–5 A twenty-seven-year-old woman with pyelonephritis. Sonography shows urothelial thickening of the right renal pelvis (**arrows**).

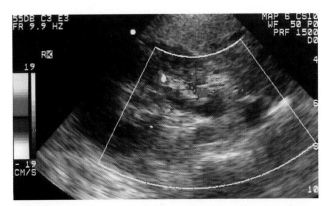

Figure 7–6 A forty-year-old woman with systemic lupus erythematosis. Sonography shows renal vein thrombosis. Collateral veins are present indicating that the thrombosis is chronic (**Figure 2 c**).

vein thrombosis. Sonography is valuable in detecting an abdominal aortic aneurysm in the hemodynamically unstable patient with abdominal pain. CT and MR imaging are often superior to sonography in the diagnosis of retroperitoneal diseases. Sonography, however, may be the first test ordered, as the initial presenting symptoms are often vague and nonspecific. Sonographic findings, while nonspecific, may demonstrate a retroperitoneal abnormality. Sonography is important in diagnosing many of the intraabdominal diseases that may uncommonly present with flank pain, but is of no value in the evaluation of musculoskeletal causes of flank pain or the Münchhausen syndrome.

References

1. Hendricksen D, Eshelman B, Dill L, Frederick R. Unusual etiology for left flank pain in a 29 year old man. *Ann Emerg Med* 1993;22:2455—1462.
2. Wiener SL. Acute unilateral costovertebral area and flank pain, acute bilateral costovertebral area and flank pain. In: Wiener SL, ed. *Differential Diagnosis of Acute Pain by Body Region.* New York, NY: McGraw-Hill, Inc., 1993, p. 245—257, 311—317.
3. Wiker AW. Standard diagnostic considerations. In: Gillenwater JY, Grayhack JT, Howards SS, Duckett JW, eds. *Adult and Pediatric Urology,* 2nd ed. St. Louis, Mo: Mosby Yearbook, 1991, p. 68—69.
4. Pahira JJ. Renal calculi. In: Schwartz GR, Cayten CG, Mayer TA, Mangelsen MA, Hanke BK, eds. *Principles and practice of Emergency Medicine,* 3rd ed. Philadelphia, Pa: Lea & Febieger, 1992, p. 1664—1668.
5. Schaeffer AJ. Renal infection. In: Gillenwater JY, Grayhack JT, Howards SS, Duckett JW, eds. *Adult and Pediatric Urology,* 2nd ed. St. Louis, Mo: Mosby Yearbook, 1991, p. 751—756.
6. Hayes WS, Hartman DS, Sesterbenn IA. Archives of AFIP Xanthogranulomatous pyelonephritis. *RadioGraphics* 1991;11:45—498.
7. Williams RD. Renal, perirenal, and ureteral neoplasms. In: Gillenwater JY, Grayhack JT, Howards SS, Duckett JW, eds. *Adult and Pediatric Urology,* 2nd ed. St. Louis, Mo: Mosby Yearbook, 1991, p. 578—580.
8. Hillman BJ. Disorders of the renal arterial circulation and renal vascular hypertension. In: Pollack HM, ed. *Clinical Urography.* Philadelphia, Pa: W.B. Saunders Co, 1990, p. 2140—2141.
9. Badr KF, Brenner BM. Vascular injury to the kidney. In: Wilson JD, Braunwald E, Isselbacher KJ, et al., eds. *Harrison's Principles of Internal Medicine,* 12th ed. New York, NY: McGraw-Hill, Inc, 1991, p. 1192—1193.
10. Mellins HZ. Renal vein obstruction. In: Pollack HM, ed. *Clinical Urography.* Philadelphia, Pa: W.B. Saunders Co, 1990, p. 2119.
11. Bengtsson H, Bergqvist D. Ruptured abdominal aortic aneurysm: a population based study. *J Vasc Surg* 1993;18:74—80.
12. Marston WA, Ahlquist R, Johnson G, Meyer AA. Missed diagnosis of ruptured abdominal aortic aneurysms. *J Vasc Surg* 1992;16:17—22.
13. Amis ES. Retroperitoneal fibrosis. *AJR* 1991;157:321—329.
14. Hirschmann JV. Localized infections and abscesses. In: Wilson JD, Braunwald E, Isselbacher KJ, et al, eds. *Harrison's Principles of Internal Medicine,* 12th ed. New York, NY: McGraw-Hill, Inc, 1991, p. 517.
15. Mankin HJ. Back and neck pain. In: Wilson JD, Braunwald E, Isselbacher KJ, et al, eds. *Harrison's Principles of Internal Medicine,* 12th ed. New York, NY: McGraw-Hill, Inc, 1991, p. 121.
16. Naitove A, Almy TP. Diverticular disease of the colon. In: Sleisinger MH, Fordtran JS, eds. *Gastrointestinal Disease, Pathophysiology Diagnosis Management,* 4th ed. Philadelphia, Pa: W.B. Saunders Co, 1989, p. 1427.
17. Greenberger NJ, Toskes PP, Isselbacher JK. Acute and chronic pancreatitis. In: Wilson JD, Braunwald E, Isselbacher KJ, et al, eds. *Harrison's Principles of Internal Medicine,* 12th ed. New York, NY: McGraw-Hill, Inc, 1991, p. 1372—1375.
18. Schrock TR. Acute appendicitis. In: Sleisinger MH, Fordtran JS, eds. *Gastrointestinal Disease, Pathophysiology Diagnosis Management,* 4th ed. Philadelphia, Pa: W.B. Saunders Co, 1989, p. 1382—1385.
19. Ellenbogen PH, Scheible FW, Talner LB, Leopold GR. Sensitivity of gray scale ultrasound in detecting urinary tract obstruction. *AJR* 1978;130:731—733.
20. Amis ES, Cronan JJ, Pfister RC, Yoder IC. Ultrasonic inaccuracies in diagnosing renal obstruction. *Urology* 1982;14:101—105.
21. Curry NS, Gobien RP, Schabel SI. Minimal-dilation obstructive nephropathy. *Radiology* 1982;143:531—534.
22. Maillet PJ, Pelle-Francoz D, Laville M, Gay F, Pinet A. Nondilated obstructive acute renal failure: diagnostic procecures and therapeutic management. *Radiology* 1986;160:659—662.
23. Naidich JB, Rackson ME, Mossey RT, Stein HL. Nondilated obstructive uropathy: percutaneous nephrostomy performed to reverse renal failure. *Radiology* 1986;160:653—657.
24. Kamholtz RG, Cronan JJ, Dorfman GS. Obstruction and the minimally dilated renal collecting system: ultrasound evaluation. *Radiology* 1989;170:51—53.
25. Hill MC, Rich JI, Mardiat JG, Finder CA. Sonography vs. excretory urography in acute flank pain. *AJR* 1985;144:1235—1238.
26. Laing FC, Jeffrey RB, Wing VW. Ultrasound vs. excretory urography in evaluating acute flank pain. *Radiology* 1985;154:613—616.
27. Platt JF, Rubin JM, Ellis JH. Distinction between obstructive and nonobstructive pyelocaliectasis with duplex Doppler sonography. *AJR* 1989;153:997—1000.
28. Platt JF, Rubin JM, Ellis JH. Acute renal obstruction: evaluation with intrarenal duplex Doppler and conventional ultrasound. *Radiology* 1993;186:685—688.
29. Deyoe LA, Cronan JJ, Breslaw BH, Ridlen MS. New techniques of ultrasound and color Doppler in the prosective evaluation of acute renal obstruction. Do they replace the intravenous urogram? *Abdom Imag* 1995;20:58—63.
30. Tublin ME, Dodd GE, Verdile VP. Acute renal colic: diagnosis with duplex Doppler ultrasound. *Radiology* 1994;193:697—701.
31. Platt JF. Duplex Doppler evaluation of native kidney dysfunction: obstructive and nonobstructive disease. *AJR* 1992;158:1035—1042.
32. Terry JD, Rysavy JA, Frick MP. Intrarenal Doppler: characteristics of aging kidneys. J Ultrasound Med 1992;11:647—651.
33. Keogan MT, Kaliewer MA, Hertzberg BS, et al. Renal resistive indexes: variability and Doppler ultrasound measurement in a healthy population. *Radiology* 1996;199:165—169.
34. Haddad MC, Sharif HS, Shahed MS, et al. Renal colic: diagnosis and outcome. *Radiology* 1992;184:83—88.
35. Mallek R, Bankier AA, Etele-Hainz A, Kletter K, Mostbeck GH. Distinction between obstructive and nonobstructive hydronephrosis: value of diuresis duplex Doppler sonography. *AJR* 1996;166:113—117.
36. Laing FC, Benson CB, DiSalvo DN, et al. Distal ureteral calculi: detection with vaginal ultrasound. *Radiology* 1994;192:545—548.
37. Baker SM, Middleton WD. Color Doppler sonography of ureteral jets in normal volunteers. Importance of the relative specific gravity of urine in the ureter and bladder. *AJR* 1992;159:773—775.
38. Burge HJ, Middleton WD, McClennan BL, Hildebolt CF. Ureteral jets in healthy patients and in patients with unilateral ureteral calculi: comparison with color Doppler ultrasound. *Radiology* 1991;180:437—442.
39. Cox IH, Erickson SJ, Foley WD, Dewire DM. Ureteral jets: evaluation of normal flow dynamics with color Doppler sonography. *AJR* 1992;158:1051—1055.
40. Sommer FG, Jeffrey RB, Rubin GD. Detection of ureteral calculi in patients with suspected renal colic: value of reformated non-contrast helical CT. *AJR* 1995;165:509—513.

41. Smith RC, Verga M, McCarthy S, Rosenfield AT. Diagnosis of acute flank pain: value of unenhanced helical CT. *AJR* 1996;166:97—101.

42. Hertzberg BS, Carroll BA, Bowie JD, et al. Doppler ultrasound assessment of maternal kidneys: analysis of intrarenal resistivity indexes in normal pregnancy and physiologic pelvicaliectasis. *Radiology* 1993;186:689—692.

43. Renal inflammatory disease. In: Dunnick NR, McCallum RW, Sandler CM. *Textbook of Uroradiology*. Baltimore, Md: Williams & Wilkins, 1991; p. 135—146.

44. Jeffrey RB, Laing FC, Wing VW, Hoddick W. Sensitivity of sonography in pyonephrosis: a reevaluation. *AJR* 1985;144:71—73.

45. Talner LB, Davidson AJ, Lebowitz RL, Dalla Palma L, Goldman SM. Acute pyelonephritis: can we agree on terminology. *Radiology* 1994;192:297—305.

46. Soulen MC, Fishman EK, Goldman SM, Gatewood OMB. Bacterial renal infection: role of CT. *Radiology* 1989;171:703—707.

47. Hoddick W, Jeffrey RB, Goldberg HI, Federle MP, Laing FC. CT and sonography of severe renal and perirenal infections. *AJR* 1983;140:517—520.

48. Rigsby CM, Rosenfield AT, Glickman MG, Hodson J. Hemorrhagic focal bacterial nephritis: findings on gray scale sonography and CT. *AJR* 1986;146:1173—1177.

49. Lee JKT, McClennan BL, Melson GL, Stanley RJ. Acute focal bacterial nephritis: emphasis on gray scale sonography and computed tomography. *AJR* 1980;135:87—92.

50. Rosenfield AT, Glickman MG, Taylor KJW, Crade M, Hodson J. Acute focal bacterial nephritis (acute lobar nephronia). *Radiology* 1979;132:553—561.

51. Nicolet V, Carignan L, Dubuc G, et al. Thickening of the renal collecting system: a nonspecific finding at ultrasound. *Radiology* 1988;168:411—413.

52. Babcock DS. Sonography of wall thickening of the renal collecting system. A nonspecific finding. *J Ultrasound Med* 1987;6:29—32.

53. Morehouse H, Darwish M, Ginsberg M, Kreutzer E, Koenigsberg M. Abstract, Society of Uroradiology, Palm Beach, Florida, January 14—19, 1995.

54. Keogan MT, Hertzberg BS, Kliewer MA, et al. Doppler sonography in the diagnosis of antepartum pyelonephritis: value of intrarenal resistive index measurements. *J Ultrasound Med* 1996;15:13—17.

55. Hilton S, Bosniak MA, Raghavendra N, et al. CT findings in acute renal infarction. *Urol Radiol* 1984;6:158—163.

56. Wong WS, Moss AA, Federle MP, Cochran ST, London SS. Renal infarction: CT diagnosis and correlation between CT findings and etiologies. *Radiology* 1984;150:201—205.

57. Glazer GM, Francis IR, Brady TM, Teng SS. Computed tomography of renal infarction: clinical and experimental observations. *AJR* 1983;140:721—727.

58. Platt JF, Ellis JH, Rubin J. Intrarenal Doppler sonography in the detection of renal vein thrombosis of the native kidney. *AJR* 1994;162:1367—1370.

59. Schuman WP, Hastrup W, Kohler TR, et al. Suspected leaking abdominal aortic aneurysm: use of sonography in the emergency room. *Radiology* 1988;168:117—119.

60. Patel SK. Retroperitoneal tumors and cysts. In: Pollack HM, ed. Clinical Urography. Philadelphia, Pa: W.B. Saunders Co, 1990; p. 2413—2416.

61. Lane RH, Stephens DH, Reiman HM. Primary retroperitoneal neoplasms: CT findings in 90 cases with clinical and pathologic correlation. *AJR* 1989;152:83—89.

8 Renal Failure

John J. Cronan

Renal failure refers to inadequate renal function with the accumulation of nitrogen waste to a toxic level that is incompatible with life. A distinction is made between renal failure and **renal insufficiency**. Renal insufficiency is the abnormal accumulation of nitrogen waste with preservation of sufficient renal function to sustain life. **End-stage renal disease** is chronic and irreversible renal failure — renal dialysis or transplantation is necessary for survival. The prevalence of renal failure is approximately 65 cases per million in the United States. Less than 20% of acute renal failure patients eventually require dialysis. At autopsy, approximately 25% of uremic patients have obstructive uropathy as either a contributory or major cause of renal insufficiency.[1]

Differential Diagnosis

Renal dysfunction, whether it be insufficiency or failure, produces the clinical state of uremia. The final common pathway for numerous disparate disease processes affecting the kidney is renal failure. During the initial clinical evaluation, it is essential to quickly determine if the renal failure is reversible. Thus, determining the etiology is crucial, in order to identify reversible causes of renal dysfunction. Diagnosis depends on evaluation and integration of the clinical history, physical exam, and laboratory data.

Maintenance of the normal internal milieu of the body is dependent on the ultrafiltration of blood by the kidney, followed by the secretory and resorptive functions of renal tubules. Renal function leads to the excretion of urine via the ureters, bladder, and urethra. Based on the physiology of renal function, renal failure is classified as **prerenal** — due to diminished renal blood flow; **intrinsic** — caused by renal parenchymal damage; and **postrenal** — due to blockage of urine flow (**Fig. 8–1**). For the referring clinician and radiologist, the initial step in assessing renal failure is to categorize the etiologic event as prerenal, renal, or postrenal. The ability to intervene and provide prompt improvement in defective renal function is limited to prerenal and postrenal processes. While intrinsic renal processes may be ameliorated, the possibility of an immediate cure is unlikely.

Diagnosis of prerenal failure focuses on levels of the blood urea nitrogen (BUN) and serum creatinine. Both

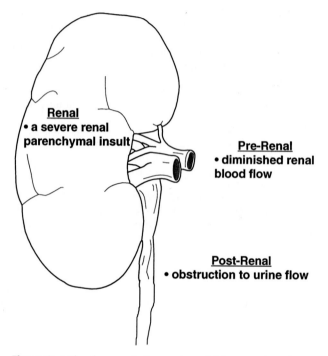

Figure 8–1 The three main types of renal failure are based on an etiologic classification.

BUN and creatinine are filtered freely at the glomerulus. Normally, urea, but not creatinine, is reabsorbed at the tubules in peritubular capillaries. With decreased renal blood flow, capillary flow decreases and more BUN is resorbed. The resulting disproportionate elevation of blood levels of BUN compared to creatinine can be used as a diagnostic indicator of prerenal renal dysfunction, related to renal blood flow decrease.

Postrenal acute renal failure has a variable clinical presentation depending on the site and completeness of the obstruction. Urine volumes in the setting of obstruction are quite variable. Reduced urine volume and azotemia usually develop only when the obstruction is located at the level of the bladder or below. Azotemia from ureteral obstruction develops only when the obstruction is bilateral or there is a solitary kidney. Obstruction is usually reversible. When the kidney becomes obstructed, renal function changes with time. Paralleling the alteration in renal function is an alteration of the composition of urine as a result of impaired water reabsorption and electrolyte transport.

Intrinsic disorders affecting the renal parenchyma cause decreased glomerular filtration rate (GFR) and resultant elevation of the BUN and creatinine. There is a difference between hospital-acquired and non-hospital-acquired intrinsic (acute renal failure) renal failure. Most hospital-acquired acute renal failure is caused by acute tubular necrosis (ATN). Intrinsic acute renal failure acquired outside the hospital is usually caused by acute glomerular, interstitial, or vascular disease. When prerenal and postrenal acute renal failure are excluded, the cause of acute renal failure must be an acute renal parenchymal insult.

Diagnostic Evaluation

Nonimaging Evaluation

The clinical difficulty in diagnosing the cause of acute renal failure arises from the plethora of potential etiologies and the difficulty distinguishing among them. It is often difficult or impossible to determine if the cause is prerenal, intrinsic, or postrenal. Compounding the diagnostic confusion is the possibility that several different causes of renal dysfunction may interact to produce acute renal failure.

Prerenal acute renal failure should be considered if there is a history of congestive heart failure or hypotension. Changes in the patient's weight can indicate fluid shifts, caused by hypoperfusion, either from dehydration or "third spacing" of fluid. Physical examination to assess skin turgor, edema, blood pressure, and pulse are helpful. The referring clinician will usually be able to diagnose or exclude prerenal acute renal failure without imaging assistance.

Postrenal acute renal failure due to obstruction is easily corrected if promptly diagnosed. For this reason, it is important to consider the possibility of obstruction as a cause of renal failure in every patient. Sonography can usually diagnose obstruction quickly and simply. It is important to evaluate the clinical history, as the presence of a single kidney or preexisting renal disease will alter the presentation. A history of stone disease or malignancy suggests possible causes of obstruction.

Urine volume is a nonspecific test for acute renal failure. Anuria, defined as a 24-hour volume of 100 mL or less, can be seen with prerenal, obstructive, and intrinsic renal disease. The urine-specific gravity or osmolality are measured to assess the concentration of solute in the urine. With hypovolemia, water is reabsorbed, and the urine becomes concentrated. With urine osmolalities below 350 mOsm, intrinsic renal disease is most likely and with osmolalities above 500 mOsm, the likely etiology is prerenal acute renal failure. There is great overlap, however, between the range of 350 and 500 mOsm. The normal specific gravity of urine is 1.002—1.028.

Creatinine is formed from the breakdown of muscle creatinine phosphate. Daily production is proportional to muscle mass. With acute renal failure, creatinine can rise 1—2 mg per dL per day. The normal range of creatinine in females is approximately 0.6—1 mg/dL and in males 0.8—1.3 mg/dL. Plasma levels of urea may also be used to assess renal function. Blood urea levels, unlike serum creatinine values, are commonly influenced by external factors; for example, an increased dietary load of protein or intestinal bleeding increases the plasma urea levels. Normal BUN is 7—18 mg/dL and may rise 10—25 mg/dL per day in acute renal failure.

Renal biopsies should be performed in only a small subset of patients with intrinsic renal disease. In most situations, the diagnosis and likely etiology of intrinsic renal disease is sufficiently certain with clinical history, urinalysis, and physical exam that appropriate treatment can be instituted. Less than 20% of patients with intrinsic renal disease require a kidney biopsy to establish the cause of acute renal failure.

Imaging Other than Ultrasound

Plain Film

A plain film of the abdomen can be useful in assessing renal size and shape and identifying radiopaque stones and renal calcification (**Fig. 8–2**). Normal renal size is 3.7 ± 0.37 x the height of the second lumbar vertebral body. Approximately 90% of renal stones are

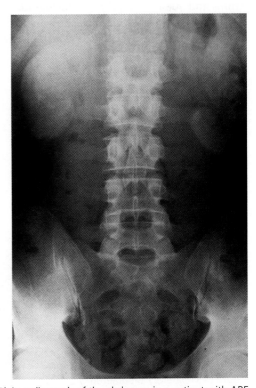

Figure 8–2 Plain radiograph of the abdomen in a patient with ARF demonstrates diffuse bilateral cortical nephrocalcinosis.

radiopaque. Thus, potentially obstructing stones can often be identified on plain radiographs. Renal osteodystrophy, a complication of chronic renal failure, or metastatic bone disease, may also be identified on the plain film.

Excretory Urography

Excretory urography is usually not performed in patients with acute renal failure because of the risks that contrast material may exacerbate renal failure or cause a hypersensitivity reaction. The utility of renal sonography has also contributed to decreased demand for excretory urography. When renal function is normal, 25 mg of iodine per kilogram body weight is appropriate for the excretory urogram. With acute renal failure, 40—60 mg of iodine per kg is necessary to achieve opacification of the collecting system. The urogram can provide information regarding the size and shape of the kidneys. With severe azotemia, tomography is necessary to assess the renal contour (**Fig. 8–3**). Small kidneys with smooth or scarred contours indicate chronic renal failure. Bilaterally normal or large kidneys are suggestive of ATN, obstruction, renal vein thrombosis, or infiltrative disease. When renal obstruction is present, contrast excretion and collecting system opacification are delayed, which often permits determination of the site and etiology of obstruction.

Retrograde Pyelography

The retrograde pyelogram is rarely employed in acute renal failure because of the reliability of excretory urography and renal sonography. Retrograde pyelography can opacify the ureter directly, showing excellent radiographic detail. The ureteral access also provides the urol-

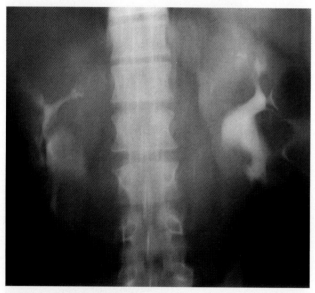

Figure 8–3 Excretory urogram in a 24-year-old man with renal failure. Kidneys are large bilaterally, with masses caused by polycystic disease of the kidneys.

ogist a means to pass a stent. Hence, the retrograde pyelogram is employed when there is a high probability of ureteral obstruction requiring stent placement.

Renal Scintigraphy

Intravenous injection of a radioisotope permits assessment of renal blood flow, filtration, and urinary excretion. A major limitation of renal scintigraphy is poor delineation of the anatomy. This makes it difficult to assess the etiology of acute renal failure with renal scintigraphy.

Computed Tomography

Computed tomography is rarely used as the primary imaging technique in renal failure. CT should be considered, however, when sonography is inconclusive. Even without intravenous contrast material, CT permits evaluation of the presence of the kidneys, their size, and location. Renal stones are readily visualized. A dilated collecting system can easily be recognized and the ureters can be followed from the kidneys to the bladder or to the point of obstruction.[2]

Aortography

Placement of a pig-tail catheter into the aortic lumen followed by the injection of contrast material provides excellent opacification of the renal arteries and is most useful when there is concern regarding the integrity of renal blood flow. Visualization of the renal arteries eliminates arterial occlusion as a cause of prerenal failure. Similarly, delayed filming following aortic injection will often permit visualization of the renal veins. On occasion, however, direct selective injection of the renal veins is necessary to properly establish venous patency.

Magnetic Resonance Imaging

MRI's role in evaluating acute renal failure is poorly defined. However, with heavily T2-weighted fast imaging techniques, MR urograms can be produced that visualize the ureters.[3] The MR urogram is particularly helpful in assessing postrenal processes (**Fig. 8–4**). Similarly, MR angiography can assess the presence and patency of the renal arteries. MRI will probably become more important in the assessment of renal failure as faster imaging sequences evolve.

Ultrasound Imaging

Postrenal causes of acute renal failure are likely to be reversible. Sonography is the optimal imaging technique in renal failure patients as it is a quick and simple tool to diagnose or exclude obstruction. Sonography rapidly provides useful information about the kidney, both noninvasively and independent of renal function. Sonography can establish the presence of the kidneys, their size, and shape. If the kidneys are small, renal failure is chronic (**Fig. 8–5**). If the kidney size is normal or enlarged, acute renal failure is likely.[4] Although prerenal

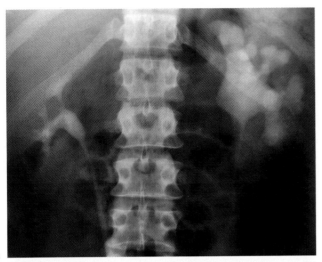

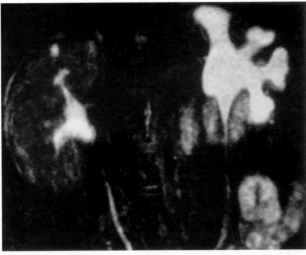

Figure 8–4 Comparison of (**A**) 5-min excretory urogram with (**B**) maximum intensity pixel image of MR urogram using three-dimensional fast-spin echo technique. The patient had undergone a left pyeloplasty. (Case courtesy of Martin E. O'Malley, MD, Department of Radiology, Boston University Medical Center, Boston, MA, USA).

acute renal failure is likely to be diagnosed by the clinician, renal blood flow can be evaluated with color Doppler or spectral Doppler, assessing the patency of renal arteries bilaterally (**Fig. 8–6**). Renal veins can also be evaluated with Doppler sonography.

Normal renal size is quite variable. Using ultrasound measurements, two standard deviations above and below the mean yields a normal renal length of 8.4—13.1 cm. It is very important to assess the amount of renal parenchyma, which can best be determined by noting the thickness of the renal cortex (**Fig. 8–7**). A thin renal cortex provides an excellent indication of renal tissue loss. Normal renal parenchyma is greater than 1 cm thick, as measured from the outer margin of the renal pyramids. The normal kidney surface is smooth. Indentations between the calyces (renal pyramids) are usually due to fetal lobulation or scarring from vascular occlusion, often caused by analgesic nephropathy. Renal size is usually normal with lobulation. Scarring of any etiology is usually accompanied by some reduction in size. It is important to note that in assessing renal tissue loss, renal length is often preserved, even when there is a reduction of overall weight or volume of the kidney, because lost parenchyma is replaced with renal sinus fat — so-called replacement lipomatosis.[5] The telltale indicator of tissue loss is the decreased parenchymal thickness.

Increased echogenicity of the renal cortex indicates intrinsic acute renal failure. Normal echogenicity of the kidney is less than or equal to that of the liver.[6] Renal echogenicity greater than that of the liver or spleen suggests intrinsic renal disease. Similarly, the resistive index, a measure of the systolic and diastolic variability of the arterial signal, can be measured in order to suggest the presence of intrinsic renal disease. Because of slight variation in flow, several measurements of the RI should be

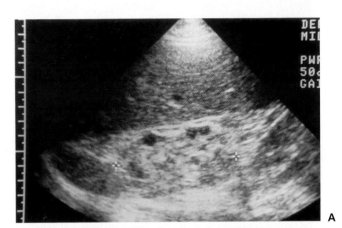

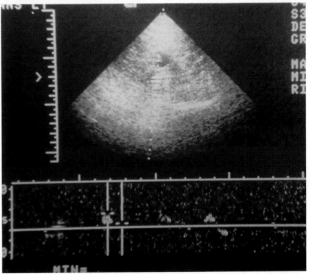

Figure 8–5 Chronic renal failure. (**A**) Sagittal view demonstrates a small dense kidney (8 cm). (**B**) Pulsed Doppler of left kidney demonstrates an elevated resistive index (RI) of 90%, comparative with intrinsic renal disease.

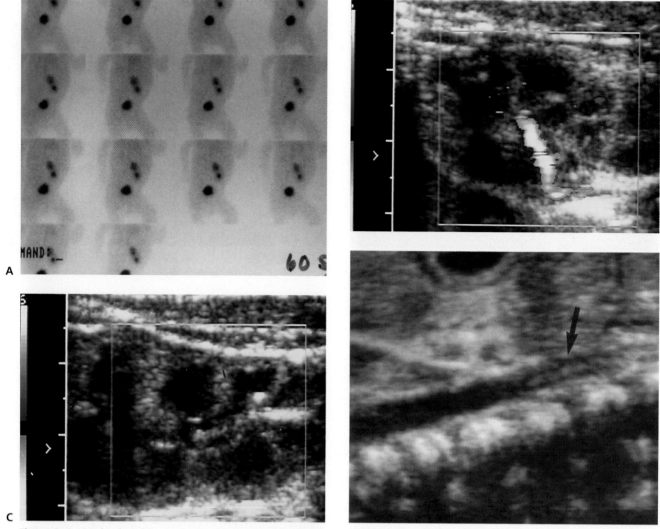

Figure 8–6 ARF developed in a neonate after placement of an intraaortic line. (**A**) Nuclear medicine scan obtained with diethyl-enetriamine-pentacetic acid injection shows no flow or function of left kidney. (**B**) Color Doppler of right kidney shows normal flow. (**C**) Color Doppler of left kidney demonstrates no flow. (**D**) US image of aorta shows catheter (**arrow**) in distal aorta with clot extending into left renal artery.

taken and averaged.[7] In the absence of hydronephrosis, an elevated RI greater than 0.70 is suggestive of intrinsic renal disease.[8] Elevation of the RI in the setting of renal disease is unpredictable. For example, the RI is more likely to become elevated with tubular interstitial processes and is less likely to rise when isolated glomerular disease is present. A normal RI does not exclude intrinsic renal disease.

Sonography's sensitivity in detecting postrenal acute renal failure in the azotemic patient is 94%. False negatives occur in some patients with stone disease or when minimal dilatation of the collecting system is ignored.[9] When assessing obstruction in a general population, sonography has a reported sensitivity of 98%.[10] However, the false-positive rate of sonography is 10—26%. False-positive images are due to pseudohydrone-phrosis, which may be caused by blood vessels or a parapelvic renal sinus cyst mimicking the appearance of hy-

dronephrosis.[11] Another problem is that hydronephrosis can occur in the absence of obstruction. It is essential, therefore, to determine if hydronephrosis is obstructive or nonobstructive in nature. Nonobstructive hydrone-phrosis can be related to a prior episode of obstruction or damage from reflux. The resistive index has been advocated as a technique to distinguish obstructive versus nonobstructive hydronephrosis.[11] If the RI is greater than 0.70, then this suggests an obstructive etiology for the hydronephrosis. Unfortunately, the reliability of the RI in diagnosing obstruction is suspect.[14] Of note is the fact that sonographically observed hydronephrosis is more likely to be caused by obstruction when clinical evaluation suggests the presence of obstruction.[15, 16]

As peristalsis expels urine from the ureter into the bladder, it creates a "jet." This ureteral jet may be detected with color Doppler. The presence of a ureteral jet indicates patency of that ureter (**Fig. 8–8**).[17] Color Dop-

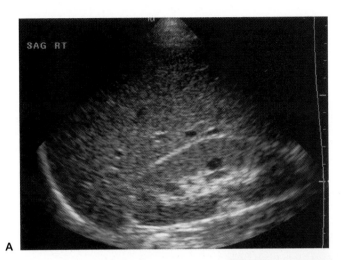

A

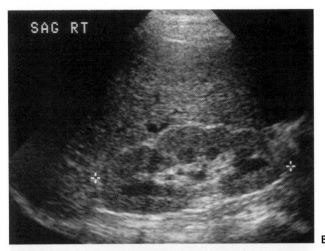

B

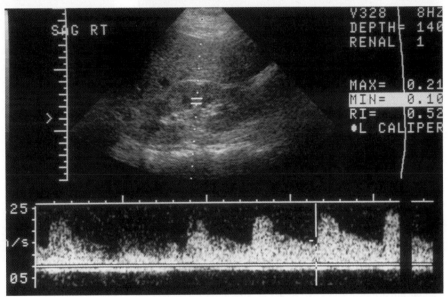

C

Figure 8–7 Images of a kidney from a 20-year-old female patient with a history of analgesic abuse and early nephrotic syndrome. Kidneys are scarred because of persistent analgesic abuse. (**A**) initial scan demonstrates smooth renal parenchyma; (**B**) two years later, the kidney is diffusely scarred; (**C**) Note the lobulated renal contour. The RI remains normal at 52%.

pler visualization of a ureteral jet requires a difference in specific gravity between the urine in the bladder and the urine passing into the bladder from the ureter. If there is no difference in specific gravity between the ureteral urine and urine in the bladder, no jet will be seen with color Doppler. Thus bilateral absence of jets has no significance. Unilateral absence of a ureteral jet is highly significant and indicates total obstruction on the affected side. If a jet is seen on one side only after ten minutes of observation, obstruction of the ureter on the side with the absent jet is almost certain. Unfortunately, a ureteral jet can be present with partial obstruction, although it is usually diminished in magnitude compared to the normal side. In addition to scanning the bladder searching for ureteral jets, signs of bladder outlet obstruction (**Fig. 8–9**) should be sought. Outlet obstruction is suggested when the bladder wall is thickened and trabeculated and the bladder is distended. Tumors such

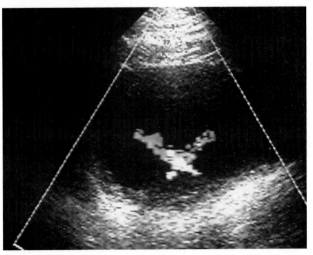

Figure 8–8 Transverse color Doppler image of bladder demonstrates bilaterally patent ureters indicated by the ureteral jets.

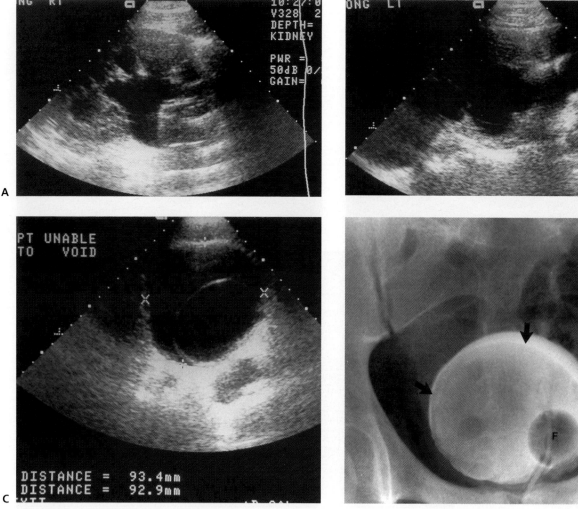

Figure 8–9 A 19-year-old male presented with a recent history of hypertension and acute onset of anuria. A ureterocele was causing bladder outlet obstruction. (**A, B**) Renal ultrasound demonstrates bilateral hydronephrosis. (**C**) Bladder US shows a 9-cm cystic mass that proved to be a ureterocele. (**D**) Contrast-enhanced cystogram reveals Foley (F) and mass (**arrows**) that represents the ureterocele.

as transitional cell carcinoma or prostate carcinoma may obstruct the bladder and can often be visualized sonographically.

In summary, sonography should be the initial imaging tool used to evaluate the kidney in patients with acute renal failure. If all ultrasound techniques are employed, including color and pulsed Doppler, the radiologist should be able to assist in excluding pre- and postrenal obstruction. On occasion, the presence of echogenic small kidneys will indicate chronic intrinsic renal disease — end-stage renal disease. It is important that the radiologist not limit the use of sonography to ruling out obstruction. If other etiologies of renal failure are sought, a diagnosis can be achieved in most patients. The American College of Radiology Appropriateness Criteria (UR-10.1, Renal Failure-Acute)[18] suggests sonography as the primary imaging technique in acute renal failure. All other techniques, for example, CT or scintigraphy play a distinctly secondary role. Their use depends

upon the experience and preferences of individual institutions.

A diagnosis of chronic renal failure implies that the process is not reversible. Acute obstructive processes causing acute renal failure must be diagnosed quickly and corrected if renal function is to be preserved. Prerenal processes are readily evident clinically and the patient will not likely be sent for imaging. Intrinsic renal disease is more difficult to diagnose but it may be suggested by excluding postrenal acute renal failure or diagnosing echogenic kidneys with an increased RI.

References

1. Klahr S, Buerkert J, Pakerson ML. The kidney in obstructive uropathy. *Contr Nephrol* 1977;7:220—249.

2. Webb JAW, Reznek RH, White FE, et al. Can ultrasound and computed tomography replace high dose urography in patients with impaired renal function? *Q J Med* 1986;211:411—425.

3. Regan F, Bohlman M, Khazan R, Rodriguez R, Schultz-Haakh H. MR urography using HASTE imaging in the assessment of ureteric obstruction. *AJR* 1996;167:1115—1120.

4. Systic A, Mauric Z, Fuckar Z, et al. Kidney length in postoperative acute renal failure. *J Clin Ultrasound* 1998;26:251—255.

5. Simon AI. Normal renal size: an absolute criterion. *AJR* 1964;92(2):270—272.

6. Platt JF, Rubin JM, Bowerman R, Marn CS. The inability to detect kidney disease on the basis of echogenicity. *AJR* 1988;151:317—319.

7. Keogan MT, Kliewer MA, Hertzberg BS, et al. Renal resistive indexes: variability in Doppler US measurement in a healthy population. *Radiology* 1996;199:165—169.

8. Platt JF, Rubin JM, Ellis JH. Acute renal failure: possible role of duplex Doppler US in distinction between acute prerenal failure and acute tubular necrosis. *Radiology* 1991;179:419—423.

9. Talner LB, Scheible W, Ellenbogen PH, Beck JR, CH, Gosink BB. How accurate is ultrasonography in detecting hydronephrosis in azotemic patients? *Urol Radiol* 1981;3:1—6.

10. Ellenbogen PH, Scheible FW, Talner LB, Leopold GR. Sensitivity of gray scale ultrasound in detecting urinary tract obstruction. *Am J Roentgenol* 1978;130:731—733.

11. Scola FH, Cronan JJ, Schepps B. Grade I hydronephrosis: pulsed Doppler evaluation. *Radiology* 1989;171:519—520.

12. Platt JF, Rubin JM, Ellis JH, DiPietro MA. Duplex Doppler US of the kidney: differentiation of obstructive from nonobstructive dilatation. *Radiology* 1989;171:515—517.

13. Platt JF, Rubin JM, Ellis JH. Acute renal obstruction: evaluation with intrarenal duplex Doppler and conventional US. *Radiology* 1993;186:685—688.

14. Lee HJ, Kim SH, Jeong YK, Yeun KM. Doppler sonographic resistive index in obstructed kidney. *J Ultrasound Med* 1996;15:613—618.

15. Kamholtz RG, Cronan JJ, Dorfman GS. Obstruction and the minimally dilated renal collecting system: US evaluation. *Radiology* 1989;170:51—53.

16. Curatola G, Mazzitelli R, Monzani G, Cozzupoli P, Maggiore Q. The value of ultrasound as a screening procedure for urological disorders in renal failure. *J Urol* 1983;130:8—10.

17. Burge HJ, Middleton WD, McClennan BL, Hildebolt CF. Ureteral jets in healthy subjects and in patients with unilateral ureteral calculi: comparison with color Doppler US. *Radiology* 1991;180:437—442.

18. American College of Radiology Appropriateness Criteria. 1995;UR-10.1.

9 Hematuria: Guidelines for Evaluation

Robert L. Bree

Hematuria is a very common clinical problem, which challenges both primary care and specialty physicians. *Hematuria* may be defined as gross or microscopic and symptomatic or asymptomatic. Asymptomatic hematuria occurs in about 13% of both men over 35 and women over 55.[1] *Asymptomatic hematuria* is defined as microscopic hematuria (three to five or more red blood cells (RBCs) per high power field) seen on three urinalyses; one episode of 100 RBCs per high power field; or gross hematuria[2]. One or two RBCs per high power field are found in about 15% of asymptomatic persons.[1] Unfortunately, the degree of hematuria does not necessarily correlate with its significance. All hematuria requires evaluation. This discussion will include both gross and microscopic hematuria. Patients suspected of having a renal or ureteral calculus, who present with flank pain and hematuria, will not be discussed in this chapter.

Causes of Hematuria

Only about 20% of patients with microscopic hematuria have a *significant* abnormality as the cause and only 4% have life-threatening lesions[1, 3-6]   (**Table 9–1**).

Table 9–1   Common causes of hematuria

Life threatening and significant diseases
Bladder cancer
   Renal cell carcinoma
   Transitional cell carcinoma of ureter or kidney
   Ureteral calculus
   Abdominal aortic aneurysm
   Prostate cancer
   Generalized renal parenchymal disease

Moderately significant diseases
   Pyelonephritis
   Cystitis
   Hydronephrosis
   Bladder calculus
   Bladder diverticulum
   Urethral stricture
   Neurogenic bladder
   Prostatitis

Insignificant diseases
   Renal cyst
   Benign prostatic hyperplasia
   Urethritis
   Bladder diverticulum
   Caliceal diverticulum

When gross hematuria occurs, almost 60% have significant abnormalities and 20% have life-threatening disorders.[7] When lower abdominal symptoms are associated with hematuria, the cause is commonly in the lower urinary tract — a significant percentage will have treatable pathology.[2, 3] **Table 9–1** lists the more common diseases, stratified by severity, that are associated with hematuria. It is not always clear that the associated diagnosis is the cause of the hematuria. In fact, only about one-half of the patients investigated for hematuria have a related diagnosis discovered in the initial evaluation. When the remaining, undiagnosed patients with persistent hematuria are followed, a small percentage will have a cause for hematuria detected within three years of the discovery of hematuria. These diseases include glomerulonephritis, calculi, and, rarely, bladder or prostate cancer.[6]

Because transient hematuria is common, the insistence on multiple positive tests is important when trying to separate disease from no disease. It can be useful to try to separate glomerular from nonglomerular hematuria. Findings that favor a glomerular source include cola-colored urine, renal insufficiency, red-cell casts, dysmorphic red cells, and proteinuria. Methods to assess red cell morphology have not been widely accepted in medical practice.[8-9]

Older patients and patients with frankly bloody urine are at higher risk for a significant lesion. 60% of patients with painless gross hematuria will have a diagnosis made by a combination of imaging and cystoscopy. The majority of these diagnoses are not life threatening. Conversely, 40% of patients with gross hematuria have no diagnosis made.[5, 7] The vast majority of patients over the age of 50 who present with hematuria will have significant diseases. As urologic cancer is more common in males, those men over 50 who present with hematuria should have a complete and thorough evaluation of the urinary tract (**Fig. 9–1**).[5, 10]

Evaluation of Hematuria

Nonimaging Tests

In addition to imaging evaluations, common testing performed in patients with hematuria include 1) search for proteinuria (seen in glomerulopathies); (2) urine cytology; (3) urine culture; (4) renal function tests; and (5) endoscopic evaluations including evaluation of the bladder, ureter, and renal collecting system.[11] Appropriate sequencing of these procedures is important. The frequency with which invasive and more expensive procedures (e.g., ureteroscopy or retrograde pyelography) are used depends on the quality and reliability of the less invasive studies, particularly the imaging studies. Risk—benefit choices must be made when deciding whether to administer iodinated intravenous contrast media to a patient of a certain age or sex. This evaluation is made relative to the extent of hematuria and the chances of finding a significant or life-threatening abnormality. In general, meta-analyses and clinical decision-making models suggest that patients with hematuria who harbor a urologic malignancy over 90% are curable, while the risk of adverse events from the evaluation is about 1%. Therefore, evaluation is always warranted except in women under 40 where the yield of pathology is less than the risk of adverse events.[5, 11–14]

Imaging Examinations other than Ultrasound:

Imaging tests for hematuria range from non-invasive to invasive. The intravenous pyelogram (IVP) has been the standard examination for many years. Other examinations that are capable of making a diagnosis in more difficult or enigmatic cases are retrograde pyelography, computed tomography (CT) (**Fig. 9–2**), magnetic resonance imaging (MRI), renal scintigraphy, renal arteriography (**Fig. 9–1**), renal venography, and antegrade pyelography. When the IVP is inadequate, ureteral evaluation can be enhanced with retrograde pyelography. For

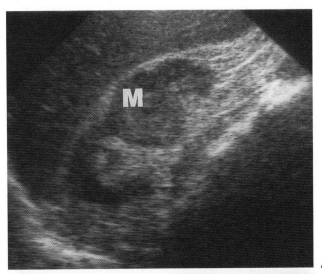

A

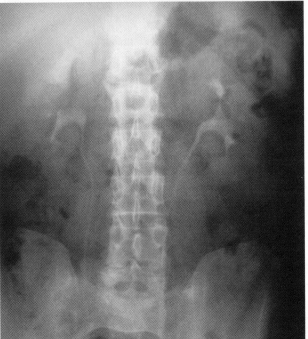

B

Figure 9–1 Central renal cell carcinoma in a 60-year-old man. (**A**) ▷ IVP shows very subtle dilatation of upper pole collecting system on the right. Tomograms did not suggest a mass. (**B**) Right renal ultrasound shows a large solid mass (M) in the mid portion of the kidney. (**C**) Arteriogram confirms typical findings of renal cell carcinoma.

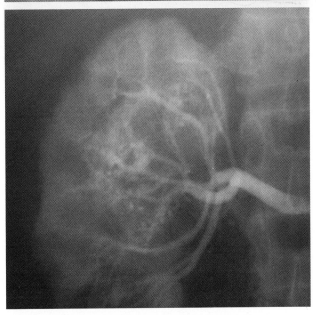

C

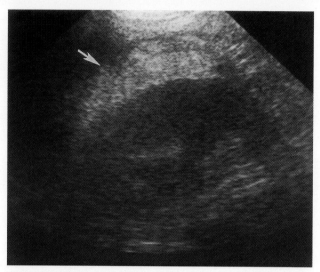

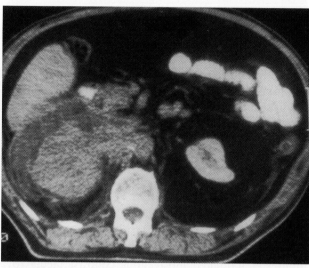

Figure 9–2 Infiltrative transitional cell carcinoma. (**A**) Ultrasound of the right kidney in a patient with gross hematuria. Normal renal architecture is absent and there is increased echogenicity in the perirenal space (**arrow**). (**B**) Computed tomogram demonstrates infiltrative neoplasm with perirenal hemorrhage. The kidney was surgically removed and contained extensive transitional cell carcinoma with spontaneous perirenal hemorrhage.

conditions such as infiltrative tumors (**Fig. 9–2**), small carcinomas (**Fig. 9–3**), or pyelonephritis (**Fig. 9–4**), contrast-enhanced CT, or MRI may be necessary to make the diagnosis.[15-17] DMSA renal scintigraphy can define renal masses when an IVP cannot be performed.[18] Renal arteriography may be the best technique capable of identifying vascular causes for hematuria, such as arteriovenous malformations or hemangiomas, although newer ultrasound techniques such as power Doppler can rival conventional or MR angiography. Vascular lesions such as this are most commonly found in young patients with gross hematuria (**Fig. 9–5**). Renal venography may be necessary to diagnose venous abnormalities, primarily renal vein varices. Finally in the patient with a nonfunctioning or obstructed kidney, antegrade pyelography may be the best choice, particularly when urothelial cancer is suspected.[2, 11]

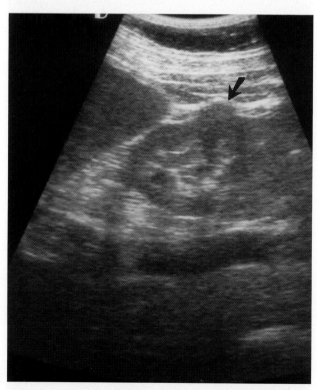

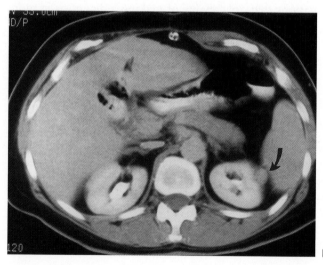

Figure 9–3   Small renal cell carcinoma. (**A**) A 55-year-old woman was initially investigated with ultrasound and a small solid mass (**arrow**) was discovered on the lateral cortex of the left kidney. (**B**) Computed tomogram confirms the solid nature of the mass (**arrow**) and suggests a neoplasm. A small renal cell carcinoma was removed surgically.

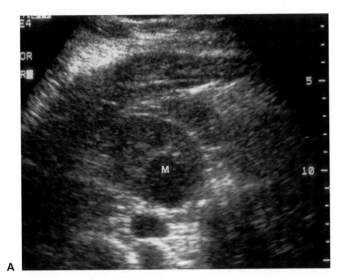

A

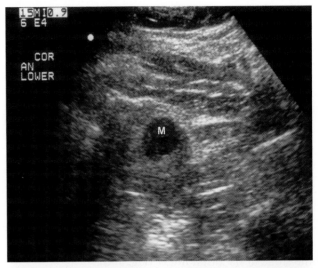

B

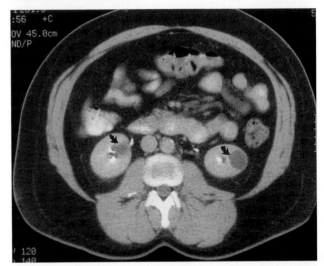

C

Figure 9–4 Bilateral focal pyelonephritis. A 45-year-old man presented with hematuria and fever. Ultrasound of the right (**A**) and left (**B**) kidneys reveals bilateral hypoechoic masses with internal echoes (M). (**C**) Computed tomogram performed at the same admission shows similar bilateral masses (**arrows**) which are nonspecific. In view of the suspected infection and lack of strong evidence of abscess, treatment with antibiotics commenced, and the symptoms resolved. Followup ultrasound was normal.

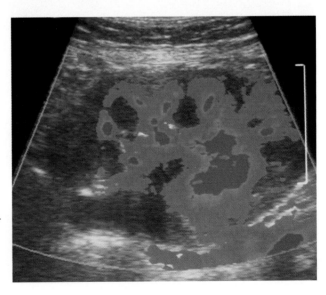

Figure 9–5 Renal arteriovenous fistula with power doppler. A ▷ patient who underwent a biopsy of a renal transplant and who subsequently developed hematuria was examined with ultrasound. Gray scale imaging was not revealing. Power Doppler examination shows turbulent flow in the renal hilus, proven to represent an arteriovenous fistula.

Role of Ultrasound in Hematuria:

The role of ultrasound in the evaluation of hematuria is controversial and has not been studied extensively.[19,20] Because the IVP remains a standard and reliable examination, ultrasound has not received much attention. There are, however, many advantages to ultrasound in this patient population. Ultrasound requires no preparation and does not use intravenous contrast material. That eliminates the possibility of an adverse event, particularly in a population at low risk for significant disease. The actual cost of ultrasound is lower than IVP, particularly if low-osmolar contrast is used for the IVP. Even in an asymptomatic patient who is suspected of having a ureteral calculus, ultrasound can identify the obstructed collecting system and, occasionally identify the stone in the distal ureter (**Fig. 9–6**).[21]

Mokulis et al.[22] in a study of 101 patients who had ultrasound after a normal IVP found that 20% of patients had an abnormal ultrasound study. All of these proved to be false-positive ultrasounds when subsequent evaluation was done. Therefore, they conclude that ultrasound is unnecessary in patients with a normal IVP and microscopic hematuria. On the other hand, IVP can miss anterior and posterior renal masses that can be seen with ultrasound.[17] In a more extensive review of 193 patients with microhematuria, Aslaksen et al.[21] demonstrated a clear advantage for ultrasound in detecting significant abnormalities, especially renal masses. Unfortunately, some stones were missed by both modalities (**Fig. 9–7**).

An additional advantage of ultrasound is the evaluation of the bladder. In the current practice standard, the bladder is included in the examination of the retroperitoneum when the urinary tract is suspected of being abnormal. Bladder tumors, hemorrhagic cystitis, calculi, and diverticula can be found with ultrasound, but are sometimes not seen well with IVP (**Fig. 9–8**).[21-23]

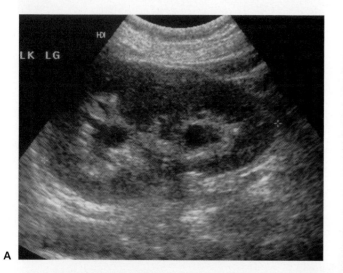

A

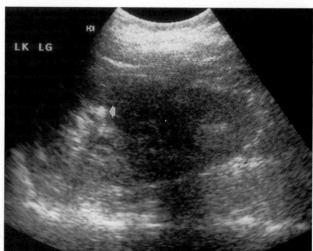

B

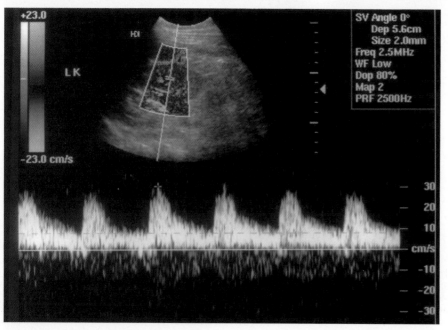

C

Figure 9–6 Obstructing distal ureteral calculus. A young woman presented to her physician after recovering from an episode of left flank pain and hematuria, but no stone was passed. An ultrasound was requested. The right kidney ultrasound was normal. (**A**) Hydronephrosis is demonstrated on the left. (**B**) Left renal Doppler indicates an elevated resistive index (0.74) indicating obstruction. (**C**) A calculus with shadowing (**arrow**) is seen in the upper pole of the left kidney.

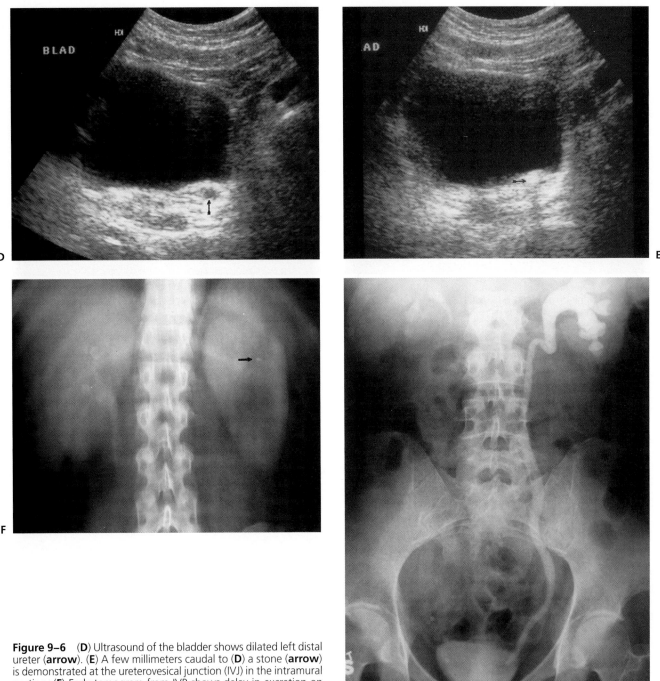

Figure 9–6 (**D**) Ultrasound of the bladder shows dilated left distal ureter (**arrow**). (**E**) A few millimeters caudal to (**D**) a stone (**arrow**) is demonstrated at the ureterovesical junction (IVJ) in the intramural portion. (**F**) Early tomogram from IVP shows delay in excretion on the left and an upper pole calculus (**arrow**) (**G**) Delayed film from IVP after voiding demonstrates obstructing calculus at the UVJ.

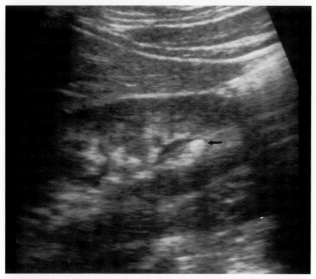

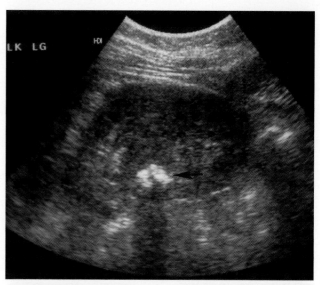

Figure 9–7   Nephrolithiasis without obstruction. (**A**) Sagittal scan of the right kidney in a patient with hematuria demonstrates a small nonobstructing calculus (**arrow**) in a lower pole calyx. This stone was not identified on an IVP. (**B**) Large left renal calculus (**arrow**) in the midportion of the kidney which was identified on a plain abdominal radiograph.

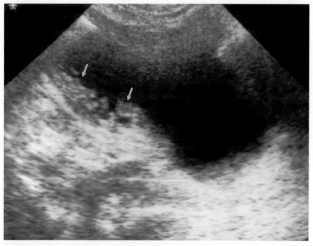

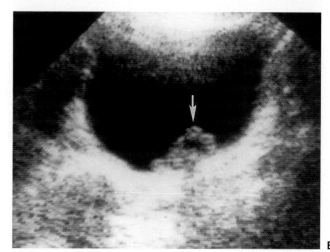

Figure 9–8   Bladder pathology. (**A**) Bullous cystitis. Focal mucosal thickening with cystic change (arrows) in a woman with chronic bullous cystitis and hematuria. (**B**) Bladder cancer. Focal polypoid mass (**arrow**) discovered in a patient being evaluated with ultrasound for hematuria. The bladder should be included in all scans directed to the retroperitoneum for suspected urinary tract abnormalities.

In the patient with known or suspected renal parenchymal disease, the most common cause of gross or microscopic hematuria is the renal disease itself. When a glomerulopathy is evident because of proteinuria, red cell casts, and red cell dysmorphism, hematuria can be attributed to the underlying disease. In these patients, IVP may be contraindicated because of the risk of provoking renal failure. Ultrasound is warranted to confirm the findings of generalized renal disease, as well as to exclude other superimposed pathology (**Fig. 9–9**).[2, 4, 9, 11]

In the patient who is known to have an acute hemorrhagic cystitis, imaging is typically not warranted unless there is failure of therapy. In this circumstance, an underlying additional cause must be investigated, particularly in men and women over 40 years of age. In the young women, because hemorrhagic cystitis is very common, imaging is only necessary in a very severe or refractory case.[2, 10]

In some patients with hematuria, economic savings result when ultrasound is used instead of IVP. In Corwin and Silverstein's series,[12] the expense of finding one renal cell carcinoma with ultrasound was one-half the cost of finding a renal cell carcinoma using IVP. Even if additional IVPs must be performed in patients with caliectasis and stones seen with ultrasound, significant cost

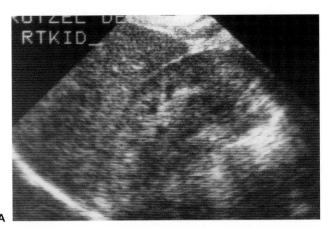

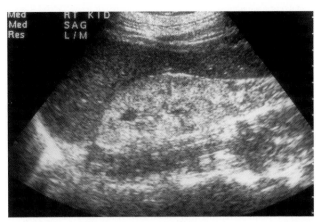

Figure 9–9 Two patients with renal parenchymal disease. **(A)** Acute glomerulonephritis. Ultrasound of the right kidney showing normal size but increased echogenicity compatible with the clinical and biopsy diagnosis of glomerulonephritis. The patient had hematuria and other urinalysis features of glomerulonephritis.

(B) Chronic renal failure. Patient with hematuria and renal failure. The kidney is small, echogenic, and has a thin cortex. No other reasons for hematuria were found, and further evaluation was not deemed necessary.

savings resulted if patients were screened with ultrasound.[21]

The most significant limitations of ultrasound are the inability to evaluate the ureters and, in some instances, the inability to define urothelial lesions. The sensitivity of ultrasound can be enhanced, particularly when blood is found coming from an individual ureter at the time of cystoscopy, by adding plain abdominal radiography, cystoscopy, and retrograde pyelography.[3, 12, 21]

Recommendations

Although there is scant literature on the role of ultrasound in hematuria, the American College of Radiology Task Force on Appropriateness guideline for hematuria[25] suggests ultrasound and IVP as the first-line imaging tests. When imaging is indicated, the choice of IVP or ultrasound may depend upon factors such as age, extent of hematuria, and result of urinary cytology, which, if positive, would suggest IVP and risk factors for contrast administration. Both IVP or ultrasound can, on occasion, miss significant disease — further evaluation with other imaging tests may be warranted. The American College of Radiology Task Force on Appropriateness Guidelines recommendations below are meant to guide the initial evaluation of hematuria and may not apply to difficult or complex patient problems.

1. *Hematuria in patients other than young women with cystitis or patients with generalized renal parenchymal disease*
   IVP: Indicated
   Urologic ultrasound: Probably indicated
   CT/angiography: Probably not indicated
   Other imaging examinations: Not indicated

2. *Hematuria in patients with generalized renal parenchymal disease*
   Urologic ultrasound: Indicated
   Other urologic imaging exams: Not indicated

3. *Hemorrhagic cystitis in woman under 40 which clears with treatment*
   All imaging tests: Not indicated.

References

1. Mohr DN, Offord KP, Owen RA, Melton LJ. Asymptomatic microhematuria and urologic disease: a population-based study. *JAMA* 1986;256:224—229.
2. Abuelo JG. The diagnosis of hematuria. *Arch Intern Med* 1983;143:967—970.
3. Bryden AAG, Paul AB, Kyriakides C. Investigation of haematuria. *Br J Hosp Med* 1995;54(9):455—458.
4. Golin AL, Howard RS. Asyptomatic microscopic hematuria. *Urology* 1980;124:389—391.
5. Mariani AJ, Mariani MC, Macchoini C, et al. The significance of adult hematuria: 1,000 hematuria evaluations including a risk-benefit and cost-effectiveness analysis. *Urology* 1989;141:350—355.
6. Murakami S, Igarashi T, Hara S, Shimazaki J. Strategies for asymptomatic microscopic hematuria: a prospective study of 1,034 patients. *J Urol* 1990;144:99—101.
7. Barkin M, Lopatin W, Herschorn S, Comisarow R. Unexplained hematuria. *Can J Surg* 1983;26(6):501—503.
8. Ahmed Z, Lee J. Asymptomatic urinary abnormalities; hematuria and proteinuria. *Med Clin North Am* 1977;81(3):641—650.
9. Webb JAW. Imaging in haematuria. Editorial. *Clin Radiol* 1997;52:167—171.
10. Froom P, Ribak J, Benbassat J. Significance of microhaematuria in young adults. *Br Med J* 1984;288:20—22.
11. Sutton JM. Evaluation of hematuria in adults. *JAMA* 1990;263(18):2475—2480.
12. Corwin HL, Silverstein MD. The diagnosis of neoplasia in

patients with asymptomatic microscopic hematuria: a decision analysis. *J Urol* 1988;139:1002—1006.

13. Green LF, O'Shaughnessey EJ, Jr, Hendricks ED. A study of five hundred patients with asymptomatic microhematuria. *JAMA* 1956;161:610.

14. Thompson IM. The evaluation of microscopic hematuria: a population-based study. *J Urol* 1987;138:1189.

15. Amendola MA, Bree RL, Pollack HM, et al. Small renal cell carcinomas: resolving a diagnostic dilemma. *Radiology* 1988;166:637—641.

16. Bree RL, Schultz SR, Hayes R. Large infiltrating renal transitional cell carcinomas: CT and ultrasound features. *J Computer Assist Tomogr* 1990;14(3):381—385.

17. Glen DA, Gilbert FJ, Bayliss AP. Renal carcinomas missed by urography. *Br J Urol* 1989;63:457—459.

18. Chisholm RA, Millet B, Sherwood T, Wraight EP, Doyle PT. The investigation of painless haematuria — a comparison of intravenous urography and DMSA scintigraphy. *Clin Radiol* 1988;39:494—495.

19. Spencer J, Lindsell D. Mastorakou I. Ultrasonography compared with intravenous urography in the investigation of adults with haematuria. *Br Med J* 1990;301:1074—1076.

20. Stonelake PS, Wallace DMA. Investigation of adults with haematuria. *Br Med J* 1990;301:1396.

21. Aslaksen A, Gadeholt G, Göthlin JH. Ultrasonography versus intravenous urography in the evaluation of patients with microscopic haematuria. *Br J Urology* 1990;66:144—147.

22. Mokulis JA, Arndt WF, Downey JR, Caballero RL, Thomason IM. Should renal ultrasound be performed in the patient with microscopic hematuria and a normal excretory urogram? *J Urol* 1995;154:1300—1301.

23. Bree RL, Silver TM. Sonography of bladder and perivesical abnormalities. *AJR* 1981;136:1101—1104.

24. Brun B, Gammelgaard J, Christoffersen J. Transabdominal dynamic ultrasonography in the detection of bladder tumors. *J Urol* 1984;132:19—20.

25. American College of Radiology Task Force on Appropriateness Criteria. American College of Radiology: Appropriateness Criteria for Imaging and Treatment Decisions. 1995:UR5.1-UR5.6.

Additional Suggested Reading

1. Abuelo JG. Evaluation of hematuria. *Urology* 1983;21(3):215—225.

2. Benson GS, Brewer ED. Hematuria: algorithms for diagnosis. II. Hematuria in the adult and hematuria secondary to trauma. *JAMA* 1981;246(9):993—995.

3. Copley JB. Review: Isolated asymptomatic hematuria in the adult. *Am J med Sc* 1986;291(2):101–111.

4. Fairley KF. Clinical evaluation of the kidney. *Urinalysis.* 359—390.

5. Lowe FC, Brendler CB. Evaluation of the urologic patient. *History, Physical Examination, and Urinalysis.* 307–331.

6. Messing EM, Young TB, Hunt BV, Emoto SE, Wehbie JM. The significance of asymptomatic microhematuria in men 50 or more years old: findings of a home screening study using urinary dipsticks. *J Urology* 1987;137:919—922.

10 Hypertension and Bruit

Laurence Needleman

The vast majority of patients with hypertension have essential hypertension; only a minority has renovascular hypertension (RVH). Despite this fact, the impetus to identify this minority exists because there is a possibility of curing their disease.

It is impractical to screen all hypertensive patients; therefore, it is important to identify the subset of patients who are at higher risk for renovascular hypertension and might benefit from screening. It is equally important to identify the imaging tests that can be applied consistently and safely to this group.

Renal artery stenosis (RAS) is the most common cause of RVH. RAS is also associated with renal insufficiency.[1-3] If revascularization were shown to consistently reverse or slow down the progression to renal failure, then identification of RAS would be important in this group of patients as well. Interest in applying diagnostic tests and therapeutic interventions to this risk group is growing.[4]

Differential Diagnosis

The recognition that a renal lesion could cause hypertension was established by Goldblatt and co-workers[5] when hypertension and renal atrophy followed renal artery constriction in a dog. In the years that followed, understanding of the renin—angiotensin system of blood pressure control has led to an understanding of RVH. Although RAS produces RVH, the two entities are not equivalent. RAS may not produce hypertension or it may coexist with essential hypertension. Processes other than RAS, such as Page kidney or dissecting aneurysm of the renal artery may also produce RVH. Other etiologies of secondary hypertension include renal disease, hyperaldosteronism, pheochromocytoma, Cushing's syndrome, sleep apnea syndrome, and coarctation of the aorta. Renal aneurysms may be associated with hypertension.[6]

The diagnosis of RVH is established retrospectively after the patient undergoes treatment: those whose hypertension responds to revascularization of RAS have RVH. The absence of a response to revascularization may be due to a variety of factors: technical failure of the intervention, incidental RAS in a patient with essential hypertension, or irreversible renal disease superimposed

on RAS or RVH. There may be no way to distinguish these groups, so it may not be possible to find a gold standard that establishes the presence or absence of RVH.

Most tests used to evaluate the hypertensive patient are anatomical — they detect RAS. A physiological test for RVH is one that bases its diagnosis on the determination of whether the renal blood flow is abnormal. Physiologic tests are theoretically more likely to predict the response to therapy, and therefore, RVH.

The prevalence of RVH is quite variable but only represents around 0.5—5% of the hypertensive population.[7, 8] Suggestive clinical clues may raise the likelihood of RVH to 5—15%.[7] Certain groups will have even greater incidence of RVH. For example, 31% of patients with accelerated hypertension may have RVH.[7]

The Cooperative Study of Renovascular Hypertension evaluated clinical features that might distinguish RVH from essential hypertension. The study compared 175 patients with RVH (91 cases of arteriosclerotic stenosis and 84 cases of fibromuscular dysplasia) that had been cured by surgery to 339 patients with essential hypertension.[9] Fibromuscular dysplasia was shown a disease of younger, predominantly female patients with no family history of hypertension. Arteriosclerotic patients were profiled as older, with higher systolic blood pressure, and often showed evidence of arterial disease at sites other than the kidney.

Although this study showed differences between the groups, no criteria was sufficiently sensitive or specific to distinguish the groups completely (**Table 10–1**). For instance, although a bruit was more often associated with RVH, a bruit is heard as frequently in essential hypertension. This is true because while a lower percentage of patients with essential hypertension have bruits, essential hypertension is much more common than RVH. Still this and other studies do point out some characteristics of patients that suggest RVH.

Mann and Pickering produced indexes of clinical suspicion that can guide the evaluation of patients with hypertension.[7] Those with borderline, low or moderate hypertension and no clinical clues have a low index of suspicion and do not require a workup. For patients with a high index of suspicion, diagnostic testing is indicated. Angiography may be the appropriate first diagnostic imaging test. Mann identified patients at high risk, includ-

Table 10–1 Clinical characteristics of 131 matched cases of essential and renovascular hypertension*

	Hypertension (%)	
	Essential (%)	Renovascular (%)
Duration of hypertension		
less than one year	12	24
greater than 10 years	15	6
Age of onset greater than 50	9	15
Family history of hypertension	71	46
Grade 3 or 4 fundi	7	46
Bruit		
Abdomen	9	46
Flank	1	12
Both	9	48
BUN greater than 20 mg/100 mL	8	15
Serum K less than 3.4 mEq/L	8	16
Serum CO_2 greater than 30 mEq/L	5	17
Urinary casts	9	20
Proteinuria trace or more	32	46

Note: 131 cases in each group matched by age, sex, race, and blood pressure. Only statistically significant differences are noted.
Reprinted with permission from Detection, evaluation, and treatment of renovascular hypertension: final report of the working group on renovascular hypertension. *Arch Intern Med* 1987;147:820—829.

ing those with (1) severe hypertension and either progressive renal insufficiency or lack of response to therapy, (2) accelerated or malignant hypertension, (3) grade 3 or 4 retinopathy, (4) hypertension with recent unexplained elevation of serum creatinine, (5) hypertension with elevation of serum creatinine reversibly induced by angiotensin-converting enzyme inhibitor, or (6) moderate or severe hypertension with asymmetrical renal size.

The workup of those with moderate risk such as those with refractory hypertension or moderate hypertension with a bruit or occlusive vascular disease elsewhere may require additional testing. Noninvasive tests may be helpful in this group if they identify patients for angiography.

The DRASTIC study is a large multicenter Dutch study looking at RVH.[10] Angiography was performed in those who did not respond to two-drug therapy in two months. Up to 25% of persistently hypertensive patients had RAS.[11] The investigators concluded that drug resistance is a simple and useful clinical criterion to identify patients for angiography. Furthermore, a calcium antagonist and a β blocker were a better combination to determine this than an ACE inhibitor/diuretic combination. It is not known how much RVH is present in the group that responded to drug therapy. Furthermore, a large number of patients, 35—49%, needed to go on to angiography and only one out of four angiograms demonstrated RAS.

Although clinical criteria may determine some characteristics that suggest RVH, using a noninvasive screening test to identify a subgroup with an even higher likelihood of a positive angiogram is another widely utilized strategy. No satisfactory outcome analysis studies evaluating the different strategies have been performed.

Noninvasive tests must be applied to a subset of hypertensives with a greater likelihood of RVH. No matter how accurate the noninvasive screening test is, it will be ineffective if it is used on an unselected population of hypertensives. For example, suppose a test is quite accurate — 100% sensitive and 95% specific. If this is applied to all hypertensives (3% incidence of RVH), the predictive value for RVH is only 6%. Only six of 100 angiograms will demonstrate RAS. If the population is preselected to have more RVH, the predictive value is higher. If applied to a population with 25% RVH "the test will have a predictive value of 87%, and will increase to 93% if 40% of patients have RVH. Indices of clinical suspicion are necessary to define a population that would reasonably benefit from screening.

The clinician's view about therapy also affects their workup. The results of revascularization are not entirely clearcut in favor of subjecting patients to this treatment. In the absence of consensus, the diagnostic workup and referrals for treatment vary. The arguments made for repair of RAS cite the potential for removing people from a lifetime dependency on medication and for stopping or slowing the development of renal failure and other complications of hypertension. The argument against repair cites the morbidity and mortality of the procedures, the absence of cure in some patients, the difficulty and expense of determining who actually has RVH, and the view that modern medical treatment may effectively reduce patient's long-term risks. Those who favor medical therapy may see no need to put patients through tests that will not alter their therapy. Those who favor revascularization are more aggressive in their efforts to detect RAS. Dean[12] has all operative candidates with diastolic blood pressure above 105 mm Hg evaluated for secondary hypertension.

Diagnostic Workup

Nonimaging Diagnostic Tests for RVH

Peripheral plasma renin activity and its evaluation after captopril (captopril test) are nonimaging screening tests used to determine whether hypertension is renin dependent. These tests do not localize the disease.

Vaughan's group advocates that all patients at high risk for RVH receive an ambulatory plasma renin activity level test[13] to determine the functional impact of an anatomical lesion that might be found. They find that low plasma renin activity levels are rare in untreated patients who do not have renal disease. The reported usefulness of plasma renin levels varies widely in other studies, probably due to such factors as patient preparation, medications, and assay techniques.[14, 15]

Another blood test is provocative testing with captopril to elicit a hyperreninemic response. A wide range of sensitivities (34—100%) and specificities (72—95%) has been reported.[11, 14, 15] To perform the test correctly patients should discontinue antihypertensive medications and have an adequate amount of salt intake. Renal insufficiency, bilateral disease, and restrictive conditions make the test difficult to perform correctly. Derkx et al. reported sensitivity of 84% and specificity of 93%, but the test was performed in the hospital.[11]

Renal vein determinations can be done with or without captopril stimulation. These invasive tests showed excellent results in early studies and results that are more modest on follow-up.[15]

Imaging Tests other than Ultrasonography

Scintigraphy

Captopril renal scintigraphy (CRS) is the most widely studied noninvasive imaging test for RVH. It is used in suspected RVH, not as a general screening study. Captopril inhibits angiotensin-converting enzyme, thereby blocking angiotensin II conversion. This, in turn, prevents postglomerular efferent arteriolar vasoconstriction and decreases the glomerular filtration rate (GFR) in the stenotic kidney. The contralateral normal kidney shows an increase in GFR. This disparity in renal function can be detected by scintigraphy. Most studies have used diethylenetriaminepentaacetic acid (DPTA), but some have also evaluated radiopharmaceuticals secreted by the tubules.

Prigent has pooled the results of several series of nuclear scans.[15] The sensitivity for RAS of this pooled data was 73% with specificity of 85% for evaluating differences between baseline and postcaptopril scans. If only the postcaptopril scans are used, the sensitivity rises to 85% and specificity becomes 83%. The value of captopril is questioned by other investigators.[11]

Pooled data also exist on how well captopril predicts a response to revascularization, and, therefore, RVH rather than RAS. Scintigraphy has a sensitivity of 76%, with a specificity of 92%, for the prediction of a cure or improvement.[15] If only postcaptopril scans are evaluated, then the test's ability to detect kidneys that will improve rises, but specificity drops off dramatically to a disappointing 66%.

Captopril renal scintigraphy is less accurate if patients have a small kidney. In the European multicenter trial,[16] abnormal renal function markedly diminished the test's specificity and accuracy (from 93% to 55% and 90% to 68%, respectively). When this trial removed the results of patients with small kidneys and abnormal renal function, the specificity for response to treatment rose from 82% to 100%.

Magnetic Resonance and Computed Tomography Angiography

Magnetic resonance (MR) angiography is being actively investigated as a means of diagnosing RAS.[17—29] A variety of tests are being evaluated, including time-of-flight and phase-contrast techniques (**Fig. 10–1**). Protocols using gadolinium enhancement are also being investigated. Gadolinium has the potential to speed the examination, improve spatial resolution and diminish artifacts. Results in the various studies have reported sensitivities from 92% to 100% with specificities of 71—96%.[18, 25, 29, 30] MR angiography misses accessory vessels. In one recent study, gadolinium enhancement did allow detection of more accessory vessels but did not improve upon the accuracy of the phase-contrast study for RAS detection.[18]

MR may also be used to evaluate some physiological aspects of RVH similar to nuclear scanning. Ros et al. is using the passage of gadopentetate dimeglumine to determine glomerular filtration rate.[31]

CT angiography using spiral CT is being evaluated for a variety of abdominal vascular diseases including RAS.[32—35] The spiral technique produces volumetric data that can produce three-dimensional reconstructions of arterial structures (**Fig. 10–2**). Thin-section axial scans can also be interpreted. A variety of reconstruction

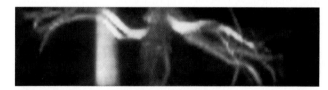

Figure 10–1   Three-dimensional recontruction of phase-contrast MR angiography of normal renal arteries.

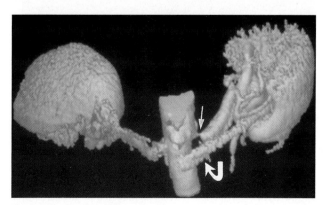

Figure 10–2   Three-dimensional reconstruction of CT angiogram of left RAS. Stenosis is at origin of left renal artery (**straight arrow**). Left renal vein (**curved arrow**) and normal right renal artery are also shown.

schemes are possible. With some thresholding techniques, stenoses may be misinterpreted.[36] The examination takes little time, and the collection of data is operator independent. Initial studies show sensitivity ranging from 88% to 98% with specificity from 94% to 98%.[32-34] Olbricht et al. found some loss of accuracy when there was impaired renal function but the numbers were too small for statistically evaluation.[34] Accessory vessels were missed if they were outside of the volume. A potential drawback to CT angiography is the requirement of a relatively large volume of iodinated contrast medium.

Both MR and CT angiography are promising techniques. Larger clinical trials and standardization of techniques (particularly for MR) are needed to determine their role. Their final place may also depend on outcome and economic issues as these are high-cost procedures.

Ultrasonography

Kidney atrophy and loss of mass over time are related to RAS.[37] In patients suspected of RVH, kidney size should be measured. In serial studies, it should be determined if there is a loss of renal mass. The demonstration of a small kidney is important because the shrunken kidney is unlikely to respond to revascularization. Testing should not spend much time on a small kidney but should concentrate on detecting a potentially curable lesion in the normal-sized kidney.

The role of Doppler ultrasound (US) in evaluating a patient for RAS is far from clear. While some investigators have shown superb results with Doppler US imaging, others have failed to duplicate these results. Successful groups and skeptics all agree the test is technically challenging. Investigations to diagnose Doppler examinations to diagnose RAS have fallen into two broad techniques: those that evaluate the renal arteries directly and those that evaluate the intrarenal vasculature.

Direct Doppler Evaluation of the Renal Artery

In this test, the renal artery is insonated along its course, and spectral Doppler tracings are obtained from the origin of the vessel to their entry into the kidney. Scanning is typically directed by color Doppler scanning (**Fig. 10–3**). For examination of the renal arteries, lower frequency transducers are often preferable, especially those at 2—2.5 MHz. Although resolution decreases with lower frequency transducers, attenuation also decreases, and this is the more critical factor. Filter settings should be set low, yet high enough to suppress peristalsis, noise, and respiratory movement.

The left renal artery is found behind the left renal vein. The right renal artery originates at a similar level, or it can be found behind the inferior vena cava. Although the vessels travel posteriorly, their origins are typically from the middle, or even the anterior third, of the aorta. In certain patients, a decubitus view is helpful to move bowel out of the way. One can detect the renal origins in a coronal plane (**Fig. 10–4**).

Localization of the site of RAS is based on the detection of a high-velocity jet at the stenosis (**Fig. 10–5**). The velocity is maximal at the site of the tightest stenosis. Distal to the jet, secondary flow disturbances may exist. These include spectral broadening, shift of the distribution of blood velocities toward the baseline and away from the envelope and simultaneous forward and reverse flow (**Fig. 10–6**). Velocities downstream from the stenotic jet are diminished. In some patients a bruit may be seen or heard. It appears on the spectrum as a low velocity signal which is symmetrically above and below the baseline (**Fig. 10–7** through **10–8**). Color Doppler may demonstrate a bruit as random color appearing in the adjacent soft tissues. Spectral or color bruits are usually detected in systole.

Color Doppler flow imaging can help detect stenoses as well as show the course of the vessels. Stenoses may be

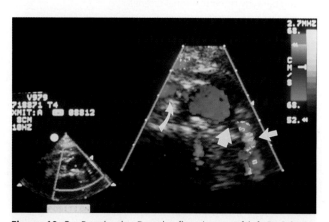

Figure 10–3 Renal color Doppler flow image of left RAS (same case as Fig. 10–2) shows marked narrowing of origin of the left renal artery (**thick straight arrow**). Red in the left renal artery, just after color is detected, represents aliasing (**thin straight arrow**). Normal right renal artery is also noted (**curved arrow**).

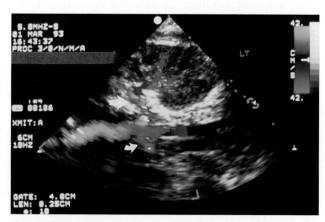

Figure 10–4 Coronal color Doppler flow image of renal artery origins. Left renal artery (**straight arrow**) can be traced in its entirety into the kidney. Proximal right renal artery (**curved arrow**) can also be seen.

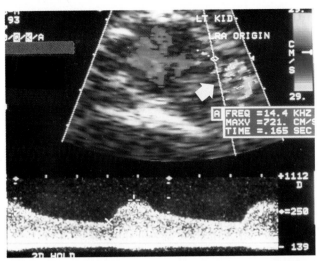

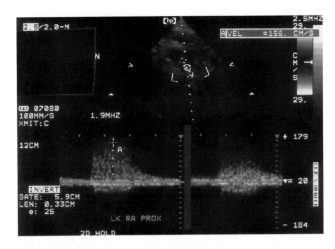

Figure 10–5   Left RAS. Spectral color Doppler flow image shows marked narrowing of color column at origin of left renal artery. Sample volume within the narrowing yields a peak systolic velocity of 721 cm/s. Poststenotic dilatation (**arrow**) is seen distal to the narrowing. Note mosaic pattern, a mixture of colors in poststenotic regions that indicates aliasing.

Figure 10–6   Spectral duplex Doppler image demonstrates downstream flow disturbances distal to a site of RAS. Edge of the waveform is poorly seen. Whiter shades near the baseline indicate that more blood is moving at the lower velocities. Many different velocities are represented, which produces spectral broadening. Note simultaneous forward and reverse flow, probably the result of vortices and flow in many directions.

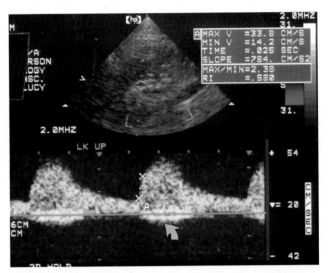

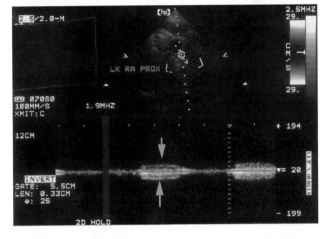

Figure 10–7   Spectral duplex Doppler intrarenal waveform with bruit. A strong, low-frequency symmetric signal above and below the baseline indicates a bruit (**arrow**). The bruit is pansystolic. Early systolic acceleration is measured as the slope in the fastest accelerating part of systole. Its value is 7.8 m/s². It is not measured to the peak systolic frequency, which occurs later in systole.

Figure 10–8   Spectral duplex Doppler image demonstrates bruit. Because bruits (**arrows**) travel through tissue, they can be detected even where no blood is flowing, as in this case. Bruits detected with Doppler imaging may not necessarily be auscultated and vice versa.

seen as narrowing of the color lumen (**Fig. 10–3, 10–5**). Poststenotic dilatation may also be appreciated (**Fig. 10–5**). The edge of the color does not exactly correspond to the edge of the flow since it may over- or under estimate the lumen, depending on the unit settings. The high-velocity jet is seen as a change in color that reflects the change in velocity. The jet could be seen to a different intensity of the same color but more frequently, it is seen as aliased color. Aliasing is produced by an inadequate sampling rate for the velocity that is being sampled. Color aliasing may be seen in a variety of ways: it may

appear as a region where flow appears reversed (**Fig. 10–3**), as bands of color changes (an onion skin appearance), or as a wilder "mosaic" a pattern (**Fig. 10–5**).

Because the normal renal artery has no fixed velocity, many investigators have chosen to compare the velocity of the jet to that of the aorta where the renal arteries originate. The diagnosis of RAS is made when the value of the "renal—aortic ratio" is elevated. The ratio is calculated by dividing the highest velocity obtained in the renal artery jet by the peak systolic velocity (PSV) of the aorta. A ratio over 3.5 has been correlated to RAS above

60% diameter reduction.[38—40] Other studies have looked at absolute velocities in the renal artery jet. Although earlier studies used lower values,[41] studies that are more recent consider values exceeding 180 as abnormal[42] and exceeding 200 cm/s as indicating a stenosis greater than 60%.[39]

In an early prospective evaluation of US duplex scanning of the main renal artery duplex scanning, Taylor et al.[38] found a sensitivity of 84%, specificity of 97%, and positive predictive value of 94%. Twelve percent of the scans were technically inadequate.

Olin et al.[39] reported detection of 98% of stenoses and occlusions (31/32 cases with stenoses of 60% to 79%, 67/69 cases with stenoses of 80% to 99%, and 22/23 cases with occlusions). Specificity was 99%. One hour was allowed for the studies that were performed by vascular technologists. Because only main renal arteries were reported, the analysis did not evaluate any accessory renal vessels.

Hoffman et al.[42] had a 10% failure rate. In this study sensitivity was 92% (44 of 48 cases with stenoses) but the specificity was only 62% for 60% stenoses. Ten of 11 patients with occlusions were correctly identified.

Hansen et al.[43] showed excellent results for cases where there was one renal artery (sensitivity 93%, specificity 98%). However, only 49% of accessory vessels were detected. When all kidneys were considered, the resultant sensitivity was 88%.

Halpern et al.[44] used similar techniques and employed experienced vascular technologists, taking as long as necessary to produce an examination. The sensitivity for the renal—aortic ratio was 71% with a specificity of 91%. This is also identical to the results of Krumme et al.[45] who showed 71% sensitivity and 96% specificity for abnormal PSV greater than 200 cm/s.

Spies et al.[46] evaluated 135 consecutive patients using color duplex sonography. Although they had trouble identifying all segments of the renal arteries, in those with adequate scans (75% of patients, 195 arteries), the sensitivity was 93% and specificity 92%. All 12 stenosis above 75% were detected, although one was considered a 50% to 74% stenosis.

Scanning the main renal artery is time consuming and does not reliably detect accessory vessels. Technical failure continues to be a problem because bowel gas can obscure the vessels. An overnight fast and bowel prep can help minimize this.[43]

Van de Hulst et al.[47] validated the use of PSV and renal artery ratios for RAS. Using a Doppler guidewire, this group compared the renal artery parameters to hemodynamically significant RAS as determined by transstenotic pressure gradients in 30 vessels. This group determined that PSV and velocity ratios did correlate with RAS. Furthermore, the receiver operating characteristic curves produced by absolute velocity measurements were equal to those generated by digital subtraction angiography.

Intrarenal Artery Evaluation

Handa et al.[48, 49] described abnormal waveforms in vessels downstream from renal stenoses. His group described a series of indices using frequency: the acceleration index, acceleration time, and a comparison of acceleration time in the renal artery compared to the aorta. Several years later Martin et al.[50] described successful results with a flank rather than translumbar approach. This Australian group described the initial systolic (the so-called *compliance*) peak but did not use its appearance to make a diagnosis. The work of Stavros et al.[51] resulted in more widespread interest in the technique in the United States. Several European groups were also pursuing intrarenal evaluation at that time.[52—54]

Normal intrarenal signals show a rapid rise during early systole and continuous flow through diastole (**Fig. 10–9** through **10–10**). To be accurate when one measures intrarenal waveforms, the scale should be diminished so the waveform fills the spectrum. The sweep rate should be fast so only one or two waveforms are in the image. Measurement errors are reduced if the size of the spectral display is larger. The highest frequency transducer that can give an adequate signal is used, preferably 3—5 MHz. Position and Doppler settings should be optimized to maximize signal to noise. The Doppler angle should be minimized. Doppler parameters such as acceleration are angle-dependent because they require velocity measurements. One should attempt along the plane of the intrarenal arteries, and angles should be routinely less than 30 degrees.

Intrarenal waveforms are taken from the hilus and from segmental waveforms from the upper, middle, and lower kidney (**Fig. 10–9**). Interlobar or interlobular arteries can be used,[55] although it is not known if the same normal values will apply because waveform shapes can vary along the vessels.[56]. Differences in the appearance between segmental waveforms may indicate stenosis of an accessory artery supplying the abnormal segment.[55, 57]

In distinction to the main renal artery test, which may take an hour or more, intrarenal scanning usually takes around 20 min. Technical failures rarely occur because the kidney can usually be insonated. Martin et al.[50] reported a failure rate of 1.5%, although a recent investigation had a 16% failure rate.[58] Patient's inability to hold their breath is the most common cause of technical difficulties. A small kidney or poor flow caused by severe occlusive disease are other causes.

In stenosis, there is a slow rise to the peak velocity distal to the stenosis, the so-called *pulsus tardus*. The slope (which is the systolic acceleration) of the systolic rise is diminished and the time to the first peak velocity is lengthened (diminished acceleration time) (**Fig. 10–10** through **10–11**). The arterial stenosis "filters" the normally complex arterial pulse. In early systole, this filtering accounts for diminished acceleration. The stenosis evens out the changes between systole and diastole and produces diminished pulsatility. In extreme cases, pulsatility is so diminished the artery may resemble a vein (**Fig. 10–12**).

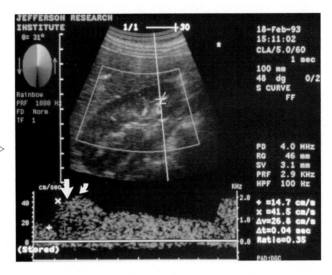

Figure 10–9 Normal intrarenal spectral Doppler waveform. The ▷ spectrum has been optimized so that one waveform fills the whole spectrum. Sweep speed is rapid so only one complete cardiac cycle is displayed. Doppler angle is determined by direction of blood flow on the color image. The angle of 31 degrees is acceptably low. Early systolic acceleration is the slope from the + marker to the x marker. In early systole, the fast-moving flow hesitates (**straight arrow**), slows down, then speeds up to peak systole (**curved arrow**). The acute angle at the hesitation marks the early systolic compliance peak/reflective wave complex (ESP).

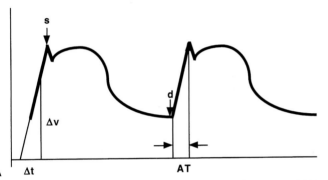

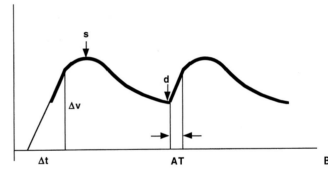

Figure 10–10 Intrarenal waveform parameters in a normal (**A**) and abnormal (**B**) waveform. Early systolic acceleration is the slope of the fastest moving portion of the systolic component (v/t). It is not the slope of the waveform to peak systole (s) unless there is one continuous straight line to peak systole [as is the case in waveform (**B**) but not waveform (**A**)]. Acceleration time (AT) is the time it takes to get to the first inflection of the waveform (**between two arrows**). In the normal case (**A**) this is the time to peak systole. In the abnormal waveform (**B**) this is the time to the first inflection which occurs earlier than peak systole. The early systolic compliance peak/reflective wave complex (ESP) is identified in waveform (**A**) at the acute angle in the waveform just after the first peak (s). The ESP is not present in waveform (**B**). Resistance index is calculated by the (peak systolic velocity — end diastolic velocity)/peak systolic velocity or (s-d)/s. The pulsatility index uses the mean velocity (not shown) as the denominator.

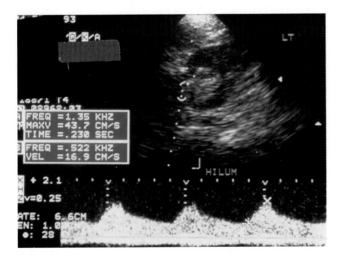

Figure 10–11 Abnormal intrarenal hilar spectral Doppler waveform. The slope of systolic acceleration is diminished, and the time to peak systole is prolonged (0.23 s), indicating proximal stenosis.

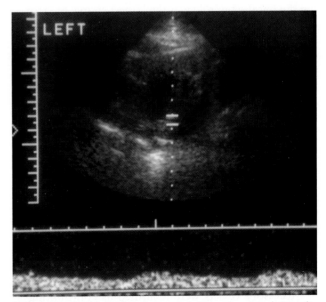

Figure 10–12 Markedly abnormal intrarenal spectral Doppler waveform shows greatly diminished systolic acceleration. Pulsatility is markedly low, to the extent that the artery might be mistaken for a vein. Note loss of the ESP.

Martin et al. et al.[50, 51] described a normal early systolic compliance peak (ESP) which is an acute angle formed after the early systolic rise (**Fig. 10–9,10–10**). ESP was associated with normal upstream vessels and was lost if there was proximal RAS. Halpern et al. evaluated this phenomenon with a phantom.[56] Their results suggest the early peak is caused by transmitted systole. Following this the blood slows and may speed up again. It is this region, in the later part of systole, which is the produced by compliance. Furthermore, phantom studies suggested that changes in compliance could significantly affect the appearance of renal waveforms.[56, 59]

In Martin's study, acceleration time and acceleration index were 87% sensitive and 98% specific.[50] Stavros et al.[51] found the acceleration time to be only 78% sensitive and 94% specific, and the acceleration index to be 89% sensitive and 83% specific. Kliewer et al.[60] found that the acceleration time and index distinguished normal from abnormal vessels only when the stenosis was severe (80—95%) but not when all the stenoses above 50% were considered. The result is not entirely unexpected as 50% diameter-reducing lesions are not hemodynamically significant in the kidneys. Higher-grade lesions of 60% to 75% may actually be necessary to produce downstream changes.[55, 61, 62]

Halpern et al.[44] found the best intrarenal test to be early systolic acceleration, which is the slope of the fastest moving part of the early waveform. Early systolic acceleration is not always the slope to the PSV (**Fig. 10–7, 10–10**). Values of less than 3 m/s^2 were considered abnormal. Minimum early systolic acceleration had 86% sensitivity and 91% specificity. Halpern et al.[44] concluded that a slope was better than acceleration time because the onset of acceleration is not precisely defined. Gottlieb et al.[63] also determined that difficulty determining the onset of systole was the largest source of error in intrarenal measurements.

Stavros et al.[51] found that a visual estimate of an abnormal waveform, as determined by the loss of the ESP, was better than any calculated measure. This loss had a sensitivity of 95% and a specificity of 97%. Because recognition of ESP is a visual parameter that describes the waveform shape, it does not require any calculation. Visual estimates of waveform shape were unsuccessful in the study by Halpern et al.,[44] with the exception of a truly blunted waveform, which had a specificity of 100%. Kliewer et al.[64] also found the interpretation of waveform morphology to be unsuccessful in predicting the presence or severity of RAS. However, in another study using pattern recognition before and after captopril, Rene et al.[65] found this technique useful after captopril. Pattern recognition was only 68% sensitive at baseline, but rose to 100% after captopril.

Accessory vessels were identified as contributing to the misses in several of the studies.[50, 60, 66] Increased pulsatility in renal vessels are also associated with missed diagnosis[50, 55, 67] which may be due to diminished compliance or elevated resistance.[59]

Pulsatility parameters evaluate the shape of a Doppler waveform by evaluating the relationship between peak systolic velocity and end diastolic velocity. Two common indices are the pulsatility index (PI) which is (peak systolic velocity — end diastolic velocity)/mean velocity and the resistance index (RI) which is (peak systolic velocity — end diastolic velocity)/end diastolic velocity.

Soulen et al.[68] showed that the intrarenal RI changed significantly from baseline following angioplasty. Ozbek et al.[54] showed there were significant differences in PI and RI between normal kidneys and those with RAS. Bardelli et al.[52] used side to side PI differences to diagnose unilateral RAS. In initial trials, Schwerk et al.[69] determined that a difference of the RI of greater than 5% between the kidneys was 82% sensitive and 92% specific for RAS greater than 50% and 100% sensitive and 94% specific for stenoses greater than 60% diameter reduction. The group conceded the test might not be as good for bilateral stenoses, and they recommended considering bilaterally low indices as suggesting bilateral RAS.

Follow-up studies using pulsatility have not been as encouraging. Burdick et al.[70] evaluated acceleration, acceleration time, PI, RI, and side to side differences of PI and RI. This group found acceleration and acceleration time to be superior to any of the pulsatility parameters. Side to side RI differences were only 73% sensitive and 86% specific. Bilateral disease accounted for some of the errors in using RI or PI. Acceleration time was significantly correlated with the degree of narrowing while RI and PI correlated with age rather than RAS. Both acceleration time and pulsatility worked better in those with fibromuscular dysplasia than atherosclerosis. The authors postulated that changes in pulsatility due to age and atherosclerosis reduced the accuracy of the pulsatility parameters. This was probably due to resistance and compliance differences in the older, stiffer vessels. Pedersen et al.[71] found a kidney length difference of 1 cm or a PI difference of greater than 0.1 to be only 75% sensitive and 76% specific for stenoses above 50% and 84% sensitive and 73% specific for stenoses above 70%. Krumme et al.[45] had a sensitivity of only 51% for bilateral stenosis.

Baseline pulsatility parameters have not always correlated with blood pressure response or RVH. Although Frauchiger et al.[72] showed intervention was less successful if diastole was less than 30% of systole, Hansen et al.[43] did not find a relationship between end diastolic values and the response of blood pressure or renal function to revascularization. Krumme et al.[45] was also unable to show a relationship between preoperative side to side differences of RI and blood pressure response after successful treatment.

Pulsatility parameters do change after successful revascularization for RVH.[54, 55, 68] Further studies will be necessary to determine if these intrarenal indices can be used to follow patients after revascularization.[66]

Renal Artery or Intrarenal Artery Evaluation

Van der Hulst et al.[47] seriously challenged the validity of all the intrarenal Doppler analysis. In his study using pressure gradients as a gold standard, no intrarenal parameter (acceleration time, acceleration, RI, PI, or loss of ESP) correlated with the presence of RAS. His group also found that the receiver operating characteristic curve of PSV is equal to angiography. This indicates that the direct renal artery study is potentially as accurate as an angiogram. However, in the real world transabdominal scanning is not as accurate as the Doppler guidewire. The changing Doppler angle, bowel gas, deep position, and diminished signal from flow-reducing lesions all contribute to transabdominal inaccuracies and technical failures.

It is the technical difficulties encountered in certain patients rather than the interpretation of the test that makes direct renal artery duplex difficult. The criteria of a renal—aortic ratio above 3.5 or a PSV of greater than 180—200 cm/s is reproducible. In technically adequate examinations, renal artery duplex scanning can reliably detect and exclude main renal artery stenosis. An adequate amount of time must be allowed to perform the study. The experience of the sonographer or vascular technologist is crucial; the more experienced sonographer will make fewer mistakes and produce fewer inadequate examinations. An experienced examiner will also be able to determine if the study is reliable or limited. When color or spectral Doppler evaluation does not demonstrate substantial portions of the renal arteries, the results should be reported as less reliable unless there is unequivocal evidence for RAS in the region seen. Those with limited examinations may need additional testing with another modality.

Intrarenal Doppler parameters are easier to produce but their significance is more difficult to interpret. The degree of stenosis,[61] etiology of the lesion,[45] resistance and compliance,[56,59] age of the patient, presence of parenchymal disease,[55] and the arterial pressure[53] all affect the final waveform shape. It is unknown if medical therapy itself affects waveform shape. Severe stenoses are correlated with the intrarenal indices but less severe stenoses are not. Some investigators feel this is because those lesser stenoses are not hemodynamically significant based on some experimental data.[55] The results of van der Hulst, which used a gold standard in human arteries, appear to refute this concept.[47]

The slope of the early systolic acceleration is more reproducible than acceleration time.[44,63] Acceleration and acceleration time are less accurate in pulsatile renal arteries, presumably due to intrinsic renal disease. Determining if there is loss of ESP is operator dependent[55] and not reproducible.[44,60,64,73] Pulsatility parameters are not accurate enough and miss many bilateral stenoses.

A very blunted waveform[44] or a very long acceleration time (above 0.12 s)[58] have a high predictive value for RAS. Intrarenal waveform analysis is most predictive when the waveforms are very abnormal. Normal intrarenal waveforms and mildly abnormal measurements are less reliable. Direct renal artery evaluation should be performed if there are equivocal intrarenal results. This is particularly true if there is diminished diastolic flow.

Future research efforts should be made to make direct renal evaluation simpler and diminish the number of inadequate studies. It is hoped that by increasing the signal from the blood, intravenous microbubble contrast agents can improve the accuracy of renal Doppler. In two initial studies of direct renal artery evaluation,[74] and intrarenal evaluation,[67] contrast enhancement improved the results and shortened the examination time.

The etiology of suspected RAS helps determine if Doppler should be performed and how it should be interpreted. Direct renal artery duplex scanning detects RAS in large, typically main vessels. Accessory vessels are routinely missed.[27,42,43,46,75,76] This may be less important in atherosclerotic patients, as some investigators feel renal artery stenosis in small accessory vessels rarely cause hypertension in this group.[75] Fibromuscular dysplasia is different — patients may have RVH from main or intrarenal stenoses. In those suspected of fibromuscular dysplasia, the significance of a normal Doppler study is not reassuring because accessory and branch disease may be missed. Patients with suspected fibromuscular dysplasia might require angiography as angiography is currently the only examination that has the resolution to evaluate intrarenal stenoses well.

Other Causes of Abdominal Bruit

Significant stenoses in any vessel may produce a bruit. In the abdomen, common locations for occlusive disease are the celiac axis and superior mesenteric artery. In patients who present with a bruit, and in whom the renal arteries are not stenotic, evaluating the celiac axis and superior mesenteric artery may be worthwhile to determine if they are stenosed (**Fig. 10–13**). Bruits from stenoses in the iliac artery are heard lower in the abdomen than the bruit from upper abdominal vessels. Bruits from arteriovenous fistulas usually have a continuous quality. Epigastric bruits are more common from the celiac axis or SMA while flank bruits are more typical for a renal origin.

Renal arteriovenous fistulas (**Fig. 10–14**) are associated with bruits.[6] They often appear as a cystic mass, typically in a hilar location. Color flow imaging demonstrates flow in these lesions. Arteriovenous fistulas have a typical high-velocity spectral waveform with low pulsatility. Fistulas are often congenital, although they are found in renal carcinoma and after trauma. Parenchymal arteriovenous fistulas may be seen after kidney biopsy.

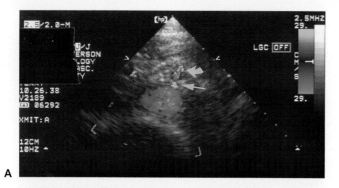

A

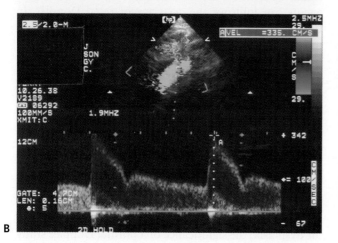

B

Figure 10–13 Celiac axis stenosis producing abdominal bruit. Patient had a bruit, and a diagnosis of RAS had been ruled out. (**A**) Color Doppler flow image shows celiac stenosis with narrowing of color column immediately after the celiac origin (**straight arrow**). Distal to the stenosis, a mosaic pattern of color can be seen (**curved arrow**), which represents aliasing. (**B**) Spectral Doppler image shows celiac stenosis with high-velocity jet (335 cm/s) at origin of the celiac axis. Jet has a well-defined envelope and no spectral broadening because jets have laminar flow. A second, smaller waveform, superimposed on the celiac waveform, is the aortic signal, which is partially in the sample volume. (**C**) Spectral Doppler image shows celiac stenosis with bruit. Downstream from the jet, the velocity diminishes (238 cm/s). Note the spectral broadening. Systolic bruit is shown (**arrow**) as a symmetrical, low-velocity waveform above and below the baseline.

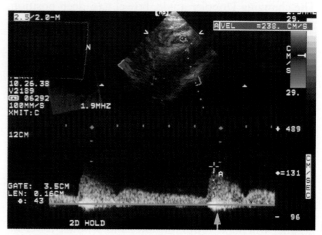

C

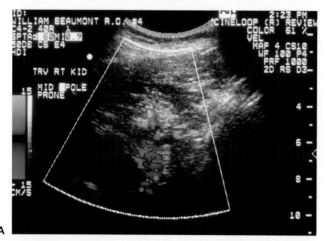

A

Figure 10–14 Renal arteriovenous fistula. (**A**) Transverse color Doppler flow image of the right renal hilum shows a large area of color not conforming to normal vessels indicating a vascular malformation.

Mid-aortic syndrome may cause hypertension and bruit. In this case, the aorta is narrowed, possibly affecting the renal, celiac, or superior mesenteric arteries. More commonly the aorta alone is narrowed. Because the renal arteries are downstream from the stenosis, their waveforms are abnormal showing diminished pulsatility and systolic upstroke. A jet may be identified in the aorta at the site of the narrowing. Distal flow disturbances such as spectral broadening can be identified in the aorta beyond the narrowing.

Summary

Although clinicians can identify some patients at greater risk for RVH, there is no consensus on whom should be tested. A noninvasive test cannot be applied to all hypertensives. Rather, clinical criteria should establish a subgroup of patients with a high prevalence of RVH. Part of the reluctance to study patients results from the lack of well-defined criteria to define who will benefit from revascularization and the lack of a clearly effective screening test. Angiography is the standard, but it is invasive and carries some risk. Nuclear scanning after captopril has some appeal for it reflects the pathophysiology of RAS. However, the ability of scintig-

Figure 10–14 (**B**) Spectral Doppler image shows an increased velocity and markedly increased diastolic velocity indicating diminished pulsatility from arteriovenous shunting. Systolic acceleration is normal and there is spectral broadening. A continuous bruit can be seen as a symmetrical, low-velocity waveform above and below the baseline (**arrow**). Flow below the baseline is renal vein in the early portion of the spectrum (**thick arrow**) and disturbed flow in the later portion. (**open arrow**). Case courtesy of Beatrice Madrazo, M.D., William Beaumont Hospital, Royal Oak, MI.

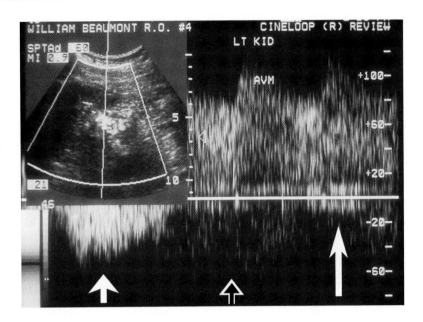

raphy to predict the outcome after revascularization is not as good as might be expected. Nuclear scanning is not warranted if there is renal insufficiency or a small kidney.

US studies show wide variations. Although there are technical failures, direct evaluation is generally accurate if the technical quality of the study is adequate. Intrarenal waveform analysis has not been the panacea it was hoped to be.

MR and CT angiography are more accurate than nuclear medicine or US, however, not all patients are candidates for these tests for reasons such as renal insufficiency, claustrophobia, or allergy. Technical failures also occur with these tests, and they are far more expensive than ultrasound.

Outcome analyses incorporating the accuracy, cost, technical success, and complication rates are not available and need to be performed. Various diagnostic pathways should be evaluated including proceeding straight to angiography, directly to CT or MR angiography, and using US. Decision analyses should not simply use positive and negative results but should evaluate technically limited studies to determine how they might be handled.

In high-risk groups, it may not be appropriate to use a screening test. In some patients, for instance, those with suspected fibromuscular dysplasia and normal renal function, it is appropriate to go directly to angiography.

References

1. Schreiber MJ, Pohl MA, Novick AC. The natural history of atherosclerotic and fibrous renal artery disease. *Urol Clin North Am* 1984;11:383—392.
2. Meyrier A. Renal vascular lesions in the elderly: nephrosclerosis or atheromatous renal disease? *Nephrology, Dialysis, Transplantation* 1996;11(Suppl 9):45—52.
3. O'Neil EA, Hansen KJ, Canzanello VJ, Pennell TC, Dean RH. Prevalence of ischemic nephropathy in patients with renal insufficiency. *Am Surg* 1992;58(8):485—490.
4. Palmaz JC. The current status of vascular intervention in ischemic nephropathy. *JVIR* 1998;9:539—543.
5. Goldblatt H, Lynch J, Hanzal RF, Summerville WW. Studies on experimental hypertension. I. The production of persistent elevation of systolic blood pressure by means of renal ischemia. *J Exp Med* 1934;59:347—378.
6. Van Way CW. Renal artery aneurysms and arteriovenous fistulas. In: Rutherford RB, ed. *Vascular Surgery,*. 4th ed. Philadelphia: W.B. Saunders Company, 1995, p. 1274—1286.
7. Mann S, Pickering T. Detection of renovascular hypertension. State of the art: 1992. *Ann Intern Med* 1992;117(10):845—853.
8. Detection, evaluation, and treatment of renovascular hypertension: final report of the working group on renovascular hypertension. *Arch Intern Med* 1987;147:820—829.
9. Simon N, Franklin SS, Bleifer KH, Maxwell MH. Clincal characteristics of renovascular hypertension. *JAMA* 1972;220(9):1209—1218.
10. van Jaarsveld BC, Derkx FH, Krijnen P, et al. Hypertension resistant to two-drug treatment is a useful criterion to select patients for angiography: the Dutch Renal Artery Stenosis Intervention Cooperative (DRASTIC) study. *Contrib Nephrol* 1996;119:54—58.
11. Derkx FH, van Jaarsveld BC, Krijnen P, et al. Renal artery stenosis towards the year 2000. *J Hypertens* Supplement 1996;14(5):S167—72.
12. Dean RH. Renovascular hypertension: an overview. In: Rutherford RB, ed. *Vascular Surgery*, 4th ed. Philadelphia: W.B. Saunders Company, 1995, p. 1371—1377.
13. Vaughan ED. Pathophysiology of renovascular hypertension. In: Rutherford RB, ed. *Vascular Surgery*, 4th ed. Philadelphia: W.B. Saunders Company, 1995, p. 1377—1390.

14. Nally JV. Provocative captopril testing in the diagnosis of renovascular hypertension. *Urol Clin North Am* 1994;21(2):227—234.

15. Prigent A. The diagnosis of renovascular hypertension: the role of captopril renal scintigraphy and related issues [see comments]. *Eur J Nucl Med* 1993;20(7):625—644.

16. Fommei E, Ghione S, Hilson AJ, et al. Captopril radionuclide test in renovascular hypertension: a European multicentre study. European Multicentre Study Group. *Eur J Nucl Med* 1993;20(7):617—23.

17. Borrello JA, Li D, Vesely TM, et al. Renal arteries: clinical comparison of three-dimensional time-of-flight MR angiographic sequences and radiographic angiography. *Radiology* 1995;197(3):793—799.

18. De Cobelli F, Mellone R, Salvioni M, et al. Renal artery stenosis: value of screening with three-dimensional phase-contrast MR angiography with a phased-array multicoil. *Radiology* 1996;201(3):697—703.

19. Debatin JF, Spritzer CE, Grist TM, et al. Imaging of the renal arteries: value of MR angiography. *AJR* 1991;157:981—990.

20. Gedroyc WM, Neerhut P, Negus R, et al. Magnetic resonance angiography of renal artery stenosis. *Clin Radiol* 1995;50(7):436—439.

21. Loubeyre P, Revel D, Garcia P, et al. Screening patients for renal artery stenosis: value of three-dimensional time-of-flight MR angiography. *AJR* 1994;162(4):847—852.

22. Kim D, Edelman RR, Kent KC, Porter DH, Skillman JJ. Abdominal aorta and renal artery stenosis: evaluation with MR angiography. *Radiology* 1990;174:727—731.

23. Kent KC, Edelman RR, Kim D, et al. Magnetic resonance imaging: a reliable test for the evaluation of proximal atherosclerotic renal arterial stenosis. *J Vasc Surg* 1991;13(2):311—318.

24. Postma CT, Hartog O, Rosenbusch G, Thien T. Magnetic resonance angiography in the diagnosis of renal artery stenosis. *J Hypertens* Suppl 1993.

25. Rieumont MJ, Kaufman JA, Geller SC, et al. Evaluation of renal artery stenosis with dynamic gadolinium-enhanced MR angiography. *AJR* 1997;169(1):39—44.

26. Servois V, Laissy JP, Feger C, et al. Two-dimensional time-of-flight magnetic resonance angiography of renal arteries without maximum intensity projection: a prospective comparison with angiography in 21 patients screened for renovascular hypertension. *Cardiovasc Intervent Radiol* 1994;17(3):138—142.

27. Strotzer M, Fellner CM, Geissler A, et al. Noninvasive assessment of renal artery stenosis. A comparison of MR angiography, color Doppler sonography, and intraarterial angiography. *Acta Radiol* 1995;36(3):243—247.

28. Yucel EK, Kaufman JA, Prince M, et al. Time of flight renal MR angiography: utility in patients with renal insufficiency. *Magn Reson Imag* 1993;11(7):925—930.

29. Bakker J, Beek FJ, Beutler JJ, et al. Renal artery stenosis and accessory renal arteries: accuracy of detection and visualization with gadolinium-enhanced breath-hold MR angiography. *Radiology* 1998;207(2):497—504.

30. Postma CT, Joosten FB, Rosenbusch G, Thien T. Magnetic resonance angiography has a high reliability in the detection of renal artery stenosis. *Am J Hypertens* 1997;10(9 Pt 1):957—963.

31. Ros PR, Gauger J, Stoupis C, et al. Diagnosis of renal artery stenosis: feasibility of combining MR angiography, MR renography, and gadopentetate-based measurements of glomerular filtration rate. *AJR* 1995;165(6):1447—1451.

32. Kaatee R, Beek FJA, de Lange EE, et al. Renal artery stenosis: detection and quantification with spiral CT angiography versus optimized digital subtraction angiography. *Radiology* 1997;205:121—127.

33. Elkohen M, Beregi JP, Deklunder G, et al. A prospective study of helical computed tomography angiography versus angiography for the detection of renal artery stenoses in hypertensive patients. *J Hypertens* 1996;14(4):525—528.

34. Olbricht CJ, Paul K, Prokop M, et al. Minimally invasive diagnosis of renal artery stenosis by spiral computed tomography angiography. *Kidney Int* 1995;48(4):1332—1337.

35. Zeman RK, Fox SH, Silverman PM, et al. Helical (Spiral) CT of the Abdomen. *AJR* 1993;160:719—725.

36. Halpern EJ, Wechsler RJ, DiCampli D. Threshold selection for CT angiography shaded surface display of the renal arteries. *J Digit Imag* 1995;8(3):142—147.

37. Guzman RP, Zierler RE, Isaacson JA, Bergelin RO, Strandness DJ. Renal atrophy and arterial stenosis. A prospective study with duplex ultrasound. *Hypertension* 1994;23(3):346—350.

38. Taylor DC, Kettler MD, Moneta GL, et al. Duplex ultrasound scanning in the diagnosis of renal artery stenosis: a prospective evaluation. *J Vasc Surg* 1988;7:363—369.

39. Olin JW, Piedmonte MR, Young JR, et al. The utility of duplex ultrasound scanning of the renal arteries for diagnosing significant renal artery stenosis. *Ann Intern Med* 1995;122(11):833—838.

40. Kohler TR, Zierler RE, Martin RL, et al. Noninvasive diagnosis of renal artery stenosis by ultrasonic duplex scanning. *J Vasc Surg* 1986;4(5):450—456.

41. Desberg AL, Paushter DM, Lammert GK, et al. Renal artery stenosis: evaluation with color Doppler flow imaging. *Radiology* 1990;177(3):749—753.

42. Hoffmann U, Edwards JM, Carter S, et al. Role of duplex scanning for the detection of atherosclerotic renal artery disease. *Kidney Int* 1991;39(6):1232—1239.

43. Hansen KJ, Tribble RW, Reavis SW, et al. Renal duplex sonography: evaluation of clinical utility. *J Vasc Surg* 1990;12:227—236.

44. Halpern EJ, Needleman L, Nack TL, East SA. Renal artery stenosis: should we study the main renal artery or segmental vessels? *Radiology* 1995;195(3):799—804.

45. Krumme B, Blum U, Schwertfeger E, et al. Diagnosis of renovascular disease by intra- and extrarenal Doppler scanning. *Kidney Int* 1996;50(4):1288—1292.

46. Spies KP, Fobbe F, El-Bedewi M, et al. Color-coded duplex sonography for noninvasive diagnosis and grading of renal artery stenosis. *Am J Hypertens* 1995;8(12 Pt 1):1222—1231.

47. van der Hulst VP, van Baalen J, Kool LS, et al. Renal artery stenosis: endovascular flow wire study for validation of Doppler US [see comments]. *Radiology* 1996;200(1):165—168.

48. Handa N, Fukanaga R, Etani H, et al. Efficacy of echo-Doppler examination for the evaluation of renovascular disease. *Ultrasound Med Biol* 1988;14:1—15.

49. Handa N, Fukanaga R, Uehara A, et al. Echo-Doppler velocimeter in the diagnosis of hypertensive patients: the renal artery Doppler technique. *Ultrasound Med Biol* 1986;12:945—952.

50. Martin RL, Nanra RS, Wlodarczyk J, DeSilva A, Bray AE. Renal hilar Doppler analysis in the detection of renal artery stenosis. *J Vasc Tech* 1991;15(4):173—180.

51. Stavros AT, Parker SH, Yakes WF, et al. Segmental stenosis of the renal artery: pattern recognition of tardus and parvus abnormalities with duplex sonography [see comments]. *Radiology* 1992;184(2):487—492.

52. Bardelli M, Jensen G, Volkmann R, Aurell M. Non-invasive ultrasound assessment of renal artery stenosis by means of the Gosling pulsatility index. *J Hypertens* 1992;10(9):985—989.

53. Veglio F, Provera E, Pinna G, et al. Renal resistive index after captopril test by echo-Doppler in essential hypertension [see comments]. *Am J Hypertens* 1992;5(7):431—436.

54. Ozbek SS, Aytac SK, Erden MI, Sanlidilek NU. Intrarenal

Doppler findings of upstream renal artery stenosis: a preliminary report. *Ultrasound Med Biol* 1993;19(1):3—12.

55. Stavros T, Harshfield D. Renal Doppler: renal artery stenosis, and renovascular hypertension: direct and indirect duplex sonographic abnormalities in patients with renal artery stenosis. *Ultrasound Quart* 1994;12(4):217—263.

56. Halpern EJ, Deane CR, Needleman L, Merton DA, East SA. Normal renal artery spectral Doppler waveform: a closer look. *Radiology* 1995;196(3):667—673.

57. Hall NJ, Thorpe RJ, MacKechnie SG. Stenosis of the accessory renal artery: Doppler ultrasound findings. *Australas Radiol* 1995;39(1):73—77.

58. Baxter GM, Aitchison F, Sheppard D, et al. Colour Doppler ultrasound in renal artery stenosis: intrarenal waveform analysis. *Br J Radiol* 1996;69(825):810—815.

59. Bude RO, Rubin JM, Platt JF, Fechner KP, Adler RS. Pulsus tardus: its cause and potential limitations in detection of arterial stenosis. *Radiology* 1994;190(3):779—784.

60. Kliewer MA, Tupler RH, Carroll BA, et al. Renal artery stenosis: analysis of Doppler waveform parameters and tardus-parvus pattern. *Radiology* 1993;189(3):779—787.

61. Lafortune M, Patriquin H, Demeule E, et al. Renal arterial stenosis: slowed systole in the downstream circulation—experimental study in dogs. *Radiology* 1992;184(2):475—478.

62. Strandness DJ. Duplex imaging for the detection of renal artery stenosis. *Am J Kidney Dis* 1994;24(4):674—678.

63. Gottlieb RH, Snitzer EL, Hartley DF, Fultz PJ, Rubens DJ. Interobserver and intraobserver variation in determining intrarenal parameters by Doppler sonography. *AJR* 1997;168(3):627—631.

64. Kliewer MA, Tupler RH, Hertzberg BS, et al. Doppler evaluation of renal artery stenosis: interobserver agreement in the interpretation of waveform morphology. *AJR* 1994;162(6):1371—1376.

65. Rene PC, Oliva VL, Bui BT, et al. Renal artery stenosis: evaluation of Doppler US after inhibition of angiotensin-converting enzyme with captopril [see comments]. *Radiology* 1995;196(3):675—679.

66. Nazzal MMS, Hoballah JJ, Miller EV, et al. Renal hilar Doppler analysis is of value in the management of patients with renovascular disease. *Am J Surg* 1997;174:164—168.

67. Missouris CG, Allen CM, Balen FG, et al. Non-invasive screening for renal artery stenosis with ultrasound contrast enhancement. *J Hypertens* 1996;14(4):519—524.

68. Soulen MC, Benenati JF, Sheth S, Merton D, Rothgeb J. Changes in renal artery Doppler indexes following renal angioplasty. *J Vasc Intervent Radiology* 1991;2(4):457—461.

69. Schwerk WB, Restrepo IK, Stellwaag M, Klose KJ, Schade-Brittinger C. Renal artery stenosis: grading with image-directed Doppler US evaluation of renal resistive index [see comments]. *Radiology* 1994;190(3):785—790.

70. Burdick L, Airoldi F, Marana I, et al. Superiority of acceleration and acceleration time over pulsatility and resistance indices as screening tests for renal artery stenosis. *J Hypertens* 1996;14(10):1229—1235.

71. Pedersen EB, Egeblad M, Jorgensen J, et al. Diagnosing renal artery stenosis: a comparison between conventional renography, captopril renography and ultrasound Doppler in a large consecutive series of patients with arterial hypertension. *Blood Pressure* 1996;5(6):342—348.

72. Frauchiger B, Zierler R, Bergelin RO, Isaacson JA, Strandness DE, Jr. Prognostic significance of intrarenal resistance indices in patients with renal artery interventions: a preliminary duplex sonographic study. *Cardiovasc Surg* 1996;4(3):324—330.

73. Postma CT, Bijlstra PJ, Rosenbusch G, Thien T. Pattern recognition of loss of early systolic peak by Doppler ultrasound has a low sensitivity for the detection of renal artery stenosis. *J Human Hypertens* 1996;10(3):181—184.

74. Melany ML, Grant EG, Duerinckx AJ, Watts TM, Levine BS. Ability of a phase shift US contrast agent to improve imaging of the main renal arteries. *Radiology* 1997;205(1):147—152.

75. Miralles M, Cairols M, Cotillas J, Gimenez A, Santiso A. Value of Doppler parameters in the diagnosis of renal artery stenosis. *J Vasc Surg* 1996;23(3):428—435.

76. Antonica G, Sabba C, Berardi E, et al. Accuracy of echo-Doppler flowmetry for renal artery stenosis. *J Hypertens* Suppl 1991;9(6).

11 Sonography in Acute Abdominal Trauma

W. Dennis Foley

The most common cause of morbidity and mortality in the second, third, and fourth decades of life is trauma. The leading cause is automobile accidents with penetrating injury, battery, and sports-related injury also important factors. The prevalence of trauma and cost to society are increasing. The spectrum of major trauma encompasses neurological, thoracic, abdominal, and musculoskeletal injuries. Life-threatening consequences may result from injury to any body region. Blunt abdominal injury poses a particular problem, as there may be minimal physical findings, particularly if the patient's state of consciousness is impaired. In addition, blunt abdominal injury may coexist with other significant trauma including intracranial hemorrhage, ruptured thoracic aorta and pneumothorax, and musculoskeletal injury, e.g., major spinal, pelvic and long bone fractures. An accurate evaluation of abdominal injury is required to select the patients' management appropriately.

With the advent of sequential CT scanning for blunt abdominal injury in the late 1970s and early 1980s, surgeons began to refine their indications for exploratory laparotomy based on an evolving understanding of the natural history of blunt abdominal injury.[1,2] In a hemodynamically stable patient, both major and minor lacerations of the liver, spleen, and kidneys will usually resolve with conservative management and no sequelae. Hepatic and splenic lacerations with intraperitoneal blood are not primary indications for laparotomy. Intervention, either angiographic or surgical, is usually reserved for lacerations associated with active bleeding, manifest as vascular contrast extravasation at the time of emergency CT scanning.[3] Other CT findings in a hemodynamically stable patient that may prompt immediate laparotomy include duodenal rupture, central renal pedicle injury, significant pancreatic transection and intraperitoneal bladder rupture. The major indication for laparotomy in a hemodynamically unstable patient is hemoperitoneum (without obvious extraabdominal blood loss) and hypotension unresponsive to intravenous fluid resuscitation. In the past, clinical evaluation and diagnostic peritoneal lavage determined the need for laparotomy.[4] Sonography has largely supplanted diagnostic peritoneal lavage for detecting hemoperitoneum.[5—9]

CT is the preferred technique for evaluating normotensive patients with documented abdominal injury.[10] It provides accurate global diagnostic information about abdominal and pelvic injury. However, the relatively high rate of negative abdominal and pelvic CT scans following blunt trauma, particularly in patients who are neurologically impaired, has prompted the use of sonography as a more cost-effective and efficient screening study.[5, 6, 8, 9] Hemodynamically stable patients with documented intraperitoneal fluid on sonography should proceed to CT evaluation. An abdominal sonogram that is negative for intraperitoneal fluid has been assumed to be sufficient to exclude significant blunt abdominal trauma in a patient without hematuria, and with no clinical evidence of occult injury following six hours of observation.[11]

This chapter will discuss the role of abdominal sonogaphy and CT scanning in evaluating patients with suspected blunt abdominal injury. Both hemodynamically unstable and hemodynamically stable patients will be discussed. The goal of sonographic imaging in trauma is to provide a cost-effective triage with high sensitivity and negative predictive value that leads to appropriate patient management and outcome.

Differential Diagnosis — Abdominal Trauma

Intraperitoneal Fluid

Intraperitoneal fluid may be blood, bile, urine, pancreatic juice, lymph, intestinal content, or preexistent ascites. Intraperitoneal fluid following blunt trauma is most often intraperitoneal blood resulting from hepatic, splenic, or mesenteric laceration. A periportal liver laceration or gallbladder rupture may cause leakage of bile into the peritoneal cavity. In acutely injured patients, bile is usually not the predominant component of intraperitoneal fluid. Other types of intraperitoneal fluid in the patient with blunt trauma are unusual. Urinary ascites usually results from intraperitoneal rupture of the bladder. The dome of the bladder is the most common site of rupture. Pancreatic ascites may result when there is pancreatic transection associated with disruption of the posterior parietal peritoneum. Pancreatic ascites is usually caused by delayed intraperitoneal rupture of a pancreatic pseudocyst. Chylous ascites is very uncommon. It results from transection of the cisterna chyli or proximal thoracic duct. Patients with underlying liver disease with portal hypertension and hypoproteinemia may have preexisting ascites.

Injuries to the liver and spleen result from compression or shearing force.[12] The resultant lacerations may be localized or multifocal and may or may not be associated with a capsular tear. Grading schemes — CT injury severity scores — have been used to classify the extent of solid organ injury.[13] However, there is no direct correlation between the injury severity score and the likelihood of delayed bleeding.[13]

Parenchymal and capsular tears usually result in a localized perihepatic or perisplenic hematoma — sentinel clot[14] — as well as intraperitoneal bleeding in the perihepatic or perisplenic spaces, paracolic gutters or pelvis. This common pattern of hemoperitoneum distribution means that a rapid four quadrant sonographic assessment will usually detect intraperitoneal fluid associated with hepatic or splenic injury.

Injuries to the mesentery or bowel are more problematic. Hematoma may be confined to the bowel wall or mesentery without lateral or inferior distribution into the dependent intraperitoneal spaces.[15] As there may be no hemoperitoneum, an emergency sonogram may not detect these injuries.

Extraperitoneal organ injury usually does not result in intraperitoneal bleeding. Injuries to the kidneys, pancreas, duodenum, and disruption of the aortoiliac arterial system (caused by seat belt injury or pelvic fracture) are in this category. Thus, a negative sonogram for intraperitoneal fluid in patients with a central abdominal compression injury or hematuria does not exclude the possibility of significant injury. Patients with hematuria and those with lumbar spine or pelvic fractures should have abdominal pelvic CT scan to exclude injuries even when sonography is negative.[16, 17] In addition, care must be taken to avoid missing traumatic pneumothorax, which has a relatively high association with blunt abdominal injury.[16, 17]

Diagnostic Evaluation

Nonimaging Evaluation and Management

Patients with abdominal injury are assessed for hemodynamic stability and the presence of associated injuries including neurological, thoracic, and orthopedic. Patients should be triaged into a hemodynamically unstable or hemodynamically stable category to guide further evaluation.

If patients are unresponsive, either due to neurological injury or alcoholism, then external signs of abdominal trauma including body wall contusion should be assessed on a clinical examination. For patients who are conscious and responsive, clinical evaluation for focal guarding and rebound tenderness is vital.

Plasma expanders are usually infused via intravenous lines. Bladder catheterization is used to evaluate for hematuria and measure urine output. Tube thoracostomy is performed if any significant hemopneumothorax is present. Endotracheal intubation may be required for neurologically impaired patients or those in respiratory difficulty following aspiration or tube thoracostomy. The early triage diagnostic evaluation by sonography is usually performed concurrent with these diagnostic or resuscitative procedures.

The Hemodynamically Unstable Patient

The hemodynamically unstable patient with suspected abdominal injury requires urgent evaluation for possible hemoperitoneum. Diagnostic peritoneal lavage can fulfill this role with very high reported sensitivity and specificity.[4] Limitations of diagnostic peritoneal lavage include its inability to detect intracapsular hemorrhage in the liver or spleen and its relative insensitivity to bowel perforation or mesenteric hemorrhage. Diagnostic peritoneal lavage is insensitive to retroperitoneal injury including pancreatic, duodenal, and renal injuries. A false-positive diagnostic peritoneal lavage may result from a traumatic peritoneal tap.

Sonography can be performed as an alternative test to diagnostic peritoneal lavage.[5—9] In general, sonography and diagnostic peritoneal lavage share the same limitations: suboptimal detection of solid organ injury, mesenteric hemorrhage, bowel perforation, and retroperitoneal injury.

A positive diagnostic peritoneal lavage or positive sonogram in the hemodynamically unstable patient should result in urgent laparotomy. It may be appropriate to delay laparotomy in some patients with multiorgan injuries. Severe associated neurological injury may require early evaluation by neurological CT. Thoracic injury may require portable chest radiography, tube thoracostomy, or thoracic aortography. A negative diagnostic peritoneal lavage or negative sonogram in a hemodynamically unstable patient should lead to urgent evaluation of the thorax, abdominal retroperitoneum, pelvis or extremities as sources of continuing blood loss.

Hemodynamically Stable Patient

The hemodynamically stable patient may be assessed by sonography. Detection of intraperitoneal fluid or sentinel clot should be an indication for an abdominal pelvic CT study. A negative emergency abdominal sonogram, in the hemodynamically stable patient, does not exclude the possibility of contained intrahepatic or intrasplenic hematoma, mesenteric or bowel wall injury or retroperitoneal injury.[16] McKenney et al. believe that patients with a negative emergency abdominal sonogram who have no extra abdominal injuries and lack hematuria should be discharged after an uneventful six-h observation period.[11] Nevertheless, a number of these patients may return with delayed presentation of abdominal injuries including splenic rupture, diaphragmatic rupture, mesenteric, and bowel injury.

Ultrasound Imaging

Small footprint 3 to 5-MHz sector transducers, either linear phased array or curved array, are the most appropriate choice for an abdominal trauma sonographic study. As with all sonographic studies, attention to appropriate depth and width of field, gain and TGC curve and focal zones is important for image quality.

A four-quadrant rapid survey sonographic technique is recommended. This involves evaluation of the perihepatic and perisplenic spaces, the paracolic gutters, and posterior deep pelvis. The right and left pleural spaces are evaluated concurrent with imaging of the perihepatic and perisplenic spaces. Operator speed and expertise are essential. Examination time to assess for fluid in the four abdominal quadrants, right and left pleural space and, in selected instances, the pericardial space should be limited to less than five min. While examination speed is critical, adequate documentation of findings is also important. This includes annotated hard copy recordings either obtained on-line at the time of examination or subsequently retrieved from playback of videotape.

In the right upper quadrant, the hepatorenal space and subphrenic spaces should be evaluated. Parasagittal and coronal imaging planes, using intercostal and subcostal access, are used to evaluate this region (**Fig. 11–1**).

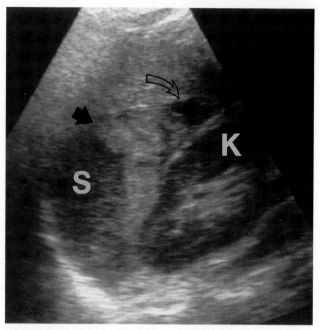

Figure 11–2 Splenic laceration with intrasplenic and perisplenic blood clot. Oblique coronal image of left upper quadrant (S, spleen, K, left kidney). There is echogenic blood clot (**arrow**) extending from the region of the splenic hilum anterior to the upper pole of the left kidney (splenorenal recess) and toward the diaphragm. This is a perisplenic "sentinel clot." An adjacent more inferior hypoechoic defect (**curved open arrow**) represents an adjacent intrasplenic laceration containing unclotted blood.

A similar approach is used in the left upper quadrant to define the left anterior subphrenic and perisplenic spaces (**Fig. 11–2, 11–3**). The lesser sac is frequently obscured

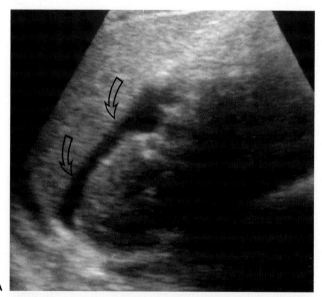

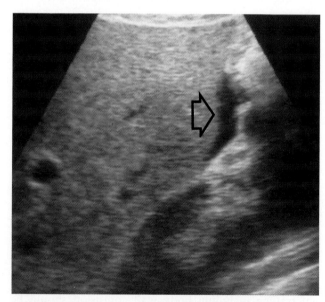

Figure 11–1 Hemoperitoneum in the hepatorenal space following blunt injury. (**A**) Fluid (**curved arrows**) is present in the posterior right subhepatic space and extends to the diaphragm. (**B**) Longitudinal sonogram in a more medial plane demonstrates contiguous fluid in the anterior right subhepatic space (**arrow**) between the right colon and the inferior surface of the liver.

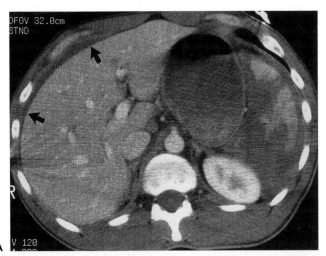 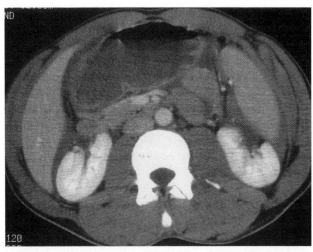

Fig. 11–3 Dynamic helical CT scan of patient illustrated in **Fig. 11–2** with splenic laceration and hemoperitoneum. (**A**) Scan at a more cephalad level demonstrates splenic laceration with a perisplenic fluid collection containing relatively high attenuation coagulum and relatively low attenuation presumed unclotted blood. Perihepatic hemoperitoneum (**arrows**), lower in attenuation than the perisplenic blood clot, is noted. (**B**) A more inferior level scan demonstrates subhepatic and perisplenic hemoperitoneum.

by gas and ingested material in the stomach. Hepatic and splenic lacerations can be recognized as linear or branching hypoechoic defects in the parenchyma (**Fig. 11–4**). Subcapsular and perihepatic and perisplenic hematomas — "sentinel clots" — may be relatively echogenic because of the aggregated red cells and blood products in the coagulum (**Fig. 11–2, 11–5**).

The spectrum of renal injuries following blunt trauma includes laceration, fracture, vascular pedicle disruption (laceration and/or thrombosis), infarction, and pyelocalyceal/ureteric disruption. Sonography is less sensitive in detecting renal injury than hepatic or splenic injury, probably because acoustic access is more difficult in a supine patient in the trauma setting (**Fig. 11–4**).

The pleural spaces and diaphragm are evaluated by cephalad tilt of the transducer probe in both the parasagittal and coronal imaging plane. Pleural space fluid is anechoic and demarcated by the diaphragm inferiorly, the costal pleural surface and chest wall peripherally, and the lower lobe of the lung superiorly (**Fig. 11–6**). Frequently, compression atelectasis of the lower lobes can be seen within the pleural fluid, moving during inspiration and expiration. Sonography cannot be relied on to exclude diaphragm rupture because it is insensitive in the detection of diaphragmatic defects. Direct ultrasonic findings of rupture of the diaphragm include focal diaphragmatic disruption, and herniation of liver, spleen or bowel loops through the diaphragmatic defect. A "floating diaphragm," the appearance of the free edge of a disrupted diaphragm outlined by pleural and peritoneal fluid, may be noted. In the hemodynamically stable patient, diagnosing rupture of the diaphragm is not urgent. It can be diagnosed in a more elective setting using reformatted coronal or sagittal images from helical CT data or by direct coronal MRI. On the left side, gastric and colonic herniation can be recognized by radiography.

Intraperitoneal fluid in the lower abdomen will usually collect in the posterior deep pelvis (retrovesical or retrouterine space) (**Fig. 11–7**). In the acute setting, in which the patient is examined without bladder distension, sonography may not be able to image this compartment of the peritoneal cavity.[18] The lower-quadrant examination evaluates the inferior aspect of the paracolic gutters and the perivesical spaces (**Fig. 11–8**).

Midline compression injuries may result in myocardial contusion or pericardial tamponade. A post-trauma echocardiogram limited to evaluation of the pericardium can be performed utilizing a subxyphoid approach with parasagittal and coronal imaging planes directed to the cardiac apex.

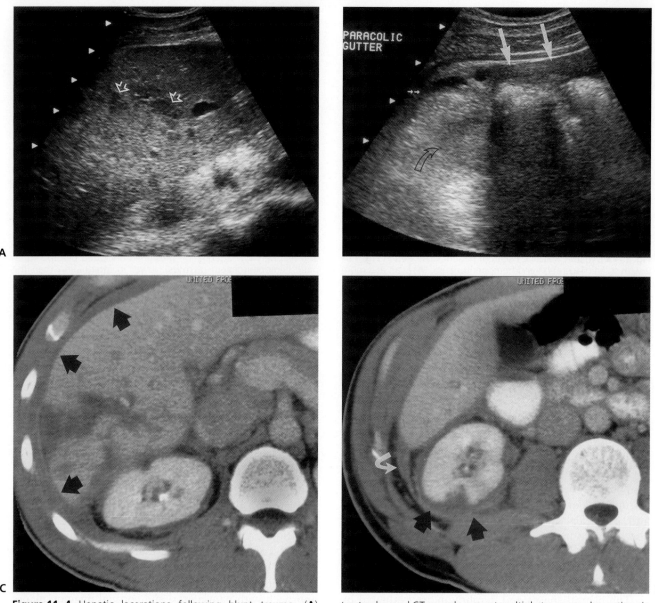

A

B

C

D

Figure 11–4 Hepatic lacerations following blunt trauma. (**A**) Coronal plane right upper quadrant sonogram demonstrates linear hypoechoic defects in the hepatic parenchyma (**arrows**).(**B**) Coronal scan at a more inferior and posterior level demonstrates fluid in the paracolic gutter between the abdominal wall and right colon (**arrows**). Note the inferior tip of the liver (**straight arrows**) and the upper pole of the right kidney (**curved arrow**). (**C**) Con-trast enhanced CT scan document multiple transverse lacerations in the right hepatic lobe extending to the capsule with perihepatic hematoma (**arrows**). (**D**) More caudal level CT scan through the inferior right hepatic lobe demonstrates hemoperitoneum (**curved arrow**) and perinephric hematoma (**arrowheads**) related to a small posterior margin renal laceration. The renal injury was not detected by abdominal sonogram.

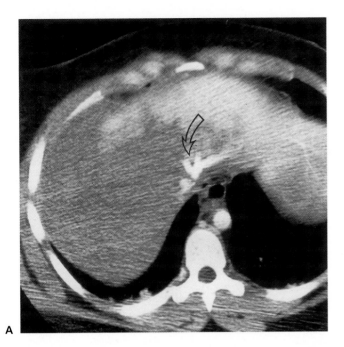

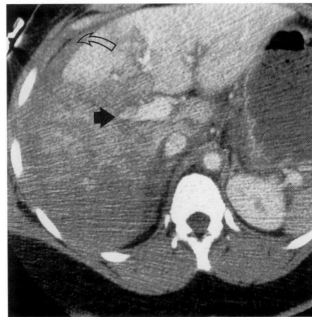

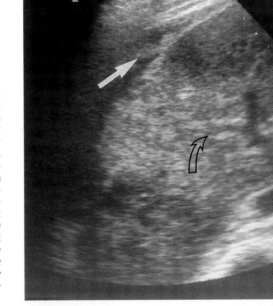

Figure 11–5 Right hepatic lobe laceration with interruption of the right hepatic vein and right portal vein. (**A**) CT scan at a cephalic level demonstrates a patent conjoint left and middle hepatic vein (**arrow**) and absent right hepatic vein at the hepatic vein/inferior vena cava confluence. Laceration margin is adjacent to the major fissure. No enhancement of the right hepatic lobe is seen at this level. (**B**) CT scan at the level of the hepatic hilum shows an amputated right portal vein (**arrow**) and relatively high attenuation coagulum in the anterior right hepatic lobe extending to the capsule. There is a high attenuation perihepatic hemoperitoneum — "sentinel clot" (**curved arrow**). The more posterior right hepatic lobe is hypoattenuating reflecting infarction. (**C**) Sonogram of the right upper quadrant using an oblique transverse plane. Echogenic intrahepatic coagulum is identified in the anterior right hepatic lobe and the heterogeneous hypoechoic posterior right hepatic lobe corresponds to infarction. Perihepatic hematoma and coagulum are identified (**arrow**). The right portal vein (**curved arrow**) was amputated.

A

B

C

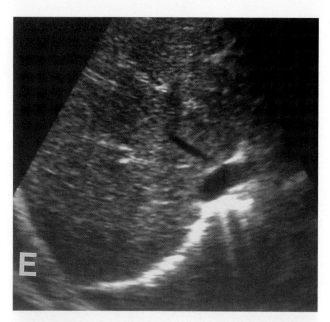

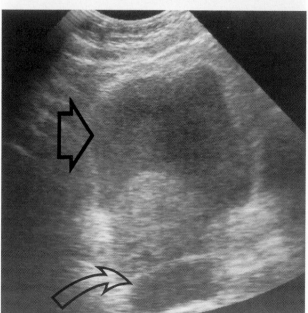

A

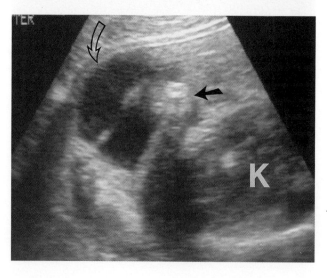

◁ **Figure 11–6** Transverse sonogram through the cephalad liver demonstrates a small right pleural effusion (E). The diaphragm was intact and moved appropriately with respiration.

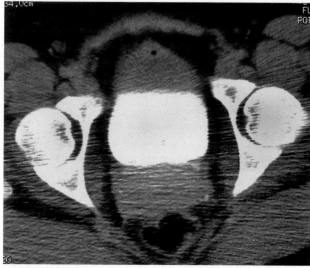

B

Figure 11–7 Hemoperitoneum in the posterior deep pelvis. (**A**) Transverse sonogram through the bladder (**straight open arrow**) demonstrates a fluid collection with low level internal echoes in the rectouterine space (**curved arrow**). Patient was examined after bladder catheterization allowing acoustic access through a relatively distended bladder. (**B**) CT scan through the distended bladder confirms relatively high-attenuation hemoperitoneum in the posterior deep pelvis. Contrast layers in the urinary bladder. A small anterior gas bubble was related to bladder catheterization.

◁ **Figure 11–8** Transverse imaging of the paracolic gutter. Transverse imaging of the right paracolic gutter at the level of the inferior right kidney (K) demonstrates paracolic gutter fluid (**curved arrow**) lateral and posterior to the collapsed right colon (**straight arrow**). The quadratus muscle is posterior to the paracolic gutter.

Evaluation of Sonographic Imaging in Blunt Abdominal Trauma

Publications in the surgical and emergency medicine literature attest to the interest and potential utility of emergency abdominal sonography in the blunt trauma patient.[19, 20] The use of sonography as a replacement for diagnostic peritoneal lavage in the hemodynamically unstable patient following blunt injury appears well supported.[5—9] Sonography can be performed more expeditiously and avoids potential false-positive results from traumatic peritoneal taps. Both techniques are insensitive to contained intracapsular hepatic or splenic injury, localized mesenteric hematoma or bowel wall injury, and injury to extraperitoneal structures including pancreas, duodenum, and kidneys. If the hemodynamically unstable patient has no free intraperitoneal fluid, then attention should be directed to possible bleeding in the extraperitoneal spaces or bleeding associated with thoracic, pelvic or long bone injury. This appraisal may require combinations of radiography (portable chest, spine and pelvis, lung bones) and tube thoracostomy.

Sonography as a screening test in the hemodynamically stable patient is a more controversial issue. A positive sonogram with documented intraperitoneal fluid is valuable information and should lead to an abdominal pelvic CT study. CT studies should be performed on patients with negative abdominal sonograms who have hematuria, spinal or pelvic fractures, or suspicion of midline compression injury that could result in trauma to the duodenum, pancreas, central renal vascular pedicle or aortoiliac vessels. In other circumstances, the value of a negative sonographic study is more problematic. Studies comparing emergency abdominal sonography to diagnostic peritoneal lavage, CT, and surgery have demonstrated sensitivity of sonography in detecting free intraperitoneal fluid to vary between 63 and 80%.[5—9, 18] The most common cause for false-negative sonographic studies has been free fluid in the pelvis detectable on CT but not on sonography owing to a collapsed bladder.[18] In addition, in Chiu et al.'s large series, in which 7% of blunt trauma victims had abdominal injury, one-third of those with documented abdominal injury had no hemoperitoneum by CT study or emergency abdominal sonography.[16] All these patients had contained intrasplenic or intrahepatic hematomas detected only on CT study and were at risk for delayed bleeding. Some of these patients with contained intracapsular hematomas and lacerations and negative abdominal sonograms underwent laparotomy.

Reported patient studies utilizing emergency abdominal sonography have high accuracy rates and high negative predictive values. However, the vast majority of patients had negative studies with good outcomes. Only a small proportion of blunt trauma victims has abdominal injury with intraperitoneal bleeding or is found to have contained intraparenchymal hematomas on CT study. Sensitivity values for blunt abdominal injury varying between 63 and 80% are relatively poor — critical diagnostic information will not be obtained in up to one-third of patients with blunt abdominal injury. Thus, claims that sonography is a cost-effective tool in the evaluation of blunt trauma are suspect because the overwhelmingly negative patient population masks a significant false-negative rate.

There are two possible approaches in hemodynamically stable patients. Triage CT could be performed instead of triage sonography in all patients. This would require lower-cost CT and/or refining the indications for CT as compared to the almost universal application of sonography to trauma patients in the emergency room. The second option is the continued liberal use of sonography with close clinical observation of those patients with negative sonograms and without hematuria. Even under the circumstances of a six-hour post sonographic clinical observation in the emergency room, a small proportion of patients are likely to represent with delayed internal bleeding. There has been no reported mortality in such patients.

Summary

The role of abdominal trauma ultrasound is to document the presence or absence of intraperitoneal fluid — a parameter that is critical in patient management decisions. In the hemodynamically unstable abdominal trauma patient, intraperitoneal fluid is an indication for exploratory laparotomy. In the hemodynamically stable abdominal trauma patient, intraperitoneal fluid is an indication for abdominal pelvic CT scan to document the site and extent of solid and/or hollow viscus injury. Used in this fashion, sonography replaces diagnostic peritoneal lavage. Sonography provides equivalent sensitivity and specificity for the detection of intraperitoneal fluid. Sonography can be performed expeditiously and fluid can also evaluate the pleural spaces and pericardium.

A negative sonogram does not exclude the possibility of contained intracapsular hemorrhage in the liver or spleen, mesenteric or bowel injury or injury to the extraperitoneal structures — the pancreas, duodenum, and kidneys. Patients with suspicious clinical findings, hematuria, and spinal or pelvic fractures should have abdominal pelvic CT scans. Patients with negative sonography can be observed for a short period and, if clinically stable, discharged. A few of these patients may re-present with delayed internal bleeding.

Effective use of sonography in abdominal trauma requires 24-h coverage on site by experienced sonologists or sonographers competent in abdominal scanning techniques. Experienced scanners can rapidly adapt scanning parameters to different patients to provide the requisite diagnostic information.

References

1. Knudson MM, Lin RC, Oakes DD, Jeffrey RB. Nonoperative management of blunt liver injuries in adults: the need for continued surveillance. *J Trauma* 1990;30:1494—1500.
2. Foley WD, Cates JD, Kellmann GN, et al. Treatment of blunt hepatic injuries: role of CT. *Radiology* 1987;164:635—638.
3. Federle MP, Courcoulas AP, Powell M, Ferris, JV, Peitzman AB. Blunt splenic injury in adults: clinical and CT criteria for management with emphasis on active extravasation. *Radiology* 1998;206(1):137—142.
4. Gomez GA, Alvarez R, Poasencia G, et al. Diagnostic peritoneal lavage in the management of blunt abdominal trauma: a reassessment. *J Trauma* 1987;27(1):1—5.
5. McKenney M, Lentz K, Nunez D, et al. Can ultrasound replace diagnostic peritoneal lavage in the assessment of blunt trauma? *J Trauma* 1994;37(3):439—441.
6. McKenney MG, Martin L, Lentz K, et al. One thousand consecutive ultrasounds for blunt abdominal trauma. *J Trauma* 1996;40(4):607—610.
7. Wherrett LJ, Boulanger BR, McLellan BA, et al. Hypotension after blunt abdominal trauma: the role of emergent abdominal sonography in surgical triage. *J Trauma* 1996;41(5):815—820.
8. Boulanger BR, McLellan BA, Brenneman FD, et al. Emergent abdominal sonography as a screening test in a new diagnostic algorithm for blunt trauma. *J Trauma* 1996;40(6):867—874.
9. Lentz KA, McKenney MG, Nunez DB Jr., Martin L. Evaluating blunt abdominal trauma: role for ultrasonography. *J US Med* 1996;15(6):447—451.
10. Foley WD. Abdominal trauma, In: Bradley N, Stevenson, GW, eds. *Margulis and Burhenne's Alimentary Tract. Radiology*, 5th ed. Philadelphia: Mosby Inc. 1994, p. 2120—2142.
11. McKenney KL, Nunez DB, McKenney MG, et al. Sonography is the primary screening technique for blunt abdominal trauma: experience with 899 patients. *AJR* 1998;170:979—985.
12. Anderson CB, Ballinger WF. Abdominal injuries, In: Zuidema GD, Rutherford RB, Ballinger WF, eds. *The Management of Trauma*; 4th ed. Philadelphia: WB Saunders, 1985 p. 449—504.
13. Mirvis SE, Whitley NO, Gens DR. Blunt splenic trauma in adults: CT based classification and correlation with prognosis and treatment. *Radiology* 1989;171(1):33—39.
14. Orwig D, Federle MP. Localized clotted blood as evidence of visceral trauma on CT: the sentinel clot sign. *AJR* 1989;153(4):747—749
15. Levine CD, Gonzales RN, Wachsberg RH, Ghanekar D. CT findings of bowel and mesenteric injury. *JCAT* 1997;21(6):974—979.
16. Chiu WC, Cushing BM, Rodriguez A, et al. Abdominal injuries without hemoperitoneum: a potential limitation of focused abdominal sonography for trauma (FAST). *J Trauma* 1997;42(4):617—623.
17. Miller JA, Ghanekar D. Pneumothoraces secondary to blunt abdominal trauma: aids to plain film radiographic diagnosis and relationship to solid organ injury. *Am Surg* 1996;62(5):416—420.
18. McGahan JP, Rose J, Coates TL, Wisner DH, Newberry P. Use of ultrasonography in the patient with acute abdominal trauma. *J US Med* 1997;16(10):653—662.
19. Rozycki GS, Ochsnner MG, Jawfin JH, Champion HR. Prospective evaluation of surgeons use of ultrasound in the evaluation of trauma patients. *J Trauma* 1993;34(4):516—526.
20. Bode PJ, Niezen RA, van Vugt AB, Schipper J. Abdominal ultrasound as a reliable indicator for conclusive laparotomy In blunt abdominal trauma. *J Trauma* 1993;34(1):27—31.

12 Right Lower-Quadrant Pain: Rule Out Appendicitis

R. Brooke Jeffrey

Although the incidence of appendicitis appears to be declining slightly in the Western world, it nonetheless remains the most common cause of acute abdominal pain requiring surgery[1,2] In the United States each year, approximately 250,000 patients undergo appendectomies for presumed appendicitis.[1,2] The differential diagnosis of acute appendicitis is extremely broad, and appendicitis often mimics the presentation of other gastrointestinal, genitourinary, or gynecologic abnormalities. Historically, clinical misdiagnosis is common, and approximately 20% of patients presumed to have appendicitis undergo a nontherapeutic laparotomy with removal of a normal appendix. The rate of negative appendectomy is even higher in women of reproductive age in whom 30% to 40% of surgeries are unnecessary.[3,4]

Until quite recently, surgeons have relied entirely on the patient's history and physical examination to determine the need for surgery. Preoperative imaging has not been the standard of care in patients with possible appendicitis. In part, this is due to the fact that before 1986, conventional radiologic studies such as plain abdominal radiographs and barium studies were of only limited value due to their lack of specificity.[5,6] One noted surgical authority put this into perspective by stating, "the diagnosis of acute appendicitis is the classic example of the application of clinical skills. Ancillary laboratory and radiologic tests are not essential in making the diagnosis".[7]

Several large clinical series have documented a high degree of sensitivity and specificity for CT and sonography in the evaluation of patients with right lower-quadrant pain and possible acute appendicitis.[8,9] The accurate noninvasive imaging of acute appendicitis now makes obsolete the complete reliance upon the patient's history and physical examination to determine the need for surgery.

Differential Diagnosis

In patients with acute right lower-quadrant pain, appendicitis is only one of a large number of gastrointestinal, genitourinary, and gynecologic disorders.[10–12] Classic mimics of acute appendicitis include mesenteric adenitis, pelvic inflammatory disease, ureteral calculi, and viral gastroenteritis. In his classic monograph on the early diagnosis of the acute abdomen, Sir Zachary Cope listed a total of 34 different disorders that may clinically mimic acute appendicitis.[13]This list has greatly expanded in the past several decades with advances in medical knowledge and newer disease entities such as AIDS associated with immunosuppressive states. One factor contributing to the overall complexity of acute right lower-quadrant pain as a clinical problem is that the differential diagnosis ranges from benign self-limited disorders (e.g., mesenteric adenitis or viral gastroenteritis) to lesions that carry significant morbidity if not treated promptly including bowel obstruction, perforation, infarction, or abscesses of various etiologies.

In women of reproductive age, it is often difficult to clinically differentiate appendicitis from any acute gynecologic disorders. Pelvic inflammatory disease, ovarian torsion, and ruptured or hemorrhagic functional cysts may all mimic the clinical presentation of acute appendicitis.[4] In patients over 50 years of age, cecal or sigmoid diverticulitis or perforated cecal neoplasm should also be considered in the differential diagnosis.[14]

Clinical Assessment

The "classic history" for acute appendicitis is diffuse abdominal or midepigastric pain that after a period of time, localizes to the right lower-quadrant.[1,2] Pain is frequently accompanied by anorexia and at times nausea and vomiting. Of note is the fact that this classic history is present in only 55% of patients with acute appendicitis.[2] The most characteristic physical finding is guarding and rebound tenderness over McBurney's point in the right iliac fossa. The early diagnosis of acute appendicitis is often difficult in pediatric patients due to problems in obtaining an adequate history. Some elderly or immunocompromised patients may have relatively minimal pain with acute appendicitis.

The location of the appendiceal tip is highly variable and may be a major factor in contributing to the patient's symptoms and localization of pain. Flank pain may be the most striking finding in a patient with a retrocecal appendix that extends along the right lateral flank. In patients with a pelvic appendix, suprapubic tenderness or deep pelvic pain may be the most predominant clinical symptom. In female patients this may closely mimic symptoms of salpingitis, ovarian torsion, or other acute gynecologic abnormalities. In patients with a pelvic appendix, a rectal examination may reveal tenderness along the right lateral wall of the rectum.

Diagnostic Workup

Laboratory values in appendicitis are highly variable and often nonspecific.[15] While leukocytosis with bandemia is common, up to one-third of adult patients with acute appendicitis have a normal leukocyte count.[15] Elderly patients, in particular, are well known to have relatively normal laboratory values with acute appendicitis. A high fever with leukocytosis is characteristic, but not invariable with a periappendiceal abscess.

Imaging Tests Other Than Sonography

In addition to graded compression sonography, a variety of computed tomography (CT) techniques have been developed that are extremely valuable in the evaluation of patients with suspected appendicitis.[16—20] The differences in CT methodology relate to whether or not there is administration of oral, intravenous, or rectal contrast. In patients with ample intraperitoneal fat, unenhanced CT (no oral and no intravenous contrast) is an accurate technique.[17,18] Scans that are performed without oral contrast facilitate identification of appendicoliths. It is important to note, however, that patient selection is key to the success of noncontrast CT for appendicitis. One significant limitation of noncontrast scans is that in very thin patients with appendiceal perforation, it may be difficult to distinguish liquefied pus from indurated soft tissue inflammation. Intravenous contrast should, therefore, be routinely administered in patients with perforated appendicitis. Another limitation is that in very thin patients without ample intraperitoneal fat, edema of the mesoappendix which is an important diagnostic criterion may not be evident. Therefore, in thin patients, oral and intravenous contrast may be of significant value.

Scans performed with rectal contrast only have been shown to be highly accurate for the diagnosis of appendicitis.[19] The value of this technique is to clearly identify the cecal tip, therefore making it easier to visualize the abnormal appendix. In general, the CT criteria for acute appendicitis include identification of an appendix 7 mm or greater in diameter with adjacent edema of the mesoappendix. Secondary findings include appendicoliths and adjacent abscesses.

Ultrasound Imaging

Graded compression sonography is based on the principle that when pressure is applied to a normal bowel loop with a transducer, it will readily compress.[9] Any inflammatory or neoplastic process infiltrating the bowel wall alters its compliability making it relatively noncompressible. Whenever possible, it is important to use the highest resolution linear ray transducer that affords adequate penetration to visualize the key anatomic landmarks of the psoas muscle and external iliac artery and vein. The study should be considering nondiagnostic if these normal structures cannot be visualized. In general, a 5- to 10-MHz linear array transducers are adequate for most pediatric and adult patients.

At the outset of the examination the patient is asked to point with a single finger to the site of maximal pain or tenderness. This maneuver often is helpful in identifying a potentially aberrantly located appendix. Sonographic imaging is then initiated in the transverse plane using light pressure to first identify the abdominal wall musculature and the right colon. The right colon is the largest structure in the right flank with a sonographic signature bowel (echogenic submucosal layer) that has no peristalsis. The right colon is then followed caudally to its termination as a cecal tip. Pressure is gradually applied to the cecal tip to express all the gas and fecal contents from its lumen to enhance visualization of the noncompressible appendix. It is very important to vary the acoustic window to obtain the optimal view to demonstrate the appendix.

Although other published reports have suggested that the normal appendix can be visualized in a high percentage of patients that has not been true in my own personal experience.[21] I am able to find the normal appendix in only approximately 15% to 20% of patients. In general, the normal appendix measures 5 m or less in maximal anteroposterior diameter and is readily compressible.[22] Often there is a small amount of echogenic residual fecal debris within the normal appendix.

The diagnosis of acute appendicitis can be established with confidence if a noncompressible appendix with a maximal outer diameter of 7 mm or greater is identified (**Fig. 12–1**). An appendix that measures in the range of 5 mm to 6 mm should be considered equivocal.[23]. These patients should be observed clinically because there is no risk of morbidity from perforation. Many of these patients will not prove to have appendicitis and, therefore, a trial period of observation is clearly warranted. Patients with right lower-quadrant pain and a visualized appendicolith are often taken to surgery even with a borderline size appendix due to the concern for the potential morbidity of perforation in such patients.

Benefits of Sonography

Despite the fact that appendiceal sonography may be technically challenging, it has a number of clear imaging advantages.[24—27] Sonography is readily available, inexpensive to perform, and has no ionizing radiation. Unlike CT, it is a real-time, interactive study. Sonographic findings are relatively easy to correlate with the patient's anatomic site of maximal pain and tenderness. In addition, sonography can display visualize bowel peristalsis and can identify discrete anatomic layers of the bowel wall such as the echogenic submucosa.

In the past several years, there have been substantial improvements in color Doppler sensitivity to enable visualization of blood flow to bowel without the use of contrast agents.[28, 29] Hyperemia, which is characteristic of inflammatory lesions, can thus be differentiated from ischemic disorders that cause a decreased flow to the bowel. As with CT, sonography can effectively survey the remainder of the abdomen and pelvis if the appendix is normal.[30] With the use of endovaginal probes, sonography excels at diagnosing gynecologic disorders. Sonography may also be useful in identifying mesenteric adenitis, inflammatory bowel disease (**Fig. 12–2**), pyosalpinx (**Fig. 12–3**), small bowel obstruction (**Fig. 12–4**) and ovarian torsion.[30]

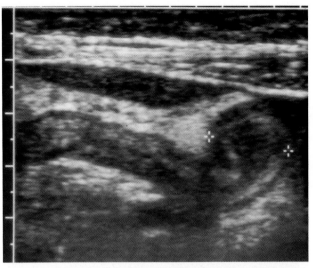

Figure 12–1 Typical US findings in early uncomplicated appendicitis. Note dilated appendix with distal tip (**cursors**) measuring 1 cm. Reprinted with permission from Acute appendicitis: the radiologist's role (editorial), JJ Brown, **Radiology** 1991;180:13—14.

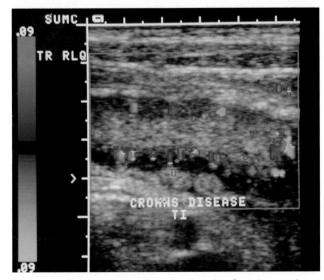

Figure 12–2 Crohn's disease. Color Doppler flow image shows marked hyperemia associated with bowel wall thickening of terminal ileum in a patient clinically thought to have appendicitis. The condition was subsequently confirmed to be Crohn ileitis.

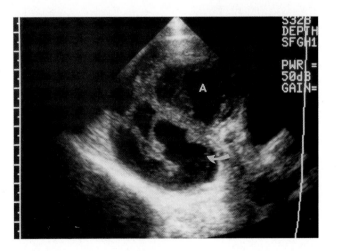

Figure 12–3 Pelvic inflammatory disease mimicking acute appendicitis. US scan shows dilated fallopian tube with low-level echoes representing pyosalpinx (**arrow**). Note adjacent anechoic tuboovarian abscess (**A**).

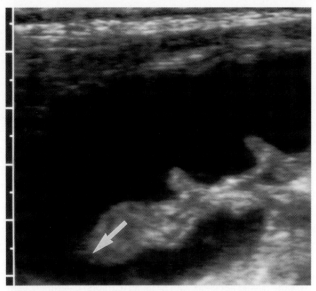

Figure 12–4 Small bowel obstruction mimicking acute appendicitis. US scan shows transition zone (**arrow**) between dilated small bowel and nondilated small bowel and nondilated small bowel, representing focal point of obstruction. Partial small bowel obstruction resulted from adhesions at surgery.

Pitfalls in the Sonographic Diagnosis of Appendicitis

The entire length of the appendix must be visualized to its termination as a blind tip to avoid false-negative diagnoses. Unless the tip is identified, one cannot conclude that the appendix is normal. This is of importance clinically because appendicitis may be entirely confined to the distal appendix (**Fig. 12–5**). In rare occasions, a mildly dilated fallopian tube may be misconstrued as the appendix (**Fig. 12–6**). Another pitfall is that the linear muscle fibers of the psoas muscle may superficially mimic the appearance of the echogenic submucosal layer of the appendix (**Fig. 12–7**). This pitfall can be readily avoided by merely obtaining transverse images of the psoas muscle. Secondary thickening of the appendix may be due to extrinsic periappendiceal inflammatory processes such as tuboovarian abscesses or Crohn's disease (**Fig. 12–8**). The diagnosis of the periappendiceal abscess can only be established with confidence if there is an associated appendicolith or if the abscess is in con-

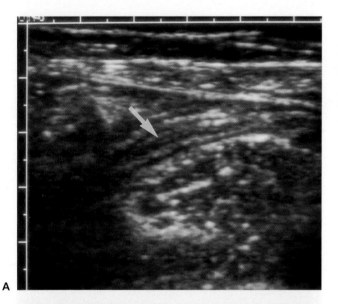

A

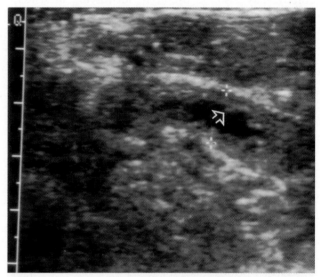

△

Figure 12–6 Dilated fallopian tube mimicking acute appendicitis. US scan shows slightly dilated fallopian tube (**cursors**). Note undulating mucosal folds (**arrow**), which are not typical of a dilated appendix. Reprinted with permission from Acute appendicitis: the radiologist's role (editorial), JJ Brown, **Radiology** 1991;180:13—14.

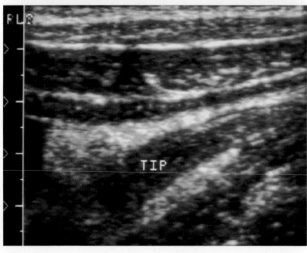

B

◁ **Figure 12–5** Appendicitis confined to distal tlp of appendix. US scans show (**A**) normal base of appendix (**arrow**) and (**B**) distention of tip (TIP) of appendix, with poor definition of echogenic submucosal layer. Surgery indicated necrosis of the distal tip of the appendix, but the proximal appendix was normal. Reprinted with permission from Acute appendicitis: the radiologist's role (editorial), JJ Brown, **Radiology** 1991;180:13—14.

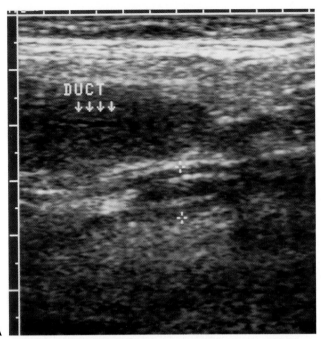

A

Figure 12–7 Muscle fibers of psoas mimicking echogenic submucosal layer of appendix. **A:** US scans shows normal pancreatic duct (**DUCT**) from pancreatic transplant. **Cursors** indicate linear echogenic structures that represent muscle fibers of the psoas muscle. **B:**

B

Transverse US scan confirms that these structures are within psoas muscle (**arrow**). Reprinted with permission from Acute appendicitis: the radiologist's role (editorial), JJ Brown, **Radiology** 1991;180:13—14.

tinuity with mural necrosis of the appendix (**Fig. 12–9**). A rare pitfall is that inspissated stool in the right colon may cause acoustic shadowing and might be misconstrued as an appendicolith (**Fig. 12–10**).

Spontaneous resolution of acute appendicitis may be observed in a small subset of patients (abortive appen-

dicitis) (**Fig. 12–11**). These patients may have imaging criteria for acute appendicitis in the absence of abdominal pain. This underscores the importance of always interpreting the imaging abnormalities in light of the clinical setting.

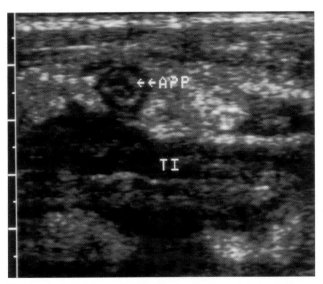

Figure 12–8 Periappendicitis due to Crohn's disease. US scan shows marked thickening of terminal ileum (**TI**) secondary to Crohn disease. Secondary edema of appendix (APP) is due to periappendicitis. Reprinted with permission from Acute appendicitis: the radiologist's role (editorial), JJ Brown, **Radiology** 1991;180:13—14.

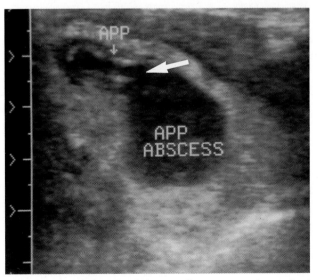

Figure 12–9 Periappendiceal abscess adjacent to mural necrosis of appendix. US scan shows interruption of echogenic submucosal layer (**arrow**) at site of mural necrosis of the appendix (**APP**). Large hypoechoic periappendiceal abscess (**APP ABSCESS**) is also seen.

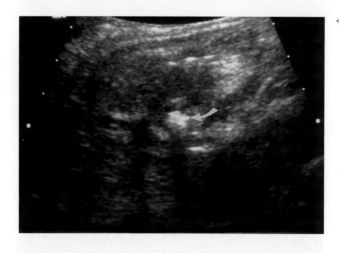

◁ **Figure 12–10** Inspissated stool in ascending colon mimicking appendicolith. Echogenic focus on US scan casts an acoustic shadow that resembles an appendicolith (**arrow**) in the cecum.

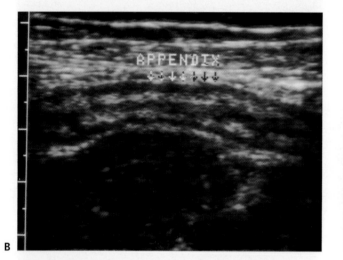

B

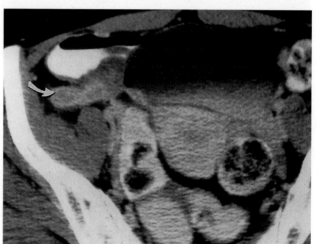

A

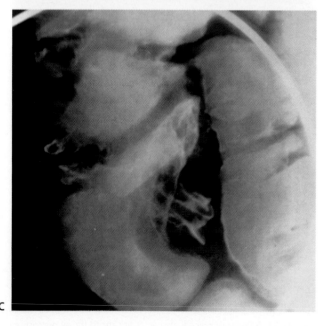

C

Figure 12–11 Abortive Appendicitis. **A**: Transverse US scan of right lower-quadrant demonstrates thickened appendix consistent with acute appendicitis. **B**: Contrast-enhanced CT scan confirms enlarged appendix (**arrow**). **C**: Barium enema study confirms lack of filling of the appendix. Despite clear-cut evidence of appendicitis based on imaging studies, the patient made an uneventful recovery without surgery.

For the most part, the diagnosis of acute appendicitis is based entirely on the gray scale imaging findings. In equivocal cases hyperemia of the inflamed appendix demonstrated by color Doppler sonography may be helpful in establishing the diagnosis. It is important to use low volume flow settings in order to visualize the small intramural appendiceal blood vessels. Other potential uses of color Doppler sonography are in the evaluation of focally thickened bowel wall segments that may assimilate appendicitis. These include ileitis, thrombosis of the ovarian vein (**Fig. 12–12**), the degenerating myomas (**Fig. 12–13**) and other focal gastrointestinal abnormalities (**Fig. 12–14**).

Numerous reports have established the sensitivity of sonography in the range of 76—89%. This is clearly an operator-dependent technique that requires a dedicated sonologist willing to spend the time and effort to master the graded compression technique. Some institutions have much greater experience with CT diagnosis of appendicitis and have relegated sonography to a second-line imaging study.

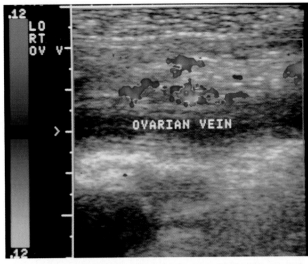

Figure 12–12 Postpartum ovarian vein thrombosis. Color Doppler flow image shows tubular noncompressible structure representing an ovarian vein coursing longitudinally in the right lower-quadrant. One week after delivery, this patient had right lower-quadrant pain that mimicked acute appendicitis.

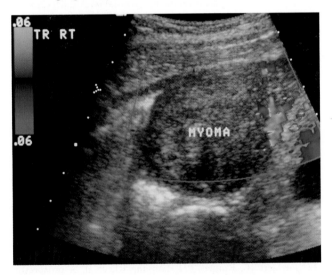

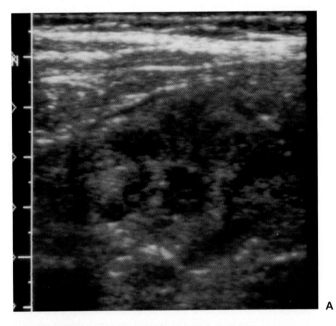

△
Figure 12–13 Degenerating myoma mimicking acute appendicitis. Color Doppler flow image shows avascular myoma in right lower-quadrant with no evidence of flow. Patient had severe pain directly over myoma that required intravenous narcotics, but made an uneventful recovery.

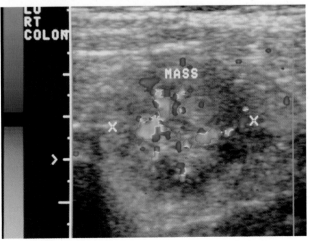

Figure 12–14 Neoplasm mimicking acute appendicitis. **A**: US scan ▷ shows hypoechoic mass involving ascending colon. **B**: Color Doppler flow image demonstrates stellate pattern of vascularity consistent with intrinsic mass. At surgery, a large villoglandular polyp was removed.

A

B

Limitations of Sonography

Graded compression sonography is often quite difficult to perform in either obese patients or in those with severe abdominal pain. It may be difficult in patients with perforation to adequately compress the cecal tip. Obese patients and patients with perforated appendicitis, however, are ideal candidates for CT.

Summary

Sonography and CT play an increasingly important role in the reducing the number of negative surgical explorations for acute appendicitis. Although at times technically challenging, sonography has a number of distinctive advantages in imaging patients with right lower-quadrant pain. At our institution sonography is the method of choice for imaging pediatric patients, women of reproductive age, and thin male patients. CT is complimentary to sonography and it excels in imaging patients who are poor candidates for sonography, namely, obese patients or patients with appendiceal perforation.

References

1. Schrock TR. Acute appendicitis. In: Sleisenger MH, Fordtran JS, eds. *Gastrointestinal Disease: Pathophysiology, Diagnosis, Management*, 4th ed. Philadelphia, Pa: Saunders, 1989, p. 1382—1389.
2. Telford GL, Condon RE. Appendix. In: Zuidema GD, ed. *Shackelford's Surgery of the Alimentary Tract*, 3rd ed. Philadelphia, Pa: Saunders, 1991, p. 133—141.
3. Velanovich V, Satava R. Balancing the normal appendectomy rate with the perforated appendicitis rate: implications for quality assurance. *Am Surg* 1992;58:264—269.
4. Lewis FR, Holcroft JH, Boey J, et al. Appendicitis: a critical review of diagnosis and treatment in 1,000 cases. *Arch Surg* 1975;110:677—684.
5. Sakover RP, Del Fava RL. Frequency of visualization of the normal appendix with the barium enema examination. *AJR* 1974;121:312—317.
6. Olutola PS. Plain film radiographic diagnosis of acute appendicitis: an evaluation of the signs. *Can Assoc Radiol J* 1988;39:254—256.
7. Condon RE. Appendicitis. In: Sabiston DC, ed. *Textbook of Surgery*, 13th ed. Philadelphia, PA: Saunders, 1986;967—982.
8. Balthazar EJ, Megibow AJ, Siegel SE, Birnbaum BA. Appendicitis: prospective evaluation with high-resolution CT. *Radiology* 1991;180:21—24.
9. Puylaert JB. Acute appendicitis: US evaluation using graded compression. *Radiology* 1986;158:355—360.
10. Anderson M, Lilja T, Lundell L, et al. Clinical and laboratory findings in patients subjected to laparotomy for suspected acute appendicitis. *Acta Chir Scand* 1980;146:55—63.
11. Pieper R, Kager L, Nasman P. Acute appendicitis: a clinical study of 1018 cases of emergency appendectomy. *Acta Chir Scand* 1982;148:51—62.
12. Dunn EL, Moore EE, Elderling SC, et al. The unnecessary laparotomy for appendicitis: can it be decreased? *Arch Surg* 1975; 110:677—684.
13. Cope Z. *Cope's Early Diagnosis of the Acute Abdomen*. New York, NY: Oxford University Press, 1987.
14. Sumpio BE, Ballantyne GH, Zdon MJ, Modlin IM. Perforated appendicitis and obstructing colonic carcinoma in the elderly. *Dis Colon Rectum* 1986;29:668—670.
15. Dueholm S, Bagi P, Bud M. Laboratory aid in the diagnosis of acute appendicitis: a blinded, prospective trial concerning diagnostic value of leukocyte count, neutrophil differential count, and C-reactive protein. *Dis Colon Rectum* 1989;32:855—859.
16. Balthazar EJ, Birnbaum BA, Yee J, et al. Acute appendicitis: CT and US correlation in 100 patients. *Radiology* 1994;190:31—35.
17. Malone AJ Jr, Wolf CR, Malmed AS, Melliere BF. Diagnosis of acute appendicitis: value of unenhanced CT. *AJR* 1993;160:763—766.
18. Lane MJ, Katz DS, Ross BA, et al. Unenhanced helical CT for suspected acute appendicitis. *AJR* 1997;168:405—409.
19. Rao PM, Rhea JT, Novelline RA, et al. Helical CT technique for the diagnosis of appendicitis: prospective evaluation of a focused appendix CT examination. *Radiology* 1997;202:139—144.
20. Rao PM, Rhea JT, Novelline RA, Mostafavi AA, McCabe CJ. Effect of computed tomography of the appendix on treatment of patients and use of hospital resources. *N Engl J Med* 1998;338(3):141—146.
21. Rioux M. Sonographic detection of the normal and abnormal appendix. *AJR* 1992;158:773—778.
22. Jeffrey RB Jr, Laing FC, Townsend RR. Acute appendicitis: sonographic criteria based on 250 cases. *Radiology* 1988;167:327—329.
23. Jeffrey RB Jr, Jain KA, Nghiem HV. Sonographic diagnosis of acute appendicitis: interpretive pitfalls. *AJR* 1994;162:55—59.
24. Jeffrey RB Jr, Ralls PW. *CT and sonography of the acute abdomen*, 2nd ed. Philadelphia, PA: Lippincott-Raven, 1995, p. 289—295.
25. Brown JJ. Acute appendicitis: the radiologist's role (editorial). *Radiology* 1991;180:13—14.
26. Schwerk WB, Wichtrup B, Ruschoff J, Rothmund M. Acute and perforated appendicitis: current experience with ultrasound-aided diagnosis. *World J Surg* 1990;14:271—276.
27. Puylaert JB, Rutgers PH, Lalisang RI, et al. A prospective study of ultrasonography in the diagnosis of appendicitis. *N Engl J Med* 1987;317:666—669.
28. Jeffrey RB Jr, Sommer FG, Debatin JF. Color Doppler sonography of focal gastrointestinal lesions: initial clinical experience. *J Ultrasound Med* 1994;13:473—478.
29. Clautice-Engle T, Jeffrey RB Jr, Li KCP, Barth RA. Power Doppler imaging of focal lesions of the gastrointestinal tract: comparison with conventional color Doppler imaging. *J Ultrasound Med* 1996;15:63—66.
30. Gaensler EH, Jeffrey RB Jr, Laing FC, Townsend RR. Sonography in patients with suspected acute appendicitis: value in establishing alternative diagnoses. *AJR* 1989;152:49—51.

Male Genital System

13 Color Duplex Sonography of Acute Scrotal Pain

Tom Stavros, Cindy Rapp, and Jon McGrath

The Clinical Picture

The differential diagnosis for acute scrotal pain includes testicular torsion (spermatic cord torsion), infection (epididymitis, orchitis, epididymoorchitis), torsion of the appendix testis, trauma, incarcerated inguinal hernia, hemorrhage into a testicular tumor, vasculitis, and spermatic cord thrombosis or occlusion (during inguinal hernia surgery). The most common causes vary with age, but in all age groups, spermatic cord torsion and infection are, by far, the leading causes of acute scrotal pain. In adults, infection is more common than torsion. However, in children (including neonates), torsion is more common. Torsion of the appendix is also relatively common in children. The remaining causes of acute scrotal pain are relatively rare in all age groups (Table 13–1).

Differentiating torsion from infection is an urgent problem. Torsion can lead to infarction of the testis within a few hours, so rapid reduction of the torsion is necessary. The mechanism of infarction is initially venous and lymphatic obstruction, later followed by arterial obstruction. The soft lymphatic and venous structures are prone to obstruction at lower degrees of torsion than are the testicular arteries. The rapidity with which torsion causes infarction varies with the degree of torsion. Infarction may not occur for days if there is only 90 degrees of torsion. On the other hand, 720 degrees of torsion may cause infarction in two h. Intermediate degrees of torsion lead to infarction in intermediate lengths of time.

An underlying anatomic abnormality, the "bell-clapper deformity," usually predisposes a patient to torsion. In the bellclapper deformity, the normal, "low, broad attachment of the tunica vaginalis to the posterior surface of the testis is absent. Instead, the tunica vaginalis attaches in an abnormally high position to the spermatic cord, and the mesorchium is abnormally long. The lack of attachment of the testis to tunica vaginalis predisposes the testis to torsion around the high point of attachment to the spermatic cord. Thus, testicular torsion should more properly be termed *spermatic cord torsion*. The bellclapper deformity is usually bilateral, predisposing both sides to torsion.

The urgent reduction of torsion may be performed surgically or nonsurgically under local anesthetic. Regardless of whether reduction of torsion is surgical or nonsurgical, orchiopexy is required to prevent repeat torsion at a later date. Orchiopexy is almost always performed bilaterally, as the bell-clapper deformity, which is the underlying predisposition to torsion, is usually bilateral.

The patient's clinical history may be helpful, but often is atypical. The precipitating factor is often an unusually strong contraction of the cremasteric muscle, which may be caused by trauma, strenuous exercise, or sexual activity. However, in many patients the onset of pain occurs during sleep, without any apparent cause for forceful contraction of the cremasteric muscle. The onset of pain in spermatic cord torsion is usually acute. Gradual onset of pain is more typical of infection, but up to 25% of torsion patients also have gradual onset of pain. Patients may spontaneously detorse, and careful questioning sometimes reveals a history of repeated episodes of scrotal pain due to torsion. Urinary symptoms such as dysuria are relatively rare in torsion in comparison to epididymitis.

Like the clinical history, the patient's physical examination may not reveal the classical signs of torsion. The torsed testis is usually swollen, painful, and tender, but may be nontender. Swelling of the testes and scrotal skin is usually present in both torsion and infection. The torsed testis usually is in an abnormally high, transverse position, with the epididymis rotated anteriorly, but in some cases it is not. The high, transverse testicular position is probably related to the degree of torsion. It is said that the pain from infection improves if the testis is elevated and supported, although the pain due to torsion

Table 13–1 Differential diagnosis of acute scrotal pain

Children	Torsion >	Infection > Appendage Torsion	Tumor Trauma Hernia Spermatic versus occlusion Vasculitis
Adults	Infection >	Torsion >	Appendage torsion Tumor Trauma Hernia Spermatic versus occlusion Vasculitis

does not. This statement is untrue in many patients. The physical examination may be suboptimal because of pain, although injection of the spermatic cord in the inguinal canal with lidocaine may allow a more thorough and accurate physical examination and facilitate nonsurgical external reduction.

In patients in whom the history and physical examination do not reveal classical symptoms, ultrasound (US), and radionuclide flow studies have been used to help differentiate between torsion and infection. The sensitivity of color duplex sonography and power Doppler sonography for demonstrating the relatively slow, sparse flow within the testes has improved markedly in the past few years. Our ability to demonstrate specific patterns of edema within the testis, epididymis, and spermatic cord has also improved. The combination of improved imaging and Doppler capabilities has increased the role of color Doppler examination, which is now the imaging procedure of choice for evaluation of acute scrotal pain in most imaging centers.

Ultrasound Equipment and Machine Setup

Scrotal sonography requires excellent high-resolution, near-field imaging equipment and excellent Doppler sensitivity. Color Doppler flow imaging must be able to depict relatively slow flow in vessels too small to see on the US image, which require a high-frequency (7.5 MHz to 10 MHz), electronically focused linear probe. A 5-MHz linear probe can be used, but its sensitivity to flow in intratesticular arteries will be much less than that of the higher frequency probes. A 5-MHz transducer will more frequently fail to show normal flow than will a 7.5-MHz transducer, especially in children. Most 5-MHz probes also have short-axis fixed focal zones too deep for optimal scanning of the scrotal contents. However, in patients with large hydroceles or hematoceles, severe testicular enlargement, a large testicular mass, or severe skin swelling, the greater focal length of the 5-MHz linear probe may be an advantage.

Power Doppler imaging is more sensitive than color Doppler flow imaging for showing relatively slow flow in small vessels, such as those within the normal testis. Power Doppler US imaging has improved our ability to demonstrate normal blood flow within the testis, especially in young boys and very old men who have less flow within the testes. Being able to demonstrate flow within the normal contralateral asymptomatic testis is critical to the diagnosis of torsion, because failure to do so makes lack of demonstrable flow in the symptomatic testis meaningless.

Some US equipment enables the user to downshift the Doppler frequency to a lower frequency than is normally used for imaging (i.e., the Doppler frequency on a 7-MHz linear transducer might be 5 MHz rather than 7 MHz). This downshift allows better penetration for peripheral vascular applications and also allows a greater degree of beam steering to optimize angles of incidence in peripheral vessels, such as the carotid and femoral arteries. However, downshifted Doppler frequencies and beam steering both reduce Doppler sensitivity and should not be used for evaluating intratesticular blood flow. If the vessels of interest within the scrotum are coursing at an obtuse angle of incidence, then it is easy to move the probe on the surface of the testis to a position in which the angle of incidence is more acute. Angles as close to 0 degrees as possible should be sought and are usually possible. Sliding the probe to a different location on the surface of the scrotum is a better way to improve angles of incidence than is beam steering. Some units may have default settings of downshifted Doppler frequency. On such units, if the steering options are visible in the left lower corner of the video monitor, the Doppler frequency is downshifted. Using these default settings may adversely affect results. Such equipment usually allows the user to create present programs with optimal parameters for a given application. It is best to use such present programs for applications such as testicular scanning to quickly optimize the settings and minimize the changes of interpretive error due to incorrect selection of parameters.

The probe and unit should be set to maximize sensitivity to blood flow. High Doppler sensitivity is especially important in young children and old men, who have less flow and slower flow than young adult and middle-aged men. Full color and pulsed Doppler power, low-velocity scales, low wall filters, and high gray-scale-write-priorities maximize sensitivity. Many units, due to U.S. Food and Drug Administration requirements, boot up at low-power settings for safety purposes. These low-power settings adversely affect Doppler sensitivity for the detection of flow, especially in children. The risk-to-benefit ratio of Doppler imaging in these patients demands full power. Low-velocity scales (pulse repetition frequency) and low wall-filter settings also maximize our chances of demonstrating flow. The US unit can write either color or gray scale to each pixel, but not both. The write-priority tells the unit how white a gray-scale pixel can be overwritten with color. Peripheral vascular applications, with large lucent vessels require low write-priority settings (that is, toward the black end of the gray scale). In such cases, high write-priorities (toward the white end of the gray-scale spectrum would result in too much artifactual color being written into echogenic tissues outside of the vessels. In contrast to large peripheral vessels, the testis and epididymis are relatively echogenic. Many of the vessels within them that are being interrogated are too small to resolve on the B-mode image. Therefore, color flow must be displayed on a relatively white background by using a high write-priority (**Fig. 13–1**). If the write-priority settings are too low (like those used for peripheral vascular imaging), color may not be written in the image of the testis, even when the unit has correctly detected it. Some units do not have a separate control for write-priority, and have combined control of this parameter with other parameters (threshold control).

In most cases, color Doppler or power Doppler imaging alone is sufficient to distinguish between infection and torsion. Sometimes, it may be helpful to perform pulsed Doppler spectral analysis. In such cases, the pulsed Doppler evaluation should be used without steering. In our experience, it is possible to maneuver the probe so that the angle of incidence of the pulsed Doppler beam is near 0 degrees without steering. We have also found that using a wider sample volume improves the quality of the spectral tracing when the vessel being interrogated is small and the angle of incidence is near 0 degrees (**Fig. 13–2**).

Occasionally, the length of the testis is too great to measure with a 7,5-MHz linear array transducer. In such cases the 5-MHz linear probe usually offers no advantage, as it is usually the same length as the 7.5-MHz probe. In such patients, a 5-MHz curved linear probe usually enables us to obtain an accurate length.

Sonographic and Duplex Technique

US examination of the scrotum in patients with acute scrotal pain should always include Doppler studies in addition to gray-scale imaging. On the other hand, Doppler evaluation is usually not necessary when the patient has a palpable nodule or mass. In patients in whom the clinical index of suspicion of torsion is high and in those who have gross enlargement of the testis, color Doppler flow imaging should be used early in the examination to make as prompt a diagnosis of torsion as possible. A color or power Doppler examination of the symptomatic testis can usually be performed in a few minutes.

The entire testis and epididymis should be scanned in real time to get an overall picture of the scrotal contents and alignment of the testis and epididymis. The contralateral asymptomatic side is also quickly surveyed to get an idea about symmetry in size and echogenicity between the two sides and also to assess the position and alignment of the contralateral testis and epididymis. The spermatic cord should be inspected from a few centimeters superior to the epididymal head to the tail of the epididymis. The presence of a complex hydrocele and debris or adhesions within it should be noted. Intratesticular nodules or masses should be excluded, and the testes measured. The presence of a solid mass or nodule within the testis suggests the presence of a neoplasm. A complex cyst within the testis may represent an abscess resulting from orchitis or necrosis resulting from infarction or tumor.

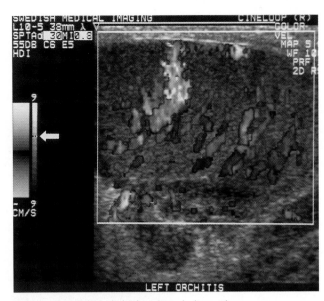

Figure 13–1 Relatively high write-priority setting.

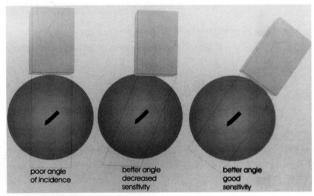

poor angle of incidence

better angle decreased sensitivity

better angle good sensitivity

Figure 13–2 Illustration showing that intratesticular vessels should be scanned at a nearly zero angle of incidence. The probe has great freedom in position and angle with respect to the surface and contents of the testis. This allows the sonographic approach to be changed to achieve Doppler angles of incidence near zero. These angles can also be accomplished by electronically steering the Doppler beam, however, steering is to be discouraged, because Doppler sensitivity is virtually always adversely affected by it.

One advantage of scrotal–testicular color duplex sonography is that there is almost always a mirror-image contralateral normal structure with which the painful side may be compared. This advantage should be employed to its fullest extent. When the color Doppler findings do not indicate torsion and the need for immediate surgery, we make this comparison by obtaining split-screen images of corresponding right and left intrascrotal contents. We always obtain transverse and longitudinal split-screen images of the testes (**Fig. 13–3** through **13–4**), epididymal heads (**Fig. 13–5**), and epididymal tails (**Fig. 13–6**). The epididymal tails are usually best seen from an inferior (**Fig. 13–6** through **13–8**) or coronal approach (**Fig. 13–9** through **13–11**). Transverse split-screen images of the testes and spermatic cords just superior to the epididymal heads are also ob-

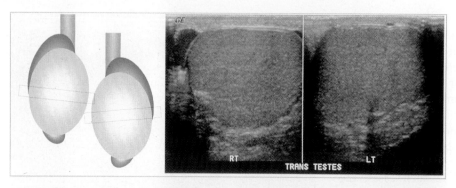

Figure 13–3 Split-screen short-axis views of right and left testes.

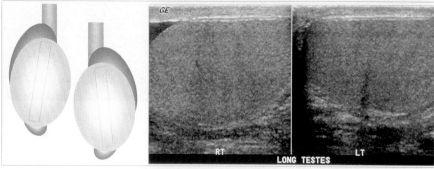

Figure 13–4 Split-screen long-axis views of right and left testes.

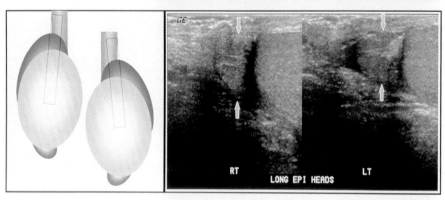

Figure 13–5 Split-screen long-axis view of epididymal head viewed from anteriorly.

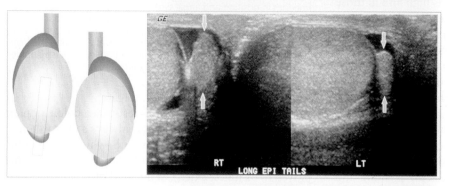

Figure 13–6 Split-screen long-axis views of the epididymal tails viewed from inferiorly.

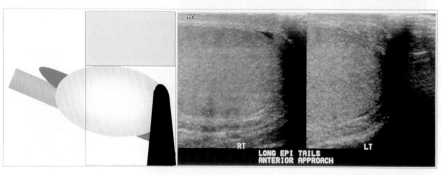

Figure 13–7 Attempted split-screen long-axis views of the epididymal tails. The epididymal tails are obscured by critical angle shadowing created by the curved lower poles of the testes. This occurs because the epididymal tails do not extend inferiorly beyond the lower poles. Obscuration of the tails by shadowing can be avoided by using an inferior or coronal approach to show the epididymal tails.

tained (**Fig. 13–12**). Occasionally, scanning the spermatic cords in the inguinal canals can be helpful. If the appendices testes or appendices epididymie are visible split-screen images of them are also obtained, especially if any asymmetry is found. It is important to make sure that the split-screen images are obtained symmetrically through the widest part of the structures being imaged and that the angles of incidence be as close to 90 degrees as possible to minimize artifactual shadowing and errant assessment of relative echogenicity. The right and left organs should be symmetrical in size and echogenicity. Demonstrating symmetrical sections through right and left sides may require grossly different probe orientations on the right and left sides, because the position of the tests within the scrotal sac in normal individuals are usually asymmetrical. In torsion, this asymmetry of position is even more pronounced. The relative position of the right and left sides is ascertained at the time of the initial survey. Because the testes are freely mobile within the scrotal sac, the alignment of the testis may change during the examination. The goal of this systematic imaging approach is to detect a pattern of swelling or abnormal echogenicity that favors a diagnosis of either infection or torsion. For example, swelling of the epididymal tail and spermatic cord in the absence of testicular swelling strongly suggests epididymitis. Furthermore, systematic scanning minimizes the chances of missing the key findings of infection. For example, epididymitis may affect only the spermatic cord and epididymal tail, sparing the epididymal head and testis. Failure to evaluate the spermatic cords and epididymal tails will cause these findings to be missed.

We also obtain a short axis view through the median raphe of the scrotum in order to compare the echogenicity of the testes on a single image (**Fig. 13–13**). It is important that the angle of incidence of the beam into the testes be bilaterally symmetrical on this view to minimize the chance that critical angle shadowing will make a testis artifactually look hypoechoic. Usually the left end of the probe must be angled inferiorly, as the left testis usually lies lower than the right, but this relationship may be altered in torsion.

A Doppler US examination begins with color or power Doppler interrogation of the testes. We usually quickly evaluate the asymptomatic testis first, to make sure that flow is detectable on the side in which torsion is not suspected. If no flow exists in the asymptomatic side,

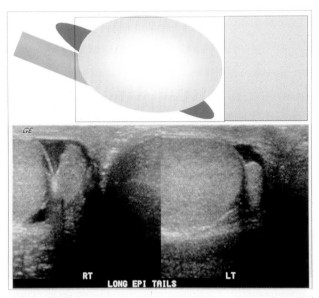

Figure 13–8 When scanned from an inferior approach, the tail of the epididymis is not obscured by critical angle shadowing created by the curved lower pole of the testis.

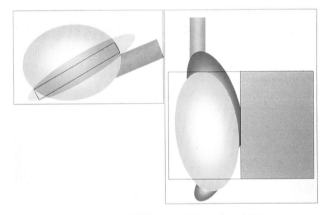

Figure 13–9 Coronal or "C" view of the left epididymis as seen from anteriorly (right illustration) and from the left side (top illustration). The epididymal tail usually lies more inferiorly and laterally than the head.

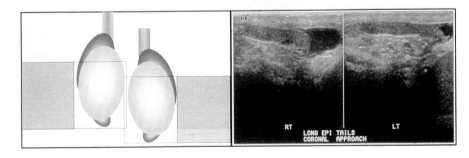

Figure 13–10 Split-screen coronal images of the right and left epididymal tails.

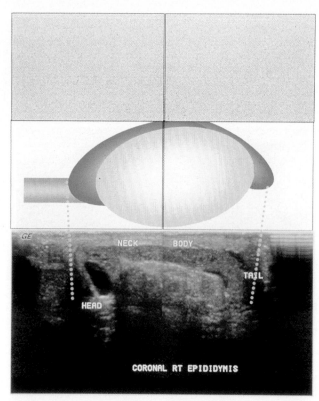

Figure 13–11 Coronal or "C" dual screen view of the entire epididymis. The "C" stands for coronal view and for the shape of the epididymis as seen from the coronal approach.

decreased or absent flow in the symptomatic side will have no meaning. On the other hand, increased flow in the symptomatic testis is always important, regardless of the contralateral findings. It indicates inflammatory hyperemia, which is usually due to orchitis. However, reactive hyperemia can also occur after spontaneous detorsion.

If flow is present in the asymptomatic testis, but *absent or decreased* in the symptomatic testis, then torsion is likely. Duplex sonographic interrogation with spectral tracings and complete color Doppler and duplex sonographic studies of the remainder of the intrascrotal contents are usually not performed because it is important for the patient to undergo surgery as soon as possible. Additional examinations in such patients may waste valuable time in which the patient could be prepared for surgery. It should be kept in mind, however, that severe infection, trauma, and inguinal hernia surgery can lead to ischemia of a testis, which appears similar to torsion on color Doppler flow imaging or power Doppler imaging. In most instances of ischemia caused by conditions other than torsion, the ischemic changes are focal or patchy rather than diffuse.

If flow is present in both testes, but increased in the symptomatic testis or if there appears to be normal and symmetrical flow in both testes, torsion is unlikely. Complete color Doppler and duplex sonographic examination of the epididymal heads and tails and spermatic

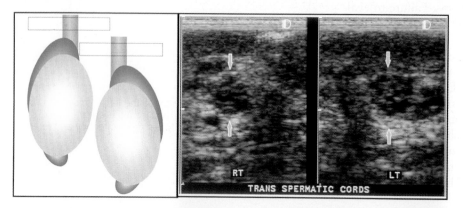

Figure 13–12 Short-axis views of spermatic cords just superior to epididymal heads.

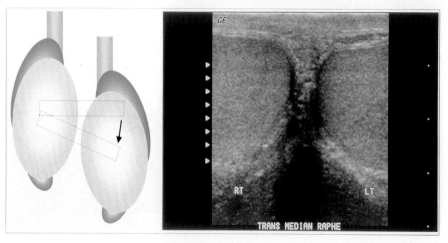

Figure 13–13 Short-axis median raphe view is usually angled inferiorly on the left because the left testis is lower.

cord can then be performed. In some cases, spectral Doppler analysis will show asymmetries in velocities and resistivity indexes, even when color Doppler appears symmetrical. The goal of complete color Doppler or duplex sonographic examination of the testes, epididymi, and spermatic cords, like the goal of a gray scale US examination of these structures, is to detect a pattern of hyperemia that suggests a specific diagnosis. For example, abnormally high velocities and low resistivity indexes in the epididymis, but normal velocities in the testes, strongly favor a diagnosis of epididymitis over other causes.

It is very important to look at and interrogate the intratesticular vessels as well as the more easily seen capsular vessels. In cases of missed torsion, marked hyperemia may exist in the tunica vaginalis, which is immediately adjacent and adherent to the testis. This flow may be mistaken for testicular capsular artery flow, causing the diagnosis of torsion to be missed. This mistake will not be made, however, if normal and symmetrical flow is seen within intratesticular arteries. By moving the probe along the surface of the scrotum, it is possible to create an optimal angle of incidence of near 0 degrees. As mentioned earlier, this approach is preferable to electronically steering the ultrasound beam, which decreases Doppler sensitivity.

In most cases the combined pattern of swelling, altered echogenicity, and increased or decreased flow on Doppler US examination suggest the exact cause of scrotal pain.

Normal Imaging and Doppler Findings

Normal testes, epididymi, and spermatic cords are bilaterally symmetrical in size and texture. The epididymi and testes are normally relatively homogenous and have midlevel echogenicity. The spermatic cords, on the other hand, are very tortuous, which makes it difficult to obtain exact longitudinal or transverse cuts and makes comparisons with the contralateral side more difficult. The spermatic cords also have heterogeneous texture due to the venous plexus and abundant loose connective tissues they contain. The tortuosity makes it virtually impossible to get exact measurements of the spermatic cord dimensions, but an eyeball estimate of size is usually possible. Asymmetries in size, shape, homogeneity, and echogenicity between right and left sides are abnormal.

With current equipment, flow is demonstrable within the capsular arteries, the intratesticular vessels (centripetal and sometimes, recurrent rami), and within the spermatic artery in the spermatic cord in adult patients (**Fig. 13–14**). However, flow can be more difficult to demonstrate in children, particularly very young children and newborns, and in very elderly men. Demonstrable color Doppler flow is symmetrical in the right

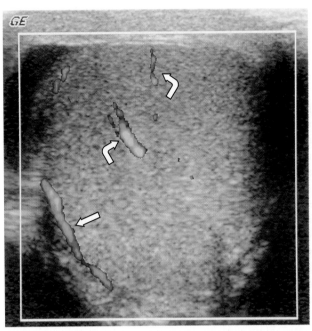

Figure 13–14 Power Doppler image of left testis showing a capsular artery (**straight arrow**) along the medial surface of the testis and portions of two centripetal arteries (**curved arrows**) within the substance of the testis. Intratesticular vessels rather than capsular arteries should be relied upon to exclude torsion.

and left testes. The intratesticular vessels are not evenly distributed through the substance of the testis, however; they pass through the testis in a few discrete tissue planes. If the US probe is parallel to the plane in which the intratesticular vessels pass on one side, but not parallel to the plane in the contralateral testis, the flow may appear falsely asymmetrical. Every effort should be made to compare comparable tissue planes within the two testes. The vascular planes of the testis are oriented in the long axis of the testis. Therefore, errors in assessment of vascularity are more likely to occur in the longitudinal planes than in transverse plans. The capsular arteries are usually best seen in segments that course at nearly a 0 degree angle of incidence to the beam. This most commonly occurs on the lower medial surface of the testis. Multiple intratesticular vessels are visible in most adult testes, but may be more or less evident, depending upon the angle of incidence and scan plane.

With current equipment, some flow is demonstrable within the epididymal head in a majority of adult patients. Flow is not demonstrable within the epididymal head in a small percentage of adults and in most children. Flow within the epididymal tail is demonstrable in a larger percentage of adult patients than flow within the epididymal head but, once again, generally not demonstrable in children. In color Doppler flow imaging it is often difficult to determine whether flow is from the epididymal head or the adjacent spermatic cord. In these patients, the pattern of flow on duplex sonographic spectral analysis can help determine whether the interrogated vessel is within the spermatic cord or epididymal head. Normal epididymal head has very low velocity and lacks an early diastolic notch. However, flow within the testicular artery or supratesticular artery has higher systolic flow velocity with prominent early diastolic notches.

Normal testicular spectral tracings for the right and left sides should be symmetrical if the vessels being interrogated are of symmetrical size, angle of incidence, and depth. Every attempt should be made to compare symmetrical vessels on the two sides. Some diastolic flow is usually present within the capsular and intratesticular arteries in normal individuals. Velocities are usually, but not always higher, within the capsular than within the intratesticular arteries. If the intratesticular arteries have higher velocities than the capsular arteries on one side, the same is usually true of the contralateral side. Peak systolic velocities in testicular arteries usually range from about 5 to 14 cm/s. Peak end-diastolic velocities vary from 2 to 3 cm/s. In severe epididymitis, the velocities in the epididymal head may exceed those within the testis. Flow with the testicular artery in the spermatic cord just posterior and superior to the epididymal head has a higher systolic velocity, which may exceed 15 cm/s, and low diastolic flow, which is similar to those of the epididymal head. The waveform shape in the testicular artery and supratesticular artery is markedly different from those seen within the epididymal head.

Epididymal tail waveforms look more like spermatic cord waveforms than epididymal head or testicular waveforms. Their peak systolic velocities are intermediate between the higher velocities of the main testicular artery within the spermatic cord and the lower velocities within the substance of the epididymal heads.

Findings in Testicular Torsion

Imaging Findings

The testis, epididymis, and spermatic cord below the point of torsion are all abnormally enlarged (Fig. 13–15 through 13–16). The enlargement increases over time, so patients who are very early in the course of torsion may have only minimal enlargement. The echogenicity of the testis is usually decreased, although late in the process, after infarction has occurred, hemorrhage into the testis may cause heterogeneously increased echogenity. The echogenicity of the epididymis and spermatic cord also vary, depending on whether hemorrhage has occurred. If the spermatic cord is carefully examined, an abrupt increase in the size and alteration of the spermatic cord may be noted below the point of torsion (Fig. 13–17). Enlarged acutely thrombosed pampiniform plexus veins within the spermatic cord may also be visible. The literature mentions enlargement and increased echogenicity within the epididymal head in torsion. However, in our experience, in most cases of torsion the epididymal head is only mildly enlarge, but the spermatic cord, which passes just superiorly and posteriorly to the epididymal head is grossly enlarged. We think that the swollen spermatic cord immediately adjacent to the epididymal head has been mistaken for an enlarged epididymal head in many reports in the literature.

Doppler Findings

In a large majority of cases, flow within the substance of the torsed testis is absent, but demonstrable flow exists in the contralateral asymptomatic testis (Fig. 13–18). In cases with lesser degrees of torsion (90 degree), however, some flow may still be present within the torsed testis. In such cases the peak systolic velocities will be abnormally low compared to the contralateral asymptomatic testis. These abnormally low velocities may be associated with either abnormally high or abnormally low resistivity indexes. Because of cases such as

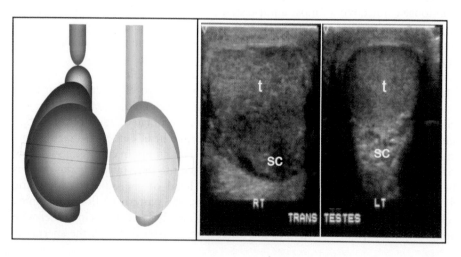

Figure 13–15 Short-axis views of right and left testes (t) and spermatic cords (sc) in a patient with right spermatic cord torsion. The right testis is swollen and mildly hyperechoic, and the right spermatic cord is swollen and mildly hypoechoic.

Figure 13–16 Long-axis views of the epididymal heads and proximal spermatic cords in a patient with right spermatic cord torsion show the right epididymal head to be mildly enlarged and hyperechoic and the right spermatic cord to be enlarged and mildly hypoechoic.

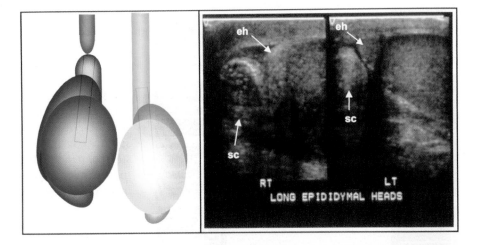

Figure 13–17 Long-axis view of the right spermatic cord in a patient with right spermatic cord torsion shows a marked difference in the size of the spermatic cord above and below the point of spermatic cord torsion. Note that the enlargement of the cord below the torsion is manifested by multiple prominent hypoechoic structures that represent enlarged thrombosed veins within the pampiniform plexus.

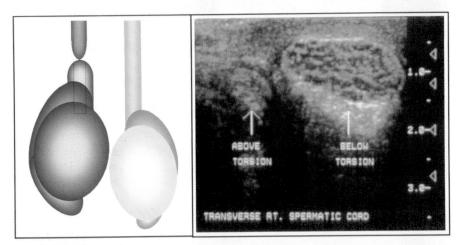

Figure 13–18 Color Doppler images of the right and left testes in a patient with torsion of the right spermatic cord show absent flow within the right testis, but normal capsular and centripetal artery flow in the contralateral asymptomatic left testis.

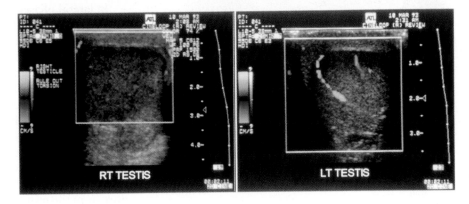

these, simply showing some flow within a torsed testis does not completely exclude a diagnosis of torsion. It is still necessary to compare the flow to that in the contralateral side. Flow on the surface of the testis also does not exclude a diagnosis of torsion. Flow must be shown within the intratesticular branches of the testicular artery, the centripetal arteries, and recurrent rami. Demonstrating this flow is necessary because the tunica vaginalis may adhere to the surface of the testis, and reactive hyperemia within tunica vaginalis may be mistaken for testicular capsular artery flow, which causes the diagnosis of torsion to be missed.

Obviously, no significance can be attributed to a lack of demonstrable flow in the painful testis if flow is not demonstrable in the contralateral asymptomatic testis.

In torsion, flow within the swollen spermatic cord and within the epididymis is also reduced or absent (**Fig. 13–19**). The presence of hyperemia within the epididymis and spermatic cord strongly favors a diagnosis of infection over one of torsion.

In some patients, spontaneous detorsion may occur before a color duplex sonographic examination. If infarction has already occurred, the findings will be the same as if torsion still exists. However, in patients in

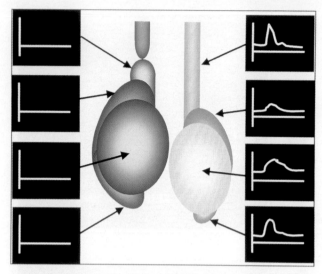

Figure 13–19 Illustration shows example of pulsed Doppler spectral analysis findings in right spermatic cord torsion. Flow is completely absent in both the right capsular and centripetal arteries within the testis, and from the epididymis and spermatic cord.

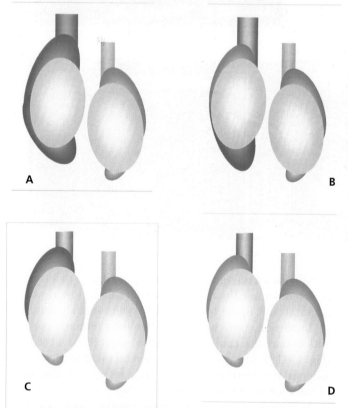

Figure 13–20A: Right epididymitis — entire epididymis and spermatic cord involved. **B**: right epididymitis — tail and spermatic cord involved. **C**: right epididymitis — head and spermatic cord involved. **D**: right funiculitis (vasitis) — spermatic cord involved alone.

whom spontaneous detorsion occurs before infarction, the US scan and Doppler findings may be either normal or show residual swelling with reactive hyperemia, findings absolutely identical to those seen in patients with epididymoorchitis. In such patients, the history may he helpful. Decreasing pain before sonographic examination raises the question of whether spontaneous detorsion has occurred. A history of previous episodes of spontaneously resolving pain may also be elicited from such patients. Most untreated patients with epididymoorchitis, on the other hand, will have not any abatement of pain before scanning.

Findings in Epididymitis, Orchitis, and Epididymoorchitis

Imaging Findings

Most cases of infection ascend from the prostate or urinary tract. The infection ascends, in order, through the vas deferens, the spermatic cord, to the epididymal tail, the epididymal body, the epididymal head, and finally into the testis. The patient may undergo a sonographic examination at any point in this progressive process. The pattern of swelling and altered echogenicity will reflect the pattern of infectious involvement (**Fig. 20 A,B,C,D**).

With isolated vasitis or funiculitis, which occurs very early in the course of ascending infection, only the spermatic cord may be swollen.

In lateral phases, the spermatic cord and epididymal tail may be infected and swollen, with sparing of the epididymal head and body. This pattern of presentation is actually quite common. It is, therefore, very important to evaluate the epididymal tails in those patients with acute scrotal pain who do not show immediate evidence of torsion. In some cases, the swelling of the epididymal tail may be so massive that the tail indents and distorts the testis and simulates a primary testicular mass. In such cases, liquefactive necrosis and abscess formation may also be found within the epididymal tail. Such very severe cases of epididymitis may obstruct venous outflow from the testis, leading to a venous infarction similar to that caused by torsion.

Some cases of epididymitis will more severely affect the head rather than the tail. In such cases, the degree of swelling and textural abnormality in the head will exceed that of the tail. From the US literature and from our daily experience it would seem that epididymitis involves the head more frequently and severely than it involves the tail. The reverse is actually true, however, clinical findings of epididymitis of the tail are more easily distinguished from those of torsion than findings of epididymitis of the head. Patients with predominant involvement of the tail are diagnosed clinically, and, therefore, less frequently require imaging studies for definitive diagnosis.

In all cases of epididymitis, the degree of swelling in the affected part of the epididymis will exceed the swelling and textural abnormality in the testis. This pattern is so typical of epididymitis that it virtually excludes a diagnosis of torsion, even before Doppler US examination is performed.

Untreated cases of epididymitis may eventually lead to orchitis, resulting in epididymoorchitis. In such cases the spermatic cord, epididymis, and testis will all be enlarged and have altered echogenicity (**Fig. 13–21** through **26**). This pattern of involvement is very similar to that caused by torsion. In these cases, color, power, or pulsed Doppler findings enable us to distinguish epididymoorchitis from torsion.

The pattern of swelling parallels the pattern of inflammation. In epididymoorchitis the testes, epididymal heads and tails, and spermatic cords are all swollen. However, in epididymitis, the spermatic cord and all or part of the epididymis is swollen. In vasitis or funiculitis, only the spermatic cord is swollen.

Doppler Findings

Acute inflammation leads to arteriolar, venular, and capillary dilatation. This dilatation, in turn, increases blood flow within vessels supplying the inflamed organ. The inflammatory hyperemia of vasitis, funiculitis, epididymitis, and orchitis is readily demonstrable by color duplex sonography. Compared with the contralateral uninfected side, the inflamed organ shows more numerous and larger vessels on color or power Doppler imaging.

The pattern of hyperemia parallels the pattern of swelling — that is, when epididymitis involves primarily the tail, the greatest and most obvious degree of hyperemia will be within the swollen epididymal tail (**Fig. 13–20** through **13–21**). When epididymoorchitis exists, both the testis and the epididymis will be hyperemic (**Fig. 13–27** through **30**). In some patients, the development of inflammatory hyperemia will precede any demonstrable enlargement.

In most cases, the increased flow in the inflamed organ will be so obvious that duplex sonographic spectral analysis is not necessary. In cases, where color Doppler evidence of increased flow is less evident, spectral analysis may be helpful. This is especially true in children and elderly adults, in whom velocities are normally lower. In these patients, a peak systolic velocity that is 4 cm/s more than a corresponding mirror image contralateral peak systolic view suggests testicular hyperemia. A ratio of the peak systolic velocity of 1.7 or greater between symptomatic and asymptomatic testes indicates the presence of hyperemia on the symptomatic side (**Fig. 13–31**).

Peak systolic velocities in the epididymal head over 5 cm/s and end diastolic velocities over 3 cm/s usually indicate epididymitis. The peak systolic velocity of the epididymal tail and spermatic cord is more variable, and

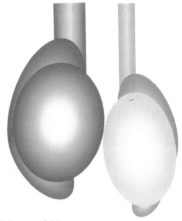

Figure 13–21   Right epididymoorchitis.

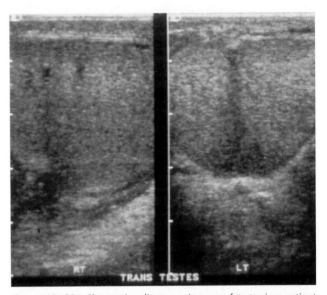

Figure 13–22   Short-axis split-screen images of testes in a patient with right epididymoorchitis shows swelling of the right testis, but normal echogenicity.

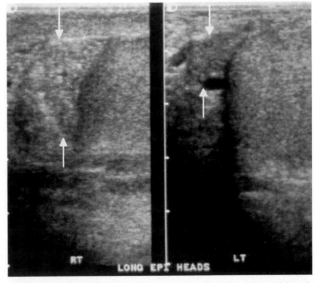

Figure 13–23   Long-axis split-screen images of epididymal heads in a patient with right epididymoorchitis shows swelling and hyperechogenicity on the right.

comparison with contralateral asymptomatic side is more important than an absolute value of the velocity. A ratio of the peak systolic velocity of 1.9 or greater between the symptomatic and the asymptomatic epididymitis indicates hyperemia on the symptomatic side (Fig. 13–32).

Most adults with acute scrotal pain have infection rather than torsion and will show obviously increased color flow. Inflammatory hyperemia is a positive finding, as opposed to torsion-induced oligemia, which is a negative finding. Positive findings are inherently more believable and reliable than negative findings. The presence of hyperemia is, therefore, very predictive that the testis is not torsed.

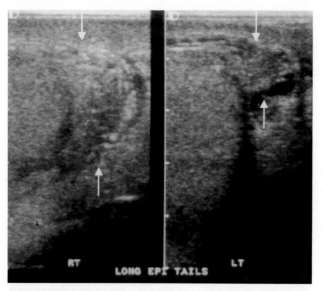

Figure 13–24 Long-axis split-screen images of the epididymal tails in a patient with right epididymoorchitis shows swelling and hyperechogenicity on the right.

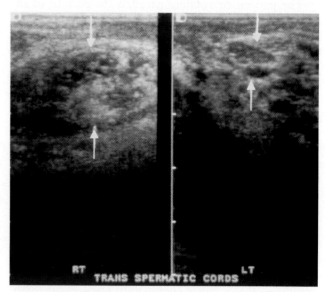

Figure 13–25 Short-axis split-screen images of the spermatic cords in a patient with right epididymoorchitis shows swelling and hyperechogenicity on the right.

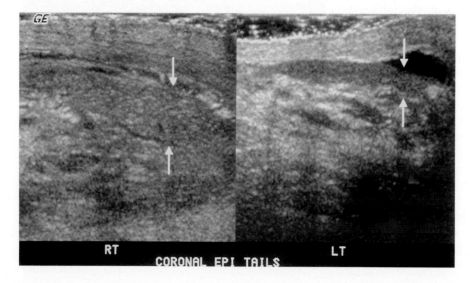

Figure 13–26 Coronal views of epididymal tails in a patient with acute right epididymoorchitis shows swelling of the right epididymal tail, but normal echogenicity.

Figure 13–27 Acute right epididymoorchitis — long-axis power Doppler views of testes show marked inflammatory hyperemia on the right.

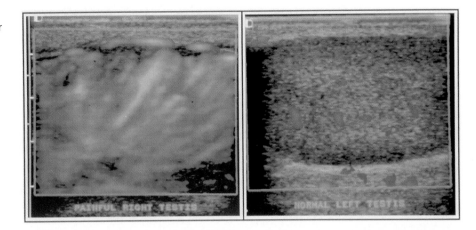

Figure 13–28 Acute right epididymoorchitis — long-axis power Doppler views of epididymal heads show marked hyperemia on the right.

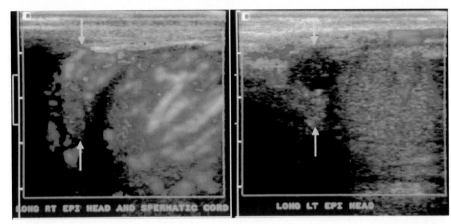

Figure 13–29 Acute right epididymoorchitis — long-axis power Doppler views of epididymal tails show marked hyperemia on the right.

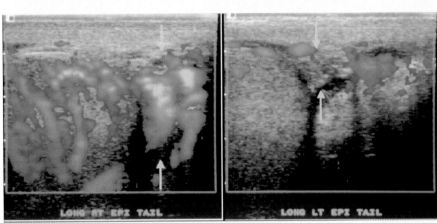

Figure 13–30 Acute right epididymoorchitis — short-axis power Doppler views of spermatic cords shows marked hyperemia on the right.

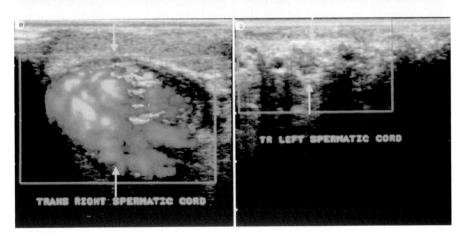

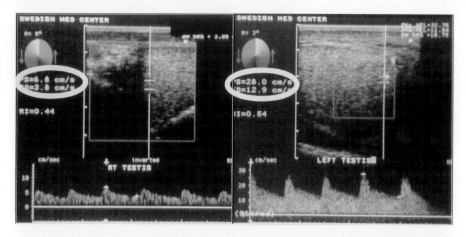

Figure 13–31 Spectral Doppler waveforms in a patient with acute left epididymoorchitis show higher peak systolic and end diastolic velocities on the painful left side than on the asymptomatic right side. The peak systolic velocity (PSV) exceeds 15 cm/s and the ratio of PSV on the left to the right exceeds 1.7.

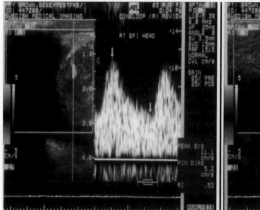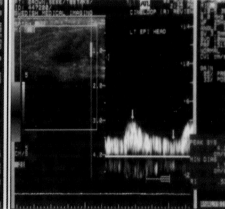

Figure 13–32 Spectral Doppler waveforms obtained from the epididymal heads in a patient with acute right epididymitis show increased velocity on the right. The PSV exceeds 5 cm/s and the ratio of right to left PSV exceeds 1.9.

Findings in Torsion of the Appendix Testis

Imaging Findings

Torsion of the appendix is more common than epididymitis in children and may present with clinical findings indistinguishable from torsion or epididymoorchitis. Few cases have been reported in the US literature. The torsed appendix testis will be visible as a small hyperechoic or mixed hyperechoic and hypeoechoic nodule medial to the epididymal head. The enlargement and alteration in echotexture of the torsed appendix testis is due to hemorrhagic infarction. The epididymal head and spermatic cord immediately adjacent to the torsed appendix testis are usually sympathetically swollen and altered in echogenicity. The testis is usually sonographically normal. An associated reactive hydrocele often exists. If no specific attempts are made to image the appendix testis, then the diagnosis will usually be missed. The swelling of the epididymal head and spermatic cord will lead to a mistaken diagnosis of epididymitis with predominant involvement of the had (**Fig. 13–33**). Longitudinal split-screen imaging of the appendices testes is definitive, but not always possible (**Fig. 13–34**). As a practical matter, the misdiagnosis of a torsed appendix testis as epididymitis is not very important because both epididymitis and torsion of the appendix testis are managed medically. Rarely is surgery necessary for torsion of the appendix testis, except to make the diagnosis. The pain eventually spontaneously abates and the hemorrhagic infarcted appendix testis may slough into the scrotal sac, calcify, and form a "scrotal pearl".

Doppler Findings.

No demonstrable flow exists within the enlarged, infarcted, and hemorrhagic torsed appendix testis. Unfortunately, we virtually never are able to demonstrate flow within a normal appendix testis, so no importance can be attached to a lack of flow. However, sympathetic hyperemia will usually be found in the enlarged epididymal head and spermatic cord, immediately adjacent to the torsed appendix testis (**Fig. 13–35**). As for imaging findings, the pattern of inflammatory hyperemia may mimic that of epididymitis that predominantly involves the head.

Figure 13–33   Short-axis split-screen images of the epididymal heads and adjacent spermatic cords show reactive inflammation and swelling on the right in this young boy with a torsed right appendix testis. In young prepubertal boys who do not have concurrent urinary tract infection, the sonographic appearance of epididymitis involving primarily the head almost always represents torsion of the appendix testis. The torsed appendix testis can usually be found just medial to the epididymal head.

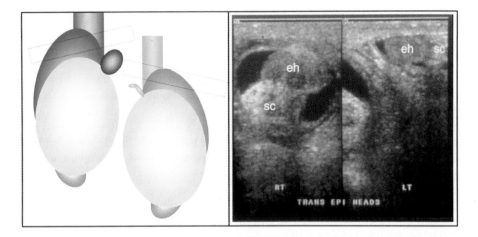

Figure 13–34   Long-axis split-screen images of the appendices testes in this patient with a torsed right appendix testis show the torsed appendix to be larger, rounder, and more echogenic than the contralateral normal-sized appendix testis. The typical torsed appendix testis has an appearance similar to an echogenic "snow pea" in comparison to the normal iscoechoic "grain of rice"-sized and-shaped contralateral normal appendix testis.

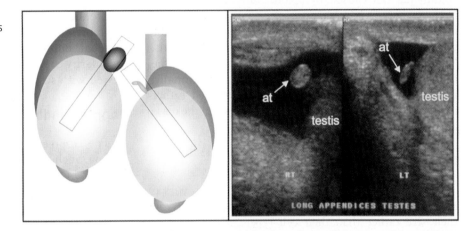

Figure 13–35   Short-axis view of a torsed appendix testis (at) and the adjacent inflamed epididymal head (eh), which is markedly hyperemic. There is also a reactive hydrocele.

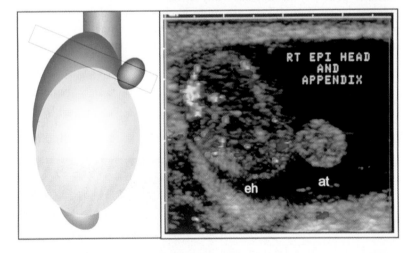

Findings in Testicular Tumors

Imaging Findings

Occasionally, necrosis and hemorrhage into a testicular tumor may result in acute scrotal pain. In fact, about 10% of testicular tumors cause pain and swelling, findings similar to those of infection or infarction. Smaller masses or nodules within the testis are usually easily recognized. Very large tumors, which almost completely replace the testicular substance, can be mistaken for an edematous testis due to orchitis or torsion. However, careful inspection will usually show a thin rim of compressed testicular tissue on one side of the mass (**Fig. 13–36**). Care must be taken not to mistake a hugely swollen epididymal tail caused by epididymitis for a primary testicular tumor. In some cases, the tail may be so swollen that it compresses and indents the lower pole of the testis sufficiently that it appears to arise from the testis. With a coronal approach, US imaging can show that the tail is connected to the epididymal body. Additionally, the borders of the indented testis are rounded rather than pointed and claw shaped, as they are when the mass arises from within the testis.

Doppler Findings

Whether abnormally increased flow exists within neoplastic testicular masses depends almost entirely on their size rather than their cell type. Small testicular nodules generally do not have any demonstrable flow. Masses larger than 1.5 cm are more likely to have demonstrable tumor flow. In general, color Doppler imaging is not very useful in assessing intratesticular masses.

Findings in Testicular Trauma

Imaging Findings

Trauma may increase the risk of torsion, lead to epididymoorchitis, or may result in fracture of the testis with or without a large hematocele. Because the differential diagnosis for trauma is essentially the same as for acute scrotal pain in the absence of trauma, the standard scrotal pain workup for scrotal pain should be used. The only difference is that a specific attempt should be made to identify testicular fracture or hematocele. Large hematoceles may make it difficult to determine whether or not testicular fracture exists. Foci of abnormal echotexture within the substance of the testis may merely indicate contusion or occult fracture, especially if they extend to the tunica albuginea. It is prudent to assume such foci represent occult fracture, however, since early surgical repair improves salvage rate and recovery time. Any irregularity or flap of the tunica albuginea should also be viewed with suspicion (**Fig. 13–37**).

Doppler Findings

The Doppler findings, like the imaging findings of trauma, include the entire gamut of causes of scrotal pain. The Doppler workup should be the same for any other patient with acute scrotal pain.

Findings in Spermatic Cord Thrombosis Due to Venous Occlusion

Imaging Findings

The imaging findings of spermatic cord occlusion, whether due to severe epididymitis, inguinal hernia surgery, or spontaneous thrombosis (in patients with varicocele) are similar to those of testicular torsion. The findings are a manifestation of venous and lymphatic oc-

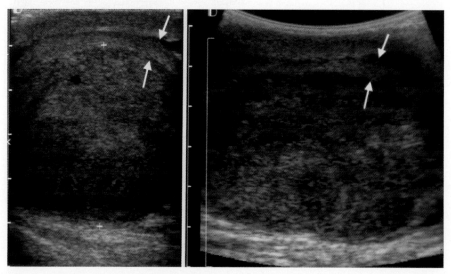

Figure 13–36 Short- and long-axis views of the left testis in a patient with a large embryonal cell tumor that replaces most of the testicular substance. In such cases it is important to try to demonstrate a thin rim of compressed normal testicular tissue (**arrows**) to distinguish between diffuse edema from infection or torsion and tumor.

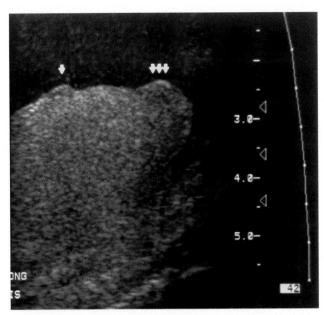

Figure 13–37   Fractured testis. This patient had been hit in the scrotum with a soccer ball, producing a large left hematocele. Although internal texture of the testis was normal irregularities of the tunica albuginea correctly suggested loss of integrity and presence of testicular fracture (**arrows**).

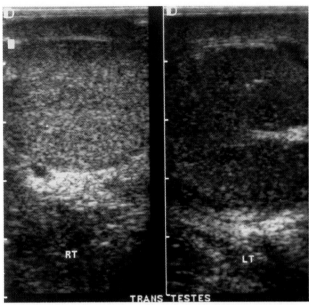

Figure 13–38 Spermatic cord thrombosis due to recurrent left inguinal hernia repair. This patient had a recurrent left inguinal hernia that was successfully repaired. The day after surgery, the patient developed acute left hemiscrotal pin and swelling. US imaging and color Doppler flow imaging showed severe edema of left testis and markedly diminished flow within the left testis and spermatic cord. Surgical exploration revealed thrombosis of the spermatic cord from the hernia repair site distally.

clusion. The ultimate result, if not treated promptly, is hemorrhagic venous infarction, the same pathological result caused by torsion. The only imaging difference between spermatic cord thrombosis and torsion is the level at which the spermatic cord swelling and hemorrhage begin. The testicular and epididymal findings are indistinguishable from those of torsion. In most adult cases of torsion, the level of torsion is in the spermatic cord slightly above the testis, whereas in cases of spermatic cord occlusion due to inguinal hernia repair, the level of obstruction is at the internal inguinal ring or within the inguinal canal. The spermatic cord within the inguinal

canal lateral to the penis will, therefore, be normal in size in most cases of torsion, but abnormal in cases of testicular venous thrombosis resulting from inguinal hernia surgery (**Fig. 13–38**). Severe epididymitis may impede venous outflow from the testis leading to venous infarction. This infarction is usually patchy, but may be global. If global, then this condition may be indistinguishable from torsion on Doppler portions of the examination. In such cases, evaluation of the spermatic cord for flow, twist, or abrupt change in size and the presence or absence of loose connective tissue edema provide the only clues to the correct diagnosis (**Fig. 13–39**).

Figure 13–39   Patchy ischemia of left testis due to severe epididymitis. Enlargement and heterogeneous appearance of the testis makes it difficult to distinguish this condition from either testicular tumor or torsion with hemorrhagic infarction. In cases of infection severe enough to impede venous outflow, the flow within the testis may be decreased rather than increased.

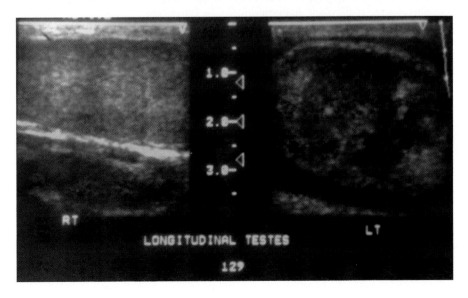

Doppler Findings

Doppler findings of testicular vein occlusion are identical to those of torsion.

Summary

Color duplex sonography is the procedure of choice for evaluation of acute scrotal pain. The initial goal is to quickly determine whether torsion is the cause of pain. If torsion is present, then the patient undergoes surgery immediately. Once a diagnosis of torsion has been excluded, complete imaging and Doppler evaluation of the testes, epididymi, and spermatic cords will usually enable a specific diagnosis to be made and the most appropriate treatment to be instituted.

References

1. Rifkin MD, Kurtz AB, Goldberg BB. Epididymitis examined by ultrasound: correlation with pathology. *Radiology* 1984;151:187—190.
2. Leopold GR, Woo VL. Scheible FW, Nachtsheim D, Gosink BB. High-resolution ultrasonography of scrotal pathology. *Radiology* 1979;131:719—722.
3. Martin B, Conte J. Ultrasonography of the acute scrotum. *J Clin Ultrasound* 1987;15:37—44.
4. Phillips GN, Schneider M, Goodman JD, Macchia RJ. Ultrasonic evaluation of the scrotum. *Urol Radiol* 1980;1:157—163.
5. Benson CB, Doubilet PM, Richie JP. Sonography of the male genitcal tract. *AJR* 1989;153:705—713.
6. Kissane JM, ed. *Anderson's Pathology* (8 th ed., vol. 1), St. Louis: CV Mosby, 1985, p. 796—811.
7. Symmers WStC, ed. *Systemic Pathology* (2 nd ed., vol. 4), London: Churchill Livingstone, 1979.
8. Burks DD, Marky BJ, Burkhard TK, et al. Suspected testicular torsion and ischemia: evaluation with color Doppler sonography. *Radiology* 1990;175:815—821.
9. Ralls PW, Jensen MC, Lee KP, et al. Color Doppler sonography in acute epididymitis and orthicitis. *J Clin Ultrasound* 1990;18:383—386.
10. Horstman WG, Middleton WD, Melson GL. Scrotal inflammators disease: color Doppler US findings. *Radiology* 1991;179:55—59.
11. Horstman WG, Middleton WD, Melson GL, Siegel BA. Color Doppler US of the scrotum. *Radiographics* 1991;11:941—957.
12. Fitzgerald SW, Erickson S, DeWire DM, et al. Color Doppler sonography in the evaluation of the adult acute scrotum. *J Ultrasound Med* 1992;11:543—548.
13. Kass EJ, Stone KT, Cacciarelli AA, Mitchel B. Do all children with an acute scrotum require exploration? *J Urol* 1993;150:667—669.
14. Tumeh SS, Benson CB, Richie JP. Acute diseases of the scrotum. *Semin Ultrasound CT MR* 1991;12:115—130.
15. DeWire DM, Begun FP, Lawson RK, Fitzgerald S, Foley WD. Color Doppler ultrasonogarphy in the evaluation of the acute scrotum. *J Urol* 1992;147:89—91.
16. Middleton WD, Siegel BA, Melson GL, Yates CK, Andriole GL. Acute scrotal disorders: prospective comparison of color Doppler US and testicular scintigraphy. *Radiology* 1992;177:177—181.
17. Wilbert DM, Schaerfe CW, Stern WD, Strohmaier WL, Bichler KH. Evaluation of the acute scrotum by color-coded Doppler ultrasonography. *Urol* 1993;149:1475—1477.
18. Lerner RM, Mevorach RA, Hulbert WC, Rabinowitz R. Color Doppler US in the evaluation of acute scrotal disease. *Radiology* 1990;176:355—358.
19. Mevorach RA, Lerner RM, Greenspan BS, et al. Color Doppler ultrasound compared to a radionuclide scanning of spermatic cord torsion in a canine model. *J Urol* 1991;145:428—433.
20. Holder LE, Martire JR, Holmes ER, Wagner HN. Testicular radionuclide angiography and static imaging: antatomy, scintigraphic interpretation and clinical indications. *Radiology* 1977,125:739—752.
21. Dunn EK, Macchia RJ, Chauhan PS, Laugani GB, Solomon NA. Scintiscan for acute intrascrotal contents. *Clin Nucl Med* 1986;11:381—388.
22. Bird K, Rosenfield AT. Testicular infarction secondary to acute inflammatory disease: demonstration by B-scan ultrasound. *Radiology* 1984;152:785—788.
23. See WA, Mack LA, Krieger JN. Scrotal ultrasonography: a predictor of complicated epididymitis requiring orchiectomy. *J Urol* 1988;139:55—56.
24. Brown JM, Hammers LW, Barton JW, et al. Quantitative Doppler assessment of acute scrotal inflammation. *Radiology* 1995;197:427—431.
    Luke GD, Siegel MJ. Color Doppler sonography of the scrotum in children. *AJR* 1994;163:649—655.

14 Elevated PSA and/or Abnormal Prostate Physical Exam

Ulrike M. Hamper

Carcinoma of the prostate is the most common malignancy in western men and the second leading cause of cancer death among men in the United States. It is estimated that 179,300 new cases will be diagnosed in the U.S.A. during 1999. An estimated 37,000 men will die from the disease during the same year. Prostate cancer and incidence rates vary among ethnic and racial groups. Prostate cancer incidence rates are 37% higher for black than white men, and mortality rates are more than two times higher for black than white men. The disease is common in North America and Northwestern Europe and rare in Asia, Africa, and South America. According to recent genetic studies an inherited predisposition may account for 5—10% of prostate cancers. In addition, international studies suggest that dietary fat and high plasma testosterone levels may also be a factor. The incidence of prostate cancer increases with age, and approximately 80% of all prostate cancers are diagnosed in men over the age of 65. Between 1980 and 1992 the prostate cancer incidence rate increased by 65%, mostly due to improved detection. A decline in prostate cancer incidence began in 1992 for white men and in 1993 for African Americans.[1] This trend is likely related to the effects of prostate specific antigen (PSA) screening. Prostate cancer incidence rates are expected to continue to decline and stabilize at rates which were in effect prior to the widespread use of PSA screening.[1] In order to detect prostate cancer early, every man aged 40 and older should undergo a digital rectal examination (DRE) as part of their annual physical checkup. In addition, the American Cancer Society recommends that all men aged 50 or over should have an annual prostate specific antigen blood test. Earlier screening is recommended for men at increased risk for prostate cancer, such as men with a positive family history or African Americans. These patients should undergo annual DRE and PSA screening starting at age 40. If either one of these test results are suspicious, further evaluation with a transrectal ultrasound (TRUS) should be performed.[1]

The Clinical Problem — Differential Diagnosis

Both prostate cancer and benign processes such as prostate hyperplasia (BPH) or prostatitis may cause elevation of serum PSA levels and can cause an abnormal DRE. The most troublesome differentiation is between cancer and BPH. Elevated PSA levels are found in 16—86% of men with BPH (average one-third of men with BPH) and in 60—70% of patients with prostate cancer. Recent studies have shown that the measurement of PSA serum concentration is well established in the diagnosis and follow-up of patients with prostate cancer and may better identify patients with organ-confined, potentially curable disease.[2—6] Over 30% of men over the age of 50 will have small cancers in their gland, which remain clinically insignificant and may never require treatment.[7,8] Therefore, skeptics of PSA testing have raised the issue of increased detection of biologically insignificant tumors. Most prostate cancers are detected when the patient has symptoms of bladder outlet obstruction or when routine DRE or PSA tests detect abnormalities.[6] Systemic symptoms such as weakness, bone pain or azotemia may be the presenting features; however, most of the time patients presenting with these symptoms have more advanced and usually metastatic disease. In general, survival of the disease has an inverse relationship with the stage of the cancer at time of detection. Survival rates also vary with race and ethnicity with African American men having a decreased five-year survival compared to white men.[1] In order to decrease the mortality rate from prostate cancer it will be necessary to: (1) detect cancers that are still organ confined and, therefore, potentially curable and (2) initiate definitive therapy, either radical prostatectomy or radiation therapy.

Diagnostic Workup

Nonimaging Tests

Prostate Specific Antigen Testing

Serum PSA testing (cost $10—$50) has become a valuable tool in the diagnosis of prostate cancer, emerging as the best single test for early detection of prostate cancer and its routine use results in a higher percentage of patients with pathologically organ confined disease at diagnosis.[2, 4, 9—11] PSA is an objective measurement unlike DRE or TRUS which are operator dependent and subjective examination techniques. Prostate specific antigen is a serum protease originally isolated from prostate tissue by Wang et al.in 1979.[12] The most commonly used radioimmune assays to measure PSA levels are

- the monoclonal Tandem-R or Tandem-E (Hybritech, San Diego, CA), antibody essay, or
- the monoclonal-polyclonal IMX (Abbott Laboratories, Abbott Park, IL) — normal value 0—4 ng/mL, and
- Pros-check (Yang, Laboratories, Bellevue, WA) polyclonal antibody essay — normal 0—2.5 ng/mL.

The synthesis of PSA is restricted to prostatic epithelium. Elevated serum PSA protein levels can be found in both benign and malignant diseases of the prostate and is not only caused by prostate cancer, but also by BPH, bacterial prostatitis, prostatic intraepithelial neoplasia (PIN), prostatic infarction and following selective manipulations, i.e., TRUS, prostate massage, prostate biopsy, catheterization, and cystoscopy.[13, 14] In benign glands, the factors that affect PSA levels most are prostatic volume and patient's age. It has been estimated that one g of prostatic hyperplastic tissue will elevate the PSA level by 0.3 ng/mL, whereas cancer will cause an about tenfold increase (3.5 ng/mL) compared to BPH. Limitation of PSA sensitivity include the fact that not all patients with prostate cancer have elevated PSA concentrations. In some series 14—27% of patients with organ-confined cancer had elevated PSA levels.[15] Likewise, nearly 33% of cancers are detected in men who had PSA levels in the normal range.[16] A large study by Catalona et al.[10] evaluated 1,653 over age 50 without cancer or prostatitis with PSA levels in the 4—10 ng/mL range with DRE and TRUS, followed by TRUS-guided biopsy if an abnormality was found. Twenty-two percent of patients with mid-range PSA values (4—10 ng/mL) had cancer on their biopsy compared to 67% with PSA-levels > 10 ng/mL. DRE alone would have missed 32% and TRUS alone 43% of cancers in this series. Therefore, elevated PSA levels greater than 10 ng/mL warrant a prostate biopsy regardless of the findings on DRE.[3, 10, 17] A recent study by Rietbergen et al.[11] concluded that if PSA levels had not been used as part of the screening regimen, DRE would have missed 52.9% of cancers and TRUS would

have missed 54.7%. Another controversial aspect of PSA testing for prostate cancer detection is that over 30% of men over the age of 50 will have small cancers in their gland, which remain clinically insignificant and may never require treatment.[7] Although the serum PSA levels correlate with the extent of disease in patients with prostate cancer, it is impossible to accurately predict occult metastatic disease except in individuals with extreme serum PSA elevations.

Because a substantial overlap in serum PSA levels in men with prostate cancer and those with BPH exists, better methods of using serum PSA in the diagnosis and management of patients with prostate cancer have been explored including but not limited to the determination of PSA density, excess PSA, PSA velocity, age-specific PSA ranges, and most recently, the use of molecular forms of PSA.

PSA Density (PSAD) and Excess PSA

As previously mentioned, increased levels of PSA are not specific for prostate cancer. Therefore, attempts have been made to correct for an elevated PSA level contributed by benign prostate enlargement through the use of PSAD, especially in the intermediate range (4—10 ng/mL), where such elevations may occur in patients with BPH or prostate cancer.[18—24] PSAD is calculated as the quotient of the serum PSA level divided by the estimated volume of the prostate gland as measured by TRUS. This technique may be useful to determine which patients with ambiguous PSA findings should undergo prostate biopsy. For tests using monoclonal antibody to detect PSA, PSAD values of 0.10,[24] 0.12[23] and 0.14[22] have been recommended. A PSAD of 0.12 has been shown to maximize the sensitivity of PSAD while maintaining a moderate specificity.[24—26] Some papers have advocated that a combination of PSAD and PSA values is more sensitive and specific for the detection of prostate cancer.[20, 23, 24] However, another study showed that the combination of PSAD and PSA did not have a higher predictive value than PSA alone.[18, 27] A recent study by Rubens et al.[28] advocates the use of only excess PSA (serum PSA level minus predicted PSA level [prostate volume x 0.12]) and concludes that in their experience the use of only excess PSA ≥ 0 ng/mL to initiate prostate biopsy results in the best combination of sensitivity and specificity compared with the other standard parameters.

PSA Velocity

A recent case-controlled study of 54 men showed that serial PSA measurements which followed the rate of change over time allowed a more accurate correlation between the serum PSA and the clinical status of the prostate than was possible with a single reading.[29] Because daily variations of PSA values up to 10% can occur, only PSA changes of at least 0.75 ng/mL per year are considered significant.

Age-Specific PSA

Age-related reference ranges for PSA in combination with DRE findings were introduced by Oesterling et al.[14] a few years ago in an attempt to improve specificity for biopsy in older men, while improving sensitivity in younger patients. Littrup et al.[26] have shown that minimal cost reductions are achieved with age-related PSA when combined with universal systematic biopsy; this was in contrast to potential savings achieved with tailored biopsies.[25,26] The increase in PSA levels with age most likely merely reflects a contribution from the increased incidence of BPH in older men.

Molecular forms of PSA

(Total PSA, Free PSA, and Complexed PSA)

Recent studies have shown that PSA can be detected in different molecular forms in sera of men. PSA is predominantly bound by α-1-antichymotrypsin (PSA-ACT), may exist in a "free" or unbound form or be bound to α-2-macroglobulin (PSA-A$_2$M).[5,31,32] Current commercially used assays for PSA measure total PSA, detect free PSA, and PSA-ACT. There is evidence that PSA bound to ACT may be higher in men with prostate cancer than in men with BPH. Determining a ratio of free PSA to total PSA may help decrease the number of unnecessary biopsies in men with diagnostically vague serum PSA levels between 4.0 and 10.0 ng/mL. Extensive prospective studies are needed and in progress to evaluate the clinical utility of these methods for early and optimal prostate cancer detection.[5,27,30,31,32]

Enhanced Reverse Transcriptase (RT) Molecular Polymerase Chain Reaction (PCR) Assay for PSA

The RT-PCR assay for PSA is a molecular assay specific for the human prostate specific antigen. This assay identifies PSA-synthesizing cells from reverse transcribed mRNA and is a marker for circulating tumor cells in the blood of patients with prostate cancer.[33,34] It has been reported to be a more sensitive modality to identify patients with extracapsular extension of disease (sensitivity 86%, specificity 84%) and positive surgical margins (sensitivity 87%, specificity 84%). It is superior to the DRE, CT, endorectal coil magnetic resonance imaging, PSA, PSAD, or Gleason score to stage correctly apparently localized prostate cancer prior to surgery.[34] However, further work is needed and currently in progress to validate this method for routine use in daily clinical practice.

Prostate Acid Phosphatase (PAP)

The determination of PAP levels, whether performed by enzymatic or radioimmune assays, has severe limitations because the levels may be normal in 57—73% of patients with localized prostate cancer.[35] In addition, most patients with elevated PAP levels have advanced disease, severely limiting its specificity.[30,31,36] Therefore this test is rarely used anymore in daily practice.

Digital Rectal Examination

The DRE, is relatively cheap (cost $10—$50) and easy to perform, however has significant limitations for the detection of prostate cancer, because it is a very subjective and operator-dependent test with a high interobserver variability. An abnormal feeling prostate gland on DRE may be caused by prostate cancer but also by benign processes, such as asymmetric prostatic enlargement or asymmetry, calcifications, cystic lesions, or chronic inflammatory changes (**Fig. 14–1—14–4**). The detection rate for prostate cancer by DRE has been reported to be only about 50% in several studies.[7,11,13,37,38] Tumors occurring anterior to midline, which comprise about 40—50% of prostate cancer, are usually not detected by DRE which predominantly allows palpation of the posterolateral aspects of the gland. Lesion size is an important factor for detection by DRE. For lesions less than 1.5 cm, the sensitivity of DRE has been reported to be only 41%.[39] The discrepancy between the clinical and surgical stage in several series[4,7] illustrates the limitations of DRE. Studies by Catalona et al.[2,3,10] showed that DRE alone would have missed 32% of biopsy-proven cancers. In the large European series by Rietbergen et al., DRE alone would have missed about 53% of cancers.[11] Screening with DRE alone also fails to increase the proportion of pathologically organ-confined cancers detected and clinical staging of prostate cancer has resulted in a 30—70% understaging of stage B disease.[4,7]

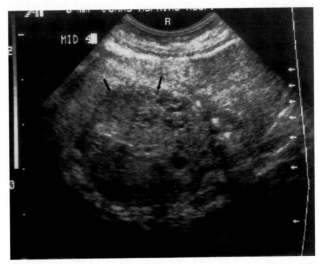

Figure 14–1 A 73-year-old man with a right-sided palpable nodule on physical exam. Coronal transrectal ultrasound (TRUS) shows an asymmetric nodule of benign prostatic hypertrophy (**arrows**) accounting for the abnormal DRE. R, rectum.

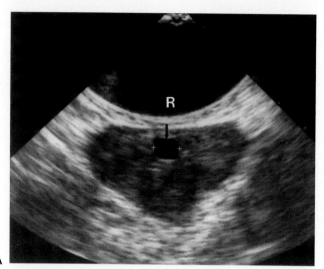

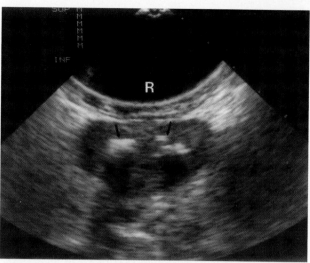

Figure 14–2 A: An 82-year-old man with a midline mass and induration felt on physical exam. Coronal TRUS demonstrates a cystic mass (**arrow**), compatible with a small utricular cyst.

B: Bilateral peripheral zone calcifications (**arrows**), causing the findings on physical examination. R, rectum.

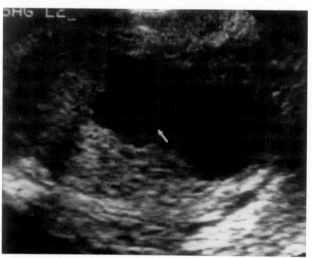

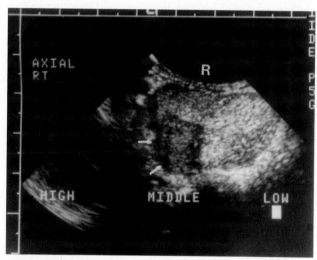

Figure 14–3 A 71-year-old man with an enlarged and hard left lobe on physical exam. Sagittal TRUS shows an ill-defined hypoechoic mass in the left central gland with fluid-filled components and internal echoes (**arrow**). This mass was aspirated transrectally and proved to be a prostatic abscess.

Figure 14–4 A 46-year-old man with a right-sided nodule felt on physical exam. Axial TRUS shows hypoechoic mass in the mid- and anterior portion of the right prostate lobe (**arrows**). TRUS-guided biopsy of this area showed benign prostatic hyperplasia. R, rectum.

Imaging Tests Other Than Ultrasound

Computed tomography (CT) and magnetic resonance imaging (MRI) with a body coil have not proven to be valuable for the detecting and staging of prostate cancer and are not recommended for the initial evaluation of patients with a prostate problem.[40, 41] In terms of detection and localization of cancerous lesions larger than 5 mm, MRI only identified 60% of the tumors in one series.[40] The staging accuracy of body coil MRI in this series was 57% for localized and 77% for advanced disease.[40] Magnetic resonance imaging with endorectal

coils however seems to be superior to other imaging techniques in the preoperative assessment of local tumor stage. Staging accuracies between 52% and 82% have been reported. Achieving high accuracies is directly related to the technique used and the experience of the reader.[41] Nuclear medicine bone scans and optional CT and/or body coil MRI are used as staging radiographic studies for metastatic disease prior to the implementation of therapy. A recent study by Huncharek and Muscat[42] questions the need for staging bone scans in asymptomatic patients with newly diagnosed prostate cancer and PSA levels of less than 10 ng/mL and staging CT/

MRI with PSA levels of less than 20 ng/mL, resulting in potentially significant economic savings. New developments in the field of nuclear medicine such as hormone receptor scintigraphy or positron emission tomography are emerging. These techniques allow in vivo characterization of tumors, which may have important implications for the diagnosis of prostate cancer in the future.[43] Work in progress in these areas is currently underway.

Ultrasound (US) Imaging

TRUS with high-frequency (6—9 MHZ) transducers is a valuable diagnostic tool for the workup of patients with a prostate problem. TRUS is performed in sagittal and transverse or coronal planes to evaluate glandular changes, delineate, and measure focal lesions and primarily guide biopsies. It is used to calculate the size of the prostate gland and can accurately assess prostate volume in glands less than 50 g. Gland volume is important for PSAD analyses which can be used to select patients for a TRUS-guided biopsy. Furthermore, TRUS in patients with an abnormal DRE can identify mimics of carcinoma such as prostatic calculi, cysts, or other benign processes (**Fig. 14–1** through **14–4**) or clarify equivocal findings on DRE especially when the physical examination was not performed by an experienced urologist or practitioner. In addition, TRUS has become the routine guidance modality for a prostate biopsy. Abnormal PSA levels and/or an abnormal DRE usually initiate the performance of a TRUS-guided biopsy (cost $200—$800), which is simple, safe, and accurately performed with automatically triggered core biopsy devices (**Fig. 14–5**). Because cancers detected before they spread beyond the confines of the prostate gland have an excellent cure rate, many authorities believe that any patient with an elevated serum PSA, especially when the DRE is also abnormal, should undergo a biopsy. Focal lesions are targeted followed by systematic usually sextant or octant biopsies of the remainder of the gland.[13, 17] Some series have shown that 61% of cancers would have been missed if only the site of palpable induration had been biopsied, and 40—52% if only the site of a hypoechoic lesion had been biopsied.[3, 17] Some authors recommend tailored sextant biopsies or targeting areas of increased flow in the absence of focal hypoechoic lesions.[25, 26, 44] In addition, staging biopsies of the seminal vesicles, ejaculatory ducts, and apex can be performed.

At some institutions, patients with PSA between 4.0 and 10.0 ng/mL undergo DRE plus TRUS-guided biopsy. Others use PSAD to determine who should undergo biopsy. Patients with PSA levels of greater than 10 ng/mL should definitely be biopsied.[18]If the biopsy shows insignificant tumor, defined as cancer cells found only in one or two needle cores with tumor present in less than half of these cores, a Gleason score of 6 or lower, and a PSAD of less than 0.1—0.15, then it has been advocated that the patient be followed by "watch-ful-waiting", serial PSA testing, and repeat prostate biopsies.[45] In addition, patients with an initially negative biopsy however increasing PSA velocity usually undergo repeat biopsy. Some studies have shown an incremental detection rate of cancers on second and even third biopsies.[21, 46] Patients with early prostate carcinoma may have a good survival without therapy, however aggressive screening should be limited by the patient's age and require a life expectancy of at least 10 years.[47]

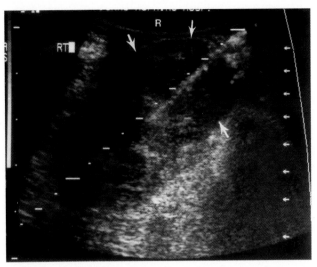

Figure 14–5 A 65-year-old man with mild elevation of PSA and prominent right lobe on physical exam. TRUS-guided biopsy of a well-defined hypoechoic right apical lesion (**arrows**) yielded benign prostatic hyperplasia. R, rectum.

Accuracy of TRUS

TRUS can document areas of abnormalities in the prostate gland that may be suspicious for cancer, such as focal hypoechoic lesions.[48, 49] The sonographic appearance of early prostate cancer is a hypoechoic lesion in the peripheral zone, (**Fig. 14–6** through **14–7**). This sonographic appearance is, however, not specific because not all cancers are hypoechoic and not all hypoechoic lesions are malignant. Sonographic pathologic correlation studies have shown that approximately 70—75% of tumors are hypoechoic whereas 25—30% of tumors are isoechoic and blend with the surrounding tissues.[48, 50] These lesions are usually not detected by TRUS. A small number of cancers are echogenic or have a heterogeneous echotexture with small echogenic foci within hypoechoic lesions (**Fig. 14–8**).[42, 51] The positive predictive value (PPV) of a hypoechoic lesion to be cancer increases with the size of the lesion, a palpable nodule, and an elevated PSA.[13, 14, 38] Overall, the incidence of malignancy in a sonographically suspicious lesion is approximately 20—25%.[13, 52] Various benign lesions mimic the sonographic appearance of early prostate cancer including inflammatory conditions, granulomatous prostatitis, dilated acinar glands, hyperplasia, scarring and fibrosis

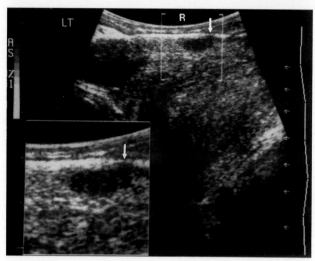

Figure 14–6 A 77-year-old man with elevated PSA and normal physical exam. Sagittal TRUS shows a hypoechoic lesion in the left peripheral zone. Note thinning and irregularity of the bright periprostatic fat line (**arrow**). Biopsy of this lesion yielded prostatic adenocarcinoma, Gleason grade 3+4=7 with capsular penetration. R, rectum.

from previous transurethral resection of the prostate (**Fig. 14–1** through **14–4**).[53,54] Normal variants such as prominent vessels in the peripheral gland (**Fig. 14–9**) or smooth muscle near the apex and ejaculatory ducts as well as positional "pseudolesions" may be mistaken for carcinoma.[54] Even with high-resolution equipment, many potentially clinically significant tumors are not visualized by TRUS. A large multicenter study[40] showed that up to 40% of significant cancers were missed by gray scale US. The overall sensitivity of TRUS to detect neurovascular bundle invasion has been reported to be 66% with a specificity of 78%.[55] To improve lesion detection and differentiate by TRUS, secondary signs such as bulging and contour abnormalities, and increased flow on color Doppler US (CDUS) have been advocated, especially for isoechoic lesions (**Fig. 14–10**).[56—59] Small tumors (< 2 mm) have been reported to be avascular and

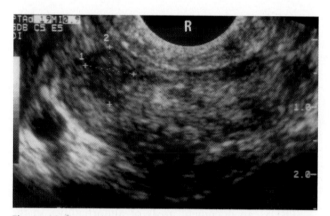

Figure 14–7 A 50-year-old man with elevated PSA of 13 ng/mL and palpable nodule on the right side. Axial TRUS shows mildly hypoechoic nodule in the right peripheral zone (between calipers). TRUS-guided biopsy yielded prostatic adenocarcinoma, Gleason 3+3=6 with perineural invasion. R, rectum.

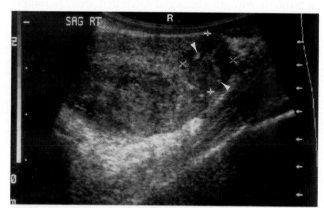

Figure 14–8 A 74-year-old man with a right-sided palpable nodule on physical exam. Sagittal TRUS shows hypoechoic apical lesion (between calipers) with bright echogenic foci (**arrowheads**). TRUS-guided biopsy showed adenocarcinoma, Gleason 3+2=5. R, rectum.

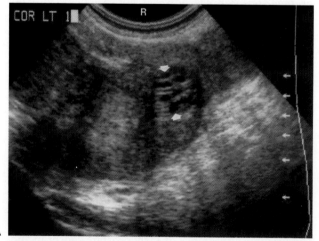

A

Figure 14–9 A: A 56-year-old man with induration of the left lobe felt on physical exam. Coronal TRUS shows hypoechoic lesion in the left peripheral zone with small cystic components (**arrows**).

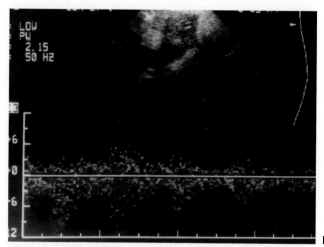

B

R, rectum. **B:** Spectral Doppler of this area demonstrates arterial flow in prominent vessels. R, rectum.

tumors of at least one cm³ demonstrate vascularity.[60] Results of recent CDUS studies[9, 56–59, 60–62] are conflicting and demonstrate a problematic overlap between increased flow detected in cancers, inflammatory condition, or benign lesions (**Fig. 14–11** through **14–15**). Also, not every cancer may demonstrate sufficient flow to be detected by CDUS.[58] CDUS will and should not replace gray scale US, but CDUS findings have been advocated to initiate a TRUS-guided biopsy which otherwise may not have been performed thus tailoring the biopsy to target isoechoic, yet hypervascular areas of the prostate gland (**Fig. 14–16**). Some investigators have suggested that tumor vascularization may allow correlation with the biological behavior of a lesion, especially its potential for rapid growth and distant metastases.[63] If this holds true, CDUS may have potential in identifying an important subgroup of patients. Further research in

this area however is needed. Newer color flow techniques such as power Doppler ultrasound may be helpful in this respect due to its increased sensitivity to flow allowing visualization and demonstration of vascularity in even smaller vessels (**Fig. 14–13 C**). Other recent developments such as intravenous ultrasound contrast agents and harmonic imaging have shown in preliminary studies a possible role for these agents and techniques to delineate subtle prostate cancers when used in combination with CDUS, power Doppler Ultrasound, or harmonic imaging. Further research in this area, however, needs to be performed and is currently underway.

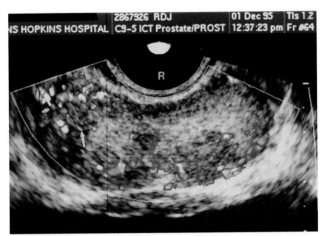

Figure 14–10 A 56-year-old man with normal DRE and mild PSA elevation to 5.4 ng/mL. Coronal TRUS with color Doppler ultrasound shows marked increased flow in hypoechoic right lesion (**arrow**) and minimal flow in isoechoic left prostate. Biopsy and subsequent prostatectomy showed extensive bilateral prostate adenocarcinoma, Gleason 3+4=7 with right-sided capsular penetration. R, rectum.

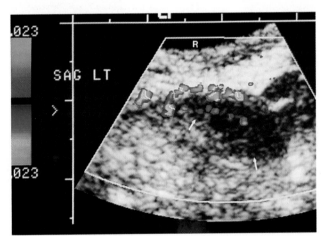

Figure 14–11 A 71-year-old man with elevated PSA (14.3 ng/mL) and negative DRE. Sagittal TRUS demonstrates left-sided hypoechoic lesion (**arrows**) with increased flow on CDUS. Biopsy revealed prostate adenocarcinoma, Gleason 4+3=7. R, rectum.

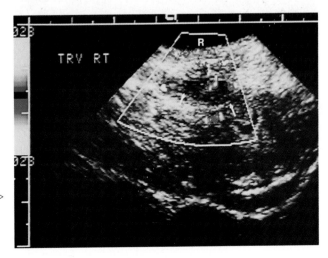

Figure 14–12 A 62-year-old man with elevated PSA level and ▷ questionable right nodule felt on PE. Axial TRUS shows hypoechoic right peripheral zone nodule (**arrows**) with locally increased flow on CDUS. TRUS-guided biopsy showed benign hyperplasia. R, rectum.

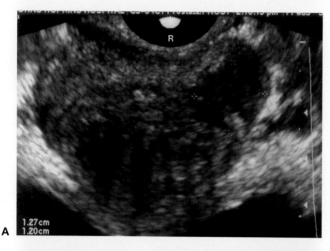

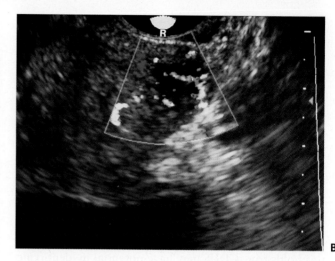

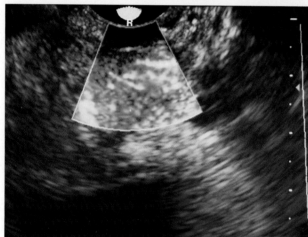

Figure 14–13 A: A 71-year-old man with elevated PSA (11.2 ng/mL) and palpable nodule on the left side. Gray scale axial TRUS shows hypoechoic left peripheral zone lesion (between calipers). **B:** CDUS. **C:** Power Doppler ultrasound demonstrates increased flow in the lesion, which pathologically proved to be adenocarcinoma, Gleason 5+3=8. R, rectum.

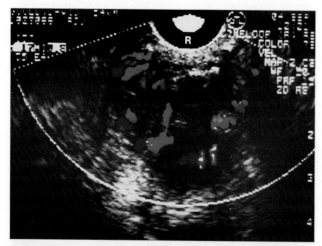

Figure 14–14 A 54-year-old man with markedly elevated PSA and negative physical exam. Axial transrectal color Doppler ultrasound shows diffusely increased bilateral flow. Biopsy yielded extensive bilateral adenocarcinoma, Gleason 5+5=10. R, rectum.

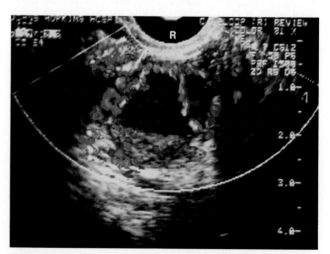

Figure 14–15 A 59-year-old man with elevated PSA and bulging prostate on physical exam. Color Doppler TRUS demonstrates diffuse increased flow in addition to centrally hypoechoic areas, which proved to be acute prostatitis with abscess formation on aspiration. R, rectum.

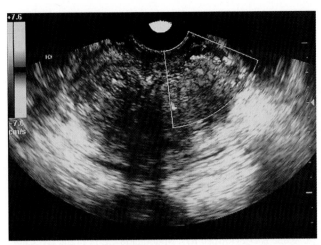

Figure 14–16 A 60-year-old man with elevated PSA (9.1 ng/mL) and negative DRE. Axial TRUS shows isoechoic, yet hypervascular area in the left mid-gland. TRUS-guided biopsy yielded adenocarcinoma, Gleason 3+3=6 with perineural invasion. R, rectum.

Limitations of Ultrasound

TRUS has been shown to be too insensitive and not specific enough to be used as a screening tool in patients with either a normal DRE or a normal PSA test. The American College of Radiology (ACR), the American Urological Association (AUA), and the American Cancer Society (ACS) have made recommendations to limit TRUS to patients with abnormal DRE and/or PSA elevation.[64] TRUS, however, is useful to delineate possible prostate pathology in patients with abnormal PSA or DRE results. As previously mentioned, however, not all gray scale abnormalities represent tumor, and similar hypoechoic lesions may be caused by cancer, atrophy, inflammation, infarction, and other benign processes, therefore, limiting its specificity.[51,53] Likewise isoechoic lesions are usually not detected unless secondary tumor signs such as focal bulge or contour irregularity are identified. As mentioned before color flow Doppler US may be useful in those patients. Small cancers (less than 5 mm) are rarely detected by TRUS, and very extensive tumors involving the entire peripheral zone are difficult to identify because comparison with normal tissue is not possible.[48] Almost 50% of cancers are located in the anterior half of the prostate, and 20—30% of tumors arise from the central or transition zone and usually remain undetected by TRUS.[57,65] Estimation of tumor volume by TRUS has been shown to be inaccurate.[66] Likewise, as previously mentioned, the detection and staging accuracy of TRUS for prostate cancer have been shown to be too inaccurate to advocate its use as a screening modality.[40] Further advances in equipment and transducer technology with increased resolution and operator experience may alter these previously reported disappointing results regarding the detection and/or staging of prostate carcinoma; however, because of the currently tight economic climate in the health care industry and declining funding by government or other agencies, prospective multicenter studies will be difficult to perform in the future.

Summary

Screening and detection of prostate cancer with PSA, DRE, and/or TRUS remains a controversial and complex issue with many open and still unanswered questions. Present data suggest that the use of PSA testing detects more and earlier cancers, however, no data are available to demonstrate improved survival for men with prostate cancer. The combination of DRE and PSA markedly improves sensitivity and currently represents the least costly detection approach to potentially decrease the mortality from prostate cancer.[16] For the future, the availability of a more cancer-specific PSA assay, other cancer-related proteins or molecular staging could become the most potent factor in lowering prostate cancer detection costs.

Currently, a combination of tests is probably still the best way to detect prostate cancer: a reasonable regimen would include the performance of DRE and PSA measurements according to the above-mentioned guidelines. TRUS with or without biopsy should be reserved for those patients with abnormal test results.[3,10,16,37,38,67,68] Local staging with magnetic resonance endorectal coils seems most accurate. In experienced hands, its staging accuracy should approach 80%. Further staging with nuclear medicine bone scans and optional tests such as CT or body coil MRI can be performed to detect lymph node and distant metastases prior to implementation of definitive therapy. Today's screening and diagnostic tools — even with biopsy, however have limits. Most importantly it is essential that we have yet to prove through prospective studies that early diagnosis of prostate cancer actually leads to an improvement in morbidity and reduction in mortality in patients with the disease.[7,8]

References

1. Cancer Facts and Figures 1998. American Cancer Society, Atlanta, GA 1998;20—24.
2. Catalona WJ, Smith DS, Ratliff TL, Basler JW. Detection of organ-confined prostate cancer is increased through prostate-specific antigen-based screening. *JAMA* 1993;270(8):948—954.
3. Catalona WJ, Richie JP, Ahmann FR, et al. Comparison of digital rectal examination and serum prostate specific antigen in the early detection of prostate cancer: results of a multicenter clinical trial of 6,630 men. *J Urol* 1994;151(5):1283—1290.
4. Stamey TA, Yang N, Hay AR, et al. Prostate-specific antigen as a serum marker for adenocarcinoma of the prostate. *N Engl J Med* 1987;317(15):909—916.

5. Leung HY, Lai LC, Day J, et al. Serum free prostate-specific antigen in the diagnosis of prostate cancer. *Br J Urol* 1978;80:256—259.

6. Clark TWI, Goldenberg SL, Cooperberg PL, Wong AD, Singer J. Stratification of prostate-specific antigen level and results of transrectal ultrasonography and digital rectal examination as predictors of positive prostate biopsy. *Can Ass Radiol J* 1997;48:252—258.

7. Gerber GS, Chodak GW. Routine screening for cancer of the prostate. *J Natl Cancer Inst* 1991;83(5):329—335.

8. Brawer MK, Catalona WJ, McConnell JD. Prostate cancer: is screening the answer? *Patient Care* 1992;Oct:55—68.

9. Santucci RA, Brawer MK. Correlation of prostate-specific antigen and ultrasonography in the evaluation of patients with carcinoma of the prostate. *Semin Urol* 1994;12(4):252—264.

10. Catalona WJ, Smith DS, Ratliff TL, et al. Measurement of prostate-specific antigen in serum as a screening test for prostate cancer [published erratum appears in *N Engl J Med* 1991; Oct 31;325(18):1324]. *N Engl J Med* 1991; 324(17):1156—1161.

11. Rietbergen JBW, Kranse R, Kirkels WJ, De Koning HJ, Schroder FH. Evaluation of prostate-specific antigen, digital rectal examination and transrectal ultrasonography in population-based screening for prostate cancer: improving the efficiency of early detection. *Br J Urol* 1997;79:57—63.

12. Wang MC, Valenzuela LA, Murphy GP, Chu TM. Purification of a human prostate specific antigen. *Invest Urol* 1979;17(2):159—163.

13. Ellis WJ, Chetner MP, Preston SD, Brawer MK. Diagnosis of prostatic carcinoma: the yield of serum prostate specific antigen, digital rectal examination and transrectal ultrasonography. *J Urol* 1994;152:1520—1525.

14. Oesterling JE, Jacobsen SJ, Chute CG, et al. Serum prostate-specific antigen in a community-based population of healthy men. Establishment of age-specific reference ranges. *JAMA* 1993;270(7):860—864.

15. Lange PH, Ercole CJ, Lightner DJ, Fraley EE, Vessella R. The value of serum prostate specific antigen determinations before and after radical prostatectomy. *J Urol* 1989;141(4):873—879.

16. Mettlin C, Murphy GP, Ray P, et al. American Cancer Society — National Prostate Cancer Detection Project. Results from multiple examinations using transrectal ultrasound, digital rectal examination, and prostate specific antigen. *Cancer* 1993;71:891—898.

17. Flanigan RC, Catalona WJ, Richie JP, et al. Accuracy of digital rectal examination and transrectal ultrasonography in localizing prostate cancer. *J Urol* 1994;152:1506—1509.

18. Van Iersel MP, Witjes WP, de la Rosette JJ, Oosterhof GO. Prostate-specific antigen density: correlation with histological diagnosis of prostate cancer, benign prostatic hyperplasia and prostatitis. *Br J Urol* 1995;76(1):47—53.

19. Van Andel G, Vleeming R, Kurth K, de Reijke TM. Incidental carcinoma of the prostate. *Semin Surg Oncol* 1995;11(1):36—45.

20. Kane RA, Littrup PJ, Babaian R, et al. Prostate-specific antigen levels in 1695 men without evidence of prostate cancer. Findings of the American Cancer Society National Prostate Cancer Detection Project. *Cancer* 1992;69(5):1201—1207.

21. Olson MC, Posniak HV, Fisher SG, et al. Directed and random biopsies of the prostate: indications based on combined results of transrectal sonography and prostate-specific antigen density determinations. *AJR* 1994;163(6):1407—1411.

22. Rommel FM, Augusta VE, Breslin JA, et al. The use of prostate specific antigen density to enhance the predictive value of intermediate levels of serum prostate specific antigen. *J Urol* 1994;151:88—93.

23. Lee F, Littrup PJ, Loft-Christensen L, et al. Predicted prostate specific antigen results using transrectal ultrasound gland volume. Differentiation of benign prostatic hyperplasia and prostate cancer. *Cancer* 1992;70:211—220.

24. Benson MC, Whang IS, Pantuck A, et al. Prostate specific antigen density: a means of distinguishing benign prostatic hypertrophy and prostate cancer. *J Urol* 1992;147:815—816.

25. Littrup PJ, Sparschu R. Transrectal ultrasound and prostate cancer risks. The "tailored" prostate biopsy. *Cancer* 1995;75:1805—1813.

26. Littrup PJ, Goodman AC. Economic considerations of prostate cancer. The role of detection specificity and biopsy reduction. *CA Cancer J Clin* 1995;75:1987—1993.

27. Brawer MK, Aramburu EA, Chen GL, Preston SD, Ellis WJ. The inability of prostate specific antigen index to enhance the predictive the value of prostate specific antigen in the diagnosis of prostatic carcinoma. *J Urol* 1993;150:369—373.

28. Rubens DJ, Gottlieb RH, Maldonado CE Jr, Frank IN. Clinical evaluation of prostate biopsy parameters: gland volume and elevated prostate-specific antigen level. *Radiology* 1996;199:159—163.

29. Carter HB, Pearson JD, Metter EJ, et al. Longitudinal evaluation of prostate-specific antigen levels in men with and without prostate disease. *JAMA* 1992;267(16):2215—2220.

30. Partin AW, Carter HB. The use of prostate specific antigen and free/total PS in the diagnosis of localized prostate cancer. *Urol Clin North Am* 1996;23(4):531—540.

31. Bangma, CH, Riebergen JB, Ranse R, et al. The free-to-total prostate specific antigen ratio improves the specificity of prostate specific antigen in screening for prostate cancer in the general population. *J Urol* 1997;157:2191—2196.

32. Van Gangh PJ, De Nayer P, De Vischer L, et al. Free to total prostate-specific antigen (PSA) ratio improves the discriminaiton between prostate cancer and benign prostatic hyperplasia (BPH) in the diagnostic gray zone of 1.8 to 10 ng/mL total PSA. *Urology* 1996;48:67—70.

33. Seiden MV, Kantoff PW, Krithivas K, et al. Detection of circulating tumor cells in men with localized prostate cancer. *J Clin Oncol* 1994;12(12):2634—2639.

34. Katz AE, Olsson CA, Raffo AJ, et al. Molecular staging of prostate cancer with the use of an enhanced reverse transcriptase-PCR assay. *Urology* 1994;43(6):765—775.

35. Cooper JF. The radioimmunochemical measurement of prostatic acid phosphatase: current state of the art. *Urol Clin North Am* 1980;7(3):653—665.

36. Burnett AL, Chan DW, Brendler CB, Walsh PC. The value of serum enzymatic acid phosphatase in the staging of localized prostate cancer. *J Urol* 1992;148(6):1832—1834.

37. Cooner WH. Rectal examination and ultrasonography in the diagnosis of prostate cancer. *Prostate* Suppl 1992;4:3—10.

38. Cooner WH, Mosley BR, Rutherford CL Jr, et al. Prostate cancer detection in a clinical urological practice by ultrasonography, digital rectal examination and prostate specific antigen. *J Urol* 1990;143(6):1146—1152; discussion 1152—1154.

39. Lee F, Littrup PJ, Torp-Pedersen ST, et al. Prostate cancer: comparison of transrectal US and digital rectal examination for screening. *Radiology* 1988;168(2):389—394.

40. Rifkin MD, Zerhouni EA, Gatsonis CA, et al. Comparison of magnetic resonance imaging and ultrasonography in staging early prostate cancer. Results of a multiinstitutional cooperative trial. *N Engl J Med* 1990;323(10):621—626.

41. Milestone BN, Seidman EJ. Endorectal coil magnetic resonance imaging of prostate cancer. *Semin Urol* 1995;13(2):113—121.

42. Huncharek M, Muscat J. Serum prostate-specific antigen as a predictor of radiographic staging studies in newly diagnosed prostate cancer. *Cancer Invest* 1995;13(1):31—35.

43. Hoisaeter PA, Norlen BJ, Norming U, et al. Imaging in the diagnosis and assessment of prognosis in localized prostate cancer. Consensus conference on diagnosis and prognostic parameters in localized prostate cancer. *Scand J Urol Nephrol* Suppl 1994;162:89—106.

44. Newman JS, Bree RL, Rubin JM. Prostate cancer: diagnosis with color Doppler sonography with histologic correlation of each biopsy site. *Radiology* 1995;195(1):86—90.

45. Epstein JI, Walsh PC, Carmichael M, Brendler CB. Pathological and clinical findings to predict tumor extent of nonpalpable (stage T1c) prostate cancer. *JAMA* 1994;271(5):368—374.

46. Keetch DW, Catalona WJ, Smith DS. Serial prostatic biopsies in men with persistently elevated serum prostate specific antigen values. *J Urol* 1994;151(6):1571—1574.

47. Johansson JE, Adami HO, Andersson SO, et al. High 10-year survival rate in patients with early, untreated prostatic cancer. *JAMA* 1992;267(16):2191—2196.

48. Dahnert WF, Hamper UM, Walsh PC, Eggleston JC, Sanders RC: Prostatic evaluation by transrectal sonography with histopathologic correlation: the echogenic appearance of early carcinoma. *Radiology* 1986;158:97—102.

49. Lee F, Gray JM, McLeary RD, et al. Prostatic evaluation by transrectal sonography: criteria for diagnosis of early carcinoma. *Radiology* 1986;158(1):91—95.

50. Salo JO, Rannikko S, Makinen J, Lehtonen T. Echogenic structure of prostatic cancer imaged on radical prostatectomy specimens. *Prostate* 1987;10(1):1—9.

51. Hamper UM, Sheth S, Walsh PC, Epstein JI. Bright echogenic foci in early prostatic carcinoma: sonographic and pathologic correlation. *Radiology* 1990;176(2):339—343.

52. Rifkin MD, Choi H. Implications of small, peripheral hypoechoic lesions in endorectal US of the Prostate. *Radiology* 1988;166(3):619—622.

53. Sheth S, Hamper UM, Walsh PC, Holtz PM, Epstein JI. Transrectal ultrasonography in stage A adenocarcinoma of the prostate: a sonographic-pathologic correlation. *Radiology* 1991;179:35—39.

54. Hamper UM, Sheth S, Walsh PC, Holtz PM, Epstein JI. Stage B adenocarcinoma of the prostate: transrectal US and pathologic correlation of nonmalignant hypoechoic peripheral zone lesions. *Radiology* 1991;180:101—104.

55. Hamper UM, Sheth S, Walsh PC, Holtz PM, Epstein JI: Carcinoma of the prostate: value of transrectal sonography to detect extension into the neurovascular bundle. *AJR* 1990;155:1015—1019.

56. Rifkin MD, Sudakoff GS, Alexander AA. Prostate: techniques, results, and potential applications of color Doppler US scanning. *Radiology* 1993;186(2):509—513.

57. Alexander AA. To color Doppler image the prostate or not: that is the question. *Radiology* 1995;195(1):11—13.

58. Kelly IM, Lees WR, Rickards D. Prostate cancer and the role of color Doppler US. *Radiology* 1993;189(1):153—156.

59. Rifkin MD, Sudakoff GS, Alexander AA. Prostate: techniques, results, and potential applications of color Doppler US scanning. *Radiology* 1993;186(2):509—513.

60. Folkman J, Cotran R. Relation of vascular proliferation to tumor growth. *Int Rev Exp Pathol* 1976;16:207—248.

61. Decarvalho V, Kulijowska E. The role of color Doppler for improving the detection of cancer in the isoechoic prostate gland. *J Ultrasound Med* 1996;15:542.

62. Newman JS, Bree RL, Rubin JM. Prostate cancer: diagnosis with color Doppler sonography with histologic correlation of each biopsy site. *Radiology* 1995;195(1):86—90.

63. Weidner N, Semple JP, Welch WR, Folkman J. Tumor angiogenesis and metastasis—correlation in invasive breast carcinoma. *N Engl J Med* 1991;324(1):1—8.

64. Mettlin C, Jones G, Averette H, Gusberg SB, Murphy GP. Defining and updating the American Cancer Society guidelines for the cancer-related checkup: prostate and endometrial cancers. *CA Cancer J Clin* 1993;43(1):42—46.

65. McNeal JE. Normal anatomy of the prostate and changes in benign prostatic hypertrophy and carcinoma. *Semin Ultrasound CT MRI* 1988;9(5):329—334.

66. Terris MK, McNeal JE, Stamey TA. Estimation of prostate cancer volume by transrectal ultrasound imaging. *J Urol* 1992;147(3 Pt 2):855—857.

67. Babaian RJ, Dinney CP, Ramirez EI, Evans RB. Diagnostic testing for prostate cancer detection: less is best. *Urology* 1993;41(5):421—425.

68. Littrup PJ, Goodman AC, Mettlin CJ. The benefit and cost of prostate cancer early detection. The Investigators of the American Cancer Society — National prostate cancer detection project. *CA Cancer J Clin* 1993;43(3):134—149.

15 The Evaluation of Erectile Dysfunction

Harvey L. Nisenbaum and Gregory A. Broderick

Clinical Scenarios

Clinical Scenario 1 (Fig. 15–1)

A 23-year-old male who has had erectile dysfunction (ED) for approximately 2 years. Patient states that his problem is difficulty in getting and maintaining an erection. The remainder of the medical history is noncontributory.

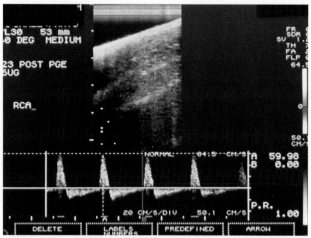

Figure 15–1   Clinical Scenario 1. Following intracavernosal injection (Figs. 15.**1A** through 15.**1E**) of 6 µg of Prostaglandin E$_1$ (Caverject®), erectile response was 5/5.
Figure 15–1A   RCA (PSV – 60 cm/sec; EDV– 0 cm/sec; RI – 1.0; reversal of diastolic flow).

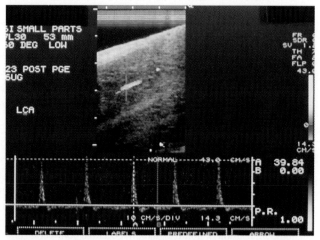

Figure 15–1B LCA (PSV – 39.8 cm/sec; EDV – 0 cm/sec; RI – 1.0; reversal of diastolic flow).

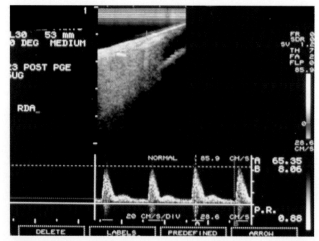

Figure 15–1C   RDA (PSV – 65.4 cm/sec; PED – 8.1 cm/sec; RI – 0.88).

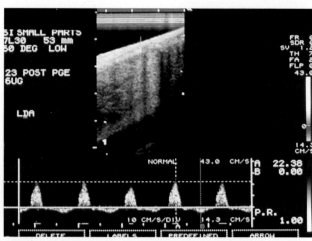

Figure 15–1D   LDA (PSV – 22.4 cm/sec; EDV – 0 cm/sec; RI – 1.0).

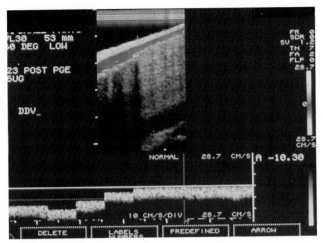

Figure 15–1E DDV (Peak velocity – 10.3 cm/sec).

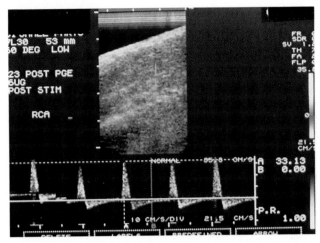

Figure 15–1F Following self-stimulation (Figs. 15–**1F** through 15–**1J**), erectile response was 5/5. RCA (PSV – 33.1 cm/sec; EDV – 0 cm/sec; RI – 1.0; reversal of diastolic flow).

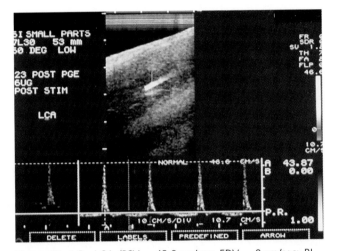

Figure 15–1G LCA (PSV – 43.9 cm/sec; EDV – 0 cm/sec; RI – 1.0; reversal of diastolic flow).

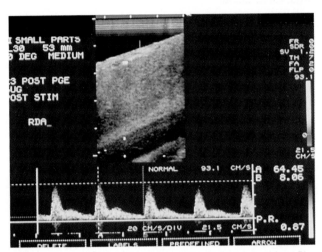

Figure 15–1H RDA (PSV – 64.5 cm/sec; EDV – 8.1 cm/sec; RI – 0.87).

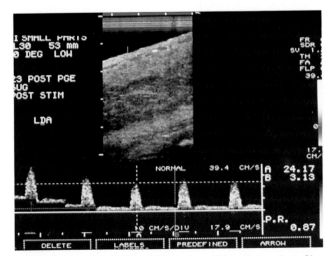

Figure 15–1I LDA (PSV – 24.2 cm/sec; EDV – 3.1 cm/sec; RI – 0.87).

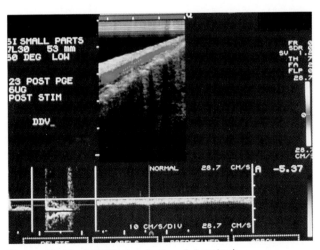

Figure 15–1J DDV (Peak velocity – 5.4 cm/sec).
Figure 15–1K, L ▷

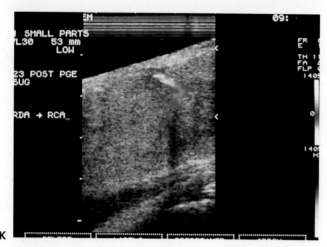

K

Figure 15–1 K RDA to RCA collateral.

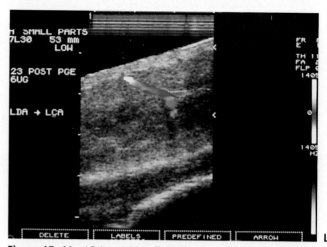

L

Figure 15–1 L LDA to LCA collateral.

Organize as below

Results – normal study.
Diagnosis – psychogenic erectile dysfunction.

Abbreviations:
RCA – right cavernous artery
LCA – left cavernous aretery
RDA – right dorsal artery
LDA – left dorsal artery
DDV – deep dorsal vein
PSV – peak systolic velocity
EDV – end–diastolic velocity
RI – resistive index.

Clinical Scenario 2 (Fig. 15–2)

A 75-year-old male who has had erectile dysfunction since radiation therapy for prostate cancer three years ago. Patient is hypertensive and is on oral medication. There is a question of heart disease, but no history of diabetes, smoking, Peyronie's disease, or pelvic trauma.

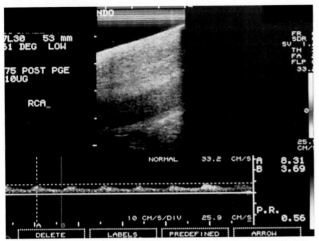

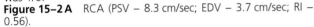

Figure 15–2 Clinical Scenario 2. Following intracavernosal injection of 10 µg of Prostaglandin E₁, (Caverject®), erectile response was 1/5.
Figure 15–2 A RCA (PSV – 8.3 cm/sec; EDV – 3.7 cm/sec; RI – 0.56).

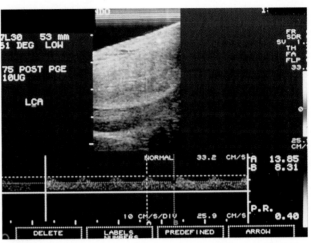

Figure 15–2 B LCA (PSV – 13.9 cm/sec; EDV – 8.3 cm/sec; RI – 0.40).

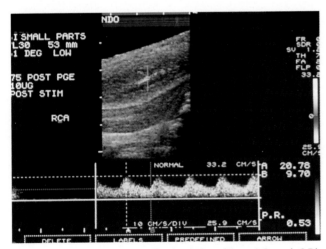

Figure 15–2 C Following self–stimulation (Figs. 2 **C** and 2 **D**), erectile response was 1/5. RCA (PSV – 20.8 cm/sec; EDV – 9.7 cm/sec; RI – 0.53).

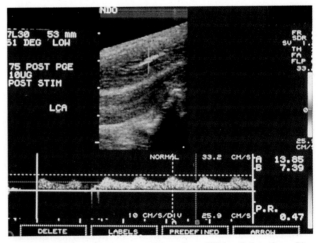

Figure 15–2 D LCA (PSV – 13.9 cm/sec; EDV – 7.4 cm/sec; RI – 0.47). **Results:** bilateral cavernosal arterial insufficiency; cannot exclude cavernosal venous occlusive dysfunction.
Diagnosis: arteriogenic erectile dysfunction.

Clinical Scenario 3 (Fig. 15–3)

A 45-year-old male who has had difficulty in getting and maintaining an erection for the last six or seven years. It has increased in severity recently. The patient has a history of prior alcohol and drug abuse and prior episode of prostatitis which was treated with antibiotics. When he was younger, he did a considerable amount of bicycle riding and did develop transient numbness in the genital area.

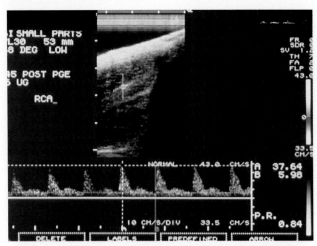

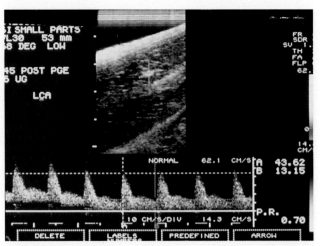

Figure 15–3   Clinical Scenario 3. Following intracavernosal injection of 6 µg of Prostaglandin E₁ (Caverject®), erectile response was 2/5.
Figure 15–3 A   RCA (PSV – 37.6 cm/sec; EDV – 6 cm/sec; RI – 0.84).

Figure 15–3 B   LCA (PSV – 43.6 cm/sec; EDV – 13.2 cm/sec; RI – 0.70).

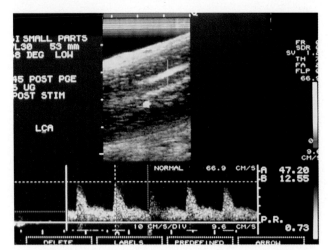

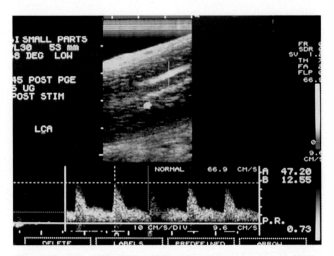

Figure 15–3 C   Following self-stimulation, (Figs. 3 **C** and 3 **D**) erectile response was 3/5. RCA (PSV – 38.2 cm/sec; EDV – 7.8 cm/sec; RI – 0.80).

Figure 15–3 D   LCA (PSV – 47.2 cm/sec; EDV – 12.6 cm/sec; RI – 0.73). **Results:** cavernosal venous occlusive dysfunction.
Diagnosis: venogenic erectile dysfunction.

Clinical Scenario 4 (Fig. 15–4)

A 56-year-old male who has had erectile dysfunction progressing for several years. The patient denies hypertension, smoking, coronary artery disease, diabetes, Peyronie's disease, pelvic trauma, or prostate cancer.

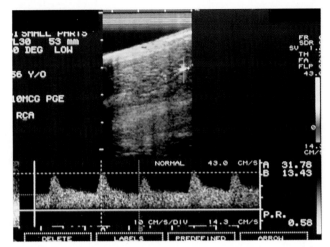

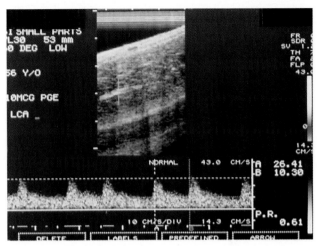

Figure 15–4   Clinical Scenario 4. Following intracavernosal injection of 10 μg of Prostaglandin E₁ (Caverject®), erectile response was 2/5.
Figure 15–4 A   RCA (PSV – 31.8 cm/sec; EDV – 13.4 cm/sec; RI – 0.58).

Figure 15–4 B   LCA (PSV – 26.4 cm/sec; EDV – 10.3 cm/sec; RI – 0.61; irregular heart rhythm).

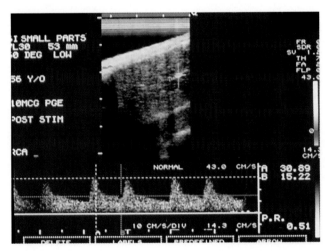

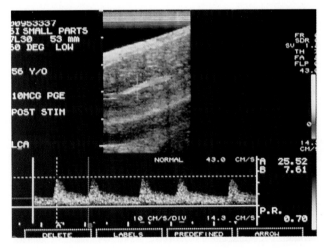

Figure 15–4 C   Following self-stimulation, (Figs. 4 **C** and 4 **D**) erectile response was 2/5. RCA (PSV – 30.9 cm/sec; EDV – 15.2 cm/sec; RI – 0,51).

Figure 15–4 D   LCA (PSV – 25.5 cm/sec; EDV – 7.6 cm/sec; RI – 0.70). **Results:** mild bilateral cavernosal arterial insufficiency with cavernosal venous occlusive dysfunction.
Diagnosis: venogenic erectile dysfunction with mild arteriogenic component and cardiac arrhythmia.

Clinical Scenario 5 (Fig. 15–5)

A 71-year-old male who has had erectile dysfunction for 20 years. Patient has had two previous transurethral resections of the prostate. Patient has unstable angina. There is no history of hypertension, smoking, diabetes, Peyronie's disease, pelvic trauma, or prostate cancer.

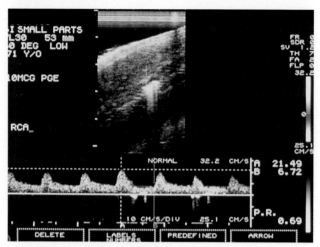

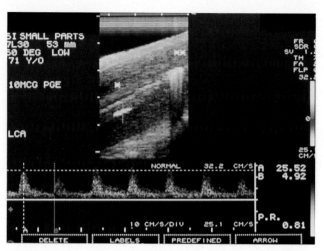

Figure 15–5   Clinical Scenario 5. Following intracavernosal injection of 10 µg of Prostaglandin E$_1$ (Caverject®), erectile response was 1/5.
Figure 15–5 A   RCA (PSV – 21.5 cm/sec; EDV – 6.7 cm/sec; RI – 0.69).

Figure 15–5 B   LCA (PSV – 25.5 cm/sec; EDV – 4.9 cm/sec; RI – 0.81).

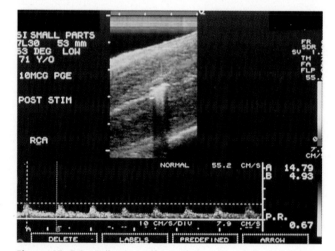

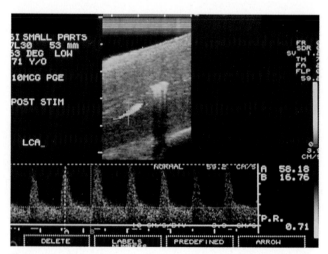

Figure 15–5 C   Following self-stimulation, (Figs. 5 **C** and 5 **D**) erectile response was 3/5. RCA (PSV – 14.8 cm/sec; EDV – 4.9 cm/sec; RI – 0.67).

Figure 15–5 D   LCA (PSV – 58.2 cm/sec; EDV – 16.8 cm/sec; RI – 0.71).

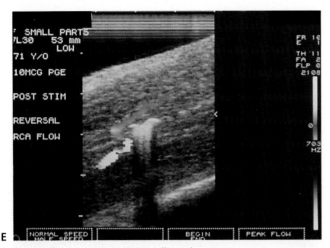

Figure 15–5 E   LCA to RCA collateral

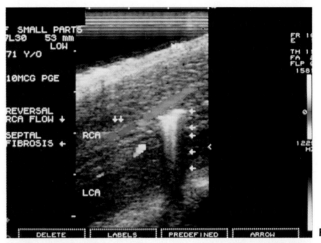

Figure 15–5 F   Reversal of flow in proximal RCA and septal fibrosis without Peyronie's deviation. Results – right cavernosal arterial insufficiency with cavernosal venous occlusive dysfunction. Diagnosis – mixed arteriogenic and venogenic erectile dysfunction.

Clinical Scenario 6 (Fig. 15–6)

A 51-year-old male who has had erectile dysfunction for approximately 5 years associated with Peyronie's dis-ease. The patient denies hypertension, smoking, coronary artery disease, diabetes, pelvic trauma, or prostate cancer.

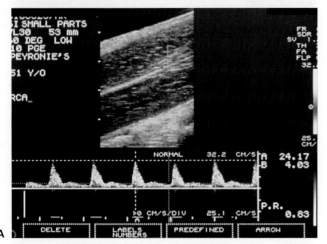

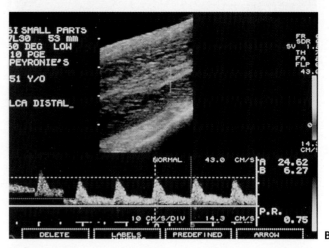

Figure 15–6   Clinical Scenario 6. Following intracavernosal injection of 10 µg of Prostaglandin E$_1$ (Caverject®), erectile response was 3/5. No self-stimulation study was performed.
Figure 15–6 A   RCA (PSV – 24.2 cm/sec; EDV – 4 cm/sec; RI – 0.83).

Figure 15–6 B   LCA (PSV – 24.6 cm/sec; EDV – 6.3 cm/sec; RI – 0.75).

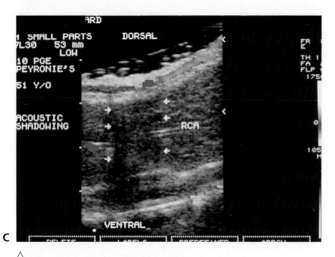

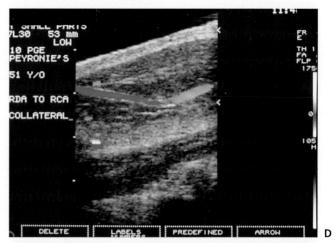

Figure 15–6 C   Distal dorsal plaque with acoustic shadowing (arrows) causing a dorsal penile curvature of approximately 45 degrees.

Figure 15–6 D   RDA to RCA collaterals.

Figure 15–6 E   RCA to LCA collaterals.
Results: penile curvature with dorsal plaque; mild bilateral cavernosal arterial insufficiency.
Diagnosis: Peyronie's disease.

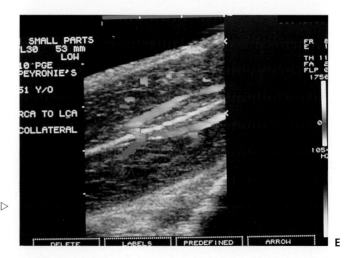

Differential Diagnosis

Prevalence

In December 1992, the National Institute of Health conducted a consensus development panel on impotence and suggested that a more precise term is erectile dysfunction.[1] They defined *erectile dysfunction* as the inability to achieve or maintain an erection sufficient for satisfactory sexual performance. Recent estimates of the number of men in the United States suffering from erectile dysfunction is 10—20 million. If one included partial erectile dysfunction, the incidence increases to approximately 30 million. The ratio of organic to psychological causes contributing to erectile dysfunction varies with age: 70% of patients under 35 years of age have psychogenic etiology and 85% of men over 50 years of age have organic causes.[2]

Erectile dysfunction is commonly associated with aging.[3] In 1948, Kinsey found that erectile dysfunction (ED) was an age-dependent disorder with a prevalence of 0.1% at 20 years of age, 0.9% at 30, 1.9% at 40, 6.7% at 50, 18.4% at 60, 27% at 70, 55% at 75, and 75% at 80 years of age. However, since only 5% of the population evaluated were older than 55 years, data for men above that age must be interpreted with caution. Martin (1981) reported 7% ED at age 20—30 years and 57% at age 70—79 years. Furlow (1985) reported 2% at age 40 years and 25—30% at 65 years. In geriatric patients, Mulligan et al. (1988) reported 26% ED at age 60—65 years, and 50% at 75—85 years. Similarly, Diokno et al. (1990) also reported age dependence of ED, with 29% at 60—64 years and 64% in men age 80 or older. Modebe (1990) showed a significant correlation between ED and age; the frequency of impotence increasing progressively from 17% in men aged 30—39 years to 75% in those aged 70 years or older. The Massachusetts Male Aging Study (MMAS) showed that the probability of complete impotence increased from 5% to 15% between the ages of 40 and 70 years, moderate impotence doubled from 17% to 34%, whereas minimal impotence remained constant at 17%.[4]

After adjustment for age, a higher probability for erectile dysfunction was directly correlated with heart disease, hypertension, diabetes, associated medications, and depression. Cigarette smoking was associated with a greater probability of complete impotence in men with heart disease, and hypertension.[5]

Anatomy

The penis comprised of three columns of spongy tissue: two dorsally located corpora cavernosa, and one ventrally located corpus spongiosum. The corpus spongiosum contains the anterior urethra. Distally, the corpus spongiosum expands to become the glans penis. Blood supply to the corpus spongiosum and glans is through bilateral dorsal arteries (**Fig. 15–1 C,D**), which arise on each side from the penile artery, itself a branch of the internal pudendal artery. The primary blood supply to each corpus cavernosum is through a cavernous artery (Figs. 15–1 A,B), a branch of the common penile artery. The cavernosal tissue is sponge-like and composed of a meshwork of interconnected cavernosal spaces that are lined by vascular endothelium and separated by trabeculae containing bundles of smooth muscle in a framework of collagen, elastin, and fibroblasts. The terminal helicine arteries are multiple muscular and corkscrew-shaped arteries that open directly into the cavernous spaces. These sinusoids in the corpora cavernosa fill and expand with blood to form an erection. The spongy tissues of the corpora cavernosa are encapsulated by a two-layered fibrous sheath called the *tunica albuginea*. The proximal ends of the corpora cavernosa, the crura, originate at the undersurface of the puboischial rami as two separate structures but merge under the pubic arch and remain attached up to the glans. The septum between the two corpora cavernosa is incomplete in men.[2, 5]

The venous drainage from the corpora originates in tiny venules leading from the peripheral sinusoids immediately beneath the tunica albuginea. These venules travel in the trabeculae between the tunica and the peripheral sinusoids to form the subtunical venous plexus before exiting as the emissary veins. The emissary veins usually take an oblique course between the two layers of the tunica albuginea. Emissary veins draining the proximal corpora cavernosa join to form cavernous and crural veins. These veins join the periurethral veins from the urethral bulb to form the internal pudendal veins. The emissary veins from the more distal corporus cavernosum and spongiosum drain dorsally to the deep dorsal vein, laterally to the circumflex vein, and ventrally to the periurethral vein. Beginning at the coronal sulcus, the prominent deep dorsal vein (DDV) (**Fig. 15–1 E**) comprises the main venous drainage of the glans penis, corpus spongiosum, and distal two-thirds of the corpora cavernosa. Usually one, but sometimes more than one, deep dorsal vein runs upward behind the symphysis pubis to join the periprostatic venous plexus. Variations in the number, distribution, and termination of the venous systems are common.[5]

The innervation of the penis is both autonomic (sympathetic and parasympathetic) and somatic (sensory and motor). The parasympathethic (S2—S4) activity is responsible for tumescence and the sympathetic (T11—L2) activity causes detumescence.[5]

Physiology of Erection

The penile erectile tissue, specifically the cavernous smooth musculature and the smooth muscles of the arteriolar and arterial walls, plays a key role in the erectile process. In the flaccid state, these smooth muscles are chronically contracted by the sympathetic discharge, allowing only for a small amount of arterial flow for nutritional purposes.[5]

Sexual stimulation triggers the release of neurotransmitters from the cavernous nerve terminals. This results in relaxation of the smooth muscles and the following events: (1) dilatation of the arterioles and arteries with increased blood flow in both the diastolic and systolic phases; (2) trapping of the incoming blood by the expanding sinusoids; (3) compression of the subtunical venous plexuses between the tunica albuginea and the distended sinusoids, reducing the venous outflow; (4) stretching of the tunica to its capacity, which encloses the emissary veins between the inner circular and the outer longitudinal layers of the tunica and further decreases the venous outflow to a minimum; (5) an increase in intracavernous pressure (maintained at around 100 mm Hg), which raises the penis from the dependent position to the erect state (the full erection phase); and (6) a further pressure increase (to several hundred mm Hg) with contraction of the ischiocavernosus muscles (rigid erection phase).[5]

There are three types of erection: psychogenic, reflexogenic, and nocturnal.[5] Psychogenic erection is the result of sensory input (sight, sound, smell) or fantasy. These stimuli are processed by the hypothalamus which orchestrates the sympathetic (T11—L2) and parasympathetic (S2—S4) response.[6] The medial preoptic area (MPOA) and the paraventricular nucleus of the hypothalamus are important integration centers for sexual drive and penile erection.[5,7] With stimulation, there is decreased sympathetic activity and increased parasympathetic activity to the penis. Activation of the nonadrenergic—noncholinergic neurons causes an increased formation of nitric oxide (NO) and secondary neuropeptides. Nitric oxide stimulates the production of cyclic guanosine monophosphate (cGMP), resulting in the depletion of intracellular calcium and thereby inducing relaxation of smooth muscles.[5—7] The new oral drug Sildenafil Citrate (Viagra, Pfizer, New York, NY) is a selective inhibitor of cGMP phosphodiesterase type 5, which is largely responsible for the breakdown of cGMP. Thereby, Viagra enhances and prolongs the effects of cGMP.

Reflexogenic erection is produced by tactile stimuli to the genital organs. The impulses reach the spinal erection centers; some of them follow the ascending tract, resulting in sensory perception, and others activate the autonomic nuclei to send messages via the cavernous nerves to the penis to induce erection. This type of erection is preserved in patients with upper spinal cord injuries.[5]

Nocturnal erections occurs mostly during rapid-eye-movement (REM) sleep. The central mechanism is as yet unknown but the end-organ physiologic responses are the same.[5]

Classification of Erectile Dysfunction

Erectile dysfunction can be classified as: psychogenic, neurogenic, endocrinologic, vasculogenic, or drug-induced.[5]

Psychogenic

Sexual behavior and penile erection are controlled by the hypothalamus, limbic system, and the cerebral cortex. Therefore, stimulatory or inhibitory messages can be related to the spinal erection centers to facilitate or inhibit erection. Two possible mechanisms have been proposed to explain the inhibition of erection in psychogenic dysfunction: direct inhibition of the spinal erection center by the brain as an exaggeration of the normal suprasacral inhibition and excessive sympathetic outflow or elevated peripheral catecholamine levels, which may increase penile smooth muscle tone and thus prevent the relaxation necessary for erection.

Neurogenic

Because erection is a neurovascular event, any disease or dysfunction affecting the brain, spinal cord, cavernous and pudendal nerves, or receptors in the terminal arterioles and cavernous smooth muscles can induce dysfunction. Pathologic processes involving the brain such as Parkinson's disease, stroke, tumors, Alzheimer's disease, and trauma can be associated with partial or complete erectile dysfunction. Spinal cord injuries, spina bifida, disc herniation, syringomyelia, tumor, and multiple sclerosis can affect the afferent or efferent neural pathways involving the spine and be associated with erectile dysfunction.

Because of the close of relationship between the cavernous nerves and the pelvic organs, surgery on these organs is a frequent cause of impotence. The incidence of iatrogenic erectile dysfunction resulting from radical prostatectomy has ranged from 43% to 100% and for abdominal perineal resection, 15—100%. The introduction of nerve-sparing radical prostatectomy has dramatically reduced the incidence of impotence from nearly 100% to between 30% and 50%.

Alcoholism, vitamin deficiency, or diabetes may affect the cavernous nerve terminals, resulting in a deficiency of neurotransmitters. In diabetics, impairment of neurogenic and endothelium-dependent relaxation results in inadequate nitrous oxide (NO) release.

Endocrinologic

The endocrine disorders that are associated with ED are hypopituitarism, nonfunctioning pituitary tumors, prolactin-secreting pituitary tumors, hyperthyroidism, and hypothyroidism. Hyperprolactinemia, whether resulting from a pituitary adenoma or drugs, leads to both reproductive and sexual dysfunction. Symptoms may include loss of libido, erectile dysfunction, galactorrhea, gynecomastia, and infertility. Hyperprolactinemia is associated with low circulating levels of testosterone, which appear to be secondary to inhibition of gonadotropin-releasing hormone secretion by the elevated prolactin levels.

Hyperthyroidism is commonly associated with diminished libido, which may be due to the increased circulating estrogen levels and less often with erectile dysfunction. In hypothyroidism, low testosterone secretion and elevated prolactin levels contribute to erectile dysfunction.

Diabetes mellitus, although the most common endocrinologic disorder, causes erectile dysfunction through its vascular, neurologic, endothelial, and psychogenic complications rather than through hormone deficiency per se.

Vasculogenic

Arteriogenic

Atherosclerotic or traumatic arterial occlusive disease of the hypogastric-cavernous-helicine arterial tree can decrease the perfusion pressure and arterial flow to the sinusoidal spaces, thus increasing the time needed to attain maximal erection and decreasing the rigidity of the erect penis. One study found that the incidence and age at onset of coronary disease and erectile dysfunction are parallel. In the majority of patients with arteriogenic erectile dysfunction, the impaired penile perfusion is a component of the generalized atherosclerotic process. Common risk factors associated with arterial insufficiency include hypertension, hyperlipidemia, cigarette smoking, diabetes mellitus, blunt perineal, or pelvic trauma, and pelvic irradiation. Focal stenosis of the common penile or cavernous artery is most often seen in young patients who have sustained pelvic fracture or direct perineal trauma.

Venogenic

Veno-occlusive dysfunction has been proposed as one of the most common causes of vasculogenic impotence. Veno-occlusive dysfunction may result from several possible pathophysiologic processes: (1) the presence or development of large venous channels draining the corpora cavernosa, frequently seen in patients with primary erectile dysfunction; (2) degenerative changes (Peyronie's disease, old age, and diabetes) or traumatic injury to the tunica albuginea (penile fracture), resulting in inadequate compression of the subtunical and emissary veins; (3) structural alterations in the fibroelastic components of the trabeculae, cavernous smooth muscle, and endothelium; (4) insufficient trabecular smooth muscle relaxation, causing inadequate sinusodal expansion and insufficient compression of the subtunical venules, occuring in an anxious individual with excessive adrenergic tone or in a patient with inadequate neuorotransmitter release from the parasympathetic nerves; and (5) acquired venous shunts (the result of operative correction of priapism), causing persistent glans-cavernosum or cavernosum-spongiosum shunting.

Peyronie's disease is characterized by a lesion in the tunica albuginea of the corpora cavernosa (**Fig. 15–6C**). During erection, this lesion causes functional shortening and curvature of the involved aspect of the tunica. The lesion has commonly been called a *plaque*. Peyronie's disease is seen in about 1% of white men. Although the disease has been reported in younger patients, there is a clear predominance between the ages of 45 and 60 years. The plaque is a focal scar that may result in susceptible individuals from an inflammatory reponse to microtrauma from bending and buckling of the erect penis during sexual intercourse. In the flaccid penis, the plaque is usually palpable as a nodule or thickening, often on the doral aspect of the penis.

Peyronie's disease is also associated with the development of erectile dysfunction in some patients. It appears that in most cases, however, erectile dysfunction precedes the development of Peyronie's disease.

Drug-induced

In general, drugs that interfere with central neuroendocrine or local neurovascular control of penile smooth muscle have a potential for causing erectile dysfunction. Central neurotransmitter pathways and dopaminergic pathways involved in sexual function, may be disturbed by antipsychotics, antidepressants, and some centrally acting antihypertensive drugs.

Centrally acting sympatholytics include methyldopa, clonidine (inhibition of the hypothalamic center by a alpha$_2$-receptor stimulation), and reserpine (depletion of the stores of catecholamines and serotonin). Guanethidine, a peripheral sympatholytic, has been reported to cause erectile as well as ejaculatory dysfunction. Alpha-adrenergic blocking agents such as phenoxybenzamine and phentolamine also reportedly cause ejaculatory inhibition. Prazosin, a selective alpha$_1$-adrenergic blocking agent, may cause erectile dysfunction. Beta-adrenergic blockers have been reported to depress libido. Thiazide diuretics have been credited with widely differing effects on potency, and spironolactone produces erectile failure in 4—30% of patients and has been associated with decreased libido, gynecomastia, and mastodynia.

Major tranquilizers or antipsychotics can decrease libido, causing erectile failure and ejaculatory dysfunction. The mechanisms involved may include sedation, anticholinergic action, a central antidopaminergic effect, alpha-adrenergic antagonist action, and release of prolactin. Among antidepressants, tricyclic antidepressants and monamine oxidase (MAO) inhibitors reportedly cause erectile dysfunction through central and peripheral actions. The sexual side effects seen in patients taking minor tranquilizers may well be a result of the central sedative effects of these agents.

Cigarette smoking may induce vasoconstriction and penile venous leakage because of its contractile effect on the cavernous smooth muscle. In a study of nocturnal penile tumescence in cigarette smokers, there was an inverse correlation between nocturnal erection, both rigidity and duration, and the number of cigarettes smoked per day. Men who smoked more than 40 cigarettes a day had the weakest and shortest nocturnal erections. Alcohol in small amounts improves erection and sexual drive because of its vasodilatory effect and suppression of anxiety; however, large amounts can cause central sedation, decreased libido, and transient erectile dysfunction. Chronic alcoholism may result in liver dysfunction, decreased testosterone, and increased estrogen levels and alcoholic polyneuropathy, which also effects penile nerves. Cimetidime, a histamine H_2 receptor antagonist, has been reported to suppress the libido and produce erectile failure. It is thought to act as an antiandrogen and increase prolactin levels.

Other drugs known to cause erectile dysfunctions are estrogens and drugs with antiandrogenic actions such as ketoconazole and cyproterone acetate. Finally, many anticancer drugs may be associated with a progressive loss of libido and erectile dysfunction.

Erectile Dysfunction Associated with Systemic Disease and Other Causes

Chronic renal failure has frequently been associated with diminished erectile function, impaired libido, and infertility. In one study, by the time patients with uremia began maintenance dialysis, 50% were impotent. The mechanism is probably multifactorial: depressed testosterone levels, diabetes mellitus, vascular insufficiency, multiple medications, autonomic and somatic neuropathy, and psychological stress. After successful renal transplantation, 50—80% of patients have returned to their pre-illness potency.[5]

Patients with severe pulmonary disease often fear aggravating dypsnea during sexual intercourse. Patients with angina, heart failure, or myocardial infarction can have erectile dysfunction from anxiety, depression, or arterial insufficiency. Other systemic diseases such as cirrhosis of the liver, scleroderma, chronic debilitation, and cachexia are also known to cause erectile dysfunction.

Diagnostic Workup

Nonimaging Tests

In the last decade, minimally invasive therapies such as the vacuum constriction device and intracavernous injection have replaced the penile prosthesis as the gold standard of treatment for erectile dysfunction. Recently, effective oral medication became available. The introduction of these highly effective but nonspecific treatments have raised questions about the need for more sophisticated diagnostic tests. In these days of cost-conscious managed-care competition, the diagnosis and treatment of erectile dysfunction will likely be dictated by insurance companies and government agencies rather than by the patient or his or her physician.

Lue and Broderick propose a two-level diagnostic approach, depending on the patient's and the partner's goal and the patient's age, general health, and medical condition.[8] The first level consists of a detailed medical and psychosexual history, physical examination, and hormonal and laboratory testing followed by a discussion of treatment options and further diagnostic tests. The patient is then given the choice of either a therapeutic trial (with oral medication, a vacuum constriction device, or intracavernous injection) or a second level of evaluation. The latter level is designed to elucidate the cause of the dysfunction and entails one or more of the following tests: psychological consultation, nocturnal penile tumescence and rigidity testing, advanced neurological testing, and functional arterial and venous studies.

The objectives of diagnostic evaluation are to (1) identify medical and psychosexual causes, (2) assess the degree and reversibility of the dysfunction, and (3) solicit motivation and treatment goals from the patient and his partner.

To begin the evaluation, a careful medical history with knowledge of concurrent illnesses and medications is essential. Because erectile dysfunction may have multiple causes, a detailed history and physical examination may help determine whether the dysfunction is a result of anatomic, psychogenic, endocrinologic, neurologic, or vascular abnormalities and/or medication induced.

The psychosexual history is a very important part of the diagnostic evaluation and should include the duration of erectile dysfunction and level of libido. The assessment of the onset of dysfunction, the presence of morning erection, intermittency, and any psychological conflict may help determine whether the dysfunction is mostly psychogenic or organic.

Because erectile dysfunction is known to be associated with many common medical conditions and medications, careful questioning may yield insights. A history of peripheral vascular or coronary artery disease, diabetes, renal failure, tobacco and alcohol use, psychologic, neurologic or chronic debilitating disease can direct further evaluation.

Similarly, patient's past surgical history is important. Pelvic surgery (prostatectomy, distal colectomy, abdominoperineal resection), radiation therapy, and pelvic trauma may be associated with impotence.

Careful physical examination with particular attention to sexual and genital development may occasionally reveal an obvious cause such as micropenis or Peyronie's plaque. The finding of small soft atrophic testes or gynecomastia should prompt an endocrine evaluation for hypogonadism or hyperprolactinemia. Patients with certain genetic syndromes, such as Klinefelter's syndrome, may present with obvious physical signs of hypogonadism or distinctive body habitus. A careful neurologic examination should also be performed. Patients with diabetes or degenerative neurologic disorders may show evidence of peripheral neuropathy. Testing for genital or perineal sensation and the bulbocavernosus reflex is also useful in assessing possible neurogenic impotence. One study showed that a careful history and physical examination had a 95% sensitivity but only a 50% specificity in diagnosing organic erectile dysfunction.

The laboratory investigation is directed at identifying treatable conditions or previously undetected metabolic illnesses that my be contributory, e.g., metabolic disturbances such as renal insufficiency, diabetes, and endocrine abnormalities (e.g., hypogonadism, hyperprolactinemia). A complete laboratory evaluation includes serum chemistries, renal function, complete blood count, urinalysis and hormonal evaluation (generally, serum testosterone, prolactin, and thyroid function). Prostate specific antigen (PSA) level is recommended in all men 50 years of age or older or starting at age 40, if there is a family history of prostate cancer.

After the patient has had a careful history and physical and laboratory testing, the results are discussed with the patient (and partner) and available treatment options are discussed. If further testing is performed, they may include psychological consultation, nocturnal penile tumescence and rigidity testing, advanced neurological testing and functional arterial and venous studies.

Psychometry and Psychologic Interview

There are three groups of psychometric instruments available for the evaluation of erectile dysfunction: (1) the standardized personality questionnaires; (2) the depression inventory and; (3) questionnaires for sexual dysfunction and relationship factors.[8]

A skillful diagnostic interview remains the mainstay of psychologic evaluation. The interview should be focused on the following: (1) the current sexual problem and its history; (2) deeper causes of sexual dysfunction; (3) the relationship with the partner; and (4) psychiatric symptoms.

Nocturnal Penile Tumescence and Rigidity Testing (NPTR)

Nocturnal penile erection — or sleep-related erection — is a recurring cycle of penile erections associated with rapid eye movement sleep in virtually all potent men. Patients documented to have normal NPTR are presumed to have normal capacity for spontaneous erotically induced erections. The primary goal of NPTR testing is to distinguish psychogenic from organic impotence. This study consists of nocturnal monitoring devices that measure the number of erectile episodes, maximum penile rigidity, tumescence (circumference) and duration of the nocturnal erections. Traditionally, NPTR is recorded in conjunction with recording of electroencephalographic, electro-occulographic, and electromyographic (EMG) activities. Laboratories now also monitor sleep-related breathing and movement patterns because erectile dysfunction is prevalent in patients with sleep apnea and periodic limb movement disorder.[7,8]

Many investigators have advocated the use of NPTR studies, particularly in identifying patients with psychogenic impotence. A normal study in a patient in whom a psychological causes is suspected will help reduce the cost of the evaluation by preventing unnecessary endocrine and vascular evaluations. Abnormal NPTR testing does not specify the etiology of erectile dysfunction.

Sexual Stimulation (Audiovisual and Vibratory)

Another alternative to NPTR testing for differential diagnosis is the use of vibrotactile or visual sexual stimulation, or both. This test is designed to elicit penile responses during visual and vibrotactile stimulation in conjunction with cognitive tasks (distraction and monitoring of erections). It has been found that about one-third of patients with purely psychogenic erectile dysfunction have an average increase in penile girth of more than 30 mm as a response to combined vibration and film. None of the patients with organic involvement exceeded this 30-mm criteria; however, one study analyzed the scientific communities attitude toward sexual stimulation, video testing, and warned that many factors may effect the outcome such as the physician's fear of being accused of voyeurism, the physician's feelings about his or her own erotic fantasies and about pornography, and the castrating effects of a hospital environment. Therefore, further studies are needed before visual and vibrotactile stimulation can be used as a screening test for differential diagnosis of erectile dysfunction.[8]

Neurologic Testing

Neurologic testing should assess peripheral, spinal, and supraspinal centers and both somatic and autonomic pathways associated with erection.

Somatic Nervous System

Biothesiometry

This test is designed to measure the sensory perception threshold to various amplitudes of vibratory stimulation produced by a handheld electromagnetic device (biothesiometer) placed on the pulp of the index fingers, both sides of the penile shaft, and the glans penis. At least, one study found no relationship between results of penile glans biothesiometry and neurourophysiologic tests of the dorsal penile nerve, probably owing to the fact that vibration is not an adequate stimulus to the glanular skin, which contains free nerve endings only and hardly any vibration receptors. The biothesiometric investigation of penile glans innervation is probably unsuited for the evaluation of penile innervation and cannot replace neurourophysiologic tests.[8]

Sacral Evoked Response-bulbocavernosus Reflex Latency

This test is performed by placing two stimulating ring electrodes around the penis, one near the corona, and the other 3 cm proximal. Concentric needle electrodes are placed in the right and left bulbocavernosus muscles to record the response. Square-wave impulses are delivered via direct current stimulator. The latency period for each stimulus response is measured from the beginning of the stimulus to the beginning of the response. An abnormal bulbocavernosus reflex (BCR) latency time, defined as a value greater than 3 standard deviations above the mean (30—40 ms), carries a high probability of neuropathology. In a study of diabetic patients, a significant clinical and neurophysiologic correlation between the absence of the bulbocavernosus reflex on clinical examination and its prolonged latency on electrophysiologic measurements was shown.[8]

Dorsal Nerve Conduction Velocity

In patients with adequate penile length, it is possible to use two BCR latency measurements, one from the glans and one from the base of the penis, to determine the conduction velocity of the dorsal nerve (i.e., by dividing the distance between the two stimulating electrodes by the difference in latency between the base and the glans).[8]

Genitocerebral-evoked Potential Studies

This test involves electrical stimulation of the dorsal nerve of the penis, as described with a BCR latency test. Instead of recording electromyogram (EMG) responses, the study records the evoked potential waveforms overlying the sacral spinal cord and cerebral cortex. The cerebral response to peripheral nerve stimulation is one of the potentials of extremely low amplitude, and complex electronic equipment is used to store and average data of thousands of waveforms recurring as often as every 10th of a millisecond. The first latency recorded is the time of stimulation to the first replicated spinal response—the peripheral conduction time. The second is from the time of the stimulation to the first replicated cerebral response — the total conduction time. The difference between the two is the central conduction time. Unlike BCR latency, this is a purely sensory evaluation. This study is not useful as a routine test, but it can provide an objective assessment of the presence, location, and nature of afferent penile sensory dysfunction in patients with subtle abnormalities on neurological examination.[8]

Autonomic Nervous System
Heart Rate Variability

Although autonomic neuropathy is an important cause of erectile dysfunction, direct testing is not available. However, many diseases that involve the autonomic nervous system affect innervation to multiple organ systems, and many tests have been developed to assess the integrity of the sympathetic and parasympathetic nervous system.

The test of heart rate control (mainly parasympathetic) consists of measuring heart rate variations during quiet breathing, during deep breathing, and response to rising to one's feet. The normal parameters are (1) heart rate variation coefficient of the mean RR variation during quiet breathing is less than 1.88 in the 41- to 60-year-old group and 2.52 for adults less than 40 years old; (2) the maximal average difference between the minimal heart rate of inspiration and maximal rate of expiration during three successive breathing cycles should be higher than 15 beats per minute in the younger group and 9 beats per minute in the older group; and (3) the ratio of the longest RR interval of the bradycardiac phase and the shortest RR interval of the tachycardiac phase should be greater than 1.11.[8]

The test of blood pressure control (mainly sympathetic) measures the blood pressure response to standing up. The decrease in systolic blood pressure should be less than 13 mm Hg. Because heart rate and blood pressure responses can be affected by many external factors, these tests must be conducted under standardized conditions.

Sympathetic Skin Response (SSR)

Sympathetic Skin Response measures the skin potential evoked by electric shock stimuli. For example, the electrical stimuli can be applied to the median or tibial nerve and the evoked potential recorded at the contralateral hand or foot or the penis. One study evaluated 50 men with erectile dysfunction with the SSR and other neurophysiologic tests and found that the SSR was absent in 11 of 30 cases but was normal in all patients with nonneurogenic erectile dysfunction. The SSR, especially if recorded from the penis, seems to be a useful method of testing penile autonomic innervation.[8]

Smooth Muscle EMG

Direct recording of cavernous electrical activity with a needle electrode during flaccidity and with visual sexual stimulation was first reported by Wagner and co-workers. The normal resting flaccid electrical activity from the corpora cavernosa was a rhythmic slow wave with an intermittent burst of activity. These bursts virtually ceased during visual sexual stimulation or after intracavernous injection of a smooth muscle relaxant. The electrical activity returned during the detumescence phase. Patients with suspected autonomic neuropathy demonstrated a discoordination pattern with continuing electrical activity during visual sexual stimulation or after intracavernous injection of a smooth muscle relaxant. The cavernous EMG is characterized by reproducible waveforms (potentials) but highly variable in the individual subject. More studies are needed to find the clinical utility of cavernous EMG and better understand how it works.[8]

Vascular Evaluation

Penile Brachial Pressure Index (PBI)

The penile brachial index represents penile systolic blood pressure divided by the brachial systolic blood pressure. The technique involves applying a small pediatric blood pressure cuff to the base of the flaccid penis and measuring the systolic blood pressure with a continuous-wave Doppler probe. Penile brachial index of 0.7 or less has been used to indicate arteriogenic impotence.

This test has many inherent limitations. Measurement in the flaccid state does not reveal the full functional capacity of the cavernous arteries in the erect state, and errors may also occur from improper fitting of the blood pressure cuff.

Second, the continuous-wave Doppler probe does not discriminately select the arterial flow of the paired cavernous arteries, which are primarily involved in producing erections. In the flaccid state, the probe detects all pulsatile flow within its path and usually detects the higher blood flow of the dorsal artery, which is located superficially and supplies the glans penis, rather than the deeper flow of the cavernous arteries. This error sometimes leads to finding of a normal PBI in a patient with true arteriogenic impotence (false negative). Therefore, a normal PBI cannot be relied upon to exclude arteriogenic impotence.[8]

Cavernous Arterial Occlusion Pressure

This variation of penile blood flow pressure determination involves infusing saline solution into the corpora at rates sufficient to raise the intracavernous pressure above the systolic blood pressure. A pencil Doppler transducer is then applied to the side of the penile base. The saline infusion is stopped and the intracavernous pressure is allowed to fall. The pressure at which the cavernous arterial flow becomes detectable is defined as the cavernous arterial systolic occlusion pressure (CASOP). The gradient between the cavernous and brachial artery pressure of less than 35 mm Hg and equal pressure between the right and left cavernous arteries have been defined as normal. This technique offers several advantages over the traditional PBI measurements. First, because a blood pressure cuff is not required, a Doppler probe can be directly applied to the base where the cavernous arteries are less likely to have branched. Second, continuous monitoring of the intracavernous pressure appears to be a more accurate way of determining the systolic arterial pressure of the cavernous artery than the pressure cuff. Last, unlike the PBI (which is performed on a flaccid penis), CASOP performed after intracavernous injection of a vasodilating agent allows assessment of the functional capacity of the cavernous arteries in the erect state. Results have been shown to correlate well with those of arteriography and peak systolic velocity obtained by high-resolution duplex Doppler ultrasound. However, despite these advantages, dynamic infusion cavernosonometry is nonetheless an invasive procedure and more prone to psychologic inhibition because of discomfort. It is not feasible if the intracavernous pressure cannot be raised above the systolic blood pressure (e.g., in patients with severe venous leakage).[8]

Penile Plethysmography (Penile Pulse Volume Recording)

This test is performed by connecting a 2.5- or 3-cm cuff to an air plethysmograph. The cuff is inflated to a pressure above brachial systolic pressure, which is then decreased by 10-mm Hg increments, and tracings are obtained at each level. The pressure demonstrating the best waveform is recorded. The normal waveform is similar to a normal arterial waveform obtained from a finger: a rapid upstroke, a sharp peak, a lower downstroke, and occasionally, a dicrotic notch. In patients with arteriogenic erectile dysfunction, the waveform shows a slow upstroke; a low, rounded peak; slow downstroke; and no dicrotic notch. The proponents of this method argue that because penile pulse volume recording measures contributions of all the vessels at the root of the penis, it is more accurate than recording the pressure in individual arteries (as in PBI). However, this study is performed with the penis in the flaccid state and cannot distinguish whether the dorsal or the cavernous artery is impaired.[8]

Combined Intracavernous Injection and Stimulation Test

Differentiation among psychogenic, neurogenic, and vascular cause is often difficult, even with a complete history, physical exam, and endocrine evaluation. Intracorporeal injection of a vasodilating agent is a useful diagnostic tool, both inexpensive and minimally invasive, in patients with suspected vasculogenic impotence. The pharmacologic screening test allows the clinician to bypass neurogenic and hormonal influences and evaluate the vascular status of the penis directly and objectively.

To produce a normal erection, arterial vasodilitation, sinusoidal relaxation, and decreased venous outflow must all occur in response to a vasodilating agent. In the past, a number of agents were used, including papavarine, a smooth muscle relaxant, and phentolamine, an alpha-adrenergic blocking agent. Currently, the most commonly used agent is alprostadil [prostaglandine $E_1(PGE_1)$], a potent vasodilating agent that is metabolized locally in the penis. The technique involves injecting 10 µg through a 28-gauge needle into the corpus cavernosum. The needle site is compressed manually to prevent hematoma formation. Erectile response is periodically evaluated for both rigidity and duration. If full erection has not occurred by 10 min, the patient performs manual self-stimulation.

The pharmacologic test yields important information regarding penile vascular status. A normal finding rules out the possibility of venous leakage. Although some patients (about 20%) with mild arterial insufficiency may achieve a rigid erection owing to an intact venoocclusive mechanism. A normal erectile response (unbending rigidity of at least 20 min duration) following pharmacologic testing rules out venoocclusive dysfunction and severe arterial insufficiency and, generally, increases suspicion for psychogenic or neurogenic erectile dysfunction.

An abnormal pharmacologic test suggests penile vascular disease and warrants further evaluation. The patient's fear of injection often produces a heightened sympathetic response, which inhibits the response of the cavernous smooth muscle to the intracavernous agent. This problem may produce a false-positive result. To avoid this error, we have found it helpful to give patients as much privacy as possible during the study. They are also instructed to perform self-stimulation if a rigid erection does not result within 15 min. This technique is known as the combined injection and stimulation (CIS) test. In our experience, many patients (about 75%) who initially have a subnormal response to an intracavernous injection have significant improvement in erection after self-stimulation. Some physicians, using audiovisual sexual stimulation after pharmacologically induced

erection, also reported that 56.5 % of the patients experience improved erection with their technique. Others will simply ask the patient if the pharmacologically induced erection is similar to or better than his best home erection. If the answer is no, then a second injection may be administered.[8]

Cavernosometry

The standard nonimaging diagnostic study for veno-occlusive dysfunction is pharmacologic cavernosometry. Cavernosometry involves simultaneous saline infusion and intracorporeal pressure monitoring. A more physiological refinement is the addition of intracavernous injection of a vasodilating agent such as papavarine or PGE_1. The saline infusion rate necessary to maintain an erection is thus directly related to the degree of venous leakage. One study compared plain and pharmacologic cavernosometry and reported that plain cavernosometry gave false-positive results in 6% and false-negative results in 16% and that pharmacologic cavernosometry was much more reproducible. Veno-occlusive dysfunction is indicated by either the inability to increase intracorporeal pressure to the level of the mean systolic blood pressure with saline infusion or a rapid drop of intracorporal pressure at the cessation of infusion.

In 1990, a modification of the pump infusion cavernosometry technique by replacing the infusion pump mechanism with a gravity saline infusion set (gravity cavernosometry) was introduced. The infusion source is placed approximately 160 cm above the penis (equivalent to 120 mm Hg pressure). With an intact veno-occlusive mechanism, the steady-state intracavernous pressure will closely approximate the pressure of the infusion source (above 110 cm water); with a defective mechanism, it will remain significantly lower. Gravity infusion cavernosometry correlates well with pump infusion cavernosometry and may provide a more economic alternative.[8]

Many technical factors may influence the findings on cavernosometry. The study is performed in a nonsexual setting with little privacy, leading to patient anxiety and an adverse effect on erectile response. The phenomenon of incomplete trabecular smooth muscle relaxation will falsely suggest veno-occlusion dysfunction in some normal patients. In the clinical setting, this may lead a clinician to diagnosis venous leakage in patients who may have another underlying cause of impotence. It has been suggested that to avoid overdiagnosis, cavernosometry should ideally be performed under the condition of compete trabecular smooth muscle relaxation. In one study, in only 17% of patients with a single dose of vasoactive agent was there complete trabecular smooth muscle relaxation. Repeated doses were required in the majority of patients. The normal maintenance rate in patients with complete smooth muscle relaxation is reported to be less than 5 mL per min, with a pressure decrease from 150 mm Hg of less than 45 mm Hg in 30 s.[8]

Imaging Tests Other Than Ultrasonography

Arteriography

Penile arteriography was introduced in 1978. At present, selective pudendal arteriography performed with the aid of intracavernous injection is considered by many the gold standard for evaluating penile arterial anatomy. The study is performed by intracavernous injection of a vasodilating agent (e.g., papavarine, papavarine and phentolamine, or PGE_1), followed by selective cannulation of the internal pudendal artery and injection of a diluted contrast solution of low osmolarity. Anatomy and radiograph appearance of the cavernous arteries are then evaluated according to an established criteria.

Arteriography provides the best anatomic information about the origin of the common penile arteries, but this data has been difficult to correlate with patient complaints and with erection dynamics. The common penile artery typically arises from the third segment of the internal pudendal artery (IPA) as it passes through the urogenital diaphragm. The paired common penile arteries may originate from either one internal pudendal artery or an accessory internal pudendal artery. The common penile artery trifurcates, giving off the bulbourethral, the cavernous, and dorsal arteries. The accessory IPA takes origin from the hypogastric artery, remnant of the umbilical, ischial, or obturator arteries. An accessory IPA is reportedly more common on the right; its presence has been variably described from 4% to 70% of pelvic angiograms. Therefore, performing selective internal pudendal arteriography, and possibly missing an accessory IPA, has an inherent false-positive rate for diagnosing penile inflow disease. Also confounding interpretation is the anatomic fact that deviations from paired common penile arteries have been documented in 50% of normally potent volunteers; unilateral absence or hypoplasia of a dorsal artery has been shown in up to 30% of volunteers. Anatomic variation of intrapenile arterial anatomy appears to be the rule rather than the exception: with unilateral or bilateral origin of the cavernous arteries, distal shaft communications between the dorsal and central cavernous arteries and anastomoses between the corpus spongiosum and cavernous body.[2]

Although angiography is likely the most accurate single test for evaluating anatomy of the cavernous arteries, significant limitations to its application have been pointed out. Like all invasive radiographic tests the study is performed under artificial conditions which may produce a significant sympathetic response that inhibits erectile response. Inadequate vasodilitation of the cavernous arteries, vasospasm induced by cannulation, and injection of contrast solution may result in an abnormal radiographic appearance.

Arteriography is most useful in providing anatomic rather than functional information. It can detect vascular anomalies relatively easily, but it cannot provide information on blood flow velocity or acceleration within the cavernous arteries. Some investigators have also reported poor correlation between angiographic findings and those of other imaging studies, such as duplex sonography, suggesting that one or both techniques may contain significant limitations. Lastly, owing to the relatively high cost and invasive nature of the study, only a small percentage of impotent patients are appropriate candidates; (generally, only those who are candidates for arterial revascularization).[8]

Cavernosography

The standard imaging study to better define veno-occlusive dysfunction is pharmacologic cavernosography. Cavernosography involves infusion of radiocontrast solution into the corpora cavernosa during an artificial erection to visualize the site of venous leakage. It should always be performed after activation of the veno-occlusive mechanism by intracavernous injection of a vasodilator. Various leakage sites to the glans, corpus spongiosum, superficial and deep dorsal veins, cavernous and crural veins can be detected. In a majority of patients more than one site can be visualized by cavernosography. Although many impotent men studied with this technique are found to have venous leakage, initial enthusiasm for venous ligation procedures have waned because of poor long-term results. The development of collateral leakage sites is presumably one reason for the high failure rate. Also, it is becoming increasingly clear that venous leakage is also the consequence of intrinsic sinusoidal disease.[8]

Radioisotopic Penography

The original studies used Xenon 133 washout technique during visual sexual stimulation. Several investigators have modified the technique and use pharmacologic erection as well as different radioisotopes with a measurement of blood flow. A method was developed for measuring flow to the dependent portion of the penis with Technetium-labeled red blood cells. None of the subjects with arterial disease achieved flows greater than 20 mL per min per 100 mg of tissue, whereas flow in patients without arterial disease exceeded this value. Hwang et al. reported a technique combining penography with intracavernous injection. The skin test and corporal Xenon 133 penile washout test were conducted on each patient before 5 and 60 min after the intracavernous injection of alprostadil (PGE_1). The authors found the Xenon 133 penile washout test helpful in assessing the hemodynamics of the cavernous and dorsal arteries.[8]

Magnetic Resonance Imaging

Another technique of assessing penile function was reported by Kaneko and coworkers in 1994. They use sequential contrast-enhanced magnetic resonant images of the penis in a flaccid state. They noted that subjects with normal erectile function showed gradual and centrifugal enhancement of the corpora cavernosa, whereas those with erectile dysfunction showed poor enhancement with abnormal progression.[9]

Ultrasound Imaging

Color Duplex Doppler Testing: Penile Blood Flow Study (PBFS)

In 1982, during the course of a vascular reconstructive procedure, Ronald Virag noted that infusion of papaverine into the hypogastric artery produced erection. In 1983, a dramatic demonstration of the efficacy of penile self-injection was offered by Charles Brindley, who injected himself.[10] Brindley subsequently popularized the use of alpha blockers (phenoxybenzamine and phentolamine) and intracorporal injection in the management of organic and psychogenic erectile dysfunction. In 1985, Lue et al. introduced the technique of high-resolution sonography and quantitative Doppler spectrum analysis.[11] Duplex Doppler allowed real-time imaging of the central cavernous arteries with measurement of dynamic changes in cavernous arterial diameter and flow following intracorporal injection of papaverine.

Zorgnioti and Lefleur promoted penile self-injection with the drug combination: papaverine and phentolamine.[12] In 1986, Ishii published the first clinical series on prostaglandin E₁ for self-injection.[13] Clinicians subsequently turned to the benefits of combination therapy: exploiting the specific pharmaco-relaxing properties of different intracavernous agents, reducing the pain sometimes associated with PGE₁ (20—33%), reducing the risk of corporal fibrosis and hepatic dysfunction (8%) associated with papaverine, and minimizing the cost and volume of penile injections. Bennett et al. (1991) first described the clinical efficacy of trimix: papaverine, phentolamine and PGE₁.[14] In July of 1995, Upjohn Company (Kalamazoo, Michigan) received Food and Drug Administration approval to market injectable PGE₁ (Caverject) specifically for the diagnosis and treatment of "male impotence". PGE₁, because of its efficacy and safety (low priapism rates), is the drug of choice for the first penile injection. The demonstration that vasoactive injections could produce penile erection without benefit of psychic or tactile stimuli revolutionized the diagnosis and treatment of ED by providing a direct test of end organ integrity and offering an etiology-specific therapy.

The formula for Resistive Index is RI = Peak systolic velocity (PSV) minus End-diastolic velocity (EDV) divided by PSV. The value of RI depends on the resistance to arterial inflow, and in the context of corporal physiology, is a function of changing intracorporal pressure during the various phases of erection following either natural or pharmacological stimulation. As penile pressure equals or exceeds diastolic systemic pressure, diastolic flow in the corpora will approach zero and the value for RI approaches 1.0; in full rigidity the diastolic flow may reverse (flow is transiently retrograde). During tumescence or with a partial erection, diastolic flow persists and the value for RI remains <1.0. The RI correlates very well with visual rating of erectile responses. Both EDV and RI are useful parameters in predicting adequacy of veno-occlusion.

The hemodynamic parameters of a normal erection on color duplex Doppler ultrasound (CDDU) vary with age. In a retrospective review of over 600 cases, 150 were documented in patients of various ages where intracavernous challenge with PGE₁ produced excellent well-sustained rigidity of at least 20 min. Penile blood flow study parameters were recorded five — ten min following PGE₁ injection and repeated following privacy and self-stimulation. Mean PGE₁ dosages producing excellent erections by age group were 5 µg, (20—49 years); 6 µg, (50—59 years); 10 µg, (60—79 years). Rigid erection following privacy and self-stimulation was associated with RI/PSV of 0.95/54 (cm/s) in men 20—29 years old; 0.93/45 (cm/s) in men 30—49 years old; 0.94/33 (cm/s) in men 50—69 years old; and 0.96/32 (cm/s) in men 70—79 years old. The data suggests that cavernous arterial flow may decrease with age, but normal corporal dynamics permit penile rigidity across a wide range of PSVs. RI parameters did not statistically vary with age, suggesting the dynamics of veno-occlusion are the critical factor in the aging erection.[15, 16]

Technique

The examination should be performed in a secure setting to reduce patient anxiety and reduce sympathetic cavernous smooth muscle tone. Following the intracavernosal injection of PGE₁ (Caverject, Upjohn, Kalamazoo, Michigan) (6 µg if < 50 years old; 10 µg if ≥ 50 years old), the erection is graded at 10 min as follows: 1-no erection; 2-slight tumescence; 3-full volume without rigidity; 4-incomplete rigidity but sufficient for sexual intercourse; and 5-full erection with unbending rigidity. The penis is scanned using color Doppler imaging with a 7- to 10-Mhz linear transducer and Doppler waveforms are obtained from both cavernous arteries in their longitudinal plane with the sampling angle being 60 degrees or less. The peak systolic velocity is a good indicator of arterial function. Peak velocities below 25 cm/s indicate severe arterial insufficiency (**Fig. 15–2**). Velocities of 25 to 34 cm/s indicate some degree of arterial compromise.

Peak velocities of 35 cm/s and above indicate normal arterial function.[17]

The dorsal arteries are not subjected to the intracorporal pressure changes of each progressive erection phase and therefore, antegrade diastolic flow persists even in well-sustained rigidity (**Fig. 15–1 C,H**). Dorsal to cavernous (**Fig. 15–1 K, L, 6 D**) and cavernous to cavernous (**Fig. 15–5 E, 6 E**) arterial collaterals are common normally and are important in the presence of cavernous arterial insufficiency. Deep dorsal vein (**Fig. 15–1 J**) flow persists during rigid erection as a function of dorsal arterial flow and should not be interpreted as evidence of corporal venous leakage.[2]

In patients with normal venous competence, the cavernous arterial waveform has significant diastolic flow as the erection is developing. Once an erection is achieved, diastolic flow ceases or may become reversed (Figs. 15–1 A,B,F,G). In cases of significant venous leakage, there is persistent diastolic flow in the cavernosal artery despite expansion of the sinusoids.

Failure of the veno-occlusive mechanism is reflected in the Doppler waveforms of the cavernous arteries. End-diastolic velocity (EDV) greater than 5 cm/s is abnormal (**Fig. 15–3, 15–4**). The suspicion of venous leakage is raised when the patient has an excellent arterial response ($\geq$ 30—35 cm/s, PSV), but with a well maintained EDV (> 3—5 cm/s), accompanied by partial erection after self-stimulation. Among patients with PSV > 25 cm/s, venous leakage on cavernosometry was predicted with a sensitivity of 90% and specificity of 56% when end diastolic flow was > 5 cm/s. In Japan, Naroda found RI > 0.9 was associated with normal dynamic infusion cavernosometry in 90% and RI < 0.75 was associated with venous leakage in 95% of patients.[18] Once a venous leak has been diagnosed, cavernosography, using radiographic contrast, is used to define the abnormal veins, if surgery is contemplated.

If the patient does not achieve a full erection (grade 5), the measurements are repeated following 5 min of privacy and self-stimulation. Evaluation of veno-occlusive dysfunction requires intact arterial inflow.

The corporal bodies should be scanned in the transverse plane from the base to the tip. The echotecture should be homogeneous with fibrotic areas being relatively hyperechoic. Peyronie's plaques will appear as linear echogenic thickenings of the tunica and if associated with acoustic shadowing may be calcified. If there is evidence of Peyronie's Disease, the degree of curvature is estimated, and the plaque is evaluated (**Fig. 15–6**).

Percent Arterial Dilatation

An increase in penile arterial blood flow velocity after the intracavernous injection is accompanied by an increase in cavernous arterial diameter. Lue and associates have determined that a mean increase in diameter of the cavernous artery following injection should exceed 75%. Patients with arterial insufficiency will show minimal or no vasodilitation.

The accuracy of this particular criteria has been disputed by other investigators. Some have found poor correlation between the percentage of arterial vasodilation and arteriographic evidence of arterial insufficiency.[8] We do not use it.

New Techniques

Lencioni et al. used contrasted-enhanced power Doppler in addition to conventional CDDU. In normal volunteers, dynamic contrasted-enhanced power Doppler imaging enabled accurate demonstration of the arteriolar structures of the penis (helicine arteries). Following the intracavernosal injection of prostaglandin E_1, the diagnosis of arteriogenic erectile dysfunction in a group of patients was confirmed by low-peak systolic velocity in the cavernous arteries by standard CDDU. These patients were also studied with power Doppler following the intravenous injection of an ultrasound contrast agent (Levovist, Schering AG, Berlin, Germany). Among these patients, two different subgroups were identified by contrasted-enhanced power Doppler imaging: group A showed normal or almost normal helicine arteries and group B with marked reduction of these vessels. In group B, a significantly higher number of patients had a history of diabetes, smoking, and hypertension. They concluded that the identification of patients with relatively intact arteriolar structures might help select patients for revascularization procedures.[19]

Benefits of Ultrasound

In contrast to pudendal arteriography, duplex sonography is not invasive and can be performed in the office setting. Second, the high-resolution duplex ultrasound probe allows the sonographer to image the individual cavernous arteries selectively and perform Doppler blood flow analysis simultaneously within these vessels. Color Doppler imaging provides an additional advantage of easier assessment of direction of blood flow (**Fig. 15–5 F**) and collaterals among the cavernous and dorsal arteries, which are crucial in penile vascular and reconstructive surgeries.

High-resolution sonography is used to image the corpora cavernosa, corpus spongiosum, and the tunica albugenia. The cavernous body should have a homogeneous, uniform echogenicity. The finding of echogenic areas or calcification within the corporal bodies or the tunica albuginea may represent intrinsic sinusoidal disease, fibrosis, or Peyronie's disease.

Pulsed Doppler analysis of the cavernous arteries provides a quantifiable functional assessment of the penile arterial flow during pharmacologic erection. In this respect, duplex sonography is superior to arteriography, which relies on radiographic criteria and provides mainly anatomical rather than functional information. Arteriography is most useful as a detailed road map of the penile arterial system in patients who are candidates for penile revascularization. Duplex sonography, on the other hand, when properly employed provides the clinician with useful objective criteria with respect to blood flow velocity and arterial vasodilitation, both of which have been demonstrated to correlate with arterial health.

Pitfalls of Sonography

Although sonography has been shown to be perhaps the most versatile technique for evaluating vasculogenic erectile dysfunction, significant limitations have been pointed out. The fact that, like all radiographic testing, it is performed in a nonsexual setting with little privacy can increase the patients anxiety level and cause a sympathetic response that will inhibit the response to injection. This may then reduce both the peak systolic blood flow velocity and arterial vasodilitation and lead the clinician to discern an incorrect diagnosis of arteriogenic impotence. We recommend that manual stimulation in a private setting after intracavernous injection be part of the test or a repeat injection be given.

The results of the sonographic study may also be influenced by the temporal response to the intracavernous injection. Arterial flow decreases significantly during the full erection phase, and sonography performed during this time will yield a deceptively low peak velocity. On the other hand, other investigators have found a small but significant number of patients who will show a delayed and eventually normal arterial response to intracavernous injection. Some have suggested that a sonographic examination be extended for up to 30 min after injection to detect these late responders. However, it is unclear if the delayed arterial response represents a normal variant or more likely, a mild form of arteriogenic impotence.[8]

While a few studies have used normal volunteers in a standardized technique to establish a normal arterial response, most criteria regarding peak systolic velocity and vasodilitation have been established with patients with nonarteriogenic impotence. Lee et al. studied a group of potent volunteers to arrive at similar criteria for their subjects.[20]

Lastly, sonography is operator dependent. A thorough understanding of erectile physiology and anatomy is necessary to perform and interpret the examination properly. The experience of the clinician is critical to arriving at the correct diagnosis and avoiding pitfalls.

Summary

Patients with erectile dysfunction should consult with a physician who is knowledgeable about the subject. They should have a complete evaluation including a detailed medical and psychosexual history, physical examination, and hormonal and laboratory testing. This should be followed by a discussion of treatment options and further diagnostic tests, if needed.

Currently, there is great enthusiasm for oral agents in the management of erectile dysfunction. If indicated, a trial of an oral agent, like Sildenafil Citrate (Viagra, Pfizer, New York, NY), could be offered. Failure of an oral agent to produce the desired effect would be an indication to initiate a diagnostic evaluation including CDDU.

In the near future, we will have a variety of orally active agents to treat erectile dysfunction. As the choices for therapy increase or become more etiology specific, clinicians may look to testing, like color duplex Doppler ultrasound, to develop vascular profiles to help predict treatment success with one or a combination of several agents (e.g., oral, intraurethral, or intracorporal).

References

1. Consensus development conference statement: impotence. National Institutes of Health. *JAMA* 1993;270(1):83—90.
2. Broderick GA. Color duplex Doppler ultrasound: penile blood flow study. In Hellstrom WJG, ed. *Male Infertility and Sexual Dysfunction*, New York, NY: Springer-Verlag, 1997, p. 367—395.
3. Bortolotti A, Parazzini F, Colli E, et al. The epidemiology of erectile dysfunction and its risk factors. *Int J Androl* 1997 Dec;20(6):323—334.
4. Feldman HA, Goldstein I, Hatzichristou DG, Krane RJ, McKinlay JB. Impotence and its medical and psychosocial correlates: results of the Massachusetts male aging study. *J Urol* 1994;151:65—61.
5. Lue TF. Physiology of penile erection and pathophysiology of erectile dysfunction and priapism. In Walsh PC, Retik AB, Vaughan ED, Jr, Wein AJ, eds. *Campbell's Urology*,7th ed, vol. 2. Philadelphia, PA: Saunders, 1998, p. 1157—1179.
6. Godschalk MF, Sison A, Mulligan T. Management of erectile dysfunction by the geriatrician. *J Am Geriatr Soc* 1997 Oct;45(10):1240—1246.
7. Fabbri A, Aversa A, Isidori A. Erectile dysfunction: an overview. *Hum Reprod Update* 1997 Sep—Oct;3(5):455—466.
8. Lue TF, Broderick G: Evaluation and nonsurgical management of erectile dysfunction and priapism. In Walsh PC, Retik AB, Vaughan ED, Jr, Wein AJ, eds. *Campbell's Urology*, 7th ed, vol 2. Philadelphia, Pa: Saunders, 1998, p. 1181—1214.
9. Kaneko K, De Mouy EH, Lee BE. Sequential contrast-enhanced MR imaging of the penis. *Radiology* 1994;191:75—77.
10. Brindley GS. Cavernosal alpha-blockade: a new technique for investigating and treating erectile impotence. *Br J Psych* 1983;143:332—337.
11. Lue TF, Hricak H, Marich KW, Tanagho EA. Vasculogenic impotence evaluated by high resolution ultrasonography and pulsed Doppler spectrum analysis. *Radiology* 1985;155:777—781.

12. Zorgniotti AW, Lefleur RS. Auto-injection of the corpus cavernosum with a vasoactive drug combination for vasculogenic impotence. *J Urol* 1985;133(1):39—41.

13. Ishii N, Watanabe H, Irisawa C, et al. Intracavernous injection of prostaglandin E_1 for the treatment of erectile impotence. *J Urol* 1989;141(2):323—325.

14. Bennett AH, Carpenter AJ, Barada JH. An improved vasoactive drug combination for a pharmacological erection program. *J Urol* 1991;146(6):1564—1565.

15. Broderick GA, Arger PA. Penile blood flow study: age specific reference ranges. *J Urol* 1994;151(5):A371.

16. Broderick GA, Arger PA. Normal values for penile blood flow studies: distinguishing prepenile from intrapenile disease. *J Urol* 1997;157(4):A694.

17. Benson CB, Aruny JE, Vickers MA. Correlation of duplex sonography with arteriography in patients with erectile dysfunction. *AJR* 1993;160:71—73.

18. Naroda T, Yamanaka M, Matsushita K, et al. Evaluation of resistance index in the cavernous artery with color Doppler ultrasonography for venogenic impotence. *Intern J Impot Res* 1994;6(1):D62.

19. Lencioni RA, Paolicchi A, Sarteschi M, et al. Dynamic contrast-enhanced power Doppler imaging in the assessment of arteriogenic impotence. *Radiology* 1997 Nov;205(P) Supplement:335.

20. Lee B, Sikka SC, Randrup ER, et al. Standardization of penile blood flow parameters in normal men using intracavernous prostaglandin E_1 and visual sexual stimulation. *J Urol* 1993:149:49—52.

Female Pelvis

16 Asymptomatic Palpable Adnexal Masses

Peter H. Arger

Various disease processes can present as a clinical problem when a patient comes to a physician's office for a routine gynecologic examination and an asymptomatic palpable adnexal mass is felt. Among these various clinical processes are cystic masses secondary to the female hormonal cycle. This is the most common etiologic likelihood. The differential diagnosis will likely include endometriosis, dermoids, and ovarian tumors. Benign ovarian tumors, when present, are more common than a malignant process in this clinical situation. Exophytic fibroids may present as an asymptomatic palpable adnexal mass but uterine problems are discussed in another chapter in this book.

Important clinical parameters bear on the diagnostic workup of the mass. Included are the patients' age, the apparent size of the mass, and the feel of the mass. The examining physician may decide to evaluate the premenopausal patient with only a follow-up physical examination after one or two menstrual cycles. The clinical-only evaluation follow-up is frequently done in premenopausal patients when the mass is < 5—6 cm in size and has a cystic or soft feel. If on follow-up clinical evaluation, the mass has not disappeared or has increased in size, then an imaging study, usually a pelvic ultrasound with transvaginal evaluation, is done. A C-125 or other nonradiologic tests are usually deferred until the imaging characteristics of the mass are determined by an ultrasound imaging study.

Other imaging studies such as computed body tomography or magnetic resonance imaging are rarely done unless the ultrasound imaging characteristics and findings suggest the possibility of a malignancy or are problematic on ultrasound examination.

In the postmenopausal patient with an asymptomatic palpable adnexal mass, the examining physician is not likely to wait, and an ultrasound examination is generally obtained. When the examining physician decides that an imaging study is needed, the radiologist becomes a consultant and can give useful clinical guidance based on the imaging evaluation of the masses using their ultrasound characteristics.

A variety of authors have used the grey scale characteristics and spectral Doppler analysis of various ovarian masses to determine the sensitivity and specificity of ultrasound to characterize adnexal masses. Two more recent articles found a sensitivity of 0.89 for transvaginal ultrasound and a specificity of 0.84. Accuracy in this series was 85%.[1]

A second recent series stated that adding color Doppler with pulsed Doppler, added an improved specificity and positive predictive value over conventional grey scale imaging. Specificity increased from 82% to 97% (p < 0.001) and positive predictive value increased from 63% to 91%. Resistive indices and pulsatility indices were of limited value.[2] (See chapter by Dr. Andrew M. Fried for a more detailed discussion on this.)

The benefit of ultrasound lies in its ability to characterize the mass and give significant insight as to the probable nature of the mass. The characteristics of various etiologic aspects of the mass are described in the following sections of this chapter and relate to the differential diagnosis.

Simple Cysts

An asymptomatic cyst is the most common finding in this clinical situation. A cystic mass must have the same characteristics in the pelvis on pelvic ultrasound that cysts have elsewhere in the body. It must be anechoic, smoothly marginated, and unilocular. Good through sound transmission causing acoustic enhancement deep to the actual cystic mass in comparison to the adjacent soft-tissues must be seen (**Fig. 16–1**).

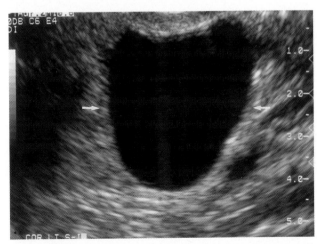

Figure 16–1 Simple ovarian cyst. Ovary evaluation shows smooth walled, anechoic mass (**white arrows**) with good sound transmission.

When a simple cyst is found on ultrasound, it can be followed with just clinical observation or a follow-up imaging study after one or two menstrual cycles. This depends upon the size of the cyst and the menstrual status of the woman. This approach is appropriate for pure cysts of 6 cm or less in premenopausal women and cysts of 5 cm or less in postmenopausal women.

Oral contraceptives may be used to help resolve the cyst but usually are not. Whether oral contraceptives really help cyst resolution is uncertain.[3] Oral contraceptives decrease follicle stimulating hormones, and some physicians feel that this can help.[4] Others have found no effect.[5]

Oral contraceptives are believed to help prevent the development of other functional ovarian cysts[3,4] during the follow-up analysis time. Advances in the development of oral contraceptives however, may now not prevent cyst formation depending upon the drug utilized. Regardless of treatment, most benign cysts will disappear on follow-up.[4,6] Benign simple cysts larger than 6 cm in a premenopausal woman or 5 cm in a postmenopausal woman is unusual. Normal follicular regression may be prevented by increased hormonal stimulation. Failure of involution of the follicles or the corpora lutea associated with changes in the menstrual cycle, can result in functional ovarian cysts. The likelihood of spontaneous regression decreases with increasing size of the cyst, therefore, though benign cysts may rarely become as large as 8—10 cm, their likelihood of disappearing decreases with the increasing size. These functional cysts are likely to be asymptomatic unless they become quite large or have an acute hemorrhage within them.

A cyst greater than 6 cm is more likely to be a benign ovarian neoplasm even in premenopausal women.

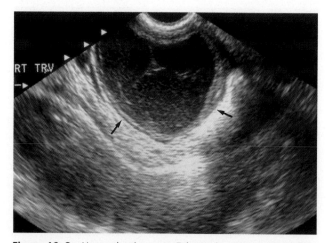

Figure 16–2 Hemorrhagic cyst. Echogenic mass with debris, thickened wall and thin septations (**black arrows**). Mass completely disappeared after 2 menstrual cycles.

Hemorrhagic Cysts

Bleeding in a cyst complicates the diagnosis. Variable characteristics can be seen in hemorrhagic cysts because of clot formation, lysis, and retraction. Because of this, the cyst may have the appearance of a solid component, mural nodularity, septations, focal wall thickening, or fluid debris levels. Thin, fibrous strands, clot retraction with convex borders, fluid levels and homogeneous low echoes throughout the mass with good sound transmission suggest the presence of hemorrhage in this cystic mass (**Fig. 16–2**).

Mild wall thickening may also be present. These cysts may appear similar to other adnexal masses including malignancies. In 90% of hemorrhagic cysts,[7-9] increase through transmission has been reported. Ruptured cysts may show some cul-de-sac fluid or even intraperitoneal fluid. Most hemorrhagic cysts will resolve spontaneously over time (**Fig. 16–3**) but surgical excision may be necessary. A changing complicated mass suggests a hemorrhagic cyst and indicates the need for further follow-up before deciding upon surgery. This is especially true when the mass size decreases over several cycles.

These hemorrhagic cysts may be complex and have the various ultrasonographic characteristics as described. Some of these give clues as to the etiology of the mass and help the radiologists advise the referring physician on the best course of action.

Theca Lutein Cyst

Theca lutein cysts are functional and are usually associated with some form of gestational trophoblastic disease. However they can result from ovarian hyperstimulation with drugs or hormones especially in infertility cases. These cysts are usually bilateral and multilocular. Their cause is not known but human chorionic gonadotropin (HCG) levels are high in these cases. Elevated pituitary follicular stimulating hormone (FSH) or increased HCG sensitivity may be involved. They can remain for weeks after removing the initial stimulus, and, therefore, the patient may be asymptomatic at the time of physical examination revealing the mass.

Polycystic Ovarian Disease

The ovaries may be of normal or increased size and may have large follicular cysts over 3 cm in polycystic ovarian disease. Polycystic ovarian disease is part of a complex clinical, laboratory and ultrasound picture. Obesity, infertility, and hirsutism may be present clinically.[10,11] As a result of this complex imbalance of the normal ovarian cycles, chronic anovulation may result. Most women with this disease have a high luteinizing

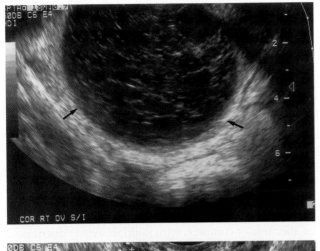

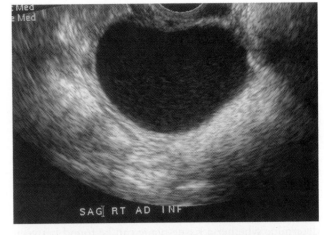

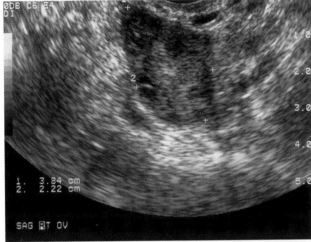

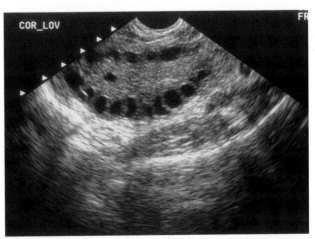

Figure 16–3 Hemorrhagic cyst evaluation. **A:** May — note very complex mass of right ovary with multiloculated areas, thin septations, echogenic areas, and echogenic debris (**black arrows**). **B:** June—mass characteristics have changed. Now have smooth walled mass with low-level echogenic debris. Marked change sig-

nals benign aspect of the mass. **C:** August — right ovary being measures[(12)] shows minimal to no residual of the mass. **D:** May — color-guided duplex Doppler shows tracing from wall of mass. PI = 0.50 and RI = 0.37 are in malignant range for a benign lesion.

hormone (LH) and a low or decreased FSH with a high LH/FSH ration and increased androgens.

On the ultrasound examination, there is a bilateral increased number of follicular cysts, usually as many as 10 in the periphery of large spherical ovaries (**Fig. 16–4**). The follicles are small, usually under 8 mm. Follicles ranging in size from 1.5—3 cm as mature follicles are rare but can be seen in up to 15% of the patients. Large follicular cysts over 3 cm may be seen and can be a presenting physical examination finding. Wedge biopsy is usually necessary to make the diagnosis.

Increased ovarian echogenicity was the most sensitive and specific sign of polycystic ovaries in an article by Pache et al.[12] in an recent evaluation. However this is a purely subjective evaluation. Because considerable overlap exists between normal and polycystic ovaries, the number of follicles and ovarian volume are not good criteria for this disease. A combination of follicular size and

Figure 16–4 Polycystic ovaries. Multiple small cysts in periphery of normal sized ovaries.

ovarian volume is the most sensitive objective parameter. The upper limit of normal ovarian volume is 15 cubic cm.[13]

Para Ovarian Cysts

Para ovarian cysts arise in the broad ligament as derivatives of mesothelial or perimesothelial structures. They mimic other ovarian masses being most often seen in middle-aged women. Though these cysts are frequently simple cysts, they may be complicated by bleeding, rupture, torsion, or infection. When the cyst does not regress over time, an attempt should be made to determine whether a tissue-plane can be found between the normal ovary and the adjacent mass (**Fig. 16–5**). This is the clue as to the etiology of these para ovarian masses. Follow-up or hormonal therapy does not cause regression of these masses. The usual treatment is surgical excision. Up to 10% of adnexal cystic masses are para ovarian in origin.[14, 15]

Tubal Ovarian Abscesses

An asymptomatic probable adnexal mass may result from a tubal ovarian abscess that did not completely resolve previously. The ultrasound appearance varies according to their appearance at the time of stabilization of the inflammatory process. The mass may be purely cystic, have multiple loculations, have thick septations, and contain complex debris (**Fig. 16–6**). A more serious diagnosis such as a benign or malignant neoplasm must be considered when these variable ultrasound characteristics are found in an asymptomatic patient. These are usually surgically removed because these masses do not change over time.

Endometriosis

Usually seen in women between the ages of 25 and 35, endometriosis is an inflammatory process. Usually, systemic systems are not present in these women but on closer evaluation they may have dysmenorrhea, dyspareunia, or infertility. Because the deposits are commonly small and widely disbursed, on ultrasound the pelvic examinations may appear normal. However, these patients may present with an asymptomatic palpable adnexal mass. Complex and primarily cystic masses due to larger deposits may occur after repeated bleeding episodes during menses. These focal blood collections may be anechoic or complex, with multiple evenly distributed echoes, clot nodules, or debris levels. There is usually good through sound transmission. The walls are usually thickened or irregular (**Fig. 16–7 A,B**). Septations are unusual. In more severe cases, multiple collections can be seen. Many of these cases come to surgery[16, 17] despite these characteristics which suggest endometriosis.

In problematic cases, magnetic resonance imaging evaluation can demonstrate the hemorrhagic characteristics of this entity.

Ovarian Neoplasms

Eighty percent of ovarian tumors are benign. Approximately 10—15% are malignant and 5% are due to ovarian metastases. Benign lesions are more common in women between the ages of 20 and 45 years and malignant lesions are more common in women between the ages of 40 and 65 years.[18-20]

Ovarian cancer is less common than either cervical or endometrial cancer comprising approximately 6% of all cancers in women. However ovarian cancer tends to be discovered late and 50% of deaths from cancer in the

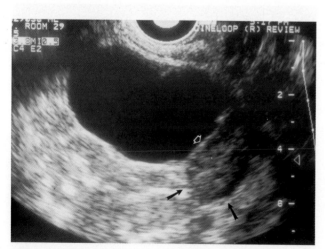

Figure 16–5 Paraovarian cyst. Simple cystic mass which did not change over 6 to 7 month follow-up. Endovaginal exam shows tissue plane (**open arrow**) separating mass from ovary (**closed arrows**).

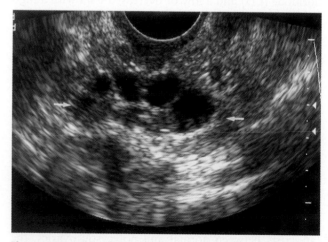

Figure 16–6 Old tuboovarian abscess (TOA). Post menopausal female with complex mass (**white arrows**). Concern was asymptomatic cystadenoma. At surgery, old TOA was found.

female genital tract result from ovarian malignancies. The surface epithelium, germ cells, and the stroma are the three different sites from which ovarian neoplasms originate. Most ovarian tumors are clinically similar though a minority may secrete a hormone such as estrogen. When they reach a large size, ovarian tumors usually produce symptoms. Most malignant tumors have spread at the time of initial diagnosis. Therefore, patients with ovarian cancer may be asymptomatic at the time of initial presentation. The surface epithelium is the primary source of ovarian neoplasms in 70—75% of patients. These neoplasms are serous, mucinous, and endometroid. They are usually discovered late as they grow very slowly. Eighty percent of serous and endometroid cancers can be detected by a CA125 analysis.

Serous fluid-containing tumors comprise about 30% of all ovarian tumors. These tumors occur usually in the age group from 20 to 50 years of age. Serous cyst adenomas are the most common benign tumors in this group. They are usually unilocular, sometimes have thin septations, and infrequently have papillary projections (**Fig. 16–8**). Serous cystadenocarcinomas usually have multiple loculations, multiple papillary projections, and septations (**Fig. 16–9**). Echogenic material may be present within the locules. Serous tumors are more likely to be bilateral than mucinous tumors (20% versus 5%). Ascites is more common in the malignant tumors. Twenty to twenty-five % of ovarian tumors are mucinous in origin. Most of these are unilateral. Mucinous-producing tumors are usually multiloculated masses with papillary excrescence's and contain echogenic material (**Fig. 16–10**). Fine gravity-dependent echoes on ultrasound examinations are due to the thick contents of this material. Metastasis or rupture of these tumors can cause pseudomyxoma peritonei.

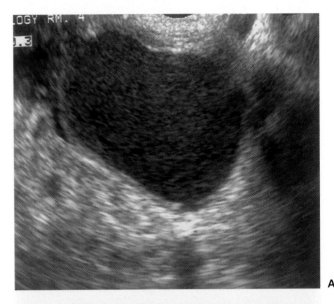

A

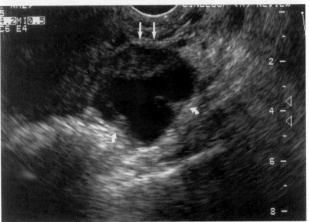

B

Figure 16–7 Endometriosis. **A:** Generalized low echogenic internal echoes throughout. Good sound transmission consistent with endometrioma. **B:** Complex mass with solid plaque-like area (**white arrows**), nodularity, and septation (**curved white arrows**). Shows variable appearance of endometrioma when compared to "usual" findings shown in an endometrioma found at surgery.

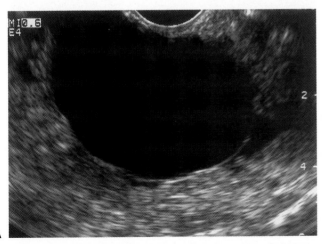

A

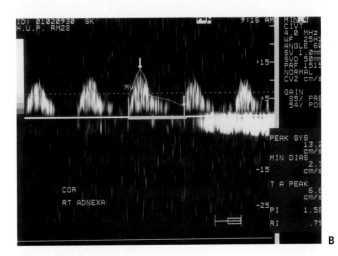

B

Figure 16–8 Benign serous cystadenoma. **A:** Benign appearance mimicking a simple cyst. Walls are minimally irregular and no loculations or nodules are seen. **B:** Color-guided duplex Doppler in wall of mass shows PI = 1.58 and RI = 0.79 in benign range.

Approximately 10—15% of ovarian tumors are germ cell tumors. Benign cystic teratomas comprise 95% of this etiology (**Fig. 16–11**). The other 5% are more likely to be malignant and include dysgerminomas, teratomas, endodermal sinus tumors, choriocarcinomas, embryonal cell carcinomas, and mixed germ cell tumors.

Dysgerminoma is the most common malignant germ cell tumor. These are usually solid tumors, unilateral and are comparable to seminomas in the male patients. These patients are candidates for surgery due to the solid aspect of these tumors.

"Dermoid cysts" are teratomas which are frequently cystic. They are bilateral in 10—15% of patients. Depending upon their composition, the ultrasound findings may vary. The mixture of sebum, fat, hair, and epithelial tissue produces an entire ultrasound spectrum. This spectrum ranges from purely cystic to fat fluid levels, hair fluid levels, echogenic mural nodules, thick septations, purely solid appearing densely echogenic masses, dense echoes with acoustic shadowing resulting from calcifications and mixed, solid, and cystic components (**Fig. 16–12**). One must be very careful to recognize the "tip of the iceberg" presentation when visualizing these lesions (**Fig. 16–13**). This is a curvilinear interface with acoustic shadowing mimicking a stool-filled rectosigmoid and may result from the presence of echogenic hair or calcium.[21–23]

Hormonally active tumors that originate from the gonadal mesenchyme are sex chord stromal tumors. These tumors are less likely to be asymptomatic. In this group are granulosa cell tumors, thecomas, fibromas, and Sertoli-Leydig cell tumors. On ultrasound scan, these tumors appear as solid echogenic tumor masses (**Fig. 16–14** through **16–15**).

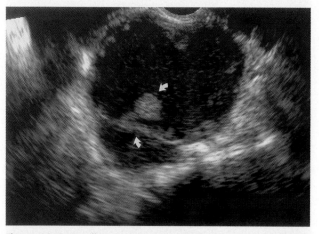

Figure 16–9 Papillary serous cystadenocarcinoma. Nodularity, thick septation (**curved white arrows**) and low echogenic debris.

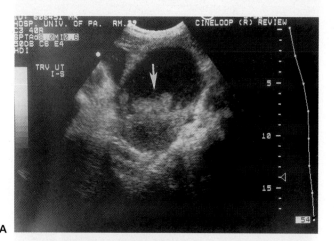

A

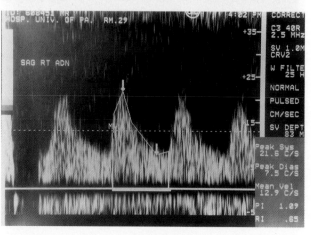

C

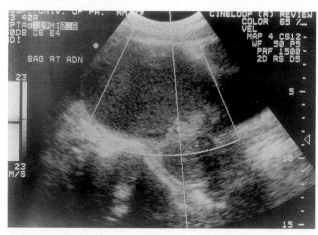

B

Figure 16–10 Mucinous cystadenocarcinoma. **A:** Mass shows solid component (**arrow**) and dependent debris. **B:** Doppler of vessel in solid component shows cursor location. **C:** Doppler of vessel in solid component of mass show PI = 1.09 and RI = 0.66 both well into the benign range. **This case illustrates the overlapping values of Doppler PI and RI between benign and malignant disease.**

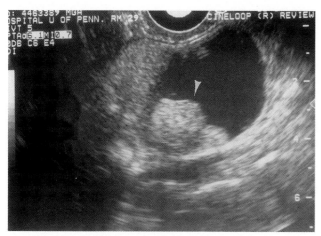

Figure 16–11 Cystic teratoma. Mass shows large cystic component with irregular solid wall mass (**arrow**).

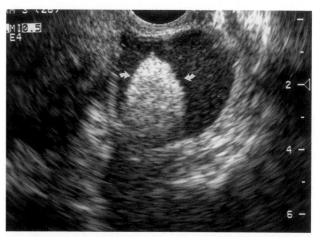

Figure 16–12 Dermoid. Complex characteristics of dermoid including echogenic area due to hair, etc (**curved white arrows**) and low-level echoes in fluid part.

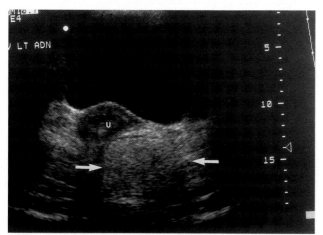

Figure 16–13 Dermoid. Echogenic rounded area mimicking bowel stool (**white arrows**) adjacent to uterus (u). This "tip of the iceberg" type appearance must not be thought to be due to bowel.

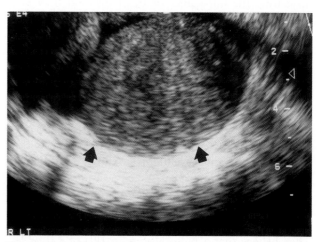

Figure 16–14 Fibroma. Echogenic mass in left ovary (**black arrows**). Surgery done because of strong family history of ovarian carcinoma. Fibroma found at surgery.

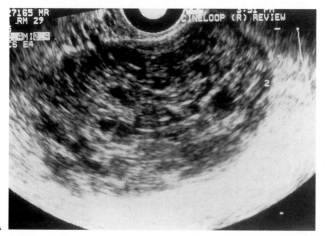

A

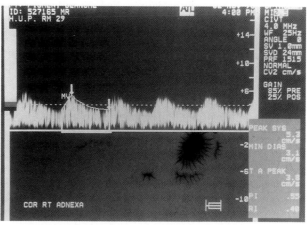

B

Figure 16–15 Granulosa cell tumor. **A:** Mass is primarily solid with small cystic areas. **B:** Doppler of internal vessels of solid mass shows PI = 0.55 and RI = 0.40 both in malignant range.

Doppler Ultrasound Evaluation of Ovarian Lesions

There is a wide variety of lesions that occur within the ovary which have overlapping imaging characteristics. Because of this, a method is needed for distinguishing between benign and malignant masses, if possible. The fact that malignant masses tend to elicit a vascular response has generated investigations into whether Doppler ultrasound imaging can distinguish between benign and malignant tumors to help avoid unnecessary surgery.

Abdominal ultrasound studies when combined with a pelvic examination and an elevated CA125 level can have a specificity for ovarian cancer of 99%.[9,20] Abdominal ultrasound alone has been reported as having a sensitivity of 80% for the detection of ovarian cancer.[24] In a series of articles by Bourne et al.[20,25,26] those authors indicate that transvaginal ultrasound can be improved by measuring the impedance of ovarian blood flow with color Doppler flow imaging. According to these authors, this measurement improves specificity. Other authors investigating the use of Doppler ultrasound imaging for this purpose have found mixed results.[27-29]

The neovascularity which ovarian cancers produce causes low impedance to blood flow. Flow within a mass seen by color Doppler flow imaging is more common in malignant tumors than in benign ones (93—35%).[30] Thus, pulse Doppler images of these tumors show flow velocity waveforms that differ from those of normal vessels. It has been stated that stage I ovarian cancers can show the same reduction and impedance. The same authors state that benign and malignant ovarian tumors showed different patterns of blood flow impedance.[24,27] They believe that a pulsatility index (PI) of 1.0 or less and a resistive index (RI) under 0.4 indicate the presence of malignant neovascularity. There is however overlap in the flow velocity waveforms of benign and malignant ovarian masses as shown by other authors[28,30] (**Fig. 16–3, 16–8**). Low-impedance flow is suggestive of malignancy, but benign abnormalities such as inflammatory masses, endometriomas, hemorrhagic corpus luteum cysts, and others may also show this pattern.

A relatively high-impedance flow pattern occasionally occurs in malignant tumors as well as benign lesions. Further flow studies need to be done to realize the promise as a noninvasive tool for characterizing adnexal masses by color Doppler ultrasound and power Doppler imaging. A large group of malignant lesions must be analyzed to determine the situations in which false-negative Doppler images would be present.

A large multiinstitutional study was done under the sponsorship of the Radiology Diagnostic Oncology Group to compare ultrasound, computed tomography, and magnetic resonance imaging in the evaluation of ovarian masses. Comparison of the ability to distinguish benign from malignant masses and the ability to stage malignant masses was done.

Two-hundred and eighty patients with 118 malignancies were included in the study. In separating non-advanced (benign and stage I and II cancers) from advanced malignancy, the data showed a specificity of 96% for ultrasound, 89% for computed tomography and 88% for magnetic resonance imaging. The sensitivity in this classification of lesions was 75% for ultrasound, 93% for computed tomography, and 98% for magnetic resonance imaging based on ROC analysis.[31]

Management Guidelines

For proper management of asymptomatic palpable adnexal masses, various guidelines need to be followed as described below. The minimal necessary clinical data includes age and hormonal status (i.e., premenopausal with or without birth control pills and postmenopausal).

Unilocular cysts are overwhelmingly benign both in the pre- and postmenopausal. Cysts of 6 cm or less in a premenopausal woman or 5 cm or less in a postmenopausal woman can be followed as described previously. Cystic lesions larger than these sizes are more likely to be benign tumors such as cyst adenomas. The finding of small mural nodules or solid plaque areas changes the whole evaluation. Careful transvaginal ultrasound imaging is most helpful in determining the presence of these nodules or areas. Even though benign solid masses such as fibromas do exist, the presence of a solid ovarian mass is uncommon and needs to be removed in a woman of any age.

Definite identification of bleeding occurs more frequently in benign masses than in malignant masses and it may be helpful in deciding to follow these patients. Hormonal suppression can be used to stop new cysts from forming though the more recently used hormones may not have this effect. Cysts may take up to 3 months to resolve over several menstrual cycles. Hormonal suppression is not usually used in patients who have cysts of less than 2.5—3 cm.

The findings which usually require surgery include masses with thick septations, irregular wall thickening, mural nodules and hyperechogenic areas or solid components. Although masses with these findings are frequently benign, surgery usually occurs.

In a recent morphological review,[32] the most consistent ultrasound characteristic of malignant ovarian tumors was abnormality of the wall structures, that is papillary projections or protruding solid wall components. No malignant tumor had a volume of less than 10 cubic cm. The authors note that what is needed is an understanding of the various types of masses to help guide the referring physician in the clinical management of asymptomatic palpable adnexal masses. The radiologist can use these characteristics and an understanding of the various types of masses to help guide the referring physician in this clinical management.

References

1. Yamashita Y, Torashima M, Hatanaka Y, Harada M, et al. Adnexal masses: accuracy of characterization with transvaginal US and pre contrast and post contrast MR imaging. *Radiology* 1995;194:557—565.

2. Buy JN, Ghossain MA, Hugal D, et al. Characterization of adnexal masses: combination of color Doppler and conventional sonography compared with spectral Doppler analysis alone and conventional sonography alone. *AJR* 1996;166:385—393.

3. Speroff L, Glass RH, Kase NG. Oral contraception. In: Speroff L, Glass RH, Kase NG, eds, *Clinical Gynecologic Endocrinology and Infertility, th ed., vol. 22.* Baltimore: Williams and Wilkins, 1994, p. 747.

4. DiSaia PJ: Ovarian neoplasms. In:, Scott JR, DiSaia PJ, Hammond CB, et al., eds, *Danforth's Obstetrics and Gynecology,* 7th ed., vol. 51. Philadelphia: JB Lippincott, 1994, p 973.

5. Turan C, Zorlu CG, Vgur M, et al. Expectant management of functional ovarian cycst: An alternative to hormonal therapy. *Internat J Gyn Obstet* 1994;47:257—260.

6. Filly RA. Ovarian masses...what to look for...what to do. In: Callen PW, ed. *Ultrasonography in Obstetrics and Gynecology,* 3rd ed., vol. 31. Philadelphia: WB Saunders, 1994, p. 625—639.

7. Baltarowich OH, et al. The spectrum of sonographic findings in hemorrhagic ovarian cysts. *Am J Roentgenol* 1987;148:901.

8. Reynolds T, Hill MC, Glassman LM. Sonography of hemorrhagic ovarian cysts. *JCU* 1986;14:449—453.

9. Deppe G, et al. Ovarian cancer: Advances in management. *Surg Clin N Amer* 1991;71:1023—1039.

10. Nicolini J, Ferrazzi E, Bellotti M, et al. The contribution of sonographic evaluation of ovarian size in patients with polycystic ovarian disease. *J Ultrasound Med* 1985;4:437—351.

11. Yeh HC, Futterweit W, Thornton JC. Polycystic ovarian disease: US features in 104 patients. *Radiology* 1987;163:111—116.

12. Pache TD, et al. How to discriminate between normal and polycystic ovaries: transvaginal study. *Radiology* 1992;183:421—423.

13. Cohen HL, Tire HM, Mandel FS. Ovarian volumes measured by US: bigger than we think. *Radiology* 1990;177:189—192.

14. Alpern MB, Sandler MA, Madrazo BL. Sonographic features of parovarian cysts and their complications. *AJR* 1984;143:157—160.

15. Athey PA, Cooper NB. Sonographic features of parovarian cysts. *AJR* 1985;144:83—86.

16. Athey PA, Diment DD. The spectrum of sonographic findings in endometriomas. *J Ultrasound Med* 1989;8:487—491.

17. Kupfer MC, Schwimmer SR, Lebovic J. Transvaginal sonographic appearance of endometriomas: spectrum of findings. *J Ultrasound Med* 1992;11:129—133.

18. Sutton CL, et al. Ovarian masses revisited: radiologic and pathologic correlation. *Radiographics* 1992;12:853—877.

19. Mendelson E, Bohm-Velez M. Transvaginal ultrasonography of pelvic neoplasms. *Rad Clin N Amer* 1992;30:703—704.

20. Bourne T, et al. Ovarian cancer screening. *Eur J Cancer* 1991;27:655—659.

21. Fried AM, Cosgrove DO. Uterus and ovaries. In: Goldberg BB, ed. *Textbook of Abdominal Ultrasound.* Baltimore, MD: Williams and Wilkins 1993, p. 452—479.

22. Sheth S, Fishman EK, Buck JL, et al. The variable sonographic appearances of ovarian teratomas: correlation with CT. *AJR* 1988;151:331—334.

23. Gutman PH, Jr. In search of the elusive benign cystic ovarian teratoma: application of the ultrasound "tip of the iceberg" sign. *JCU* 1977;5:403—406.

24. Kurjak A, et al. Evaluation of adnexal masses with transvaginal color Doppler ultrasound. *J Ultrasound Med* 1991;10:295—297.

25. Bourne T, et al. Transvaginal color Doppler in gynecology. *Ultrasound Obstet Gynecol* 1991;1:359—373.

26. Bourne T, et al. Transvaginal color flow imaging: A possible new screening technique for ovarian cancer. *BMJ* 1989;299:1367—1370.

27. Kawai M, et al. Transvaginal Doppler ultrasound with color flow imaging in the diagnosis of ovarian cancer. *Obstet/Gynecol* 1992;79:163—167.

28. Hamper UM, et al. Transvaginal color Doppler sonography of adnexal masses: differences in blood flow impedance in benign and malignant lesions. *AJR* 1993;160:1225—1228.

29. Fleischer AC, et al. Assessment of ovarian tumor vascularity with transvaginal color Doppler sonography. *J Ultrasound Med* 1991;10:563—568.

30. Fried AM, Kenney III CM, Stigers KB, et al. Benign pelvic masses: sonographic spectrum. *Radiographics* 1996;16:321—334.

31. Kurtz AB, Tsimikas JV, Tempany CM, et al. The comparative values of Doppler/US, CT and MR in ovarian cancer diagnosis and staging: correlation with surgery and pathology. A report of the Radiology Diagnostic Oncology Group. In press.

32. DePriest PD, Shenson D, Fried AM, et al. A morphology index based on sonographic findings in ovarian cancer. *Gynecol Oncol* 1993;51:7—11.

17 Acute Pelvic Pain

John S. Pellerito

Acute pelvic pain is a common problem seen in everyday practice. There are multiple possible causes of acute pelvic pain and a quick, cost-effective evaluation is desirable for timely diagnosis. Because ultrasound can distinguish between many of the diagnostic possibilities noninvasively, it is the preferred initial imaging modality performed to evaluate this condition. This chapter addresses the role of ultrasound in the clinical evaluation of acute pelvic pain. The value of other diagnostic modalities will also be discussed.

Differential Diagnosis

Causes of acute pelvic pain can be divided into gynecologic and nongynecologic etiologies. Gynecologic causes of pelvic pain include ovarian cysts, pelvic inflammatory disease, ectopic pregnancy, and ovarian torsion. Less commonly, benign or malignant adnexal masses such as fibroids or ovarian cancer, and endometriosis may produce acute pelvic pain. Nongynecologic causes of pelvic pain include appendicitis, urinary calculi, mesenteric adenitis, inflammatory bowel disease, bowel obstruction, metastatic disease, or diverticulitis.

Diagnostic Workup

The evaluation of the patient with acute pelvic pain begins with the clinical history and physical examination. The value of any imaging technique is enhanced by the addition of clinical information. Because multiple disease processes may present with a similar clinical syndrome, the differential diagnosis is constructed from data obtained from the clinical history including the age of the patient and menopausal status. The duration and recurrence of the problem as well as current medications are important considerations. Significant historical information concerning prior urinary or gynecologic problems also guide the diagnostic evaluation. For example, a prior history of ectopic pregnancy will focus the workup to exclude recurrence of the disease.

This diagnostic evaluation is also supported by the physical examination. The location of pain as well as signs of pelvic mass limit the differential diagnoses. Signs of infection including fever and rebound tenderness suggest inflammatory etiologies such as appendicitis or tuboovarian abscess. Sudden decrease in blood pressure or change in mental status portend more serious conditions prompting immediate diagnostic or surgical examinations.

The differential diagnosis is also informed by laboratory information. Hematologic and blood chemistry studies are obviously important tools to determine the origin of pain. An elevated white blood cell count and sedimentation rate support an infectious or inflammatory etiology for pain. Abnormal renal or liver function tests may suggest a specific cause for pain or point to a generalized process such as diffuse metastatic disease. Urine or serum pregnancy tests are essential in premenopausal patients, whereas serum tumor markers may be helpful in postmenopausal women.

Ultrasound Imaging

Ultrasound is the primary imaging modality utilized to distinguish between the different causes of acute pelvic pain. It is a noninvasive examination with no known adverse effects. Other advantages of ultrasound include ready availability, low cost, and high sensitivity for many disease processes.

Endovaginal sonography (EVS) has proven highly accurate for the diagnosis of many gynecologic conditions. EVS offers improved visualization of the pelvic structures compared to the transabdominal approach. EVS demonstrates adnexal masses, collections, free fluid, hydroureter, and other important clues to diagnosis.

Duplex and color flow Doppler techniques demonstrate physiologic as well as anatomic information and may provide important diagnostic clues. Detection of tissue vascularity and characterization of specific flow patterns improve diagnostic accuracy and provide specific diagnoses not possible with gray scale imaging alone.

Ovarian Cysts

The most common gynecologic cause of acute pelvic pain is the growth of ovarian cysts. The occurrence of pain is closely associated with follicular rupture during the midportion of the menstrual cycle.[1] Mittelschmerz or "middle pain" was initially thought to be due to peritoneal irritation from release of blood and follicular contents during ovulation. This coincides with FSH/LH surge during days 14—16 of the menstrual cycle. Sonographic monitoring of midcycle ovaries has shown that the symptoms precede follicular rupture in 97% of cases.[2,3] The pain is usually noted on the side of the dominant follicle and is probably related to follicular enlargement.

Characteristic sonographic findings are associated with the periovulatory period. Prior to ovulation, the mature follicle demonstrates a mean diameter of 20—24 mm.[4,5] The cyst will demonstrate an echogenic rim (**Fig. 17–1**). Irregularity of the inner lining of the cyst may be seen when ovulation is imminent.[1] A small echogenic focus or rim may be seen along the wall of the mature follicle. This represents the cumulus oophorus and confirms that the follicle contains the oocyte. Ovulation usually occurs within 36 h of visualization of the cumulus oophorus.

Following ovulation, there is usually a decrease in size of the follicular cyst. Fluid is commonly seen in the cul-de-sac and surrounding adnexae. This is thought to be due to exudation from the ovary and has been measured to be about 15—25 mL at laparoscopy.[6]

Color and pulsed Doppler examination of the mature follicle demonstrates a rim of increased vascularity surrounding the cyst (**Fig. 17–2**). This is best visualized during endovaginal color flow imaging and is helpful in the identification of the corpus luteum.[7] The ring of vascularity ("ring of fire") is initially seen during day 8 of the menstrual cycle and continues through day 24. Peripheral vascularization of the corpus luteum may persist through the first trimester.

Color Doppler aids in the identification of the hemorrhagic corpus luteum. The cystic component may not be visualized due to hemorrhage within the cyst which appears isoechoic to the adjacent ovarian parenchyma.

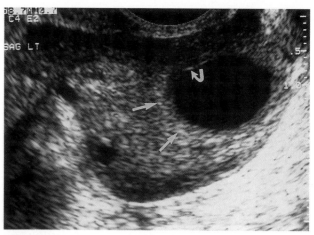

Figure 17–1 Ovarian cyst. A well-circumscribed cyst is identified within the ovary. Note the thickened rim (**arrows**) surrounding the cyst and the echogenic focus (**curved arrow**) consistent with the cumulus oophorus.

Increased vascularity is identified around the periphery of the isoechoic ovarian mass (**Fig. 17–3**).

Pulsed Doppler sampling of the corpus luteum reveals higher-velocity, low-impedance flow from the vascular ring.[8] Dillon et al. demonstrated a peak systolic velocity of 27 +/– 10 cm/s and RI = 0.44 +/– 0.09 for corpus luteal flow.[9] This low-impedance flow pattern should not be confused with low-resistance flow associated with ovarian cancer. The pain associated with formation of the dominant follicle and ovulation is self-limited, not requiring treatment in most cases.

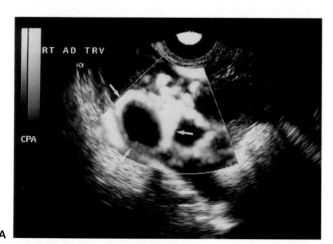

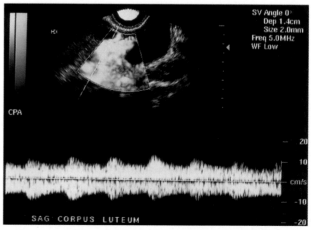

Figure 17–2 Corpus luteum. **A:** Color power angiography demonstrates typical "ring of fire" pattern (**arrows**) around the corpus luteum. **B:** Pulsed Doppler reveals low impedance flow during sampling of the corpus luteum.

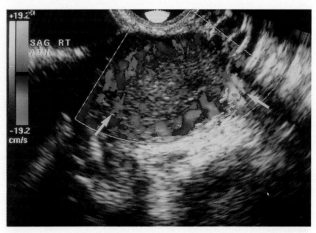

Figure 17–3 Hemorrhagic luteal cyst. A ring of vascularity (**arrows**) surrounds the hemorraghic corpus luteum which is isoechoic to the ovarian parenchyma.

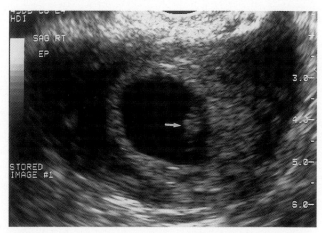

Figure 17–4 Ectopic embryo. An embryo (**arrow**) is identified within the ectopic gestational sac. Cardiac activity was noted.

Ectopic Pregnancy

Ectopic pregnancy is one of the most common indications for pelvic sonography in patients with acute pelvic pain. Ectopic pregnancy represents approximately 1.4% of all reported pregnancies with 75,000 cases occurring in the United States each year.[10] The risk of maternal death from ectopic pregnancy is ten times greater compared to that from natural childbirth.

Important risk factors include pelvic inflammatory disease, endometriosis, prior tubal surgery and prior ectopic pregnancy. This is probably related to mechanical obstruction of the Fallopian tube. Other risk factors include in vitro fertilization and embryo transfer as well as ovulation induction with gonadotropins.

Less than 50% of patients present with the classic clinical presentation of adnexal pain, pelvic mass, and vaginal bleeding.[11, 12] Patients typically present with one or more of these nonspecific signs or symptoms. The menstrual history and pregnancy test are essential in the evaluation for ectopic pregnancy. A positive pregnancy test increases the suspicion for ectopic pregnancy. The differential diagnosis includes threatened abortion and gestational trophoblastic neoplasia.

Prompt sonographic examination is indicated to diagnose ectopic pregnancy as delayed diagnosis may result in life-threatening hemorrhage from tubal rupture. Endovaginal sonography is the preferred initial examination because it can diagnose intrauterine and ectopic pregnancy earlier than the transabdominal approach.[13–15] Culdocentesis is no longer considered a first-line diagnostic examination as a negative test does not exclude ectopic pregnancy. Uterine curettage and laparoscopy are useful but should be delayed pending the sonographic results.

The definitive diagnosis of ectopic pregnancy is made based on the observation of an extrauterine embryo or fetal cardiac pulsations (**Fig. 17–4**). If these findings are not identified, then a thorough evaluation of the uterus, adnexae, and cul-de-sac is performed to look for other evidence of pregnancy.

The uterus is evaluated first for evidence of an intrauterine pregnancy. If an intrauterine pregnancy is identified, then the likelihood of a concomitant or heterotopic ectopic pregnancy is low, occurring in one of 30,000 spontaneous pregnancies. The frequency of heterotopic pregnancy increases if the patient underwent ovulation induction with clomid or pergonal. If the uterus fails to demonstrate evidence of pregnancy, the adnexae are carefully surveyed for signs of ectopic pregnancy. Other possibilities include a complete abortion or very early intrauterine pregnancy (less than 5 weeks gestational age). Careful correlation with menstrual data and serum HCG titers is helpful in distinguishing these entities. A subnormal rise or plateau of the serum HCG titers suggests a diagnosis of ectopic pregnancy.

An abnormal sac in the endometrial canal may represent an abnormal intrauterine pregnancy such as an incomplete abortion or a pseudogestational sac associated with an ectopic pregnancy. Duplex and color Doppler can distinguish these entities by demonstrating placental flow.[16] Endovaginal color flow imaging demonstrates placental flow as an area of increased vascularity around the periphery of the true gestational sac. Taylor et al. described placental flow as a relatively high-velocity, low-impedance signal localized to the site of placentation during pulsed Doppler sampling.[17] He theorized that placental flow is related to the invasion of maternal tissues by trophoblastic villi. As the developing placenta invades the myometrium, maternal spiral arteries shunt blood into the intervillous space across a pressure gradient of approximately 60 mm Hg. This results in the low-resistance flow pattern observed during color and pulsed Doppler imaging.

Dillon et al. showed that placental flow is noted in an intrauterine pregnancy approximately 36 days after the last menstrual period.[16] A velocity cut-off value of 21 cm/s was found to distinguish an intrauterine pregnancy from a pseudogestational sac. Pulsed Doppler sampling is performed with 0 degrees angle correction with manual manipulation of the transducer to obtain maximal Doppler velocity shifts.

The pseudogestational sac appears as an irregular sac-like structure or thickening of the endometrial canal. This is related to a decidual reaction from an associated ectopic pregnancy. Unlike a normal gestational sac, the pseudogestational sac does not exhibit a double decidual lining, yolk sac, fetal pole, or placental flow.

The most common sonographic appearance for ectopic pregnancy is an extrauterine sac (**Fig. 17–5**). The

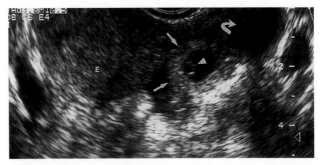

Figure 17–5 Ectopic gestational sac. An extrauterine gestational sac (**straight arrows**) with a yolk sac (**arrowhead**) is identified. Also note endometrial thickening (E) and left corpus luteal cyst (**curved arrow**).

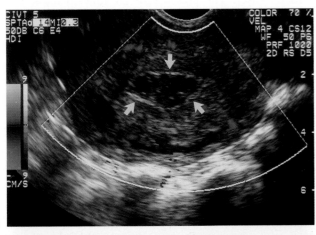

A

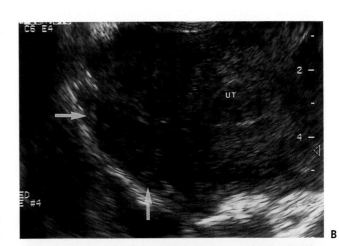

B

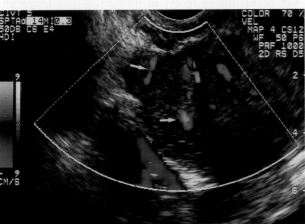

C

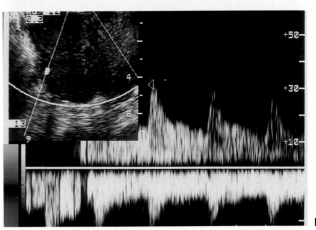

D

Figure 17–6 Solid ectopic with placental flow. **A:** A pseudogestational sac (**arrows**) is seen in the uterus. Color flow imaging demonstrates no flow within the pseudogestational sac. **B:** An ill-defined mass (**arrows**) is seen adjacent to the uterus (UT). The findings suggest small bowel, hematoma, or ectopic pregnancy. **C:** Color flow imaging reveals flow (**arrows**) within the mass confirming the location of the ectopic pregnancy. **D:** Spectral analysis demonstrates low-impedance flow consistent with placental flow.

sac usually demonstrates a thick echogenic ring and may contain a yolk sac or fetal pole. The mass should be separate from the ovary to avoid confusion with a corpus luteum cyst. If the mass is not separate from the ovary, then follow-up endovaginal scans and serum HCG titers may be necessary for diagnosis.

Solid and complex adnexal masses may also represent an ectopic pregnancy in conjunction with an empty uterus and positive serum HCG titer. Placental flow may be demonstrated within these complex masses during endovaginal color flow imaging[7] (**Fig. 17–6**). These masses usually represent hemorrhage into the ectopic gestational sac or a ruptured ectopic pregnancy in the fallopian tube. They may also present as free intraperitoneal hematomas.

In a recent study, placental flow was found in 55 (85%) of 65 ectopic pregnancies.[7] There was a sensitivity of 95% and specificity of 85% for the diagnosis of ectopic pregnancy with endovaginal color flow imaging. Detection of placental flow in an adnexal mass separate from the ovary is diagnostic of ectopic pregnancy. A velocity cutoff value is not required for the detection of placental flow in the adnexae.

Treatment of ectopic pregnancy is primarily surgical excision, preferably under laparoscopic guidance. Salpingectomy or salpingostomy are the most commonly performed procedures. Nonsurgical treatment utilizing methotrexate has been found to be efficacious in several series.[18, 19] The risk of recurrent ectopic pregnancy is increased following tubal surgery, and close surveillance is recommended in subsequent pregnancies.

Ovarian Torsion

Ovarian torsion accounts for approximately 3% of gynecologic emergencies. Torsion usually occurs in premenopausal patients and is often associated with an ovarian mass. The mass serves as the focal point for the torsion which involves both the ovary and fallopian tube. Twenty percent of patients are pregnant at the time of diagnosis. Torsion can also occur in postmenopausal patients and may be associated with an ovarian neoplasm. Torsion of normal adnexa is uncommon.

Patients with ovarian torsion present with acute, severe onset of unilateral pelvic pain. The right ovary is more commonly involved than the left.[20] Pain may be accompanied with nausea and vomiting which mimics other conditions including appendicitis or small bowel obstruction. Recurrent, intermittent bouts of pain may precede the current episode by days to weeks.

Sonography is the primary noninvasive examination for the diagnosis of ovarian torsion. Sonographic findings in ovarian torsion are variable. Most patients with torsion present with an enlarged ovary or mass. The sonographic appearance of the mass can vary from cystic to complex to completely solid.[20] The torsed ovary may contain hypoechoic areas representing hemorrhage

or infarction. Venous and lymphatic obstruction produce edema and free intraperitoneal fluid. With partial torsion, the ovary can attain massive size due to edema from lymphatic obstruction. In pediatric patients, two sonographic patterns have emerged. In prepubertal girls, torsion tends to occur in enlarged, complex cystic masses whereas pubertal girls torse predominantly solid, enlarged adnexal masses.[21]

The diagnosis of ovarian torsion is confirmed by the failure to detect arterial or venous flow from within ovarian parenchyma with color and pulsed Doppler (**Fig. 17–7**). The absence of flow within the torsed ovary during color flow, power, and pulsed Doppler is diagnostic. All color flow parameters must be optimized to ensure that the absence of flow is not related to technical factors such as high PRF, high wall filter or low color gain settings. Arterial flow may be seen only around the periphery of the ovary with chronic torsion due to reactive inflammation. Decreased vascularity may be seen within the ovary with partial torsion. Several authors have described the presence of venous and arterial signals within surgically proven torsed ovaries.[21—23]Thus, it is necessary to incorporate clinical and sonographic information to consider the diagnosis of ovarian torsion in difficult cases. The presence of an adnexal mass in a patient presenting with acute or recurrent pelvic pain should suggest the diagnosis of ovarian torsion.

Diagnostic laparoscopy is usually performed for ovarian torsion following sonographic evaluation. If the ovary appears viable, it is detorsed with removal of ovarian mass, if present. The ovary may be secured to prevent recurrent torsion. The ovary is removed if found to be nonviable or gangrenous.

Pelvic Inflammatory Disease

Most cases of pelvic inflammatory disease (PID) are due to an ascending infection from the cervix to the endometrium. Continued spread to the fallopian tubes may occur due to reflux of menstrual blood with the eventual spill of exudate into the peritoneal cavity. Signs of a lower genital tract infection usually precede symptoms of PID. Most patients are premenopausal with a typical history of multiple sexual partners and gonococcal or chlamydial infection.

Tuboovarian abscess (TOA) represents a severe complication of PID, occurring in approximately 15% of cases. This results from exudation of pus and microorganisms from the tube to the adjacent ovary or surrounding pelvic structures. This leads to tissue destruction and the formation of loculations or abscess cavities affecting the tube, ovary, uterus, and bowel.

The most frequent symptom is bilateral lower abdominal or pelvic pain or tenderness. There may be associated nausea, vomiting, and fever which reflect peritoneal inflammation. Physical examination may demonstrate cervical motion tenderness, palpable, tender

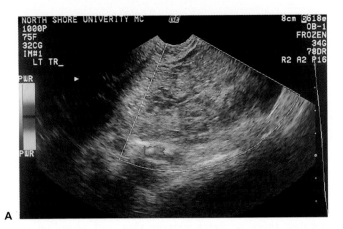

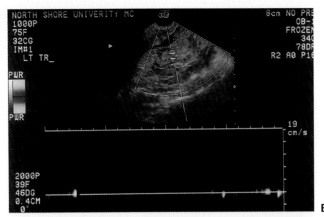

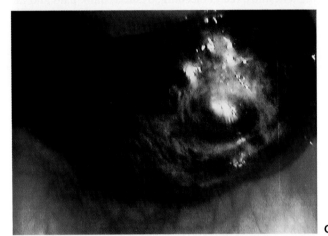

Figure 17–7 Ovarian torsion. **A:** An enlarged solid adnexal mass is seen. No flow is identified within the mass during power Doppler imaging. **B:** Pulsed Doppler evaluation fails to demonstrate arterial or venous flow within the mass suspicious for ovarian torsion. **C:** An enlarged gangrenous ovary is identified at laparoscopy.

adnexae, and leukorrhea. Laboratory data consistent with PID include leukocytosis, elevated erythrocyte sedimentation rate, and positive cultures for Neisseria gonorrhoeae or Chlamydia trachomatis.

Ultrasound is not reliable to detect subtle signs of salpingitis but can identify other signs of inflammation including endometritis, pyosalpinx, tuboovarian abscess, and pelvic collections. Sonographic signs of endometritis include fluid or gas within the endometrial cavity. Fluid or debris within the fallopian tube is suspicious for pyosalpinx. The tube typically tapers as it enters the uterus and distends distally. Tuboovarian abscess appears as a cystic mass which may demonstrate fluid levels or echogenic debris within the collection (**Fig. 17–8**). Occasionally, they may have a complex appearance with solid regions, nodularity, and septations. The ovary may not be identified separate from the mass.

Endometrial biopsy and laparoscopy are useful for confirming the diagnosis and obtaining cultures of the upper genital tract. These studies are particularly useful for patients failing antibiotic therapy due to severe disease or incorrect diagnosis.

Treatment for PID requires antibiotic therapy. Severe PID and TOA require hospitalization and intravenous administration of broad-spectrum antibiotics. Surgical

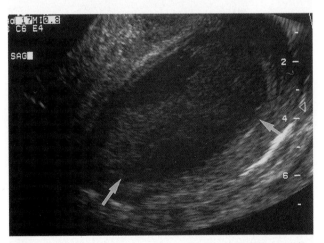

Figure 17–8 Tuboovarian abscess. A large complex mass (**arrows**) is filled with echogenic debris. The ovary was not identified separate from the mass.

exploration is considered for patients who do not respond to medical therapy within 72 to 96 h. Surgical drainage or TAH-BSO may be performed for impending abscess rupture or overwhelming sepsis. US or CT-guided abscess drainage has proven valuable in selected cases.

Endometriosis

Endometriosis results from ectopic location of endometrial tissue outside the uterus within the peritoneal cavity and on the surfaces of pelvic organs and ligaments. Endometriosis less commonly presents with acute pelvic pain. The pain is described as aching and constant, beginning 2—7 days before the onset of menses and increasing in severity during menstruation. The patient may give a history of similar prior episodes of dysmenorrhea. Patients may also complain of infertility, dyspareunia, back pain, and uterine bleeding. Symptoms may relate to endometriosis at multiple sites causing tenesmus, rectal bleeding, dysuria, flank pain and urgency. Physical findings are variable and may include tenderness, nodularity, parametrial thickening, and adnexal masses.

Endometriosis is difficult to detect sonographically when the implants are small (< 5 mm). These implants

may bleed and produce cystic or complex masses which can be seen with ultrasound. These represent endometriomas and may contain low-level internal echoes consistent with hemorrhage (**Fig. 17–9**). The masses may contain nodules or septations that may simulate ovarian neoplasms. They may wax and wane in size and vascularity from cycle to cycle. These periodic changes are seen when comparing serial examinations and are diagnostic for this disease. Magnetic resonance imaging (MRI) confirms the presence of blood products within these adnexal masses and may find smaller implants in locations difficult to assess with ultrasound. Laparoscopy is considered the gold standard for this diagnosis because there is direct visualization and sampling of small implants.

The choice of treatment depends on the severity of symptoms and the extent of disease. Implants may be cauterized and adhesions lysed at laparoscopy. Hormonal suppression is reserved for invasive disease or cases resistant to laparoscopic treatment. Hysterectomy and oophorectomy are also an option for severe cases.

Adnexal tumors

Adnexal tumors are another uncommon cause of acute pelvic pain. Pain usually results from infection, torsion, or hemorrhage into the pelvic mass. Both benign and malignant ovarian tumors may torse. Acute pain and adnexal swelling with a decrease in the hematocrit are consistent with hemorrhage into a pelvic mass. Similarly, an elevated white blood cell count, fever, and pelvic tenderness associated with an adnexal mass suggest superimposed infection.

Uterine fibroids can also undergo torsion, infection, or hemorrhage. MRI is helpful for identification of an adnexal mass as a fibroid. It is necessary to identify the uterine pedicle attachment of a pedunculated fibroid to distinguish a torsed fibroid from other adnexal mass.

Appendicitis

Appendicitis is one of the most common causes of acute abdominal/pelvic pain and is the most common indication for emergency laparotomy. Patients present with right lower-quadrant pain which may be accompanied by fever, leukocytosis, and tenderness. Unfortunately, the clinical features are not specific. Thirty percent of patients will have an atypical presentation resulting in a high (20—46%) negative appendectomy rate.[24, 25] The differential diagnosis includes all the gynecologic problems discussed earlier as well as urolithiasis, diverticulitis, bowel obstruction, and other inflammatory conditions. A pregnancy test and endovaginal sonography are helpful to exclude other conditions.

Because appendicitis can mimic other clinical entities, the diagnostic evaluation should include the abdomen and pelvis. Radiography, ultrasound, and com-

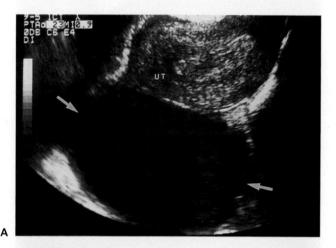

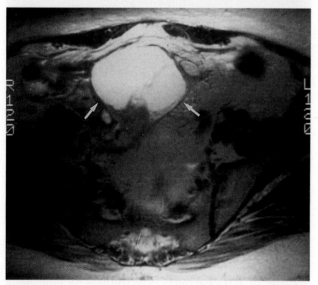

Figure 17–9 Endometrioma. **A:** A complex cystic mass (**arrows**) is noted adjacent to the uterus (UT). **B:** MRI image demonstrates increased signal within the mass (**arrows**) consistent with hemorrhage.

puted tomography (CT) are useful in the imaging workup. Plain-film radiographs may demonstrate right lower-quadrant calcification consistent with an appendicolith or findings suggestive of another process such as obstruction, ileus, or ureteral calculus.

Sonography is effective in the diagnosis of acute appendicitis with sensitivity of 80—89% and accuracy of 90—95%.[26—28] A graded compression technique is performed to demonstrate a distended, noncompressible appendix. A high-frequency (5—7 MHz) linear array transducer is used to gradually compress and disperse overlying bowel loops over the site of maximum tenderness. The inflamed appendix will appear as a noncompressible, apersistaltic blind loop on sagittal and transverse views (**Fig. 17–10**). The inflamed appendix demonstrates a "target" appearance on the transverse view with a diameter greater than 6 mm. An appendicolith is occasionally seen within the appendix. Sonography will also detect loculated periappendiceal fluid consistent with perforation and abscess formation. Gas can be seen within the appendix or adjacent abscess. Loss of the echogenic submucosal ring is associated with advanced infection and perforation.

CT is recommended for patients with suspected appendiceal perforation on clinical or sonographic grounds. CT can better define the extent of inflammation compared to ultrasound and help guide percutaneous drainage procedures. Similarly, CT can better define abscesses or collections related to diverticulitis or Crohn's disease. CT should also be performed in patients with persistent symptoms without a diagnosis.

Ureteral calculus

Patients with urinary obstruction related to ureteral calculus may also present with acute lower quadrant or pelvic pain. The pain is unilateral and may radiate to the back, flank, or pelvis. There may be associated hematuria, fever, and leukocytosis.

When the clinical presentation is nonspecific, the diagnostic evaluation should include the abdominal and pelvic organs. A KUB may demonstrate renal or ureteral calculi. Like appendicitis, sonography is employed to distinguish between gynecologic and nongynecologic processes. Although ultrasound may demonstrate dilatation of the renal collecting system, there may be minimal or no hydronephrosis with early obstruction.[29] Ultrasound is less sensitive than intravenous urography for the diagnosis of acute renal obstruction. Sonography and KUB may replace intravenous urography in patients with renal insufficiency or contrast allergy.[30] Unenhanced helical CT has proven accurate and reliable for the detection of ureteral calculi in patients with flank pain. A recent study demonstrated a 98% sensitivity and 100% specificity for the detection of ureteral calculi with noncontrast-enhanced spiral CT in patients referred with acute flank pain.[31]

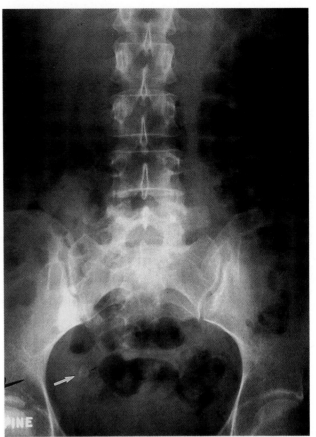

A

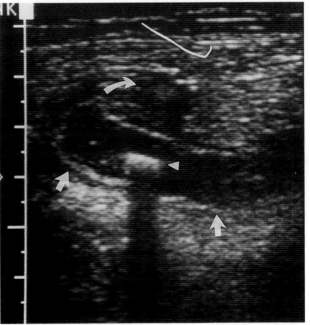

B

Figure 17–10 Appendicitis. **A:** Abdominal radiograph demonstrates focal calcification (**arrow**) in the right lower quadrant consistent with an appendicolith. **B:** A noncompressible, distended loop (**arrows**) is identified at the site of maximal tenderness. Note periappendiceal fluid (**curved arrow**) and fecalith (**arrowhead**).

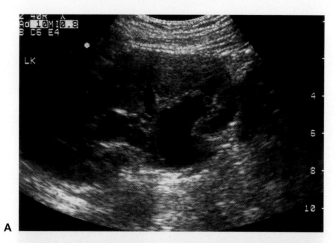

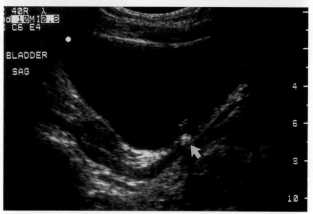

Figure 17–11 Ureteral calculus. **A:** There is moderate left hydronephrosis. No obstructing calculus is seen. **B:** Transvesical examination of the pelvis reveals a calculus (**arrow**) at the ureterovesical junction.

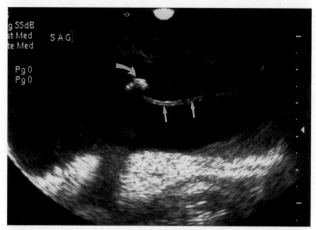

Figure 17–12 Ureteral calculus. Endovaginal sonogram reveals a calculus (**curved arrow**) in the distal ureter (**straight arrows**).

When renal colic is suspected, a search for the level of obstruction should be performed. Careful sonographic examination of the pelvis, including the region of the ureterovesical junction (UVJ) may reveal the obstructing calculus (**Fig. 17–11**). Endovaginal sonography may be helpful in identification of the distal ureteral stone. The transducer is directed toward the posteroinferior aspect of the bladder at the level of the UVJ. A dilated distal ureter can be followed to the level of obstruction. An obstructing calculus appears as an echogenic structure with acoustic shadowing (**Fig. 17–12**). In patients without obstruction, a ureteral jet can be identified at the UVJ with color flow imaging.

Summary

Acute pelvic pain is a common clinical problem with many possible etiologies. The clinical history, physical examination, and laboratory data are necessary to formulate the differential diagnosis. Ultrasound is the preferred first-line noninvasive imaging examination due to ready availability, low cost, and high diagnostic accuracy. Ultrasound can distinguish between gynecologic and nongynecologic causes of pelvic pain. Duplex and color Doppler may add important diagnostic information to improve diagnosis.

References

1. Ritchie WGM. Sonographic evaluation of normal and induced ovulation. *Radiology* 1986;161:1.
2. Hackeloer BJ, Fleming R, Robinson HP, et al. Correlation of ultrasonic and endocrinologic assessment of human follicular development. *Am J Obstet Gynecol* 1979;135:122.
3. O'Herlihy C, Robinson HP, deCrispigny LJ. Mittelschmerz is a preovulatory symptom. *Br Med J* 1980;280:986.
4. Kerin JF, Edmonds DK, Warnes GM, et al. Morphological and functional relations of graafian follicle growth to ovulation in women using ultrasonic, laparoscopic and biochemical measurements. *Br J Obstet Gynecol* 1981;88:81.
5. Queenan JT, O'Brien GD, Bains LM, et al. Ultrasound scanning of ovaries to detect ovulation in women. *Fertil Steril* 1980;34:99.
6. Koninckx PR, Renaer M, Brosens IA. Origin of peritoneal fluid in women: an ovarian exudation product. *Br J Obstet Gynecol* 1980;87:177.
7. Pellerito JS, Taylor KJW, Quedens-Case C, et al. Ectopic pregnancy: evaluation with endovaginal color flow imaging. *Radiology* 1992;183:407.
8. Taylor KJW, Burns P, Wells PNT. Ultrasound Doppler flow studies of the ovarian and uterine arteries. *Br J Obstet Gynecol* 1985;92:240.
9. Dillon EH, Quedens-Case C, Ramos IM, et al. Endovaginal pulsed and color flow Doppler in first trimester pregnancy. *Ultrasound Med Biol* 1993;19:517.
10. Centers for Disease Control. Ectopic pregnancy: United States, 1986. *MMWR* 1989;38:481.

11. Weckstein LN. Clinical diagnosis of ectopic pregnancy. *Clin Obstet Gynecol* 1987;30:236.
12. Halpin TF. Ectopic pregnancy: the problem of diagnosis. *Am J Obstet Gynecol* 1970;106:227.
13. Nyberg DA, Mack LA, Jeffrey RB, Laing FC. Endovaginal sonographic evaluation of ectopic pregnancy: a prospective study. *AJR* 1987;149:1181.
14. Dashefsky SM, Lyons EA, Levi CS, et al. Suspected ectopic pregnancy: endovaginal and transvesical US. *Radiology* 1988;169:181.
15. Cacciatore B, Stenman UH, Ylostalo P. Comparison of abdominal and vaginal sonography in suspected ectopic pregnancy. *Obstet Gynecol* 1989;73:770.
16. Dillon EH, Feyock AL, Taylor KJW. Pseudogestational sacs: Doppler US differentiation from normal or abnormal intrauterine pregnancies. *Radiology* 1990;176:359.
17. Taylor KJW, Ramos IM, Feyock AL, et al. Ectopic pregnancy: duplex Doppler evaluation. *Radiology* 1989;173:93.
18. Stovall TG, Ling FW, Carson SA, Buster JE. Nonsurgical diagnosis and treatment of tubal pregnancy. *Fertil Steril* 1990;54:537.
19. Kojima E, Abe Y, Morita M, Ito M, et al. The treatment of unruptured tubal pregnancy with intratubal methotrexate injection under laparoscopic control. *Obstet Gynecol* 1990;75:723.
20. Warner MA, Fleischer AC, Edell SL, et al. Uterine adnexal torsion: sonographic findings. *Radiology* 1985;154:773.
21. Stark JE, Siegel MJ. Ovarian torsion in prepubertal and pubertal girls: sonographic findings. *AJR* 1994;163:1479.
22. Rosado WM, Trambert MA, Gosink BB, Pretorius DH. Adnexal torsion: diagnosis by using Doppler sonography. *AJR* 1992;159:1251.
23. Fleischer AC, Stein SM, Cullinan JA, Warner MA. Color Doppler sonography of adnexal torsion. *J Ultrasound Med* 1995;14:523.
24. Abu-Yousef MM, Franken EA. An overview of graded compression sonography in the diagnosis of acute appendicitis. *Semin Ultrasound CT MRI* 1989;10(4):352.
25. Lewis FR, Holcroft JW, Boey J, et al. Appendicitis. A critical review of diagnosis and treatment in 1,000 cases. *Arch Surg* 1975;110:677.
26. Abu-Yousef MM, Bleicher JJ, Maher JW, et al. High-resolution sonography of acute appendicitis. *AJR* 1987;149:53.
27. Puylaert JBCM. Acute appendicitis: US evaluation using graded compression. *Radiology* 1986;158:355.
28. Jeffrey RB, Laing FC, Lewis FR. Acute appendicitis: high-resolution real-time US findings. *Radiology* 1987;163:11.
29. Laing FC, Jeffrey RB, Wing VW. Ultrasound versus excretory urography in evaluating acute flank pain. *Radiology* 1985;154:613.
30. Haddad MC, Hassan SS, Shahed MS. et al. Renal colic: diagnosis and outcome. *Radiology* 1992;184:83.
31. Fielding JR, Steele G, Fox LA, et al. Spiral computerized tomography in the evaluation of acute flank pain: a replacement for excretory urography. *J Urol* 1997 June;157(6):2071—2073.

18 Family History of Ovarian Carcinoma

Andrew M. Fried

The prevalence of ovarian carcinoma in the United States has been estimated at 30—50 cases per 100,000 women translating into a lifetime incidence of one case per 70 women in the general population. With an anticipated 24,000 new cases and 13,600 deaths from the disease each year, the National Institutes of Health has recently determined ovarian cancer to be the leading cause of death from gynecologic malignancies in this country.[1]

The preponderance (95%) of cases of ovarian carcinoma are sporadic in nature with no discernible pattern of inheritance. Some 5% occur in women considered at increased risk for the disease by virtue of first-degree relatives with ovarian cancer or a family history of one of three heritable syndromes discussed below.

As ovarian cancer in its early stages produces few symptoms (and those are nonspecific), some 70% of these tumors are detected at advanced stages (stages III and IV) when the process has already spread beyond the ovaries. Only about 20% are discovered while still in stage I. Since the five-year survival rate for stage III or IV disease is 15%, whereas that for stage I exceeds 90%, the impetus for early detection is obvious.[2—4]

Certain general factors contribute to an increased risk for ovarian cancer: advancing age, nulliparity, North American or Northern European descent, family members with documented ovarian cancers, and a personal history of cancer of the colon, endometrium, or breast. Forty-five percent of masses removed from postmenopausal patients proved to be malignant as opposed to 13% from premenopausal women in one large study.[5] In another report, 85% of all cases were found in women over 45 years of age.[6] Conditions that seem to impart a measure of protection against ovarian cancer include more than one full-term pregnancy, oral contraceptive use, and breast feeding. The physiologic factor common to all these is the interruption of incessant ovulation.

A woman with one first- or second-degree relative with ovarian cancer faces a risk of developing the disease which is 3.1 times that of the general population (5% lifetime risk); the risk increases to 4.6-fold (7% lifetime risk) with two or three affected relatives;[7] van Nagel and DePriest offer annual screening to all women 25 years old and above with such a family history.[8] A very small number of women (0.05% of the population) are known to be at marked, increased risk for the development of ovarian cancer by virtue of a family history of one of three hereditary syndromes. Patients with a family history of hereditary nonpolyposis colorectal cancer (Lynch II Syndrome), breast and ovarian cancer syndrome, or site-specific ovarian cancer incur a lifetime risk of developing ovarian cancer approaching 40%. In this small group of high-risk women, in addition to annual screening, comes the recommendation for prophylactic oophorectomy at age 35 or whenever childbearing is complete.[7,9] This is not applied to women who simply have a history of affected relatives without one of the defined syndromes.

Familial Ovarian Cancer

Malignant ovarian neoplasms are found with much higher frequency in women with three heritable syndromes than in the general population. They also occur at significantly younger ages in this small group. Women with hereditary nonpolyposis colorectal cancer syndrome develop ovarian cancer at a mean age of 40 years; with hereditary breast—ovarian cancer syndrome at 52 years. This is in contrast to the general population in whom sporadic cases of ovarian carcinoma occur at a mean age of 59 years.

Lynch II syndrome (hereditary nonpolyposis colorectal carcinoma syndrome) is transmitted by an autosomal dominant pattern with high penetrance and produces colorectal cancers in women under 45 years old as well as an increased incidence of endometrial carcinoma. Women with this syndrome have a risk of developing ovarian carcinoma which is 3.5 times that of the general population.[10] Histologically, these tumors are most likely to be cystadenocarcinomas.

The recently identified BRCA 1 gene (on the long arm of chromosome 17) is the marker for the hereditary breast and ovarian cancer syndrome which carries with it a 50% lifetime risk of developing ovarian cancer.[11,12] BRCA 2 is similarly implicated. The BRCA 1 gene is characterized as a tumor-suppressor gene; it is considered responsible for disease in 45% of families with multiple cases of breast carcinoma and the preponderance of the families with both breast and ovarian malignancies.[13]

The site-specific ovarian cancer syndrome is much less common than either the Lynch II syndrome or the breast/ovarian cancer syndrome. Only an increased incidence of ovarian neoplasm is seen without involvement of breast, colon, or other organs.[12]

Screening

The decision to implement a screening program is based on estimates of prevalence of the disease, cost per case discovered, altered clinical outcomes and availability of a practical, sensitive screening test among other factors. Despite its obvious morbidity and mortality, ovarian cancer has a relatively low incidence and prevalence (as compared, for example, with breast cancer whose prevalence and incidence unquestionably make mammographic screening worthwhile). Current recommendations, therefore, are for screening only a small subset of the population considered at increased risk for the disease by virtue of a family history of ovarian cancer or the presence of one of the syndromes known to confer a substantially increased risk of ovarian malignancy. Screening of the general population is not advocated by any authorities at this time.

Certain caveats with respect to screening bear mention. The detection of ovarian cancer by screening may still not be early enough in the evolution of the disease to affect ultimate outcome despite prompt intervention. The duration of preclinical disease has not been established; if it is short, screening at sufficiently close intervals to affect outcome may not be practically possible. There is also no assurance that tumors detected at an early stage by a screening program will exhibit the same biological behavior as those that are clinically manifested at the same stage.[8] That said, there is still a perceived benefit to be derived from screening a selected population.

Screening the high-risk patient is considered appropriate and advisable despite the current lack of definitive data to confirm improved outcomes from early detection. Logic dictates, however, that, because there is such a vast gap in five-year survivals between early and advanced stages of disease (90% versus 15%, respectively), discovering and treating ovarian cancer in stage I will inevitably be of benefit. The goal in a screening program would understandably be the highest possible positive predictive value (PPV) for the process (i.e., true-positive results/true-positive × false-negative) × 100. Clinical investigators have suggested that a PPV of less than 10% (i.e., 9 negative surgeries for the discovery of each ovarian cancer) would not be acceptable to either clinician or patient.[14] For this reason, some researchers have explored the efficacy of combining screening modalities. One such study using CA 125 levels in concert with ultrasound examinations produced an overall specificity of 99.9% and a positive predictive value of 26.8%.[15] For

the at-risk patient, annual screening should begin by 25—30 years of age and include bimanual rectovaginal physical examination, serum CA 125 determination, and transvaginal ultrasound.[13,16] Here follows a discussion of each screening element with its advantages and shortcomings.

Physical Examination

The targeted family history is actually a critical element in the physical examination process and identifies the patient at increased risk for ovarian cancer. Those patients with a pertinent history for familial or syndromic predisposition to ovarian malignancy should undergo a careful bimanual rectovaginal examination yearly. This is a universally available, noninvasive, and an inexpensive approach that would seem intuitively to be the appropriate first step in a screening program.[15] Indeed, it is so used. Unfortunately, the physical examination is relatively nonspecific as well as of limited sensitivity. In one study, physical examination detected only 30% of ovarian masses identified by ultrasound.[16] Limitations include examiner experience, patient body habitus, and a variety of pelvic pathologies that can produce masses or mass-like effects on the physical examination. Nonetheless, physical examination continues to be viewed, rightly so, as the proper starting point in the screening process.

CA 125

Serum CA 125 levels are not considered sufficiently sensitive by themselves to provide effective screening for ovarian malignancy. A level of greater than 30—35 U/mL is generally considered abnormal.[15,17,18] Overall, CA 125 is elevated in more than 90% of patients with epithelial cancers of the ovary of FIGO stages II, III, and IV; unfortunately, fewer than 50% of women with stage I disease are found to have abnormal levels.[19,20] This is, understandably, the very group in which early detection would have a profound effect upon outcome. Another difficulty encountered with CA 125 is that mucinous neoplasms of the ovary often do not produce this high-molecular weight surface glycoprotein.[19,21]

In an effort to improve sensitivity of serum detection of ovarian malignancy, Woolas et al. examined three serum markers (CA 125, M-CSF, and OVX1); they found at least one marker elevated in 98% of patients with stage I disease.[22] The specificity of this approach is, however, compromised by the fact that at least one marker was elevated in 11% of healthy women and in 51% of patients with nonmalignant disease. DePriest and van Nagell used the serum CA 125 level in conjunction with transvaginal ultrasound and attained an encouraging specificity of 0.995.[16] Specificity of CA 125 levels has been shown to be less in premenopausal women than in the postmenopausal group by virtue of a variety of physiologic (e.g., menstruation, pregnancy) and benign pathologic (e.g., endometriosis) variations and conditions.[14, 15, 23]

Ultrasound Screening

The basis for ultrasound (US) screening for ovarian neoplasm was established by transabdominal techniques available at the time with transducer frequencies in the range of 3.5 MHZ. Although these studies form the basis for the current approach, it is essentially universally recognized that transvaginal US is the only acceptable method of evaluating the ovary for early-stage tumors.[24—27] Three parameters are considered in the sonographic assessment of the ovary: gray scale morphology, spectral Doppler wave forms and quantification, and color flow Doppler imaging. All three have been extensively studied for specificity, sensitivity, and predictive value in screening for ovarian cancer; each will be discussed and its overall contribution to effective screening outlined.

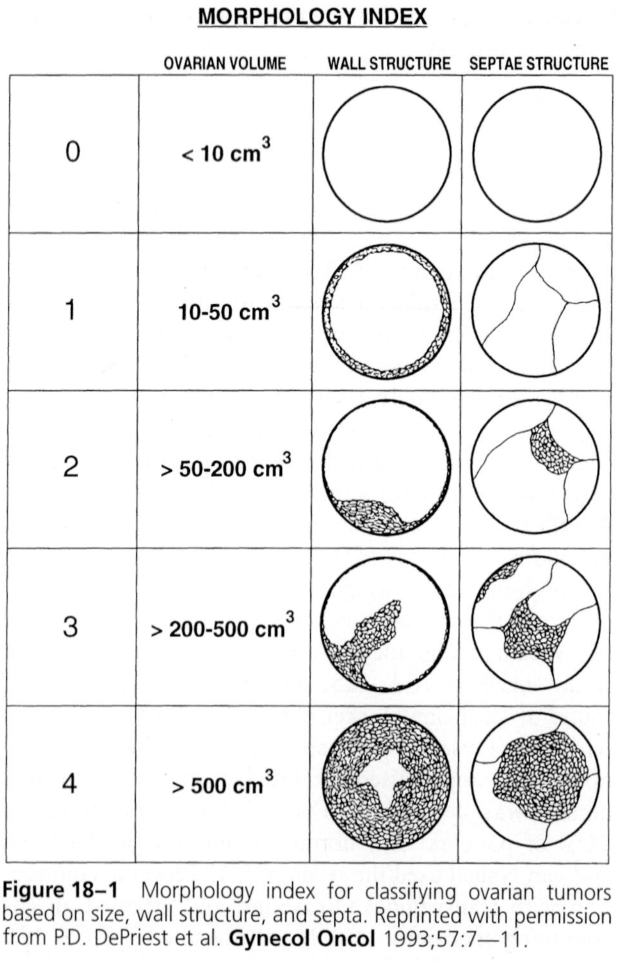

MORPHOLOGY INDEX

Figure 18–1 Morphology index for classifying ovarian tumors based on size, wall structure, and septa. Reprinted with permission from P.D. DePriest et al. **Gynecol Oncol** 1993;57:7—11.

Gray Scale Morphology

Essentially all investigators attempting to define gray scale characteristics of benign versus malignant ovarian neoplasms have established some form of morphologic classification that assesses several parameters; size, wall thickness, number and thickness of septa, soft tissue excrescences (from walls or septa, and overall echogenicity are the factors common to most studies.[20, 28, 29] Most investigators assign numerical values to each characteristic and derive a composite score that is taken to reflect the likelihood of malignancy or benignancy (**Fig. 18–1**).

Size

Estimation of ovarian size is accomplished with the formula for the volume of a prolate ellipsoid (oval with flattened ends): volume = length x width x height x 0.5233 (or, by approximation, one-half the product of the three dimensions). The accepted upper limits for normal ovaries vary somewhat with different authorities but are generally felt to fall in the range of 15—18 cm³ for the premenopausal subject and 5—8 cm³ for the postmenopausal woman. Some observers have found no relationship between the size of an ovarian mass and the likelihood of malignancy; Jain et al. however, reported a series of ovarian masses in which the mean size of benign lesions was 3.6 cm +/– 1.9 and that of malignant masses 8 cm +/– 3.8.[35] Likewise, DePriest et al. found no tumors with a volume of less than 10 cm³ to be malignant.[28] Although Sassone et al found ovaries larger than 5 cm on transvaginal US to have a risk of malignancy greater than 2.5 times smaller ovaries, they concluded that the inclusion of this factor in their scoring system did not result in improved sensitivity[29] (**Fig. 18–2** through **18–6**).

Wall Features

Virtually all observers place significant emphasis on the thickness and contours of the walls of an ovarian mass relying heavily on these factors for predicting malignancy.[31, 32] Solid-tissue excrescences from the inner walls of a cystic mass, and focal or diffuse thickening of the walls (exceeding 3 mm.) are worrisome for malignancy.[29, 30, 33—35] Indeed, DePriest et al. found morphology of the wall of an ovarian mass to be the most reliable morphologic indicator in distinguishing between benign and malignant processes.[36] Several authors have devised morphologic classification systems that take into account size, wall characteristics, number, and thickness of internal septa and debris and assign numerical values to each factor evaluated. These allow for at least a semiquantitative assessment of the likelihood of a benign versus malignant process, although, admittedly, there is necessarily some measure of subjectivity which is inescapable. For example, some systems distinguish be-

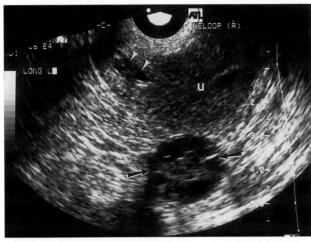

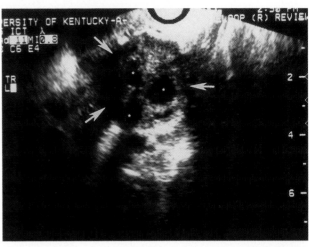

Figure 18–2. A,B: Transvaginal views of normal ovaries in two different patients (**arrows**). Note multiple small follicles in both (asterisks in **B**). The peripheral arrangement of the follicles in **A** is said to be suggestive of ovarian torsion, but is seen incidentally with some frequency. U, uterus; arrowheads, Nabothian cysts in cervix.

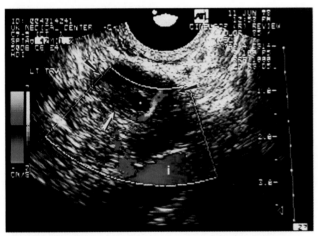

Figure 18–3 Color flow study of normal ovary (**arrows**) demonstrates intraparenchymal flow, sometimes difficult to confirm even in the normal ovary and small follicle (asterisk). I, internal iliac vein.

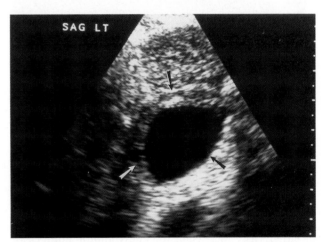

Figure 18–4 Normal ovary (**arrows**) contains a simple cyst measuring approximately 33 mm in maximum diameter. This represents a functional (corpus luteum) cyst and will regress spontaneously. Follicles can range up to 24 mm.

Figure 18–5 This cyst with multiple septa (**open arrowheads**) in the cul-de-sac is a theca lutein cyst secondary to endogenous hyperstimulation from circulating HCG levels in a patient with gestational trophoblastic disease. Similar cysts are encountered in patients with exogenous hyperstimulation from fertility drugs. The morphology is very similar to that of a benign epithelial neoplasm. u, uterus; b, urinary bladder.

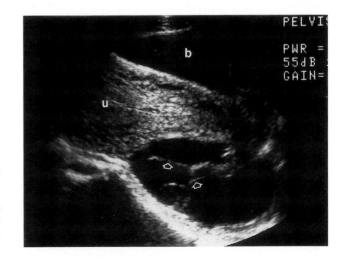

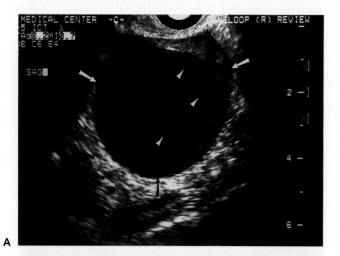

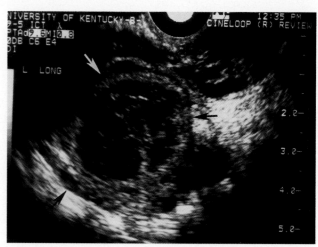

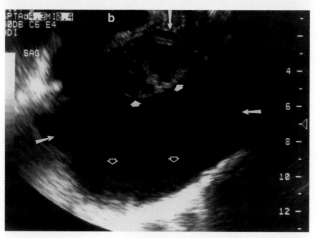

Figure 18–6 Three examples of hemorrhagic ovarian cysts. **A:** The ovary (**arrows**) demonstrates a 4-cm cyst with almost imperceptible low-level echoes within (**arrowheads**) representing small fragments of clot. **B:** Normal ovarian tissue (**arrows**) surrounds a complex cyst with multiple septa composed of clot and fibrin. **C:** This large ovarian cyst (**long arrows**) contains both gravity-dependent particulate matter (open arrowheads) and a mural clot (**solid arrowheads**). It is important to confirm lack of flow by either color or spectral doppler as a soft tissue nodule in a neoplasm could produce a similar appearance.

tween papillary excrescences of less than or greater than 3 mm where others assess such thicknesses subjectively. In either case, increasing thickness and/or number of soft tissue projections raises the suspicion of malignancy. Most of the classification systems have considerable common ground; we have chosen that published by De-Priest et al. by way of example[36] (**Fig. 18–1**).

Septa

Septa occurring within an ovarian mass are evaluated with respect to number, thickness, and irregularity; with an increased number (relatively subjective judgement) and/or increased thickness or irregularity of one or more septa (either focal or diffuse) beyond 3 mm, comes an increased chance of malignancy.[29, 30, 33, 37] Most investigators agree that the more septations present within a cystic mass, the more the likelihood of malignancy; however, none has yet offered a specific number (or ratio of septations to tumor volume, for example) to be used as a discriminator between benign and malignant. It is generally acknowledged that mucinous neoplasms, whether benign or malignant, will usually display more septations than serous tumors. Again, there is no abso-

lute number that allows consistent distinction between mucinous and serous as the overlap is considerable.

Echotexture

The majority of primary neoplasms of the ovary are epithelial in origin; they are, to a greater or lesser degree, cystic. There is considerable variation in the amount of solid tissue within an epithelial tumor of the ovary as well as the echotexture of the material within the cystic and solid elements in the mass. Tumors with a higher proportion of solid tissue admixed with the cystic components or substantial amounts of echogenic internal debris show an increased likelihood of malignancy. As would be expected, mucin-producing tumors often demonstrate low-level internal echoes, sometimes with fluid/debris levels, presumed to represent the mildly echogenic mucin itself. Quantification of the amount of solid tissue present in any given tumor is subjective at best; classification systems which assign numerical values to this factor do so on the basis largely of the subjective assessment of an experienced sonologist.[29, 33, 38] Diagrammatic representation of the spectrum of solid tissue proportions is provided by charts such as the one in Fig. 18–1 to serve as a reference guideline (**Fig. 18–7** through **18–14**).

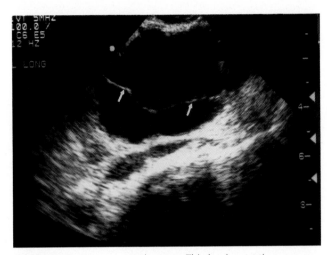

Figure 18–7 Serous cystadenoma. This benign cystic mass contains a few thin septa (**arrows**) less than 3 mm thick, but is otherwise purely cystic.

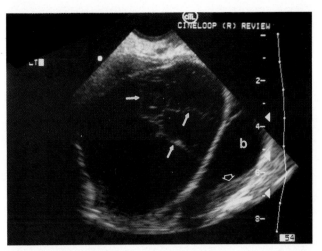

Figure 18–8 Another benign serous cystadenoma, this cystic mass contains more septatations (**arrows**) than are seen in **Fig. 18–7** but they are still quite thin. b, urinary bladder with artifactual echoes (**open arrowhead**).

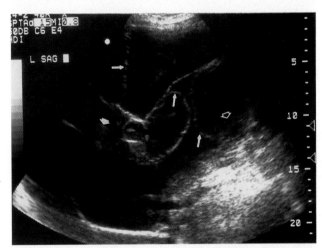

Figure 18–9 Mucinous cystadenomas, while still benign, tend to ▷ have more septations (**arrows**) than their serous counterparts. Despite the presence of artifactual echoes (**solid arrowhead**) in this lesion, there do appear to be low-level echoes representing mucin (**open arrowhead**) as are frequently seen with mucin-producing tumors both benign and malignant.

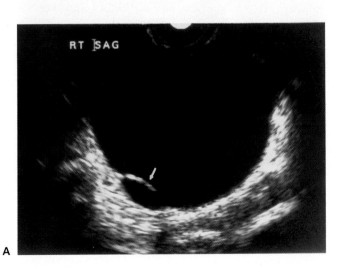

A

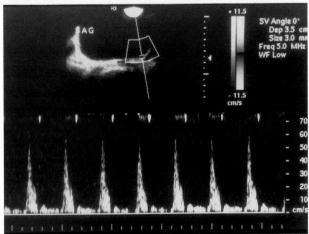

B

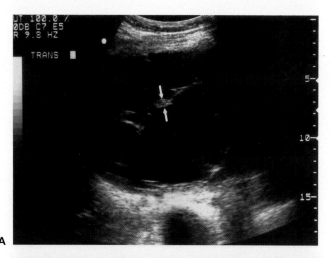

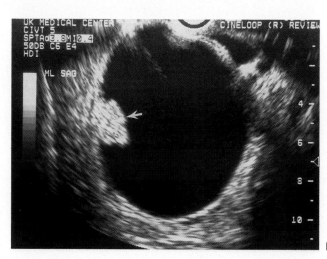

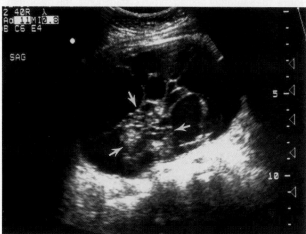

Figure 18–11   Three examples of cystic neoplasms of "low malignant potential" (LMP) which, in effect, represent a middle ground between clearly benign and definitely malignant lesions. **A:** The septum (**arrows**) in this mucinous cystic neoplasm of LMP exceeds the criterion (3 mm) for benignancy. **B:** The mural nodule (**arrow**) in this serous cystic neoplasm of LMP contained flow (excluding a resolving clot) and therefore required excision. **C:** The multiplicity of septa and areas of soft tissue excrescences (**arrows**) within this mucinous cystic neoplasm of LMP raise suspicions of malignancy based on morphology.

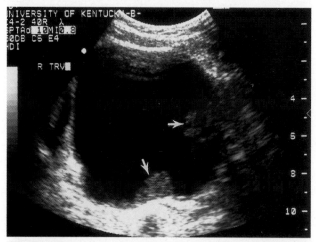

Figure 18–12   This histologically malignant ovarian neoplasm has at least two solid mural nodules in the range of 2 cm in width (**arrows**) making it suspect by morphologic criteria.

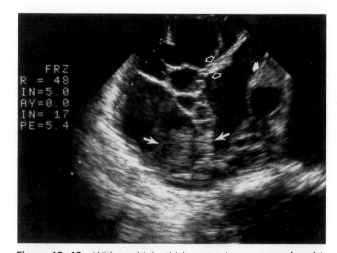

Figure 18–13   With multiple thick septa (**open arrowheads**), soft tissue excrescences from the septa (**arrows**) and solid tissue mural nodules (**solid arrowhead**), this cystadenocarcinoma of the ovary fulfills virtually all the criteria for malignancy.

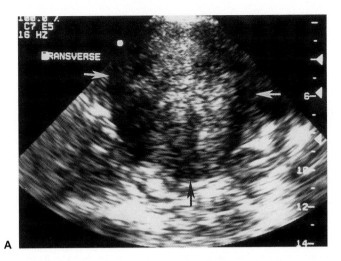

A

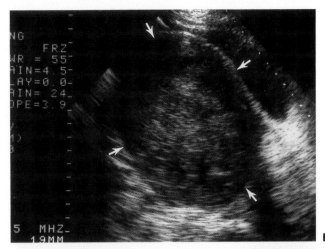

B

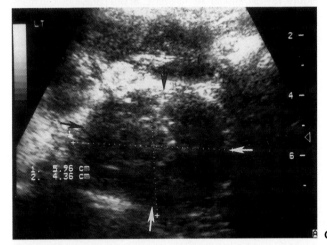

C

Figure 18–14 Several examples of nonepithelial neoplasms of the ovary, both benign and malignant. Predominantly solid tumors such as these are generally differentiable from epithelial neoplasms by their sonographic morphology. **A:** Benign fibroma. **B:** Malignant mixed Mullerian tumor. **C:** Germ cell (yolk sac) tumor.

Ovarian teratomas constitute a significant exception to the correlation between internal echogenicity of an ovarian mass and its malignant potential. This is usually a benign tumor although there are no reliable sonographic criteria for differentiating benign from malignant (save identification of metastases). Teratomas commonly have substantial internal echogenicity in the form of a highly echogenic mural nodule of tissue (the "Rokitansky nodule" or "dermoid plug") or considerable amounts of highly echogenic material representing fat or hair, often oriented in fluid/debris or debris/fluid levels depending upon which component is floating.[39—42] It should be noted that the hair or fat found in a dermoid will be considerably more echogenic than the low-level reflectivity of mucin in an epithelial neoplasm. The finding of a highly echogenic focus producing shadowing within a cystic mass strongly suggests calcification and reinforces the impression of a dermoid (**Fig. 18–15** through **18–17**).

Several studies have addressed prediction of benignancy versus malignancy of an ovarian mass based on its internal echotexture. In one such recent study those masses found to have morphologies considered benign

(i.e., completely anechoic cysts, cysts with smooth, thin septations — less than 3 mm, or complex cysts with internal echoes thought to represent hemorrhagic cysts, cystic teratomas or endometriomas) had a negative predictive value of 99%.[37] The positive predictive value for malignancy for those thought to represent malignant tumors was, however, only 50%.

Filly has outlined criteria for the practical approach to ovarian cysts.[43] He considers a simple unilocular cyst of less than 6 cm in the premenopausal woman to be benign and requiring only follow-up scans at 1- to 2-month intervals to confirm spontaneous resolution. The same is true for simple cysts of less than 5 cm diameter in the postmenopausal patient; this may be safely followed with periodic ultrasound examinations.

Several other neoplastic processes in the ovary (both primary and secondary) demonstrate high proportions of solid tissue. Endometrioid carcinoma of the ovary, metastatic tumors from a number of different primary malignancies (e.g., breast, lung, gastrointestinal tract) grouped under the broad heading of Krukenberg tumors, germ cell tumors, and lymphoma all produce predominantly solid enlargement of the ovary.[44—49] It is

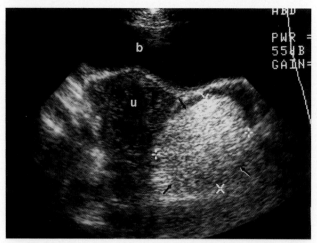 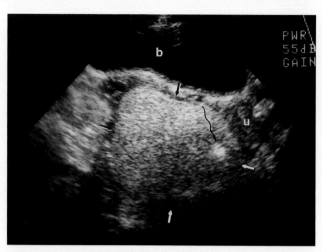

Figure 18–15 Dermoid. **A:** Transverse. **B:** Left parasagittal. In many cases, the echotexture of an ovarian mass will strongly suggest dermoid. This highly echogenic mass (**arrows**) containing mostly fat is seen to have an even more echogenic focus (wavy arrow in **B**) representing calcification. b, urinary bladder; u, uterus.

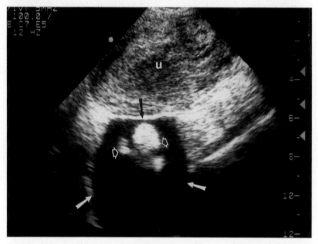 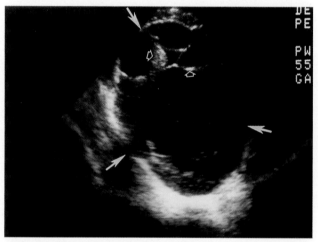

Figure 18–16 This dermoid (**arrows**) is largely cystic with a cluster of calcifications (**open arrowheads**), another characteristic pattern. u, uterus.

Figure 18–17 Dermoid. The almost infinite variability of the components of a dermoid make it the almost universal pelvic mimic. Here a largely cystic benign dermoid (**arrows**) contains septa with soft tissue excrescences (**open arrowheads**) and internal debris, closely simulating an epithelial neoplasm, very possibly malignant.

uncommon for these processes to resemble epithelial carcinomas of the ovary sonographically and they will not be discussed in detail here other than to point out the morphologic differences.

Spectral Doppler Imaging

The neovascularity produced by malignant neoplasms lacks both vasomotor control and muscular walls. The sonographic consequences are the production of a high-flow, low-resistance perfusion pattern that translates into a large passive forward diastolic flow component. This effect will be reflected in measurements of both the resistive index (RI) and pulsatility index (PI). The RI = (peak systolic flow — end diastolic flow/peak systolic flow) as calculated from the spectral Doppler shifts; the PI= (peak systolic flow — end diastolic flow/mean Doppler shift). Most investigators have adopted an RI of < 0.40 and PI of < 1.0 as suggestive of malignant vascularity; both are indicative of increased diastolic flow. Benign neoplasms, on the other hand, generally display little passive diastolic flow as they have high-resistance vascular beds and, therefore, produce higher RI and PI values.[31, 33, 34, 50—56]

The overwhelming majority of recent studies attempting to distinguish between benign and malignant ovarian neoplasms on the basis of the spectral Doppler calculations have unfortunately determined a sufficiently broad overlap of values as to preclude effective discrimination on this basis alone.[30, 35, 37, 38, 57, 58—60] None of the recent studies could combine an acceptable sensitivity with an equally acceptable specificity for the spectral Doppler findings. Spectral Doppler is, therefore, not currently considered to be adequate by itself to distinguish between benign and malignant ovarian processes.

Color Flow Doppler Imaging

Logic dictates that the neovascularity generated by a neoplasm would produce a significant increase in the color flow Doppler pattern. This premise has led a number of investigators to evaluate the presence, distribution, and prevalence of color flow signals in ovarian masses in an attempt to distinguish between benign and malignant processes.[37,50,60] A negative predictive value of 94% (for malignancy) has been cited for masses with absent central or peripheral flow.[33,37] Others have concluded that peripheral flow may still be compatible with a benign process but that central flow indicates malignancy.[61,62] Unfortunately, still other observers have found that even apparently complete absence of color flow does not exclude malignancy.[58] Conversely, Stein et al. found complete absence of flow in only 10% of masses proved to be benign; absence of flow, therefore, is relatively insensitive as a hallmark of benignancy.[37] They did demonstrate vascularity in all malignant vegetations greater than 1 cm, however. Buy et al. likewise reported color flow in all malignant ovarian masses in their series.[33]

In short, the basic premise that malignant tumors of the ovary will generally demonstrate increased color flow, low-resistance spectral tracings with high-passive diastolic flow and lower RI (< 0.4) and PI (< 1.0) values as contrasted with benign masses, appears to be valid. However, attempts thus far to establish discriminatory parameters that result in adequate specificity and/or sensitivity have not been successful. Studies are ongoing and there is reason to believe that practical, applicable criteria will be developed to allow separation of benign from malignant ovarian masses. At present, findings of increased vascularity of low resistance by either spectral or color flow techniques will at least serve to raise the sonologist's suspicion of a malignant process and prompt further workup. It should be remembered that a number of nonmalignant processes (e.g., pelvic inflammatory disease, ectopic pregnancy) may also produce hypervascularity with relatively strong passive diastolic flow.

Summary

The role of US in screening for ovarian malignancy is currently still evolving with respect to technique, criteria, and application. Screening of the general population is not felt to be justified by virtue of the low prevalence of the disease and the unfavorable cost-per-case-discovered ratio. Extensive experimental screening protocols now in progress will yield strong objective data in the next several years by which our current approach can be reassessed.

A population considered at high risk by virtue of family history of ovarian malignancy (more than one first-degree relative) or the presence of a heritable syndrome which predisposes to the disease has been clearly identified and is considered appropriate for annual screening. Screening should begin at age 25—30 and include physical examination, serum CA 125 determination, and transvaginal ultrasound. Women deemed to be at intermediate risk (single first-degree relative, several more distant relatives or personal history of breast cancer) may be offered screening with CA 125 determination followed by ultrasound only if the serum CA 125 is elevated.[8]

The mainstay of sonographic evaluation of ovarian masses is currently their morphologic characteristics. Enlargement of the ovary beyond 15—18 cm^3 in the premenopausal patient or 5—8 cm^3 in the postmenopausal subject is generally considered abnormal and deserving of further evaluation. Jacobs, van Nagell, and DePriest have selected 20 cm^3 in the premenopausal woman and 10 cm.^{3} in the postmenopausal as exceeding two standard deviations above the accepted norm and, therefore, as the threshold values.[8,27] Any patient with an abnormal volume at initial screening is scheduled for repeat examination in 4—6 weeks. Any ovarian mass that exhibits a wall thickness, focal or diffuse, of greater than 3 mm, or mural soft tissue excrescences of greater than 3 mm projecting into the cystic components is suspect. Likewise, the mass with multiple or thickened (greater than 3 mm. focal or diffuse) septa demands at least close follow-up, if not excision.

Several morphologic classification systems are available, providing a means of summarizing and, to some extent, quantifying characteristics to arrive at a numerical scoring value; from this the level of suspicion with respect to malignancy is established. Although certain clinical situations allow for close follow-up of borderline lesions by rescanning in 6—8 weeks, the bias in cases in which the ultrasound morphology suggests malignancy overwhelmingly favors surgical excision. Percutaneous biopsy is not considered an acceptable alternative at this point. The tendency toward early surgery for suspicious lesions is justifiably predicated on the excellent prognosis for early-stage ovarian malignancy (stage I and II) with a greater than 90% five-year survival, and the discouraging outcomes (15—20% five year survival) for those with advanced (stage III and IV) disease. Several authors now advise prophylactic oophorectomy at age 35 or when childbearing is complete for women with two first-degree relatives with ovarian cancer or the inherited conditions discussed above.[7,13]

Both spectral and color flow Doppler are currently felt to be of adjunctive value in the assessment of ovarian masses; findings with these modalities influence levels of suspicion but are currently of insufficient discriminatory value to be used as stand-alone criteria to characterize a mass as clearly benign or malignant.

References

1. Boring CC, Squires TS, Tong T. Cancer statistics. *CA Cancer J Clin* 1994;43:7—26.
2. Young RC, Decker DG, Wharton TJ, et al. Staging laparotomy in early ovarian cancer. *JAMA* 1983;250:3072.
3. Ozols RF, Rubin SC, Dembo AJ, Robboy SJ. Epithelial ovarian cancer. In: Hoskins WJ, Perez CA, Young RC, eds. *Principles and Practice of Gynecologic Oncology*. Philadelphia, PA: Lippincott, 1992, p. 731—781.
4. Morrow CP. Malignant and borderline epithelial tumors of the ovary: clinical features, staging, diagnosis, intraoperative assessment and review of management. In: Coppleson M, ed. *Gynecologic Oncology*. Edinburgh, Scotland: Churchill Livingston, 1992. p. 889—915.
5. Koonings PP, Campbell K, Mishell D, et al. Relative frequency of primary ovarian neoplasms: a ten-year review. *Obstet Gynecol* 1989;74:921—925.
6. Westoff C, Randall MC. Ovarian cancer screening: potential effect on mortality. *Am J Obstet Gynecol* 1991;165:502—505.
7. Kerlikowske K, Brown JS, Grady DG. Should women with familial ovarian cancer undergo prophylactic oophorectomy? *Obstet Gynecol* 1992;80:700—707.
8. Jacobs I, van Nagell JR, Jr., DePriest PD. Screening for epithelial ovarian cancer. In: Gershenson DM, McGuire WP, ed. *Controversies in Management of Ovarian Cancer*. New York, NY: Churchill Livingston 1998, p. 1—16.
9. National Institute of Health. Ovarian cancer: screening, treatment and followup: Consensus Development Conference statement. Washington, DC: National Institute of Health, 1994, 1—29.
10. Lynch HT, Kimberling WJ, Albano WA, et al. Hereditary non-polyposis colorectal cancer: Lynch syndrome I + II. *Cancer* 1985;56:939—951.
11. Lynch HT, Harris RE, Guirgis HA, et al. Familial association of breast/ovarian carcinoma. *Cancer* 1978;41:1543—1548.
12. Lynch HT, Albano WA, Black L, et al. Familial excess of cancer of the ovary and anatomic sites. *JAMA* 1981;245:261—264.
13. Gallion HH, Smith SA. Hereditary ovarian carcinoma. *Semin Surg Oncol* 1994;10:249—254.
14. Jacobs I, Bridges J, Reynolds C, et al. Multimodal approach to screening for ovarian cancer. *Lancet* 1988;1:268—271.
15. Jacobs I, Davies AP, Bridges J, et al. Prevalence screening for ovarian cancer in postmenopausal women by CA 125 measurement and ultrasonography. *BMJ* 1993;306:1030.
16. DePriest PD, van Nagell JR, Jr. Transvaginal ultrasound screening for ovarian cancer. *Clin Obstet Gynecol* 1992;35:40—44.
17. Helzlsouer KJ, Bush TL, Alberg AJ, et al. Prospective study of serum CA 125 levels as markers of ovarian cancers. *JAMA* 1993;269:1123—1126.
18. Zurawski VR Jr. Orjaseter H, Andersen A, Jellum E. Elevated serum CA 125 levels prior to diagnosis of ovarian neoplasia: relevance for early detection of ovarian cancer. *Int J Cancer* 1988;42:677—680.
19. Jacobs I, Bast RC. The CA 125 tumour associated antigen: a review of the literature. *Hum Reprod* 1989;4:1—12.
20. van Nagell JR Jr, Higgins RV, Donaldson ES, et al. Transvaginal sonography as a screening method for ovarian cancer: a report of the first 1000 cases screened. *Cancer* 1990;65:573—577.
21. Bast RC, Klug TL, St John E, et al. A radioimmunoassay using a monoclonal antibody to monitor the course of epithelial ovarican cancer. *N Engl J Med* 1983;309:883—887.
22. Woolas RP, Xu F-J, Jacobs IJ, et al. Elevation of multiple serum markers in patients with stage I ovarian cancer. *J Natl Cancer Inst* 1993;85:1748—1751.
23. Jacobs IJ, Oram DH, Bast R, Jr. Strategies for improving the specificity of screening for ovarian cancer with tumor-associated antigens CA 125, CA 15–3, and TAG 72.3. *Obstet Gynecol* 1992;80:396.
24. Campbell S, Bhan V, Royston P, et al. Transabdominal ultrasound screening for early ovarian cancer. *Br Med J* 1989;299:1363—1367.
25. Davies AP, Jacobs I, Woolas R, Fish A, Oram D. The adnexal mass: benign or malignant? Evaluation of a risk of malignancy index. *Br J Obstet Gynecol* 1993;100:927—931.
26. DeLand M, Fried A, van Nagell JR, Donaldson ES. Ultrasonography in the diagnosis of tumors of the ovary. *Surg Gynecol Obstet* 1979;148:346—348.
27. Goswamy RK, Campbell S, Whitehead MI. Screening for ovarian cancer. *Clin Obstet Gynecol* 1983;10:621—643.
28. DePriest PD, van Nagell JR, Gallion HH, et al. Ovarian cancer screening in asymptomatic postmenopausal women. *Gynecol Oncol* 1993;51:205—209.
29. Sassone AM, Timor-Tritsch IE, Artner A, et al. Transvaginal sonographic characterization of ovarian disease: evaluation of a new scoring system to predict ovarian malignancy. *Obstet Gynecol* 1991;78:70—76.
30. Jain KA. Prospective evaluation of adnexal masses with endovaginal gray-scale and duplex and color Doppler US: correlation with pathologic findings. *Radiology* 1994;191:63—67.
31. Kurjak A, Zalud I. Transvaginal colour Doppler in the differentiation between benign and malignant ovarian masses: In: Sharp F, Mason WP, Creasman W, eds. *Ovarian Cancer*. London, England: Chapman & Hall, 1992, p. 249—264.
32. Rottem S, Levit N, Thaler I, et al. Classification of ovarian lesions by high-frequency transvaginal sonography. *JCU* 1990;18:359—363.
33. Buy JN, Ghossain MA, Hugol D, et al. Characterization of adnexal masses: combination of color Doppler and conventional sonography compared with spectral Doppler analysis alone and conventional sonography alone. *AJR* 1991;166:385—393.
34. Bourne TH, Campbell S, Reynolds KM, et al. Screening for early familial ovarian cancer with transvaginal ultrasonography and colour blood flow imaging. *Br Med J* 1993;306:1025—1029.
35. Bromley B, Goodman H, Benacerraf BR. Comparison between sonographic morphology and Doppler waveform for the diagnosis of ovarian malignancy. *Obstet Gynecol* 1994;83:434—437.
36. DePriest PD, Shenson D, Fried A, et al. A morphology index based on sonographic findings in ovarian cancer. *Gynecol Oncol* 1993;51:7—11.
37. Stein SM, Laifer-Narin S, Johnson MB, et al. Differentiation of benign and malignant adnexal masses: relative value of gray-scale, color Doppler, and spectral Doppler sonography. *AJR* 1995;164:381—386.
38. Taylor KJW, Schwartz PE. Screening for early ovarian cancer. *Radiology* 1994;192:1—10.
39. Quinn SF, Erickson S, Black WC. Cystic ovarian teratomas: the sonographic appearance of the dermoid plug. *Radiology* 1985;155:477—478.
40. Sisler CL, Siegel MJ. Ovarian teratomas: a comparison of the

sonographic appearance in prepubertal and postpubertal girls. *AJR* 1990;154:139—141.

41. Guttman PH Jr. In search of the elusive benign cystic ovarian teratoma: application of the ultrasound "tip of the icerberg" sign. *JCU* 1977;5:403—406.

42. Sheth S, Fishman EK, Buck JL, et al. The variable sonographic appearance of ovarian teratomas: correlation with CT. *AJR* 1988;151:331—334.

43. Filly FA. Ovarian masses…What to look for…what to do. In: Callen PW, ed. *Ultrasonography in Obstetrics and Gynecology.* Philadelphia, PA: Saunders, 1994, p. 639.

44. Diakoumakis E, Vieux U, Seife B. Sonographic demonstration of thecoma: report of two cases. *Am J Obstet Gynecol* 1984;150:787—788.

45. Yaghoobian J, Pinck RL. Ultrasound findings in thecoma in the ovary. *JCU* 1983;11:91—93.

46. Talerman A. Mesenchymal tumors and malignant lymphoma of the ovary. In: Blaustein A, ed. *Pathology of the Female Genital Tract*, 2 nd ed. New York, NY: Springer-Verlag, 1982, p. 705—715.

47. Athey PA, Malone RS. Sonography of ovarian fibromas/thecomas. *J Ultrasound Med* 1987;6:431—436.

48. Athey PA, Siegel MF. Sonographic features of Brenner tumor of the ovary. *J Ultrasound Med* 1987;6:367—372.

49. Young RH, Scully RE. Metastatic tumors of the ovary. In: Kurman RJ, eds. *Blaustein's Pathology of the Female Genital Tract.* 4 th ed. New York, NY: Springer-Verlag, 1994,939—974.

50. Kurjak A, Shalan H, Kupesic S, et al. An attempt to screen asymptomatic women for ovarian and endometrial cancer with transvaginal color and pulsed Doppler sonography. *J Ultrasound Med* 1994;13:295—301.

51. Hata T, Hata K, Senoh D, et al. Doppler ultrasound assessment of tumor vascularity in gynecologic disorders. *J Ultrasound Med* 1989;8:309—314.

52. Bourne T, Campbell S, Steer C, et al. Transvaginal colour flow imaging: a possible new screening technique for ovarian cancer. *Br Med J* 1989;299:1367—1370.

53. Fleischer AC, Rodgers WH, Kepple DM, et al. Color Doppler sonography of benign and malignant ovarian masses. *RadioGraphics* 1992;12:879—885.

54. Hamper UM, Seth S, Abbas FM, et al. Transvaginal Doppler sonography of adnexal masses: differences in blood flow impedance in benign and malignant lesions. *AJR* 1993;160:1225—1228.

55. Weiner Z, Thaler I, Beck D, et al. Differentiating maligant from benign ovarian tumors with transvaginal color flow imaging. *Obstet Gynecol* 1992;79:159—162.

56. Bonilla-Musoles F, Ballester MJ, Simon C, et al. Is avoidance of surgery possible in patients with perimenopausal ovarian tumors using transvaginal ultrasound and duplex color Doppler sonography? *J Ultrasound Med* 1993;12:33—39.

57. Levin D, Feldstein VA, Babcook CJ, Filly RA. Sonography of ovarian masses: poor sensitivity of resistive index for identifying malignant lesions. *AJR* 1994;162:1355—1359.

58. Brown DL, Frates MC, Laing FC, et al. Ovarian masses: can benign and malignant lesions be differentiated with color and pulsed Doppler US? *Radiology* 1994;190:333—336.

59. Hata K, Hata T, Manabe A, et al. A critical evaluation of transvaginal Doppler studies, transvaginal sonography, magnetic resonance imaging, and CA 125 in detecting ovarian cancer. *Obstet Gynecol* 1992;80:922—926.

60. Carter J, Saltzman Z, Hartenbach E, et al. Flow characteristics in benign and malignant gynecologic tumors using transvaginal color flow Doppler. *Obstet Gynecol* 1994;83:125—130.

61. Tekay A, Jouppila P. Validity of pulsatility and resistance indices in classification of adnexal tumors with transvaginal color Doppler ultrasound. *Ultrasound Obstet Gynecol* 1992;2:338—344.

62. Fleischer AC, Rodgers WH, Kepple DM, et al. Color Doppler sonography of ovarian masses: a multiparameter analysis. *J Ultrasound Med* 1993;12:41—48.

19 Abnormal Premenopausal Vaginal Bleeding: From Menarche to Menopause

Edward A. Lyons

The Initial Assessment

Bleeding in a patient during her reproductive years is more commonly than not, associated with a pregnancy. The clinician will first assess the likelihood of pregnancy and will do a qualitative or quantitative pregnancy test to detect the presence of the beta subunit of human chorionic gonadotrophin (HCG).

The Pregnancy Test

HCG is produced by the syncytiotrophoblast of the chorionic sac as it invades and implants in the decidual layer of the endometrium. Implantation takes place on or about day 22 or 8 days after fertilization and HCG can be detected in maternal serum as early as 9 days postfertilization. The commonly used tests in the office and those available as "home pregnancy tests" are immunologic tests based on the antigenic properties of the HCG protein, and are positive 4—7 days after the first missed period. Testing time varies from 2 min to 2 h. The most sensitive test is a radioimmunoassay for HCG which can detect serum levels as low as 2—4 mU/mL. It requires 24—48 h of incubation time and gives a quantitative analysis.

It is important to remember that the half-life of beta HCG in maternal serum is 1.5 days. After termination of pregnancy, spontaneous or induced, the test will remain positive for a period of time relative to the initial level. At 10 weeks menstrual age the level of beta HCG may be as high as 100,000 mIU/mL and will be detectable for 24 days after termination.

The Clinician's Evaluation of Abnormal Uterine Bleeding

Bleeding during the reproductive years is a common occurrence. The gynecologist can evaluate the patient completely in the office, and the patient may never present to the radiologist.

History

The history should focus on the potential or actuality of pregnancy, the date of the last normal menstrual period, the volume, duration and color of the bleeding, associated pain, cramps, mass, infection or intrauterine contraceptive device (IUCD).

Physical Exam

The physical exam of the gynecologist may detect uterine enlargement commonly from pregnancy, fibroids, or adenomyosis but also possibly from endometrial carcinoma. A mass lesion in the adnexa or localizing tenderness may indicate the presence of blood in the peritoneal cavity. Vulvar, vagina, and cervical lesions will be visualized directly upon speculum exam as well as the type of bleeding and any cervical dilatation. Pain on cervical motion may be an important indicator of an ectopic pregnancy.

Cytological Exam

The cervical or Pap smear may detect abnormal cervical mucosal changes or in some cases abnormal endometrial cells from carcinoma.

Endometrial Biopsy

As an office procedure the introduction of a fine endometrial curet or suction curet (Pipelle) may sample abnormal sites of endometrium but more often than not, misses *focal* abnormalities or mass lesions. The currettes are flexible polypropylene cannulas with an outer diameter of 3.1 mm, which are introduced without the need for cervical dilatation or anesthesia. These have replaced a large number of procedures known as dilation and curettage (D&C) as the method of choice for the diagnosis of abnormal uterine bleeding. Histological examination is carried out on the tissue obtained.

Hysterosalpingography

This has been used for a wide variety of conditions but is being requested less commonly in favor of ultrasound and direct hysteroscopy.

D & C

This has always been the gold standard for abnormal bleeding. It is done mainly on an outpatient basis with local anesthesia or conscious sedation.

Ultrasound

This is being used to advantage by some knowledgeable clinicians in the office in addition to the clinical exam. Office-based ultrasound is frequently limited by a less expensive, lower-resolution scanner that often lacks color doppler. One should begin with a transabdominal exam with or without a full bladder, which is clearly desirable but may not always be present. This portion of the exam is focused on finding large masses that may be obscured during the endovaginal study or will be out of the field of view. Solid ovarian dermoid tumors may not be appreciated during the endovaginal study because of the echogenic fat that may resemble bowel.

The endovaginal exam is essential for the most complete evaluation of the nongravid uterus. It provides the operator with a magnified view of the uterus, myometrium, endometrial canal, and adnexa. The endovaginal probe also provides a unique opportunity to palpate the pelvic organs and "visualize" the site of any pain or tenderness. It is also useful in assessing mobility of structures and therefore their relationship. With pressure on the uterine fundus, one may see an echogenic endometrial polyp move within the canal. This is very helpful in making the diagnosis and correlating the ultrasound and clinical findings.

Bleeding in the Nonpregnant Patient

Abnormal uterine bleeding includes abnormal menstruation as well as bleeding due to pregnancy, systemic, or local disease. Patients may present with bleeding which they misinterpret as vaginal but actually arises from the urinary or gastrointestinal tracts. The radiologist should be aware of this when evaluating the pelvis sonogram.

Abnormal Menstrual Flow[1]

Menorrhagia or Hypermenorrhea

Increased volume or duration of menstrual flow is sometimes associated with clots. Sudden heavy flow or "gushing" is always abnormal. The usual causes are adenomyosis, early pregnancy loss, submucous fibroids or just dysfunctional bleeding. Endometrial hyperplasia, malignant tumors are less common.

Fibroids or *leiomyomata* are said to be present in 20—25% of women in the reproductive age group, increasing with age, decreasing with parity and increased in blacks[2]. The age-standardized rates of ultrasound- or hysterectomy-confirmed diagnoses per 1000 woman-years were 8.9 among white women and 30.6 among black women. There has also been reported a 2.2-fold increase in the incidence of fibroids among first-degree relatives[3].

Fibroids are often asymptomatic and grow only during the reproductive years under the influence of estrogen. During pregnancy they may enlarge, become tender while postpartum, then shrink, and may calcify. In menopause they tend to shrink and may even disappear. There are frequently multiple fibroids of varying size. Abnormal uterine bleeding is said to be present in 30% of patients with fibroids.

A fibroid located in the submucous region is the likely site when bleeding occurs and may be due to vascular engorgement and/or erosion of the overlying endometrial membrane.

Pathologically, a fibroid is a rounded, firm gray-white tumor with the characteristic whorled pattern of smooth muscle bundles. As they grow, they push the myometrium aside and compress it forming a pseudocapsule. This provides a cleavage plane for a fibroid to be shelled out at surgery. When the uterus is incised, the fibroid tends to pop out but not detach, as the myometrium tries to assume its normal configuration (**Fig. 19–1**).

Sonographically, the features of fibroids include the following:

1. A *discrete, well-defined* mass with a hypoechoic periphery. The fibroid displaces and not invades normal myometrium. The hypoechoic periphery may only be a few millimeters thick and represents compressed myometrium.(**Fig. 19–2**) They may distort the endometrial cavity or the serosal surface (**Fig. 19–3**) or extend partially (**Fig. 19–4**) or even lie entirely within the endometrial canal, occasionally prolapsing out of the cervix (**Fig. 19–5**).
2. They may be hypo, iso- or hyperechoic. The hyperechoic masses are usually due to hyaline degeneration, are soft on palpation, and easily distorted by the endovaginal probe (**Fig. 19–6**).
3. Cystic areas of degeneration are uncommon in fibroids, although they certainly do occur.
4. Diffuse shadowing or distal attenuation of sound. This is commonly seen.
5. Vessels are usually seen in the periphery of fibroids and occasionally within the fibroid as well (**Fig. 19–3 C**). Tsuda et al.[4] found in 70 women that only 6.1% of fibroids without a visible peripheral artery on endovaginal exam increased in volume over a one-year period. This is compared with an increase in 46.2% of those with an artery. Of the 101 leiomyomata, an artery was detected in 51.5%.

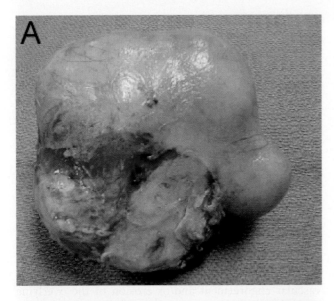

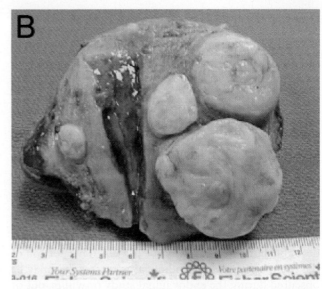

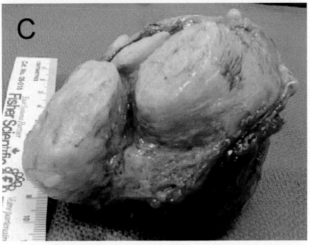

Figure 19–1 Fibroid uterus at pathology. This enlarged uterus contains four fibroids. **A:** The intact uterus showing the typical lobulated appearance. **B:** The uterus sectioned in the coronal plane. The large fibroids are seen displacing the endometrial canal to the right.

C: A side view of the sectioned uterus is showing the bulging of the fibroids above the cut surface. **D:** A close-up view of a fibroid showing the typical disorganized and whorled appearance of the muscle bundles.

6. Fibroids are seldom tender, except those that have undergone red degeneration often associated with pregnancy.

7. Calcification, likely dystrophic, is common especially after a pregnancy and in postmenopausal women. It may have a curvilinear or flocculate appearance. The calcific deposits are usually clumps about 0.5—1 cm and seldom small.

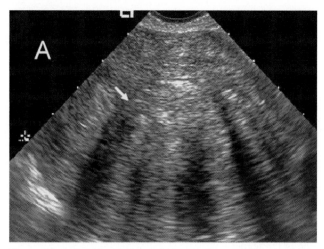

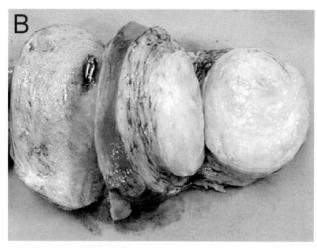

Figure 19–2 Fibroid with hypoechoic periphery. **A:** There is a large, relatively isoechoic mass within the uterus on this coronal scan. A hypoechoic line (**arrow**) can be seen around the periphery. This also exhibits distal shadowing, another characteristic feature. **B:** The gross specimen is showing the well-defined fibroid.

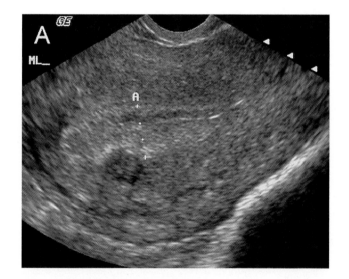

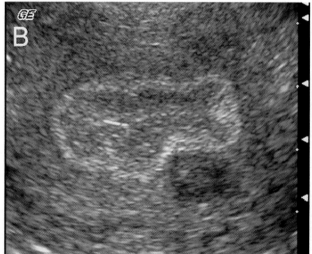

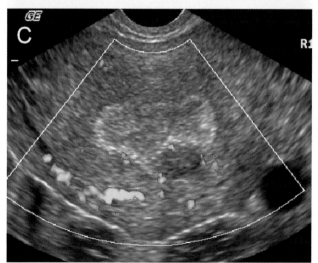

Figure 19–3 Submucous fibroid shown on **(A)** sagittal and **(B)** coronal scans that is distorting the echogenic endometrium posteriorly. The fibroid is 9 mm in diameter and shows a typical hypoechoic pattern. Notice the subtle shadow behind the fibroid on the sagittal scan. **(C)** This color flow coronal scan shows the vessels that surround the fibroid, none are seen within it.

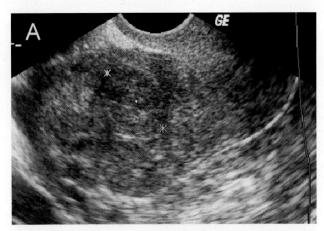

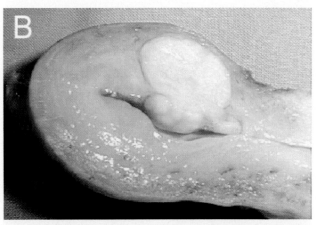

Figure 19–4 Submucous fibroid shown in **(A)** a sagittal scan and **(B)** the gross specimen. The sonogram shows an isoechoic mass (calipers) distorting the anterior myometrium and displacing the en-dometrial canal. The gross specimen shows the intraluminal extension of the fibroid.

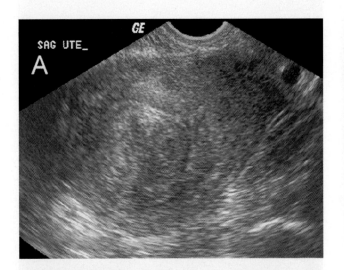

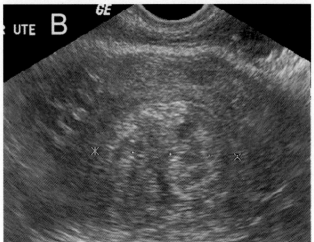

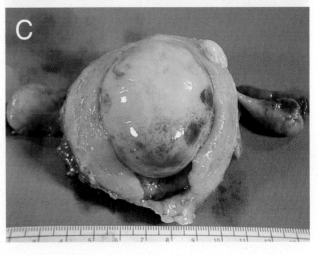

Figure 19–5 This is a submucous fibroid that lies entirely within the endometrial canal and is attached only by a short stalk (not visible). **A:** Sagittal scan showing the somewhat heterogeneous fibroid within the fundal portion of the endometrial canal. **B:** A coronal scan through the body shows the fibroid (calipers) situated centrally. **C:** The gross specimen shows the 5-cm polypoid fibroid mass. Notice the ecchymotic areas that may have been the site of the patient's spotting.

In the past, sonologists have often dictated reports that read "the myometrium is diffusely inhomogeneous. This may be due to the presence of multiple small fibroids." The author cannot yet say that this statement is never true, but the occurrence is certainly close to never. Fibroids are discrete masses and do not give an ill-defined, inhomogeneous appearance. This appearance is almost certainly due to adenomyosis, *not* fibroids.

Treatment of fibroids in general, is done on a basis of symptomatology. If there is a large mass causing pressure, pain, or bleeding, a hysterectomy may be done in women who have completed their childbearing. To preserve the uterus and its reproductive capacity, a myomectomy may be done. The initial therapy is often medical with the administration of gonadotropin-releasing hormone (GnRH) agonists to shrink the mass enough to relieve symptoms or in preparation for surgery. GnRH agonist therapy is used only temporarily as it induces an artificial menopause.

Fibroids in a submucous location that are either causing bleeding or contributing to recurrent spontaneous abortion can be removed under direct visualization with hysteroscopy. This is becoming a more commonplace procedure. A newer technique involves angiographic embolization with polyvinyl alcohol, a powder-like plastic material that is injected into the uterine arteries and selectively fills the fibroid. Success rates of 88% have been reported with an average decrease in size by 39% and relief of symptoms.[5]

The accuracy of the ultrasound diagnosis of fibroids has not been recently published. Ultrasound is currently the most sensitive and cost-effective diagnostic modality for fibroid detection. They can be detected by magnetic resonance imaging and computed tomography but these are less commonly used for the evaluation of pelvic pathology in the reproductive years. The gold standard would be pathological confirmation. It is recognized that the very small masses of less than 1 cm and those that are isoechoic with normal myometrium, will be harder to identify. If these masses are not distorting the endometrial cavity or the serosal surface, they may go unrecognized, on the other hand, they are unlikely to be causing any symptoms and would not need therapy.

Adenomyosis or endometriosis interna is a condition characterized pathologically by nests of endometrial glands and stroma within the myometrium at least one high-power field (2 mm) deep to the endomyometrial junction. This must also be associated with compensatory hypertrophy of the myometrium surrounding the ectopic endometrium. Grossly, the uterus is enlarged and feels boggy. The cut surface through the adenomyosis is often congested with a focal bulging (**Fig. 19–7**). It is more infiltrative and does not have the discrete mass effect of a fibroid. Adenomyosis is a common finding varying from 5 to 70% in routine sampling of uteri following hysterectomy.[6] This wide variation may depend on the age of the patients and on how meticulous the uterus

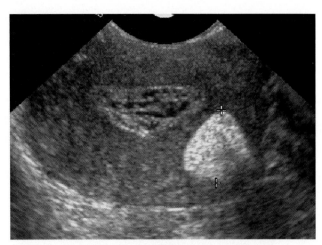

Figure 19–6 This coronal scan through the uterine body of a 50-year-old woman with cystic hyperplasia of the endometrium shows a brightly echogenic mural mass on the left with distal shadowing. This is due to hyaline degeneration of the fibroid.

was sectioned. It may be focal or diffuse and may be totally asymptomatic.

The cause is unknown, although it is likely related to pregnancy or childbirth, as it is uncommon in nulliparous women. It is most common in multiparous women over 30 years of age with the majority being in the fourth and fifth decades of life. There is no relationship between the incidence and the type of delivery, vaginal or Caesarian but does tend to be higher in women reporting abortions either spontaneous or induced.[7]

The most common complaints are reported as menorrhagia (40—50%), dysmenorrhea (15—30%), and dyspareunia or pelvic tenderness (7%).[6] Personally, the author feels that these percentages may be lower than the true incidences.

1. Menorrhagia or heavy periods. These are often associated with clots and may even be reported as gushing of blood. Onset of these can usually be traced back to a time after childbirth.
2. Dysmenorrhea or painful periods. These may vary in length from 1 or 2 days to lasting throughout the cycle. They may be cramping or continuous in nature.
3. Pelvic tenderness or dyspareunia. Painful intercourse is often an indication of a tender uterus or adnexa. One should try to elicit tenderness during the endovaginal exam applying pressure to different parts of the uterus. Tenderness is very common in women not on any medication.

Diagnosis may be difficult and it is important to take a good history at the time of scanning.

Magnetic resonance imaging may show ill-defined areas of low-signal intensity and/or focal or diffuse thickening of the junctional zone greater than 5 mm.

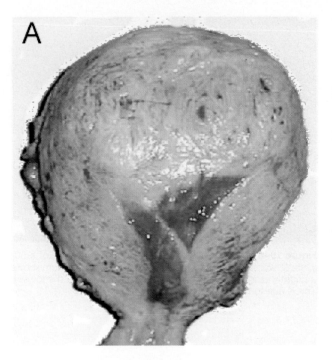

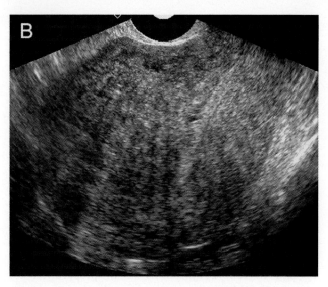

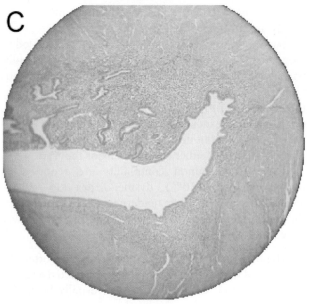

Figure 19–7 Adenomyosis involving the anterior myometrium and fundus. **A:** A gross specimen showing the fundal myometrial thickening. Numerous vessels can be seen throughout the involved area. There is also a bulging of the myometrium, commonly seen in adenomyosis. This is an infiltrative process and is easily differentiated from fibroids. **B:** A sagittal sonogram of the same uterus showing the thick inhomogeneous anterior myometrium, streaky shadowing and small cysts. **C:** A photomicrograph showing a dilated endometrial gland, seen as a cyst on a sonogram.

Sonographically, the characteristic features are as follows:

1. Ill-defined areas of abnormally decreased or increased echogenicity. They vary in size from a few millimeters to a large mass of several centimeters. There can be numerous areas or a single mass, referred to as an adenomyoma. This is an infiltrative process as compared to a fibroid that is a well-defined mass (**Fig. 19–7 and 19–8**).

2. Asymmetrical myometrial thickening. This is commonly seen and may be quite pronounced. It has been reported that the posterior uterus is more often involved than the anterior portion.

3. Myometrial cysts. They may be single or multiple, often in a subendometrial location and ranging in size from 0.2 to 1.5 cms (**Fig. 19–9**). Around menstruation, there may be echogenic blood filling the cyst making it more difficult to visualize. The presence of myometrial cysts has been shown to be highly specific for adenomyosis. Reinhold[8] found cysts in 13 (46%) of 28 patients with histologically proven adenomyosis. No cysts were found in the group without adenomyosis. Most important was that in all patients with cysts, they all had adenomyosis. The author wonders if all or almost all patients with adenomyosis will therefore have sonographi-

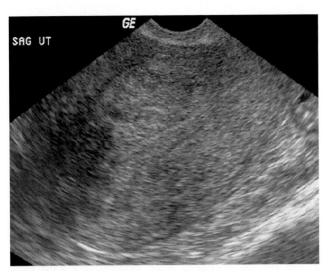

Figure 19–8 A midsagittal scan of the uterus with a more focal area of inhomogeneity just anterior to the endometrial canal. This was a focal area of adenomyosis at hysterectomy.

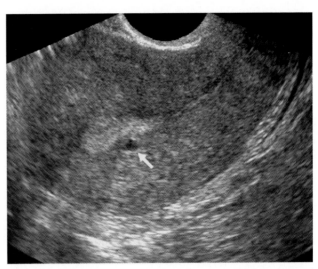

Figure 19–9 A sagittal scan of a uterus on day 19 of the menstrual cycle. The subendometrial cyst (**arrow**) is seen with an echogenic periphery.

cally visible cysts if examined in the second half of the menstrual cycle. The cysts were shown to be dilated endometrial glands, which would be most prominent in the secretory phase. We now examine all patients with a suggestive history or myometrial inhomogeneity in the secretory phase around day 19.

4. Central vascularity. The vessels are spread throughout the mass and are less well organized than those in normal myometrium. The cysts seen are not vessels (**Fig. 19–10**).

5. Streaky shadowing. There is a streaky type of shadow with small bands of shadow interspersed between more normal areas. Some of this may be associated with cysts, but not all. The audience is cautioned to note that in sagittal section at the lateral aspect of the uterus, one may normally get some irregular shadowing.

6. Tender on palpation. This is an important sign to elicit. During the endovaginal exam, push lightly on the uterus in various areas and ask the patient if it feels tender. The patient may well feel the same discomfort she experiences during intercourse. Tenderness may be felt in some areas and not others. Often the areas with cysts or inhomogeneity are tender. After treatment or at different times during the normal cycle, the tenderness may subside.

7. Do not calcify. Adenomyosis is seldom seen with calcification. Fibroids, on the other hand, may calcify.

Endometriosis is associated with adenomyosis in only about 15% of cases and may also be associated with fibroids.

The results of Reinhold et al.[8] for the detection of adenomyosis are impressive (**Table 19–1**). They are based on histopathologic correlation with a 95% confidence

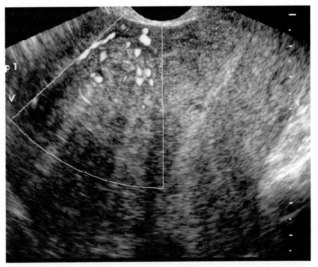

Figure 19–10 A midsagittal color doppler scan of the uterus with diffuse adenomyosis in Fig. 19–7 showing vascularity within the involved area.

Table 19–1   Sensitivity of detection of adenomyosis by endovaginal ultrasound and MRI

Detection of adenomyosis (Reinhold[8])				
	Sensitivity	Specificity	PPV	NPV
Endovaginal US (%)	89	89	71	96
MRI (%)	86	86	65	95

interval. Their criteria are as follows: *Endovaginal ultrasound*: a poorly defined area of abnormal echotexture (increased, decreased, mixed, and/or myometrial cysts), central vasculature, tender. *MR imaging*: a subjective opinion of localized or diffuse thickening of the uterine junctional zone or the presence of a low-signal intensity myometrial mass with ill-defined borders.

In North America the diagnosis of adenomyosis is seldom made with ultrasound. Sonologists should now look on the endovaginal exam for the myometrial inhomogeneity and cysts, should ask the patient about menorrhagia and dysmenorrhea and should be making the diagnosis.

The sonographic differences between fibroids and adenomyosis are important to remember and have been summarized in **Table 19–2**.

Treatment is ultimately by hysterectomy or menopause as it naturally regresses after menopause with the lack of estrogen. It may be reactivated with hormone replacement therapy and tamoxifen therapy for breast cancer. The use of GnRH agonists such as danazol are being used successfully with low doses relieving the symptoms. This is generally used only for six months at a time.

Chemotherapy has generally not been successful and oral contraceptives tend to only accentuate the pain or bleeding.

Dysfunctional uterine bleeding is defined as the absence of an identifiable pathology and is a diagnosis of exclusion. The endometrium likely outgrows its blood supply and is sloughed in an irregular manner. It occurs more commonly in adolescents and perimenopausal women. A higher than normal dose of oral contraceptives are commonly used for 3 to 6 cycles.

Hypomenorrhea

Decreased volume or duration of menstrual flow may be normal in women on oral contraceptives. A mechanical obstruction such as an imperforate hymen or cervical stenosis may occur although rarely in the premenopausal female.

Metrorrhagia

Intermenstrual bleeding occurs any time between normal menstrual periods. The most common cause is spotting associated with ovulation, which can be documented with a rise in basal body temperature. Endometrial polyps are the next most common cause followed by carcinoma of the endometrium or cervix.

Endometrial polyps are protruding stromal cores with mucosal surfaces projecting into the endometrial canal. Histologically, they are of two types: (1) functional endometrium that mimics the adjacent endometrium in its cyclic changes, and (2) hyperplastic endometrium which is the most common. They respond to the growth effects of estrogen but do not regress with progesterone. They may be sessile or polypoid on a stalk. They are common at all ages but increase in frequency after 50 years of age. They may be single or multiple and generally measure 0.5—3 cm in diameter. Most arise in the fundus and project downward. Adenocarcinoma rarely develops in a polyp.

The diagnosis can be made sonographically. The transvesical examination is least sensitive. Endovaginal features include the following:

Table 19–2   Sonographic characteristics of uterine fibroids and adenomyosis

Fibroids	Adenomyosis
Often in nulliparous women	Usually multiparous
Discrete mass	Ill-defined
Hypoechoic periphery	Asymmetric myometrial thickening
Hypo, iso- or hyperechoic	Mixed echogenicity
Cysts are uncommon	Cysts are common
Vessels peripheral	Vessels usually central
Diffuse shadowing	Streaky shadowing
Nontender on palpation	Tender on palpation
Calcify late or after pregnancy	Do not calcify

1. An oblong echogenic mass occasionally with fluid around it. It is best visualized in the first half of the menstrual cycle, the secretory phase when the endometrium is less echogenic (**Fig. 19–11 and 19–12**).
2. Cyst or cysts in the endometrium. These are most often within a polyp.
3. A prominent artery or feeding vessel on color doppler. The vessel is less apparent in postmenopausal women and may be absent.
4. Nothing at all. Occasionally, the mass may not be apparent on the sonogram.

Hysterosonography or fluid installation into the endometrial canal is helpful and usually diagnostic. This will detect even small polyps that are virtually invisible by other sonographic studies.

Hysteroscopy is also an excellent method of visualization and diagnosis. It is being used more frequently and in place of radiographic hysterosalpingography.

Treatment may be with dilatation and curettage, with a special Overstreet polyp forceps or under direct visualization by hysteroscopy.

Polymenorrhea

Periods that occur too frequently are usually associated with anovulation.

Menometrorrhagia

Bleeding at irregular intervals with varying amounts of bleeding. It may be caused by things that result in intermenstrual bleeding, i.e., polyps and carcinoma. The complications of pregnancy may also present this way.

Oligomenorrhea

Menses that occur more than 35 days apart are infrequent. The causes are generally systemic (like excessive weight loss) or endocrine (pregnancy, menopause or estrogen secreting tumors).

Contact bleeding

The most common history is of postcoital spotting. Although cervical cancer can be a cause, it is most commonly secondary to infection, vaginal, or cervical.

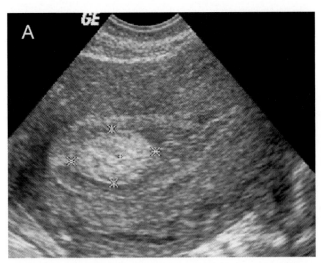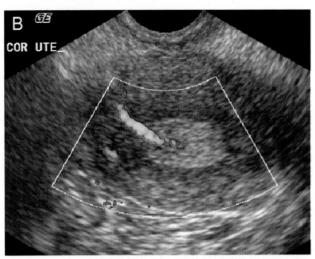

Figure 19–11 Endometrial polyp in a women at mid-cycle presenting with spotting. **A:** A sagittal scan showing an echogenic mass (calipers) in the endometrial canal. This patient is **B:** A color doppler scan showing the prominent feeding artery.

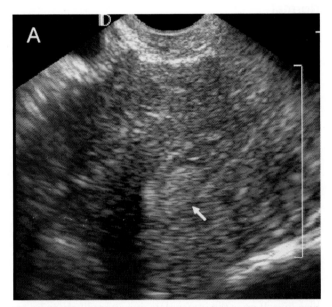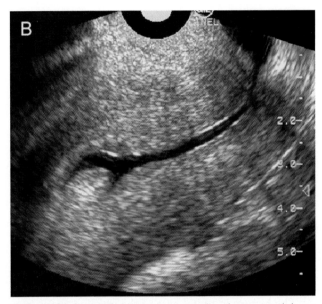

Figure 19–12 Endometrial polyp in a 48-year-old woman with heavy metrorrhagia. **A:** The echogenic polyp (**arrow**) is visible in the endometrial canal but could not be appreciated three months earlier. **B:** A hysterosonogram was done to outline the mass and shows it to be attached to the fundal portion of the cavity.

The Local Causes of Nonmenstrual Bleeding in the Nonpregnant Patient

Discussion of the specific disease entities occurs elsewhere in this chapter or in others on postmenopausal bleeding.

Vulva and vagina

Atrophic vaginitis, vulvitis, trauma, infection (*Trichomonas*, *Chlamydia*), cancer (uncommon in this age group)

Cervix

Polyps, cancer, and pedunculated fibroids.

Uterus

Endometritis particularly after instrumentation (D & C), hyperplasia, cancer, polyps, adenomyosis, submucous fibroids, oral contraceptives, intrauterine contraceptive devices (IUCDs).

Fallopian tubes

Salpingitis, tumors, ectopic pregnancy

Ovaries

Estrogen-producing tumors, other cancers, functional ovarian cysts.

Systemic, Nongynecologic Causes of Bleeding

Hypothyroidism, liver disease which interferes with estrogen metabolism, blood dyscrasias or coagulopathies, administration of anticoagulants or steroids.

Bleeding in the Pregnant Patient

Many people recommend the routine use of ultrasound in early pregnancy. The differential diagnosis of bleeding in the first trimester includes:

1. Intrauterine gestation
   Normal
   Normal with a subchorionic bleed
   Early failure
2. Extrauterine (ectopic) gestation
3. Heterotopic pregnancy

To differentiate these, the ultrasound study and, in particular, an endovaginal exam is almost 100% diagnostic. The recognition of an intrauterine sac alone or with a yolk sac confirms an intrauterine gestation. It does not guarantee the "viability" of the gestation, i.e., whether or not the pregnancy will go to term. It does, on the other hand rule out an ectopic pregnancy in all but 1 out of 6000 cases when a "heterotopic" gestation will occur. The heterotopics are much more common in cases of assisted reproduction especially in vitro fertilization and embryo transfer where the incidence can be as high as 1%.[9] This information must be part of the history taking for the imaging specialist as the information may fail to be transmitted or appreciated if the patient presents to the emergency room.

The history is a vital part of the imaging exam, particularly an ultrasound exam where the studies rely so heavily on the individual performing it. In fact, if the sonographer fails to document the key diagnostic images then the interpreting physician may not be able to make the correct interpretation. Should the imaging physician then scan all patients him or herself?

Tessler[10] in 1996 examined the result of a selective second look where a fully trained ultrasound physician scanned the patient after the sonographer had completed the study. In a total of 392 patients, 28 cases (7%) the radiologist made important new findings and in 24 (6%) refuted initial positive sonographers findings. They do not record the cases in which the radiologist was in error and the sonographer was correct, possibly an insignificant number. Is it really worth the time of the radiologist to scan all patients? They found that if the sonographer was confident of his or her diagnosis then the yield from the radiologist scan was generally low.

This study focuses on the results gleaned from a tertiary care imaging facility with dedicated, trained imaging physicians and sonographers. This is not always the case in the general imaging world. There are imaging facilities where the radiologist never sees any patients but only reviews the scans after the fact. There are realities to consider, some of these facilities are in private offices or small communities where there is not always a radiologist in attendance. Throughout North America, the level of training, interest and commitment of radiologists and sonographers varies widely. The paper does make a good argument for at least selective scanning of some patients, which in their laboratory would involve 175/392 or 44% of cases. They would have missed significant findings in 6% of the cases not scanned.

Intrauterine gestation

Normal

First trimester bleeding is one of the most common obstetrical complications, occurring in 15—25% of all pregnancies.[11] Even in a normal pregnancy, spotting can occur from bleeding at the implantation site 6 days after fertilization and last until 29—35 days after the last normal period.

Sonographically, a pregnancy presenting with bleeding can have an entirely normal-looking gestational sac, yolk sac and embryo (**Fig. 19–13**).

Normal with a Subchorionic Hemorrhage (SCH)

Subchorionic hemorrhage can be seen in a pregnancy that continues to term but there is an increased risk of pregnancy failure depending on the size of the bleed (**Fig. 19–14**). Not all patients with SCH will present with bleeding. If near the internal os, it is more likely to be associated with vaginal bleeding than if it is near the fundus and remains concealed.

Sonographically, there may be a small fluid collection elevating the edge of the placenta that is the cause of the vaginal bleeding. The collection of blood can look echogenic initially, become echo-free, and may then disappear as the blood in reabsorbed. A small degree of placental elevation is common if not always seen with an SCH (**Fig. 19–15**).

This is also discussed later in relation to early pregnancy failure.

Early failure

Bleeding is also the hallmark of the abnormal pregnancy, occurring in most cases of early pregnancy failure. Approximately half of women who bleed in early pregnancy will ultimately abort. In almost 40% of

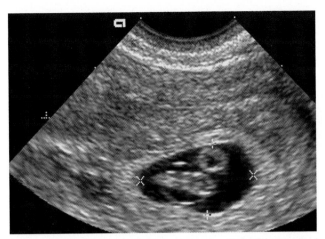

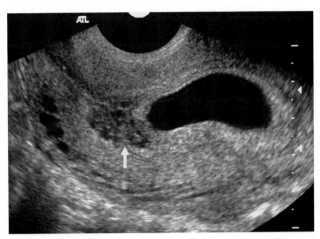

Figure 19–13 Normal intrauterine gestation 7 weeks menstrual age. The patient presented with spotting but went on to a full-term delivery. The fetus can be seen with the amniotic membrane surrounding it and the yolk sac anterior to it.

Figure 19–14 Normal intrauterine gestation 7 weeks menstrual age with a small echogenic subchorionic hemorrhage (**arrow**). The pregnancy carried on to term.

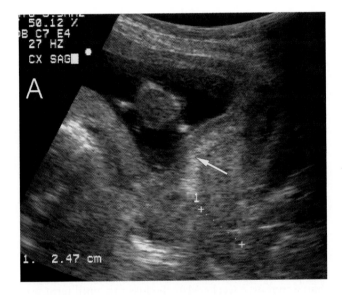

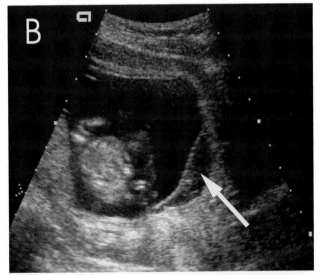

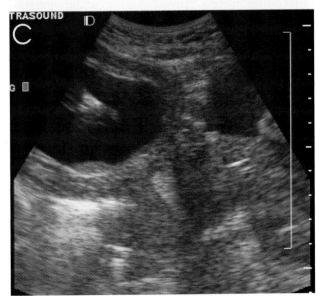

Figure 19–15 Subchorionic hemorrhage. Mid-sagittal scans of a 12.5-, 14-, and 17.5- week pregnancy. **A:** Demonstrates a posterior placenta with an echogenic area (**arrow**) in the lower uterine segment anteriorly. This is a recent subchorionic bleed. **B:** The amnion and chorionic membranes are elevated but the space (**arrow**) is now echo-free. This is liquefied blood. **C:** This scan at 17.5 weeks shows that in the anterior lower uterine segment, the subchorionic bleed is now gone.

patients, a failed early pregnancy will be diagnosed by the initial ultrasound examination.[12]

Bleeding, alone, has a better prognosis than bleeding with pain and cramps. The pain of abortion may simulate that of labor, being anterior and rhythmic. It may, however, be only an ache or simulate low back pain.

The treatment of nonlife threatening bleeding in early pregnancy is mostly expectant. The physical exam will rule out local, more superficial causes. An ultrasound examination will identify the site and size of the gestation and may indicate the likelihood for a successful outcome. In the otherwise uncomplicated gestation with bleeding, bed rest, and occasionally intramuscular injections of progesterone is used. The scientific efficacy for the use of synthetic progestational agents is not strong.

The etiology of first-trimester pregnancy loss is still not fully understood. There is a multitude of known and suspected causes. Including all causes, the spontaneous failure rate is about 75% of all pregnancies. About 15% of fertilized ova fail to divide, 15% are lost prior to implantation, 30% during implantation, 13—16% after implantation and before the first missed period[13] and 9—10% following the first missed period. Multiple authors have found a postimplantation failure rate of 18—31%. The higher numbers may reflect the use of a more sensitive pregnancy test to detect a greater number of preclinical losses that have an otherwise normal period following implantation and spontaneous abortion.

Causes of First Trimester Pregnancy Loss

Fetal (70%)

1. Non recurring chromosomal abnormalities. This is the most common cause. X monosomy or trisomy may be seen due to errors at the time of gonadogenesis during meiosis. Triploidy may occur during fertilization with two sperm entering the egg. Tetraploidy or mosaics will occur during the first division of the zygote.
2. Abnormal placental formation

Maternal (30%)

1. Maternal age over 35 years.[14]
2. Paternal age over 35 years
3. Systemic influences, i.e., insulin dependent diabetes, smoking, alcohol consumption
4. Luteal phase defect or corpus luteum failure.[15]
5. Immunologic disorders, i.e., antisperm or anticonceptus antibodies
   Antiphospholipid antibodies (APA)
   Anticardiolipin antibodies

The role of antiphospholipid antibodies and anticardiolipin antibodies is a matter of some discussion. Simpson[16] found that in 238 women these antibodies were present before and at 21 days of gestation, the time of implantation. He found no increase in the levels comparing women who delivered normally with those who had single or recurrent abortions.
   Lupus anticoagulant
   Thyroid-thyroglobulin and microsomal antibodies (TGT)
   Embryotoxic factor (ETA)
   Natural killer cells, i.e., systemic CD56 and CD16 cell
   Deficiency in transforming growth factor beta-2 producing suppressor cells in uterine tissue near the placental attachment site

6. Uterine defects that affect implantation, i.e., scarring, myomata,[17] congenitally small or distorted cavity.

7. Unknown

First-trimester Pregnancy Loss

Without Bleeding

Goldstein[18] studied 232 first trimester private practice patients with an endovaginal scan at the first visit to determine the incidence of pregnancy loss. All patients had a positive urinary pregnancy test and no history of vaginal bleeding. All patients were followed to delivery or spontaneous abortion. In the embryonic period, (i.e., 70 days from last menstrual period), 27 (11.5%) losses occurred and 4 (1.7%) losses in the fetal period. Specifically, the losses during the first 10 weeks can be further broken down based on what was visible sonographically by endovaginal scanning (**Table 19–3**). With each landmark there was a reduction in the loss rate. Once an embryo had achieved a CRL (crown rump length) of greater than 6 mm or 7 weeks MA, the loss rate until term was between 0 and 3%.

Table 19–3 First-trimester pregnancy loss in private patients with no bleeding[18]

Sonographically visible	Loss rate (%)
Gestational sac	11.5
Yolk sac	8.5
Embryo < 5 mm CRL	7.2
Embryo 6—10 mm CRL	3.3
Embryo > 10 mm CRL	0.5
From 8.5 to 14 weeks	0
Fetal period 14—20 weeks	2

With Bleeding

In the world of the primary care physician, bleeding in early pregnancy is still defined in terms of the amount of bleeding, passage of tissue, size of the uterus, and whether or not the external cervical os is open. Nonetheless, it is important for the radiologist to understand the traditional definitions and classification. (It is important to note that these designations are used only *before* the sonographic evaluation.

Clinical Classification of First-trimester Bleeding and Potential Pregnancy Loss:[19]

Spontaneous abortion: termination of a pregnancy prior to the 20th week gestation or 139 days. It implies the expulsion of any or all of the products of conception.
Complete abortion: expulsion of all of the products of conception before the 20th week of gestation
Incomplete abortion: the expulsion of only some of the products of conception up to the 20th week
Threatened abortion: uterine bleeding before the 20th week with or without uterine contractions, expulsion of products of conception, and without dilatation of the cervix.
Inevitable abortion: uterine bleeding before the 20th week of gestation with continuous and progressive cervical dilatation and without expulsion of products of conception.
Missed abortion: the embryo or fetus dies in utero before the 20th week and is retained for 8 weeks or more.
Subclinical spontaneous abortion: the pregnancy is aborted or resorbed before it has been recognized. The incidence is about 16% in the normal fertile population.
Infected abortion: abortion associated with infection of the genital organs
Septic abortion: an infected abortion with generalized spread through the maternal circulation.

Studies of Pregnancy Loss with Bleeding

In 1987, Stabile[12] reported on 624 women referred to an emergency gynecological clinic with a provisional diagnosis of threatened abortion. They all had a history of amenorrhea and vaginal bleeding, with or without pain. No pregnancy was present in 25% (158/624) with the most common causes of bleeding being follicular/luteal cyst (32) and pelvic inflammatory disease (26). Ectopic pregnancy was diagnosed in 9.6% (60/624). The remaining 406 patients were pregnant and of these, 61.5% (250/406) presented between 7 and 10 weeks. All women underwent a transabdominal ultrasound study through a full urinary bladder with a 3.5-MHz transducer. The clinical outcome resulted in 55.9% live births and 44.1% failed pregnancies, a significantly higher proportion than the 11.5% abortion rate of nonbleeding patients in the Goldstein[18] study (**Table 19–4**).

Table 19–4 Clinical outcome of 406 pregnant patients with bleeding[12]

Clinical outcome of 406 patients with bleeding	Number	Percent	US findings
Normal pregnancy	227	55.95	Live fetus
Anembryonic pregnancy	67	16.5%	
Incomplete abortion	41	10.1%	
Missed abortion	34	8.4%	
Therapeutic abortion	26	6.4%	Live fetus
Spontaneous abortion	6	1.5%	Live fetus
Complete abortion	4	1.0%	
Molar pregnancy	1	0.2%	

US, ultrasound

If one discounts the patients who had a subsequent abortion (therapeutic or spontaneous), then 36% (146/406) of patients with a threatened miscarriage had a nonviable pregnancy (i.e., no live fetus) diagnosed at first presentation by transabdominal ultrasound. This study is 9 years old and does not include studies investigated with the more sensitive endovaginal technique.

Falco et al.[20] prospectively studied a group of 270 patients with transvaginal ultrasound between 5 and 12 weeks gestation with first-trimester bleeding. Of these, 45% were excluded revealing a nonviable pregnancy, a sac without an embryo, or multiple gestation. The exact numbers of each were not recorded. Of the 149 remaining with demonstrable fetal cardiac activity, 15% (23/149) aborted. They predicted the probability of abortion based on the following abnormal sonographic findings:

1. Slow embryonic heart rate (less than —1.2 SD from the mean). This varied with CRL from 90 beats per min at 10 mm to 120 bpm at 30 mm and was the best criterion. This sign was not very sensitive (0.30), but when present, was highly specific (0.93).
2. Mean gestational sac diameter minus crown rump length less than — 0.5 SD of the mean. Small sac size was the next most important finding although it was seldom present (sensitivity of 0.39 and specificity of 0.88). A difference of less than 5 mm were associated with abortion in 80—90% of cases[21]. A discrepancy of 5—8 mm also had an increased risk.
3. Discrepancy between menstrual and sonographic age of > 1 week due to slow embryonic growth.
4. Subchorionic hematoma was seen in 17% of cases, equally common in continuing and aborted pregnancies being of no value in predicting outcome.

Bennett[22] found that the presence of a subchorionic bleed was associated with a higher incidence of pregnancy failure. In a retrospective study of 516 first-trimester patients with bleeding, a live fetus and a subchorionic hematoma, they found a loss rate of 18.8% for a large hematoma involving two-thirds of the chorionic sac. This was double their overall loss rate of 9.3%. Pandya[23] supported this association in a screening study finding a prevalence of pregnancy failure with bleeding of 5.1% with spotting and 10.5% with heavy bleeding. The risk of spontaneous abortion was increased over normal by 2.3 times for spotting and 4.7 times for heavy bleeding.

In a recent screening study of 17,870 women between 10 and 13 weeks gestation, Pandya at al.[23] found the prevalence of early pregnancy failure in London, England to be 2.8%. Of the 501 cases, 313 (62.5%) were missed abortions with a dead embryo visible and 188 (37.5%) were anembryonic with an empty sac. These were patients invited to participate in a study of fetal nuchal fold thickness and included patients with and without bleeding. A transabdominal study was routinely done and if no fetal heart was detected, then a transvaginal exam was performed. The risk of spontaneous abortion compared to the normal group was increased with vaginal bleeding and maternal age over 40 years (2.48 times). The risk was not significantly affected by previous pregnancy loss or smoking and was decreased with increasing gestational age. The latter association (i.e., gestational age) is understandable if one remembers that there is a high incidence reported (45—70%) of chromosomal abnormalities, most commonly autosomal trisomies in miscarriages. The lethal forms will abort early in pregnancy giving a decreasing rate of failure later in the first trimester.

The rate of spontaneous abortion in the studies of women with and without bleeding is summarized in Table 19–5.

Table 19–5 Summary of the rates of spontaneous abortion in women with and without bleeding[18, 12, 23, 20]

Gestational age Author	Weeks	Number	Indication	Abortion rate (%)
Goldstein (1994)	5–10	232	Routine	11.5
Pandya et al. (1996)	10–13	17,870	Routine	2.8
Stabile et al. (1987)	5–16	624	Bleeding	45
Falco et al. (1996)	5–12	270	Bleeding	51.5
Falco et al. (1996)	5–12	149	Bleeding + live fetus	15
Pandya et al. (1996)	10–13	17,870	Bleeding	15.6

Sonographic Findings of Early Pregnancy Failure

1. No embryonic cardiac activity with a CRL > 5 mm[24]
2. Embryonic bradycardia relative to CRL.[25] There is a 100% loss rate if the CRL < 5 mm and the rate is < 80 beats per min (bpm), or with a CRL of 5—9 mm a rate < 100 bpm, and a CRL of 10—15 mm with a rate <110 bpm.

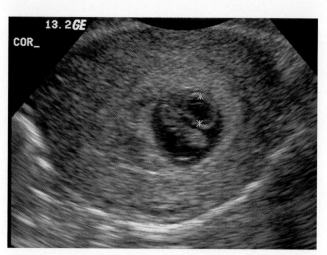

Figure 19–16 This is a scan of a 7-week gestation with a normal sized embryo but a small mean gestational sac diameter. The yolk sac is also larger than normal. There was cardiac activity that ceased one week later.

3. Gestational sac larger than 8 mm without a yolk sac.
4. Gestational sac larger than 16 mm without an embryo.
5. Mean sac diameter minus CRL is less than 5 mm (**Fig. 19–16**)
6. Poor sac growth. The sac grows normally at a rate of 1 mm mean sac diameter per day. If followed for 4—7 days most failed pregnancies will fail to grow appropriately
7. Large yolk sac (> 5.6 mm prior to 10 weeks)
8. Abnormally large or floppy, amniotic sac.[26]

Extrauterine Gestation (Ectopic Pregnancy)

Abnormal uterine bleeding occurs in 75% of ectopics and is due to involution of the endometrium and sloughing of the decidua. It may be associated with pain and the presence of an adnexal mass. The pregnancy test is not always available to the radiologist at the time of the study and when available, is not always helpful or positive.

The sonographic signs of an ectopic are an empty nongravid uterus and the following:

1. A live embryo in the adnexa
2. An adnexal mass with a tubal ring (gestational sac) +/– yolk sac
3. An adnexal mass with no definite tubal ring
4. Echogenic free fluid
5. Decidual cyst (Ackerman[27])

The utility of the various signs is listed in **Table 19–6** with the sensitivity, specificity, negative predictive value (NPV), and positive predictive value (PPV) of each. The data has been derived principally from two authors[27, 28].

Table 19–6 Sensitivity and specificity of sonographic criteria for ectopic pregnancy

Sonographic criterion for ectopic pregnancy	Sensitivity	Specificity	PPV	NPV
Adnexal embryo with heart beat	20.1	100	100	78.5
Adnexal mass with yolk sac or embryo	36.1	100	100	82.2
Adnexal mass with tubal ring	64.6	99.5	97.8	89.1
Any adnexal mass, not a simple cyst	84.4	98.9	96.3	94.8
Decidual cyst (from Ackerman[27])	21	92	80	42

Heterotopic pregnancy

The heterotopic gestation with an intrauterine and extrauterine gestation is uncommon at a rate of 1 per 6000 pregnancies. In our lab we can expect to see one case a year. The incidence increases to 1% in cases of in vitro fertilization and embryo transfer.[9]

They may be difficult to recognize as one seldom has the increased level of suspicion, as with an ectopic where there is a positive pregnancy test and an empty uterus, so there must be a pregnancy somewhere. In addition, any ectopic may be either difficult to visualize due to location, associated with a hemorrhagic mass or be very small. In a Danish survey of 13 cases, five were diagnosed by ultrasound at 6—9 week gestation and eight were diagnosed at surgery for acute abdominal pain. Of all of the cases, 4 (30%) presented with vaginal bleeding. Ten (77%) of these cases ended satisfactorily in a term pregnancy.

The overall incidence of bleeding is hard to determine as the literature contains mostly case reports.

Bleeding during the reproductive years can pose a dilemma for the imaging specialist. Most often the patient has already been assigned to a pregnant or non-pregnant category. It is then up to the imaging team to detect the exact cause of the bleeding using ultrasound as the primary diagnostic modality as it is still the least invasive and most informative in this situation.

References

1. Gerbie MV. Complications of menstruation: Abnormal uterine bleeding. In: Decherney AH, Pernoll ML, eds. *Current Obstetric and Gynecologic Diagnosis & Treatment* 8th ed. East Norwalk, Connecticut: Appleton & Lange 1994; p. 662—669.
2. Marshall LM, Spiegelman D, Barbieri RL, et al. Variation in the incidence of uterine leiomyoma among premenopausal women by age and race. *Obstet Gynecol* 1997;90:967—973.
3. Vikhlyaeva EM, Khodzhaeva ZS, Fantschenko ND. Familial predisposition to uterine leiomyomas. *Int J Gynaecol Obstet* 1995;51:127—131.
4. Tsuda H, Kawabata M, Nakamoto O, Yamamoto K. Clinical predictors in the Natural History of uterine leiomyoma: Preliminary study. *J Ultrasound Med* 1998;17:17—20.
5. Goodwin et al. Reported at the Society of Cardiovascular and Interventional Radiology 1998.
6. Azziz R. Adenomyosis: current perspectives. *Obstet Gynecol Clinics North Am* 1989;16:221—232.
7. Vercellini P, Parazzini F, Oldani S, et al. Adenomyosis at hysterectomy: a study on frequency distribution and patient characteristics. *Hum Reprod* 1995;10:1160—1162.
8. Reinhold C, McCarthy S, Bret P, et al. Diffuse adenomyosis: comparison of endovaginal US and MR imaging with histopathologic correlation *Radiology* 1996;199:151—158.
9. Svare J, Norup P, Grove Thomsen S, et al. Heterotopic pregnancies after in-vitro fertilization and embryo transfer — a Danish survey. *Hum Reprod* 1993;8:116—118.
10. Tessler F, Tublin ME, Peters JC, Jie T, Peters T. Value of selective second-look sonography by radiologists. *Radiology* 1996;199:551—553.
11. Editorial. Vaginal bleeding in early pregnancy. *Br Med J* 1980;280:470.
12. Stabile I, Campbell S, Grudzinskas JG. Ultrasonic assessment of complication during first trimester of pregnancy. *Lancet* 1987;2:1237—1240.
13. Bateman BG, Felder R, Kolp LA, Burkett B, Nunley WC Jr. Subclinical pregnancy loss in clomiphene citrate treated women. *Fertil Steril* 1992;57:25—27.
14. Sterzik K, Dallenbach C, Schneider V, Sasse V, Dallenbach-Hellweg G. In vitro fertilisation: the degree of endometrial insufficiency varies with the type of ovarian stimulation. *Fertil Steril* 1988;50:457—462.
15. Blumenfeld Z, Ruach M. Early pregnancy wastage: the role of repetitive human chorionic gonadotrophin supplementation during the first 8 weeks of gestation. *Fertil Steril* 1992;58:19—23
16. Simpson JL, Carson SA, Chesney C, et al. Lack of association between antiphospholipid antibodies and first trimester spontaneous abortion: prospective study of pregnancies detected within 21 days of conception. Fertil Steril 1998;69:814–820.
17. Benson CB, Doubilet PM, Cooney MJ, Frates MC, David V, Hornstein MD. Early singleton pregnancy outcome: effects of maternal age and mode of conception. *Radiology* 1997;203:399—403.
18. Goldstein SR. Embryonic death in early pregnancy: a new look at the first trimester. *Obstet Gynecol* 1994;84:294—297.
19. Pernoll ML and Garmel SH. Early pregnancy risks. In: DeCherney AH, Pernoll ML, eds. *Current Obstetric and Gynecologic Diagnosis & Treatment* East Norwalk, Connecticut: Appleton & Lange, 1994, p. 306–330.
20. Falco P, Milano V, Pilu G, David C. Sonography of pregnancies with first trimester bleeding and a viable embryo: a study of prognostic indicators by logistic regression analysis. *Ultrasound Obstet Gynecol* 1996;7:165—169.

21. Bromley B, Harlow BL, Laboda LA, Benacerraf BR. Small sac size in the first trimester: a predictor of poor fetal outcome. *Radiology* 1991;178:375—377.

22. Bennett GL, Bromley B, Lieberman E, Benacerraf BR. Subchorionic hemorrhage in first-trimester pregnancies: prediction of pregnancy outcome with sonography. *Radiology* 1996;200:803—806.

23. Pandya PP, Snijders RJM, Psara N, Hilbert L, Nicolaides KH. The prevalence of non-viable pregnancy at 10—13 weeks of gestation *Ultrasound Obstet Gynecol* 1996;7:170—173.

24. Levi CS, Lyons EA, Zheng XH, et al. Endovaginal ultrasound: demonstration of cardiac activity in embryos of less than 5 mm in crown—rump length. *Radiology* 1990;176:71—74.

25. Doubilet PM, Benson CB. Embryonic heart rate in the early first trimester; what rate is normal? *J Ultrasound Med* 1995; 14:431—434.

26. Horrow MM. Enlarged amniotic cavity: a new sonographic sign of early embryonic death. *Am J Roentgenol* 1992;158:359—62.

27. Ackerman, TE, Levi, CS, Lyons EA, et al.: Decidual cyst: endovaginal sign of ectopic pregnancy. *Radiology* 1993;189:727—731.

28. Brown DL, Doubilet PM. Transvaginal sonography for diagnosing ectopic pregnancy: positivity criteria and performance characteristics. *J Ultrasound Med* 1994;13:259—266.

20 Vaginal Bleeding — Postmenopausal

Peter M. Doubilet

Postmenopausal vaginal bleeding is an important, and fairly common, problem in older women. It can be the presenting symptom of endometrial cancer, the fourth most common malignancy in women in the United States,[1] and the most common pelvic gynecologic malignancy.[2] Because of this, "unscheduled" postmenopausal bleeding (i.e., any bleeding other than that occurring at the expected time in the cycle of a woman on sequential hormone replacement therapy[3]) merits diagnostic evaluation. Henceforth, we shall use the term *postmenopausal bleeding* to refer to unscheduled bleeding.

Conventional teaching, until recently, has been that any woman with postmenopausal bleeding should undergo endometrial sampling (via one of the methods described below).[2,3] With the advent of transvaginal sonography, done on its own or following the instillation of saline into the uterine cavity, the endometrium can be examined with exquisite detail in a minimally invasive fashion. This permits a more selective and directed approach to biopsying the endometrium in women with postmenopausal bleeding.

Differential Diagnosis

There are a number of etiologies of postmenopausal bleeding. The most common cause is endometrial atrophy.[4,5] The endometrium in a postmenopausal woman typically becomes thin and atrophic. This atrophic endometrium is prone to develop superficial ulcers that bleed. Bleeding can also be caused by a number of endometrial lesions, including endometrial carcinoma, which accounts for approximately 7—30% of cases of postmenopausal bleeding,[4—6] endometrial hyperplasia, and endometrial polyps. These lesions are somewhat interrelated, in that polyps may contain foci of malignancy or hyperplasia, and endometrial hyperplasia (especially in the presence of cytological atypia) may progress to carcinoma. In one series, 23% of women with atypical hyperplasia subsequently developed endometrial carcinoma, as did 1.6% of women with simple hyperplasia.[7] In addition to endometrial lesions, submucosal fibroids can be a cause of postmenopausal bleeding.

Diagnostic Tests

Nonimaging Tests

There are a number of different ways to obtain an endometrial tissue specimen for pathological evaluation. Endometrial tissue can be obtained by dilatation and curettage (D & C), usually performed in an operating room, or via an "office biopsy." The latter is substantially lower in cost and morbidity.[8,9] Both of these procedures obtain tissue from only a portion of the endometrium, and so may miss lesions due to sampling error. In a study of 50 patients who had D & C immediately preceding hysterectomy, examination of the hysterectomy specimen revealed that in 16% of patients less than one quarter of the cavity had been sampled, and in 60% of patients less than one-half the endometrium had been sampled.[10] Office biopsies are likely to obtain even more limited samples.

Both D & C and office biopsy have been shown to have sensitivities below 100% for endometrial pathology, with polypoid lesions being missed most frequently. The false-negative rate of D & C is often found to be in the range of 2—6%, with somewhat higher rates for office biopsy.[11] Some studies have found even higher false-negative rates. Grimes estimated office biopsy to have a sensitivity of 96% for endometrial cancer and 80% for endometrial hyperplasia.[8] In 407 patients undergoing D & C prior to hysterectomy, Stovall found that D & C correctly diagnosed 28 of 30 cancers (93%) and 28 (55%) of 51 cases of hyperplasia.[12] While the reported sensitivity of office biopsy and D & C varies from study to study, it is clear that both of these sampling procedures miss some cases of endometrial pathology.

Another method of obtaining endometrial tissue for pathological examination is hysteroscopically guided biopsy. Because the biopsy is not performed blindly, but instead can be directed to sites of grossly visible abnormalities, this approach is less prone to sampling error. In particular, focal lesions such as polyps, or a small patch of malignant tissue, are less likely to be missed by hysteroscopically guided biopsy than by blind biopsy techniques (office biopsy or D & C). However, the cost of this procedure, and the skill required to carry it out expertly, limits its applicability to selected cases. Furthermore, some hysteroscopes do not have an operating channel through which biopsy can be performed, which necessitates removing the scope prior to biopsy.

Imaging Tests Other than Ultrasound

Hysterosalpingography and magnetic resonance imaging can provide diagnostic information about the endometrium. The former can play a useful role in the workup of infertility,[13] and the latter may contribute to preoperative staging in cases of proven endometrial carcinoma.[14, 15] Neither, however, plays a significant role in the workup of postmenopausal bleeding.

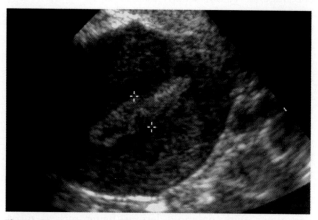

Figure 20–1 Endometrial thickness measurement technique. The measurement is done on a sagittal transvaginal image, measuring from the anterior endometrial—myometrial interface to the posterior endometrial—myometrial interface (calipers). This is a double-layer measurement, as it includes both the anterior and the posterior layers of endometrium.

Ultrasound Imaging

The literature on ultrasound of the postmenopausal uterus is extensive and has focused on several questions. Is there an endometrial thickness below which significant endometrial pathology can be confidently excluded? How is endometrial thickness affected by various regimens of hormone replacement therapy? Besides endometrial thickness, can other sonographic features (e.g., echotexture of the endometrium, Doppler waveforms) identify pathology and distinguish among various pathological conditions? Can sonohysterography aid in the differential diagnosis of postmenopausal bleeding?

Postmenopausal endometrial thickness, and its relationship to endometrial pathology, has been fairly extensively studied.[16—25] While the technique for measuring endometrial thickness varies somewhat among different authors, most use double-layer endometrial measurements (anterior and posterior layers) obtained via transvaginal sonography. The endometrium is imaged sagittally and is measured at its thickest point from the anterior to the posterior endometrial—myometrial junction (**Fig. 20–1**). Each of these junctions is generally easy to identify, as the endometrium is typically hyperechoic and the inner myometrium hypoechoic. If there is fluid in the endometrial cavity, then the anterior and posterior layers of endometrium are measured separately, and the two values are summed. A number of studies have demonstrated the endometrial thickness, measured by sonography, has little intra- or interobserver variability.[26, 27]

Table 20–1 summarizes the results of several studies examining whether there is a thickness cutoff below which significant endometrial pathology can be excluded in women with postmenopausal bleeding. In each study, patients underwent sonography shortly before endometrial tissue sampling, usually by D & C or hyster-

Table 20–1   Endometrial pathology in women with postmenopausal bleeding and endometrial thickness <4—8 mm: literature review

Reference	Endometrial thickness cut-off (mm)	Number of cases below cutoff	Histological findings	Minimal thickness of endometrial carcinoma (mm)
16	< 8 a	46	Negative b: 32 (70%) Hyperplasia or polyps: 14 (30%)	—
17	≤ 5	11	Negative: 11 (100%)	—
18	≤ 5	117	Negative: 117 (100%)	9
19	≤ 4	60	Negative: 60 (100%)	—
20	≤ 5	150	Negative: 150 (100%)	9
21	≤ 5	58	Negative: 57 (98%)Endometrial carcinoma 1 (2%)	5
22	≤ 4	54	Not malignant: 51 (94%) Malignant: 3 (6%)	2
23	≤ 5	11	Negative: 10 (91%) Polyp 1 (9%)	10
24	≤ 4	46	Negative: 44 (96%) Endometrial polyp: 1 (2%) Endometrial carcinoma: 1 (2%)	3
25	≤ 4	518	Negative: 491 (95%) Endometrial polyp: 6 (1%) Endometrial hyperplasia: 6 (1%)	

a   Was reported as a < 4 mm single-layer measurement.
b   "Negative" includes histological readings of "atrophic endometrium," "inactive endometrium," "tissue insufficient for diagnosis," and related findings.

ectomy. Most of the studies employ a cutoff of 4 or 5 mm. While the findings vary somewhat among studies, the overall pattern of results suggests that post-menopausal bleeding is rarely due to significant endometrial pathology (carcinoma, hyperplasia, or polyp), and almost never due to carcinoma, when the endometrial thickness is ≤ 4—5 mm. Using a conservative cutoff of ≤ 4 mm (**Fig. 20–2**), postmenopausal bleeding can be attributed to endometrial atrophy with a high degree of confidence when the endometrial thickness is below this cutoff.

It should be noted that, while a thickness below 4—5 mm largely excludes significant pathology, a greater measurement does not exclude endometrial atrophy. In the 1995 Karlsson study, for example, among 245 women with endometrial thicknesses of 6—10 mm, 88 (36%) had endometrial atrophy.[25]

In a small fraction of cases, the endometrial margins are obscure, so that the thickness cannot be measured. This is most likely to occur when there are uterine fibroids distorting the endometrium. In these cases, the sonogram provides no information about the presence or nature of endometrial pathology.[17]

Most studies have found that the endometrial thickness in cases of endometrial carcinoma is larger, on average, than it is with polyps or hyperplasia.[16, 18, 20, 21, 23—25] In the largest study, for example, the mean thickness with endometrial cancer was 21.1 mm, as compared to 12.9 mm for polyps and 12 mm for hyperplasia.[25] However, there is considerable overlap in endometrial thickness among these three lesions, so that the degree of thickening cannot be used to make a specific diagnosis.

Endometrial thickness in postmenopausal women is somewhat affected by hormone replacement therapy, which many women take to counter the effects of menopause. Several treatment regimes are available, employing estrogen with or without progesterone. Estrogen suppresses "hot flashes" and reduces the risk of osteoporosis and cardiovascular disease in postmenopausal women. It has the drawback of increasing the likelihood of endometrial hyperplasia or carcinoma, and so is often given in combination with progesterone, which decreases the risk of endometrial pathology. Progesterone, when used, can be given either continuously or periodically (e.g., the first 10—14 days of each month), leading to three types of treatment regimen: estrogen only, continuous estrogen/progesterone, and sequential estrogen/progesterone. On the last of these regimens, "withdrawal" bleeding is expected each month and is not associated with endometrial pathology, so that bleeding in women on sequential therapy merits diagnostic workup only when unscheduled.[3, 28]

Hormone replacement therapy tends to increase endometrial thickness, by approximately 1—1.5 mm for continuous estrogen or estrogen/progesterone, and by 3 mm for sequential therapy.[29] Women on sequential

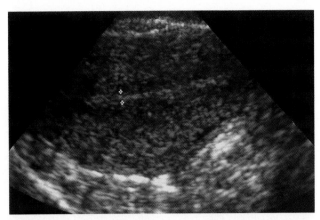

Figure 20–2 Thin endometrium. The endometrial thickness (calipers) is 2 mm.

therapy also have more variation in thickness during each month than do those on continuous or no therapy, with the thinnest endometrium following progesterone withdrawal.

A number of studies have examined whether sonographic features other than endometrial thickness, such as echotexture or Doppler indices, may be useful in the diagnosis of endometrial pathology. Several studies have found that the sonographic finding of cystic spaces in the postmenopausal endometrium suggests polyps, a heterogeneous appearance suggests malignancy (**Fig. 20–3**), and a homogeneously thickened endometrium suggests hyperplasia (**Fig. 20–4**).[30—32] There is too much overlap in the sonographic appearance of the various pathologic entities, however, to allow a diagnosis to be made with confidence based on echotexture alone. Analysis of echotexture, therefore, has little or no practical impact on the diagnostic evaluation or management of patients with postmenopausal bleeding.

The data on Doppler for diagnosing endometrial pathology are mixed, at best. Bourne found that the uterine artery pulsatility index accurately distinguished between endometria with and without cancer,[33] but Aleem found no significant difference in uterine artery pulsatility index or resistive index in pathological versus control groups.[34] Sheth found that Doppler of endometrial vessels in postmenopausal women with thick (≥8 mm) endometria was not helpful, as there was no significant difference in mean pulsatility and resistive indices in benign versus malignant lesions.[35] It is noteworthy that the lead author of a favorable Doppler study in 1990[33] later wrote in a 1995 editorial that "Doppler has a relatively insignificant role to play in the context of evaluating the postmenopausal endometrium for the presence of carcinoma".[11]

In the last several years, sonohysterography (SHG) — transvaginal sonography immediately following saline instillation into the uterine cavity — has generated considerable interest as a technique for diagnosing endometrial lesions.[36—41] To perform the procedure, a

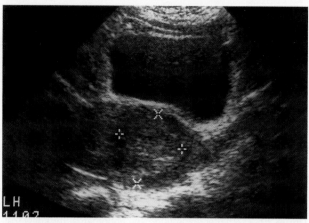

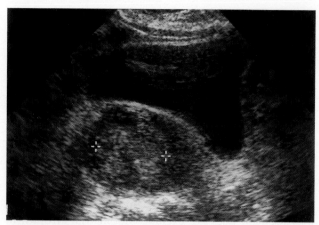

Figure 20–3 Endometrial carcinoma. The endometrium, outlined by calipers, is markedly thickened (41 mm) and heterogeneous, and has indistinct margins on (**A**) sagittal and (**B**) transverse views. D & C revealed endometrial carcinoma.

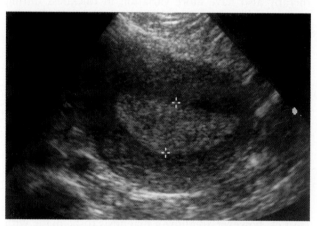

Figure 20–4 Endometrial hyperplasia. The endometrium is thick (22 mm) and homogenous, and has a distinct interface with the myometrium. Endometrial biopsy revealed hyperplasia.

speculum is inserted into the vagina and a catheter is threaded through the cervix into the uterine cavity. The speculum is removed; taking care not to dislodge the catheter, a transvaginal ultrasound transducer is inserted, approximately 10 cc of saline is instilled, and the uterus is scanned thoroughly in sagittal and transverse planes (**Fig. 20–5**). Because fluid may leave the uterus through the cervix and Fallopian tubes, several saline injections may be needed during the course of the examination. Some practitioners use a catheter with an inflatable balloon and place traction on the balloon-filled catheter to prevent fluid from escaping out of the cervix, especially in patients with a patulous cervix,[37] while others use a balloonless catheter.[38]

Sonohysterography can contribute useful diagnostic information in a number of clinical settings, including

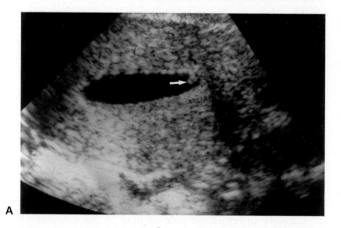

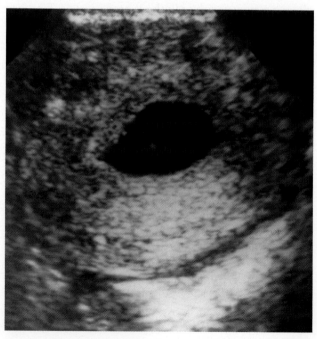

Figure 20–5 Normal sonohysterogram. Fluid in the uterine cavity delineates smooth, thin, endometrium surrounding the entire cavity. **A:** Sagittal view, with catheter tip (**arrow**) seen within the fluid-filled uterine cavity in the lower uterine segment. **B:** Coronal view.

the workup of postmenopausal bleeding. In a woman with postmenopausal bleeding in whom transvaginal sonography demonstrates endometrial thickening, an SHG can determine whether the thickening is diffuse (**Fig. 20–6**) or due to a focal lesion, such as a polyp (**Fig. 20–7**). This distinction can be used to help guide the selection of a biopsy approach.[37, 38, 40, 41] In the presence of a submucosal fibroid, SHG can aid in its diagnosis, and also assess whether it is pedunculated or superficial enough to permit transcervical resection via an operative hysteroscope.[37, 38] If the endometrial thickness cannot be measured on transvaginal sonography, SHG can clarify whether it appears normal (atrophic) or not, as well as identify one or more submucosal fibroids that may be distorting the endometrium.

Benefits of Ultrasound

Until fairly recently, the conventional teaching had been that a woman with unscheduled postmenopausal bleeding should be biopsied, either via office biopsy or

D & C.[2, 3] The main benefits of ultrasound are twofold: First, ultrasound can identify a subset of women with postmenopausal bleeding in whom the risk of significant endometrial pathology is so low that biopsy may not be necessary. Second, in patients in whom biopsy is indicated, sonohysterography can help to select the optimal biopsy technique.

The ultrasound finding of an endometrial thickness ≤ 4 mm is near-definitive proof of endometrial atrophy and excludes malignancy with very high confidence (**Table 20–1**). In fact, the false-negative rate associated with a sonographic thickness of ≤ 4 mm appears to be as low as, or lower than, that of office biopsy or D & C, so that a negative ultrasound may be at least as reliable as a negative biopsy or D & C. Transvaginal ultrasound can thus play a key role in the evaluation of postmenopausal bleeding, in one of two ways. First, it can be performed prior to biopsy, and if the endometrial thickness is found to be ≤ 4 mm, it is reasonable to attribute the bleeding to endometrial atrophy and not perform a biopsy. In one study, this diagnostic strategy led to a 46% reduction in the number of biopsies performed, without loss of diag-

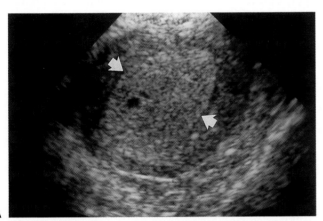
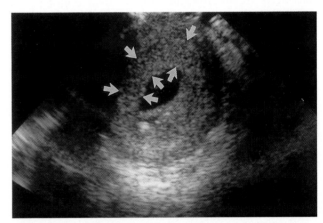

Figure 20–6 Diffuse endometrial thickening. **A:** Sagittal sonogram demonstrates thickened (24 mm) endometrium (**arrows**) with small cyst. **B:** Sonohysterogram demonstrates diffuse endometrial thickening (between **arrows**).

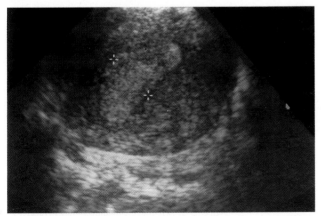
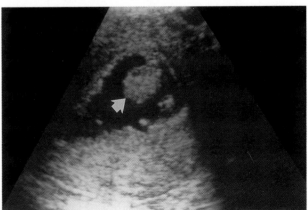

Figure 20–7 Endometrial polyp. **A:** Sagittal sonogram demonstrates thickened endometrium (17 mm). **B.** Sonohysterogram demonstrates polyp (**arrow**) surrounded by fluid. Blind endometrial biopsy prior to the sonohysterogram had been negative. Hysteroscopically guided biopsy following the sonohysterogram revealed endometrial polyp with focal simple hyperplasia.

nostic accuracy.[25] Second, if endometrial biopsy has been performed (without prior ultrasound) and if there is "insufficient tissue for diagnosis," ultrasound can then help to decide whether to believe the result (i.e., attribute the bleeding to endometrial atrophy) or to proceed to D & C or hysteroscopy.[42,43] If the sonographically measured endometrial thickness is ≤ 4 mm, then the biopsy result can be accepted, and if > 4 mm, then further tissue sampling should be considered.

Ideally, diagnostic strategies for postmenopausal bleeding should involve a combination of sonography, SHG, and tissue sampling. Sonography, using the ≤ 4 mm cutoff, can guide the decision concerning whom to biopsy or whether to accept the result of an office biopsy that yields scanty tissue. Sonohysterography can help to choose the best biopsy approach — office biopsy or D & C for diffuse endometrial thickening (**Fig. 20–6**), hysteroscopically-guided biopsy for focal or polypoid lesion (**Fig. 20–7**) — as well as to clarify the significance of an unmeasurable endometrial thickness or identify the best way to excise a submucosal fibroid. Tissue sampling yields a specific histopathologic diagnosis.

Two reasonable diagnostic algorithms that employ these tests are an ultrasound-first strategy (**Fig. 20–8 A**) or a biopsy-first strategy (**Fig. 20–8 B**). With the ultrasound-first strategy, the sonographically measured endometrial thickness is used to decide whether further workup is needed: no if ≤ 4 mm, yes if > 4 mm. If the thickness is > 4 mm or is unmeasurable, then SHG is per-

formed and the next step is based on the SHG findings. Using the biopsy-first approach, positive biopsy results end the diagnostic workup, while ultrasound (and, in some cases, SHG) is used following a negative biopsy. Both of these algorithms will lead to decreased cost and/ or improved diagnostic accuracy when compared to relying on tissue sampling alone. A cost analysis has suggested that using ultrasound as the first test is less costly than beginning with office biopsy.[44]

These algorithms apply to any woman with postmenopausal bleeding, including those with unscheduled bleeding on hormone replacement therapy. For a woman with unscheduled bleeding on sequential therapy, the sonogram and SHG should be performed shortly after subsequent progesterone withdrawal bleeding, when the endometrium is expected to be at its thinnest. While hormone therapy tends to increase endometrial thickness, the prudent and conservative approach in the face of unscheduled bleeding is to employ the same ≤ 4-mm cutoff for the decision concerning biopsy in women on hormones as is used in women who are not taking hormones.

It is important to recognize that these algorithms apply only to postmenopausal women who have vaginal bleeding, not to asymptomatic ones. The measurement of 4 mm is not a "normal" or "upper limit of normal" value for postmenopausal endometrial thickness, but instead is an "action threshold" for women with bleeding. In the absence of bleeding, the sonographic finding of an

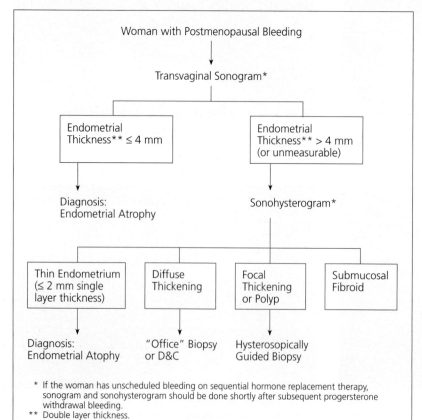

* If the woman has unscheduled bleeding on sequential hormone replacement therapy, sonogram and sonohysterogram should be done shortly after subsequent progersterone withdrawal bleeding.
** Double layer thickness.

A

Figure 20–8 Algorithms for diagnostic workup of postmenopausal bleeding using sonography, sonohysterography, and endometrial sampling. **A:** Ultrasound-first strategy.

Figure 20–8 B: Biopsy-first strategy.

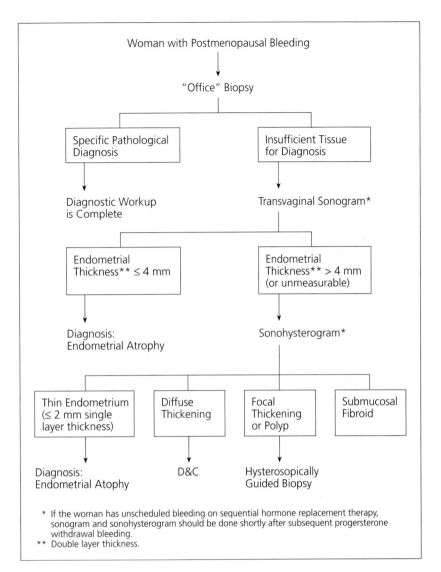

Woman with Postmenopausal Bleeding

"Office" Biopsy

Specific Pathological Diagnosis | Insufficient Tissue for Diagnosis

Diagnostic Workup is Complete | Transvaginal Sonogram*

Endometrial Thickness** ≤ 4 mm | Endometrial Thickness** > 4 mm (or unmeasurable)

Diagnosis: Endometrial Atrophy | Sonohysterogram*

Thin Endometrium (≤ 2 mm single layer thickness) | Diffuse Thickening | Focal Thickening or Polyp | Submucosal Fibroid

Diagnosis: Endometrial Atophy | D&C | Hysterosopically Guided Biopsy

* If the woman has unscheduled bleeding on sequential hormone replacement therapy, sonogram and sonohysterogram should be done shortly after subsequent progersterone withdrawal bleeding.
** Double layer thickness.

endometrial thickness >4 mm in a postmenopausal woman does not necessarily indicate that she should be biopsied. In this setting, the decision about whether or not to biopsy should take into account factors such as the degree of thickening, whether and what regimen of hormone replacement therapy she is on, the endometrial echotexture, as well as age and other risk factors for endometrial carcinoma.[45]

Summary

Postmenopausal bleeding, except that occurring at the expected time in certain hormone replacement regimens, may be a sign of malignant or premalignant endometrial lesions. Conventional teaching has been that any woman with unscheduled bleeding should undergo endometrial tissue sampling, via office biopsy or D & C. Because these tests carry costs, risk, and a chance of false-negative results, sonography and sonohysterography can contribute to the diagnostic workup. A sonographically measured endometrial thickness of ≤ 4 mm

indicates a high likelihood of endometrial atrophy being the cause of bleeding, and so may obviate the need for biopsy. When the endometrial thickness is > 4 mm, sonohysterography can determine whether the thickening is diffuse or due to a polyp or other focal lesion, and thus help guide the choice of biopsy technique. Incorporating sonography and sonohysterography into the diagnostic algorithm for postmenopausal bleeding can lead to decreased cost and morbidity with no loss of, or improvement in, diagnostic accuracy.

References

1. Parker SL, Tong T, Bolden S, Wingo PA. Cancer statistics, 1996. *CA* 1996;46:5—27.
2. American College of Obstetrics and Gynecology. Technical Bulletin 162: Carcinoma of the endometrium, December 1991.
3. American College of Obstetrics and Gynecology. Technical Bulletin 166: Hormone replacement therapy. April 1992.
4. Choo YC, Mak KC, Hsu C, Wong TS, Ma HK. Postmenopausal uterine bleeding of nonorganic cause. *Obstet Gynecol* 1985;66:225—228.

5. Lidor A, Ismajovic E, Confino E, David MP. Histopathological findings in 226 women with postemenopausal uterine bleeing. *Acta Obstet Gynecol Scand* 1986;65:41—43.

6. Rosenwaks Z, Benjamin F, Stone ML. *Gynecology: Principles and Practice*. New York: Macmillan, 1987, p. 515.

7. Kurman RJ, Kaminski PF, Norris HJ. The behavior of endometrial hyperplasia: a long-term study of "untreated" hyperplasia in 170 patients. *Cancer* 1985;56:403—412.

8. Grimes DA. Diagnostic dilation and curettage: a reappraisal. *Am J Obstet Gynecol* 1982;142:1—6

9. Feldman S, Berkowitz RS, Tosteson ANA. Cost-effectiveness of strategies to evaluate postmenopausal bleeding. *Obstet Gynecol* 1993;81:968—975.

10. Stock RJ, Kanbour A. Prehysterectomy curettage. *Obstet Gynecol* 1975;45:537—541.

11. Bourne TH. Evaluating the endometrium of postmenopausal women with transvaginal ultrasonography. *Ultrasound Obstet Gynecol* 1995;6:75—80.

12. Stovall TG, Solomon SK, Ling FW. Endometrial sampling prior to hysterectomy. *Obstet Gynecol* 1989;73:405—409.

13. Fagan CJ. Hysterosalpingography. Ins: Putman CE, Ravin CE, eds. *Textbook of Diagnostic Imaging*. Philadelphia: W.B. Saunders, 1988.

14. Yamashita Y, Mizutani H, Torashima M, et al. Assessment of myometrial invasion by endometrial carcinoma: transvaginal sonography vs. contrast-enhanced MR imaging. *AJR* 1993;161:595—599.

15. Yamashita Y, Harada M, Sawada T, et al. Normal uterus und FIGO stage I endometrial carcinoma: dynamic gadolinium-enhanced MR imaging. *Radiology* 1993;186:495—501.

16. Osmers R, Volksen M, Schauer A. Vaginosonography for early detection of endometrial carcinoma? *Lancet* 1990;335:1569—1571.

17. Goldstein SR, Nachtigall M, Snyder JR, Nachtigall L. Endometrial assessment by vaginal ultrasonography before endometrial sampling in patients with postmenopausal bleeding. *Am J Obstet Gynecol* 1990;163:119—123.

18. Nasri MN, Shepherd JH, Setchell ME, Lowe DG, Chard T. sonographic depiction of postmenopausal endometrium with transabdominal and transvaginal scanning. *Ultrasound Obstet Gynecol* 1991;1:279—283.

19. Varner RE, Sparks JM, Cameron CD, Roberts LL, Soong SJ. Transvaginal sonography of the endometrium in postmenopausal women. *Obstet Gynecol* 1991;78:195—199.

20. Granberg S, Wikland M, Karlsson B, Norstrom A, Friberg LG. Endometrial thickness as measured by endovaginal ultrasonography for identifying endometrial abnormality. *Am J Obstet Gynecol* 1991;164:47—52.

21. Karlsson B, Granberg S, Wikland M, Ryd W, Norstrom A. Endovaginal scanning of the endometrium compared to cytology and histology in women with postmenopausal bleeding. *Gynecol Oncol* 1993;50:173—178.

22. Dorum A, Kristensen B, Langebrekke B, Sornes T, Skaar O. Evaluation of endometrial thickness measured by endovaginal ultrasound in women with postmenopausal bleeding. *Acta Obstet Gynecol Scand* 1993;72:116—119.

23. Cacciatore B, Ramsay T, Lehtovirta P, Ylostalo P. Transvaginal sonography and hysteroscopy in postmenopausal bleeding. *Acta Obstet Gynecol Scand* 1994;73:413—416.

24. Conoscenti G, Meir YJ, Fischer-Tamaro L, et al. Endometrial assessment by transvaginal sonography and histological findings after D & C in women with postmenopausal bleeding. *Ultrasound Obstet Gynecol* 1995;6:108—115.

25. Karlsson B, Granberg S, Wikland M, et al. Transvagnial ultrasonography of the endometrium in women with postmenopausal bleeding — a Nordic multicenter study. *Am J Obstet Gynecol* 1995;172:1488—1494.

26. Delisle M-F, Villeneuve M, Boulvain M. Measurement of endometrial thickness with transvaginal ultrasonography: is it reproducible? *J Ultrasound Med* 998;17:481—484.

27. Wolman I, Jaffa AJ, Sagi J, et al. Transvaginal ultrasonographic measurements of endometrial thickness: a reproducible study. *J Clin Ultrasound* 1996;24:351—354.

28. Padwick ML, Pryse-Davies J, Whitehead MI. A simple method for determining the optimal dosage of progestin in postmenopausal women receiving estrogens. *New Engl J Med* 1986;315:930—934.

29. Levine D, Gosnik BB, Johnson LA. Change in endometrial thickness in postmenopausal women undergoing hormone replacement therapy. *Radiology* 1995;197:603–608.

30. Sheth S, Hamper UM Kurman RJ. Thickened endometrium in the postmenopausal woman: sonographic-pathologic correlation. *Radiology* 1993;187:135—139.

31. Hulka CA, Hall DA, McCarthy K, Simeone JF. Endometrial polyps, hyperplasia, and carcinoma in postmenopausasl women: differentiation with endovaginal sonography: *Radiology* 1994;191:755—758.

32. Atri M, Mazarnia S, Aldis AE, et al. Tansvaginal US appearance of endometrial abnormalities. *RadioGraphics* 1994;14:438—492.

33. Bourne TH, Campbell S, Whitehead MI, et al. Detection of endometrial cancer in postmenopausal women by transvaginal ultrasonography and colour flow imaging. *Br Med J*;1990;301:369.

34. Aleem F, Predanic M, Calame R, Moukhtar M, Pennisi J. Transvaginal color and pulsed Doppler sonography of the endometrium: a possible role in reducing the number of dilation and curettage procedures. *J Ultrasound Med* 1995;14:139—145.

35. Sheth S, Hamper UM, McCollum ME, et al. Endometrial blood flow analysis in postmenopausal women: can it help differentiate benign and malignant causes of endometrial thickening? *Radiology* 1995;195:661—665.

36. Syrop CH, Sahakian V. Transvaginal sonographic detection of endometrial polyps with fluid contrast augmentation. *Obstet Gynecol* 1992;70:1041—1043.

37. Parsons AK, Lense JJ. Sonohysterography for endometrial abnormalities: preliminary results. *J Clin Ultrasound* 1993;21:87—95.

38. Goldstein SR. Use of ultrasonohysterography for triage of perimenopausal patients with unexplained uterine bleeding. *Am J Obstet Gynecol* 1994;170:565—570.

39. Cohen JR, Luxman D, Sagi, et al. Sonohysterography for distinguishing endometrial thickening from endometrial polyps in postmenopausal bleeding. *Ultrasound Obstet Gynecol* 1994;4:227—230.

40. Dubinsky TJ, Parvey R, Gormaz G, Maklad N. Transvaginal hysterosonography in the evaluation of small endoluminal masses. *J Ultrasound Med* 1995;14:1—6.

41. Cullinan JA, Fleischer AC, Kepple DM, Arnold AL. Sonohysterography: a technique for endometrial evalaution. *Radio-Graphics* 1995;15:501—514.

42. Goldchmit R, Katz Z, Blickstein I, Caspi B, Dgani R. The accuracy of endometrial pipelle sampling with and without sonographic measurement of endometrial thickness. *Obstet Gynecol* 1993;82:727—730.

43. Van Den Bosch T, Vandendael A, Van Schourbroeck D, Wranz PAB, Lombard CJ. Combining vaginal ultrasonography and office endometrial sampling in the diagnosis of endometrial disease in postmenopausal women. *Obstet Gynecol* 1995;85:349—352.

44. Weber AM, Belinson JL, Bradly LD, Piedmonte MR. Vaginal ultrasonography versus endometrial biposy in women with postmenopausla bleeding. *Am J Obstet Gynecol* 1997;77:924—929.

45. Feldman S, Cook EF, Harlow BL, Berkowitz RS. Predicitng endometrial cancer among older women who present with abnormal vaginal bleednig. *Gynecol Oncol* 1995;56:376—381.

21 Tamoxifen

Beverly G. Coleman

This chapter is somewhat unique in the sense that the title does not describe a particular clinical symptom. However, the subject matter is extremely relevant and important because Tamoxifen currently is the most widely prescribed endocrine therapy for breast cancer. Dramatic findings that Tamoxifen reduced the rate of breast cancer by an estimated 45% for healthy women over age 34 at increased risk was reported by new agencies worldwide last spring when the Breast Cancer Prevention Trial was halted early.[1] This unusual step was taken so that the 13,000 participants in the U.S.A. and Canada would be unmasked and given the opportunity to take Tamoxifen if they had been randomly assigned to the placebo group. The announcement alone before reports of the detailed study results or recommended guidelines generated so much publicity because breast cancer is the second leading cause of cancer deaths in women. It has long been a major public health problem for Americans accounting for one of every three cancer diagnoses. Estimates are that more than 184,000 cases of invasive cancer will be newly diagnosed this year. In addition, there are many more women at significant risk of subsequently developing breast cancer because of genetic, reproductive, hormonal, and environmental factors. A woman in the United States has a 12.6% or a 1 in 8 risk of developing breast cancer and a 3.6% or 1 in 28 risk of dying from breast cancer over her lifetime.[2] Currently, this disease cannot be prevented and most risk factors cannot be modified. The high rate of morbidity and mortality associated with breast cancer has sparked renewed research efforts directed at the treatment and prevention of this dreaded disease. Therapeutic regimes currently include surgery, radiation, hormones, and/or chemotherapy. Tamoxifen has been one of the most widely used, yet hotly debated treatments to date. Reported serious adverse effects including an increased risk of endometrial cancer and deep venous thrombosis have raised the question of whether the net benefits outweigh the risks.

Tamoxifen: Effects and Mechanism of Action

Tamoxifen is a synthetic, nonsteroidal drug which acts primarily as an estrogen antagonist on breast tissue and as an estrogen agonist on the endometrium. It was introduced in the early 1970s and was found to be widely effective as palliative therapy for women with advanced or recurrent breast cancer. Tamoxifen competes for estrogen receptors when administered to women who produce estrogen, thereby decreasing the net estrogenic effect. It has been hypothesized that Tamoxifen deprives estrogen receptor-positive tumor cells of one of their necessary growth stimulatory factors.[3] Another theory is that Tamoxifen interacts with estrogen receptors to induce synthesis of inhibitory substances that block the growth of mammary tumor cells but do not cause death or eradication of these cells.[4—6] Tamoxifen also has a weak estrogen effect in hypoestrogenic women.[7, 8] About 50% of women with metastatic breast cancer benefit from Tamoxifen.[9] The beneficial effects are most apparent for postmenopausal women with estrogen receptor-positive tumors.

By the 1980s, success of Tamoxifen in the management of advanced breast cancer provoked interest in its utility as adjuvant therapy in the treatment of surgically resected early-stage tumors. Overall survival statistics as well as disease-free survival with reduced recurrence rates have been documented for postmenopausal women when Tamoxifen was added to other treatments. Several clinical trials also demonstrated prolonged disease-free survival for premenopausal women as well as those with estrogen receptor-negative disease.[9] The Scottish trial results suggested that postsurgical treatment with Tamoxifen is more effective in prolonging survival than treatment at first signs of relapse. This data was used to support the rationale for preventative therapy in women at increased risk of developing breast cancer.[10] Large randomized, controlled clinical trials of adjuvant therapy for early-stage breast cancer demonstrated a 35—40% decrease in contralateral breast tumors for women treated with Tamoxifen compared with controls.[11, 12]

Additional reported potential benefits derived from the estrogenic action of Tamoxifen included the stabilization of bone mineral loss which may prevent morbidity due to osteoporosis and, lowered circulating cholesterol levels which may significantly reduce the risk of death from coronary artery disease.[13, 14] However, other researchers worried that the alleged protection afforded by Tamoxifen had been overstated. The initially described effects on the lumbar vertebrae were subsequently disputed, and the controversy has not been resolved. Also, numerous studies report conflicting data on the effects of Tamoxifen on total cholesterol.[15] Experts generally agree that Tamoxifen provides very effective treatment for women with all stages of breast cancer. Evidence now supports the use of long-term adjuvant Tamoxifen therapy for extended periods of up to 5 years in order to prevent the reemergence of tumors.[16] The benefits from 5 years of Tamoxifen therapy persists through 10 years of follow-up with no additional advantage of more prolonged treatment.[17]

Tamoxifen and the Endometrium

Tamoxifen's complex mode of action is not yet completely understood, therefore, its long-term effects on the female genital tract are still being unraveled. Its dual estrogenic and antiestrogenic actions may vary among women. The mechanism of these variations is not well understood and may depend on factors such as body habitus and endogenous estrogen production. Generally, the antiestrogenic effects of Tamoxifen are believed to predominate. Initially, the drug was noted for its relatively low incidence of side effects. Adverse symptoms were believed due to a blockade of estrogen effect and included rapid pulse, hot flashes, irregular menses, and vaginal discharge.[11] Estrogenic changes in the vaginal epithelium of postmenopausal women with breast cancer were then described.[18, 19] Laboratory studies demonstrated Tamoxifen-stimulated growth of human endometrial carcinoma transplanted into athymic mice and breast cancer cells in culture medium.[20] Endometrial hyperplasia, polyps, uterine leiomyomas, uterine sarcomas, adenomyosis, and endometriosis were subsequently described in Tamoxifen-treated patients by numerous researchers who implicated the prolonged estrogenic effects on the sensitive endometrium.[11, 21, 22] The endometrial response to Tamoxifen may even vary according to the menopausal status of the patient. A small study of 46 patients described polyps mainly in younger women treated with Tamoxifen compared to predominantly hyperplastic and neoplastic lesions among postmenopausal women.[23] The first case report of endometrial carcinoma associated with continuous postmenopausal Tamoxifen exposure appeared in 1985 and many others soon followed.[11, 20—24]

The relative risk of endometrial adenocarcinoma in patients with breast cancer has been reported as 1.72, 1.0 in women younger than 50 years, and almost 2.4 in women 70 years or older.[25] In asymptomatic postmenopausal women, the estimated prevalence of endometrial cancer approaches 7 per 1000.[26] In view of these statistics and the uncertain association between these two malignancies, some authorities have suggested that a finite number of women will develop endometrial cancer, irrespective of their treatment protocol for breast cancer.[27] Similarly, several studies have been unable to show an increased risk of endometrial cancer in postmenopausal Tamoxifen-treated patients.[28, 29] Some researchers also raise the issue of whether the increase in incidence of endometrial carcinoma was a true phenomenon or perhaps due to an improved detection rate of very early tumors.[4] A randomized Swedish trial of Tamoxifen in 1846 postmenopausal patients undergoing primary surgery for early breast cancer with median follow-up for 4—5 years reported a 6.5-fold higher occurrence of endometrial cancer in the Tamoxifen group compared to that of controls. In addition, the cumulative frequency of endometrial cancer was significantly greater in those who continued on Tamoxifen compared to those who stopped treatment at 2 years.[30] Supporting data by others have shown relative risks for developing endometrial cancer ranging from 1.7 to 4.6.[31, 32] Both the dose level and duration of Tamoxifen therapy may be relevant to some degree. There may be a dose-dependency relationship associated with the proliferative effects of Tamoxifen on endometrial tissue because the higher-dose Swedish trial had a more dramatic increase in endometrial cancer than other series using Tamoxifen at lower doses of 20 mg daily.[10, 33] However, endometrial cancers have developed in patients on daily dosages ranging from 60—20 mg. In our hospital setting, most patients are prescribed the lower dose of 20 mg daily. A higher frequency of endometrial cancer with increasing duration of therapy has also been reported by other investigators.[30] Endometrial cancer occurring after Tamoxifen therapy is not of a different type with a worse prognosis than are such tumors in non Tamoxifen-treated patients.[16] One recent study advocated pretreatment screening in order to identify patients at a higher risk of developing endometrial cancer. The authors reported a 17.4% incidence of asymptomatic endometrial lesions in 264 postmenopausal women who underwent pelvic sonography before starting Tamoxifen at a daily dose of 20 mg. At 3 years of follow-up, the incidence of atypical endometrial lesions was significantly higher in women with initial lesions compared to those with a normal endometrium on pretreatment scans.[34]

Most researchers concur that there is a definite increased risk of endometrial cancer following chronic Tamoxifen therapy for invasive breast cancer. Therefore, Tamoxifen therapy should continue with close patient monitoring and timely evaluation of relevant clinical complaints. Progestational therapy has been discussed as a means of blunting the estrogen effects of Tamoxifen on the endometrium. Such treatment, however, runs the risk of negating the beneficial effects of Tamoxifen on breast cancer. Although Tamoxifen has proven valuable in the treatment of patients with various stages of breast cancer, some researchers object to its use as prophylaxis in healthy women until further information becomes available. A more stringent standard of safety is believed imperative for a primary prevention measure before it becomes acceptable for the general population.[15] Others report that the benefits of Tamoxifen in saved lives exceeds the incidence of endometrial cancer which is predominately low-grade, well-differentiated disease.[35] However, the benefit—risk ratio must be assessed for each individual especially when Tamoxifen is being considered for prophylaxis. Regardless of how the drug is administered, informed consent should be obtained and rigorous criteria used to monitor all patients. Gynecologic examination, PAP smears, endometrial biopsy, hysteroscopy, and pelvic ultrasound have been described as valuable methods in the follow-up of women on long-term Tamoxifen therapy.[21-23]

Ultrasound Imaging

The imaging approach to evaluating the female pelvis includes both transabdominal (TAS) and transvaginal (TVS) sonography. Ultrasound has undergone tremendous technological advances with the introduction of TVS, affording high-resolution scanning capability with 5—7 Mhz vaginal probes used in close proximity to the pelvic organs. In less than a decade, TVS has become an established tool in the investigation of obstetric and gynecologic pathology. Numerous reports have appeared in the literature describing how this technique supplements the pelvic examination. The role of TVS in the assessment of the uterus, ovaries, fallopian tubes, vessels, and other pelvic structures has continued to expand. The most recent improvements include the introduction of vaginal transducers with color and spectral Doppler capabilities. The ease with which pelvic vessels are demonstrated has virtually eliminated any possibility of confusion of arteries and veins with other structures. In addition, spectral Doppler can be used to analyze areas of color to determine normal and abnormal flow characteristics.

The vaginal technique is very well accepted by most premenopausal and postmenopausal women. Occasionally, we encounter patients who are hesitant about undergoing the procedure, however, the majority acquiesce once the probe and sterile technique are demonstrated. We have two intracavitary probes, and some postmenopausal patients with a narrow introitus can only tolerate the smaller-caliber transducer. TVS permits excellent visualization of the endometrium in the vast majority of women and is far superior to TAS in this regard. The endometrial—myometrial interface is better depicted than was possible with full bladder TAS

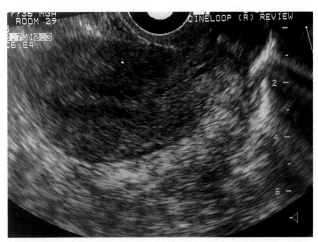

Figure 21–1 Normal postmenopausal uterus. Sagittal TVS depicts the endometrium (**arrow**) as a thin echogenic line. Note the normal surrounding hypoechoic inner myometrium (**arrowhead**).

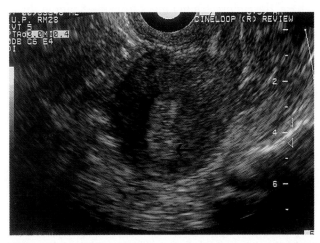

Figure 21–2 Mildly thickened endometrium in retroverted uterus. Sagittal TVS of retroverted uterus in a postmenopausal Tamoxifen-treated patient demonstrates an endometrium (**arrow**) of 10 mm thickness. Atrophy was present on biopsy.

(**Fig. 21–1**). The vaginal technique has been shown to consistently yield additional diagnostic information regarding subtle endometrial changes not detectable with TAS.[36—38] Meticulous scanning techniques may be necessary to image the endometrium of the retroverted or retroflexed uterus, which may lie at odd angles to the incident sound beam (**Fig. 21–2**).

TVS can accurately measure endometrial thickness which is the total measurement across the lumen of the endometrial cavity from one endometrial—myometrial interface to the other. This measurement should be performed with digital calipers in the sagittal plane at the site of maximal thickness which is generally at or just below the uterine fundus. The value obtained actually represents two closely opposed endometrial layers. Endometrial fluid and the hypoechoic, inner compact layer of the myometrium should be excluded in order to avoid overestimation of endometrial thickness (**Fig. 21–3**). In experienced hands, sonographic measurements of the endometrium are usually in excellent agreement among observers and have been shown to correlate well with measurements from gross specimens.[39, 40]

During the menstrual cycle in premenopausal women, the endometrium displays a wide range of appearances that can be correlated to the proliferative, secretory, or menstrual phase. Both the thickness and texture of the endometrium are influenced by the amount of circulating estrogen and progesterone. In the early proliferative phase, the endometrium appears as a slightly irregular, thin echogenic interface. It progressively thickens and develops a multilayered appearance with the opposed endometrial surfaces constituting the central echogenic line, surrounded by the hypoechoic developing functional layer with the basal endometrium as the outer echogenic layer. During the proliferative phase, the endometrium ranges from 4—8 mm in thickness. The secretory phase of the endometrium begins after ovulation and during this time the maximum thickness and echogenicity is achieved. The endometrium at this time ranges from 7—14 mm in thickness. The endometrium has a variable appearance during menses but once the functional layer has shed, it generally becomes thin with the degree of reflectivity based on the presence of blood or clots.

In postmenopausal patients, the endometrium becomes atrophic due to a lack of epithelial stimulation. It appears on sonography as a thin echogenic line that ranges in thickness from 4—8 mm normally (**Fig. 21–1**). The relatively vascular and compact inner third of the myometrium appears as a surrounding hypoechoic halo.[41] It has been shown conclusively that endometrial thickness declines with age, yet measurements may increase to 6—10 mm following hormone replacement therapy. Most experts are advocating biopsy in asymptomatic postmenopausal patients only when the endometrial thickness exceeds 8 mm. Treatment of patients with endometrial thickness from 5—8 mm should be determined on an individual case basis depending upon symptomatology and risk factors. Some women may present for evaluation because of abnormal bleeding due to the friable nature of atrophic endometrial vessels.[42] However, numerous studies have consistently shown that regardless of symptoms, an endometrial thickness of ≤ 4—5 mm is associated with benign histopathology in the vast majority of cases.[43, 44] This threshold level serves as a useful guide for determining which patients should undergo endometrial biopsy. Statistical analysis of the probability of endometrial pathology at a specific thickness indicates that the risk of missing an endometrial abnormality using a single measurement of 5 mm as a cut-off is approximately 5.5%, comparing favorably with the false-negative rate of 4—6% for dilatation and curettage.[45] Unfortunately, this cut-off value cannot be applied to patients on hormone replacement therapy, in whom abnormal bleeding occurs frequently due to breakdown of the atrophic endometrium. It is essential to ascertain which hormonal regimen a patient is actually taking. Commonly used sequential estrogen and progesterone induces the cyclical endometrial changes similar to those occurring in premenopausal patients. Endometrial thickness is, therefore, significantly greater in these women compared to controls, reaching maximum values on days 13—23. These patients should be scanned early in their cycle or near the end of withdrawal bleeding when the endometrium is most likely to be thin. Changes in endometrial thickness greater than 3 mm during a single cycle have been documented in patients on sequential hormones.[46] The use of continuous estrogen and progesterone regimens leads to endometrial atrophy and,

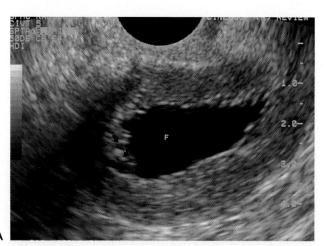
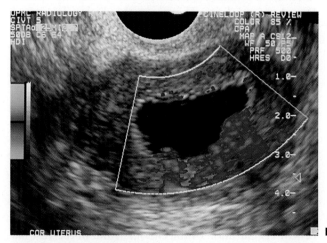

Figure 21–3 Endometrial fluid with tiny endometrial cysts. **A:** Sagittal scan of the uterus in postmenopausal patient on Tamoxifen for approximately 6 months demonstrates a large quantity of endometrial fluid (F) and numerous tiny cysts (**arrows**). **B:** Coronal power Doppler scan demonstrates no areas of hypervascularity in this asymptomatic patient in whom the endometrial abnormalities were first noted incidentally on a renal sonogram.

therefore, endometrial thickness in these patients usually measures within the normal range. Women on unopposed estrogen tend to have a greater percentage of endometrial thickening because of the cellular proliferation that occurs. Biopsy of endometria greater than 8 mm thick is required in these patients because of the known risk of endometrial cancer. Because of the accuracy of endometrial assessment with TVS, serial sonograms may be of value to closely monitor patients at high risk for malignancy. The most important sign of carcinoma, endometrial thickening, unfortunately is not very specific. In symptomatic and asymptomatic patients, benign conditions such as hyperplasia, cystic atrophy, polyps, and proliferation occur more frequently than carcinoma nevertheless, a persistently thickened endometrium is worrisome even in patients on sequential therapy and a change in hormonal regimen or biopsy is indicated. Endometrial fluid in postmenopausal patients is a more common finding than initially thought and is not unusual in women on hormone replacement therapy.[45] It is more often an indicator of benign rather than malignant disorders (**Fig. 21–4, 21–5**). The presence of a moderate degree of fluid helps in evaluating the appearance of the adjacent endometrium which is the most important consideration (**Fig. 21–3**).

Although TVS is very sensitive in visualizing endometrial morphology including abnormal thickening and small fluid collections, the differential diagnosis of such findings in postmenopausal patients includes so many benign disorders that the false-positive rate for malignancy is significant. Recent investigations have assessed uterine blood flow with color Doppler to determine if tumor neovascularity induces detectable arterial changes in endometrial cancer. Transvaginal color Doppler has been used to reproducibly measure impedance to blood flow in the uterine arteries which normally increases with years from menopause. Several researchers

have reported alterations in uterine blood flow with endometrial cancer. One study suggested that the presence of malignant tissue decreases the impedance to blood flow in the main uterine artery. In this series of postmenopausal women, the PI was < 1.8 in all cases of malignancy. The observed changes were possibly due to neoangiogenesis in the endometrial cavity. The authors concluded that the addition of color Doppler decreased the false-positive rate of malignancy while maintaining high overall sensitivity.[47] Another small series of ten cases of endometrial cancer reported low-resistance flow in the arcuate arteries with an average PI of 0.535 ± 0.158 compared to 0.679 ± 0.131 within uterine leiomyomas in twenty-one patients without evidence of cancer.[48] A much larger series of 308 patients reported RI values of 0.58 ± 0.12 for 291 cases of leiomyomas and 0.34 ± 0.03 for 17 cases of endometrial carcinoma. The authors concluded that TVS with color Doppler could be useful in discriminating benign from malignant uterine tumors and that an RI value within a tumor between 0.40 and 0.50 should be regarded as suspicious and those less than 0.40 as malignant.[49] Another large series compared color Doppler findings on TVS with endometrial biopsy which was performed after the sonogram. Of the 227 postmenopausal women investigated, 155 were asymptomatic and 72 had abnormal bleeding. The endometrium was significantly thicker in patients with cancer, compared to those with endometrial atrophy, a mean thickness of 20.2 mm versus 1.35 mm, respectively. The PI value was significantly lower in endometrial cancer compared to atrophy, mean PI 1.00 versus 3.80, respectively. It was hypothesized that estrogens may directly affect the uterine vasculature, and that women on hormone replacement therapy had a markedly decreased resistance to blood flow in the uterine arteries with a mean PI of 2.5.[50] Because the use of color Doppler in the evaluation of the uterine vascula-

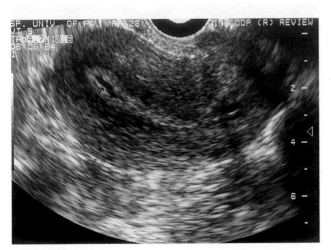

Figure 21–4 Proliferative and inactive endometrium. Sagittal TVS demonstrates a tiny amount of endometrial fluid (**arrow**) in a postmenopausal Tamoxifen-treated patient with abnormal bleeding.

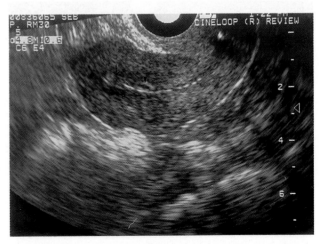

Figure 21–5 In situ cervical carcinoma. Sagittal TVS of the endometrium demonstrates a slightly heterogeneous stripe (**arrow**) with a suggestion of a tiny amount of fluid (**arrowhead**). Histopathology in this Tamoxifen-treated patient revealed inactive endometrium and squamous cell carcinoma of the cervix in situ.

ture has been described in only a few series, its overall significance in the monitoring and evaluation of postmenopausal patients exclusive of the grey scale features on TVS is yet to be determined (**Fig. 21–6**). Whether it adds diagnostic information not available without Doppler must still be answered. Unfortunately, there is likely to be significant overlap between benign and malignant tumors with color Doppler similar to the most recent reports describing problems with color Doppler in discriminating ovarian disease processes. A small series of 45 postmenopausal patients reported low-resistance arterial flow observed in various endometrial diseases with a significant overlap between PI and RI in benign and malignant conditions. In 4 of 9 endometrial cancers, arterial flow was not depicted with color or spectral Doppler presumably due to intravascular thrombosis with tumor emboli proven in two cases. Endometrial polyps were reported as the most common cause of endometrial thickening with the mean PI of polyps actually

lower than that of tumor neovessels in endometrial cancer.[51] However, the various flow patterns of the endometrium seen on color Doppler may help in the differentiation of pathologic conditions involving the postmenopausal endometrium. We have observed endometrial hypervascularity in numerous cases of endometrial polyps with the finding of a prominent feeding vessel supplying an area of endometrial thickening (**Fig. 21–7, 21–8**). Uterine leiomyomas, in my experience as well as that of others, often display low-resistance, high-velocity flow patterns in the periphery of a hypoechoic, heterogeneous, sound-attenuating mass.[52] The concomitant occurrence of leiomyomas, Tamoxifen-induced cystic change and endometrial cancer can pose a diagnostic dilemma when attempting to assess uterine blood flow (**Fig. 21–9, 21–10**). It is therefore unlikely that color Doppler will play any role other than as a complimentary tool perhaps in confusing cases to increase one's diagnostic confidence.

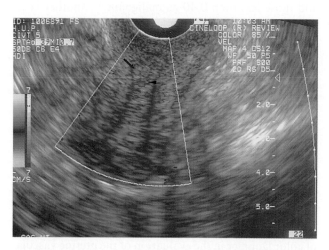

◁ **Figure 21–6** Retroverted uterus with endometrial venous flow. Sagittal TVS was performed in this postmenopausal Tamoxifen-treated patient with abnormal bleeding. The endometrium was thickened in the lower uterine segment (**arrow**) where venous flow was noted (**arrowhead**). Insufficient tissue for diagnosis was obtained on biopsy.

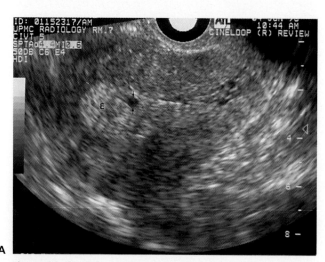

A

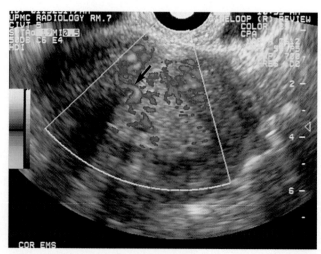

B

Figure 21–7 Endometrial polyp with large feeding vessel. **A:** Sagittal scan in a postmenopausal patient whose endometrial strip has doubled from 12 mm to 24 mm in the past 6 months. The patient has been on Tamoxifen therapy for approximately 4 years.

Endometrial polyps and cystic atrophy were noted at total abdominal hysterectomy and bilateral salpingo-oophorectomy (TAH BSO). Endometrium (E) and tiny cysts (**arrow**). **B:** Coronal power Doppler scan of large feeding vessel (**arrows**).

Figure 21–8 Endometrial polyp and atrophic endometrium. ▷ Sagittal TVS in this patient with abnormal bleeding and a four-year history of Tamoxifen therapy demonstrates a markedly thickened endometrium (E) which had high-velocity, low-resistance flow.

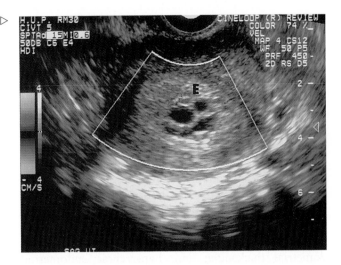

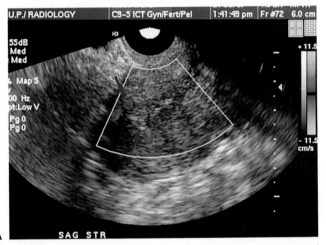

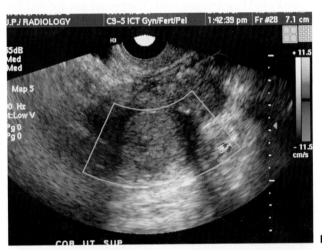

Figure 21–9 Endometrial carcinoma and leiomyomas. **A:** Sagittal color Doppler scan in a postmenopausal patient on Tamoxifen for 11 years in whom the endometrium (**arrows**) was not measured

due to heterogeneity, poor marginal definition and hypervascularity. **B:** Coronal scan of myometrial hypervascularity probably arising in a leiomyoma.

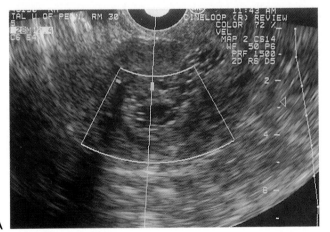

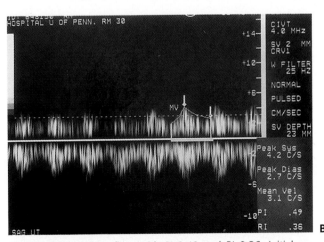

Figure 21–10 Endometrial carcinoma. **A:** Sagittal TVS in this patient on long-term Tamoxifen therapy demonstrated extensive cysts and foci of hypervascularity. **B:** Arterial waveform demon-

strates low-resistance flow with PI 0.49 and RI 0.36. Initial endometrial biopsy yielded benign tissue; however, poorly differentiated adenocarcinoma was subsequently diagnosed.

Benefits of Ultrasound

The radiologist has a pivotal consultant role to play in the utilization of TVS in evaluating symptomatic and asymptomatic Tamoxifen-treated patients. TVS is accepted as a screening tool because it affords excellent visualization of the endometrium and is less invasive than D&C, endometrial biopsy, and hysteroscopy. A normal appearance of the endometrium with TVS reliably excludes significant endometrial pathology. In Tamoxifen-treated patients with an abnormally thickened endometrium, various sonographic patterns have been described including hyperechoic, homogeneous endometrial thickening; hyperechoic, heterogeneous endometrial thickening; and, hyperechoic endometrial thickening with cystic spaces which vary in size and number.[53] These endometrial changes are not specific for Tamoxifen-treated patients and may actually be seen in asymptomatic postmenopausal patients without a contributory history. In our experience, the extensive cystic changes that may occur in and around the endometrium are unique and more typical of Tamoxifen stimulation. Careful inspection of the endometrial echotexture may be helpful in distinguishing between different endometrial processes. Although studies have correlated changes in the texture and thickness of the endometrium with histopathology, there is no particular distinguishing sonographic feature that permits a specific diagnosis (**Fig. 21–11**). One study suggested that a well-defined, thickened, very echogenic endometrial cavity was highly suggestive of hyperplasia yet we have noted similar findings in polyps (**Fig. 21–12**). Endometrial carcinoma on the other hand, appeared as an irregular, thickened, hyperechoic area of the endometrium with accompanying loss of the hypoechoic inner myometrial layer.[54] However, in our experience, Tamoxifen-treated patients not infrequently have mixed histology following biopsy and we have seen poor definition of the subendometrial layer in various conditions (**Fig. 21–13**). One report of endometrial polyps in postmenopausal patients on Tamoxifen described two cases of endometrial carcinoma actually occurring within the polyps.[55]

Perhaps one of the most intriguing aspects of endometrial abnormalities in Tamoxifen treated patients has been the finding of atrophy and insufficient tissue for diagnosis in patients with markedly thickened endometria and multiple small cysts (**Fig. 21–14** through **21–16**). These findings were originally felt to be due to atypical, complex hyperplasia or endometrial polyps with cystically dilated glands.[56,57] Sonohysterography (SHG), in which sterile saline is instilled into the endometrial cavity, has been helpful in improving the direct visualization of the endometrium. In a high percentage of cases, the associated polyps with cystic change are well outlined by the adjacent fluid (**Fig. 21–17, 21–18**). In addition, researchers have found that the heterogeneous, bizarre appearance of the endometrium was actually due to subendometrial cystic change occurring in the inner myometrial layer.[58] The endometrium in these patients is actually quite thin which explains the histologic diagnosis of benign or atrophic endometrium as well as the frequent lack of clinical signs, such as abnormal bleeding, which often heralds endometrial malignancy or hyperplasia. In some cases it may be virtually impossible to discern the exact site of diffuse cystic change (**Fig. 21–15**).

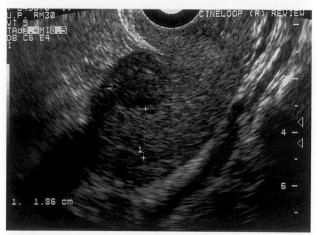

Figure 21–11 Chronic endometritis. Sagittal TVS in this postmenopausal Tamoxifen-treated patient demonstrates marked endometrial thickening (**cursors**) and fibroids (**arrow**).

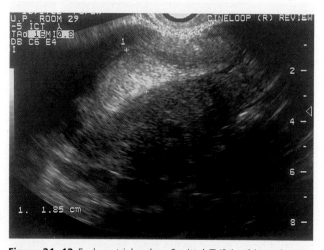

Figure 21–12 Endometrial polyp. Sagittal TVS in this patient on Tamoxifen for 2 years depicted a markedly thickened, highly reflective endometrium (**cursors**). An endometrial polyp was surgically resected.

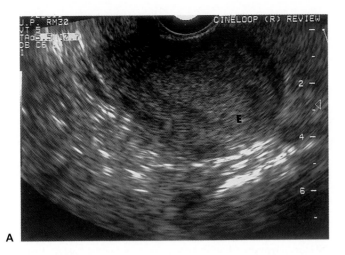

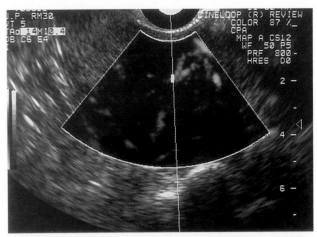

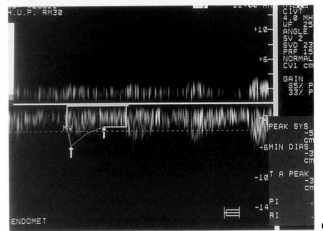

Figure 21–13 Endometrial polyp and complex hyperplasia. **A:** Sagittal TVS in patient on Tamoxifen for 4 years shows a heterogeneous, markedly thickened endometrium (E). **B:** Power Doppler scan of areas of endometrial hypervascularity. **C:** Arterial waveform of low resistance flow with PI 0.60 and RI 0.45.

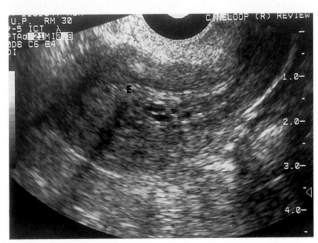

Figure 21–14 Benign inactive endometrium. Sagittal TVS of several ▷ tiny cystic spaces (**arrows**) which are most likely arising from the inner myometrium rather than the endometrium (E).

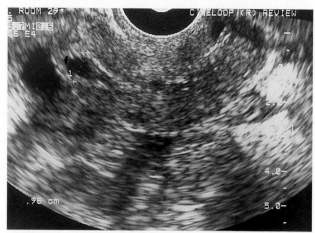

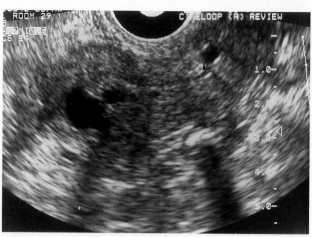

Figure 21–15 Endometrium with cystic atrophy. **A:** Sagittal TVS of thickened endometrium (**cursors**) with questionable fluid (f). **B:** At TAH BSO, multiple endometrial cysts (**arrow**) and endocervi- cal cysts (**arrowhead**) were noted. The endometrial cavity actually measured 2.5 x 2 cm.

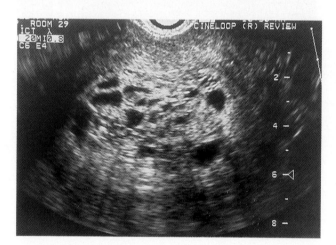

Figure 21–16 Cystic atrophy and endometrial polyp. Coronal TVS of markedly thickened, highly reflective endometrium with numerous cysts of various sizes.

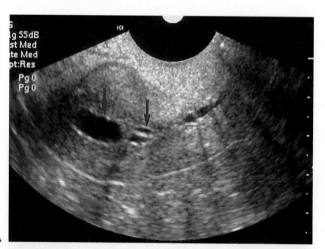

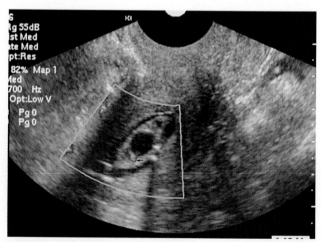

Figure 21–17 Endometrial polyp with cystic change. **A:** Sagittal TVS of one large and several tiny central cysts (**arrows**) which ob- scure the endometrium in this patient on Tamoxifen for 3.5 years with a progressively thickened stripe on serial studies. **B:** Sagittal TVS from SHG of large feeding vessel (**arrows**) within a solitary polyp with cystic change.

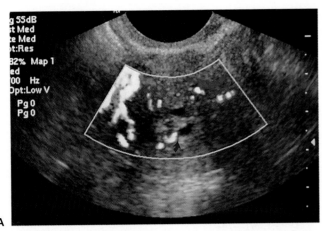

A

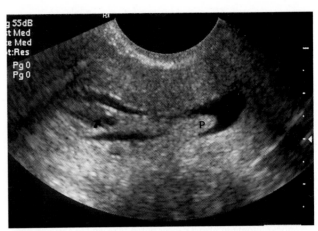

B

Figure 21–18 Endometrial polyp with cystic change. **A:** Power Doppler scan of large feeding vessel (**arrow**) supplying a focal area of thickening in the uterine fundus in this patient who has been on Tamoxifen for 4.5 years. **B:** During SHG, a large broad-based pedunculated polyp (**arrows**) originating from the fundus was noted with a tiny area of cystic change (**arrowhead**).

Summary

TVS is widely available, readily accepted by most postmenopausal patients, relatively inexpensive, and the least invasive method other than gynecologic examination for the evaluation of patients on long-term Tamoxifen. Because Tamoxifen will probably be increasingly used in more patients who will require close monitoring, the radiologist will often be responsible for the actual triage of cases. TVS with the added benefits of SHG is simple and can be performed in the office setting. Those asymptomatic patients who have a normal appearing endometrium on TVS can be conservatively referred for follow-up sonograms. On the other hand, SHG is likely the preferred method of evaluating asymptomatic Tamoxifen-treated patients with heterogeneous, markedly thickened endometria on TVS. This procedure affords excellent visualization of the endometrium and may actually obviate the need for more invasive and costly surgical procedures such as hysteroscopy. Endometrial sampling, if necessary, can be performed precisely at the site of the abnormality noted on SHG. Increasing use of this procedure will hopefully decrease the frequency of unsuccessful, "blind" endometrial biopsies in which insufficient tissue for diagnosis is obtained.

References

1. McCullough M. Breast cancer breakthrough: drug cuts rates in study. *Philadelphia Inquirer*, April 5, 1998, PC1.
2. Breast Cancer Facts and Figures, American Cancer Society Surveillance Research, 1995, p. 1—12.
3. Rutqvist LE, Cedermark B, Fornander T. The relationship between hormone receptor content, and the effect of adjuvant Tamoxifen in operable breast cancer. *J Clin Oncol* 1989;7:1474—1484.
4. Wolf DM, Jordan VC. Gynecologic complications associated with long-term adjuvant Tamoxifen therapy for breast cancer. *Gynecol Oncol* 1992;45:118—128.
5. Jordan VC, Lababidi MK, Langan-Fahey S. Suppression of mouse mammary tumorigenesis by long-term Tamoxifen therapy. *J Natl Cancer Inst* 1991;83:492—496.
6. Osborne CK, Boldt DH, Clark GM, et al. Effects of Tamoxifen on human breast cancer cell cycle kinetics: accumulation of cells in early G_1 phase. *Cancer Res* 1983;43:3583—3585.
7. Harper MJK, Walpole P. A new derivative of triphenylethelene: effect on implantation and mode of action in rats. *J Reprod Fertil* 1967; 13:101—119.
8. Jordan GV. Long-term adjuvant Tamoxifen therapy for breast cancer. *Breast Cancer Res Treat* 1990;15:125—136.
9. Early breast cancer trialists' collaborative group: effects of adjuvant Tamoxifen and of cytotoxic therapy on mortality in early breast cancer. An overview of 61 randomized trials among 28,896 women. *N Engl J Med* 1988; 319:1681—1692.
10. Breast cancer trials committee, Scottish cancer trials office (MRC), Edinburgh: adjuvant Tamoxifen in the management of operable breast cancer: the Scottish trial. *Lancet* 1987;2:171—175.
11. Nayfield SG, Karp JE, Ford LG, Door FA, Kramer BS. Potential role of Tamoxifen in prevention of breast cancer. *J Natl Cancer Inst* 1991;83:1450—1459.
12. Bonadonna G, Valagussa P, Brambilla C, et al. Adjuvant and neoadjuvant treatment of breast cancers with chemotherapy and endocrine therapy. *Semin Oncol* 1991;18:515—524.
13. Prentice RL. Tamoxifen as a potential preventive agent in healthy postmenopausal women. *J Natl Cancer Inst* 1990;82:1310—1311.
14. Turken S, Siris E, Seldin D, et al. Effects of Tamoxifen on spinal bone density in women with breast cancer. *J Natl Cancer Inst* 1989;81:1086—1088.
15. Fugh-Berman A, Epstein S. Tamoxifen: disease prevention or disease substitution? *Lancet* 1992;340:1143—1145.
16. Fisher B, Costantino J, Redmond L, et al. A randomized, clinical trial evaluating Tamoxifen in the treatment of patients with node negative breast cancer who have estrogen receptor-positive tumors. *New Engl J Med* 1989;320:479—484.
17. Fisher B, Dignam J, Bryant J, et al. Five vs. more than five years of Tamoxifen therapy for breast cancer patients with negative lymph nodes in estrogen receptor positve tumors. *J Natl Cancer Institute* 1996;88:1529—1542.
18. Ferrazzi E, Cortei G, Mattarazzo R, et al. Estrogen-like effect of Tamoxifen on vaginal epithelium. *Br Med J* 1977;1:1351—1352.

19. Boccardo F, Bruzzi P, Rubagotti A, et al. Estrogen-like action of Tamoxifen on vaginal epithelium in breast cancer patients. *Oncology* 1981;38:281—285.

20. Satyaswaroop PG, Zaino RJ, Mortel R. Estrogen-like effects of Tamoxifen on human endometrial carcinoma transplanted into nude mice. *Cancer Res* 1984;44:4006—4010.

21. Cohen I, Altaras MM, Shapira J, Tepper R, Beyth Y. Postmenopausal Tamoxifen treatment and endometrial pathology. *Obstet Gynecol Survey* 1994;49:823—829.

22. Muhieddine AFS, Johnson J, Weed JC Jr. Gynecologic tumors in Tamoxifen treated women with breast cancer. *Obstet Gynecol* 1993;82:165—169.

23. Muylder X, Neven P, DeSomer M, et al. Endometrial lesions in patients undergoing Tamoxifen therapy. *Int J Gynaecol Obstet* 1991;36:127—130.

24. Killackey MA, Hakes TB, Pierce VK, et al. Endometrial adenocarcinoma in breast cancer patients receiving antiestrogens. *Cancer Treat Rep* 1985;69:237—238.

25. Adami HO, Kruesmo UB, Bergvist L, Person I, Pettersson B. On the age-dependent association between cancer of the breast and of the endometrium: A nationwide cohort study. *Br J Cancer* 1987;55:77—80.

26. Koss L, Schreiber K, Oberlander S, et al. Detection of endometrial carcinoma and hyperplasia in asymptomatic women. *Obstet Gynecol* 1984;64:1—11.

27. Ugwumadu AHN, Bower D, Kin-Hoi Ho P. Tamoxifen induced adenomyosis and adenomyomatous endometrial polyp. *Br J Obstet Gynaecol* 1993;100:386—388.

28. Stewart HJ, Knight GM. Tamoxifen and the uterus and endometrium. *Lancet* 1989;1:375—376.

29. Ribeiro G, Swindell R. The Chrisite Hospital adjuvant Tamoxifen trial: status at 10 years. *Br J Cancer* 1988;57:601—603.

30. Fornander T, Cedermark B, Mattsson A, et al. Adjuvant Tamoxifen in early breast cancer: occurrence of new primary cancers. *Lancet* 1989;21:117—120.

31. Andersson M, Storm HH, Mouridsen HT. Incidence of new primary cancers after adjuvant therapy for early breast cancer. *J Natl Cancer Inst* 1991;83:1013—1017.

32. Cohen I, Rosen DJD, Shapira J, et al. Endometrial changes with Tamoxifen: comparison between Tamoxifen-treated and nontreated asymptomatic, postmenopausal breast cancer patients. *Gynecol Oncol* 1994;52:185—190.

33. Fisher B, Costantino JT, Redmond CK, et al. Endometrial cancer in Tamoxifen-treated breast cancer patients: findings from the National Surgical Adjuvant Breast and Bowel Project (NSABP) B-14. *J Natl Cancer Inst* 1994;86:527—537.

34. Berliere M, Charles A, Gallant C, Donnez J. Uterine side-effects of Tamoxifen: a need for systematic pretreatment screening. *Obst Gynecol* 1998;91:40—44.

35. Assikis VJ, Jordan VC. Risks and benefits of Tamoxifen therapy. *Oncology* 1997;11:21—23.

36. Love RR. Tamoxifen prophylaxis in breast cancer. *Oncology* 1992;6:33—43.

37. Mendelson EB, Bohm-Velez M, Joseph N, Neiman HL. Endometrial abnormalities: evaluation with transvaginal sonography. *AJR* 1988;150:139—142.

38. Coleman BG, Arger PH, Grumbach K, et al. Transvaginal and transabdominal sonography: prospective comparison. *Radiology* 1988;168:639—643.

39. Tessler FN, Schiller VL, Perrella RR, Sutherland ML, Grant EG. Transabdominal vs. endovaginal pelvic sonography: prospective study. *Radiology* 1989;170:553—556.

40. Karlsson B, Granberg S, Ridell B, Wikland M. Endometrial thickness as measured by transvaginal sonography: interobserver variation. *Ultrasound Obstet Gynecol* 1994;4:320—325.

41. Fleischer AC, Kalemeris GC, Machin JE, Entman SS, James AE, Jr. Sonographic depiction of normal and abnormal endometrium with histopathologic correlation. *J Ultrasound Med* 1986;5:445—452.

42. Goldstein SR, Nachtigall M, Snyder JR, Nachtigall L. Endometrial assessment by vaginal ultrasonography before endometrial sampling in patients with postmenopausal bleeding. *Am J Obstet Gynecol* 1990;163:119—123.

43. Granberg S, Wikland M, Karlsson B, Norstrom A, Fribert L-G. Endometrial thickness as measured by endovaginal ultrasonography for identifying endometrial abnormality. *Am J Obstet Gynecol* 1991;164:47—52.

44. Levine D. Postmenopausal pelvis. *Ultrasound* 1995;13:75—86.

45. Granberg S, Bourne TH. Transvaginal ultrasonography of endometrial disorders in postmenopausal women. *Ultrasound* 1995;13:61—74.

46. Levine D, Gosink BB, Johnson LA. Change in endometrial thickness in postmenopausal women undergoing hormone replacement therapy. *Radiology* 1995;197:603—608.

47. Bourne TH, Campbell S, Steer C, et al. Detection of endometrial cancer by transvaginal ultrasonography with color flow imaging and blood flow analysis: a preliminary report. *Gynecol Oncol* 1991;40:253—259.

48. Hata K, Makihara K, Hata T, Takahashi K, Kitao M. Transvaginal color Doppler imaging for hemodynamic assessment of tumors in the reproductive tract. *Int J Gynecol Obstet* 1991;38:301—308.

49. Kurjak A, Zalud I, Jurkovic D, Alfirovic Z, Miljan M. Transvaginal color Doppler for the assessment of pelvic circulation. *Acta Obstet Gynecol Scand* 1989;68:131—135.

50. Bourne TH, Crayford T, Hampson J, Collins WP, Campbell S. The detection of endometrial cancer by transvaginal ultrasonography with color Doppler. *Ultrasound Obstet Gynecol* 1992;2:75—80.

51. Sheth S, Hamper UM, McCollum ME, et al. Endometrial blood flow analysis in postmenopausal women: can it help differentiate benign from malignant causes of endometrial thickening? *Radiology* 1995;195:661—665.

52. Creighton S, Bourne TH, Lawton F, et al. Use of transvaginal ultrasonography with color Doppler imaging to determine an appropriate treatment regimen for uterine fibroids with a GnRH agonist before surgery: a preliminary study. *Ultrasound Obstet Gynecol* 1994;4:494—498.

53. Hulka CA, Hall DA. Endometrial abnormalities associated with Tamoxifen therapy for breast cancer: sonographic and pathologic correlation. *AJR* 1992;160:809—812.

54. Nasri MN, Shepherd JH, Setchell ME, Lowe DG, Chard P. The role of vaginal scan in measurement of endometrial thickness in postmenopausal women. *Br J Obstet Gynaecol* 1991;98:470—475.

55. Nuovo MA, Nuovo GJ, McCaffrey RM, et al. Endometrial polyps in postmenopausal patients receiving Tamoxifen. *Int J Gynecol Pathol* 1989;8:125—131.

56. Kedar RP, Bourne TH, Powles TJ, et al. Effects of Tamoxifen on the uterus and ovaries of women involved in a randomized breast cancer prevention trial. *Lancet* 1994;343:1318—1321.

57. Corley D, Rowe J, Curtis MT, et al. Postmenopausal bleeding from unusual endometrial polyps in women on chronic Tamoxifen therapy. *Obstet Gynecol* 1992;79:111—116.

58. Goldstein SR. Unusual ultrasonographic appearance of the uterus in patients receiving Tamoxifen. *Am J Obstet Gynecol* 1994;170:447—451.

22 The Use of Ultrasound in the Evaluation and Treatment of the Infertile Woman

Kurt Barnhart and Christos Coutifaris

Introduction

The advent of high-resolution ultrasonographic imaging has revolutionized the diagnosis and treatment of many gynecologic conditions. Perhaps one of the greatest applications of this advanced technology has been in the management and diagnosis of the infertile couple. Ultrasound imaging, and, in particular, transvaginal sonography provides a very detailed and reproducible image of the female pelvis. Most vaginal transducers operate at 5 to 7.5 MHz, which allows the use of high-frequency sound in close proximity to the organs under study.

The use of ultrasound in the management of infertility can be divided into two main categories: (1) diagnosis and (2) monitoring of treatment. Ultrasound used for diagnosis can evaluate normal pelvic anatomy and pathology, but it can also be applied for monitoring the normal menstrual cycles and endometrial and follicular development. Additionally, ultrasound is used to monitor the progression of follicular development during controlled ovarian stimulation, optimize the timing of inseminations, and reduce the potential of development of ovarian hyperstimulation syndrome. Finally, ultrasound is also an integral part of in vitro fertilization (IVF) monitoring and treatment, allowing real-time guidance for transvaginal ovum retrieval and optimizing the transfer of embryos into the uterus.

Diagnosis

Ultrasound imaging of the female pelvis allows visualization of the uterus and distinction between myometrium and endometrium.[1] Transvaginal ultrasound also allows detailed imaging of the ovaries, both in the determination of size and shape, but also provides closer scrutiny of the internal ovarian structure, such as ovarian follicles and stroma. While normal fallopian tubes cannot be visualized by ultrasound, the pathologic changes of the fallopian tubes, such as a collection of clear fluid (hydrosalpinx) or collection of inflammatory fluid and debris (pyosalpinx) are readily and reproducibly identifiable.[1] A transvaginal ultrasound examination is an important component of the workup for women with impaired fertility.

A pretreatment or baseline ultrasound starts with a structural evaluation of the uterus in the long axis and coronal planes. Uterine size consistency in the presence or absence of leiomyomata should be noted. The cervix can be evaluated by measuring its length from the internal to the external os and for any pathology. Measuring the cervix and the endometrium is accomplished on the saggital long-axis view. The endometrial lining can be visualized and characterized by its appearance and size. Ultrasound of the ovaries can be used to identify and describe their location, mobility, and appearance. Information can be obtained evaluating the number and size of ovarian follicles and the presence and characterization of a cystic, solid or complex ovarian mass. Other ultrasound findings which may assist in the diagnosis of pelvic pathology includes examination of the peritoneum for free fluid and evaluation of the urinary bladder. Small amounts of fluid in the lower pelvis can be visualized with ultrasound and is a normal finding. If a large amount of abdominal or pelvic fluid is suspected, the space between the liver and the right kidney should be examined. Examination of the urinary bladder can be used to identify extrinsic or intrinsic pathologic masses.

Evaluation of the Uterus

The normal globular shape of the fundus is easily identifiable with ultrasound. Congenital uterine malformations (lateral fusion defects) such as a didelphys or a bicornuate or septate uterus can be identified with the use of transvaginal ultrasound (**Fig. 22–1**). Tracing the hyperechoic endometrial stripe to a bifurcation identifying a left and right uterine horn can identify an abnormal shape of the uterine cavity. Additionally, a bicornuate uterus can be identified by the wide appearance of the uterine body with a fundal notch. Transvaginal ultrasound can be accurate in the identification of a uterine malformation. However, the distinction between bicornuate uterus and the presence of a uterine septum often needs to be resolved with a magnetic resonance imaging (MRI) examination or laparoscopic evaluation. Alternative techniques to better visualize the shape of the uterine cavity include hysteroscopy and hysterosalpingography. It is best to confirm suspected uterine anomalies by an ultrasonographic examination during the secretory

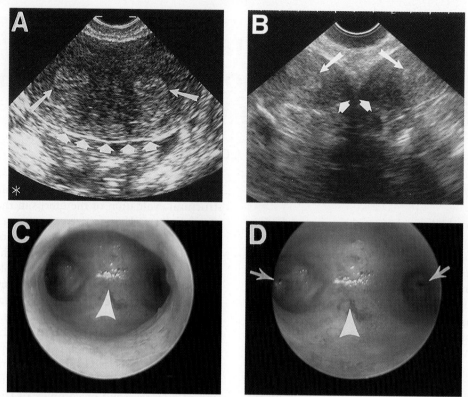

Figure 22–1 Congenital uterine anomalies. Ultrasonographic appearance of a septate (**A**) and bicornuate (**B**) uterus. The endometrium in each cavity is clearly seen (**long arrows**). Note that in the case of the septate uterus (**A**), the cavities are localized within a uniform uterine body (**short arrows**) while in the case of the bicornuate uterus (**B**), there is a notch (**short arrows**) giving the appearance of two separate fundal uterine bodies. On hysteroscopy (**C,D**) a view from the lower uterine segment (**C**) identifies the presence of two cavities separated by a thick midline structure (**arrowhead**). On closer view (**D**), the cavities continue to be distinct and the tubal ostia can be visualized (arrows). Both **C** and **D** represent a septum from the same patient but note that the hysteroscopic view of a bicornuate uterus would be identical to the one shown in the figure. Only through evaluation of the uterine body, can the two uterine malformations be distinguished.

phase of the cycle as the hyperechoic endometrium tends to delineate better the shape of the cavity or cavities.

Additional pathology of the myometrium, such as the presence of leiomyomata, can be also readily identified with ultrasound (**Fig. 22–2**). The characteristic circumferential swirling pattern of a fibroid can be noted and delineated. Frequently, calcifications obstruct the transmission of sound and produce a characteristic "shading" behind the myoma, further confirming the diagnosis. Most importantly, the location of the fibroids in relation to the endometrial cavity, lower uterine segment or uterine fundus should be evaluated. It should be noted that myomata impinging into the endometrial cavity are the ones that are of clinical significance with respect to infertility and should be carefully excluded during the preliminary workup of the woman seeking evaluation for infertility.

The endometrial cavity is a potential space identifiable on ultrasound by the convergence of the hyperechoic endometrium on the anterior and posterior surface. Sonographically, the interface of the two endometrial surfaces appears as a thin echogenic line. The endometrial stripe varies in thickness and appearance depending on the stage of the menstrual cycle or the use of exogenous hormones (**Fig. 22–3**). Measurement of the endometrial stripe thickness should be performed on the long axis with a combined anterior/posterior measurement. If fluid is found in the uterine cavity, the measurement should exclude the fluid interface. The endometrium increases in thickness throughout the follicular phase in response to the rising estrogen serum concentrations. In the days preceding ovulation, a clear, trilaminar pattern is apparent. The luteal phase of the menstrual cycle is notable for high progesterone serum concentration, which changes the endometrium into a secretory histologic pattern. The appearance of a secretory endometrium on ultrasound is characterized by increased echogenecity and a loss of the trilaminar pattern (**Fig. 22–3**). The endometrial stripe should be traced from the cervix to the uterine fundus. Irregularities or deformities of the endometrial stripe may be suggestive of intracavitary lesions such as endometrial polyps or submucosal myomata (**Fig. 22–4**).[2] Further delineation of potential intracavitary lesions can be per-

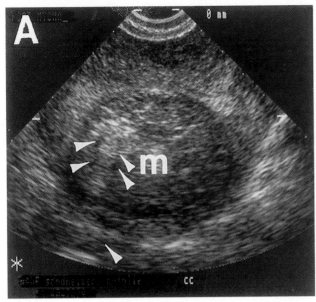
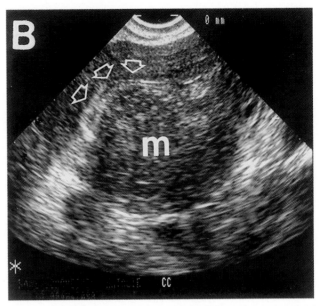

Figure 22–2   Uterine myoma. Ultrasonographic appearance of a uterine myoma (**m**) showing some calcifications with some minimal characteristic "shadowing" (**arrowheads**). Note the submucosal component of the myoma which clearly distorts the endometrial cavity (**B**; **open arrows**).

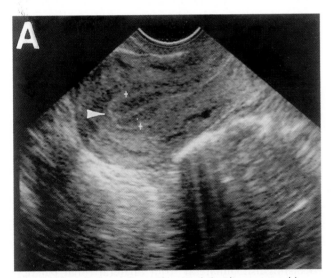
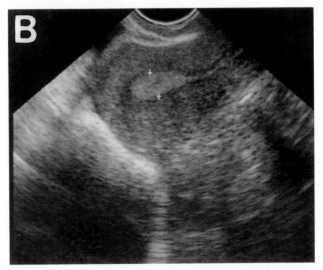

Figure 22–3   Endometrium. Characteristic ultrasonographic appearance of proliferative (**A**) and secretory (**B**) endometrium. Note the trilaminar appearance of proliferative endometrium with the echogenic line (**arrowhead**) at the point where the anterior and the posterior endometrium abut on each other. This is in contrast to the uniformly echogenic appearance of secretory endometrium during the progesterone-dominated luteal phase of the menstrual cycle (**B**).

formed by the injection of saline into the endometrial cavity while performing vaginal ultrasound, a procedure called *sonohysterography*. Sonohysterography is best performed in the early proliferative phase of a woman's menstrual cycle when there is thinner proliferative endometrium.

Evaluation of the Fallopian Tubes

Under normal circumstances, a fallopian tube cannot be visualized with ultrasound. However, in a pathologic state, the fallopian tube is readily identifiable. Ultrasonographic findings of a collection of fluid in a tubular-shaped structure suggest the presence of a hydrosalpinx (**Fig. 22–5**).

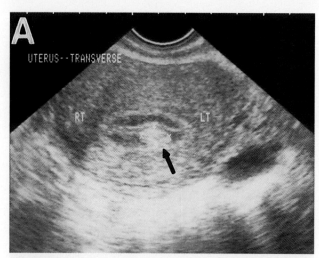

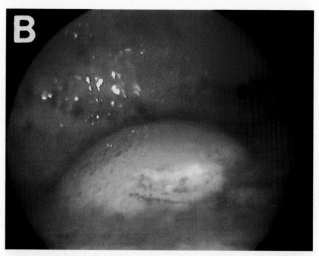

Figure 22–4 Endometrial polyp. Screening ultrasound in the proliferative phase uncovered an echogenic 1 × 2 cm focus within the endometrium (**arrow**). A sessile endometrial polyp was visualized and excised during hysteroscopic evaluation of the endometrial cavity (**B**).

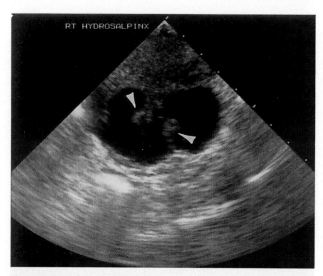

Figure 22–5 Hydrosalpinx. The presence of a hydrosalpinx can be suspected if, on ultrasound, a tubular structure is appreciated in the adnexa which frequently has the appearance of internal partial septations (**arrowheads**) as the large, fluid-filled fallopian tube is folded onto itself secondary to pelvic adhesions. It is critical to determine whether what is ultrasonographically diagnosed as hydrosalpinx is clearly separate from the ovary as ovarian neoplasms can present with similar ultrasonographic configuration. Due to the close anatomic proximity of fallopian tube and ovary, this can often be difficult.

The accurate identification of a hydrosalpinx is very important because its presence signifies a nonpatent tube. Additionally, the presence of a hydrosalpinx is negatively associated with successes with in vitro fertilization. A complex mass with fluid levels in close proximity to the ovaries suggests the possibility of a tuboovarian abscess. While the presence of an isolated fallopian tube complex mass can be identified with ultrasound, this condition, which may be suspicious for primary fallopian tube cancer, is very rare.

Recently, there has been increased interest in the assessment of fallopian tube patency with the use of ultrasound. Using high-resolution ultrasound in combination with injection of normal saline or air, the patency of the fallopian tubes can be assessed with the visualization of bubbles passing through the fallopian tube or the accumulation of air in the peritoneal cavity.[3] While technology is improving in the visualization of the fallopian tube, currently, these techniques suffer from the inability to distinguish unilateral from bilateral tubal patency. Traditional assessment of the fallopian tube with the use of hysterosalpingogram or laparoscopic chromopertubation is still considered the gold standard in assessing fallopian tube patency.

Evaluation of the Ovaries

Transvaginal ultrasound can be used to identify and describe the location, mobility, and appearance of the ovaries. Ovarian follicles are readily identified by their characteristic hypoechoic, circular appearance within the capsule of the ovary. The number and size of follicles on each ovary can easily be documented. In many cases, this may provide information about infertility, such as the presence or absence of a dominant follicle, the presence of a corpus luteum, or sonographic findings that may suggest the presence of polycystic ovarian syndrome (**Fig. 22–6**). For proper interpretation of ultrasound findings, it is of paramount importance to know the time in the menstrual cycle that the ultrasound is being performed.

The presence of ovarian follicles is a normal physiologic finding. Antral ovarian follicles can be identified when they are as small as 3 to 5 mm. As folliculogenesis progresses, a certain number of antral follicles will start to mature, and the follicular size will increase. When an ovarian follicle has reached a minimum size of approximately 1 cm it should be considered to be among the cohort of follicles that may be ovulate in the current cycle. By day nine or ten of the menstrual cycle, a dominant follicle ranging in size form 1.2 to 2 cm should be apparent. This follicle will increase in size to approximately 2 to 2.5 cm before ovulation. Ovulation usually occurs on day 14 or 15 of a 28-day menstrual cycle.

If ultrasound is performed at the time of ovulation, a collapse of the follicle can be noted. However, this follicle frequently will reexpand with fluid/blood within 24 to 48 h and eventually have the characteristics confirming its transition into that of a corpus luteum cyst (**Fig. 22–7**). Sonographic signs of ovulation include a reduction in the size of a previously seen large follicle and the simultaneous appearance of small amounts of fluid in the cul-de-sac that was not previously seen.[4] A corpus luteum has the characteristic ultrasound findings of cobwebbing or increased echogenecity and size ranging from 1.5 to 3 cm (**Fig. 22–7**).

During the evaluation of the infertile woman, frequently ultrasound examinations uncover abnormal ovarian masses. Most often, these prove to be functional follicular or corpus luteum cysts, but other pathology, such as endometriomas, dermoids or malignant ovarian neoplasms can be unexpectedly uncovered. The size and internal structures of an ovarian cystic structure should be identified and reported. Functional ovarian cysts range in size from 2 to 4 cm. Characteristic findings of a functional ovarian cyst include a simple, thin, regular cyst wall and contents without internal echoes. Findings characteristic of an endometrioma include a ground glass appearance of the internal contents of an ovarian cyst (**Fig. 22–8**). Complex ovarian masses with fluid levels, internal excrescences, multiple septations, a thick wall, and lack of mobility increase the risk that the visualized ovarian mass may be that of a neoplasm (**Fig. 22–9**).[5] It should be stressed that ultrasound is not diagnostic of a neoplastic ovarian process and further evaluation needs to be undertaken. Frequently, a repeat ultrasound

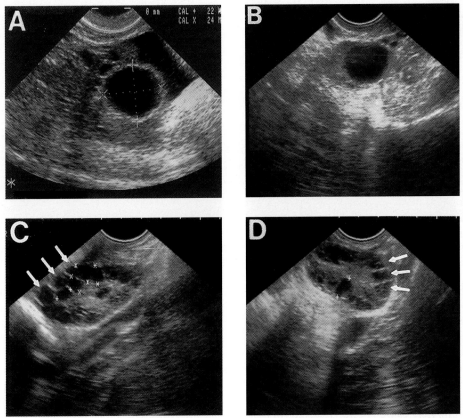

Figure 22–6 Folliculogenesis. Ultrasonographic appearance of preovulatory follicles (**A "B**) during an unstimulated menstrual cycle. Note that the diameter of a mature human follicle just prior to ovulation is between 20 and 30 mm. Characteristic appearance of the ovaries (**C,D**) of a spontaneously anovulatory patient with polycystic ovarian syndrome. Note the distribution of small (less than 8 mm), follicular structures distributed in the periphery of the ovaries (**arrows**).

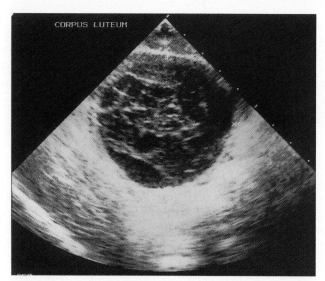

Figure 22–7 Ultrasonographic appearance of an early corpus luteum. Immediately following ovulation, frequently the follicular cavity fills with blood which eventually clots and then partially liquefies. Thus, frequently in the midluteal phase, the corpus luteum has the characteristic appearance on ultrasound shown in this figure. Note the "cobweb" appearance within the substance of the cystic structure. Upon gentle intermittent pressure with the vaginal transducer, the internal echogenic foci can be seen shaking as they represent the partially solid components of a clot.

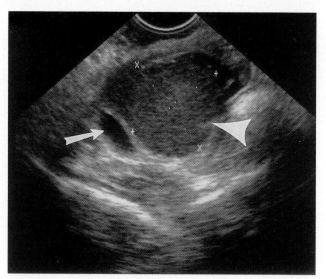

Figure 22–8 Endometrioma. The ultrasonographic appearance of the endometrioma (**arrowhead**) has uniformly increased echogenecity from old, liquefied blood and contrasts sharply to the echolucent appearance of a developing follicle (**arrow**).

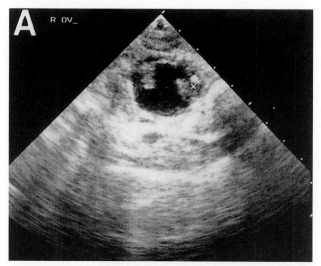

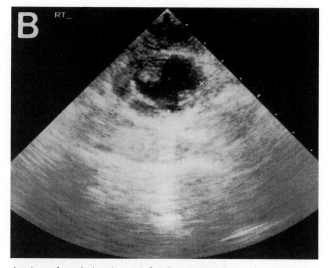

Figure 22–9 Borderline ovarian neoplasm. Ultrasonographic appearance of a 2.5-cm cystic ovarian mass with internal excrescences found on screening transvaginal ultrasound before initiation of induction of ovulation in an infertility patient (**A**). When the mass failed to regress one menstrual cycle later (**B**), surgical excision revealed an epithelial ovarian neoplasm of low malignant potential.

examination following the patient's menses or following hormonal suppression with oral contraceptives or gonadotropin releasing hormone analogs, is needed to evaluate the persistence of the mass. If, after treatment, the mass has failed to regress, or has grown, surgical excision is the preferred approach in order to obtain histologic diagnosis of the process. With the exception of thin-walled, simple cysts without internal echoes in women of reproductive years, cystic ovarian masses should not be aspirated as they usually reaccumulate the fluid. Most importantly though, cyst aspiration invariably induces some fluid spillage in the peritoneal cavity,

which, in the case of a malignant neoplasm, will change the patient's subsequent staging and possibly ultimate prognosis. It should be stressed that under no circumstances should cyst aspiration be undertaken in the postmenopausal woman as the risk of ovarian malignancy increases with age. In today's era of assisted reproduction and the possibility of achieving a pregnancy in the postmenopausal years after utilization of donor oocytes, the infertility specialist frequently evaluates women in this age group, and evaluation of their adnexae should be an integral part of the pretreatment screening.

Sonographically polycystic ovary syndrome is associated with large ovaries and multiple small subcapsulary follicles, approximately 4 to 6 mm. Characteristics of polycystic ovary include greater than 8 peripherally placed 4- to 6-mm follicles with a 15% increase in ovarian stroma (**Fig. 22–6**). The diagnostic criteria of polycystic ovarian syndrome, however, are not universally accepted in the absence of corresponding hyperandrogenism and oligoamenorrhea.

Finally, ultrasound can also be used to determine the mobility of the ovaries. The ovary can be appreciated to be fixed or mobile using real-time ultrasound with direct pressure by the transvaginal probe or monitoring of a transvaginal ultrasound while providing abdominal pressure with a free hand. A fixed ovary may suggest the presence of endometriosis.

Monitoring Infertility Treatments

One of the most powerful uses of ultrasound in the management of patients undergoing infertility treatment is the monitoring of ovulation induction techniques. Ultrasound is sensitive in identifying the process of folliculogenesis in ovaries. Ultrasound can also document the effect of increasing estrogen throughout the follicular phase on the endometrium. Monitoring the process of ovulation induction allows for assessment of the development of a dominant follicle, assessment of the number of follicles responding to ovulation induction techniques, and assessment of the optimal time of triggering ovulation. Careful monitoring of controlled ovarian stimulation allows adjustment of gonadotropin dosing in an attempt to limit the percentage of women who develop ovarian hyperstimulation syndrome.

Evaluation of the Uterus

Transvaginal ultrasound can accurately identify the thickness of the endometrium as it responds to estrogen. During the course of ovulation induction therapy, a progressive thickening of the endometrium should be noted. The endometrial stripe increases in thickness from approximately 2 to 3 mm to 12 to 14 mm. Just as important as the thickness of the endometrium is its characteristic pattern. A well-estrogenized endometrium should reflect the characteristic trilaminar pattern. This pattern has been associated with successful implantation after in vitro fertilization and ovulation induction.[6] The absence of at least an 8-mm trilaminar endometrial stripe has been associated with a decreased chance of the establishment of pregnancy during that particular cycle.

Evaluation of the Ovaries

Ultrasound is commonly used to assess the process of folliculogenesis during controlled ovarian stimulation with clomiphene citrate, or, most commonly, parenterally administered gonadotropins. Additionally, ultrasound can be used to track the development of a dominant follicle in a cycle without pharmacological intervention. Controlled ovarian stimulation begins with a baseline ultrasound examination to ensure that the process of folliculogenesis has not already selected a dominant follicle and to rule out the presence of an ovarian cyst. Controlled ovarian stimulation with either clomiphene citrate or gonadotropins is initiated on days 3 to 5 of a normal menstrual cycle. It is expected that multiple follicles will enlarge in contrast to the enlargement of a single dominant follicle in a natural menstrual cycle. Ultrasound is used to document the number as well as the growth of the follicles. Ultrasound monitoring of follicle growth is performed intermittently throughout the follicular phase. Ultrasound performed early in the follicular phase, such as days 6 to 8, will insure adequate follicular recruitment. Continued monitoring of the ovarian follicles in conjunction with serum estradiol determinations, on days 7 through 10 will help determine the optimal timing of ovulation. When ultrasound has identified this optimal follicular size, intramuscular human chorionic gonadotropin (hCG) is used as a substitute for luteinizing hormone to trigger ovulation. This allows for the optimal timing of an intrauterine insemination or oocyte retrieval for in vitro fertilization. A dominant follicle should reach approximately 2.5 cm in women stimulated with clomiphene citrate. The optimal size of the follicles in a woman stimulated with gonadotropins is at least two follicles of 18 mm diameter. In the case of in vitro fertilization, as many as 20 or more follicles are recruited, and ovulation is triggered when at least 4 follicles are 19 to20 mm or greater (**Fig. 22–10**).

During cycles of ovulation induction with gonadotropins, if too many follicles have developed, withholding hCG may prevent ovarian hyperstimulation syndrome (OHSS). If ovarian hyperstimulation does occur, ultrasound can be used to document free peritoneal fluid and ovarian size. Sometimes the vaginal probe cannot encompass the entire size of the ovaries on one screen. In this instance, a transabdominal scanning approach may be needed. As part of the treatment for OHSS, paracentesis is frequently indicated and this is performed under ultrasound guidance.

Transvaginal ultrasound has become an integral part of in vitro fertilization treatment. Follicular development is monitored in a fashion similar to that of controlled ovarian simulation. Importantly, transvaginal ultrasound also allows the real-time aspiration of ovarian follicles during ovum retrieval. The ultrasound probe is fitted with a guide for a specialized needle. Under direct

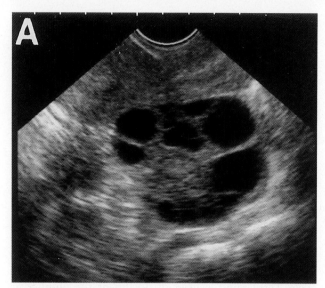

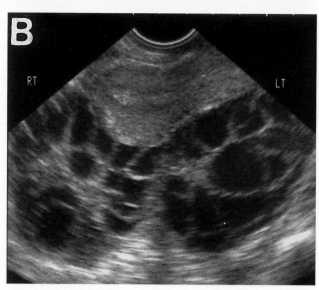

Figure 22–10 Hormonally stimulated ovaries. Parenteral gonadotropin administration induces multifollicular development (**A**) which in patients with polycystic ovarian syndrome can lead to the development of 20 to 40 follicles per ovary (**B**) and extremely high serum estradiol levels.

ultrasound guidance, the ovarian follicles are punctured and their contents aspirated and the oocyte is retrieved after microscopic examination of the aspirated follicular fluid. After fertilization, embryos are transferred into the endometrial cavity. Ultrasound is used to map the endometrial cavity and determine the optimal length and direction a catheter should be inserted to atraumatically transfer the embryos (**Fig. 22–11**). Occasionally, real-time ultrasound is used to ensure the transfer catheter has reached the optimal position in the uterus and that the embryos are replaced approximately 1 cm from the fundal apex of the endometrial cavity.

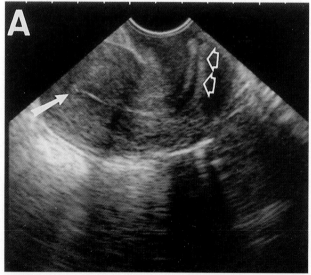

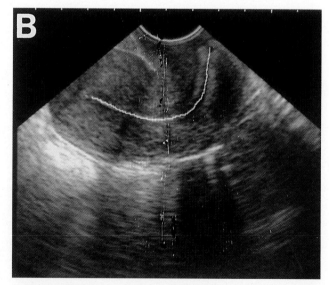

Figure 22–11 Uterine/endometrial mapping. Detailed evaluation of the endocervical and endometrial canal is critical in order to perform an embryo transfer atraumatically and within 1 cm of the apex of the endometrial cavity. During the period of induction of ovulation, both the endocervical canal (**open arrows**), the endometrial apex (**arrow**) (**A**), as well as the version and flexion of the uterine body (**B**) can be determined. Utilizing the "abdominal circumference" measurement mode, the exact length of the canal can be determined, thus providing the exact length from the external cervical os for the embryos to be transferred.

Diagnosis of Early Pregnancy

Ultrasound has revolutionized the diagnosis and management of early pregnancy. A gestational sac can be visualized with transvaginal ultrasound at 2 to 3 weeks from conception and is the first definitive sign of an intrauterine pregnancy.[7] An early pregnancy sac is characterized by a sonolucent center (the chorionic cavity) containing the amnion and eventually the embryonic disk and yolk sac. A symmetrical thick echogenic ring that is formed by primary trophoblastic invasion characterizes a true gestational sac. A double ring can be visualized which identifies both the fluid contained within the chorionic sac, as well as visualization of the remnant of the uterine cavity itself contained between the decidua capsularis and parietalis (**Fig. 22–12**). This double ring sign can be considered diagnostic of an implanted intrauterine pregnancy. In the absence of a double ring sign, discrimination between an intrauterine gestational sac and a pseudo sac cannot be completely determined (**Fig. 22–13**). Once a yolk sac or embryonic pole with cardiac activity is visualized, an intrauterine pregnancy can be confirmed.

Once an intrauterine pregnancy has been identified, its growth can be assessed by serial ultrasounds. The mean diameter of a gestational sac increases approximately 1 mm a day during early pregnancy.[8] The yolk sac is a very round and regular structure and is the next ultrasound finding to be documented. Once an embryonic pole has been identified, ultrasound can be used to assess for the presence of cardiac activity. In addition, embryonic heart rate can be assessed. If there is normal progression of the pregnancy,[9] serial examinations should show a progressive increase in the heart rate. If such an increase is not noted, a spontaneous abortion should be strongly suspected. In cases of multiple gestations, discrepancies between the embryonic heart rates or their progressive heart rate increases, may signal the impending demise of one of the embryos.

Ultrasound can also be used for the assessment of gestational age. Gestational sac size expressed as mean sac diameter can be used for correlation with menstrual age before the visualization of an embryo. However, once a fetal pole is identified, a more sensitive estimation of gestational age is performed by measuring the crown rump length of the developing embryo.[10–12] The embry-

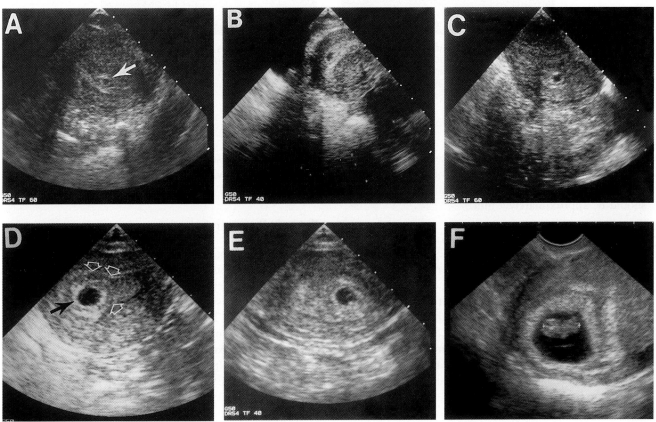

Figure 22–12 Early intrauterine pregnancy. Transvaginal ultrasonographic evaluation during early pregnancy can easily detect 2 to 5 mm intrauterine gestational sacs (A—C) at HCG serum concentrations below 3000 mIU/mL (first or third IRP). Larger gestational sacs with clear demarcation of the chorionic (**D; arrow**) and endometrial decidual (**D; open arrows**) components are easily discernible before the appearance of the yolk sac (**E**) or the fetus and fetal heart activity (**F**). Note that the chorionic and decidual layers can be distinguished even at very early stages, thus confirming the presence of an intrauterine pregnancy before visualization of the fetal pole with cardiac activity.

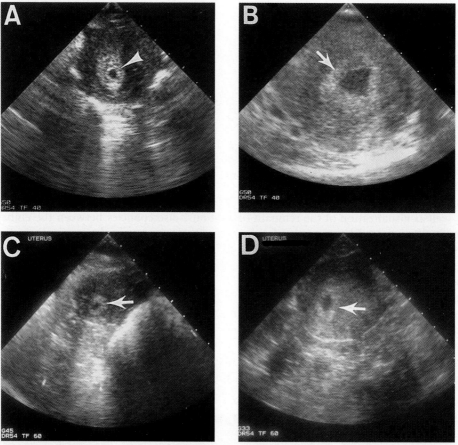

Figure 22–13 Intrauterine pseudosac. Accumulation of intrauterine fluid (usually blood) within the endometrial cavity during early pregnancy can give the appearance of an intrauterine sac-like structure that can be mistakenly interpreted as an intrauterine ges-tation (**B—D; arrows**). Note the clear double decidual sign seen in a normal early intrauterine pregnancy (**A; arrowhead**) and the pseudosacs shown in panels **B** through **D**.

onic pole begins as a straight structure until it reaches a length of 4 mm, at which point it becomes C-shaped. By 49 days of gestation, a measurement and greatest length should be approximately 7 mm.[8]

Assessment of Early Pregnancy Failure

Ultrasound can also assist the infertility physician in determining the continued well being of a pregnancy. A pregnancy complicated by bleeding through a closed cervical os is considered a threatened abortion. To assess the viability of a threatened abortion, serial ultrasounds can be used. Unless an ectopic pregnancy is still in question, following quantitative hCG values are only of limited value. Serial ultrasound examination can detect an abnormal or nonviable pregnancy by detecting a distorted gestational sac, a collapsed fragmented sac, or a lack of continued growth and expected landmarks.[4] If an embryo is no more than 4 mm long and no cardiac activity is discernible, a follow-up scan conducted at an appropriate interval will confirm the presence of a nonviable pregnancy consistent with an embryonic demise. Ad-

ditionally, the absence of cardiac activity, when it had been detected previously, confirms the presence of a nonviable pregnancy.

Ectopic Pregnancy

One of the most common complications of pregnancy that the infertility specialist faces is an ectopic pregnancy. History of infertility or infertility treatments are recognized risk factors for the development of ectopic pregnancy. Thus, all infertility patients achieving pregnancy are routinely followed until an ectopic pregnancy has been excluded. Ultrasound is very sensitive in identifying a healthy intrauterine pregnancy. Detection of an intrauterine pregnancy virtually eliminates an ectopic pregnancy with the exception of heterotopic pregnancy. The presence of simultaneous intrauterine and extrauterine pregnancies occurs in one in 30,000 spontaneous pregnancies.[13] However, in women undergoing assisted reproduction, the rate of heterotopic pregnancy has been estimated to increase to approximately one in 6000 pregnancies.[14, 15] The ability to diagnose an ectopic

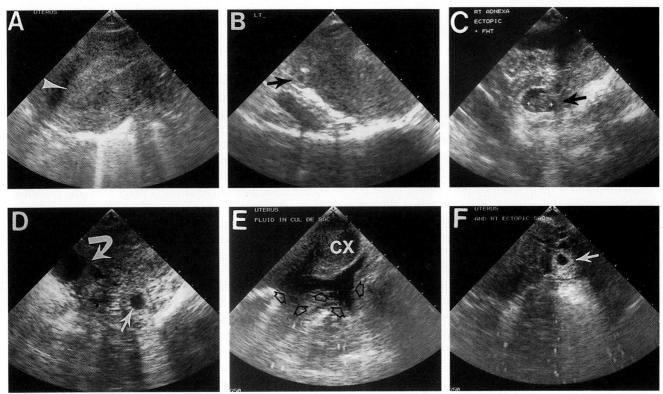

Figure 22–14 Ectopic pregnancy. The absence of an intrauterine gestational sac when the HCG serum concentration is above the discriminatory zone provides the strongest suggestion for the presence of an ectopic pregnancy (**A**). Small (2 to 5 mm) extrauterine chorionic sacs termed "**rings of fire**" can be identified frequently in the adnexa (**B, D, F; arrows**) and rarely a fetus with cardiac activity can also be visualized (**C; arrow**). During the ultrasonographic evaluation, it is critical to separate the presumed extrauterine gestational sac from the ipsilateral ovary (**D; curved arrow**). Frequently, the fluid in the cul-de-sac (**E; open arrows**) can be identified behind the lower uterine segment and cervix (cx), suggestive of accumulating blood from a bleeding ectopic pregnancy.

pregnancy relies heavily on the ability to identify a normal intrauterine pregnancy. The detection of an extrauterine pregnancy is much less sensitive and when it is detected is also less specific. A concept called a *discriminatory level* is useful when evaluating for a potential abnormal pregnancy.[16] A normal, healthy intrauterine pregnancy should always be visualized at approximately 35 days from the last menstrual period.[17] However, menstrual dating can often be inaccurate when relying on menstrual history. Therefore, a discriminatory level of human chorionic gonadotropin has been reported. This is not the level of hCG that corresponds to the earliest detection of an intrauterine pregnancy, but instead, it refers to the level at which a transvaginal ultrasonographic evaluation should identify the presence of an intrauterine pregnancy with 100% sensitivity, if it is truly present. Discriminatory levels have ranged from 935 to 2383 mIU/mL (3rd international preparation).[10, 18, 19] However, most commonly, the hCG serum concentration used for this purpose is in the 1500 to 2000 mIU/mL range.[16] The presence of leiomyomata, an intrauterine device or multiple gestations may affect this discriminatory level. When a patient has an hCG serum concentration greater than the discriminatory level and an intrauterine pregnancy is not visualized, a clinician must suspect the presence of either an abnormal intrauterine pregnancy or possibly an ectopic gestation (**Fig. 22–14**). A diagnostic algorithm combining the use of ultrasound in all cases with a hCG above an established discriminatory zone and serial outpatient hCG determinations can detect an ectopic pregnancy with 100% sensitivity and 99.9% specificity.[16]

When the hCG level is below the discriminatory zone, the interpretation of ultrasound findings, including the presence of an extrauterine pregnancy, is far less sensitive and specific and should be viewed with caution.[20] The measurement of the endometrial stripe in women with an hCG below the discriminatory zone, however, may be of some value. An endometrial stripe greater than 13.4 mm has been associated with a viable intrauterine pregnancy, while a stripe thickness of under 7.3 mm has been associated with an abnormal pregnancy including an ectopic pregnancy.[21] Once an abnormal pregnancy has been confirmed, dilatation and curettage and/or laparoscopy may be used to distinguish between an abnormal intrauterine gestation and an ectopic gestation.[22]

Ultrasound can detect an extrauterine gestation. However, in the absence of a clearly identifiable fetal pole with fetal heart activity, the presence of an extrauterine mass is not diagnostic of an ectopic pregnancy. A possible exception is the presence of a gestational sac in the adnexa ("ring of fire"), which is separate from the ovary and when the hCG serum concentration is above the discriminatory level (**Fig. 22–14**). This evaluation and diagnosis can be problematic if the person performing the ultrasound examination does not meticulously determine whether the ectopic "sac" is separate from the ovary. The ultrasonographic configuration of a corpus luteum can very easily be mistaken for an ectopic gestational sac (**Fig. 22–15**). In the absence of definitive separation of the adnexal structures, cardiac activity in the adnexa may be the only definitive finding to confirm the presence of an ectopic pregnancy by ultrasound. Unfortunately, only up to 28% of ectopic pregnancies develop a yolk sac or cardiac activity or both.[23, 24]

Conclusion

Ultrasound has become an important clinical tool in the management of a couple being evaluated and treated for infertility. Transvaginal ultrasound is perhaps the most useful ultrasound technique because of its high-resolution imaging of the pelvic structures. Ultrasound can be used to diagnose existing uterine, tubal, or ovarian anomalies. Ultrasound is also paramount in monitoring infertility treatments and assisting in ovum retrieval and embryo transfer. Pelvic ultrasound is the gold standard in the identification of an early pregnancy and assisting in the discrimination of a normal from an abnormal gestation, notably, an ectopic pregnancy.

Future directions of ultrasound include the use of Doppler ultrasound to assess blood flow to the endometrium, early antral follicles, or dominant follicles. Potentially, criteria can be created to identify the potential viability of the oocytes within these follicles.[25, 26] Doppler ultrasound may also be able to help assist in the identification of the viability of an implanted embryo. At present, these modalities are being evaluated and may add, in the near future, to the armamentarium of ultrasound tools available to the infertility specialist.

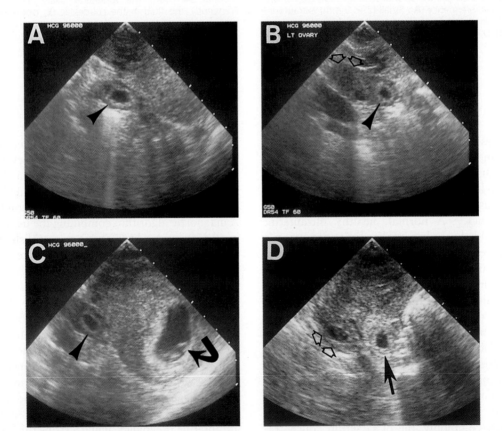

Figure 22–15 Pseudosacs in the adnexa . A small corpus luteum can assume the ultrasonographic appearance of a "ring of fire" (**A—C; arrowhead**) which, on careful evaluation, is localized within the ovary (**B; open arrows**). An intrauterine pregnancy was clearly seen in this patient (**C; curved arrow**). Note the similarities of a sac-like structure in an ovary (**D; open arrows**) in juxtaposition to an adjacent "ring of fire" (**D; arrow**) representing an ectopic pregnancy.

References

1. Timor-Tritsch IE, Rottem S, Thaler I. Review of transvaginal ultrasonography: A description with clinical application. *Ultrasound* 1988;6:1—3.
2. Granberg S, Wikland M, Karksson B. Endometrial thickness measured by ultrasonography for identifying endometrial abnormality. *Am J Obstet Gynecol* 1991;164:47—53.
3. Deichert U, Schlief R, Van de Sandt M, Juhnke I. Transvaginal hysterosalpingo-contrast-sonography (Hy-CO-Sy) compared with conventional tubal diagnostics. *Hum Reprod* 1989;4:418—424.
4. ACOG Technical Bulletin. *Gynecologic Ultrasound*, No. 215, November 1995.
5. Rodriquez MH, Platt LD, Medearis AL, Lacarra M, Lobo RA. The use of transvaginal sonography for evaluation of postmenopausal ovarian size and morphology. *Am J Obstet Gynecol* 1988;159:810—814.
6. Gonen Y, Casper R. Prediction of implantation by the sonographic appearance of the endometrium during controlled ovarian stimulation for in vitro fertilization (IVF). *J In Vitro Fertil* 1990;7:146—152.
7. Goldstein SR, Snyder JR, Watson C, Danon M. Very early pregnancy detection with endovaginal ultrasound. *Obstet Gynecol* 1988;72:200—204.
8. Goldstein SR, Wolfson R. Endovaginal ultrasonographic measurement of early embryonic sizes— a means for assessing gestational age. *J Ultrasound Med* 1994;13:25—31.
9. Howe RS, Isaacson KJ, Albert JL, Coutifaris C. Embryonic heart rate in human pregnancy. *J Ultrasound Med* 1991;10:367—371.
10. Bernaschek G, Rudelstorger R, Csaicsich P. Vaginal sonography versus serum human chorionic gonadotropin in early detection of pregnancy. *Am J Obstet Gynecol* 1988;158:606—612.
11. Hellman LM, Kobayashi M, Fillisti L, Lavenhar M. Growth and development of the human fetus prior to the twentieth week of gestation. *Am J Obstet Gynecol* 1969;103:789—800.
12. Daya S, Woods S, Ward S, Lappalainen R, Caco C. Early pregnancy assessment with transvaginal ultrasound scanning. *Can Med Assoc J* 1991;144:441—446.
13. DeVoe RW, Pratt JH. Simultaneous intrauterine and extrauterine pregnancy. *Am J Obstet Gynecol* 1948;56:1119—1126.
14. Gamberdella FR, Marrs RP. Heterotopic pregnancy associated with assisted reproductive technology. *Am J Obstet Gynecol* 1989;160:1520—1524.
15. Dimitry ES, Subak-Sharpe R, Mills M, Margara R, Winston R. Nine cases of heterotopic pregnancies in 4 years of in vitro fertilization. *Fertil Steril* 1990;174:375—378.
16. Barnhart K, Mennuti M, Benjamin I, et al. Prompt diagnosis of ectopic pregnancy in an emergency department setting. *Obstet Gynecol* 1994;84:1010—1015.
17. Fossum GT, Davajan V, Kletzky OA. Early detection of pregnancy with transvaginal ultrasound. *Fertil Steril* 1988;49:788—791.
18. Bateman BG, Nunley WC Jr, Kolp LA, Kitchin JD III, Felder R. Vaginal sonography findings and HCG dynamics of early intrauterine and tubal pregnancies. *Obstet Gynecol* 1990;75:421—427.
19. Bree RL, Edwards M, Bohm-Velez M, et al. Transvaginal sonography in the evaluation of normal early pregnancy: correlation with HCG level. *AJR* 1989;153:75—79.
20. Barnhart K, Kamelle S, Simhan H. The accuracy of ultrasound in the identification of an abnormal pregnancy above and below a discriminatory zone. *Obstet Gynecol* (In Press).
21. Spandorfer S, Barnhart K. Endometrial stripe thickness as a predictor for the diagnosis of ectopic pregnancy. *Fertil Steril* 1996;66(3):474—477.
22. Spandorfer S, Menzin A, Barnhart K, Livolsi V, Pfeifer S. Efficacy of frozen section evaluation of uterine currettings in the diagnosis of ectopic pregnancy. *Am J Obstet Gynecol* 1996;175:603—605.
23. Stiller RJ, De Regt RH, Blair E. Transvaginal ultrasonography in patients at risk for ectopic pregnancy. *Am J Obstet Gynecol* 1989;161:930—933.
24. Fleischer AC, Pennell RG, McKee MS, Worrell JA, Keefe B, Herbert CM, et al. Ectopic pregnancy: features at transvaginal sonography. *Radiology* 1990;174:375—378.
25. Zaidi J, Barber J, Kyei-Mensah A, et al. Relationship of ovarian stromal blood flow at the baseline ultrasound scan to subsequent follicular response in an in vitro fertilization program. *Obstet Gynecol* 1996;88:779—784.
26. Tekay A, Martikainen H, Jouppila P. Blood flow changes in uterine and ovarian vasculature, and predictive value of transvaginal pulsed color Doppler ultrasonography in an in vitro fertilization program. *Hum Reprod* 1995;10:688—693.

Obstetric Patient

23 Sonographic Evaluation of First-trimester Pain, and/or Bleeding

Arthur C. Fleischer

Overview

Transvaginal sonography (TVS) has a pivotal role in the evaluation of the patient presenting with first-trimester pain and/or bleeding. Along with the pregnancy test, TVS is the most important diagnostic test used to determine the cause and proper treatment of the patient presenting with pain and/or bleeding in the first trimester.

The diagnostic entities that are considered in the patient who presents with first-trimester pain and/or bleeding include ectopic pregnancy, threatened abortion, gestational trophoblastic disease, and adnexal torsion. With the improved resolution afforded by transvaginal sonography and the additional diagnostic information available through color Doppler sonography (CDS), these entities can be confidently distinguished from each other. This chapter will emphasize newly described sonographic signs, especially with color Doppler sonography, which may enable more specific diagnosis in these patients.

Ectopic Pregnancy

The improved resolution afforded by transvaginal sonography and color Doppler sonography has greatly enhanced the ability to confidently diagnose ectopic pregnancy and assess its viability. These parameters are pivotal in determining the optimal management of patients with this condition.[1]

Fortunately, the fatality rate associated with this condition has been decreasing substantially, even though its incidence has increased significantly over the last 20 years. Most patients have a clinical history of pelvic inflammatory disease. The abnormal and irregular bleeding that occurs in ectopic pregnancies is associated with abnormal hormonal fluctuations. The "classical" clinical triad for ectopic pregnancy, consisting of pain, abnormal vaginal bleeding, and an adnexal mass, occurs in less than half of patients. In fact, on pelvic examination in patients with ectopic pregnancy, only 50% of patients will have a palpable adnexal mass.

Pregnancy tests assist in establishing the presence of a pregnancy, but do not indicate whether it is intra- or extrauterine. The two major types of pregnancy tests available now consist of maternal serum radioimmunoassay (RIA) and urinary enzyme-linked immunosorbentassay (ELISA). The advantage of the serum test is that it is very sensitive, although it may not be available at the time of the patient's presentation. The urine pregnancy test is qualitative rather than quantitative but now approaches the accuracy of the maternal serum test.

In either test, the level of human chorionic gonadotropin (HCG) is assessed relative to either the Second International Standard (2nd I.S.) or the International Reference Preparation (I.R.P.). It is important to realize that HCG levels measured against the Second International Standard are approximately half those measured against the International Reference Preparation i. e., 50 ml µ/mL (2nd I.S.) ~ 100 ml µ/mL (I.R.P.).

It is important to realize that in up to 20% of ectopics examined transabdominally and 0—8% examined transvaginally, no apparent sonographic signs of an ectopic pregnancy are observed.[1] As a medicolegal precaution, it may be prudent to include a statement such as "although an ectopic pregnancy is considered unlikely, it cannot be totally excluded" in the official report in cases where no definite sonographic abnormality is seen.

Sonographic Findings in Ectopic Pregnancy

Transvaginal sonography is clearly the most accurate means for documentation of the presence or absence of an ectopic pregnancy. Color Doppler sonography can also be used as a means for detection and assessment of the vascularity of the adnexal masses detected. Occasionally, color Doppler sonography may demonstrate a "ring of fire", representing the vascularity associated with an ectopic pregnancy that it is not appreciated on transvaginal sonography.[2]

The sonographic findings in ectopic pregnancy can be divided into consideration of uterine, adnexal, and cul-de-sac findings, however, in a single patient, any combination of findings may exist.

Uterine findings focus on the presence or absence of a gestational sac with intact choriodecidua. Typically, the endometrium undergoes a decidualization, which is a microscopic change in the nuclei of the endometrial stromal cells. The endometrium may thicken and in some cases contain fluid or blood centrally having the appearance of a "pseudo-gestational sac." However, the decidua in ectopic pregnancies lacks the low-impedance flow seen on Doppler in normal early intrauterine pregnancy. In addition, the decidualized endometrium in ectopics lacks a focal thickening in the decidua basalis region seen in normal early pregnancies. In some cases of normal early (less than 6 weeks) intrauterine pregnancy, a double lining of decidua is present, representing decidua capsularis and opposing decidua vera. When this is documented sonographically, an intrauterine pregnancy is most likely (**Fig. 23–1**).

In most cases of ectopic pregnancy, the endometrium is slightly thickened similar to a secretory-phase endometrium. In more advanced ectopic pregnancies (8 weeks and more), there can be intraluminal blood and clotting due to sloughing of the endometrium secondary to poor corpus luteum support.

The adnexal findings in ectopic pregnancies form the basis for sonographic diagnosis of this entity. In most ectopic pregnancies, an adnexal ring of echogenic tissue with a hypoechoic center can be identified separately from the ovary (**Fig. 23–2**). One should be careful not to confuse a corpus luteum with the presence of an ectopic pregnancy on TVS.

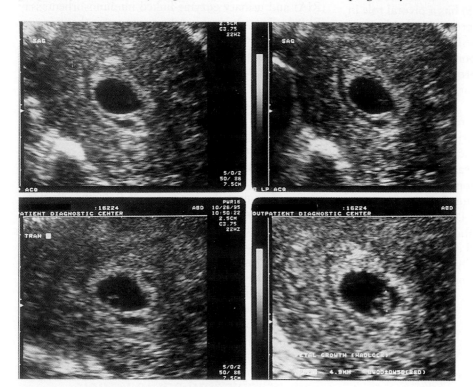

Figure 23–1 Composite TVS of normal six-week intrauterine pregnancy showing decidua capsularis and vera. A yolk sac/embryo complex is also seen in the lower right-hand image.

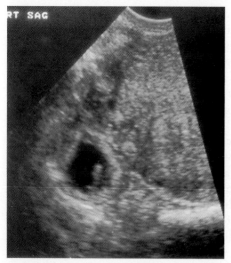

Figure 23–2 TVS of an unruptured tubal pregnancy showing a decidual ring containing an embryo.

In some cases, color Doppler sonography can be used as a "roadmap," outlining the presence of a corpus luteum as separate from the tubal mass itself (**Fig. 23–3**). The flow pattern seen in ectopic pregnancies can vary from absent diastolic flow to low-impedance, high-velocity flow, and this parameter is not accurate in determining whether or not an adnexal mass is a corpus luteum or an ectopic pregnancy (**Figs. 23–4** through **23–6**). However, using CDS, one can get a general approximation of the relative vascularity of the ectopic pregnancy (**Fig. 23–5**). Spontaneous resolution of an ectopic is most likely when there is little or no adnexal ring flow. "Bizarre" waveforms that exhibit significant reversed diastolic flow have been described in ectopic pregnancies undergoing necrosis and resorption.

Color Doppler sonography can be used in assessment of response to methotrexate treatment.[3] In most cases, there is an initial increase in flow probably due to va-

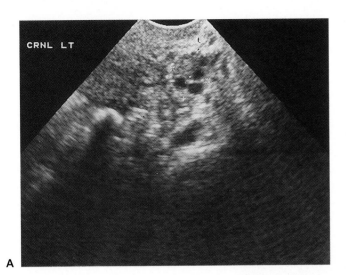

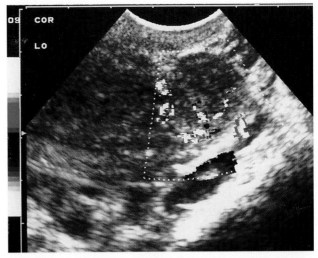

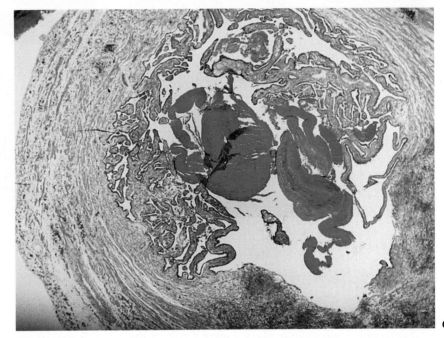

Figure 23–3 enhanced visualization of an unruptured ectopic adjacent to a corpus luteum with color Doppler sonography: **A:** TVS showing a normal left ovary (**between cursors**) with tiny cystic areas. **B:** TV-CDS showing a vascular ring adjacent to the corpus luteum, suggesting the possibility of an unruptured ectopic pregnancy. **C:** Histologic specimen showing a 3 x 4 mm unruptured ectopic pregnancy.

sodilatation, as indicated by low-impedance diastolic flow, followed by a gradual increase in resistance to flow within the adnexal mass itself.

Intraperitoneal and/or cul-de-sac fluid that has low-level echoes is highly indicative of an ectopic pregnancy. The presence of intraperitoneal fluid, however, does not always indicate that rupture is present, as bleeding can occur as the gestational sac is being passed out the fimbriated end of the tube into the peritoneum.

Uncommon types of ectopic pregnancies can be diagnosed sonographically, the most important of which include the interstitial ectopic pregnancy, where the gestational sac is extremely eccentric to the endometrium.[4] One must not overcall interstitial ectopics in normal pregnancies, as the gestational sac may be eccentrically located during early (less than 6—7 weeks) pregnancy. However, when it approximates the uterine serosa and is very eccentric to the endometrium, this condition should be suspected.

In abdominal ectopic pregnancies, the uterus can be seen as separate from the developing gestational sac. This condition may not be suspected until second and third trimester, when the finding of a "pseudo placenta previa," abnormal amniotic fluid collection, or abnormal fetal position is seen on transabdominal sonography. It is noted that over one-quarter of abdominal ectopic pregnancies may be missed sonographically.[5]

Sonography has become a means for assessing proper management of patients with ectopic pregnancies. In some centers, systemic methotrexate is used for treatment of known ectopic pregnancies, whereas in others local injection is performed utilizing transvaginal sonography as a means for guidance.[3] In some cases, ectopic pregnancies are observed and followed sonographically for changes in blood flow, as well as abnormal increases in β-HCG.

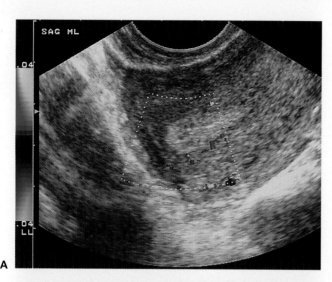

Figure 23–4 TV-CDS of an unruptured ectopic pregnancy. **A:** TV-CDS of the uterus showing mild endometrial thickening with sparse myometrial flow. **B:** TV-CDS of the right ovary showing a mostly cystic mass with low-impedance flow within the wall. This represented a hemorrhagic corpus luteum. **C:** In the left adnexa, a ring-like structure with relatively high-velocity and intermediate-impedance flow was seen. This was an unruptured ectopic pregnancy.

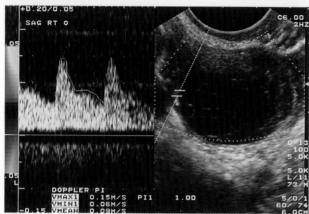

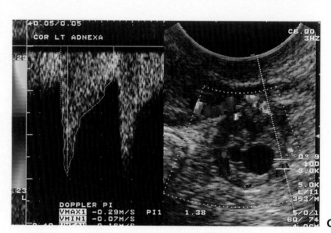

Threatened Abortion

Transvaginal sonography plays a pivotal role in the evaluation of the patient presenting with pain and/or bleeding in the first trimester. Because bleeding can occur in up to 20% of normal pregnancies in the first trimester, transvaginal sonography is used to distinguish conditions that are physiologic from those that may require surgical intervention.

Subchorionic Hemorrhage

Subchorionic hemorrhage appears as a crescent hypoechoic area adjacent to the choriodecidua in early pregnancy. Although there is significant controversy as to its importance, if it is localized to the placental edge and small (less than one-quarter of the gestational sac size), it is usually not associated with adverse pregnancy outcome. However, if it extends behind the chorion and is large (over two-thirds sac size), the prognosis for pregnancy completion is usually guarded (**Fig. 23–7**).[6—8] Other factors that seem to indiciate poor prognosis in-

clude weeks of gestation (less than 6 weeks) and more advanced maternal age (over 35 years).[9]

A similar condition involving a "blighted twin" can be encountered when two gestational sacs are observed with only one living embryo. In this condition, there is embryonic demise in one gestational sac with a living embryo or fetus in the second gestational sac. Usually, the gestational sac in the demised embryo deflates and is eventually absorbed.

Embryonic Demise

Embryonic heart activity can usually be established as early as 6 weeks when the embryo is 3—4 mm in length. Heart rate analysis indicates that slow heart rates of 85 beats per minute or less are typically associated with spontaneous demise.[10] Embryonic demise may be associated with a "deflated" yolk sac (less than 6 mm in size) or, on the other hand, an enlarged hydropic yolk sac (**Fig. 23–8**).[11]

Figure 23–5 Vascularity of ectopic pregnancies. **A:** Composite CDS showing hypervascular ectopic including flow to the embryo (lower left image). **B:** In contrast to the patient shown in (**A**), this ectopic is hypovascular, probably the result of sloughing.

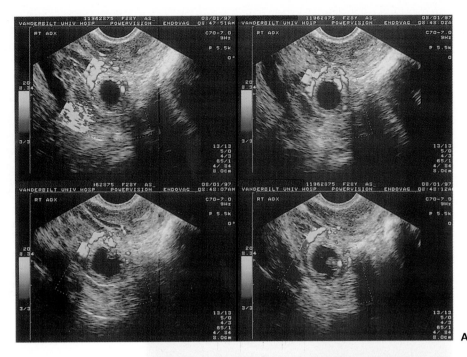

A

Incomplete versus Complete Abortion

There are certain sonographic milestones that can be used to establish normalcy of pregnancy in the first trimester. In general, these include the presence of a yolk sac within a gestational sac of 10 mm or more, the presence of an embryo at 15-mm gestational sac dimension, and heart motion seen as early as embryonic visualization. In incomplete abortion, there may be a small gestational sac, defined as less than a 5-mm difference between embryonic length and mean sac dimension, or, if there is demise, a very large gestational sac.[12] The choriodecidua is typically irregular and, on color Doppler, increased venous flow is seen within the choriodecidua.

In complete abortion, there is a thin and regular endometrium; and, on speculum examination, the cervix is closed. In these patients, conservative treatment might be indicated, with monitoring using serial β-HCG (**Fig. 23–7 C**).[13]

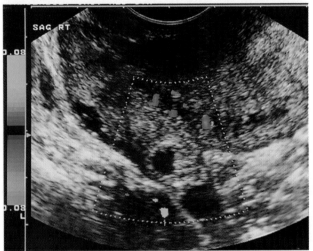

B

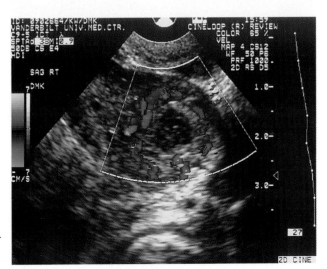

Figure 23–6 TV-CDS of a hemorrhagic corpus luteum that ▷ mimicked the appearance of an ectopic except that it could be localized to be within the right ovary.

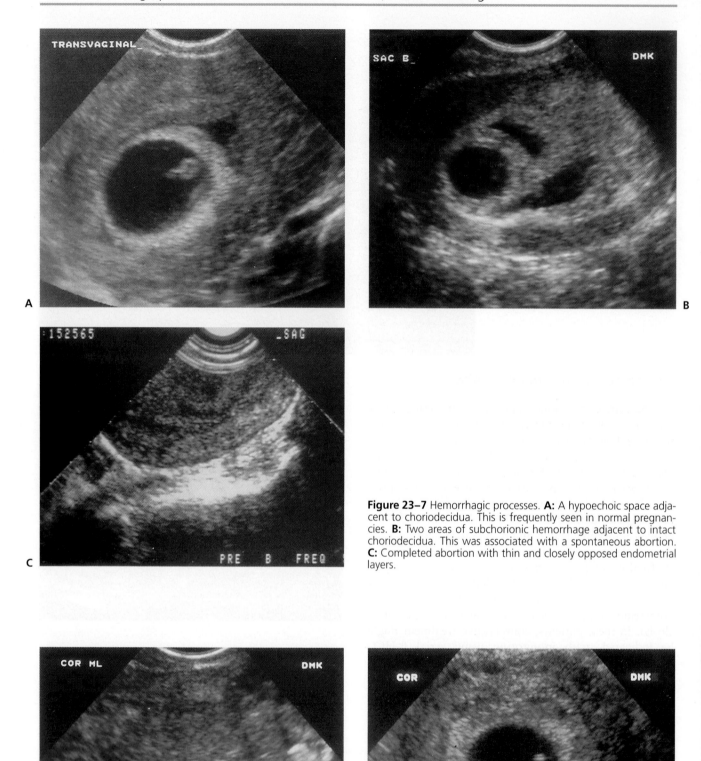

Figure 23–7 Hemorrhagic processes. **A:** A hypoechoic space adjacent to choriodecidua. This is frequently seen in normal pregnancies. **B:** Two areas of subchorionic hemorrhage adjacent to intact choriodecidua. This was associated with a spontaneous abortion. **C:** Completed abortion with thin and closely opposed endometrial layers.

Figure 23–8   Too large and too small yolk sac. **A:** Hydropic yolk sac (**between cursors**) associated with embryonic disease. **B:** Tiny, deflated yolk sac associated with long-standing embryonic demise.

Gestational Trophoblastic Disease

This rare condition occurs when there is fertilization of a chromosomally empty zygote. The typical morphologic appearance of hydropic villi may not be seen in the first trimester. In fact, only echogenic irregular tissue may be seen and occasionally associated with theca lutein cysts. If this condition is suspected, then a β-HCG will typically reveal markedly elevated values. CDs may show clustered areas of low-impedance flow (**Fig. 23–9**).

Adnexal Torsion

Approximately 20% of ovarian torsion occurs in pregnant women. This may be related to increased arterial flow to the ovary coupled with decreased venous return. These may result in diffuse ovarian edema and enlargement thereby increasing susceptibility to torsion. Because intraovarian venous flow is most sensitive to interstitial pressure changes, venous flow is typically absent and arterial flow shows high impedance in most cases of adnexal torsion.[14] As the condition progresses, intraovarian arterial flow may be absent. Sonographic depiction of the "twisted pedicle" with CDS may be diagnostic in some cases (**Fig. 23–10**).

Summary

This presentation covers the current applications of transvaginal sonography, with and without color Doppler capability, in evaluating the conditions associated with first-trimester pain and bleeding. Transvaginal sonography offers an accurate means for not only diagnosis, but also establishment of proper management of these patients.

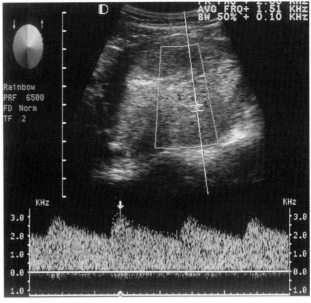

Figure 23–9 TV-CDS showing low-impedance flow within echogenic trophoblastic tissue.

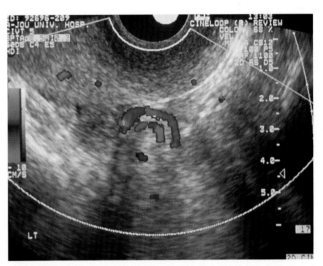

Figure 23–10 TV-CDS showing "twisted pedicle" sign associated with adnexal torsion. There is no flow within the enlarged ovary located in the cul-de-sac. (Courtesy of Dr. E. Lee).

References

1. Ackerman T, Levic C, Dashefsky D. Interstitial line: sonographic findings in interstitial (cornual) ectopic pregnancy. *Radiology* 1993;189:83—86.
2. Atri M, Bret PM, Tulandi T, Senterman MK. Ectopic pregnancy: evolution after treatment with transvaginal methotrexate. *Radiology* 1992;185:749—753.
3. Bennett G, Bromley B, Liebermans E, Bennaceraf B. Subchorionic hemorrhage in first trimester pregnancies: prediction of pregnancy outcome with sonography. *Radiology* 1996,199:447.
4. Bromley B, Harlow BKL, Laboda LA, et al. Small sac size in the first trimester: predictor of poor fetal outcome. *Radiology* 1991;178:375—377.

5. Dillon EH, Case CQ, Ramos IM, Holland CK, Taylor KJW. Endovaginal US and Doppler findings after first-trimester abortion. *Radiology* 1993;186:887—91.
6. Emerson DS, Cartier MS, Altieri LA, et al. Diagnostic efficacy of endovaginal color Doppler flow imaging in an ectopic pregnancy screening program. *Radiology* 1992;183:413—420.
7. Fleischer AC, Stein SM, Cullinan JC, Warner MA. Color Doppler sonography of adnexal torsion. *J Ultrasound Med* 1995;14:523—528.
8. Frates MC, Laing FC. Sonographic evaluation of ectopic pregnancy: an update: *AJR* 1995;165:251—259.
9. Jouppila P. Clinical consequences after ultrasonic diagnosis of intrauterine hematoma in threatened abortion. *J Clin Ultrasound* 1985;13:107—111.

10. Laboda LA, Estroff JA, Benacerraf BR. First trimester brady-cardia: a sign of impending fetal loss. *J Ultrasound Med* 1989;8:561—563.

11. Nyberg DA, Mack LA, Harvey D, Wang K. Value of the yolk sac in evaluating early pregnancies. *J Ultrasound Med* 1988;7:129—135.

12. Pedersen JF, Mantoni M. Prevalence and significance of sub-chorionic hemorrhage in threatened abortion: a sonographic study. *AJR* 1990;154:535—537.

13. Sauerbrei EE, Pham DH. Placental abruption and subchorion-ich hemorrhage in the first half of pregnancy: US appearance and clinical outcome. *Radiology* 1986;160:109—112.

14. Stanley R, Horger J, Fagon C, et al. Sonographic findings in abdominal pregnancies. *AJR* 1986;147:1043.

24 Second- and Third-Trimester Bleeding

Barbara S. Hertzberg

Ultrasound plays an important role in the workup of the patient who presents with vaginal bleeding. Bleeding is a common complication of pregnancy,[1–4] and is a frequent indication for sonography. Although the majority of patients who present with second- or third-trimester vaginal bleeding experience only slight blood loss, even minor bleeds can signal the presence of a life-threatening condition. Hemorrhage is a major source of perinatal morbidity and mortality: along with pulmonary embolism and pregnancy-induced hypertension, bleeding is one of the three leading causes of maternal death.[5]

Ultrasonography is a critical step in the evaluation for potentially life-threatening obstetric sources of hemorrhage. This discussion focuses on the role of ultrasonography in diagnosing serious obstetric causes of bleeding, including placenta previa, placental abruption, circumvallate placenta, vasa previa, and uterine rupture.

Diagnostic Considerations

The conditions causing second- and third-trimester hemorrhage fall into two main groups: obstetric and non-obstetric etiologies. Nonobstetric sources of hemorrhage are generally less hazardous and typically result in relatively little blood loss compared with the obstetric etiologies.[3] Among the nonobstetric causes of second- and third-trimester bleeding are benign vaginal and cervical lesions such as lacerations, varices, benign neoplasias, eversions, and polyps, and malignant lesions such as cervical carcinoma. Unusual nonobstetric etiologies of bleeding during pregnancy include urethral varices and condyloma acuminata.[2,6] In some patients, the source of bleeding is not found, and it is unclear whether the underlying etiology is obstetric or nonobstetric.[7]

Obstetric sources of hemorrhage tend to be more serious and can result in substantial blood loss. The most common serious obstetric causes of hemorrhage are placenta previa and placental abruption.[1,2] Other less frequent, but similarly important obstetric sources of third-trimester hemorrhage include vasa previa, circumvallate placenta, and uterine rupture.[1,3] Digital vaginal and rectal examinations are contraindicated in the patient with placenta previa, so a critical question guiding management of the patient who presents with vaginal bleeding is whether or not placental tissue overlies the cervix, a determination generally made by ultrasonography.

Near term, the most common cause of bleeding is a benign obstetric phenomenon termed the "bloody show". The bloody show occurs secondary to expulsion of the cervical plug, and is a normal phenomenon which virtually never requires medical intervention.[3,7] Despite this, it can result in sufficient blood loss that the mother seeks medical attention, and should, therefore, be considered in the differential diagnosis of bleeding late in the third trimester.

Diagnostic Workup

Nonobstetric sources of hemorrhage are assessed with nonimaging tests such as pap smear, speculum examination, and culture. Speculum examination is helpful in evaluating for a vaginal or cervical lesion such as a vaginal laceration or a cervical eversion, but should be done only after placenta previa has been excluded.

Depending on the source and severity of the hemorrhage, a variety of other laboratory and clinical tests may be needed. With large bleeds, a complete blood count, type and cross match, serial vital signs, and serial hematocrit levels may be necessary.[2] Tests for nucleated blood cells or fetal hemoglobin in the expelled blood may be indicated if vasa previa is suspected as it is the only source of pure fetal blood.[2,3] When heavy bleeding is due to placental abruption, continuous electronic fetal monitoring may be required to determine if emergent intervention is indicated for fetal distress. Additionally, coagulation profiles are followed in patients with severe degrees of placental abruption in order to assess for the development of disseminated intravascular coagulation.

Ultrasound is the primary imaging test to assess the patient with vaginal bleeding. Although angiography, radiography, and radioisotope scanning were performed in the past to assess for placenta previa, because of the potential risks of ionizing radiation and contrast, such tests are now of only historical interest in this assessment.[8] Likewise, magnetic resonance imaging has been suggested as a possible alternate imaging technique,[9] but has not received widespread acceptance, and currently appears to be necessary only in unusual situations.

Obstetric Sources of Hemorrhage: Ultrasound and Clinical Features

Placental Abruption

Placental abruption is defined as premature separation of a normally implanted placenta prior to birth of the fetus. A common and serious disorder, placental abruption complicates approximately 1% of pregnancies. Abruption is the most common cause of intrapartum fetal death, and accounts for up to 15—25% of perinatal mortality.[10—13] Other complications can include preterm delivery,[10] and neurological impairment in surviving infants.[2]

The clinical diagnosis of placental abruption can be surprisingly difficult.[2] Placental abruptions present a wide variety of clinical symptomatology which overlaps with symptoms accompanying other disorders such as placenta previa and uterine rupture. The often advanced constellation of clinical signs includes vaginal bleeding, abdominal pain and uterine tenderness, painful uterine contractions, fetal distress or demise, and coagulopathy, but occurs in only a small proportion of patients.

The variability in clinical presentation is partly attributable to the wide range of severity of placental abruption. Placental separation can be complete, partial, or involve only the margin of the placenta. Minor degrees of abruption can be self-limited events with little impact on maternal and fetal outcome, even though they can be accompanied by alarming amounts of vaginal bleeding.[13—15] Some patients have signs and symptoms that are so mild that the diagnosis is only established retrospectively after delivery of a placenta with a retroplacental clot.[2]

The sensitivity and specificity of ultrasound for diagnosing placental abruption is not well established. The wide range of clinical presentations makes such an assessment difficult, and most ultrasound reports of abruption consist of case reports and retrospective reviews.[10—12, 14, 16—19] Histopathologic confirmation of placental abruption is likewise complicated by the wide spectrum of pathologic findings, which include placental infarction, decidual necrosis, marginal thrombosis, and retroplacental blood clot.[10] Confirmation cannot always be obtained, even in cases strongly suspected by clinical and sonographic findings.[19, 20]

There is likewise a wide range of sonographic findings attributable to placental abruption,[10, 11] and ultrasonography was until recently thought to be an extremely insensitive test for diagnosing placental abruption.[17, 19] This was partly because the ultrasound evaluation focused on identification of a retroplacental hematoma: the retroplacental hematoma is not the most common sonographic presentation of placental abruption. Additionally, in some cases, imaging findings are not seen because the bleeding is predominantly external.

At ultrasonography, retroplacental hemorrhage typically results in focal elevation of the placenta by a hematoma which is less echogenic than the overlying placental tissue (**Fig. 24–1**). A number of processes can potentially be confused with a retroplacental hematoma at ultrasound.[11] For example, because the normal subplacental vascular region is less echogenic than placenta,[12] it can mimic a retroplacental hematoma. Distinguishing features are that the normal subplacental vascular complex does not exert a mass effect on the placenta,[20—22] and that high-resolution gray scale ultrasound and/or color Doppler evaluation may reveal discrete vascular spaces in the normal retroplacental space.

A retroplacental myometrial contraction can also resemble a retroplacental hematoma because it can cause a rounded soft-tissue thickening posterior to the placenta.[22] Like the retroplacental hematoma, a contraction will exert mass effect on the placenta. A contraction will, however, be transient, and is typically more homogeneous in echopattern than a retroplacental hematoma. In contrast, a hematoma exhibits a range of appearances which is dependent on the time interval since the bleed.

Finally, a retroplacental mass such as a leiomyoma should also be considered in the differential diagnosis of retroplacental hematoma (**Fig. 24–2**).[22] A leiomyoma will not exhibit the typical evolution a retroplacental hemorrhage demonstrates on follow-up sonography and may also have other characteristic findings, such as calcifications, posterior sound attenuation, and shadowing.

The acute retroplacental hemorrhage can be particularly difficult to diagnose because if it is echogenic it can resemble the overlying placenta. The placenta may then spuriously appear to be thickened because the hematoma is not perceived as being distinct from placenta.[11, 16, 20, 23, 24] Demonstration of an apparently thick placenta in a patient suspected clinically of having placental abruption should therefore suggest the possi-

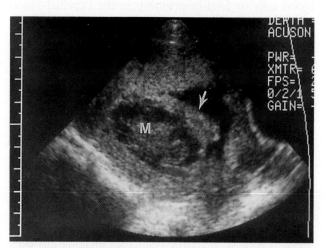

Figure 24–1 Retroplacental hematoma due to placental abruption. Longitudinal transabdominal sonogram demonstrates a heterogeneous mass (M) posterior to the placenta (**arrow**), which corresponded to a retroplacental hematoma at delivery.

bility of a retroplacental hematoma secondary to placental abruption. If definitive diagnosis is not possible at the time of the initial scan, then follow-up sonography should confirm the diagnosis by depicting interval evolution of the hematoma.[11,24]

Although the retroplacental region would intuitively seem to be a logical place to search for sonographic signs of placental abruption, in fact it is not the most commonly detected location for an intrauterine hematoma. Rather, a subchorionic hematoma is more frequently seen. The subchorionic hematoma is thought to be a consequence of detachment of the placental margin. At ultrasonography, it typically presents as a region of variable echogenicity which elevates the overlying amniochorionic membrane, and is usually contiguous with the edge of the placenta.[1] Subchorionic hematomas also exhibit a variety of other sonographic presentations which include an intrauterine membrane, an intrauterine mass, and an apparently elongated placenta.

The intrauterine membrane is the most common sonographic presentation of a subchorionic hematoma (**Fig. 24–3**). Sonography will depict a membrane projecting into the amniotic cavity when a chronic subchorionic hematoma has an echopattern similar in echogenicity to that of the amniotic fluid. With the hematoma nearly identical in appearance to amniotic fluid, only the elevated amniochorionic membrane is perceived by sonography. Increasing ultrasound gain settings can occasionally corroborate the diagnosis by depicting low-level echoes within the hematoma.

A subchorionic hematoma can mimic an intrauterine mass if it is echogenic and bulges into the amniotic cavity (**Fig. 24–4**).[11,14,18,20] This sonographic pattern could potentially be mistaken for a uterine contraction, a fibroid, an accessory lobe of the placenta, a chorioangioma, or other placental mass. When these diagnoses are contemplated in a patient clinically suspected of placental abruption, the competing diagnosis of subchorionic hematoma resembling the intrauterine mass should also be considered. Typically, a subchorionic hematoma is soft, gelatinous, and impressionable when kicked by the fetus.[14,18] When the diagnosis is in question, serial sonography may be helpful, as it can demonstrate evolution in the echo pattern of the hematoma. With time, the hematoma should become progressively less echogenic in appearance. Color Doppler and/or power Doppler imaging may also prove helpful in making this distinction, but further investigations are needed to confirm the value of Doppler in this setting.

Because a subchorionic hematoma originates near the edge of the placenta, the hematoma may not be perceived as distinct from the placenta if it is scanned at a stage in which its overall echogenicity is similar to that of the placenta. The overall sonographic pattern can then simulate that of an elongated placenta (**Fig. 24–5 A**). In the appropriate clinical setting, detection of an apparently elongated placenta should be considered cor-

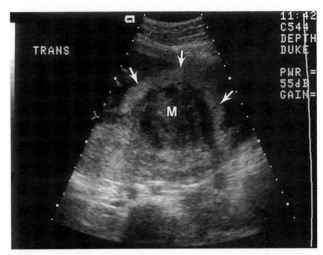

Figure 24–2   Retroplacental leiomyoma. The mass (M) elevating the placenta (**arrows**) is a leiomyoma. Note the similarity in appearance of this mass to the retroplacental hematoma in Fig. 24–1.

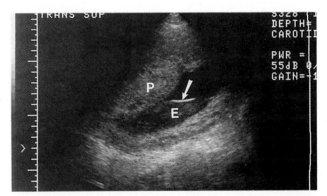

Figure 24–3   Intrauterine membrane due to subchorionic hematoma. Transabdominal sonogram demonstrates a highly echogenic membrane (**arrow**) which has been elevated by a chronic subchorionic hematoma. Although the hematoma is predominantly echopenic in sonographic pattern, note that low-level echoes (E) are seen within. The intrauterine membrane presentation of a subchorionic hematoma tends to occur in patients with chronic hematomas. (P, placenta)

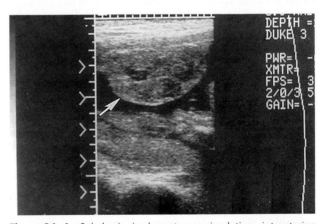

Figure 24–4   Subchorionic hematoma simulating intrauterine mass. The heterogeneous mass (**arrow**) bulging into the uterine cavity corresponds to a subchorionic hematoma. This sonographic presentation can mimic the ultrasound pattern produced by a uterine contraction, a fibroid, an accessory lobe of the placenta, or a placental mass such as a chorioangioma.

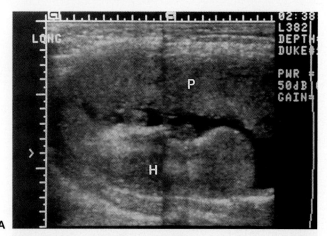

A

B

Figure 24–5 Subchorionic hematoma resembling elongated placenta. **A:** An echogenic subchorionic hematoma (H) is seen along the posterior surface of the uterus. Normal placental tissue (P) is imaged along the anterior surface of the uterus. The overall appearance is similar to that of an elongated placenta, although the edge of the subchorionic hematoma has a more rounded appearance than typical of normal placenta. **B:** Sonogram obtained 2.5 weeks after the image in (**A**) demonstrates interval evolution of the subchorionic hematoma (H) which is now considerably less echogenic than on the initial scan. (P, placenta)

roborative evidence supporting the possibility of a subchorionic hematoma. A subtle distinction in echo pattern between the true placenta and the hematoma should be sought. If the diagnosis is still not clear, serial sonography may clarify the question by showing evolution in appearance of the hematoma (**Fig. 24–5 B**).

Placental abruptions can also cause other sonographic findings, including a preplacental clot or intraamniotic echoes owing to intraamniotic hemorrhage.[18] A hemorrhage in the "preplacental" location can be in either the subamniotic or subchorionic space. Clinical symptoms include vaginal bleeding and can be remarkably similar to those arising from other sites of placental abruption. Even though such preplacental hematomas may not be associated with actual placental separation, they can be just as serious as the classic placental abruption. A preplacental hematoma can cause preterm delivery due to stimulation of uterine contractions or fetal demise from compression of the umbilical cord.[10]

Retroplacental hematomas tend to have a poorer outcome than subchorionic hematomas. In general, the greater the percentage of placental involvement, the worse the outcome tends to be.[10]

In conclusion, ultrasound can strengthen the case for a clinically suspected placental abruption. Negative findings at ultrasonography do not, however, exclude placental abruption. Indeed, in the setting of severe fetal distress or unstable maternal condition and suspected placental abruption, it may not be in the patient's best interest to perform ultrasonography, potentially losing valuable time, and delaying emergent delivery. Nevertheless, in the more common case in which symptomatology is less extreme, ultrasound can provide valuable information and definitively distinguish placental abruption from placenta previa.

Placenta Previa

Placenta previa is an abnormality of placental location in which placental tissue is implanted on the cervix. Patients with placenta previa typically present with painless third-trimester vaginal bleeding. Less than one-half of patients who experience painless vaginal bleeding, however, have placenta previa.[2] Ultrasound has long been considered a critical step in the assessment of patients with third-trimester bleeding because a vaginal or rectal examination should not be performed until placenta previa has been excluded. Indeed, ultrasound is so useful in excluding placenta previa, that it has for the most part replaced the potentially dangerous "double setup examination" traditionally used for assessing patients with third-trimester bleeding.[3]

The sensitivity of ultrasonography for detecting placenta previa approaches 100%. Even the earliest reports of placental localization by ultrasound describe an accuracy between 93% and 97%.[26—30] To optimize sensitivity, it is necessary to image both the lower edge of the placenta and the cervix. Evaluation of the cervix is needed to exclude the rare but potentially dangerous coincidence of an accessory (succenturiate) lobe of the placenta implanted over the cervical os.

Reported specificities of ultrasound for placenta previa vary widely.[31—33] The specificity depends on the severity of the condition (a complete placenta previa is less likely to resolve with advancing gestation than an incomplete placenta previa), the time in gestation at which placenta previa is detected, and on whether a concerted effort was made to avoid sources of false positives and false negatives. The reported incidence of sonographically detected placenta previa during the second trimester varies from 6–49%, but the incidence of placenta previa at term is much lower.[31—33]

Ultrasound can be used to classify the severity of placenta previa. Grading systems vary slightly from institution to institution,[8] but variations in grading systems are relatively unimportant provided the clinicians involved understand the terminology used. A typical classification defines complete placenta previa as comprising placental tissue overlying the entire internal cervical os, and a marginal or partial previa as indicating placental tissue which covers only part of the cervix and/or os.

The severity of vaginal bleeding tends to be proportional to the severity of placenta previa. Complete placenta previa is associated with earlier, more severe bleeding, and virtually always requires cesarean section. In contrast, less severe degrees of placenta previa have variable outcomes. Some patients can have a vaginal delivery, but others have such severe hemorrhage that blood transfusion and/or cesarean section must be performed.[32, 33] A true centrally implanted complete placenta previa (**Fig. 24–6**) will virtually never resolve, but many marginal and partial previas detected in the second trimester resolve later in pregnancy. In patients with an apparent placenta previa during the second trimester, the degree of symmetry of the placenta with regard to the internal os is helpful in predicting the likelihood that placenta previa will persist or resolve. A symmetrical, centrally located placenta previa predicts a much higher likelihood of persistence to delivery than an asymmetric or a marginal placenta previa.[34]

A number of potential sources of a false-positive diagnosis of placenta previa have been described. An important but avoidable explanation for a false-positive result is an overdistended urinary bladder. The bladder can cause a spurious impression of placenta previa because it compresses and distorts the lower uterine segment. If placenta previa is suspected after scans are performed with a full urinary bladder, then imaging should be repeated after the bladder has been emptied.

Another common source of false positive is a contraction in the lower uterine segment. Like the overdistended urinary bladder, a uterine contraction can distort the appearance of the lower uterus, and produce a spurious appearance of placental tissue overlying the cervix (**Fig. 24–7 A**). A contraction is recognized as a focal thickening of the myometrium with a distorted appearance to the region of the cervix and lower uterine segment. The cervix may spuriously appear to be elongated: a cervical length of 5 cm or more with an empty urinary bladder suggests that not only cervix, but also a lower uterine contraction was imaged. A rounding or bulging of the upper margin of the cervix may also be seen: in the absence of a contraction, the normal cervix is shaped like a cylinder with a flat upper surface. When a contraction is suspected, images obtained after the contraction subsides will reveal the true relationship of the placental edge to the cervix (**Fig. 24–7 B**).

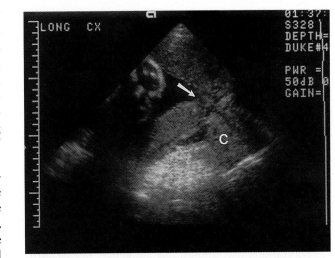

Figure 24–6 Complete central placenta previa. Transabdominal sonogram of lower uterus reveals placental tissue (**arrow**) centrally implanted on the cervix (C).

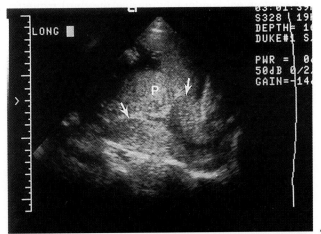

A

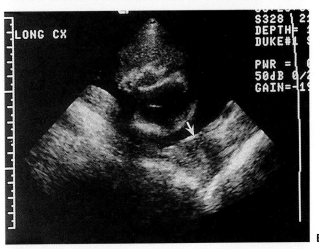

B

Figure 24–7 Lower uterine contraction simulating placenta previa. **A:** Longitudinal transabdominal sonogram of lower uterus demonstrates placental tissue (P) apparently overlying the region of the cervix. Closer scrutiny of the image, however, reveals rounding and bulging of the upper margin of the cervix (**arrows**) suggesting a lower uterine contraction. **B:** Image obtained 22 min after the scan in (**A**) after resolution of the lower uterine contraction reveals a normal appearing cervix (**arrow**) without overlying placental tissue.

A subchorionic hematoma overlying the cervix is another source of a false positive diagnosis of placenta previa. This is most likely to occur if imaging is performed soon after the bleed, when the hemorrhage may be similar in echogenicity to the adjacent placental tissue. Distinction between subchorionic hematoma overlying the cervix and placenta previa can be difficult, particularly because both disorders may present with similar symptomatology, i.e., vaginal bleeding. Color Doppler may help distinguish a hematoma from a previa because it will demonstrate blood flow in a placenta previa, whereas a hematoma will be avascular. Follow-up ultrasound should show interval evolution in the echo pattern of a subchorionic hematoma, but little change in appearance of a placenta previa.

Transabdominal sonography alone may not be sufficient to accomplish the dual goals of imaging both the lower edge of the placenta as well as the cervix. The lower edge of the placenta may be difficult to see by transabdominal sonography during the third trimester of pregnancy, particularly if it is located in the midline, directly posterior to the fetus. Moreover, though transabdominal ultrasound is usually successful in depicting the cervix during the second trimester of pregnancy, it becomes increasingly more difficult to image the cervix with advancing pregnancy, largely due to attenuation of sound by the presenting part of the fetus. Consequently, a variety of techniques have been developed in an attempt to improve transabdominal visualization of the cervix. Such maneuvers include Trendelenburg positioning, overdistention of the urinary bladder, and the application of traction to the presenting part of the fetus in an attempt to elevate it out of the pelvis.[35—37] These techniques, however, can be uncomfortable for the patient,

can distort the appearance of the cervix and lower uterus, and frequently are ineffective late in pregnancy.[35]

Transperineal and endovaginal sonography have both been used to circumvent this problem. These ultrasound approaches effectively bypass the shadowing from the presenting part of the fetus, thereby permitting cervical visualization in the vast majority of patients.[38—44] Placenta previa has the same overall appearance by transabdominal, transperineal, and endovaginal sonography, except that the orientation of the cervix varies depending on the approach used (**Fig. 24–8 A,B**). Both the transperineal and the endovaginal techniques are highly successful in visualizing the cervix and establishing the presence or absence of placenta previa.[38—45] Transperineal sonography has the relative advantage of not requiring vaginal penetration. Despite this, endovaginal ultrasound has been shown to be safe in patients with placenta previa, with the caveat that it should be performed cautiously.[42—44, 46]

The patient with placenta previa is at increased risk for aberrant placental attachment.[32] Therefore, once an ultrasound diagnosis of placenta previa has been established, the sonologist should consider the question of whether or not there is ancillary evidence to suggest a concurrent abnormality of placental attachment. The grades of abnormal placental attachment include placenta accreta, placenta increta, and placenta percreta. *Placenta accreta* refers to extension of chorionic villi into the myometrium, *placenta increta* indicates extension of villi through the myometrium, and *placenta percreta* denotes penetration of villi through the uterine serosa. These complications are most likely in the multigravid woman with a prior history of cesarean section and placenta previa during the current pregnancy. The

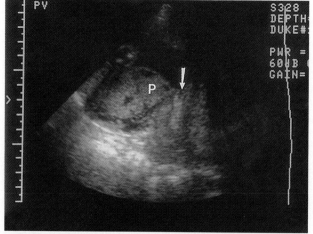

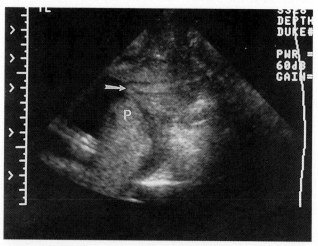

Figure 24–8 Marginal placenta previa at transabdominal and transperineal ultrasound. **A:** Transabdominal ultrasound reveals placental tissue (P) overlying a portion of the cervix (**arrow**) but not implanted on the os, consistent with marginal placenta previa. **B:** Transperineal ultrasound reveals a similar appearance, with placental tissue (P) overlying a portion of the cervix (**arrow**). Note that the transabdominal and transperineal images are depicted in different orientations: the cervix is in an approximately vertical orientation by transabdominal ultrasound, and approximately horizontal orientation by transperineal ultrasound.

risk of placenta accreta rises progressively as the number of prior cesarean sections increases.

Until recently, most cases of abnormal placental attachment were not diagnosed by ultrasonography. Sonographic features predicting an increased likelihood of abnormal placental attachment in patients with placenta previa have since been described. Recognition of these signs can alert the obstetrician to the possibility of placenta accreta, and thereby facilitate advance preparation for the possibility of severe hemorrhage and the possible need for cesarean hysterectomy at the time of delivery. Detection of large and irregular placental vascular lacunar spaces, with flow by color Doppler interrogation (**Fig. 24–9**)[47–51] has been associated with an increased likelihood of placenta accreta. Although vascular spaces can also be seen in the placentas of patients without placenta accreta, there is a tendency for them to be more numerous, larger, and more irregular in configuration in the setting of placenta accreta.[52] Other sonographic findings may include loss of the normal hypoechoic retroplacental area, thinning or disruption of the hyperechoic uterine serosa-bladder interface, and the presence of focal mass like elevations of tissue (similar in echogenicity to the placenta) projecting beyond the uterine serosa, into or adjacent to the bladder.[52, 53] In patients with placenta previa and a prior history of cesarean section, these findings provide very good, although not perfect discrimination between normal versus abnormal placental attachments.[52] If the sole finding is loss of the retroplacental hypoechoic area, however, prediction of placenta accreta is less accurate than if multiple findings are present.[52] Magnetic resonance imaging may be helpful if the placenta is suboptimally seen by ultrasound.[47]

Circumvallate Placenta

The normal placenta is completely covered by villus chorion. Circumvallate or circummarginate placenta occurs when the villus chorion ends short of the placental margin so that some villi are unprotected by membranes. Placenta circummarginate is characterized by a narrow band of exposed villi, with the transition from villus to membranous chorion marked by a flat ring of membranes.[54] Circummarginate placenta generally does not cause symptoms and is considered a variant of normal. Circumvallate placenta, in contrast, is characterized by a raised, rolled edge of tissue with a larger volume of unexposed villi. Circumvallate placenta can cause bleeding, most commonly during the second trimester of pregnancy.[54] The etiology for the bleeding is postulated to be that the exposed placental tissue is more friable so it bleeds more easily than the normal placenta. Other potential complications include inflammation, infection, and preterm delivery.

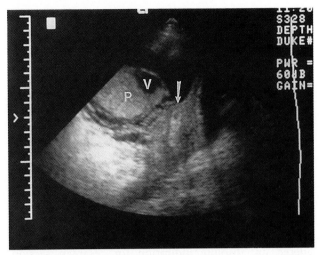

Figure 24–9   Placenta previa with placenta accreta. Transabdominal ultrasound reveals placental tissue (P) partially overlying the cervix (**straight arrow**), consistent with a marginal placenta previa. In addition, a large hypoechoic vascular space (V) is seen in the lower placenta. Similar spaces were seen throughout the inferior portion of the placenta, suggesting the possibility of placenta accreta. This diagnosis was confirmed histopathologically, and the patient required emergency cesarean hysterectomy due to profuse bleeding.

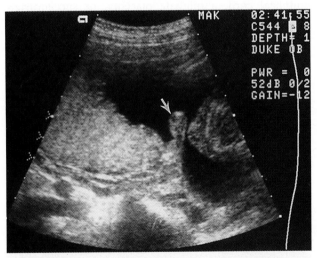

Figure 24–10   Circumvallate placenta. An elevated shelf of tissue (**arrow**) projects into the amniotic fluid at the inferior margin of the placenta. This is a typical appearance for circumvallate placenta.

At ultrasonography, circumvallate placenta is characterized by an elevated shelf of placental tissue at the placental edge, projecting into the amniotic fluid[54–56] (**Fig. 24–10**). The shelf can involve the entire perimeter of the placental margin, but frequently is only partial.[54] The elevated shelf of placental tissue can be difficult to image if it is obscured by a uterine contraction or closely apposed to the placenta.[54] Indeed, a recent study showed that the sensitivity and specificity of ultrasonography in identifying circumvallate placenta is limited.[57]

Vasa Previa

Vasa previa is a rare but dangerous condition in which placental vessels within the membranes cross the internal cervical os in advance of the presenting part of the fetus, unprotected by placenta or umbilical cord. Vasa previa occurs in patients with a bilobate or succenturiate lobe of the placenta or a velamentous insertion of the umbilical cord. The only known source of vaginal bleeding comprising pure fetal blood, it is an extremely important diagnosis to make, as fetal complications are potentially catastrophic. The vessels crossing the internal cervical os are prone to rupture at the time of rupture of the membranes, potentially leading to rapid fetal exsanguination and death. Vasa previa is therefore considered an absolute indication for cesarean section. Despite the high incidence of fetal mortality, vasa previa poses little or no risk to the mother.

The diagnosis of vasa previa should be suspected in the patient with the classic clinical presentation of bright red vaginal bleeding beginning around the time of membrane rupture. A high level of suspicion is likewise indicated in patients with a velamentous insertion of the umbilical cord, a bilobate placenta, or succenturiate placental lobes, particularly when an accessory placental lobe is implanted low in the uterus.

Until recently, the ultrasonographic diagnosis of vasa previa was rarely established antenatally. With the advent of color Doppler and endovaginal imaging, however, there have been an increasing number of reports of antenatally diagnosed vasa previa.[58—65] By gray scale ultrasound the diagnosis can be suspected if circular or linear hypoechoic structures typical of vessels are seen traversing the cervical os (**Fig. 24–11**).[58] The vascular nature of these structures can then be confirmed by color Doppler imaging. Spectral Doppler will demonstrate an arterial waveform with the fetal heart rate, confirming the fetal origin of these vessels.

The blood vessels comprising a vasa previa must be distinguished from prominent but normal cervical and lower uterine blood vessels. Cervical varices and myometrial vessels can be distinguished from vasa previa based on their location lateral to the lower uterine segment and around the periphery of the cervix. Umbilical cord presentation or umbilical cord prolapse can also present a sonographic picture resembling that of vasa previa, with blood vessels overlying the cervix, but contained within the umbilical cord structure.

The accuracy of ultrasound for vasa previa is unknown because the literature has been predominately comprised of case reports. There are well-documented cases in which antenatal ultrasonography failed to detect a vasa previa which was subsequently documented at delivery.[63, 66] Antenatal ultrasound diagnosis seems to require a high level of suspicion, and is more likely to be made in the patient with suggestive clinical signs such as bright red vaginal bleeding at the time of membrane rupture, or ultrasonographic evidence of a high risk of vasa previa based on the presence of succenturiate lobes of the placenta, a bilobate placenta, or a velamentous umbilical cord insertion.

Uterine Rupture and Uterine Dehiscence

Uterine rupture is a rare, but clinically important etiology for third-trimester bleeding. This potentially catastrophic event poses an extremely high risk both to the fetus and the mother. Maternal death rates have been reported to be as high as 2—20%, with fetal mortality in the 10—60% range.[67] The classic clinical presentation of uterine rupture includes uterine pain, vaginal bleeding, and shock. Often, however, the clinical picture is less dramatic. Clinical symptomatology can be surprisingly elusive, and signs or symptoms may be absent in up to 50% of patients, with symptoms mimicking other conditions.[60—70] For example, the pain which accompanies uterine rupture may closely resemble the pain occurring due to placental abruption. Not surprisingly then, in some cases uterine rupture is not discovered until the time of delivery.[68]

The terms *uterine rupture* and *uterine dehiscence* have been used interchangeably in the literature.[69] Strictly speaking, uterine rupture is defined as disruption of all the layers surrounding the fetus, including the membranes, myometrium, and serosa, and results in direct communication between the uterine cavity and peritoneal cavity.[67] In contrast, uterine dehiscence refers to rupture of the myometrium, but does not imply rupture of fetal membranes.[67] Dehiscence tends to be a gradual process, often with few if any symptoms, whereas rupture tends to be acute in nature and is more likely to be fatal.[69]

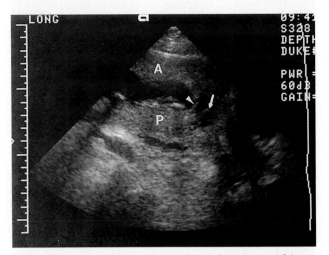

Figure 24–11 Vasa previa. Transabdominal sonogram of lower uterus reveals anterior (A) and posterior (P) lobes of the placenta, connected by a membrane (**arrowhead**) containing blood vessels (**closed arrow**) overlying the cervix (**open arrows**). The diagnosis of succenturiate lobes of the placenta with vasa previa was confirmed at delivery.

The possibility of uterine rupture should be considered in the symptomatic pregnant patient who has undergone prior uterine surgery or a complicated curettage procedure. The majority of ruptures occur in patients who have had a prior cesarean section,[67] but other predisposing conditions include myomectomy, curettage,[71] resection of cornual ectopic pregnancy,[72] and other uterine surgeries. Rupture of a low transverse cesarean section scar tends to occur during labor,[73] and should be considered in patients with prior cesarean sections who experience vaginal bleeding during labor. The classic cesarean section scar, on the other hand, tends to rupture explosively, usually before the onset of labor.[67,73] Uterine rupture also can occur secondary to intense labor induction, excessively long or difficult labor, or following blunt abdominal trauma.

A number of cases of preoperative sonographic diagnosis of uterine rupture or dehiscence have been reported. Diagnosis has typically relied on nonspecific ultrasound findings such as progressive myometrial thinning,[74] intraperitoneal or extraperitoneal hematomas or intraamniotic blood clots[68,75] detected in the appropriate clinical setting. A more specific diagnosis has been rendered based on sonographic depiction of a defect in the uterine wall, in conjunction with free or loculated abdominal fluid, a hematoma, or protrusion of the amniotic sac and/or fetal parts through the defect.[69,70,72,73,76] In one of the more extreme examples reported, ultrasound revealed an empty uterus in conjunction with hemoperitoneum and an intraabdominal placenta and fetus, creating an ultrasound picture similar to that of abdominal pregnancy.[77]

Conclusion

Second- and third-trimester bleeding occurs due to a range of obstetric and nonobstetric disorders. Obstetric sources of bleeding tend to be more serious and can pose grave risks to the health and welfare of mother and fetus. Ultrasonography plays a critical role in evaluating serious obstetric sources of hemorrhage, but is of less importance in assessing nonobstetric etiologies. Important obstetric conditions to be considered in the differential diagnosis of second- and third-trimester bleeding include placenta previa, placental abruption, circumvallate placenta, vasa previa, and uterine rupture.

The author wishes to thank Susan Murray for assistance with manuscript preparation.

References

1. Tucker SM. Perinatal protocol — Second or third trimester bleeding. *J Perinatol* 1988;8:174—177.
2. Scott JR. Placenta previa and placental abruption. In: Scott JR, DiSaia PJ, Hammond CB, Spellacy WN (eds). *Danforth's Obstetrics and Gynecology*, 7th ed.. J.B. Lippincott Co, Philadelphia: 1994, p. 489—500.
3. Pernoll ML. Third-trimester hemorrhage. In: Pernoll ML (ed). *Current Obstetric and Gynecologic Diagnosis and Treatment*, 7th ed. Appleton & Lange, Norwalk, CT: 1991, p. 388—400.
4. Spinillo A, Fazzi E, Stronati M, et al. Early morbidity and neurodevelopmental outcome in low-birthweight infants born after third trimester blooding. *Am J Perinatol* 1994;11:85—90.
5. Third-trimester bleeding. In: Dunnihoo DR (ed). *Fundamentals of Gynecology & Obstetrics*, 2nd ed. J.B. Lippincott Co, Philadelphia, PA: 1992, p. 535—538.
6. Prater JM, Warrington P. Urethral varices as an unusual cause of third-trimester bleeding — a case report. *J Reprod Med* 1988;33:664—666.
7. Obstetrical hemorrhage. In: Cunningham FG, MacDonald PC, Gant NF (eds). *William's Obstetrics*. Appleton & Lange, Norwalk, CT: 1989, p. 695—725.
8. Langlois SLP, Miller AG. Placenta praevia — a review with emphasis on the role of ultrasound. *Aust NZ J Obstet Gynaecol* 1989;29:110—116.
9. Powell MD, Buckley J, Price H, Worthington BS, Symonds EM. Magnetic resonance imaging and placenta previa. *Am J Obstet Gynecol* 1986;154:565—569.
10. Nyberg DA, Mack LA, Benedetti TJ, Cyr DR, Schuman WP. Placental abruption and placental hemorrhage: correlation of sonographic findings with fetal outcome. *Radiology* 1987;164:357—361.
11. Nyberg DA, Cyr RD, Mack LA, Wilson DA, Shuman WP. Sonographic spectrum of placental abruption. *AJR* 1987;148:161—164.
12. Jouppila P, Kirkinen P. Problems associated with the ultrasonic diagnosis of abruptio placentae. *Int J Gynaecol Obstet* 1982;20:5—11.
13. Combs CA, Nyberg DA, Mack LA, Smith JR, Benedetti TH. Expectant management after sonographic diagnosis of placental abruption. *Am J Perinatol* 1992;9:170—174.
14. Metzger DA, Bowie JD, Killam AP. Expectant management of partial placental abruption in previable pregnancies — a report of two cases. *J Reprod Med* 1987;32:789—792.
15. Sholl JS. Abruptio placentae: clinical management in non-acute cases. *Am J Obstet Gynecol* 1987;156:40—51.
16. Mintz MC, Kurtz AB, Arenson R, et al. Abruptio placentae: apparent thickening of the placenta caused by hyperechoic retroplacental clot. *J Ultrasound Med* 1986;5:411—413.
17. Ito M, Kawasaki N, Matsui K, Fujisaki S. Fetal heart monitoring and ultrasound in the management of placental abruption. *Int J Gynaecol Obstet* 1986;24:269—273.
18. Hill LM, Breckle R. Fetal outcome after intraamniotic hemorrhage with placental abruption — a report of three cases. *J Reprod Med* 1986;31:1065—1070.
19. Jaffe MH, Schoen WC, Silver TM, Bowerman RA, Stuck KJ. Sonography of abruptio placentae. *AJR* 1981;137:1049—1054.
20. McGahan JP, Phillips HE, Reid MH, Oi RH. Sonographic spectrum of retroplacental hemorrhage. *Radiology* 1982;142:481—485.
21. McGahan JP, Phillips HE, Reid MH. The anechoic retroplacental area. *Radiology* 1980;134:475—478.

22. Gottesfeld KR. The clinical role of placental imaging. *Clin Obstet Gynecol* 1984;27:327—341.

23. Kuhn W, Ulbrich R, Rath W. Changes of the clinical presentation of abruptio placentae. *Europ J Obstet Gynecol Reprod Biol* 1984;17:131—140.

24. Fleming AD. Abruptio placentae. *Crit Care Clin* 1991;7:865—875.

25. Hill LM, Breckle R, Gehrking W. Abruptio placentae: an unusual ultrasonic presentation. *Am J Obstet Gynecol* 1984;148:1144—1145.

26. Gottsfeld KR, Thompson HE, Holmes JH, Taylor ES. Ultrasonic placentography: a new method for placental localization. *Am J Obstet Gynecol* 1966;96:538—547.

27. Donald I, Abdulla U. Placentography by sonar. *J Obstet Gynaecol Br Commonw* 1968;75:993—1006.

28. Campbell S, Kohorn EI. Placental localization by ultrasonic compound scanning. *J Obstet Gynaecol Br Commonw* 1968;75:1007—1013.

29. Sunden B. Placentography by ultrasound. *Acta Obstet Gynecol Scand* 1970;49:179—184.

30. Bowie JD, Rochester D, Cadkin AV, Cooke WT, Kunzmann A. Accuracy of placental localization by ultrasound. *Radiology* 1978;128:177—180.

31. Townsend RR, Laing FC, Nyberg DA, et al. Technical factors responsible for "placental migration": sonographic assessment. *Radiology* 1986;160:105.

32. Mabie WC. Placenta previa. *Clin Perinatol* 1992;19:425—435.

33. Lavery JP. Placenta previa. *Clin Obstet Gynecol* 1990;33:414—421.

34. Zelop CC, Bromley B, Frigoletto Jr FD, Benacerraf BR. Second trimester sonographically diagnosed placenta previa: prediction of persistent previa at birth. *Int J Gynecol Obstet* 1994;44:207—210.

35. Wells SW, Anderson NG, Allan RB. Efficacy of fetal part elevation to visualise internal cervical os. *Australas Radiol* 1992;36:110—111.

36. Jeffrey RB, Laing FC. Sonography of the low-lying placenta: value of Trendelenburg and traction scans. *AJR* 1981;137:547—549.

37. Lee TG, Knochel JQ, Melendez MG, Henderson SC. Fetal elevation: a new technique for placental localization in the diagnosis of previa. *J Ultrasound Med* 1981;9:467—471.

38. Hertzberg BS, Bowie JD, Carroll BA, Kliewer MA, Weber TM. Diagnosis of placenta previa during the third trimester: role of transperineal sonography. *AJR* 1992;159:83—87.

39. Zilianti M, Azuaga A, Calderon F, Redondo C. Transperineal sonography in second trimester to term pregnancy and early labor. *J Ultrasound Med* 1991;10:481—485.

40. Farine D, Fox HE, Jakobson S, Timor-Tritsch IE. Vaginal ultrasound for diagnosis of placenta previa. *Am J Obstet Gynecol* 1988;159:566—569.

41. Timor-Tritsch IE, Monteagudo A. Diagnosis of placenta previa by transvaginal sonography. *Ann Intern Med* 1993;25:279—283.

42. Timor-Tritsch IE, Yunis RA. Confirming the safety of transvaginal sonography in patients suspected of placenta previa. *Obstet Gynecol* 1993;81:742—744.

43. Leerentveld RA, Gilberts ECAM, Arnold MJCWJ, Wladimiroff JW. Accuracy and safety of transvaginal sonographic placental localization. *Obstet Gynecol* 1990;76:759762.

44. Tan NH, Abu M, Woo JLS, Tahir HM. The role of transvaginal sonography in the diagnosis of placenta praevia. *Aust NZ J Obstet Gynaecol* 1995;35:42—45.

45. Farine D, Peisner DB, Timor-Tritsch IE. Placenta previa — is the traditional diagnostic approach satisfactory? *J Clin Ultrasound* 1990;18:328—330.

46. Hilpert PL, Kurtz AB. The role of transvaginal ultrasound in the second- and third-trimesters. *Semin Ultrasound CT MR* 1990;11:59—70.

47. Levine D, Hulka CA, Ludmir J, Li W, Edelman RR. Placenta accreta: evaluation with color Doppler US, power Doppler US, and MR imaging. *Radiology* 1997;205:773—776.

48. Silver LE, Hobel CJ, Lagasse L, Luttrull JW, Platt LD. Placenta previa percreta with bladder involvement: new considerations and review of the literature. *Ultrasound Obstet Gynecol* 1997;9:131—138.

49. Lerner JP, Deane S, Timor-Tritsch IE. Characterization of placenta accreta using transvaginal sonography and color Doppler imaging. *Ultrasound Obstet Gynecol* 1995;5:198—201.

50. Craigo S. Placenta previa with suspected accreta. *Current Opinion Obstet Gynecol* 1997;9:71—75.

51. Guy GP, Peisner DB, Timor-Tritsch IE. Ultrasonographic evaluation of uteroplacental blood flow patterns of abnormally located and adherent placentas. *Am J Obstet Gynecol* 1990;163:723—727.

52. Finberg HJ, Williams JW. Placenta accreta: prospective sonographic diagnosis in patients with placenta previa and prior cesarean section. *J Ultrasound Med* 1992;11:333—343.

53. Hoffman-Tretin JC, Koenigsberg M, Rabin A, Anyaegbunam A. Placenta accreta — additional sonographic observations. *J Ultrasound Med* 1992;11:29—34.

54. McCarthy J, Thurmond AS, Jones MK, et al. Circumvallate placenta: sonographic diagnosis. *J Ultrasound Med* 1995;14:21—26.

55. Cutillo DP, Swayne LC, Schwartz JR, Dise CA, Faux RG. Intra-amniotic hemorrhage secondary to placenta circumvallate. *J Ultrasound Med* 1989;8:399—401.

56. Bey M, Dott A, Miller Jr JM. The sonographic diagnosis of circumvallate placenta. *Obstet Gynecol* 1991;78:515—517.

57. Harris RD, Wells WA, Black WC, et al. Accuracy of prenatal sonography for detecting circumvallate placenta. *AJR* 1997;168:1603—1608.

58. Reuter KL, Davidoff A, Hunter T. Vasa previa. *J Clin Ultrasound* 1988;16:346—348.

59. Gianopoulos J, Carver T, Tomich PG, Karlman R, Gadwood K. Diagnosis of vasa previa with ultrasonography. *Obstet Gynecol* 1987;69:488—491.

60. Hsieh FJ, Chen HF, Ko TM, Hsieh CY, Chen HY. Antenatal diagnosis of vasa previa by color-flow mapping. *J Ultrasound Med* 1991;10:397—399.

61. Meyer WJ, Blumenthal L, Cadkin A, Gauthier DW, Rotmensch S. Vasa previa: prenatal diagnosis with transvaginal color Doppler flow imaging. *Am J Obstet Gynecol* 1993;169:1627—1629.

62. Hata K, Hata T, Fujiwaki R, et al. An accurate antenatal diagnosis of vasa previa with transvaginal color Doppler ultrasonography. *Am J Obstet Gynecol* 1994;171:265—267.

63. Hurley VA. The antenatal diagnosis of vasa praevia: the role of ultrasound. *Aust NZ J Obstet Gynaecol* 1988;28:177—179.

64. Harding JA, Lewis DF, Major CA, et al. Color flow Doppler — a useful instrument in the diagnosis of vasa previa. *Am J Obstet Gynecol* 1990;163:1566—1568.

65. Nelson LH, Melone PJ, King M. Diagnosis of vasa previa with transvaginal and color flow Doppler ultrasound. *Obstet Gynecol* 1990;76:506—509.

66. Eddleman KA, Lockwood CJ, Berkowitz, Lapinski RH, Berkowitz RL. Clinical significance and sonographic diagnosis of velamentous umbilical cord insertion. *Am J Perinatol* 1992;9:123—126.

67. Rooholamini SA, Au AH, Hansen GC, et al. Imaging of pregnancy-related complications. *RadioGraphics* 1993;13:753—770.

68. Gale JT, Mahony BS, Bowie JD. Sonographic features of rupture of the pregnant uterus. *J Ultrasound Med* 1986;5:713—714.

69. Shrout AB, Kopelman JN. Ultrasonographic diagnosis of uterine dehiscence during pregnancy. *J Ultrasound Med* 1995;14:399—402.

70. Osmers R, Ulbrich R, Schauer A, Kuhn W. Sonographic detection of an asymptomatic rupture of the uterus due to necrosis during the third trimester. *Int J Gynecol Obstet* 1988;26:279—284.

71. Acton CM, Long PA. The ultrasonic appearance of a ruptured uterus. *Aust Radiol* 1978;22:254—256.

72. van Alphen M, van Vugt JMG, Hummel P, van Geijn HP. Recurrent uterine rupture diagnosed by ultrasound. *Ultrasound Obstet Gynecol* 1995;5:419—421.

73. Suonio S, Saarikoski S, Kääriäinen J, Virtanen R. Intrapartum rupture of uterus diagnosed by ultrasound: a case report. *Int J Gynaecol Obstet* 1984;22:411—413.

74. Chapman K, Meire H, Chapman R. The value of serial ultrasounds in the management of recurrent uterine scar rupture. *Br J Obstet Gynaecol* 1994;101:549—551.

75. Bedi DG, Salmon A, Winsett MZ, Fagan CJ, Kumar R. Ruptured uterus: sonographic diagnosis. *J Clin Ultrasound* 1986;14:529—533.

76. Kushnir O, Tamarkin M, Barkai G, et al. Extrauterine amniotic sac (amniocele) — clinical workup in a case of silent uterine rupture. *J Ultrasound Med* 1990;9:367—369.

77. Harrison SD, Nghiem HV, Shy K. Uterine rupture with fetal death following blunt trauma. *AJR* 1995;165:1452.

25 Cervical Sonography in Premature Labor

Geoffrey Wong, Deborah Levine

Introduction

Premature delivery (delivery before 37 weeks gestational age) complicates 8 to 10% of all pregnancies in the United States and is a major cause of perinatal morbidity and mortality.[1,2] There has been a decrease in perinatal mortality rate with improvement of obstetrical and neonatal care, but prematurity is still responsible for over 70% of perinatal deaths. The cost of providing care to an extremely premature infant in the immediate neonatal period is 50 times more than that of an infant born at term, and the health care cost for the rest of the first year of life is 20 times more expensive.[3] In addition, there frequently are significant physical and neurological sequelae in children born very prematurely.

Although there have been recent advances in the prevention, detection, and treatment of premature labor, these advances have not produced a significant decrease in the incidence of premature delivery. A possible explanation for the lack of impact is an increase in the population at high risk for premature delivery. For example, with increased use of assisted reproductive technology, there is a dramatic increase in multifetal gestations. In addition, patients with significant medical or reproductive risk factors previously advised not to conceive are now attempting pregnancy under the supervision of high-risk obstetrical teams.

Obstetrical ultrasound plays an important role in the evaluation of patients in premature labor, not only in the determination of gestational age and fetal well-being, but also in the assessment of the cervix. The cervix plays a unique role in pregnancy. The closed and uneffaced cervix physically maintains the fetus in utero, and secretions from the cervix form the mucous plug that is partly responsible for preventing ascending infection. The chapter can be the cause of premature delivery in cases of incompetent cervix. An incompetent cervix results from compromised cervical strength, which may be congenital or acquired, that leads to a decrease in cervical length and painless dilatation of the cervix as early as the second trimester. Changes in cervical length, dilatation, and effacement predict and reflect the stages of premature labor (contractions causing cervical change before 37 weeks gestational age). Sonography, using a transvaginal or transperineal approach, provides an additional method beyond the traditional digital examination for the study of the uterine cervix during pregnancy. This chapter will review the use of sonography in the assessment of the cervix in premature labor and delivery.

Technical Aspects

The transabdominal approach to scanning of the cervix is less accurate than the transvaginal or transperineal approach because the cervix is poorly visualized when the maternal bladder is empty (**Fig. 25–1**),[4] yet overdistention of the bladder artificially increases the length of the cervix and can obscure the presence of a dilated cervix. Maternal body habitus or a low fetal presenting part also may limit visualization of the cervix transabdominally. Because of the problems inherent with transabdominal scanning, imaging of the cervix is best performed with either a transperineal or transvaginal approach (**Fig. 25–2**).

Transperineal scanning is performed with a 3.5- to 5-MHz sector probe. The probe should be covered by a condom or plastic wrap for hygienic reasons and infection control.[5] The probe is placed on the perineum, over the labia minora, and is aimed in the direction of the vaginal canal toward the cervix (**Fig. 25–3**). Transperineal scanning is very operator-dependent. Pitfalls include obscuration of the cervix by rectal gas, shadowing by the pelvic bones, and inadequate visualization of the external os due to direct contact of the vaginal wall with the cervix. Hertzberg et al.[6] have shown that elevating the patient's hips and buttocks off the scanning table can improve cervical visualization in cases where routine transperineal views are inadequate. Transperineal sonography has an advantage over transvaginal sonography in that the probe is not introduced into the vagina. Therefore, in patients with active bleeding or in whom ruptured membranes are suspected, transperineal scanning is our recommended approach. Additional benefits are that transperineal scanning is more comfortable for the patient than is transvaginal scanning and no artifact is produced by pressure exerted on the cervix.

A 5- to 10-MHz vaginal probe is used in transvaginal scanning of the cervix. When using the transvaginal approach, care should be taken not to insert the probe abruptly or too deeply. The ultrasound monitor should be viewed in real-time during insertion of the probe to

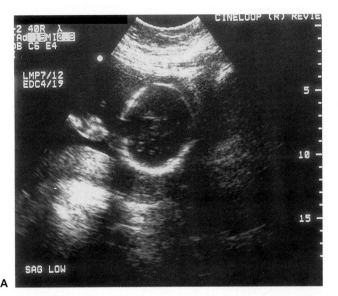

A

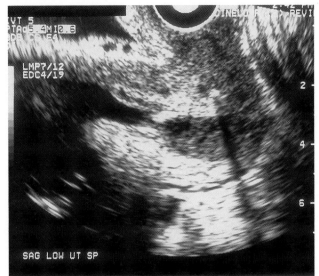

B

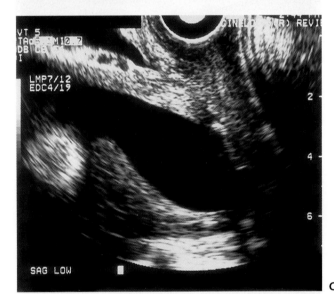

C

Figure 25–1 Abnormal cervix, not visualized on transabdominal scan. On transabdominal scan (**A**) the cervix was difficult to visualize due to nondistended bladder and position of the fetal head. On transvaginal scan (**B,C**) images seconds apart show the opening of the cervix with ballooning membranes. Note the position of the vaginal probe in image B, just at the introitus, almost like a translabial scan. When the cervix is suspected to be abnormal, the probe should be inserted gently, not to disrupt the membranes. Reproduced with permission from reference 4.

avoid traumatizing prolapsed fetal membranes or a low placenta (**Fig. 25–4**). The cervix should be identified and then the probe should be slightly withdrawn in order to obtain an accurate image of the internal os, external os, and cervical length (**Fig. 25–5**).[7] To avoid interobserver variability, Burger recommends that the image of the cervix meet the following criteria: (1) the internal os appears either flat or as an isosceles triangle; (2) the whole length of the cervical canal can be visualized; (3) a symmetric image of the external os can be obtained; and (4) the distance from the surface of the posterior lip to the cervical canal is equal to the distance from the anterior lip to the cervical canal.[8] The cervix should be observed for several minutes to detect dynamic change of the internal os and cervical length.[9] Even patients with known placenta previa can be safely scanned with a transvaginal probe, although for patients with active bleeding we recommend the transperineal approach.

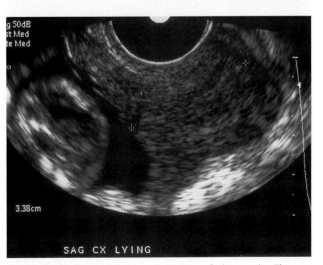

Figure 25–2 Normal transvaginal view of the cervix. The endocervical canal is indicated with calipers.

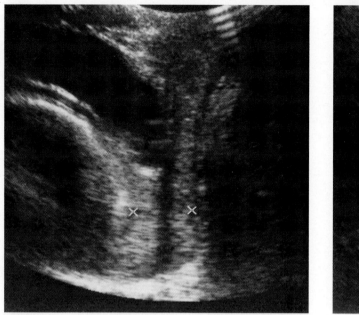

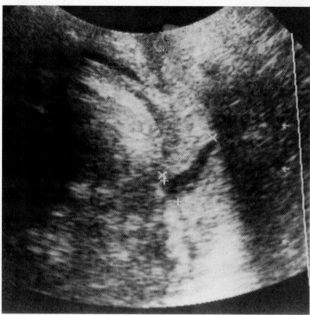

Figure 25–3 Translabial scan. (**A**) Calipers mark the internal and external os in a normal appearing cervix. (**B**) In a different patient, ballooning membranes are present.

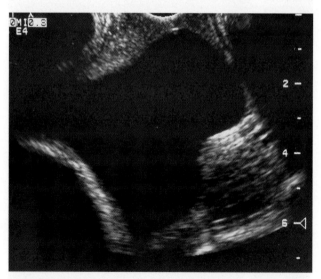

Figure 25–4 Ballooning membranes. When ballooning membranes are seen, the probe should not be inserted further into the vagina, but should be removed. The patient should be placed in Trendelenberg position and transferred to labor and delivery.

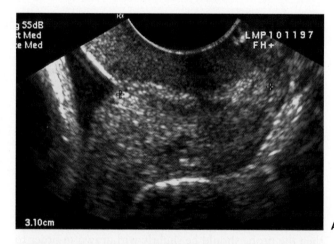

Figure 25–5 Pitfalls in measuring cervical length. Initial image (**A**) ▷ shows 3.1 cm cervical length. The transducer is withdrawn slightly and angled to demonstrate the shortest cervical length (**B**), which is 1 cm. Funneling of the internal os was obscured on the initial image due to pressure on the cervix.

The cervical length is measured from the internal os to the external os. When the internal os is open, with funneling, only the closed portion of the cervix is measured. When funneling is present, the anteroposterior diameter (at the region of the presumed internal os) and length of the funnel (from the presumed internal os to the closed portion of the cervix) also are measured.

The Cervix in Normal Pregnancy

It is difficult to distinguish the cervix from the lower uterine segment in the nonpregnant state and in the first half of pregnancy. By the middle of the second trimester, the amniotic sac provides a clear landmark for the internal cervical os. Cervical length measurements (defined as the distance between the internal and the external cervical os) have been shown to correlate well with digital examination of the cervix. Many authors suggest cervical sonography is superior to digital examination[10—16] because the measurements are reproducible, the intraabdominal portion of the cervix can be measured and the internal cervical os, where early changes from incompetent cervix and premature labor occur can be assessed. Sonography also has the theoretical advantage of less risk of infection and irritation of the cervix than digital examination.[11]

Cervical length often measures over 5 cm in the first trimester,[17] but some of this length may reflect the inability to define clearly the upper cervix from the lower uterine segment. Most studies define a normal cervical length as 3—4 cm in midpregnancy.[18—23] In a National Institute of Child Health and Human Development Network (NICHD) sponsored study, 2915 women with singleton pregnancies were studied by transvaginal cervical ultrasound examination at 22 to 24 weeks with follow-up examinations in 2531 patients at 26—28 weeks gestation.[24] The mean cervical length was 3.52 cm in the first group and 3.37 cm in the second group. The distribution of cervical lengths in the population followed a normal bell curve (**Fig. 25–6**). Other studies have shown that cervical length is the same in nulliparous and multiparous women.[17, 21]

Patients carrying multiple gestations have significantly shorter cervical lengths for matched gestational age, than singleton pregnancies. In singleton pregnancies, cervical length usually remains above 4 cm through 37 weeks, while in twin pregnancies it is often less than 3 cm by 32 weeks.[25—27] This cervical shortening is associated with an increased risk of preterm delivery.[26, 27]

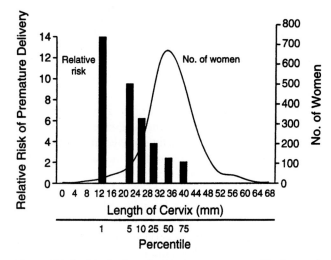

Figure 25–6 Distribution of subjects among percentiles for cervical length measured by transvaginal ultrasonography at 24 weeks of gestation (**solid line**) and relative risk of spontaneous preterm delivery before 35 weeks of gestation according to percentiles for cervical length (bars). The risks among women with values at or below the first, fifth, 10th, 25th, 50th, and 75th percentiles for cervical length are compared with the risk among women with values above the 75th percentile. Reproduced with permission from the **New England Journal of Medicine**, Copyright 1996, Massachusetts Medical Society. All rights reserved.

The Role of Cervical Sonography in Premature Labor

The most commonly used sonographic parameters in the assessment of premature labor are cervical length, dilation of the cervix, and the appearance of the internal cervical os. There is an inverse relationship between the sonographically measured length of the cervix and the risk of preterm delivery. Most studies place the at risk threshold at 2 to 3 cm.[17, 28-32] The NICHD study[24] demonstrated that a sonographically measured cervical length of less than 3.2 cm at 24 weeks gestation is associated with a sixfold increased risk of premature delivery before 35 weeks, and a cervical length of 1.2 cm at 24 weeks has a 14-fold risk of premature delivery. A transvaginally measured cervical length of less than 2 cm at 24 weeks has a sensitivity of 23% and a specificity of 97% for the prediction of preterm delivery. Cervical lengths measured sonographically at 24 weeks gestation of 3 cm, 2.5 cm, and 2 cm are associated with premature delivery in 9.3%, 18%, and 25%, respectively, of cases.

Some authors have proposed using a single transvaginal measurement of cervical length at 28 to 30 weeks will help to detect patients at risk for premature delivery.[33] However, the cost-effectiveness of such a program for the general population is questionable and the various cut-off values for cervical length have poor positive predictive values.

In twin pregnancies, a mean cervical length of 2.7 cm +/- 1 cm measured at 24 to 26 weeks is associated with either premature delivery or a necessity for obstetrical interventions to prolong pregnancy.[34,35] A cervical length of 3.5 cm at 24 to 26 weeks predicts delivery at term in the majority of cases.

In addition to cervical length, the appearance of the internal os is important in the assessment of preterm labor. The presence of funneling or wedging (dilation of the internal os with prolapse of fetal membranes into the cervical canal) is associated with preterm delivery.[36,37] Ominous signs predicting preterm delivery include a funnel length of > 1.5 cm, a funnel width of greater than 1.4 cm, a residual cervical length of less than 2 cm, and funneling over 40% of the cervical length.[36]

Recently, there has been interest in the use of fetal fibronectin[38,39] and prostaglandin[40] assays in combination with cervical sonography to identify patients at risk for premature labor and delivery. Because premature labor has multiple etiologies, these protocols may have merit, but further studies are needed to evaluate the validity and cost effectiveness of such approaches.

In addition to predicting preterm delivery, cervical sonography can be used to select patients who would benefit from treatment of preterm contractions. Premature labor is associated with a heavy economic cost, and is one of the most overdiagnosed and overtreated medical conditions.[41] Yet it is important to diagnose and treat true premature labor in order to gain time to administer antenatal steroid treatment to promote fetal lung maturation and transport the pregnant woman to a tertiary care facility when necessary.

In patients with premature contractions, sonography of the cervix can be used to direct management. In such patients, hospitalization and tocolytic therapy is usually required only in those patients whose cervical length is less than 3 cm.[42]

Incompetent Cervix

The diagnosis of cervical incompetence is based on the demonstration of cervical dilatation and prolapsed fetal membranes into the cervical canal in the absence of uterine contractions (**Fig. 25–7**). Although the etiology of premature delivery is often multifactorial, incompetent cervix is felt to be the primary cause in 16% of premature births.[2] Risk factors such as DES exposure in utero, cone biopsy of the cervix, and prior cervical laceration identify some of the patients at risk, but the diagnosis of cervical incompetence is usually made on the basis of a history of midtrimester pregnancy loss associated with painless dilatation of the cervix. Often the patient cannot give an accurate description of the events surrounding a prior pregnancy loss. In addition, it is difficult to determine the initiating cause of preterm delivery when the patient already has embarked upon the final common pathway of premature labor, premature rupture of membranes, and chorioamnionitis. The identification of patients at risk for incompetent cervix is further made difficult as many patients with an incompetent cervix are nulliparous with no identifiable risk factors.[43,44]

In the past, it was believed that the cervix was either competent or incompetent. However, recent studies have shown the cervical changes occur on a continuum. Iams showed that cervical length in the current pregnancy can be predicted by the gestational age at delivery of the pre-

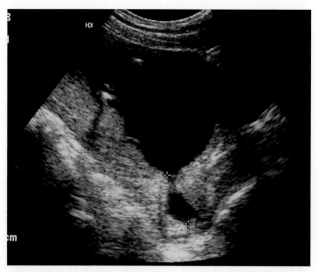

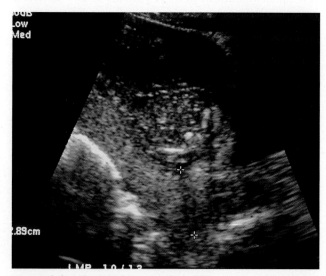

Figure 25–7 Incompetent cervix. Transabdominal view of the cervix at 19 weeks gestational age in an otherwise asymptomatic patient. The initial image (**A**) demonstrates ballooning membranes. Later in the examination (**B**), the cervix appeared normal. We rec-ommend that the initial image taken during routine obstetric sonography be the view of the cervix. This will help to identify cases of cervical incompetence that would otherwise escape detection.

vious preterm birth. For women who previously had preterm delivery before 32 weeks, the association between cervical length and preterm birth holds true in subsequent pregnancies.[45] This leads to the hope that when cervical sonography detects shortening of the cervix and/or development of membranes funneling at the internal os, timely intervention can be performed with improved perinatal outcome.

The timing of the initial examination and the frequency of follow-up examinations in patients with possible incompetent cervix have not been established. In patients with a history of pregnancy loss from an incompetent cervix, repeated loss usually occurs at the same gestational age or at an earlier gestational age. Therefore, in subsequent pregnancies, it is prudent to get an initial cervical scan to establish the baseline cervical length at a time before the gestational age at which the previous loss occurred. We recommend follow-up examinations every one to two weeks, depending on the findings of examinations and the clinical symptoms.

Conventional vaginal sonography to diagnose incompetent cervix will only detect a short cervix if some cervical changes have already taken place before the examination.[46–51] Functional maneuvers, such as transfundal pressure,[52] straining,[53] or scanning the cervix with the patient standing[54, 55] can elicit early cervical changes and identify patients at risk for incompetent cervix who otherwise would have gone undiagnosed. After a positive response is elicited from transfundal pressure, many patients have progressive cervical change 1 to 3 weeks later.[56] We prefer to examine patients standing, as this is a more physiologic reproduction of daily activity than is transfundal pressure. The standing position has no effect on the normal cervix, but patients with greater than 33% shortening in cervical length measured in the standing position after standing for 15 min are likely to deliver prematurely (**Fig. 25–8**).[55] We recommend scanning patients at risk for cervical incompetence both supine and upright and comparing the cervical measurements obtained in the two positions. This allows for identification of cervical changes in an incompetent cervix at an earlier stage than is possible with supine examination alone. It is also possible that a patient with a slightly short cervix, who does not demonstrate further shortening upon standing, will not benefit from cerclage. Further studies are needed to assess further the predictive value of functional maneuvers for detecting clinically significant changes in the cervix.

Because up to one-third of patients with cervical incompetence are nulliparous with no identifiable risk factors, when routine obstetrical sonography is performed during the second trimester, it may be beneficial to obtain the view of the cervix at the beginning of the study rather than at the end (**Fig. 25–7**). This will be a transabdominal view with the limitations mentioned above; however, it can identify an unsuspected short cervix or dilated internal os in those low-risk patients. These early cervical views, obtained just after the patient has attained the supine position, may identify a short cervix that would no longer be apparent after the patient had been lying supine for 30 or more minutes during a routine obstetric scan.

A dynamic or spontaneously changing cervix has been noted during transvaginal scanning of the cervix (**Fig. 25–1 B;C**).[57, 58] Transient, but striking dilation of the internal cervical os and cervical canal occurs in the absence of subjective symptoms and objective signs of uterine contractions. The etiology and mechanism of the dynamically changing cervix is not known. Because many patients with this finding deliver preterm, most

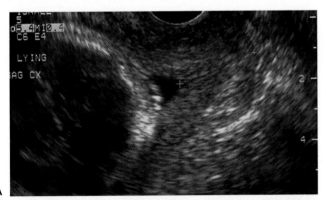

A

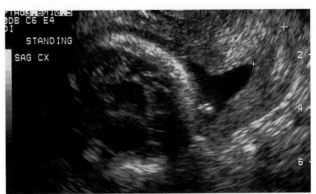

B

Figure 25–8 Changing cervix in a patient with a history of second-trimester pregnancy loss. (**A**) In the supine exam, the closed cervical length was 2.9 cm with 7 mm of wedging of the internal os. (**B**) After standing for 15 min, and being scanned upright, the closed cervical length was 1.8 cm. The patient delivered at 33 weeks gestational age. Reproduced with permission from reference 55.

patients with a changing cervix are advised to reduce their physical activities. The shorter the measurement of the cervix, the more likely the patient is to deliver pre-term.[57]

Cervical Cerclage

It is important to establish accurately the diagnosis of incompetent cervix to avoid unnecessary, costly, and potentially harmful surgical procedures aimed at correcting the condition. Cerclage placement (**Fig. 25–9**) should be considered when there is a firm diagnosis of incompetent cervix, by either historical events or current sonographic findings. Cervical cerclage is most successful when it is performed prophylactically or when there are only early cervical changes, rather than when cervical changes are pronounced.[44] The uterus and its contents are unlikely to be heavy enough to exert much pressure on the cervix before 14 to 15 weeks. Prophylactic cerclage can therefore be placed after the first trimester, after the period of maximum risk of spontaneous abortion. Sonographic guidance can be useful to assist in placement of the cerclage.[59] Follow-up cervical scans are obtained to assess the length and dilatation of the portion of cervix above the cerclage.[60–63] Shortening of the proximal cervical length (less than 1 cm) is associated with an increased risk of preterm delivery. Additional therapeutic maneuvers such as bed rest or reduced physical activities are important if there is either significant funneling above the cerclage or only a short portion of closed cervix remaining.[64]

For patients who do not have a clear history of incompetent cervix, a conservative approach without prophylactic cerclage can be successful if the cervix can be closely followed with transvaginal or translabial scans.

False-positive Incompetent Cervix

False-positive findings of incompetent cervix can be caused by uterine contractions.[9] The narrowed lower uterine segment can mimic funneling of the cervix. This can be clarified by observation of the cervix over time or with visualization of the thick myometrium associated with a contraction. Vaginal sonography will demonstrate that the cervix is of normal length. Compression of the lower uterine segment to produce an impression of funneling can also result from an overdistended urinary bladder (**Fig. 25–10**). Nabothian cysts (**Fig. 25–11**) and vaginal cysts located near the internal cervical os can create the false impression of a dilated internal os.

Premature Rupture of Membranes

When premature rupture of fetal membranes occurs before term, expectant management is often pursued to gain time for further fetal maturation. Digital examination of the cervix is contraindicated because of the risk of infection. Speculum examination is often used to help make the diagnosis of rupture of membranes, but visualization of the cervix is not accurate in determining dilatation or effacement of the cervix. Cervical sonography is helpful in assessing cervical dilation and effacement when there is premature rupture of membranes.[65] It is also useful in ruling out the presence of umbilical

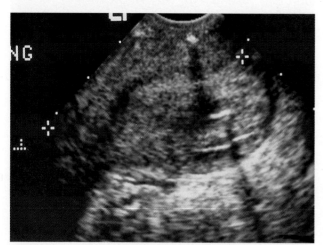

Figure 25–9   Cervical cerclage. Transvaginal view shows a normal appearing cervix with a cerclage in place.

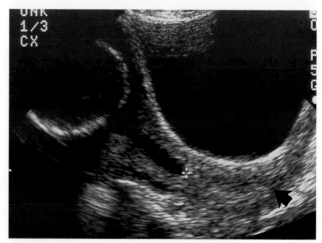

Figure 25–10   Full bladder mimicking funneling of the internal os. Transabdominal scan shows shows a normal appearing cervix (internal os, caliper; external os, arrow). The full bladder has caused compression of the lower uterine segment giving the appearance of funneling.

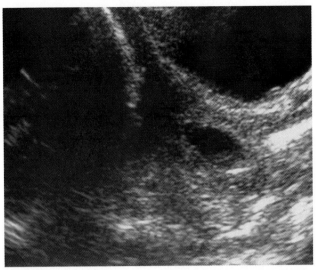

A

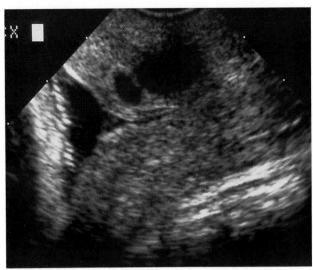

B

Figure 25–11 Nabothian cyst masquerading as funneling of the internal os. (**A**) Transabdominal view of the cervix shows an anechoic region suggestive of funneling of the internal os. This region is eccentric to the cervical canal (**arrowheads**). (**B**) Transvaginal scan shows two Nabothian cysts in the anterior cervix. A small amount of funneling of the internal os is present, however, this is not the region in question on the transabdominal scan. Reproduced with permission from reference 4.

cord in the lower uterine segment or near the cervical opening. Transvaginal sonography has not been associated with increased risk of infection when used to assess the cervix after premature rupture of membranes.[66] However, we prefer to use transperineal sonography to assess the cervix in such a setting.

Summary

Ultrasonography has emerged as an important diagnostic tool in assessment of the cervix during pregnancy. Cervical length, cervical dilation, and the status of the internal cervical os are all important prognosticators in premature labor and can be safely and accurately assessed by transvaginal and transperineal sonography. A short cervical length (less than 2 cm) and funneling of 40 to 50% of the length of the cervix places patients at high risk of premature delivery. Transvaginal sonography also can be used to diagnose and manage patients with incompetent cervix. Tests to provoke an incompetent cervix (such as transfundal pressure or scanning with the patient upright) help to detect incompetent cervix even earlier in asymptomatic patients. It is hoped that early identification of these at risk patients will lead to more effective treatment, resulting in a decrease in perinatal morbidity and mortality.

References

1. Berkowitz G, Papiernik K. Epidemiology of preterm birth. *Epidemiol Re.* 1993;15:141—143.
2. Roberts WE, Morrison JC, Hamer C. The incidence of preterm labor and specific risk factors. *Obstet Gynecol* 1990;76(Suppl 1):85 S.
3. Rogowski J. The economics of preterm deliveries. *Prenat Neonat Med* 1998;3:16—20.
4. Wong G, Levine D. Sonographic assessment of the cervix in pregnancy. *Sem Ultrasound CT MRI* 1998;19:370—380.
5. Liang F, Ryan T, Hadley K, et al. Plastic wrap for US transducer sterility or sanitization. *Radiology* 1986,160:486.
6. Hertzberg BS, Kliewer MA, Baumeister LA. Optimizing transperineal sonographic imaging of the cervix: the hip elevation technique. *J Ultrasound Med* 1994;13:933—936.
7. Confino E, Mayden K, Giglia R, et al. Pitfalls in sonographic imaging of the incompetent uterine cervix. *Acta Obstet Gynecol Scand* 1986;65:593—597.
8. Burger M, Weber-Rossler T, Willman M. Measurement of the pregnant cervix by transvaginal sonography: an interobserver study and new standards to improve the interobserver variability. *Ultrasound Obstet Gynecol* 1997;9:188–193.
9. Karis J, Hertzberg B, Bowie J. Sonographic diagnosis of premature cervical dilatation: potential pitfall due to lower uterine segment contractions. *J Ultrasound Med* 1991;10:83—87.
10. Berhella V, Tolosa J, Kuhlman K, et al. Cervical ultrasonography compared with manual examination as a predictor of premature delivery. *Am J Obstet Gynecol* 1997,177:723—730.
11. Goldberg J, Newman RB, Rust PF. Interobserver reliability of digital and endovaginal ultrasonographic cervical length measurements. *Am J Obstet Gynecol* 1977;177:853—858.
12. Gomez R, Glasso M, Romero R, et al. Ultrasonographic examination of the cervix is better than cervical digital examination as a predictor of preterm delivery in patients with premature labor and intact membranes. *Am J Obstet Gynecol* 1994;171:956—964.

13. Mahony B, Nyberg D, Luthy D, et al. Tarnslabial ultrasound of the third trimester uterine cervix correlates with digital examination. *J Ultrasound Med* 1990;9:717—723.

14. Onderoglu L. Digital examinaton and transperineal ultrasonographic measurement of cervical length to assess risk of preterm delivery. *Int J Gynaecol Obstet* 1997;59:223—228.

15. Richey S, Ramin K, Roberts S, et al. The correlation between transperineal sonography and digital examination in the evaluation of the third trimester cervix. *Obstet Gynecol* 1995;85:745—748.

16. Sonek J, Iams J, Blumenfeld M, et al. Measurement of the cervical length in pregnancy: comparison between vaginal ultrasonography and digital examination. *Obstet Gynecol* 1990;76:172—175.

17. Ayers J, DeGrood R, Compton A, et al. Sonographic evaluation of cervical length in pregnancy; diagnosis and management of preterm cervical effacement in patients at risk for premature delivery. *Obstet Gynecol* 1988;71:939—944.

18. Anderson H. Transvaginal and transabdominal ultrasonography of the uterine cervix during pregnancy. *J Clin Ultrasound* 1991;19:77—83.

19. Brown J, Thieme G, Shad D, et al. Transabdominal and transvaginal endosonography evaluation of the cervix and lower uterine segment in pregnancy. *Am J Obstet Gynecol* 1986,155:721—726.

20. Cook C, Ellwood D. A longitudinal study of the cervix in pregnancy with transvaginal ultrasound. *Br J Obstet Gynaecol* 1996;103:16—18.

21. Kushnir O, Vigil D, Izquierdo L, et al. Vaginal ultrasonographic assessment of cervical length changes during normals pregnancy. *Obstet Gynecol* 1990;162:991—993.

22. Smith C, Anderson J, Matamoros A, et al. Transvaginal sonography of cervical width and length during pregnancy. *J Ultrasound Med* 1992;11:465—467.

23. Zorzoli A, Soliani A, Perra M, et al. Cervical changes throughout pregnancy as assessed by transvaginal sonography. *Obstet Gynecol* 1994;84:960—964.

24. Iams J, Goldenberg R, Meis P, et al. The length of the cervix and the risk of spontaneous premature delivery. *N Engl J Med* 1996;334:567—572.

25. Kushnir O, Izquierdo L, Smith J, et al. Transvaginal sonographic measurement of cervical length. Evaluation of twin pregnancies. *J Reprod Med* 1995;40:380—382.

26. Eppen W, Schurz B, Frigo, et al. Vaginal sonography of the cervix in twin pregnancies. *Geburtshilfe Frauenheilkd* 1994;54:20—26.

27. Ludmir J, Abbott J, Wong G, et al. Vaginal sonography of the cervix in the management of triplet gestation. *Am J Obstet Gynecol* 1994;172:407.

28. Anderson H, Nugent C, Wanty S, et al. Prediction of risk for preterm delivery by ultrasonographic measurement of cervical length. *Am J Obstet Gynecol* 1990;163:859—867.

29. Bartolucci L, Hill W, Katz M, Gill P, Kitzmiller J. Ultrasonography in preterm labor. *Am J Obstet Gynecol* 1984;149:52—56.

30. Iams J, Paraskos J, Landon M, et al. Cervical sonography in preterm labor. *Obstet Gynecol* 1994;84:40—46.

31. Murawaka H, Utumi T, Hasegawa I, et al. Evaluation of threatened preterm delivery by transvaginal ultrasonographic measurement of cervical length. *Obstet Gynecol* 1993;82:829—832.

32. Okitus O, Mimura T, Nakayama T, et al. Early prediction of preterm delivery by transvaginal ultrasonography. *Ultrasound Obstet Gynecol* 1992;2:402—409.

33. Tongsong T, Kamprapanth P, Srisomboon J, et al. Single transvaginal sonographic measurement of cervical length early in the third trimester as a predictor of preterm deelivery. *Obstet Gynecol* 1995;86:184—187.

34. Imseis H, Albert T, Iams J. Identifying twins gestations at low-risk for preterm birth with a transvaginal sonographic measurement at 24—26 weeks gestation. *Am J Obstet Gynecol* 1997;176:(S6).

35. Crane J, Hof MVD, Armson R, Liston R. Transvaginal ultrasound in the prediction of preterm delivery: singleton and twin gestations. *Obstet Gynecol* 1997;90:357—363.

36. Berghella V, Kuhlman K, Weiner S. Cervical funneling: sonographic criteria predictive of preterm delivery. *Ultrasound Obstet Gynecol* 1997;10:161—166.

37. Timor-Tritsch I, Boozarjomehri F, Masakowski Y, et al. Can a snapshot sagittal view of the cervix by transvaginal ultrasonography predict active preterm labor. *Am J Obstet Gynecol* 1996;174:990—995.

38. Rizzo G, Capponi A, Arduini D, et al. The value of fetal fibronectin in cervical and vaginal secretions and of ultrasonographic examination of the uterine cervix in predicting premature delivery for patients with preterm labor and intact membranes. *Am J Obstet Gynecol* 1996;175:1146—1151.

39. Rozenberg P, Goffinet F, Malagrida L, et al. Evaluating the risk of preterm delivery: a comparison of fetal fibronectin and transvaginal ultrasonographic measurement of cervical length. *Am J Obstet Gynecol* 1997;176:196—199.

40. Vavra N, Eppel W, Sevelda P, et al. Serum prostaglandin F2 alpha (PGFM) and oxytocin levels correlates with sonographic changes in the cervix in patients with preterm labor. *Arch Gynecol Obstet* 1993;253:33—36.

41. Hueston W. Preterm contractions in community settings: I. Treatment of preterm contractions. *Obstet Gynecol* 1998;92:38—42.

42. Rageth J, Kernen B, Saurenmann E, et al. Premature contractions: possible influence of sonographic measurement of cervical length on clinical management. *Ultrasound Obstet Gynecol* 1997;9:183—187.

43. Ludmir J. Sonographic detection of cervical incompetence. *Clin Obstet Gynecol* 1988;31:101—109.

44. Wong G, Farquharson D, Dansereau J. Emergency cervical cerclage: a retrospective review of 51 cases. *Am J Perinatol* 1993;10:341—347.

45. Iams J, Johnson F, Sonek J, et al. Cervical incompetence as a continuum: a study of ultrasonographic cervical length and obstetrical performance. *Am J Obstet Gynecol* 1995;172:1097—1106.

46. Balde M, Stolz W, Unteregger B, et al. Transvaginal ultrasound: its value in the diagnosis of the incompetent cervix: *J Gynecol Obstet Biol Reprod* 1988;17:629—633.

47. Bernstine R, Sung H, Crawford W, et al. Sonographic evaluation of the incompetent cervix: *J Clin Ultrasound* 1981;9:417—420.

48. Brook l, Feingold M, Schwartz A. Ultrasonography in the diagnosis of cervical incompetence in pregnancy — a new diagnostic approach. *Br J Obstet Gynaecol* 1981;88:640—643.

49. Jackson G, Pendleton H, Nicol B, Wittman B. Diagnostic ultrasound in the assessment of patients with cervical incompetence. *Br J Obstet Gynaecol* 1984;91:232—236.

50. Michaels W, Schreiber F, Ager J, et al. Ultrasound surveillance of the cervix in twin gestations: management of cervical incompetence. *Obstet Gynecol* 1991;78:739—744.

51. Podobnik M, Bulic M, Smiljanic N, et al. Ultrasonography in the detection of cervical incompetence. *J Clin Ultrasound* 1988;13:383—391.

52. Guzman E, Rosenberg J, Houlihan C, et al. A new method using vaginal ultrasound and transfundal pressure to evaluate asymptomatic incompetent cervix. *Obstet Gynecol* 1994;83:248—252.

53. Sherif L, Shalan D. Detection of pregnant women at risk of cervical incompetence by transvagainal sonography during straining. *J Obstet Gynaecol Res* 1994;23:353—357.

54. Arabin B, Aardenburg R, van Eyak J. Maternal position and ultrasonic cervical assessment in multiple pregnancy. Preliminary observation. *J Reprod Med* 1997;42:719—724.

55. Wong G, Levine D, Ludmir J. Maternal postural challenge as a functional test for cervical incompetence. *J Ultrasound Med* 1997;16:169—175.

56. Guzman E, Vintzileos A, McLean D, et al. The natural history of a positive response to transfundal pressure in women at risk for incompetent cervix. *Am J Obstet Gynecol* 1997;176:634—638.

57. Hertzberg B, Kliewer M, Farrell T, et al. Spontaneously changing gravid cervix: clinical implications and prognostic featurers. *Radiology* 1995;196;721—724.

58. Parulekar S, Kiwi R. Dynamic incompetent cervix uteri. *J Ultrasound Med* 1988;7:481—485.

59. Ludmir J, Jackson G, Samuels P. Transvaginal cerclage under ultrasound guidance in cases of severe cervical hypoplasia. *Obstet Gynecol* 1991;78:1067—1072.

60. Anderson H, Karimi A, Sakala E, et al. Prediction of cerclage outcome by endovaginal sonography. *Am J Obstet Gynecol* 1994;171:1102—1106.

61. Fox R, Holmes R, James M, Tuohy J, Wardle P. Serial transvaginal ultrasonography following McDonald cerclage and repeat suture insertion. *Aust N Z J Obstet Gynaecol* 1998;38:27—30.

62. Parulekar S, Kiwi R. Ultrasound evaluation of sutures following cervical cerclage for incompetent cervix uteri. *J Ultrasound Med* 1982;1982:223—228.

63. Rana J, Davis S, Harrigan J. Improving the outcome of cervical cerclage by sonographic follow-up. *J Ultrasound Med* 1990;9:275—278.

64. Ludmir J, Cohen B, Wong G. Managing the patient with cerclage: bedrest versus ambulation based on sonographic findings. *Am J Obstet Gynecol* 1997;176:(S)147.

65. Rizzo G, Capponi A, Angelini E, Vlachopoulou A, Grassi C. The value of transvaginal ultrasonographic examination of the uterine cervix in predicting premature delivery in patients with premature rupture of membranes. *Ultrasound Obstet Gynecol* 1998;11:23—29.

66. Carlan S, Richmond L, O'Brien W. Randomized trial of endovaginal ultrasound in preterm premature rupture of membranes. *Obstet Gynecol* 1997,89:458—461.

26 Estimating Gestational Age

Alfred B. Kurtz

Gestational age can be estimated by a combination of menstrual history, physical examination, quantitative β-HCG levels, and ultrasound. Of these, menstrual history and ultrasound are more precise than the physical examination (**Table 26–1**). The β-hCG is only of value in the first trimester when it correlates within certain ultrasound landmarks.

In a comparison of the menstrual history and the ultrasound examination, ultrasound is usually better (**Table 26–1**). The expected 2 Standard Deviation (2 SD) range for women with *certain* menstrual dates is a disappointing ± 2.5 weeks.[1] Gestational age estimations by first- and second-trimester ultrasound studies are superior.[2—4] In the third trimester, an accurate menstrual history is preferred; uncertain menstrual dates are not. In most instances, menstrual history only supports the ultrasound findings.

The terms *gestational age*, *fetal age*, and *menstrual age* can be used interchangeably. They all estimate the age of the pregnancy from the first day of the last normal menstrual period. Additionally, the living conceptus is termed an *embryo* until ten menstrual weeks;[5] afterward it is called a *fetus*. For convenience, however, because the end of the twelfth week marks the end of the first trimester, 12 weeks is often used.

The American College of Radiology (ACR) first produced a Standard for the Antepartum Obstetrical Ultrasound Examination in 1985. This document has been twice updated, the last time in 1995.[6] In this update, one of the indications for the performance of a sonographic examination is to estimate gestational age. In the first trimester, the embryo's crown—rump length (CRL) measurement is preferred. If not identified, the mean gestational sac diameter (MGSD) can be substituted. In the second and third trimesters, measurements of the head and femur are used to estimate gestational age.

The abdominal measurement has value in evaluating fetal size and can be used, along the head and femur to analyze interval growth. Fetal weight and growth, however, are beyond the scope of this chapter. Additionally, less common measurements of such structures as the outer orbital diameter and the humerus have been used to estimate fetal age. Only infrequently needed and usually less precise, they too will not be discussed further.

First-trimester Sonography

The ACR Antepartum Obstetrical Standards include first-trimester sonographic guidelines. The section dealing with the estimation of gestational age is as follows: **Overall comment: Scanning in the first trimester may be performed either abdominally or vaginally. If a transabdominal examination is performed and fails to provide definitive information concerning any of the following guidelines, a transvaginal scan should be done whenever possible.**

The uterus and adnexa should be evaluated for the presence of a gestational sac. If a gestational sac is seen, then its location should be documented. The presence or absence of an embryo should be noted and the crown—rump length recorded.
Comment:

a. The crown—rump length is a more accurate indicator of gestational age than is gestational sac diameter. Comparison should be made to standard tables.

Table 26–1 Gestational age predictors

Parameters	2 SD
Ovulation induction	± 3 days
Basal body temperature	± 4—5 days
First-trimester ultrasound (CRL & probably MGSD)	± 1 week
Early second-trimester ultrasound — 14—20 weeks (BPDa & HC)	± 1—1.2 weeks
Late second-trimester ultrasound — 20—26 weeks (BPDa & HC)	± 1.9 weeks
First-trimester physical examination	± 2 weeks
"Accurate" menstrual history	**± 2.5 weeks**
Early third-trimester ultrasound — 26—32 weeks (BPDa & HC & FL)	± 3.1—3.3 weeks
Late third-trimester ultrasound — 32—42 weeks (BPDa, HC & FL)	± 3.5—3.8 weeks
Physical examination — fundal height — before 28 weeks	± 4 weeks
Uncertain menstrual history	**± 4 weeks**
Physical examination — fundal height — after 28 weeks	± 4 weeks

2 S.D., 2 Standard Deviations; MGSD, mean gestational sac diameter; CRL, crown—rump length; BPDa, area corrected biparietal diameter; HC, head circumference; and FL, femur length.

b. If the embryo is not identified, the mean diameter of the gestational sac should be calculated to estimate gestational age and the gestational sac should be evaluated for presence and size of the yolk sac.

c. Caution should be used in making the presumptive diagnosis of a "gestational sac" in the absence of a definite fetal pole or yolk sac, because without these findings an intrauterine fluid collection could represent a pseudogestational sac associated with an ectopic pregnancy.

d. During the late first trimester, biparietal diameter and other fetal measurements may also be used to establish fetal age.[6]

The CRL measurement has been thoroughly studied and is precise to within ± 1 week. Although the MGSD has had limited evaluation, its range is similar early in the first trimester.[7] Therefore, the gestational sac diameter can be used to estimate gestational age before the embryo is identified.

The gestational sac is routinely identified transabdominally by six menstrual weeks and transvaginally one week earlier. The MGSD is measured inside its hyperechoic rim. If round, only one sac measurement is needed (**Fig. 26–1**). More commonly, when oval, three orthogonal (perpendicular) measurements of the sac are averaged (**Fig. 26–2**). Even when the sac is unusually shaped, the MGSD is still accurate provided that all three measurements are taken at their largest diameters.

Transvaginally, the smallest identifiable MGSD is 2 mm, equivalent to a mean gestational age of five weeks ± 0.1 week (**Table 26–2**).[8] The MGSD increases to 30 mm, a mean gestational age of 8.5 weeks.

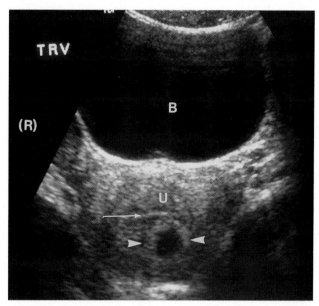

Figure 26–1 Round gestational sac at 6.0 weeks. Transabdominal transverse (TRV) ultrasound image shows a retroverted uterus (U) within which is a well-defined 10 mm round gestational sac with a uniformly thick hyperechoic rim (**arrowheads**). The sac is measured as an inner to inner diameter inside the rim. B, urinary bladder; (R), toward patient's right. **Arrow**, closed, separate, endometrial canal.

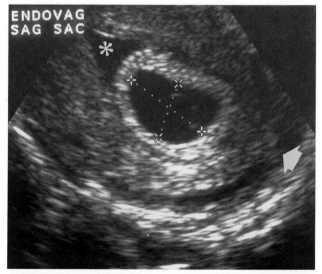

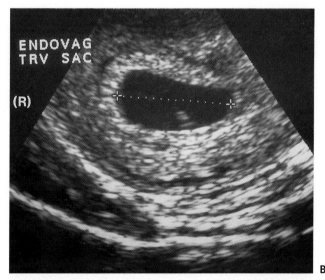

Figure 26–2 Oval gestational sac at 6.6 weeks. Transvaginal (ENDOVAG) ultrasound images show a well-defined oval gestational sac with a uniformly thick hyperechoic rim. The +'s or x's (with dotted lines) denote the three orthogonal measurements of the inner to inner diameter, and a mean gestational sac diameter (MGSD) of 15 mm is obtained. **A:** Sagittal image of a retroverted uterus (**arrowhead** denotes uterine fundus). Fluid is identified with the endometrial canal(*).**B:** Transaxialcoronal view. (R), toward patient's right.

Table 26–2 Mean diameter of gestational sac and corresponding estimates of gestational age

Mean sac diameter, mm	Gestational age, weeks (mean)
2	5.0
3	5.1
4	5.2
5	5.4
6	5.5
7	5.6
8	5.7
9	5.9
10	6.0
11	6.1
12	6.2
13	6.4
14	6.5
15	6.6
16	6.7
17	6.9
18	7.0
19	7.1
20	7.3
21	7.4
22	7.5
23	7.6
24	7.8
25	7.9
26	8.0
27	8.1
28	8.3
29	8.4
30	8.5

a   The mean gestational age was calculated from a regression equation. Reported range: ± 0.1 week at 2 SD.
b   Reprinted with permission from Table 2 in Early pregnancy assessment with transvaginal ultrasound scanning by S. Daya, S. Woods, S. Ward, R. Lappalainen, and C. Caco. *Can Med Assoc J* 1991;144:441—445.

The ACR Obstetrical Standards caution against making a predictive diagnosis of a gestational sac in the absence of a definite fetal pole or yolk sac. While this precaution is appropriate, a normal gestational sac can be confidently diagnosed when its hyperechoic rim is thick (> 2 mm) and its shape is round or oval (without unusual angulation) (**Fig. 26–1 and 26–2**). The endometrial canal is often detected separately, usually as either a double decidual sac or an intradecidual sign (**Fig. 26–1**).

Embryonic size (CRL) has an early linear acceleration followed by a curvilinear slow down. Throughout the first trimester, except when very small, the CRL is easy to identify and measure (**Fig. 26–3 and 26–4**) (**Table 26–3**).[9, 10] The early linear growth is best analyzed in a study on embryos from 2 to 25 mm, from mean gestational ages of 5.7 to 9.2 weeks with the more curvilinear slowing continuing from 26 to 54 mm, from mean gestational ages of 9.4—12 weeks. The authors of **Table 26–3** also studied fetuses in the early to mid-second trimester and proposed using the CRL measurement up to 18 weeks. There are methodological issues after 12 weeks as the fetus is more likely to flex and extend, making its CRL less accurate. Because the fetal head is easily identified and measured and its age is equally precise, it should be used after 12 weeks. Therefore, **Table 26–3** reserves the CRL measurement to the first trimester.

Studies in the first trimester often combine transabdominal and transvaginal measurements. Measurements by both methods are equally accurate and either can be used to obtain an accurate MGSD and CRL.[11] However, for diagnostic purposes, the transvaginal approach detects landmarks earlier and should be used whenever the transabdominal examination is not diagnostic.

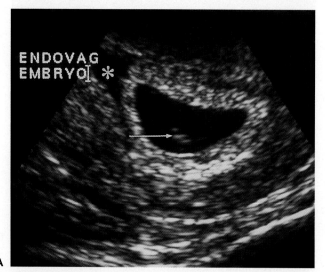

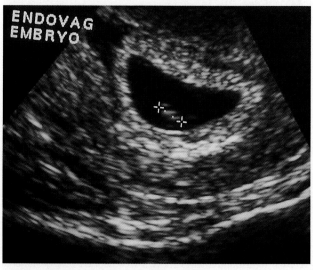

Figure 26–3 Early embryo of 6.2 weeks. **A:** Transvaginal (ENDOVAG) ultrasound image shows a small embryo (**arrow**) with heart motion within a well-defined gestational sac. *, small amount of fluid within the endometrial canal. **B:** +'s denote the crown—rump length measurement of 5 mm.

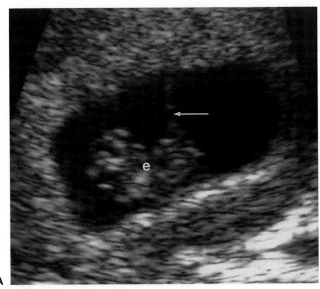

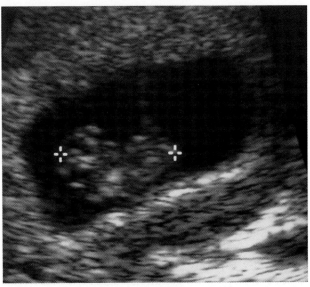

Figure 26–4 Later embryo at 8.7 weeks. **A:** Transabdominal magnified ultrasound image identifies an embryo (e) with heart motion within a well-defined gestational sac. **Arrowhead**, umbilical cord. **B:** Crown—rump length of 21 mm is measured by +'s.

Table 26–3 Predicted menstrual age (MA) from crown—rump length (CRL) from 5.7 to 12 weeks[b]

MA (Weeks)			MA (weeks)		
CRL (mm)	Mean	95% Confid. limits[a] (rounded to farther 0.1	CRL (mm)	Mean	95% Confid. limits[a] (rounded to farther 0.1)
2	5.7	5.2—6.2	31	10.0	9.2—11
3	5.9	5.4—6.4	32	10.1	9.2—11
4	6.1	5.6—6.6	33	10.2	9.3—11.1
5	6.2	5.7—6.7	34	10.3	9.4—11.2
			35	10.4	9.5—11.3
6	6.4	5.9—7	36	10.5	9.6—11.4
7	6.6	6—7.2	37	10.6	9.7—11.5
8	6.7	6.1—7.3	38	10.7	9.8—11.6
9	6.9	6.3—7.5	39	10.8	9.9—11.7
10	7.1	6.5—7.7	40	10.9	10—11.8
11	7.2	6.6—7.8	41	11.0	10.1—11.9
12	7.4	6.8—8	42	11.1	10.2—12
13	7.5	6.9—8.1	43	11.2	10.3—12.1
14	7.7	7—8.4	44	11.2	10.3—12.1
15	7.9	7.2—8.6	45	11.3	10.3—12.2
16	8.0	7.3—8.7	46	11.4	10.4—12.3.
17	8.1	7.4—8.8	47	11.5	10.5—12.5
18	8.3	7.6—9	48	11.6	10.6—12.6
19	8.4	7.7—9.1	49	11.7	10.7—12.7
20	8.6	7.9—9.3	50	11.7	10.7—12.7
21	8.7	8—9.4	51	11.8	10.8—12.8
22	9.0	8.1—9.7	52	11.9	10.9—12.8
23	9.1	8.2—9.8	53	12.0	11—13
24	9.2	8.3—9.9	54	12.0	11—13
25	9.2	8.4—10			
26	9.4	8.6—10.2			
27	9.5	8.7—10.3			
28	9.6	8.8—10.4			
29	9.7	8.8—10.5			
30	9.9	9.1—10.7			

[a] The 95% confidence interval is ± 8% of the predicted age.
[b] Reprinted with permission from Table 3 in Fetal crown—rump length: reevaluation of relation to menstrual age (5—18 weeks) with high-resolution real-time US by F.P. Hadlock, V.P. Shah, D.J. Kanon, B.Math, J.V. Lindsey. **Radiology** 1992;182:501—505.

The serum pregnancy test can be quantitated and compared to the ultrasound parameters.[12] Using the first (and now the third) International Reference Preparation, a β-hCG discriminatory level of 1000 IU/L allows identification of the gestational sac at < 5 weeks. At β-hCG levels of 7200 IU/L and 10,800 IU/L, the yolk sac and then the embryo with heart motion are detected, both between five and six weeks. The diagnostic value of the yolk sac is limited to its identification: a gestational sac with a yolk sac at 5.5 menstrual weeks and a gestational sac with both a yolk sac and embryo by 6 weeks.

It is not necessary to measure specific *fetal* parts in the late first trimester. The CRL is highly precise in establishing gestational age, can easily be measured throughout the first trimester, and is as exact as any second-trimester fetal measurement. Conversely, and more importantly, there are no well established measurement tables of fetal parts for gestational ages *before* 12 weeks.

The ACR Obstetrical Standards state the following about multiple gestations in the first trimester:

Multiple pregnancies should be reported only in those instances where multiple embryos are seen. Due to incomplete fusion between the amnion and chorion and elevation of the chorionic membrane by intrauterine hemorrhage in some patients with vaginal bleeding, more than one sac-like structure may be seen in early pregnancy and incorrectly thought to represent multiple gestations.[6]

Each CRL should be measured. Gestational sacs alone or sac-like structures should not. They could be one of the following: a blighted second sac, intrauterine hemorrhage, necrotic fibroid, fluid in the endometrial canal, or a normal chorioamniotic separation. However, multiple MGSDs can be confidentially measured when each gestational sac contains it own yolk sac.

In each multiple pregnancy, usually twins, a single gestational age and a range should be determined. For twins with the same CRLs, one gestational age is immediately available. Mild discrepancies of ≤ 2 mm are usually normal growth variants, and an *average* and gestational age range is easily computed. Instead of reporting twin embyros with CRLs of 6 and 8 mm as gestational ages of 6.4 weeks (range of 5.9 to 7 weeks) and 6.7 weeks (range of 6.1–7.3 weeks) (**Table 26–3**), they should be combined as a single *average* mean gestational age of 6.6 weeks (with a range of 5.9 to 7.3 weeks) (the lower end of the 6.4 week embryo range to the upper end of the 6.7 week range).

Embryos may still be normal with CRL discrepancies of ≥ 3 mm. However, they may not, especially when there are also MGSD discrepancies. A single gestational age can be difficult to establish sonographically but is more likely to be the age of the larger embryo. If too discrepant, however, an accurate menstrual history may be the best estimator of age. The decision of which method to use is best left to the examiner. Regardless, follow-up examinations to evaluate abnormalities in structure and growth are recommended.

Second- and Third-trimester Sonography

The ACR Antepartum Obstetrical Standards have guidelines for second- and third-trimester sonograms. The section discussing estimation of gestational age is as follows:

Assessment of gestational age should be accomplished at the time of the initial scan using a combination of femur length and biparietal diameter, corrected biparietal diameter, or head circumference.

Comment:

a. **Third-trimester measurements may not accurately reflect gestational age. Initial determination of gestational age should therefore be performed prior to the third trimester whenever possible.**

b. **If one or more previous studies have been performed, then the gestational age at the time of the current examination should be based on the earliest examination that permits measurement of crown—rump length, biparietal diameter, head circumference, and/or femur length by the equation: current fetal age = estimated age at time of initial study + number of weeks elapsed since first study.[6]**

An *initial* ultrasound study, when performed in the first or second trimester, gives the most precise gestational age of ± 1—1.2 weeks (**Table 26–1**). By the third trimester, however, the range approaches ± one month, and age estimation is of limited value. Regardless of when established, once determined, the gestational age does not change for the remainder of the pregnancy . On a follow-up study, fetal age is the *initial* age plus the number of calendar weeks between studies. For example, if a first-trimester embryo of 7.4 week (with a range of 7 to 7.8 weeks) is reexamined 10 weeks later, the fetus is 17.4 weeks (with a range of 17 to 17.8 weeks), regardless of its size on the second study. Similarly, a second-trimester fetus with a mean gestational age of 16.2 weeks (with a range of 15.2 to 17.2 weeks) is 31.2 weeks (with a range of 30.2 to 32.7 weeks) 15 weeks later.

The gestational age in the second and third trimester is usually established from a measurement of the fetal head, either the biparietal diameter (BPD) or the head circumference (HC). Both are acceptable. The ACR Obstetrical Standards state the following:

Biparietal diameter should be measured at a standard level, typically an axial plane that includes the thalamus and cavum septum pellucidum.

Comment:

If the fetal head is dolichocephalic or brachycephalic, the biparietal diameter alone may be misleading. On occasion, the computation of the cephalic index, a ratio of the biparietal diameter to frontal-occipital diameter, is needed to make this determination. In such situations, the head circumference or corrected biparietal diameter

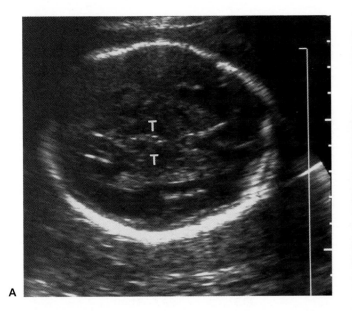

A

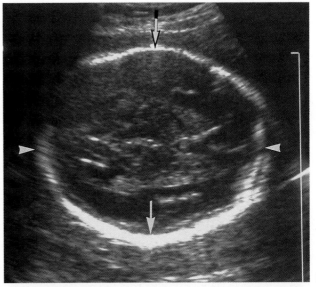

B

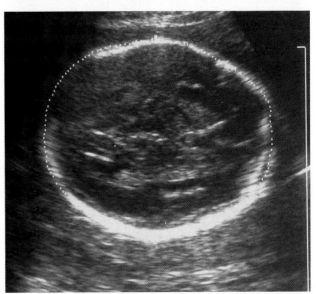

C

Figure 26–5   Late second-trimester fetal head measurements. **A:** Transaxial ultrasound image of the fetal head at the thalami (T). **B:** Same image as (**A**) showing the biparietal diameter measured from the tip of the arrows as a leading edge to leading edge measurement (outer edge of the closest temporoparietal table to inner edge of the further temporoparietal table). Note the distinct bony margins caused by the excellent axial resolution. **Arrowheads** denote the approximate place to measure the frontal-occipital diameter. Because of the lateral resolution and curve surface of the calvarium, these points are less distinct. **C:** A perimeter-traced head circumference from the same image as (A).

is required. Head circumference is measured at the same level as the biparietal diameter, around the outer perimeter of the calvarium.[6]

The BPD is measured leading edge to leading edge (from the outer edge of the closer temporoparietal bone to the inner edge of the farther temporoparietal bone) usually at the anatomic level of the thalamus (**Fig. 26–5**), but occasionally at the midbrain. The soft tissues outside the calvarium are not included. A mean gestational age and a range around this mean are reported (**Table 26–4**).[13]

The accuracy of the BPD measurement assumes a normal transaxial head shape. Typically, the head is oval. To confirm this shape, a second linear measurement called the frontal-occipital diameter (FOD) is obtained from the same BPD image, taken outer edge of the frontal bone to the outer edge of the occipital bone (**Fig. 26–5 B**). These two are then compared in an equation called the cephalic index (CI) = BPD/FOD x 100.[14] The CI defines a normal

head shape at a mean of 78 and range of 70—86 (2 SD). Theoretically, and only for this comparison, the BPD is measured outer to outer edge; however, in most cases, the standard BPD measurement is used.

There can be a technical problem in the measurement of the FOD and the HC (**Fig. 26–5 B,C**). A measurement parallel to the ultrasound beam (along its axis) uses its superior axial resolution and has distinct bony margins. Most BPD measurements are obtained this way. When a measurement is taken tangential to the ultrasound beam and uses the beam's lateral resolution, the curved margins of the calvarium are less distinct, broadened, and a "drop-out" sound after a critical angle is exceeded. These measurements can therefore be more difficult to obtain and are sometimes inaccurate. In an attempt to minimize this problem, some observers have measured the FOD as a middle to middle measurement; this technique, while interesting, has not proven superior.

Table 26–4 Composite biparietal diameter table

Biparietal diameter (mm)	Gestational age (weeks)		Biparietal diameter (mm)	Gestational age (weeks)	
	Mean[a]	Range 90% variation[b]		Mean[a]	Range 90% variation[b]
20	12.0	12.0			
21	12.0	12.0	61	24.2	22.6—25.8
22	12.7	12.2—13.2	62	24.6	23.1—26.1
23	13.0	12.4—13.6	63	24.9	23.4—26.4
24	13.2	12.6—13.8	64	25.3	23.8—26.8
25	13.5	12.9—14.1	65	25.6	24.1—27.1
26	13.7	13.1—14.3	66	26.0	24.5—27.5
27	14.0	13.4—14.6	67	26.4	25—27.8
28	14.3	13.6—15	68	26.7	25.3—28.1
29	14.5	13.9—5.2	69	27.1	25.8—28.4
30	14.8	14.1—15.5	70	27.5	26.3—28.7
31	15.1	14.3—15.9	71	27.9	26.7—29.1
32	15.3	14.5—16.1	72	28.3	27.2—29.4
33	15.6	14.7—16.5	73	28.7	27.6—29.8
34	15.9	15—16.8	74	29.1	28.1—30.1
35	16.2	15.2—17.2	75	29.5	28.5—30.5
36	16.4	15.4—17.4	76	30.0	29—31
37	16.7	15.6—17.8	77	30.3	29.2—31.4
38	17.0	15.9—18.1	78	30.8	29.6—32
39	17.3	16.1—18.5	79	31.1	29.9—32.5
40	17.6	16.4—18.8	80	31.6	30.2—33
41	17.9	16.5—19.3	81	32.1	30.7—33.5
42	18.1	16.6—19.8	82	32.6	31.2—34
43	18.4	16.8—20.2	83	33.0	31.5—34.5
44	18.8	16.9—20.7	84	33.4	31.9—35.1
45	19.1	17—21.2	85	34.0	32.3—35.7
46	19.4	17.4—21.4	86	34.3	32.8—36.2
47	19.7	17.8—21.6	87	35.0	33.4—36.6
48	20.0	18.2—21.8	88	35.4	33.9—37.1
49	20.3	18.6—22	89	36.1	34.6—37.6
50	20.6	19—22.2	90	36.6	35.1—38.1
51	20.9	19.3—22.5	91	37.2	35.9—38.5
52	21.2	19.5—22.9	92	37.8	36.7—38.9
53	21.5	19.8—23.2	93	38.8	37.3—39.3
54	21.9	20.1—23.7	94	39.0	37.9—40.1
55	22.2	20.4—24	95	39.7	38.5—40.9
56	22.5	20.7—24.3	96	40.6	39.1—41.5
57	22.8	21.1—24.5	97	41.0	39.9—42.1
58	23.2	21.5—24.9	98	41.8	40.5—43.1
59	23.5	21.9—25.1			
60	23.8	22.3—25.5			

[a] Weighted least mean square fit equation: BPD (mm) = -34.5701 + 5.0157 GA —0.00441 GA (GA = mean gestational age).

[b] For each biparietal diameter, 90% of gestational age data points fell within this range. Reprinted with permission in Analysis of biparietal diameter as an accurate indicator of gestational age. by A.B. Kurtz, R.J. Wapner, R.J. Kurtz, D.D. Dershaw, C.S. Rubhin, C. Beuglet, B.B. Goldberg. *J Clin Ultrasound* 1980;8:319—326.

Regardless, the CI is useful in predicting head shape. When the fetal head is brachycephalic (round) or doliocephalic (elongated), the CI can approach or go beyond the outer two SDs. The BPD head shape can be corrected by an area-corrected calculation (BPDa).[15] The BPDa = [BPD x FOD/1.265)]$^{1/2}$.

The HC is also obtained from the BPD transaxial image (**Table 26–5**).[16] The circumference is measured along the outer edge of the calvarium (disregarding the overlying soft tissues) by one of the following two methods: by tracing the outer perimeter of the calvarium (**Fig. 26–5 C**) or by using the formula for the circumference of a circle (BPD + FOD) x Pi/2 = (BPD + FOD) x 1.57. Neither is superior, both methods having relatively minor errors approaching 2%.

The ACR Obstetrical Standards discuss the femur length measurement as follows:

Femur length should be measured routinely and recorded after the 14th week of gestation.

Comment:

As with head measurements, there is considerable biological variation in normal femur lengths late in pregnancy.[6]

The femur length (FL) is a measure of the ossified femoral diaphysis, disregarding its cartilagenous ends (**Fig. 26–6**). This diaphysis has a straight lateral and curved medial border. Even if the medial border is imaged, the femur is measured linearly, disregarding the curvature which causes only a 1-mm error.

Typically, only one femur is measured, although an argument can be made for routinely imaging both. The FL is often compared to one of the head measurements to assess proportionality of fetal parts. An important secondary role, however, is its use in determining fetal

Table 26–5 Head circumference measurement table

| Head circumference (mm) | Gestational age (weeks) | | Head circumference (mm) | Gestational age (weeks) | |
	Predicted mean values[a]	95% confidence limits[b]		Predicted mean values[a]	95% confidence limits
80	13.4	12.1—14.7	230	24.9	22.6—27.2
85	13.7	12.4—15	235	25.4	23.1—27.7
90	14.0	12.7—15.3	240	25.9	23.6—28.2
95	14.3	13—15.6	245	26.4	24.1—28.7
100	14.6	13.3—15.9	250	26.9	24.6—29.2
105	15.0	13.7—16.3	255	27.5	25.2—29.8
110	15.3	14—16.6	260	28.0	25.7—30.3
115	15.6	14.3—16.9	265	28.1	25.8—30.4
120	15.9	14.6—17.2	270	29.2	26.9—31.5
125	16.3	15—17.6	275	29.8	27.5—32.1
130	16.6	15.3—17.9	280	30.3	27.6—33
135	17.0	15.7—18.3	285	31.0	28.3—33.7
140	17.3	16—18.6	290	31.6	28.9—34.3
145	17.7	16.4—19	295	32.2	29.5—34.8
150	18.1	16.5—19.7	300	32.8	30.1—35.5
155	18.4	16.8—20	305	33.5	30.7—36.2
160	18.8	17.2—20.4	310	32.4	31.5—36.9
165	19.2	17.6—20.8	315	34.9	32.2—37.6
170	19.6	18—21.2	320	35.5	32.8—38.2
175	20.0	18.4—21.6	325	36.3	32.9—39.7
180	20.4	18.8—22	330	37.0	33.6—40.4
185	20.8	19.2—22.4	335	37.7	34.3—41.1
190	21.2	19.8—22.8	340	38.5	35.1—41.9
195	21.6	20—23.2	345	39.2	35.8—42.6
200	22.1	20.5—23.7	350	40.0	36.6—43.4
205	22.5	20.9—24.1	355	40.8	37.4—44.2
210	23.0	21.4—24.6	360	41.6	38.2—45
215	23.4	21.8—25			
220	23.9	22.3—25.5			
225	24.4	22.1—26.7			

[a] Table 3.
[b] Table 4. Reprinted with permission in Fetal head circumference: relation to menstrual age, by FD Hadlock, RL Deter, RB Harrist, SK Park. *AJR* 1982;138:649—653.

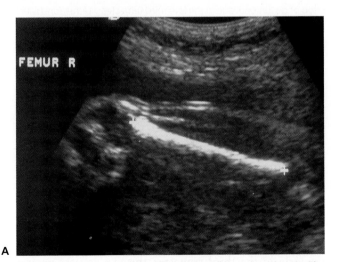

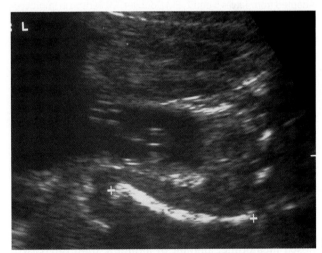

A **B**

Figure 26–6 Late second-trimester fetal femur lengths. **A:** The right femur. The straight lateral surface of its ossified shaft (diaphysis) is measured by +'s. **B:** The left femur. Its curved medial surface is measured along the +'s. The curvature is not included.

age. (**Table 26–6**).[17] While less precise than the head measurements in the first and second trimester, the FL becomes superior by the third trimester: ± 3.1 weeks at 26—32 gestational weeks (compared to ± 3.3 weeks for the BPDa) and ± 3.5 weeks at 32—42 gestational weeks (compared to ± 3.8 weeks for the BPDa).[4]

Multiple parameters have also been used to assess fetal age, with the mean fetal ages of the BPD, HC, AC and FL averaged to obtain a *composite* mean fetal age.[18] While this method initially claimed a greater accuracy than any single parameter, this optimism has not been substantiated. The main weakness of this approach ap-

Table 26–6   Gestational age (GA) prediction based on femur length (FL) measurements

FL (mm)	Predicted GA (weeks) Mean	2 SD Range[a]	FL (mm)	Predicted GA (weeks) Mean	2 SD Range[a]
10	13.7	12.5 14.9	45	24.5	22.6—26.4
11	13.9	12.7—15.1	46	24.9	23—26.8
12	14.2	13—15.4	47	25.3	23.4—27.2
13	14.4	13.2—15.6	48	25.7	23.8—27.6
14	14.6	13.4—15.8	49	26.2	23.5—28.9
15	14.9	13.7—16.1	50	26.2	23.9—29.3
16	15.1	13.9—16.3	51	27.0	24.3—29.7
17	15.4	14.2—16.6	52	27.5	24.8—30.2
18	15.6	14.4—16.8	53	28.0	25.3—30.7
19	15.9	14.7—17.1	54	28.4	25.7—31.1
20	16.2	15—17.4	55	28.9	26.2—31.6
21	16.4	15.2—17.6	56	29.4	26.7—32.1
22	16.7	15.5—17.9	57	29.9	27.2—32.6
23	17.0	15.8—18.2	58	30.4	27.7—33.1
24	17.3	16.1—18.5	59	30.9	28.2—33.6
25	17.6	16.4—18.8	60	31.4	28.7—34.1
26	17.9	16.7—19.1	61	31.9	29.2—34.6
27	18.2	17—19.4	62	32.5	28.5—36.5
28	18.5	17.3—19.7	63	33.0	29—37
29	18.8	17.6—20	64	33.6	29.6—37.6
30	19.1	17.9—20.3	65	34.1	30.1—38.1
31	19.4	18.2—20.6	66	34.7	30.7—38.7
32	19.7	18.5—20.9	67	35.3	31.3—39.3
33	20.1	18.2—22	68	35.9	31.9—39.9
34	20.4	18.5—22.3	69	36.5	32.5—40.5
35	20.7	18.8—22.6	70	37.1	33.1—41.1
36	21.1	19.2—23	71	37.7	33.7—41.7
37	21.4	19.5—23.3	72	38.3	35.1—41.5
38	21.8	19.9—23.7	73	39.0	35.8—42.2
39	22.2	20.3—24.1	74	39.6	36.4—42.8
40	22.5	20.6—24.4	75	40.3	37.1—43.5
41	22.9	21—24.8	76	40.9	37.7—44.1
42	23.3	21.4—25.2	77	41.6	38.4—44.8
43	23.7	21.8—25.6	≥ 78	42.0	38.8—45.2
44	24.1	22.2—26			

[a] 2 SD = 2 Standard Deviations
Adapted from Tables 5 and 7, PM Doubilet, CB Benson in Improved prediction of gestational age in the late third trimester. *J Ultrasound Med*. 1993;12:647—653.

pears to be in the use of the abdominal measurement. It is considerably less precise than the other parameters throughout most of the second and third trimesters. At 14—20, 20—26, 26—32, and 32—42 gestational weeks, the AC ranges are ± 2.1, 3.7, 3.0, 4.5 weeks compared to ± 1.2, 1.9, 3.3 and 3.8 weeks for the BPDa.[4]

The ACR Obstetrical Standards do not discuss gestational age estimation in multiple (typical twin) pregnancies. The Standards only state the following:
Multiple pregnancies require the documentation of additional information: placental number, sac number, comparison of fetal size, presence or absence of an interposed membrane, amount of amniotic fluid (increased, decreased, or normal) on each side of the membrane, and fetal genitalia (when visualized).[6]

The following are important statements about twin gestations.

1. Twins normally grow parallel to each other, usually within 5 mm and maintain similar sizes in utero.
2. Twins normally grow similar to normal singleton gestations until the early third trimester, at least until 30 weeks. If growth deceleration is then detected, it remains above the 10th percentile.
3. Whereas the overall size of the fetal head and body and its weight decreases toward the lower 10th percentile in the third trimester, fetal length remains relatively unaffected. Because the FL is directly proportional to fetal length, the FL remains precise even in the late third trimester.[19]

It is therefore recommended that singleton measurement tables be used to establish the fetal age of twins because singleton pregnancies have been more thoroughly studied, and their tables are based on considerably larger numbers of pregnancies. When there are measurement discrepancies in the head and body measurements, particularly in the third trimester, the FLs assume greater importance. If they remain within 5 mm throughout pregnancy, the twins are undoubtedly normal.

In the second and third trimester, it is also necessary to establish *one* gestational age for the twins. If on their initial ultrasound examination the twin gestations have the same head (and in the third trimester the same FL) measurements, then a single mean and range is readily established. If their sizes are mildly discrepant, i.e. ≤ 5 mm, then the fetuses are most likely normal and an *average* age can be calculated. For example, if twin fetuses have BPD measurements of 40 and 43 mm, corresponding to gestational ages of 17.6 and 18.4 weeks, then the age assigned should be the average of the two, 18.0 weeks with an encompassing range.

If larger discrepancies exist, then a composite age may not be accurate. In general, the fetal age is usually closer to (if not the same as) the larger fetus. The menstrual age, if accurate, however may be more appropriately used. On a follow-up study, the new age of the twins is the number of calendar weeks added to the first study.

References

1. Campbell S, Warsof SL, Little D, et al. Routine ultrasound screening for the prediction of gestational age. *Obstet Gynecol* 1985;65:613—620.

2. Kopta MM, May RR, Crane JP. A comparison of the reliability of the estimated date of confinement predicted by crown—rump length and biparietal diameter. *Am J Obstet Gynecol* 1983;145:562—565.

3. Hadlock FP, Harrist RB, Martinenz-Poyer J. How accurate is second trimester fetal dating? *J Ultrasound Med* 1991;10:557—561.

4. Benson CB, Doubilet PM. Sonographic prediction of gestational age: accuracy of second- and third-trimester fetal measurements. *AJR* 1991;157:1275—1277.

5. Moore KL, Persaud, TVN. *The Developing Human: Clinical Oriented Embryology*, 5th ed. W.B: Saunders Co., Philadelphia: 1993.

6. The Performance of Antepartum Obstetrical Ultrasound. Reston, VA: ACR, 1996, p. 1—5.

7. Jouppila PC. Length and depth of the uterus and the diameter of the gestational sac in normal gravidas during early pregnancy. *Acta Obstet Gynecol Scand* 1971;50(Suppl 15):29—31.

8. Daya S, Woods S, Ward S, et al. Early pregnancy assessment with transvaginal ultrasound scanning. *Can Med Assoc J* 1991;144:441—445.

9. Goldstein SR, Wolfson R. Endovaginal ultrasonographic measurement of early embryonic size as a means of assessing gestational age. *J Ultrasound Med* 1994;13:27—31.

10. Hadlock FP, Shah YP, Kanon DJ, Math B, Lindsey JV. Fetal crown—rump length: reevaluation of relation to menstrual age (5—18 weeks) with high-resolution real-time US. *Radiology* 1992;182:501—505.

11. Pennell RG, Needleman L, Pajak T, et al. Prospective comparison of vaginal and abdominal sonography in normal early pregnancy. *J Ultrasound Med* 1991;10:63—67.

12. Bree RL, Edwards M, Bohm-Velez M, et al. Transvaginal sonography in the evaluation of normal early pregnancy: correlation with hCG level. *AJR* 1989;153:75—79.

13. Kurtz AB, Wapner RJ, Kurtz RJ, et al. Analysis of biparietal diameter as an accurate indicator of gestational age. *J Clin Ultrasound* 1980;8:319—326.

14. Hadlock FP, Deter RL, Carpenter RJ, et al. Estimating fetal age: effect of head shape on BPD. *AJR* 1981;137:83—85.

15. Doubilet PM, Greenes RA. Improved prediction of gestational age from fetal head measurements. *AJR* 1984;142:797—800.

16. Hadlock FP, Deter RL, Harrist RB, et al. Fetal head circumference: relation to menstrual age. *AJR* 1982;138:649—653.

17. Doubilet PM, Benson CB. Improved prediction of gestational age in the late third trimester. *J Ultrasound Med* 1993;12:647—653.

18. Hadlock FP, Deter RL, Harrist RB, et al. Estimating fetal age: computer-assisted analysis of multiple fetal growth parameters. *Radiology* 1984;152:497—501.

19. Grumbach K, Coleman BG, Arger PH, et al. Twin and singleton growth patterns compared using US. *Radiology* 1986;158:237—241.

27 The Sonographic Evaluation of a Pregnancy Whose Size Is Greater than Dates

Beryl R. Benacerraf

Sonography is very helpful to evaluate pregnancies that are larger than expected based on menstrual dates. Possible explanations for a large uterine size include incorrect dates, macrosomia, multiple fetuses, as well as complications of twinning such as twin/twin transfusion syndrome or acardia. The pregnancy can be complicated by polyhydramnios which can be idiopathic, or a result of fetal growth acceleration, maternal diabetes, or fetal malformations. The fetal anomalies most often associated with polyhydramnios include those involving the gastrointestinal tract, central nervous system, thoracic and cardiac anomalies, fetal hydrops (isoimmune and nonimmune etiologies), some skeletal defects, chromosomal anomalies, and fetal tumors. When a fetus in the presence of polyhydramnios appears structurally normal sonographically, the outcome is generally excellent. Masses unrelated to the fetus may also be responsible for the clinical impression that the uterus is larger than expected for the patient's dates. These masses include uterine fibroids and adnexal enlargement such as an ovarian cyst. The evaluation of the patient whose uterine size is larger than dates includes a complete structural survey of the fetus including an echocardiogram, fetal biometry, and estimated weight assessment, as well as an evaluation of the myometrium and adnexae for possible masses.

Size/date discrepancy is one of the most common indications for obtaining an obstetrical ultrasound. Obstetricians can measure the uterus externally and compare its overall size to what is expected from the patient's dates. It is common to find that the size is either too large or too small, thus prompting further evaluation of the pregnancy. When the uterus is larger than anticipated based on the patient's dates, a sonogram will most often find the explanation.

Most commonly, the dates are incorrect. The patient may have had some spotting within the first month after she conceived. If she mistook the spotting for a true menstrual period, she would have estimated her dates at four weeks less than the actual gestation. It is not uncommon to find that the gestational age is four weeks ahead of what was expected, based on the last "menstrual" period. If the fetal biometry measures several weeks ahead of what the menstrual dates would predict, the fetus may have macrosomia or growth acceleration. Although in the first trimester the fetal size is normally within 3—5

days of the menstrual age, by the third trimester the fetal size can be as much as a month ahead of dates due to an accelerated growth. It is important not to rely on sonographic biometry for dating pregnancies in the third trimester due to differential growth rates.

Other explanations for a uterine size greater than dates include multiple pregnancy, masses, such as fibroids or adnexal masses external to the gestational sac, macrosomia or accelerated growth, as in cases of diabetes, and polyhydramnios, which can be associated with many different processes including various fetal malformations. An ultrasound investigating the reason for a size/date discrepancy of this sort is the cornerstone in managing the remainder of the pregnancy.

Multiple Pregnancy

Nowadays, it is extremely rare to make the discovery of twins at the time of delivery. In the vast majority of cases, the size of the uterus will have exceeded the expectation by dates sometime during the pregnancy — thus prompting an ultrasound to discover multiple fetuses. Once an ultrasound shows that there is more than one fetus (in most cases, twins), the pregnancy is considered at higher risk. Although multiple gestations only account for 1—2% of all births, they represent 10—15% of perinatal mortality and more than 15% of the low birth weight incidence. Higher-order multiple fetal pregnancies than twins are more common than ever before due to assisted reproduction treatments. The more fetuses present, the higher the risk of prematurity and other complications (**Fig. 27–1**).

Once a twin pregnancy is identified, its chorionicity must be determined because monochorionic twins have yet a higher morbidity and mortality than dichorionic twins.[1] The prenatal death rate has been reported as 9% for dichorionic/diamnotic twins and 26% for monochorionic/diamniotic twins. When twins are monochorionic/monoamniotic with no membrane separating them into two sacs, the incidence of nonsurvival is 50%.[1] It is crucial to search for the dividing membrane and to evaluate its morphology. Determining whether the membrane is monochorionic/diamniotic (thin) versus dichorionic/diamniotic (thick) is easier in the first trimester, when the difference in thickness is more obvious. It may be difficult to distinguish between the two types of chorionicity in the third trimester.

Monochorionic/diamniotic twins are at risk for complications based on the shared placenta, such as twin-to-twin transfusion syndrome (**Fig. 27–2**).[1—3] Deep vascular anastomoses within the placenta can result in an uneven distribution of blood flow to the two fetuses, with one fetus essentially transfusing the other. This results in one anemic fetus and one plethoric fetus. The anemic fetus is usually associated with severe oligohydramnios, whereas the fetus who has received too much blood flow tends to have severe polyhydramnios. Acute enlargement of the uterus, secondary to the development of polyhydramnios, is typical of severe twin-to-twin transfusion syndrome. When discovered at less than 22 weeks, there is a 90—100% chance of complete loss of the pregnancy — in most cases, due to premature labor before viability. [2, 3] Attempts at treating the polyhydramnios by serial removal of large quantities of amniotic fluid by amniocentesis have been helpful in some cases, although the mortality of the polyhydramnios/oligohydramnios sequence in monochorionic twins remains very high.

Another complication of the monochorionic twinning process is the development of an acardiac twin, who is kept alive by its cotwin. This phenomenon results from artery to artery shunts in the placenta and reversal of the arterial blood flow in one twin due to the over-

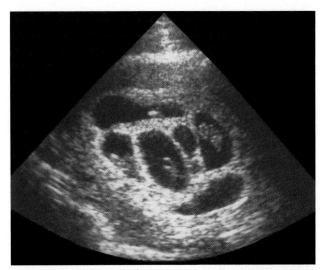

Figure 27–1 Sextuplet pregnancy at 7 weeks with 6 live embryos.

powering arterial pressure of its cotwin (pump twin). With blood flowing in reverse through its arterial system, the acardiac twin's heart fails to develop and, in most cases, the head and upper body regress, leaving an isolated, malformed lower body with edema (**Fig. 27–3**). These acardiac twins can grow very large, often larger than the pump twin and thus threatening the well being of the pump twin.

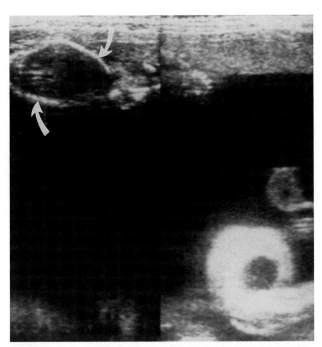

Figure 27–2 Composite image of the uterus in a monochorionic-diamniotic twin pregnancy, complicated by twin-to-twin transfusion syndrome. Note the tremendous amount of polyhdramnios associated with the twin in the dependent portion of the uterus. The twin associated with the polyhydramnios has an enlarged bladder, indicated increased perfusion (**arrow**). The stuck twin's head is noted in a superior aspect of the uterus, as indicated by **curved arrows**. It is suspended by its membrane, due to the severe oligohydramnios in its sac.

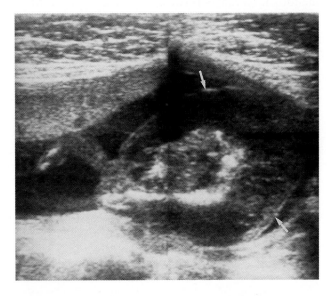

Figure 27–3 Longitudinal view of an acardiac twin. Note the very edematous rounded lower body (**arrows**) with one lower extremity visible.

Polyhydramnios

The volume of amniotic fluid normally increases throughout gestation, until approximately 24 weeks after which it declines until term. During pregnancy, the fetus swallows and excretes fluid in the form of urine. The fluid is then resorbed through the gastrointestinal tract and recirculated through the fetal kidneys. Although in the early second trimester fetal urine only represents approximately 10% of the total volume of amniotic fluid, during the second half of pregnancy the portion of amniotic fluid resulting from fetal urine increases until it is largely dependent upon fetal urination. Amniotic fluid is constantly being used and replenished, not unlike keeping a bathtub filled by constantly running the water with the drain open. Sonographic determination of the amniotic fluid volume has been attempted using various means, including the largest single pocket measurement as well as the four-quadrant measurement of amniotic fluid volume. Many experienced practitioners use subjective assessments of amniotic fluid volume rather than an actual measurement.[4] The best accepted measurement, however, is the Amniotic Fluid Index, which is based on the four-quadrant technique.[5]

The presence of absence of fetal malformations associated with polyhydramnios is largely related to the degree of excess amniotic fluid present. In pregnancies complicated by mild polyhydramnios, the risk of fetal malformation ranges between 20% and 40%. [6—8] Most of the malformations, however, are visible sonographically.

In the absence of any sonographic finding, mild polyhydramnios is usually idiopathic or is associated with macrosomia.[9—11] Several studies have shown that, when compared with pregnancies with normal amniotic fluid volumes, sonographically unexplained mild polyhydramnios was associated with a significantly higher incidence of birth weights greater than 4000 g. Birth weights were in the 90% percentile or more in 28% of fetuses with mild polyhydramnios versus 9% of normal controls. [9—11]

Diabetic women are at an increased risk for having macrosomic fetuses as well as for having their pregnancies complicated by polyhydramnios. When polyhydramnios associated with growth acceleration is detected by a prenatal sonogram, a glucose tolerance test is indicated to detect possible diabetes.

The incidence of malformations is considerably higher when the polyhydramnios is severe versus when it is mild. Fetuses associated with severe polyhydramnios have a prevalence of fetal anomalies of 75% versus 29% when the polyhydramnios is mild. [6,7]

The most common malformations associated with polyhydramnios are those involving the gastrointestinal tract.[7] Gastrointestinal obstructions, such as duodenal atresia, jejunal atresia, or esophageal atresia invariably cause polyhydramnios as early as the mid-second trimester.[7, 12, 13] Other gastrointestinal conditions sometimes associated with polyhydramnios include meconium peritonitis, anterior abdominal wall defects, and intraluminal masses such as intraoral teratomas or other obstructions to the swallowing mechanism (**Fig. 27–4**).[7] The sonographic manifestation of gastrointestinal obstruction includes marked dilatation of the bowel proximal to the obstruction, such as proximal duodenum in duodenal atresia or the duodenum and stomach as well as proximal jejunum in jejunal atresia (**Fig. 27–5 through 27–6**). More distal obstructions, such as anal

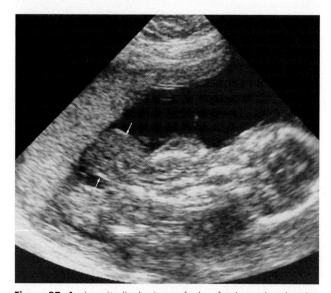

Figure 27–4 Longitudinal view of the fetal trunk, showing complete disruption of the lower aspect of the anterior abdominal wall with the entire liver (**arrows**) in an anterior abdominal wall defect.

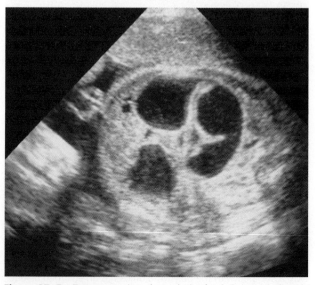

Figure 27–5 Transverse view through the fetal abdomen, directly caudad to the fetal liver. Note the marked dilatation of several loops of bowel, indicating small bowel obstruction.

atresia, may not be associated with polyhydramnios or marked bowel dilatation. Absence of the stomach bubble associated with polyhydramnios may be the result of a tracheoesophageal fistula, in particular, associated with esophageal atresia (**Fig. 27–7**).

Nonimmune hydrops is a condition almost always associated with polyhydramnios.[14] It is easily detected sonographically by a marked accumulation of fluid in various body cavities, such as ascites and pleural effusions as well as marked skin edema (**Fig. 27–8** through **27.12**). There is a large number of etiologies for nonim-

mune hydrops, including heart abnormalities such as arrhythmias and cardiomyopathies, as well as chromosomal anomalies, infectious processes such as TORCH syndromes, fetal tumors, etc. Nonimmune hydrops can be present in twin pregnancies, particularly when associated with either twin-to-twin transfusion syndrome or acardiac twinning (where one twin is responsible for pumping blood throughout the entire placenta as well as through its abnormal cotwin who does not have cardiac function). A detailed sonogram, including a fetal echocardiogram, is indicated when hydrops fetalis is de-

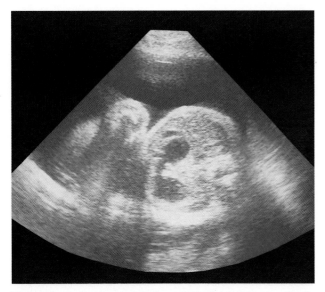

Figure 27–6 Transverse view through the fetal abdomen, directly caudad to the fetal liver. Note the double bubble appearance of the bowel, consistent with duodenal atresia.

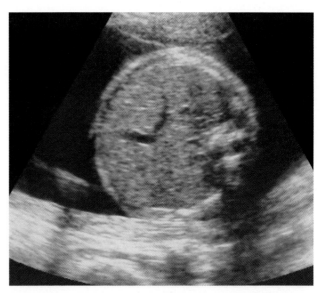

Figure 27–7 Transverse view through the fetal abdomen at the level of the stomach bubble. Note the absence of the stomach bubble in this image. This pregnancy was complicated by polyhydramnios, and the fetus had esophageal atresias at birth.

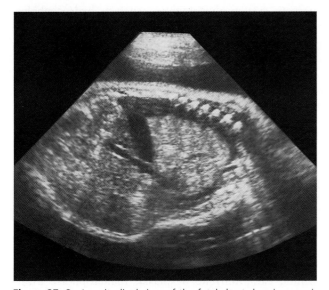

Figure 27–8 Longitudinal view of the fetal chest showing a unilateral pleural effusion.

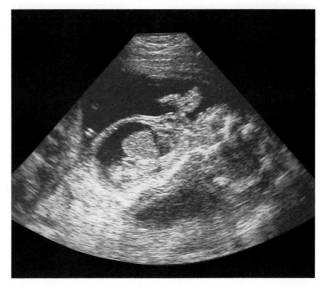

Figure 27–9 Longitudinal view of the fetal body showiong marked ascites.

tected. When hydrops is present, the fetus is considered very ill and the prognosis is guarded.[14] Workup includes umbilical blood sampling to aid in establishing a cause for the hydrops as well as to determine whether an early delivery is necessary if in utero treatment is not possible.

Hydrops may be secondary to fetal anemia, as in the patient whose exposure to the parvo virus has resulted in a reversible but profound fetal anemia. Umbilical blood sampling is necessary to determine the fetal hematocrit, both in cases of nonimmune hydrops secondary to anemia as well as isoimmune hydrops due to Rh or Kell in-

compatibility of the mother and fetus.[15] Massive fetal-to-maternal hemorrhage can also cause nonimmune hydrops. Treatment, in the form of intrauterine transfusion, is indicated for those fetuses and can be completely lifesaving.

Central nervous system abnormalities are a common group of malformations which cause polyhydramnios.[7,16] Specific anomalies, most often associated with excess amniotic fluid, include open neural tube defects such as anencephaly, encephaloceles, and meningomyeloceles (**Fig. 27–13** through **27–14**). Other central

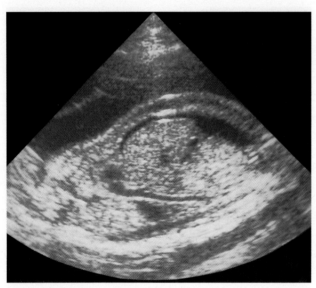

Figure 27–10 Longitudinal view of the fetal abdomen showing ascites in a fetus with hydrops. Note the skin edema.

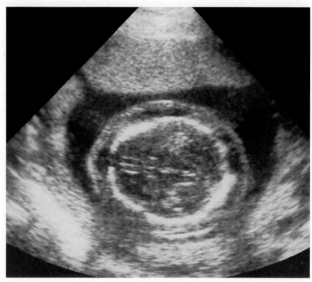

Figure 27–11 Transverse view through the fetal head, showing marked scalp edema throughout the entire scalp in a fetus with hydrops. Note the difference between the circumference of the head and the circumference of the outer aspect of the skin, caused by the edema.

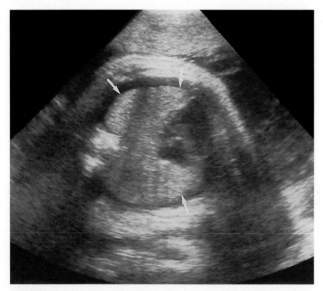

Figure 27–12 Transverse view through the fetal chest in a fetus with nonimmune hydrops. There are bilateral pleural effusions surrounding the fetal lungs (**arrows**), as well as marked soft tissue edema of the torso.

nervous system abnormalities, such as hydrocephalus, holoprosencephaly, and agenesis of the corpus callosum have been associated with polyhydramnios, although these abnormalities may be secondary to the specific etiologies of the intracranial malformations, as in chromosomal abnormalities such as trisomy 18.

Thoracic abnormalities, including diaphragmatic hernia and adenomatoid cystic malformation of the lung, invariably cause polyhydramnios, as do tracheal atresia and intrathoracic tumors such as teratomas (**Fig. 27–15** through **27–17**).[7] Isolated pleural effusions may be associated with polyhydramnios, although when polyhydramnios exists in association with pleural effusions, this is often an early stage of nonimmune hydrops.

Skeletal dysplasias may lead to nonimmune hydrops, thus, to polyhydramnios as well.[17,18] This includes bone dysplasias such as spondeloepithesial dysplasia congenita, camptomyelic dysplasia, thanatophoric dwarfism, and achondrogenesis. Although the cause of the polyhydramnios in fetuses with dwarf syndromes is unclear, the enhanced acoustic window provided by the excess amniotic fluid improves our capability of studying the fetal limbs by ultrasound.

Chromosomal abnormalities such as trisomies 21, 18, and 13 are associated with polyhydramnios.[19] Fetuses with trisomy 21 may develop polyhydramnios because of duodenal atresia and/or congenital heart defects. Those with trisomy 18 are well known to develop the combination of intrauterine growth retardation and polyhydramnios, which is often an indication for increased risk of a lethal trisomy. Fetuses with trisomy 13 and 9 are prone to having neural tube defects as well as

major intracranial facial and multiorgan abnormalities, often leading to excess amniotic fluid volume (**Fig. 27–18 through 27–19**). Even when these defects are discovered after 24 weeks' gestation, rapid karyotyping is required to aid in obstetrical management, particularly in cases of lethal trisomies (trisomies 13 and 18) so as to avoid unnecessary monitoring and operative delivery of nonviable fetuses.

Cardiac abnormalities have been associated with polyhydramnios, although most isolated cardiac malformations have normal amniotic fluid volumes The pres-

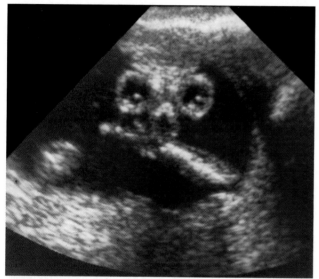

A

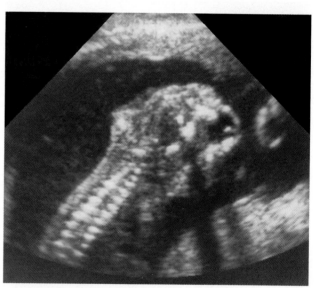

B

Figure 27–13 A: Transvaginal view of the fetal head of a fetus with ancencephaly. Note the prominent orbits without any evidence of skull formation. **B:** Longitudinal view of the same fetus, showing the relationship between the orbit and the cervical spine. Note the absence of the cranium.

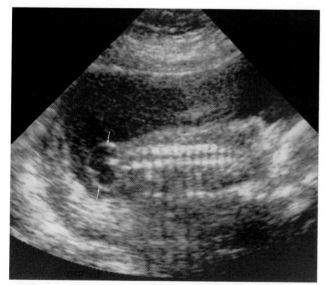

Figure 27–14 Coronal view of the fetal spine in the second trimester, showing a lumbar neural tube defect (**arrows**).

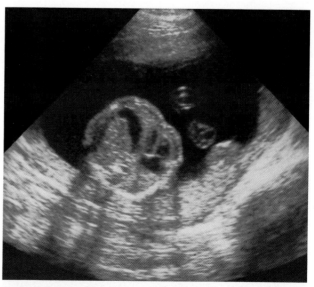

Figure 27–15 Transverse view through the fetal thorax of a second-trimester fetus, showing a left diaphragmatic hernia. Note that the stomach is at the same level as the fetal heart and the heart is displaced into the right hemithorax.

ence of polyhydramnios may be secondary to nonimmune hydrops in cases of arrhythmia or to congestive heart failure in cases of left heart outflow obstruction such as critical aortic stenosis.[20]

Fetal tumors are rare but can be a cause for an enlarged uterus and excess amniotic fluid volume (**Fig. 27–20 through 27–21**). These tumors include sacrococcygeal teratomas, intracranial teratomas, large fetal liver hemangiomas, renal hamartomas, and even placental tumors such as chorioangiomas.[21—31] These can, in turn, lead to severe polyhydramnios associated with fetal hy-

drops and fetal vascular compromise. Cystic hygromas, lymphangiomas as well as hemangiomas will also cause polyhydramnios. Any mass in the cervical region of the fetus is associated with polyhydramnios. The survival of such fetuses depends upon the location and type of tumor and the possibility of successful surgical resection, Other miscellaneous conditions sometimes associated with polyhydramnios include amniotic band syndrome, lethal multiple pterygium syndrome, facial clefts, and dysmorphia.[7]

The outcomes of fetuses who have malformations associated with polyhydramnios vary greatly, according to the types of lesions. In one study, the survival rate of all fetuses with polyhydramnios was 58%.[7] However, when idiopathic polyhydramnios was noted where no fetal abnormality could be seen sonographically, all fetuses survived. Several authors suggest that ultrasound is an excellent modality for the detection of malformations associated with polyhydramnios.[6—8, 23] If no anomalies are found sonographically, the prognosis is good.[6—8, 23] This is not surprising, as the presence of excess amniotic fluid enhances the acoustic window for viewing fetal anatomy.

Miscellaneous

Other than polyhydramnios and multiple fetuses, large masses in the uterus can lead the clinician to detect a uterus that is larger than anticipated by gestational age. These masses include tumors such as molar pregnancies or partial moles with markedly enlarged and hydropic placentae or large chorioangiomas (**Fig. 27–22**). Tumors, such as large sacrococcygeal teratomas, will cause the uterus to enlarge, both because of the tumor's

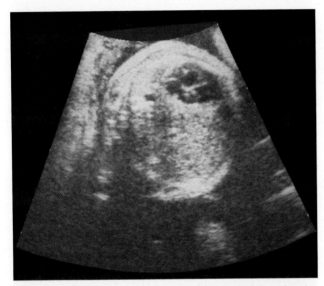

Figure 27–16   Transverse view through the fetal thorax showing a right diaphragmatic hernia. Note that the heart is displaced to the left by a part of the liver (**arrows**) in the right hemithorax.

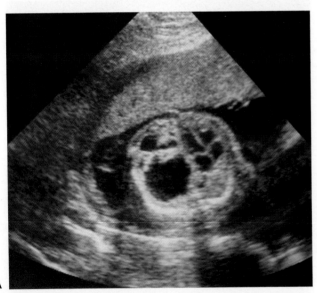

A

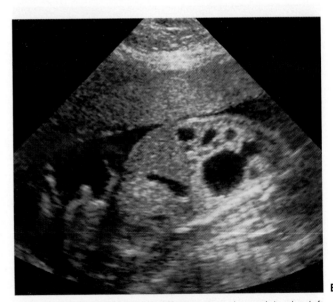

B

Figure 27–17 A, B   Longitudinal and transverse view of the fetal thorax of a fetus with a type I cystic adenomatoid malformation of the lung. Note the cysts of different sizes, located in the left hemithorax and deviating the heart and mediastinum to the right.

size and the associated polyhydramnios (**Fig. 27–21**). Fetuses with nonimmune hydrops are also subject to having enlarged placentae which can contribute to the enlargement of the uterus. Pelvic masses not associated with the pregnancy may also lead to the clinical finding of an enlarged uterus. These include fibroid tumors, which can enlarge dramatically in the first part of pregnancy (**Fig. 27–23**). Also, adnexal masses such as ovarian cysts, dermoids, and other adnexal enlargements can result in the perception of an enlarged uterus by the clinician. Part of the evaluation of the pregnant uterus includes the assessment of the adnexa as well as the surrounding myometrium and cervix.

In conclusion, ultrasound is very successful at evaluating the pregnancy which is thought by the clinician to be large for dates. In many cases, an explanation can be found (incorrect dates, multiple pregnancies, or a uterine fibroid). When polyhydramnios is detected, fetal biometry can be helpful to detect any growth acceleration leading to macrosomia, perhaps in a diabetic mother. A careful structural survey is necessary, however, when evaluating a fetus associated with polyhydramnios.

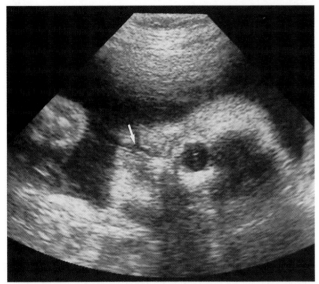

Fig. 27–18 Coronal view of the fetal lower face in a fetus with trisomy 9. Note the median cleft lip and palate (**arrow**). This was associated with polyhydramnios and multiple other congenital abnormalities.

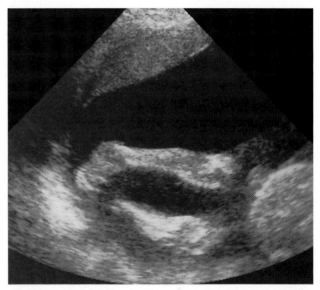

Figure 27–19 Longitudinal view of the fetal lower leg, showing congenital clubbed foot in a fetus with trisomy 18. Note the polyhydramnios associated with it.

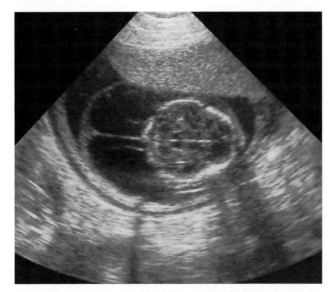

Figure 27–20 Transverse view through the fetal head, showing large septated cystic hygromas of the nuchal region in a fetus with Turner's syndrome.

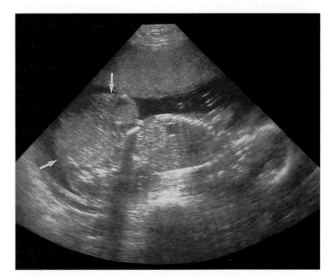

Figure 27–21 Longitudinal view of the fetal body in the second trimester showing a large sacrococcygeal teratoma (**arrows**). The fetus is at risk for hydrops an dpolyhdramnios.

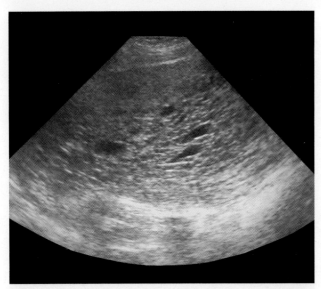

Figure 27–22 View of the uterus early in the second trimester showing no visible fetus. The uterus is filled with a solid mass with many small cystic spaces, typical of a complete mole.

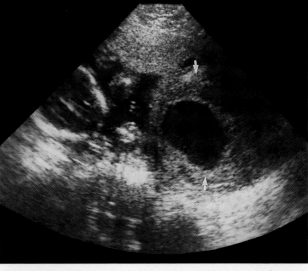

Figure 27–23 The uterus is larger than dates because of a cystic mass (**arrows**) in the wall of the uterus, typical of a degenerating fibroid.

When abnormalities are detected, it may be necessary to proceed with an amniocentesis or a percutaneous blood sampling for evaluation or treatment. In most cases, a normal structural survey — even in association with significant polyhydramnios — results in a good outcome.

References

1. Benirschke K, Kim CK. Multiple pregnancy part one. *NEJM* 1973;288:1276—1284.
2. Blickstein I. Review: the twin-twin transfusion syndrome. *Obstet Gynecol* 1990;76:714—722.
3. Bromley B, Frigoletto FD, Estroff JA, Benacerraf BR. The natural history of oligohydramnios/polyhydramnios sequence in monochorionic diamniotic twins. *Ultrasound Obstet Gynecol* 1992;2:317—320.
4. Goldstein RB, Frilly RA. Sonographic estimation of amniotic fluid volume: subjective assessment versus pocket measurements. *J Ultrasound Med* 1988;7:363—367.
5. Phelan JP, Ahn MO, Smith CV, Rutherford SE, Anderson E. Amniotic fluid index measurements during pregnancy. *J Repro Med* 1987;32(8):601—604.
6. Barkin SZ, Pretorius DH, Beckett MK, et al. Severe polyhydramnios: incidence of anomalies. *AJR* 1987;148:155—159.
7. Damato N, Filly RA, Goldstein RB, et al. Frequency of fetal anomalies in sonographically detected polyhydramnios. *J Ultrasound Med* 1993;12:11—15.
8. Stoll CG, Alembik Y, Dott B. Study of 156 cases of polyhydramnios and congenital malformations in a series of 118,265 consecutive births. *Am J Obstet Gynecol* 1991;165:586—590.
9. Benson CB, Coughlin BF, Doubilet PM. Amniotic fluid volume in large-for-gestational-age fetuses of nondiabetic mothers. *J Ultrasound Med* 1991;10:149—151.
10. Sohaey R, Nyberg DA, Sickler GK, Williams MA. Idiopathic polyhydramnios: association with fetal macrosomia. *Radiology* 1994;190:393—396.
11. Smith CV, Plambeck RD, Rayburn WF, Albaugh KJ. Relation of mild idiopathic polyhydramnios to perinatal outcome. *Obstet Gynecol* 1992;79:387—389.
12. Pretorius DH, Drose JA, Dennis MA, Manchester DK, Manco-Johnson ML. Tracheoesophageal fistula in utero: 22 cases. *J Ultrasound Med* 1987;6:509—513.
13. Heydanus R, Spaargaren MC, Wladimiroff JW. Prenatal ultrasonic diagnosis of obstructive bowel disease: a retrospective analysis. *Prenatal Diagnosis* 1994;14:1035—1041.
14. Hutchison AA, Drew JH, Yu VYH, et al. Nonimmunologic hydrops fetalis; a review of 61 cases. *Obstet Gyneco.* 1982;59:34752.
15. Chitkara U, Wilkins, Lynch L, Mehalek K, Berkowitz RL. The role of sonography in assessing severity of fetal anemia in Rh and Kell isoimmunized pregnancies. *J Obstet Gynecol* 1988;71:393—397.
16. Goldstein RB, Filly RA. Prenatal diagnosis of anencephaly: spectrum of sonographic appearances and distinction from the amniotic band syndrome. *AJR* 1988,151:547—550.
17. Pretorius DH, Rumack CM, Manco-Johnson ML, et al. Specific skeletal dysplasias in utero: sonographic diagnosis. *Radiology* 1986,195:237—242.
18. Wong WS, Filly RA. Polyhydramnios associated with fetal limb abnormalities. *AJR* 1983;140:1001—1003.
19. Brady K, Polzin WJ, Kopelman JN, Read JA. Risk of chromosomal abnormalities in patients with idiopathic polyhydramnios. *Obset Gynecol* 1992;79:234—238.
20. Jouppila P, Makarainen L, Rasanen J, Valkama M, Paavilainen T. Aggressive direct treatment of a fetus with supraventricular tachycardia and hydrops fetalis. *Ultrasound Obstet Gynecol* 1993;3:279—283.
21. Hubinont C, Bernard P, Khalil N, et al. Fetal liver hemangioma and chorioangioma: two unusual cases of severe fetal anemia detected by ultrasonography and its perinatal management. *Ultrasound Obstet Gynecol* 1994;4:330—331.
22. Williams FL, Williams RA. Placental teratoma: prenatal ultrasonographic diagnosis. *J Ultrasound Med* 1994;13:587—589.
23. Sivit CJ, Hill MC, larsen JW, Lande IM. Second-trimester polyhydramnios: evaluation with US. *Radiology* 1987;165:467—469.

24. Tonkin IL, Setzer ES, Ermocilla R. Placental chorioangioma: a rare cause of congestive heart failure and hydrops fetalis in the newborn. *AJR* 1980;134:181—183.

25. Treadwell MC, Sepulveda W, LeBlanc LL, Romero R. Prenatal diagnosis fo fetal cutaneous hemangioma: case report and review of the literature. *J Ultrasound Med* 1993;12:683—687.

26. Kangarloo H, Diament MJ. Diagnostic oncology case study: cervical mass in a fetus associated with maternal hydramnios. *AJR* 1983;140:507—509.

27. Chervanak FA, Isaacson G, Blakemore KJ, et al. Fetal cystic hygroma: cause and natural history. *N Engl J Med* 1983;309:822—825.

28. Perez-Aytes A, Sanchis N, Barbal A, et al. Short communication: non-immunological hydrops fetalis and intrapericardial teratoma: case report and review. *Prenatal Diagnosis* 1995;15:859—863.

29. Chervenak FA, Tortora M, Moya FR, Hobbins JC. Antenatal sonographic diagnosis of epignathus. *J Ultrasound Med* 1984;3:235—237.

30. Benacerraf BR, Frigoletto FD. Prenatal sonographic diagnosis of isolated congenital cystic hygroma, unassociated with lymphedema or other morphologic abnormality. *J Ultrasound Med.* 1987;6:63—66.

31. Gross SJ, Benzi RJ, Sermer M, Skidmore MB, Wilson SR. Sacrococcygeal teratoma: prenatal diagnosis and management. *Am J Obstet Gynecol* 1987;156:393—396.

28 Uterine Size Less than Dates: A Clinical Dilemma*

Frank P. Hadlock

The growth of the human fetus, a complex process resulting in an increase in size over time, has been the subject of extensive study.[1-102] Before the advent of ultrasound (US), physicians interested in the growth process of the fetus could only look at the infant at delivery and infer what had happened in utero.

Based on these observations, clinicians were able to categorize fetuses in very general terms on the basis of their age and size. For example, fetuses could be classified by birth weight as small for gestational age (SGA), appropriate for gestational age (AGA), and large for gestational age (LGA). Clinicians soon recognized that perinatal morbidity and mortality considerably increased for fetuses born preterm or postterm and for fetuses born too small or too large for menstrual age.[1-11]

Because of these observations, a considerable interest exists in monitoring fetal growth in utero. The primary clinical tool for evaluation of fetal growth is an estimate of uterine size. In the first trimester of pregnancy, this is typically done by means of pelvic examination. In the second and third trimester of pregnancy, this is generally accomplished by means of measurement of the fundal height of the uterus. When uterine size is less than expected for the number of completed menstrual weeks, the clinican must be concerned that either the dates are misleading or in error or that the fetus and intrauterine environment are compromised. In this article, we will discuss the important role that US can play in the resolution of this clinical dilemma.

Clinical Considerations of Intrauterine Growth Retardation

As consultants, it is imperative that we understand the nature of the clinical problems and the language unique to them. For example, definition of "intrauterine growth retardation" (IUGR) is problematic, as in a given case we do not know the inherent growth potential of the fetus.[13,15] For this reason, population standards have been developed, and fetuses whose weight falls below the 10th percentile for age are classified as SGA. Although some authors have used the terms SGA and IUGR synonymously, SGA and IUGR should, in fact, be considered as separate entities. For example, a fetus born at the fifth percentile for weight who has reached its genetic potential may be small in relation to the reference population, but it is not actually growth retarded. On the other hand, a full-term fetus whose weight is at the 50th percentile for age but whose genetic potential was for the 90th percentile could be considered growth retarded. As a practical matter, most authors use the 10th percentile for age as a cutoff below which fetuses must be considered small for gestational age. It is our job as ultrasonologists to help the clinician determine which fetuses are small because of IUGR, so that appropriate management may optimize fetal outcome.

The incidence of IUGR in a general, low-risk population is only about 5%, reaching a level of approximately 10% in women who can be considered at risk. In our experience, the most important maternal factors for IUGR are a previous IUGR fetus, marked maternal hypertension, smoking, a uterine anomaly (bicornuate uterus or large fibroids), and placental hemorrhage. We must remember, however, that because the low-risk population is a substantially larger group than the high-risk population, approximately one-half of all IUGR fetuses will come from the low-risk population.

Historically, the classification of IUGR has been based on the morphologic characteristics of the fetuses studied.[29-33] Symmetric IUGR, usually the result of a first-trimester insult (chromosomal abnormality, infection), results in a fetus that is proportionately small throughout pregnancy (**Fig. 28–1**). Unfortunately, although this group can often be identified in utero, very little can be done to impact fetal outcome. Asymmetrical IUGR is usually thought to be a process that begins in the late second or early third trimester and results from placental insufficiency (**Fig. 28–2**). With asymmetrical IUGR, growth of the fetal head is relatively spared at the expense of abdominal and soft tissue growth, while fetal length is compromised to varying degrees. Doppler studies have demonstrated that this pattern results from preferential blood flow to the fetal brain instead of to the other organ systems. If this process continues unabated to term, the head sparing is usually compromised, and the growth of the fetus is more symmetrically retarded.

Department of Radiology, Baylor College of Medicine, Houston, Texas, U.S.A.
* Originally published in RSNA Special Course in Ultrasound (1996; 281–293).

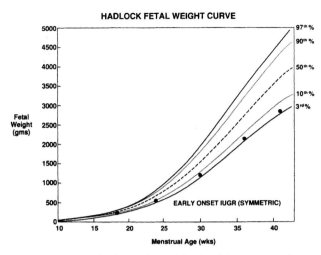

Figure 28–1 Graph plots estimated fetal weight in a case of symmetric IUGR. Note that weight approximates the third percentile throughout pregnancy. Other sonographic parameters of fetal growth (head size, abdominal girth, femur length) would show similar growth pattern throughout pregnancy. This type of growth pattern may be seen in otherwise normal fetuses that are constitutionally small, but is more commonly seen in fetuses that suffer a first-trimester insult. Reprinted, with permission, from reference 14.

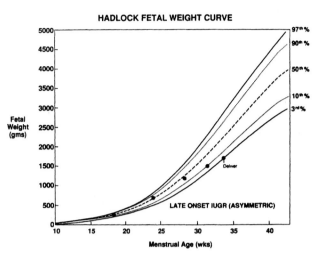

Figure 28–2 Graph plots estimated fetal weight in a case of late-onset asymmetric growth retardation. In these cases, head size and body length are compromised to varying degrees, but abdominal girth is compromised early. These cases frequently result from placental insufficiency. Early delivery at 35–35 weeks may prevent these fetuses from suffering the increased perinatal morbidity and mortality frequently seen in IUGR fetuses at term. Reprinted, with permission, from reference 14.

Although some authors have disputed the validity of the symmetric–asymmetric classification, in our experience it has proven to be a workable one, with approximately one-third of growth-retarded fetuses falling into the symmetric category and approximately two-thirds into the asymmetric category.

Finally, and most importantly, we should consider the clinical significance of IUGR. The literature has consistently indicated that fetuses with IUGR are at high risk for perinatal morbidity and mortality in comparison with the normal-weight peer population.[14-22] For example, in a recent study of 66 IUGR fetuses, Hill et al.[73] reported a perinatal mortality rate (corrected for severe congenital anomalies) of 91 per 1000 deliveries. This compares with a corrected perinatal mortality rate of approximately 4.4 per 1000 deliveries in a large, high-risk population that was closely monitored by antepartum testing, including US.[98] Other authors have emphasized that IUGR fetuses suffer long-term neurologic and intellectual impairment when delivered at term, probably because of chronic hypoxia and severe acidemia in utero.[16-20] However, it has been recognized more recently that early recognition and delivery of growth-retarded fetuses from the hostile intrauterine environment (preferably at approximately 34 to 35 weeks) result in infants whose growth and intellectual development are equivalent to those of the appropriately grown peer group at 24 months of age. For this reason, those who use US as a prenatal diagnostic tool must examine every fetus, regardless of the indication of the scan, for evidence of IUGR.

US Detection of IUGR

First-Trimester Evaluation

When evaluating a woman in the first trimester of pregnancy, we should generally use the transvaginal approach because it allows us to visualize the gestational sac, the yolk sac, the embryonic pole, and cardiac activity by 6 menstrual weeks. In our experience, the most frequent finding in a woman with clinically small uterine size is the presence of cardiac activity in a fetus whose crown-rump length (CRL) is appropriate for the dates (±5 days). This finding simply reflects the limitations of the clinical pelvic examination in establishing exact menstrual age. A second possibility is visualization of an empty sac or a fetus with a CRL smaller than expected for the dates and with no visible cardiac activity. In this situation, the small uterine size simply reflects the point at which the pregnancy ceased to develop.

The third possibility, and certainly a common one, is that a definite fetal pole and cardiac activity are demonstrated, but the CRL measurement (**Table 28–1**) is less than expected (>7 days) for the menstrual history. With these findings, the patient's history is critically important. For example, if the woman has a history of irregular cycles or previous oral contraceptive use, this may explain the discrepancy in uterine or fetal size and menstrual dates. In some cases, the woman will simply have ovulated and conceived late in the cycle, which clearly explains the discrepancy in size and dates (**Fig. 28–3**). Because cases have been reported in which the CRL growth in the first trimester has been compromised by a genetic or infectious insult,[25] it is imperative to rescan these women to evaluate interval growth. Theoretically, this can be done after a 3-week interval, but we prefer to wait until 16 menstrual weeks, because at that time we can gather information concerning anatomy, amniotic fluid volume, and fetal growth. This examination is especially important for ruling out cases of trisomy 13 and 18 (**Fig. 28–4**). It is equally important to obtain maternal serum trisomy screens in these women and

proceed with genetic amniocentesis if the size–dates discrepancy has widened or the trisomy screen is abnormal.

Consider two examples. Suppose that at a woman's initial examination, the fetus had a menstrual age of 8 weeks but a CRL age of 6.5 weeks. At the second examination, 4 weeks later, it had a menstrual age of 12 weeks and a CRL age of 10.5 weeks.

In this case, the second examination shows normal interval growth, suggesting that the woman probably ovulated and conceived late in the cycle (day 24). In our laboratory, however, we would scan this woman again at 16 weeks to confirm normal anatomy, amniotic fluid volume, and fetal growth.

Again, suppose that at a woman's initial examination, the fetus had a menstrual age of 8 weeks but a CRL age of 6.5 weeks. Six weeks later, at a second examination, it had a menstrual age of 14 weeks and a CRL age of 11.5 weeks. In this case, the second examination demonstrates suboptimal CRL growth, which suggests that the initial date-size discrepancy was due to poor growth rather than late ovulation. A genetic evaluation is warranted at this point. If this evaluation is normal, then close follow-up for growth is still warranted, as the growth compromise may be due to an infectious agent or a lethal anomaly.

Second- and Third-Trimester Evaluation

Beyond the first trimester of pregnancy, the choice of parameters for detection of IUGR is problematic. In cases of severe IUGR at term, almost any US parameter could prove useful as a diagnostic tool if the dates are known unequivocally by early CRL measurement (**Table 28–1**). As Dicke and others[26,27] have demonstrated, this is especially true for chromosomal abnormalities such as

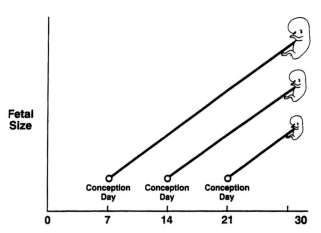

Figure 28–3 Drawing illustrates the effect of early or late ovulation on CRL size of fetus. All these women had their last normal menstrual period on the same date. Fetuses conceived late in the menstrual cycle (day 21) are smaller than fetuses conceived in midcycle because they are 1 week younger, not because they are growing abnormally. Thus, measurements of CRL growth in the first trimester should not be considered abnormal until size is at least 1 week less than expected for good dates, and follow-up evaluation is always necessary to confirm abnormal growth. Reprinted, with permission, from reference 14.

Table 28–1 Predicted menstrual age from CRL measurements*

CRL (cm)	MA (wk)	CRL (cm)	MA (wk)	CRL (cm)	MA (wk)	CRL (cm)	MA (wk)	CRL (cm)	MA (wk)	CRL (cm)	MA (wk)
0.2	5.7	2.2	8.9	4.2	11.1	6.2	12.6	8.2	14.2	10.2	16.1
0.3	5.9	2.3	9.0	4.3	11.2	6.3	12.7	8.3	14.2	10.3	16.2
0.4	6.1	2.4	9.1	4.4	11.2	6.4	12.8	8.4	14.3	10.4	16.3
0.5	6.2	2.5	9.2	4.5	11.3	6.5	12.8	8.5	14.4	10.5	16.4
0.6	6.4	2.6	9.4	4.6	11.4	6.6	12.9	8.6	14.5	10.6	16.5
0.7	6.6	2.7	9.5	4.7	11.5	6.7	13.0	8.7	14.6	10.7	16.6
0.8	6.7	2.8	9.6	4.8	11.6	6.8	13.1	8.8	14.7	10.8	16.7
0.9	6.9	2.9	9.7	4.9	11.7	6.9	13.1	8.9	14.8	10.9	16.8
1.0	7.2	3.0	9.9	5.0	11.7	7.0	13.2	9.0	14.9	11.0	16.9
1.1	7.2	3.1	10.0	5.1	11.8	7.1	13.3	9.1	15.0	11.1	17.0
1.2	7.4	3.2	10.1	5.2	11.9	7.2	13.4	9.2	15.1	11.2	17.1
1.3	7.5	3.3	10.2	5.3	12.0	7.3	13.4	9.3	15.2	11.3	17.2
1.4	7.7	3.4	10.3	5.4	12.0	7.4	13.5	9.4	15.3	11.4	17.3
1.5	7.9	3.5	10.4	5.5	12.1	7.5	13.6	9.5	15.3	11.5	17.4
1.6	8.0	3.6	10.5	5.6	12.2	7.6	13.7	9.6	15.4	11.6	17.5
1.7	8.1	3.7	10.6	5.7	12.3	7.7	13.8	9.7	15.5	11.7	17.6
1.8	8.3	3.8	10.7	5.8	12.3	7.8	13.8	9.8	15.6	11.8	17.7
1.9	8.4	3.9	10.8	5.9	12.4	7.9	13.9	9.9	15.7	11.9	17.8
2.0	8.6	4.0	10.9	6.0	12.5	8.0	14.0	10.0	15.9	12.0	17.9
2.1	8.7	4.1	11.0	6.1	12.6	8.1	14.1	10.1	16.0	12.1	18.0

* The 95% confidence interval is ± 8% of the predicted age.
 Reprinted, with permission, from reference 39.
 MA; menstrual age; CRL; crown rump length.

trisomy 13 and trisomy 18 (**Fig. 28–4**). Because our goal is to detect IUGR early enough for proper clinical management, however, we have developed a comprehensive fetal-growth profile to optimize our chances for detecting this entity early in pregnancy. This profile, which is designed to provide the same type of information gained from neonatal evaluation at delivery, evaluates head size, trunk size, soft tissue mass, weight, length, and body proportionality.[36] This wealth of information can be gained from evaluation of three high-quality images of the fetal head, abdomen, and femur (**Fig. 28–5**).

Head size—As outlined in our chapter on fetal dating, the head is imaged in an axial plane using the cavum septum pellucidum, thalamic nuclei, falx cerebri, and choroid plexus as landmarks.[14] Because the biparietal diameter of the head can be misleading in cases associated with head shape changes (e.g., dolichocephaly), the head circumference is the measurement of choice for evaluation of head growth in utero.[14] After a satisfactory image has been obtained (**Fig. 28–5**), the perimeter can be traced along the outer margin of the calvarium using a map measurer or electronic digitizer, or it can be calculated from the two outer-to-outer diameters using the formula for the perimeter of an ellipse. Our experience has indicated that these measurement techniques give equivalent results. In examining the fetal head for this measurement, it is very important to rule out anomalies, because these may be seen in association with some forms of growth retardation. The normalcy of fetal head growth can then be judged against population standards such as those shown in Table 28–2.

In symmetric IUGR, fetal head size will frequently be compromised early in pregnancy; therefore, when dates are known unequivocally, a head circumference below the third percentile for age is cause for concern. This finding could be the result of a focal process such as microcephaly, or it may be associated with more generalized growth retardation, in which case other fetal parameters will also be small for age. When this finding is observed in early pregnancy, we prefer to proceed with genetic amniocentesis and amniotic fluid cultures to rule out the possibility of a chromosomal abnormality or intrauterine infection accounting for poor head growth.

In asymmetric IUGR, the growth of the fetal head is typically normal until very late in pregnancy because of preferential blood flow to the brain at the expense of other organ systems, such as the liver. For this reason,

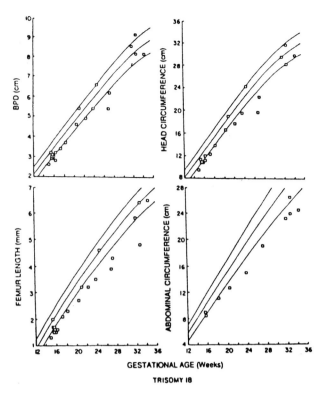

Figure 28–4   These four graphs plot biparietal diameter *(BPD)*, head circumference, abdominal circumference, and femur length in a group of fetuses with trisomy 18 at varying stages in pregnancy. Note that growth disturbances, particularly for abdominal circumference, are evident in the early second trimester of pregnancy. Reprinted, with permission from reference 26.

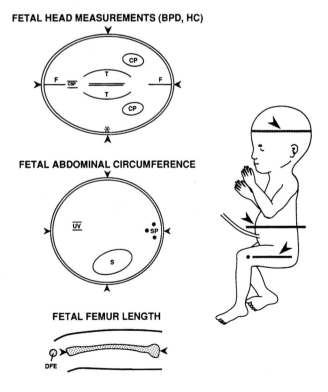

Figure 28–5   Illustration show appropriate planes of section for ▷ measurement of fetal head, fetal abdomen, and fetal femur. Landmarks in the head are the falx *(F)* anteriorly and posteriorly, cavum septum pellucidum anteriorly *(CSP)*, thalamic nuclei *(T)* in the midline, and choroid plexus *(CP)* in the atria of the lateral ventricles. Landmarks in the abdomen are the umbilical vein *(UV)*, stomach *(S)*, and spine *(SP)*. The femur is measured along the diaphyseal shaft, excluding the distal femoral epiphysis *(DFE)*. Reprinted, with permission, from reference 14.

Table 28–2 Percentile values for fetal head cirumference

Menstrual weeks	Head circumference (cm)				
	3rd	10th	50th	90th	97th
14	8.8	9.1	9.7	10.3	10.6
15	10.0	10.4	11.0	11.6	12.0
16	11.3	11.7	12.4	13.1	13.5
17	12.6	13.0	13.8	14.6	15.0
18	13.7	14.2	15.1	16.0	16.5
19	14.9	15.5	16.4	17.4	17.9
20	16.1	16.7	17.7	18.7	19.3
21	17.2	17.8	18.9	20.0	20.6
22	18.3	18.9	20.1	21.3	21.9
23	19.4	20.1	21.3	22.5	23.2
24	20.4	21.1	22.4	23.7	24.3
25	21.4	22.2	23.5	24.9	25.6
26	22.4	23.2	24.6	26.0	26.8
27	23.3	24.1	25.6	27.1	27.9
28	24.2	25.1	26.6	28.1	29.0
29	25.0	25.9	27.5	29.1	30.0
30	25.8	26.8	28.4	30.0	31.0
31	26.7	27.6	29.3	31.0	31.9
32	27.4	28.4	30.1	31.8	32.8
33	28.0	29.0	30.8	32.6	33.6
34	28.7	29.7	31.5	33.3	34.3
35	29.3	30.4	32.2	34.1	35.1
36	29.9	30.9	32.8	34.7	35.8
37	30.3	31.4	33.3	35.2	36.3
38	30.8	31.9	33.8	35.8	36.8
39	31.1	32.2	34.2	36.2	37.3
40	31.5	32.6	34.6	36.6	37.7

Reprinted, with permission, from reference 42.

Table 28–3 Percentile values for fetal abdominal cirumference

Menstrual weeks	Abdominal circumference (cm)				
	3rd	10th	50th	90th	97th
14	6.4	6.7	7.3	7.9	8.3
15	7.5	7.9	8.6	9.3	9.7
16	8.6	9.1	9.9	10.7	11.2
17	9.7	10.3	11.2	12.1	12.7
18	10.9	11.5	12.5	13.5	14.1
19	11.9	12.6	13.7	14.8	15.5
20	13.1	13.8	15.0	16.3	17.0
21	14.1	14.9	16.2	17.6	18.3
22	15.1	16.0	17.4	18.8	19.7
23	16.1	17.0	18.5	20.0	20.9
24	17.1	18.1	19.7	21.3	22.3
25	18.1	19.1	20.8	22.5	23.5
26	19.1	20.1	21.9	23.7	24.8
27	20.0	21.1	23.0	24.9	26.0
28	20.9	22.0	24.0	26.0	27.1
29	21.8	23.0	25.1	27.2	28.4
30	22.7	23.9	26.1	28.3	29.5
31	23.6	24.9	27.1	29.4	30.6
32	24.5	25.8	28.1	30.4	31.8
33	25.3	26.7	29.1	31.5	32.9
34	26.1	27.5	30.0	32.5	33.9
35	26.9	28.3	30.9	33.5	34.9
36	27.7	29.2	31.8	34.4	35.9
37	28.5	30.0	32.7	35.4	37.0
38	29.2	30.8	33.6	36.4	38.0
39	29.9	31.6	34.4	37.3	38.9
40	30.7	32.4	35.3	38.2	39.9

Reprinted, with permission, from reference 42.

measurement of the fetal head in such cases will typically fail to detect IUGR early enough to affect clinical management.

Trunk size—Fetal trunk size and soft-tissue mass are best analyzed by measurement of the fetal abdominal circumference. This measurement, first proposed by Campbell and Thoms[57] as a means of estimating fetal weight and ruling out growth retardation, is obtained from an axial section of the fetal abdomen at the level of the portal-umbilical venous complex (**Fig. 28–5**). This measurement can be traced along the outer perimeter using a map measurer or electronic digitizer, or it can be calculated from two outer diameters by using the formula for the circumference of a circle ($D_1 + D_2 \times 1.57$). In our laboratory, measurements using these two techniques have given equivalent results, and our normal data for abdominal circumference have been very reproducible (**Table 28–3**).

Remember, however, that the abdominal circumference measurement has the greatest inter- and intraobserver variability of all fetal measurements reported in the literature (**Table 28–4**). In addition to differences in imaging and measurement techniques, population differences and differences in mathematic modeling techniques may play a role in the marked differences reported in the literature for 10th percentile cutoff boundaries for abdominal circumference. For example, the data from Jeanty et al.[44] are based on a longitudinal study of 46 white fetuses examined by one physician, and the perimeter measurements were calculated from mean abdominal diameters. The data from Tamura et al.,[46] on the other hand, are from a cross-sectional analysis of 197 women of different racial origins, and the abdominal circumference was traced directly by using an electronic digitizer. The differences are dramatic, particular late in pregnancy (beyond 30 weeks), when the 50th percentile values reported by Jeanty et al. are less than the 10th percentile values reported by Tamura et al (**Table 28–4**). It is critically important, therefore, to duplicate the techniques of the original authors when using data from another source. Although one should theoretically choose tables from medical centers that have similar population characteristics, our data have not shown statistically significant differences in women of different races and socioeconomic origins.[14]

When fetal growth is compromised, the abdominal circumference is dramatically affected because of the reduction in adipose tissue and the depletion of glycogen stores in the liver. It is not surprising, then, that virtually all studies that have included this measurement have shown it to be the most sensitive single indicator of growth retardation in both symmetric and asymmetric IUGR (**Table 28–5**). In our experience, measurements below the 10th percentile for known age are highly suggestive of growth abnormality, and measurements below the third percentile for age are considered unequivocal evidence of IUGR until proven otherwise (**Fig. 28–6**).

Table 28–4 Fetal abdominal circumference at US imaging

Menstrual weeks	10th percentile (cm)			90th percentile (cm)		
	Jeanty et al[44]	Hadlock et al[42]	Tamura and Sabbegha[45]	Jeanty et al[44]	Hadlock et al[42]	Tamura and Sabbegha[45]
18	10.2	11.5	11.7	13.6	13.5	12.0
20	12.4	13.7	14.2	15.8	16.3	16.7
22	14.6	16.0	14.7	18.0	18.8	19.7
24	16.7	18.1	18.9	20.1	21.3	22.8
26	18.8	20.1	19.8	22.2	23.7	26.7
28	20.8	22.0	23.1	24.2	26.0	27.2
30	22.7	23.9	24.4	26.1	28.3	30.1
32	24.5	25.8	26.7	27.9	30.4	32.4
34	26.2	27.5	28.6	29.6	32.5	33.6
36	27.6	29.2	31.0	31.0	34.4	37.8
38	28.9	30.8	32.8	32.3	36.4	38.5
40	29.9	32.4	33.3	33.3	38.2	41.2

Table 28–5 Sensitivity of individual sonographic parameters for detecting IUGR

Parameter	Sensitivity	
	Hadlock et al[60] (37.9 wk ± 1.9)	Brown et al[61] (37.5 wk ± 2.1)
Abdominal circumference	100	96
Femur length	20	45
Head circumference/ abdominal circumference	70	ND
Femur length/abdominal circumference	63	57
Estimated weight percentile	87	63
Ponderal index	47	54

Numbers are percentages.
ND no data.

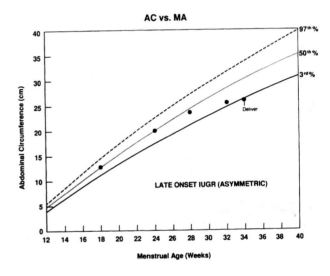

Figure 28–6 Graph plots abdominal-circumference growth against known menstrual age in a case of late-onset asymmetric IUGR. Note that abdominal growth began to decline at approximately 28 menstrual weeks and that virtually no growth occurred between 32 and 34 weeks. In such cases, intensive antenatal surveillance is mandatory, and early delivery is often indicated. Reprinted, with permission, from reference 14.

The limiting factor in the use of the abdominal circumference to predict IUGR is that the dates must be known unequivocally for proper use of this measurement. If the dates are not known, then serial evaluation at 2-week intervals can be performed to evaluate interval growth. For example, Divon and coworkers[62] have demonstrated that abdominal-circumference growth of less than 1 cm in 14 days is indicative of IUGR.

Fetal length—Neonatal crown–heel length is an important measure of growth because of its role in the ponderal index, which describes the weight-for-length relationship of the newborn at delivery. Although we can measure fetal CRL by using US in early pregnancy, it is virtually impossible to obtain a realistic measure of crown–heel length particularly beyond 18 menstrual weeks. Several authors have evaluated the fetal femur length using US, however, and have shown a consistent relationship between fetal femur length and neonatal crown–heel length.[59] Thus, US measurement of femur length can be used as a substitute variable for crown–heel length in the US growth profile (**Fig. 28–5**).

Fetal femur length in utero has been the subject of extensive US investigation, and the data across medical centers have been very reproducible (**Table 28–6**). Moreover, most authors have demonstrated no statistically significant differences in femur lengths among fetuses of different racial and socioeconomic origins. However, the degree to which the fetal femur is compromised in IUGR is less well established. Fetal femur length can be affected in early pregnancy in cases of early symmetrical growth retardation related to chromosomal abnormalities or infection, but generally the fetal femur length is not affected until very late in pregnancy in asymmetrical IUGR. For example, Hadlock et al.[60] reported the femur length to be below the third percentile in only 20% of third-trimester IUGR fetuses, and Brown et al.[61] reported the femur length to be less than the 10th percentile in 45% of growth-retarded fetuses in the third trimester. Perhaps the major role of femur length in the

Table 28–6   Percentile values for fetal femur length

Menstrual weeks	Femur length (cm)				
	3rd	10th	50th	90th	97th
14	1.2	1.3	1.4	1.5	1.6
15	1.5	1.6	1.7	1.9	1.9
16	1.7	1.8	2.0	2.2	2.3
17	2.1	2.2	2.4	2.6	2.7
18	2.3	2.5	2.7	2.9	3.1
19	2.6	2.7	3.0	3.3	3.4
20	2.8	3.0	3.3	3.6	3.8
21	3.0	3.2	3.5	3.8	4.0
22	3.3	3.5	3.8	4.1	4.3
23	3.5	3.7	4.1	4.5	4.7
24	3.8	4.0	4.4	4.8	5.0
25	4.0	4.2	4.6	5.0	5.2
26	4.2	4.5	4.9	5.3	5.6
27	4.4	4.6	5.1	5.6	5.8
28	4.6	4.9	5.4	5.9	6.2
29	4.8	5.1	5.6	6.1	6.4
30	5.0	5.3	5.8	6.3	6.6
31	5.2	5.5	6.0	6.5	6.8
32	5.3	5.6	6.2	6.8	7.1
33	5.5	5.8	6.4	7.0	7.3
34	5.7	6.0	6.6	7.2	7.5
35	5.9	6.2	6.8	7.4	7.8
36	6.0	6.4	7.0	7.6	8.0
37	6.2	6.6	7.2	7.9	8.2
38	6.4	6.7	7.4	8.1	8.4
39	6.5	6.8	7.5	8.2	8.6
40	6.6	7.0	7.7	8.4	8.8

Reprinted, with permission, from reference 42.

Table 28–7   In utero fetal sonographic weight standards

Menstrual weeks	Estimated fetal weight (g)				
	3rd percentile	10th percentile	50th percentile	90th percentile	97th percentile
10	26	29	35	41	44
11	34	37	45	53	56
12	43	48	58	68	73
13	55	61	73	85	91
14	70	77	93	109	116
15	88	97	117	137	146
16	110	121	146	171	183
17	136	150	181	212	226
18	167	185	223	261	279
19	205	227	273	319	341
20	248	275	331	387	414
21	299	331	399	467	499
22	359	398	478	559	598
23	426	471	568	665	710
24	503	556	670	784	838
25	589	652	785	918	981
26	685	758	913	1068	1141
27	791	876	1055	1234	1319
28	908	1004	1210	1416	1513
29	1034	1145	1379	1613	1724
30	1169	1294	1559	1824	1949
31	1313	1453	1751	2049	2189
32	1465	1621	1953	2285	2441
33	1622	1794	2162	2530	2703
34	1783	1973	2377	2781	2971
35	1946	2154	2595	3036	3244
36	2110	2335	2813	3291	3516
37	2271	2513	3028	3543	3785
38	2427	2686	3236	3786	4045
39	2576	2851	3435	4019	4294
40	2714	3004	3619	4234	4524

Reprinted, with permission, from reference 49.

growth profile is in the evaluation of fetal weight and body proportionality.

Fetal weight—Early efforts to evaluate fetal weight in utero demonstrated that the abdominal circumference could be used for predicting weight in normally growing fetuses at term. In preterm fetuses, however, and in fetuses with abnormalities of fetal growth, the variability of predicting fetal weight from abdominal circumference alone (2 standard deviations [SD] = 24%) was too great for general clinical use.[40] For this reason, many authors have attempted to incorporate additional parameters into models for estimating fetal weight. Some have suggested that separate fetal-weight models must be used for fetuses that are small or large for their dates. In our own experience, the use of a model that incorporates head size, abdominal size, and femur length has proved to be remarkably accurate over the entire range of weights and ages (1 SD = 7.5%).[49] With this model, estimated fetal weights below the 10th percentile in our laboratory have successfully identified 87% of IUGR fetuses scanned in the late third trimester of pregnancy (**Table 28–5**).[60] Vintzileos et al.[52] have recently reported similar results using this multiparameter approach to fetal-weight estimates.

A major problem in the evaluation of normal growth has been the application in utero of fetal-weight charts developed postnatally.[48] In a recent comprehensive review of this problem, we demonstrated that postnatal weight charts are appropriate for use in the full-term fetus (38 to 42 weeks), because over 90% of the infants in these large studies were born at term, but that the range of preterm weights is too broad to be clinically useful.[49] This is because the sample population below 38 weeks in postnatal studies is based on premature deliveries, and these fetuses may not have been growing normally prior to term. To resolve this issue, we have established normal weights and weight ranges in utero from 10 to 40 weeks and have shown that the variability is constant when expressed as a percentage of the predicted value (**Table 28–7**). Because our preterm boundaries for normal and abnormal weights are narrow compared with those of postnatal studies, we recommend that in-utero weight evaluations using our tables be applied only to fetuses whose fetal age has been verified by CRL in the first trimester of pregnancy.[49]

Body proportionality—The earliest application of US to the recognition of abnormal body proportionality was reported by Campbell and Thoms,[57] who used the ratio of head circumference to abdominal circumference to evaluate fetuses with asymmetric IUGR. In our experience, this ratio is abnormal in approximately two-thirds of all growth-retarded fetuses, but it generally fails to identify the one-third of growth-retarded fetuses that have symmetric IUGR (**Table 28–5**).[60] A major limitation of this ratio is the fact that the normal values change with time; therefore, strict knowledge of menstrual age is required to use the ratio. The second problem with the ratio is that a high number of false-positive values may result. For example, a fetus might have a 75th-percentile head size and a 50th-percentile abdominal size (yet its weight might actually be above the 50th percentile for age). In view of these findings, most authors feel that the use of abdominal circumference alone in patients with known menstrual age can be used effectively in place of this ratio.[60]

In an attempt to develop an in-utero ponderal index for evaluating the weight-length relationship of the fetus, Hadlock et al.[60] and Jeanty et al.[43] independently proposed an evaluation of the relationship between abdominal circumference (as an indicator of fetal weight) and femur length (as an indicator of the fetal length). Subsequently, several authors have found this relationship to be relatively constant beyond 20 weeks, indicating that it could be used as an age-independent indicator of IUGR. We have found this ratio to be elevated in the approximately two-thirds of IUGR fetuses with asymmetrical growth retardation, but it generally fails to detect the one-third of IUGR fetuses with symmetrical growth retardation (**Table 28–5**).[60] Given the low incidence of IUGR in the general population, we postulated that the positive predictive value of this ratio in screening the general population would be only approximately 25%, and this has been confirmed in subsequent studies.[61,64] Because this tool is age independent, we feel it will be especially useful in the evaluation of fetuses that present in the third trimester with no dates.

Vintzileos and coworkers[66,67] have reported other age-independent indices of fetal growth (tibia–abdominal circumference ratio, femur–thigh circumference ratio, and tibia–calf circumference ratio) and have suggested their use in high-risk patients who present late in pregnancy with no dates. Unfortunately, no follow-up data have demonstrated the usefulness of these ratios. Yagel and coworkers[70] evaluated an in-utero ponderal index calculated using the estimated fetal weight and the femur length (IUPI = EFW/FL^3), where IUPI = in-utero ponderal index, EFW = estimated fetal weight, and FL = femur length. Interestingly, these authors found that fetal and neonatal well-being were clearly compromised when IUGR was associated with a low in utero ponderal index. In my opinion, these more complicated approaches are less reproducible than the femur length–abdominal circumference ratio and offer no additional advantage over it.

Intrauterine environment—It is now well known that compromise of the intrauterine environment may also contribute to the reduction in uterine size detected clinically by measurement of the fundal height. For example, a reduction in amniotic fluid volume may occur secondary to ruptured membranes or severe fetal renal disease. Oligohydramnios is also a common finding in pregnancies affected by IUGR, and Manning and associates[82]

initially advocated using an estimate of amniotic fluid volume as a screening tool for IUGR. They had observed that when the largest pocket of amniotic fluid is less than 1 cm in its greatest dimension, the probability is high that the fetus is growth retarded. However, this degree of oligohydramnios is unusual until very late in pregnancy. For example, Hill and others[73] found oligohydramnios that satisfied this definition in only three of 66 growth-retarded fetuses in the third trimester of pregnancy. Moreover, they demonstrated that even a subjective decrease in amniotic fluid volume was present in only 20 of the 66 growth-retarded fetuses.[73] Because oligohydramnios is also common in postdate pregnancies (>42 weeks), it obviously cannot be specific for the detection of IUGR. Nevertheless, when one suspects oligohydramnios in patients with intact membranes and no fetal renal abnormalities, the possibility of IUGR is increased, and close monitoring of fetal growth and well-being is indicated.[84-87] Because the identification of oligohydramnios requires a great deal of experience, we recommend use of the four-quadrant technique using the normal values reported by Moore and Cayle[84] (**Table 28–8**).

Another structure that is frequently compromised in IUGR and may contribute to a reduction of uterine size is the placenta. Although measuring placental volume in utero is difficult, the finding of advanced placental senescence (grade 3 placenta) is a clue to the possible

Table 28–8 Amniotic fluid index values in normal pregnancy

Men-strual weeks	Amniotic fluid index values (cm)				
	3rd per-centile	10th per-centile	50th per-centile	90th per-centile	97th per-centile
16	73	79	121	185	201
17	77	83	127	194	211
18	80	87	133	202	220
19	83	90	137	207	225
20	86	93	141	212	230
21	88	95	143	214	233
22	89	97	145	216	235
23	90	98	146	218	237
24	90	98	147	219	238
25	89	97	147	221	240
26	89	97	147	223	242
27	85	95	146	226	245
28	86	94	146	228	249
29	84	92	145	231	254
30	82	90	145	234	258
31	79	88	144	238	263
32	77	86	144	242	269
33	74	83	143	245	274
34	72	81	142	248	278
35	70	79	140	249	279
36	68	77	138	249	279
37	66	75	135	244	275
38	65	73	132	239	269
39	64	72	127	226	255
40	63	71	123	214	240
41	63	70	116	194	216
42	63	69	110	175	192

Reprinted, with permission, from reference 84.

presence of IUGR.[88] Platt and Petrucha[89] have shown that although 20% of normal women have a grade 3 placenta at term, a grade 3 placenta is rare prior to 36 weeks; therefore, having a grade 3 placenta at that stage of pregnancy could be a marker of early placental insufficiency. Subsequently, Kazzi and associates[90] demonstrated that fetuses with a grade 3 placenta and a US fetal-weight estimate below 2700 grams have a fourfold higher incidence of IUGR than fetuses of the same size with placental grades of less than 3. Thus, the presence of oligohydramnios and a grade 3 placenta in fetuses weighing less than 2700 grams should be considered evidence of IUGR until proven otherwise. In such cases, aggressive monitoring of the pregnancy to ensure fetal growth and well-being is indicated.

New Developments

The latest developments in the US identification of IUGR have focused on using a combination of factors to detect IUGR. In independent studies, Hill et al[73] and Benson et al.[71-72] have suggested the use of models that incorporate clues from the maternal history with fetal measurements or amniotic fluid volume scores (**Table 28–9**). The Hill et al. study[73] combined the maternal history score with fetal measurements to produce a logistic IUGR score that could define the probability of IUGR in a given case. Interestingly, the authors found that the probability of IUGR was directly related to the estimated weight percentile and inversely related to femur length. Unfortunately, they did not evaluate the abdominal-circumference percentile as a potential variable in their model.

Benson and coworkers[71,72] designed an IUGR score (**Table 28–9**) so that the combination of elevated maternal blood pressure, severe oligohydramnios, and an estimated fetal weight 3 SDs below the mean for age yields a score of 100, while the combination of normal blood pressure, normal fluid volume, and an estimated weight 3 SDs above the mean for age yields a score of 0. In their initial report, an IUGR score below 50 virtually excluded the diagnosis of IUGR, with a negative predictive value of 99.1%. A score above 75 allowed confident prediction of IUGR, with a positive predictive value of 82%. A score between 50 and 75 was equivocal, in that it could be associated within a 24% likelihood of IUGR. In a subsequent follow-up study in fetuses with accurate early dating, the authors found that a score below 50 virtually excludes IUGR (3% probability), a score above 60 allows confident diagnosis of IUGR (75% probability), and a score from 50 to 60 is intermediate (13% probability). It is possible that the use of a weight curve generated in utero, such as the one recently reported from our institution, will further enhance the ability of these complex models to detect IUGR.

Other authors have compared the use of real-time US measurements with Doppler studies of the fetus or umbilical cord in detection of IUGR.[74-81] Some authors feel that Doppler studies reveal abnormalities long before the measurements in the fetal-growth profile become abnormal, but this has not been our experience when using Doppler evaluation of the umbilical artery systolic/diastolic (S/D) ratio. Other authors have suggested that Doppler studies of the fetal cerebral circulation,[79-81] especially when used in comparison with the Doppler evaluation of the umbilical cord, provide strong evidence of IUGR. Recent data suggest that biometry is the best indicator of fetal size, whereas abnormal Doppler studies, particularly those showing absent or reversed end-diastolic flow, are more predictive of poor outcome. Most authors, therefore, have concluded that the combination of fetal biometry and fetal Doppler imaging is more useful than either tool used alone.[74-77]

It is clear that the diagnosis of IUGR requires attention to a number of details, and that the diagnosis will be enhanced if maternal history, fetal biometry, intrauterine observations, and fetal Doppler studies are combined. Although on the surface such an approach would appear to be exceedingly time consuming and expensive, we routinely incorporate maternal history, fetal biometry (fetal-growth profile), and intrauterine observations in every complete obstetrical US examination, and we find that in most cases these studies can be done in 15–20 min. At the present time, we reserve the use of Doppler imaging for patients in whom an abnormality is suspected on the basis of a complete US scan (with low weight percentile, low amniotic fluid volume, or placental or uterine abnormality) or an abnormal biophysical profile score. It is likely, however, that a Dop-

Table 28–9 Multiparameter models for IUGR dedection

Benson method[71]
    IUGR score = 39.2 (constant)
    + Maternal blood pressure score (normal = 0, high = 6.8)
    + Amniotic fluid score (normal = 0, mild = 9.1, moderate or severe 14.8)
    − 13.1 × age-standardized estimated weight (SD)
    Example: maternal high blood pressure, amniotic fluid mildly decreased, estimated weight; 2 SD below mean for age)
    Score = 39.2 + 6.8 + 9.1 − (13.1 × −2 SD) = 81.3
    Conclusion: probable IUGR

Hill method[73]
    IUGR score = 15.24 (constant)
    + 1.2 × antenatal IUGR score (previous SGA = 1, blood pressure >140/90 after 34 weeks = 1, history of renal disease = 1, smoking = 2, bleeding or preterm labor = 1, poor weight gain = 1, no fundal growth or decrease in fundal height = 3)
    − 2.0 × femur length in cm
    − 0.35 × estimated weight percentile
    Example: antenatal score 1, femur length = 6.5 cm, fifth weight percentile
    Score = 15.24 + 1.2 − 13.0 − 1.75 = 1.69
    Conclusion: probability of IUGR = $e^{1.69}/(1 + e^{1.69})$ = 84%*

*e = base of the natural logarithm.

pler sample of the umbilical cord will eventually become a routine part of a complete obstetrical US examination.

Examples of Clinical Problems

Case 1—A woman whose dates were confirmed by first-trimester CRL presents at 34 menstrual weeks with fundal height small for the dates. All fetal measurements are at the ninth percentile for 34 weeks, the placenta is grade 1, the amniotic fluid index is normal, and the fetus is active. The biophysical profile and umbilical cord Doppler S/D ratio are normal. Is the fetus growth retarded?

The most likely possibility is that this fetus is small for its gestational age, based on our percentile definitions (<10th percentile), but it is probably not growth retarded. Some authors would suggest Doppler evaluation of the cerebral circulation to confirm this, but this is probably not necessary. One could repeat the study in two weeks to confirm a stable weight percentile, with clinical evaluation (nonstress test) if indicated.

Case 2—A woman whose dates were confirmed by first-trimester CRL presents at 34 menstrual weeks with fundal height small for the dates. All fetal measurements are at the ninth percentile for 34 weeks, the placenta is grade 3, the amniotic fluid index is low (<8), and the fetus is active. The biophysical profile is normal, but the umbilical cord Doppler S/D ratio is high (5.5). Is this fetus growth retarded?

The most likely diagnosis here is symmetrical IUGR due to long-standing placental insufficiency. The small fetal size, reduced amniotic fluid volume, advanced placental senescence, and increased resistance in the umbilical cord suggest a long-standing process. The real dilemma in this case is whether the fetus should be monitored closely or simply delivered at this point.

The Future

We have made great strides in the identification of abnormal fetal growth in the last decade. This advance has been due primarily to the development of normal range data for a number of individual fetal-growth parameters. It can only be enhanced by the recent development of a normal standard for the in-utero fetal weight curve[49]. Nonetheless, an inherent problem in the diagnosis of growth disturbances is not knowing the genetic growth potential of a given fetus, so the normalcy of the growth of any fetus has been judged to this point against population standards. Fortunately, great strides have been made in this area by using sophisticated mathematical modeling of growth in longitudinal studies of normally growing fetuses. Deter and colleagues[101,102] have demonstrated that a specific growth curve for any fetal-growth parameter can be developed on an in-dividualized basis from two US examinations obtained before the third trimester of pregnancy (preferably at 16 weeks and 26 weeks). By using these techniques, the authors have been able to predict birth characteristics with a high degree of accuracy 14 weeks before delivery in normally growing fetuses.[102] Based on these fetal measurements and actual birth measurements at delivery, a growth-potential realization index can be calculated for fetal weight, head circumference, abdominal circumference, and thigh circumference. Deter et al.[102] recently combined these growth-potential realization index values to form a neonatal growth-assessment score, which appears to be a sensitive indicator of third-trimester growth abnormalities. Further validation of these exciting techniques will undoubtedly enhance our ability to recognize abnormalities of fetal growth both prenatally and postnatally.

References

1. Battaglia FC, Lubcheno LO. A practical classification of newborn infants by weight and gestational age. *J Pediatr* 1967;71:159–163.
2. Gruenwald P. Growth of the human fetus. *Am J Obstet Gynecol* 1966;94:1112–1119.
3. Vorherr H. Factors influencing fetal growth. *Am J Obstet Gynecol* 1982;142:577–588.
4. Lubchenco LO, Hansman C, Dressler M, Boyd E. Intrauterine growth as estimated from liveborn birth-weight data at 24 to 42 weeks of gestation. *Pediatr* 1963;32:793–800.
5. Brenner WE, Edelman DA, Hendricks CH. A standard of fetal growth for the United States of America. *Am J Obstet Gynecol* 1976;126:555–564.
6. Williams RL, Greasy RK, Cunningham GC. Fetal growth and perinatal viability in California. *Obstet Gynecol* 1982;59:624–632.
7. Ulrich M. Fetal growth patterns in normal newborn infants in relation to gestational age, birth order, and sex. *Acta Paediatr Scand* 1982;292(suppl):5–45.
8. Robertson PA, Sniderman SH, Laros RK, et al. Neonatal morbidity according to gestational age and birth weight from five tertiary care centers in the United States, 1983 through 1986. *Am J Obstet Gynecol* 1992;166:1629–1645.
9. Altman DG, Coles EC. Nomograms for precise determination of birth weight for dates. *Br J Obstet Gynaecol* 1980;87:81–86.
10. Forbes JF, Smalls MJ. A comparative analysis of birthweight for gestational age standards. *Br J Obstet Gynaecol* 1983;99:297–303.
11. Kloosterman GJ. On intrauterine growth. *Int J Gynaecol Obstet* 1970;8:895–912.
12. Galbraith RS, Karchmar EJ, Piercy WN, Low JA. The clinical prediction of intrauterine growth retardation. *Am J Obstet Gynecol* 1979;133:281–286.
13. Hill RM, Verinaud WM, Deter RL, et al. The effect of intrauterine malnutrition on the human infant. *Acta Paediatr Scand* 1984;73:482–487.
14. Hadlock FP. Ultrasound evaluation of fetal growth. In: Callen P, ed. *Ultrasound in Obstetrics and Gynecology.* New York, NY: Saunders, 1994;8:129–143.

15. Patterson RM, Poudiot MR. Neonatal morphometrics and perinatal outcome: who is growth retarded? *Am J Obstet Gynecol* 1987;157:691–693.

16. Fitzhardinge PM, Steven EM. The small-for-date infant. II. Neurological and intellectual sequelae. *Pediatr* 1972;49:50–57.

17. Vohr BR, Oh W, Rosenfield AG, Cowett RM. The preterm small-for-gestational age infant: a two-year follow-up study. *Am J Obstet Gynecol* 1979;133:425–431.

18. Soothill PW, Ajayi RA, Campbell S, et al. Relationship between fetal acidemia at cordocentesis and subsequent neurodevelopment. *Ultrasound Obstet Gynecol* 1992;2:80–83.

19. Low JA, Galbraith RS, Muir DW, et al. Mortality and morbidity after intrapartum asphyxia in the preterm fetus. *Obstet Gynecol* 1992;80:57–61.

20. Lin CC, Su SJ, River LP. Comparison of associated high-risk factors and perinatal outcome between symmetric and asymmetric fetal intrauterine growth retardation. *Am J Obstet Gynecol* 1991;164:1535–1542.

21. Low JA, Galbraith RS, Muir D, et al. Intrauterine growth retardation: a study of long-term morbidity. *Am J Obstet Gynecol* 1982;142:670–674.

22. Sibai BM, Anderson GD, Abdella TN, McCubbin JH, Dilts PV Jr. Eclampsia. III. Neonatal outcome, growth and development. *Am J Obstet Gynecol* 1983;146:307–316.

23. Visser GHA, Huisman A, Saathof PWF, Sinnige HAM. Early fetal growth retardation: obstetric background and recurrence rate. *Obstet Gynecol* 1986;67:40–43.

24. Lang JM, Cohen A, Lieberman E. Risk factors for small-for-gestational-age birth in a preterm population. *Am J Obstet Gynecol* 1992;166:1374–1378.

25. Benacerraf BR. Intrauterine growth retardation in the first trimester associated with triploidy. *J Ultrasound Med* 1988;7:153–154.

26. Dicke J, Crane JP. Sonographic recognition of major malformations and aberrant fetal growth in trisomic fetuses. *J Ultrasound Med* 1991;10:433–437.

27. Dicke JM, Gray DL, Songster GS, et al. Fetal biometry as a screening tool for the detection of chromosomally abnormal pregnancies. *Obstet Gynecol* 1989;74:724–728.

28. Thomas D, Makhoul J, Muller C. Fetal growth retardation due to massive subchorionic thrombohematoma: report of two cases. *J Ultrasound Med* 1992;11:245–247.

29. Daikoku NH, Johnson JWC, Graf C, et al. Patterns of intrauterine growth retardation. *Obstet Gynecol* 1979;54:211–219.

30. Saintonge J, Cote R. Intrauterine growth retardation and diabetic pregnancy: two types of fetal malnutrition. *Am J Obstet Gynecol* 1983;146:194–198.

31. Villar J, Belizan JM. The timing factor in the pathophysiology of the intrauterine growth retardation syndrome. *Obstet Gynecol Survey* 1982;37:499–506.

32. Miller HC, Hassanein K. Diagnosis of impaired fetal growth in newborn infants. *Pediatr* 1971;48:511–522.

33. Woods DL, Malan AF, de V Hesse H. Patterns of retarded fetal growth. *Early Hum Dev* 1979;3:257–262.

34. Keirse MJNC. Epidemiology and etiology of the growth retarded baby. *Clin Obstet Gynaecol* 1984;11:415–436.

35. Ott WJ. The diagnosis of altered fetal growth. *Obstet Gynecol Clin North Am* 1988;1592:237–263.

36. Hadlock FP, Deter RL, Harrist RB. Sonographic detection of abnormal fetal growth patterns. *Clin Obstet Gynecol* 1984;27:342–351.

37. Matsumoto S, Nogami Y, Ohkuri S. Statistical studies on menstruation: a criticism of the definition of normal menstruation. *Gumma J Med Sci* 1962;11:294–318.

38. Waldenstrom U, Axelsosson O, Nilsson S. A comparison of the ability of a sonographically measured biparietal diameter and the last menstrual period to predict the spontaneous onset of labor. *Obstet Gynecol* 1990; 76:336–338.

39. Hadlock FP, Shah YP, Kanon DJ, Lindsey JV. Fetal crown-rump length: reevaluation of relation to menstrual age (5–18 weeks) with high-resolution real-time US. *Radiology* 1992;182:501–505.

40. Hadlock FP. Sonographic estimation of fetal age and weight. *Radiol Clin North Am* 1990;28:39–50.

41. Hadlock FP, Harrist RB, Martinez-Poyer J. Fetal body ratios in second trimester: a useful tool for identifying chromosomal abnormalities? *J Ultrasound Med* 1992;11:81–85.

42. Hadlock FP, Deter RL, Harrist RB, Park SK. Estimating fetal age: computer-assisted analysis of multiple fetal growth parameters. *Radiology* 1984;152:497–501.

43. Jeanty P, Cousaert E, Hobbins JC, et al. A longitudinal study of fetal head biometry. *Am J Perinatol* 1984;11:118–128.

44. Jeanty P, Cousaert E, Cantraine F. Normal growth of the abdominal perimeter. *Am J Perinatol* 1984; 1:129–135.

45. Tamura RK, Sabbagha RE. Percentile ranks of sonar fetal abdominal circumference measurements. *Am J Obstet Gynecol* 1980;138:475–480.

46. Tamura RK, Sabbagha RE, Pan WH, Vaisrub N. Ultrasonic fetal abdominal circumference: comparison of direct versus calculated measurement. *Obstet Gynecol* 1986;67:833–835.

47. Jeanty P, Cousaert E, Cantraine F, et al. A longitudinal study of fetal limb growth. *Am J Perinatol* 1984;1:136–144.

48. Goldenberg RL, Cutter GR, Hoffman JH, et al. Intrauterine growth retardation: standards for diagnosis. *Am J Obstet Gynecol* 1989;161:271–277.

49. Hadlock FP, Harrist RB, Martinez-Poyer J. In utero analysis of fetal growth: a sonographic weight standard. *Radiology* 1991;181:129–133.

50. Deter RL, Harrist RB, Hadlock FP, et al. Longitudinal studies of fetal growth with the use of dynamic image ultrasonography. *Am J Obstet Gynecol* 1982;143:545–554.

51. Hadlock FP, Harrist RB, Sharman RS, Deter RL, Park SK. Estimating fetal weight with the use of head, body and femur measurements: a prospective study. *Am J Obstet Gynecol* 1985;151:333–337.

52. Vintzileos AM, Campbell WA, Rodis JF, Bors-Koefoed R, Nochimson DJ. Fetal weight estimation formulas with head, abdominal, femur, and thigh circumference measurements. *Am J Obstet Gynecol* 1987;157:410–414.

53. Secher NJ, Hansen PK, Lenstrup C, Pedersen-Bjergaard L, Eriksen PS. Birthweight-for-gestational age charts based on early ultrasound estimation of gestational age. *Br J Obstet Gynaecol* 1986;93:128–134.

54. Jeanty P, Cantraine F, Romero R, et al. A longitudinal study of fetal weight growth. *J Ultrasound Med* 1984;3:321–324.

55. Ott WJ. Defining altered fetal growth by second-trimester sonography. 1990;75:1053–1059.

56. Deter RL, Harrist RB, Hadlock FP. Carpenter RJ. The use of ultrasound in the detection of intrauterine growth retardation: a review. *J Clin Ultrasound* 1982;10:9–16.

57. Campbell S, Thoms A. Ultrasound measurement of the fetal head to abdomen circumference ratio in the assessment of growth retardation. *Br J Obstet Gynaecol* 1977;84:165–174.

58. Crane JP, Kopta MM. Prediction of intrauterine growth retardation via ultrasonically measured head/abdominal circumference ratios. *Obstet Gynecol* 1979;54:597–601.

59. Hadlock FP, Deter RL, Roecker E, Harrist RB, Park SK. Relation of fetal femur length to neonatal crown-heel length. *J Ultrasound Med* 1984;3:1–3.

60. Hadlock FP, Deter RL, Harrist RB, Roecker E, Park SK. A date-independent predictor of intrauterine growth retardation: femur length/abdominal circumference ratio. *AJR* 1983;141:979–984.

61. Brown HL, Miller JM, Gabert HA, Kissling G. Ultrasonic recognition of the small-for-gestational age fetus. *Obstet Gynecol* 1987;69:631–635.
62. Divon MY, Chamberlain PF, Sipos L, Manning FA, Platt LD. Identification of the small for gestational age fetus with the use of gestational age-independent indices of fetal growth. *Am J Obstet Gynecol* 1986;155:1197–1201.
63. Ott WJ. Fetal femur length, neonatal crown-heel length, and screening for intrauterine growth retardation. *Obstet Gynecol.* 1984;65:460–464.
64. Benson CB, Doubilet PM, Saltzman DH, Jones TB. FL/AC ratio: poor predictor of intrauterine growth retardation. *Invest Radiol* 1985;20:727–730.
65. Benson CB, Doubilet PM, Saltzman DH. Intrauterine growth retardation: predictive value of US criteria for antenatal diagnosis. *Radiology* 1986;160:415–417.
66. Vintzileos AM, Neckles S, Campbell WA, et al. Three fetal ponderal indexes in normal pregnancy. *Obstet Gynecol* 1985;65:807–811.
67. Vintzileos AM, Neckles S, Campbell WA. Ultrasound fetal thigh-calf circumferences and gestational age-independent fetal ratios in normal pregnancy. *J Ultrasound Med* 1985;4:287–292.
68. Hays D, Patterson RM. A comparison of fetal biometric ratios to neonatal morphometrics. *J Ultrasound Med* 1987;6:71–75.
69. Eden RD, Seifert LS, Kodack LD, et al. A modified biophysical profile for antenatal fetal surveillance. *Obstet Gynecol* 1988;71:365–370.
70. Yagel S, Zacut D, Igelstein S, et al. In utero ponderal index as a prognostic factor in the evaluation of intrauterine growth retardation. *Am J Obstet Gynecol* 1987;157:415–419.
71. Benson CB, Boswell SB, Brown DL, Saltzman DH, Doubilet PM. Improved prediction of intrauterine growth retardation with use of multiple parameters. *Radiology* 1988;168:7–12.
72. Benson CB, Belville JS, Lentini JF, Saltzman DH, Doubilet PM. Intrauterine growth retardation: diagnosis based on multiple parameters—a prospective study. *Radiology* 1990;177:499–502.
73. Hill LM, Guzick D, Belfar HL, et al. A combined historic and sonographic score for the detection of intrauterine growth retardation. *Obstet Gynecol* 1989;73:291–296.
74. Gaziano E, Knox GE, Wager GP, et al. The predictability of the small-for-gestational-age infant by real-time ultrasound-derived measurements combined with pulsed Doppler umbilical artery velocimetry. *Am J Obstet Gynecol* 1988;158:1431–1439.
75. Miller JM, Gabert HA. Comparison of dynamic image and pulsed Doppler ultrasonography for the diagnosis of the small-for-gestational-age fetus. *Am J Obstet Gynecol* 1992;166:1820–1826.
76. Divon MY, Guidetti DA, Braverman JJ, Oberlander E, Langer O, Merkatz IR. Intrauterine growth retardation: a prospective study of the diagnostic value of real-time sonography combined with umbilical artery flow velocimetry. *Obstet Gynecol* 1988;72:611–615.
77. Berkowitz GS, Mehalek KE, Chitkara U, Rosenberg J, Cogswell C, Berkowitz RL. Doppler umbilical velocimetry in the prediction of adverse outcome in pregnancies at risk for intrauterine growth retardation. *Obstet Gynecol* 1988;71:742–746.
78. Ott WJ. Comparison of dynamic image and pulsed Doppler ultrasonography for the diagnosis of intrauterine growth retardation. *J Clin Ultrasound* 1990;18:3–7.
79. Wladimiroff JW, Tonge HM, Stewart PA. Doppler ultrasound assessment of cerebral blood flow in the human fetus. *Br J Obstet Gynaecol* 1986;93:471–475.
80. Cohn HE, Sacks EJ, heymann MA, Rudolph AM. Cardiovascular response to hypoxemia and acidemia in fetal lambs. *Am J Obstet Gynecol* 1974;120:817–824.
81. Mari G, Moise KJ, Deter RL. Doppler assessment of the pulsatility index in the cerebral circulation of the human fetus. *Am J Obstet Gynecol* 1989;160:698–703.
82. Manning FA, Hill LM, Platt LD. Qualitative amniotic fluid volume determination by ultrasound: antepartum detection of intrauterine growth retardation. *Am J Obstet Gynecol* 1981;139:254–260.
83. Vintzileos AM, Tsapanos V. Biophysical assessment of the fetus. *Ultrasound Obstet Gynecol* 1991;2:133–143.
84. Moore TR, Cayle JE. The amniotic fluid index in normal human pregnancy. *Am J Obstet Gynecol* 1990;162:1168–1173.
85. Philipson EH, Sokol RJ, Williams T. Oligohydramnios: clinical associations and predictive value for intrauterine growth retardation. *Am J Obstet Gynecol* 1983;146:271–276.
86. Hoddick WK, Callen PW, Filly RA, et al. Ultrasonographic determination of qualitative amniotic fluid volume in intrauterine growth retardation. *Am J Obstet Gynecol* 1984;149:758–762.
87. Rutherford SE, Phelan JP, Smith CV, Jacobs N. The four-quadrant assessment of amniotic fluid volume: an adjunct to antepartum fetal heart rate testing. *Obstet Gynecol* 1987;70:353–356.
88. Grannum PA, Berkoweitz RL, Hobbins JC. The ultrasonic changes in the maturing placenta and their relation to fetal pulmonic maturity. *Am J Obstet Gynecol* 1979;133:915–920.
89. Petrucha RA, Platt LV. Relationship of placental grade to gestational age. *Am J Obstet Gynecol* 1982;144:733–736.
90. Kazzi GM, Gross TL, Sokol RJ, Kazzi NJ. Detection of intrauterine growth retardation: a new use for sonographic placental grading. *J Obstet Gynecol* 1983;145:733–737.
91. Wittmann BK, Robinson HP, Aitchison T, Fleming JEE. The value of diagnostic ultrasound as a screening test for intrauterine growth retardation: comparison of nine parameters. *Am J Obstet Gynecol* 1979;134:30–35.
92. Hughey MJ. Routine ultrasound for detection and management of the small-for-gestational-age fetus. *Obstet Gynecol* 1984;64:101–107.
93. Ferrazzi E, Nicolini U, Kustermann A, Pardi G. Routine obstetric ultrasound: effectiveness of cross-sectional screening for fetal growth retardation. *J Clin Ultrasound* 1986;14:17–22.
94. Warsof SL, Cooper DJ, Little D, Campbell S. Routine ultrasound screening for antenatal detection of intrauterine growth retardation. *Obstet Gynecol* 1986;67:33–39.
95. Waldenstrom U, Nilsson S, Fall O, et al. Effects of routine one-stage ultrasound screening in pregnancy: a randomised controlled trial. *Lancet* 1988;2:585–588.
96. Rosendahl H, Kivinen S. Routine ultrasound screening for early detection of small for gestational age fetuses. *Obstet Gynecol* 1988;71:518–522.
97. Skovron ML, Berkowitz GS, Lapinski RH, Kim JM, Chitkara U. Evaluation of early third-trimester ultrasound screening for intrauterine growth retardation. *J Ultrasound Med* 1991;10:153–159.
98. De Vore GR, Herbertson RM. The temporal association of the implementation of a fetal diagnostic and surveillance program and decreased fetal mortality in a private hospital. *Obstet Gynecol* 1990;75:210–214.
99. Grumbach K, Coleman BG, Arger PH, Mintz MC, Gabbe SV, Mennuti MT. Twin and singleton growth patterns compared using US. *Radiology* 1986;158:237–241.
100. Parker AJ, Davies P, Mayho AM, Newton JR. The ultrasound estimation of sex-related variations of intrauterine growth. *Am J Obstet Gynecol* 1984;149:656–659.

101. Deter RL, Rossavik IK. A simplified method for determining individual growth curve standards. *Obstet Gynecol* 1987;70:801–806.
102. Deter RL, Harrist RB, Hill RM. Neonatal growth assessment score: a new approach to the detection of intrauterine growth retardation in the newborn. *Am J Obstet Gynecol* 1990;162:1030–1036.

29 Ruling Out Fetal Anomalies

Carol B. Benson

In the first few weeks after conception, the embryo undergoes growth, morphogenesis, and differentiation of tissues and organs. This is termed the *embryonic period* and lasts until about eight weeks gestational (menstrual) age. The remaining weeks of gestation are termed the *fetal period*, during which rapid growth occurs.[1] Fetal anomalies most often result from abnormal morphogenesis or differentiation during the embryonic period.

Ultrasound is the imaging modality of choice for evaluation of the fetal anatomy to assess for fetal anomalies. The fetus can be assessed from multiple angles in multiples planes to obtain the images required. The real-time capabilities of ultrasound permit evaluation even while the fetus is moving. In addition, real-time scanning allows identification of fetal cardiac activity before other means of assessment can document fetal life. Real-time is essential when assessing the fetal heart for structural or rhythmic abnormalities.

Fetal anomalies occur in about 2—5% of newborn infants,[2,3] and, in most cases, no prior history of a fetal malformation is present. There are, however, some conditions associated with increased risk of fetal anomaly, including a prior family history of congenital anomaly, maternal diabetes, advanced maternal age, and exposure to certain teratogens, drugs, or infections during pregnancy. Once pregnant, signs associated with increased risk of fetal malformation include abnormal amniotic fluid volume, either polyhydramnios or oligohydramnios, abnormal maternal serum alpha fetoprotein levels, and multiple gestations. Given any of these conditions, ultrasound is used to screen the developing fetus for an anomaly.

The American College of Radiology and the American Institute of Ultrasound in Medicine have published standards for Antepartum Obstetrical Ultrasound that include a list of the fetal anatomic structures that should be evaluated when performing ultrasound during the second and third trimesters (**Table 29–1**).[4,5] While it is not possible to detect all fetal anomalies prenatally, if these standards are used for fetal evaluation, most major congenital malformations will be detected. In some cases more specialized examinations may be required, and in some cases a fetal anomaly may not be visible on prenatal ultrasound.

Table 29–1 Fetal Anatomic Survey: Structures to be assessed

Cerebral ventricles
Choroid plexus
Posterior fossa to include cerebellum and cisterna magna
Heart — four-chamber view including its position in thorax
Spine — longitudinal and transverse
Stomach
Urinary bladder
Umbilical cord insertion at anterior abdominal wall
Kidneys

Images taken for fetal measurements
Biparietal diameter
Abdominal diameter/circumference
Femur length

(From Standards Published by the ACR and AIUM)

The Fetal Head

During an obstetrical ultrasound examination, three views of the fetal head are routinely obtained: the biparietal diameter, the cerebral ventricles, and the posterior fossa. The biparietal diameter view is an axial view of the fetal head at the level of the paired thalami and cavum septum pellucidum (**Fig. 29–1**). This view is ob-

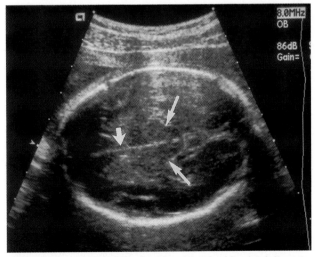

Figure 29–1 Image of the fetal head for the biparietal diameter measurement. Axial image at the level of the paired thalami (**arrows**) and the cavum septum pellucidum (**arrowhead**) is used for measurement of the biparietal diameter.

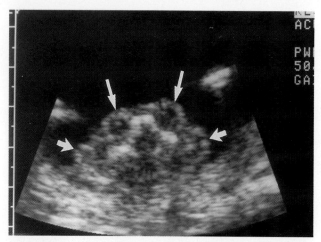

Figure 29–2 Anencephaly. Sonogram of fetal face with absence of forehead above the orbits (**arrows**). Dysplastic brain tissue is seen lateral to the face on each side (**arrowheads**).

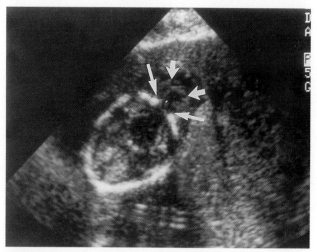

Figure 29–3 Encephalocele. Axial sonogram of fetal head demonstrating occipital defect (**arrows**) with brain tissue and meninges protruding outside the skull in the encephalocele (**arrowheads**).

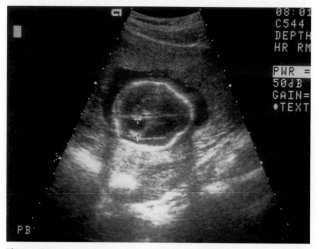

Figure 29–4 "Lemon" sign. Axial view of the fetal head in a fetus with a meningomyelocele demonstrating concavity of the frontal bones giving the head a lemon shape. There is associated hydrocephalus (**calipers**).

tained both to document that the head is present and assess the cranial contour. The normal fetal head is oval in shape with a smooth contour.

Anencephaly (**Fig. 29–2**) is a neural tube defect where the cranium and brain tissue are absent. The lower face is usually normally formed, but the forehead above the orbits and the cranium above the cervical spine are absent.

An encephalocele (**Fig. 29–3**) is a neural tube defect involving the cranium. These lesions are often identified on the biparietal diameter view. A defect in the skull is present, through which intracranial contents herniate outside the skull. Most encephaloceles are midline and posterior involving the occipital bone. Less common are frontal and parietal encephaloceles. Sonographically, the defect appears as an interruption in the calvarium with a sac containing soft tissue and sometimes fluid protruding outside the skull.

Flattening of the frontal bones in the second trimester, giving the appearance of a "lemon"-shaped head (**Fig. 29–4**) on the biparietal diameter view, is associated with meningomyeloceles. When this finding is present, the posterior fossa should be evaluated carefully for an Arnold-Chiari malformation, and the spine should be examined for spina bifida.[6]

Evaluation of intracranial contents should include assessment of the lateral ventricles, the choroid plexus, and the posterior fossa. The lateral ventricles are evaluated on axial view to assess both the size and shape of the ventricles. The width of the lateral ventricle is measured at the atrium of the lateral ventricle, perpendicular to the axis of the ventricle (**Fig. 29–5**), and should not exceed 10 mm. Excess cerebral spinal fluid in the head can be seen with dilatation of the lateral ventricles in such anomalies as hydrocephalus or the agenesis of the corpus callosum or with an abnormal configuration of the ventricles in anomalies such as holoprosencephaly or porencephaly.

Hydrocephalus is defined as dilatation of the lateral ventricles. It may be an isolated anomaly or it may result from in utero exposure to infection or a toxic agent, or it may be part of a syndrome or other complex congenital malformation. Hydrocephalus is commonly seen in association with meningomyeloceles and Dandy-Walker malformations. On ultrasound the diagnosis is made when the width of the lateral ventricle at the atrium measures more than 10 mm on axial view (**Fig. 29–6**),[7] and the choroid plexus appears to dangle away from its midline attachment.[8] If the lateral ventricles are dilated, then the third ventricle, located between the thalami on axial view, should be examined to look for dilatation. Aqueductal stenosis is a cause of hydrocephalus that leads to dilatation of the lateral and third ventricles with a normal fourth ventricle and posterior fossa.

An abnormal configuration of the cerebral ventricles is seen with holoprosencephaly (**Fig. 29–7**), an anomaly in which there is absence or incomplete cleavage of the prosencephalon. There is fusion of the lateral ventricles into a single ventricle that crosses the midline. The cerebral hemispheres are fused as well, and the falx is absent or rudimentary. This anomaly is often associated with abnormalities of the fetal face, including midline facial clefts, hypotelorism, a proboscis, or cyclops.[3]

The choroid plexus is examined for its position in the lateral ventricle and for cysts. This is best done on the same view used to assess the cerebral ventricles. A dangling choroid plexus, where the posterior end of the choroid plexus is abnormally separated from the medial wall of the lateral ventricle, is seen with hydrocephalus. Choroid plexus cysts (**Fig. 29–8**) may be seen in the second trimester and are associated with increased risk for chromosomal abnormalities, especially trisomy 18.[9] These cysts are round, anechoic, with thin, smooth walls. Sometimes in the early second trimester, the choroid plexus has a "spongy" appearance, containing lobular, hypoechoic areas. This is a normal finding that should not be confused with choroid plexus cysts.

Evaluation of the posterior fossa includes careful assessment of the cerebellum and the cisterna magna (**Fig. 29–9**). The normal cerebellum is made up of two rounded cerebellar hemispheres, separated by the echogenic vermis. The cisterna magna is a fluid space between the posterior aspect of the cerebellar vermis and the occipital bone. When a Dandy-Walker malformation is present, the vermis is hypoplastic or absent, replaced by a cystic space connecting the fourth ventricle with the cisterna magna (**Fig. 29–10**). In such cases, the cerebellar hemispheres often have an abnormal appearance, as well.[3]

Arnold-Chiari malformations are associated with meningomyeloceles and are characterized by a small posterior fossa with loss of the cisterna magna and compression of the cerebellum against the occiput. The cerebellum appears curved and flattened posteriorly against the occipital bone.[10, 11] In the second trimester, the ap-

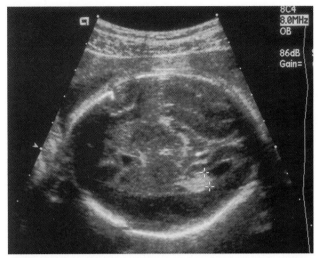

Figure 29–5   Lateral ventricular measurement. Axial view of the fetal head demonstrating measurement of a normal lateral ventricle. The measurement is taken at the level of the atrium of the lateral ventricle (**calipers**).

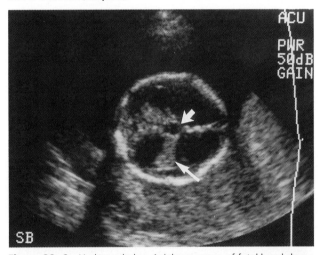

Figure 29–6   Hydrocephalus. Axial sonogram of fetal head showing dilated lateral ventricles with the choroid plexus dangling from the midline (**arrow**). The third ventricle is also dilated, seen as a cystic space in the midline between the lateral ventricles (**arrowhead**).

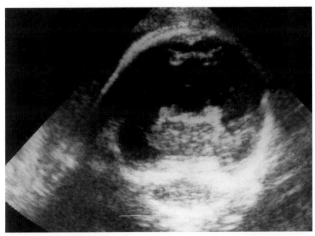

Fig-29–7   Holoprosencephaly. Vaginal sonogram of fetal head demonstrating a single cerebral ventricle between fused cerebral cortex and fused thalami.

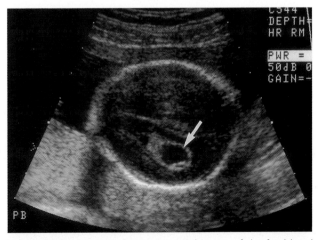

Figure 29–8   Choroid plexus cyst. Axial image of the fetal head demonstrating a cyst (**arrow**) in the choroid plexus.

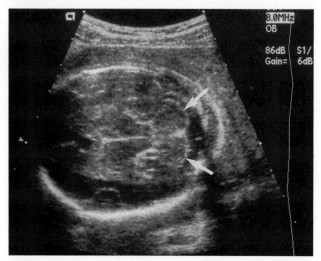

Figure 29–9 Normal posterior fossa. Angled axial view of the fetal head demonstrating a normal posterior fossa with the curved cerebellar hemispheres (**arrows**) separated by echogenic vermis and fluid in the cisterna magna posterior to the vermis.

pearance of the cerebellum has been termed the "*banana*" sign (**Fig. 29–11**). When an Arnold-Chiari malformation is identified at sonography, careful examination of the spine is warranted to locate the spina defect.

Examination of the fetal face is not listed in the published standards as a component of the fetal anatomic survey. However, when performing a thorough examination of the fetus, evaluation of the face will permit diagnosis of abnormalities, such as cleft lip or hypoplastic mandible, that would otherwise be missed. The two best views for examining the fetal face are a coronal view of the lower face demonstrating the nose and upper lip (**Fig. 29–12**), and a sagittal or profile view demonstrating the forehead, nose, lips, and chin (**Fig. 29–13**). Midline facial defects are associated with intracranial anomalies, such as holoprosencephaly. Lateral cleft lip and hypoplastic mandible are also often associated with other anomalies.

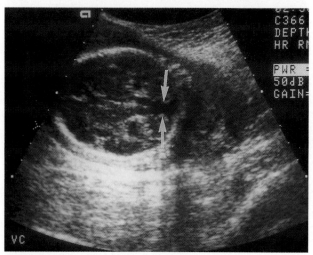

Figure 29–10 Dandy-Walker malformation. Image of posterior fossa demonstrating absence of the vermis between the cerebellar hemisphere, replaced by a cystic structure (**arrows**) connecting the fourth ventricle to the cisterna magna.

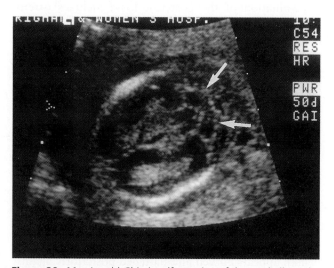

Figure 29–11 Arnold-Chiari malformation of the cerebellum, the "banana" sign. Sonogram of the posterior fossa showing small curved cerebellum (**arrows**) and no cisterna magna.

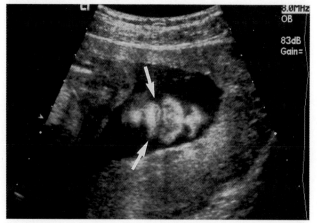

Figure 29–12 Fetal face. Coronal image of the lower face demonstrating the two nostrils and upper and lower lips (**arrows**).

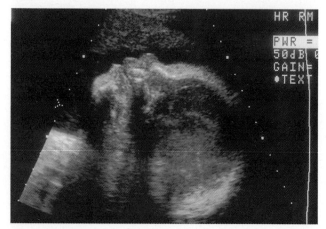

Figure 29–13 Fetal face in profile. Sagittal image of the fetal face demonstrating a normal profile of the forehead, nose, lips, and chin.

The Fetal Spine

Each vertebra of the fetal spine develops with three ossification centers, two posteriorly that form the pedicles and posterior elements and one anteriorly that forms the vertebral body. On transverse view, the three ossification centers form a C-shape, with the two posterior ossification centers toward each other (**Fig. 29–14**). On longitudinal view, the spine appears as parallel ossification centers that converge at the distal sacrum (**Fig. 29–15**). During an obstetrical ultrasound examination, the entire spine should be assessed both longitudinally and transversely.

Neural tube defects involving the spine are characterized by disruption and splaying of the posterior elements with protrusion of meninges and nerve tissue outside the spinal canal. These bony defects are visible sonographically as splaying of the posterior ossification centers. The protruding tissue forms a dorsal sac that extends posteriorly (**Fig. 29–16**). Meningomyeloceles are most commonly located in the lower lumbar spine and sacrum, but they also occur in the thoracic and cervical spine.

The Fetal Heart

The normal fetal heart is positioned in the thorax slightly to the left of midline with the apex pointing to the left (**Fig. 29–17**). Homogeneous lung tissue fills the rest of the thorax. When an intrathoracic mass is present, such as a diaphragmatic hernia or cystic adenomatoid malformation, the heart is displaced to the contralateral side (**Fig. 29–18**). Intrathoracic masses may arise from the lung, as with cystic adenomatoid malfor-

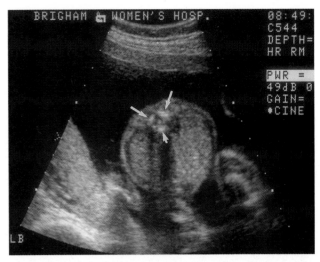

Figure 29–14   Fetal spine. Transverse view of the fetal spine demonstrating three ossification centers, two posterior (**arrows**) and one anterior (**arrowhead**), forming a C-shape or closed ring.

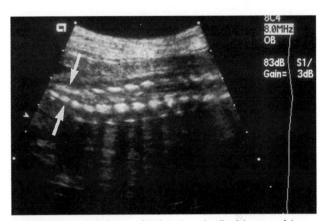

Figure 29–15   Lumbosacral spine. Longitudinal image of lower spine demonstrating converging posterior ossification centers in the lower sacrum (arrows)

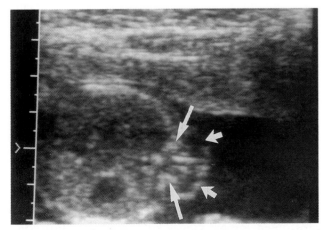

Figure 29–16   Meningomyelocele. Transverse sonogram of fetal spine demonstrating splaying of the posterior elements of the vertebral body (**arrows**) and a dorsal sac of the meningomyelocele (**arrowheads**).

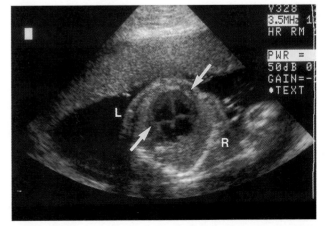

Figure 29–17   Fetal heart in the thorax. Transverse view of the fetal thorax demonstrating a normal heart (**arrows**) located in the left thorax, with the apex pointing to the left. R, right, L, left.

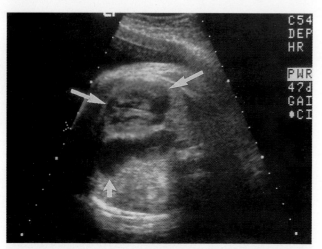

Figure 29–18   Left diaphragmatic hernia displacing heart to the right. Transverse sonogram of fetal thorax demonstrating heart (**arrows**) displaced to the right by fetal stomach (**arrowhead**) in left thorax.

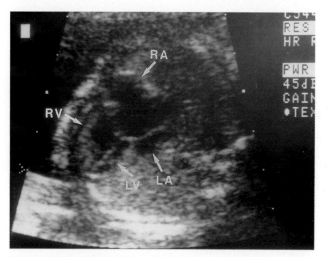

Figure 29–19   Hypoplastic left ventricle. Four-chamber view of abnormal heart with enlarged right atrium (RA, **arrow**) and right ventricle (RV, **arrow**) and small left atrium (LA, **arrow**) and left ventricle (LV, **arrow**).

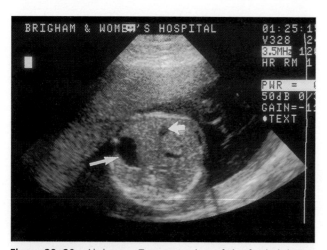

Figure 29–20   Abdomen. Transverse view of the fetal abdomen at the level of the stomach (**arrow**) and intrahepatic portion of the umbilical vein (**arrowhead**). This is the level used to measure the abdominal diameter or circumference.

mation and bronchial atresia, or they may arise in the mediastinum, as with a teratoma, or they may result from a diaphragmatic hernia.[12, 13] Secondary signs of an intrathoracic mass include polyhydramnios and hydrops.

The four-chamber view of the heart is obtained in an axial plane of the thorax. The right and left chambers should be symmetric. Asymmetry of the ventricles is usually a sign of a cardiac anomaly. Absence of one ventricle suggests hypoplastic left or right heart (**Fig. 29–19**). Enlargement of the right atrium suggests Ebstein's anomaly. Ventricular septal defects may also be diagnosed on the four-chamber view of the heart.[3, 14]

Anomalies of the great vessels can be detected if, in addition to the four-chamber view, images of the right and left ventricular outflow tracts are obtained. With these views, tetralogy of Fallot, truncus arteriosus, and transposition of the great vessels can be diagnosed.

The Fetal Abdomen

Four views of the fetal abdomen are included on the obstetrical ultrasound examination. These include images of the abdomen for measurement of the abdominal diameter or circumference, the kidneys, the bladder, and the anterior abdominal wall at umbilical cord insertion.

The image used to measure the fetal abdomen is a transverse view at the level of the fetal stomach and the umbilical vein in the liver (**Fig. 29–20**). The fetal stomach should be identified in the left upper quadrant in all normal fetuses by the beginning of the second trimester. Absence of the stomach is a sign of a fetal abnormality, the most common being esophageal atresia. Severe polyhydramnios is usually associated with this abnormality. In syndromes associated with situs inversus or situs ambiguous, the stomach may be seen in the midline or in the right upper quadrant.[15] A dilated stomach associated with a second round fluid collection in the upper abdomen is seen with duodenal obstruction from duodenal atresia or an annular pancreas (**Fig. 29–21**). As with esophageal atresia, polyhydramnios is usually severe in these cases.

If other dilated loops of bowel are present in the fetal abdomen, the diagnosis of a gastrointestinal obstruction is made. The obstruction may be at any level and result from a variety of causes, including atresia, volvulus, or meconium plug. Polyhydramnios is usually associated with the gastrointestinal obstruction.

The fetal kidneys can usually be seen in the renal fossas (**Fig. 29–22**), adjacent to the spine on each side, by the beginning of the second trimester. Failure to see one or both kidneys in their usual location should prompt a thorough examination of the fetal abdomen in search of an ectopic kidney, such as a pelvic kidney (**Fig. 29–23**) or cross-fused ectopic kidney or horseshoe kidney. Unilateral or bilateral renal agenesis may also occur. When the condition is bilateral, there is absence of renal function, leading to severe oligohydramnios and pulmonary hypoplasia. The prognosis is dismal.[16]

Dilatation of the fetal renal collecting system can occur due to obstruction at the ureteropelvic junction, distal ureter at the ureterovesical junction, or bladder outlet. Dilatation may also occur as a result of ureterovesical reflux. The diagnosis of hydronephrosis (**Fig. 29–24**) is made when there is intrarenal calyceal dilatation or when the renal pelvis measures in anteroposterior dimension at least 8 mm before 20 weeks and at least 10 mm after 20 weeks. When the measurement of the renal pelvis is 4—7 mm before 20 weeks or 5—9 mm after 20 weeks, hydronephrosis may be present, although the diagnosis is less certain. Dilatation of the ureters is seen when the obstruction is below the ureteropelvic junction or in cases of ureterovesical reflux.[16]

Severe urinary obstruction that occurs after about 10 weeks gestation or that is incomplete, such as with posterior urethral valves, causes renal dysplasia. The resulting kidneys appear small, with a thin, echogenic cortex (**Fig. 29–25**). Dilated calyces may remain visible in some cases. Complete urinary obstruction beginning early in the embryonic period causes a multicystic dysplastic kidney (**Fig. 29–26**). The kidney is replaced by multiple cysts of varying sizes that do not communicate with each other. The overall size of the kidney is larger than a normal kidney.[16]

Autosomal recessive polycystic kidney disease is an inherited disorder that leads to enlarged, echogenic kidneys with poor function and an absent urinary bladder (**Fig. 29–27**). In most cases, the prognosis is poor due to severe oligohydramnios.[16]

The fetal urinary bladder is usually visible sonographically by the end of the first trimester (**Fig. 29–28**). Absence of the bladder is seen when renal function is severely impaired or absent, such as with bilateral renal

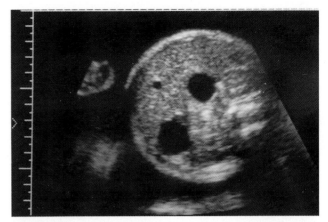

Figure 29–21 Duodenal atresia. Transverse sonogram of fetal abdomen demonstrating two fluid collections in the upper abdomen, the dilated stomach and duodenal bulb.

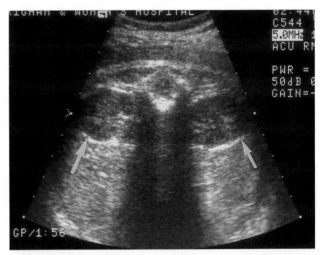

Figure 29–22 Kidneys. Transverse view of the posterior fetal abdomen at the level of the kidneys. The kidneys (**arrows**) are seen on either side of the spine, which casts an acoustic shadow.

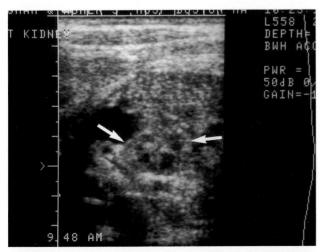

Figure 29–23 Pelvic kidney. Sonogram through the fetal pelvis demonstrating a pelvic kidney (**arrows**) adjacent to the fluid-filled bladder.

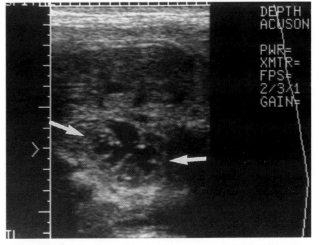

Figure 29–24 Hydronephrosis. Sonogram of fetal kidney (**arrows**) demonstrating calyceal dilatation and dilated renal pelvis.

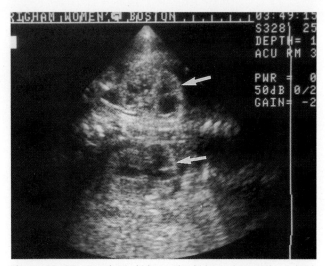

Figure 29–25   Dysplastic kidney. The kidneys (**arrows**) are both echogenic with thinned cortices and hydronephrosis, due to dysplasia from bladder outlet obstruction.

agenesis or autosomal recessive polycystic kidney disease. These conditions are associated with severe oligohydramnios. With posterior urethral valves, the bladder is very dilated and the dilated posterior urethra may be visible inferiorly (**Fig. 29–29**). Both kidneys show changes of long-standing obstruction, including hydronephrosis and renal dysplasia. Hydroureters are seen in the fetal abdomen.[16]

The normal fetal anterior abdominal wall is intact with the three vessels of the umbilical cord entering the abdomen at the umbilicus (**Fig. 29–30**). Omphaloceles (**Fig. 29–31**) are abdominal wall defects at the umbilicus through which abdominal contents, contained by a peritoneal membrane, herniate. Omphaloceles are commonly associated with other anomalies and with chromosomal abnormalities, and thus have a poor prognosis.[17] Gastroschisis (**Fig. 29–32**) is an abdominal wall defect that is paraumbilical. Herniated abdominal contents are not contained by a membrane, but are seen floating freely in the amniotic cavity. The prognosis is good, be-

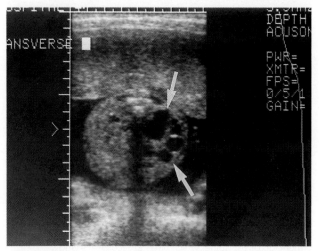

Figure 29–26   Multicystic dysplastic kidney. Transverse sonogram of fetal abdomen showing dysplastic kidney with multiple cysts (**arrows**) in the renal fossa.

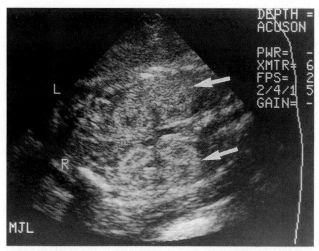

Figure 29–27   Autosomal recessive polycystic kidneys. Longitudinal sonogram of both fetal kidneys (**arrows**), which are enlarged and echogenic. The fetus is surrounded by severe oligohydramnios.

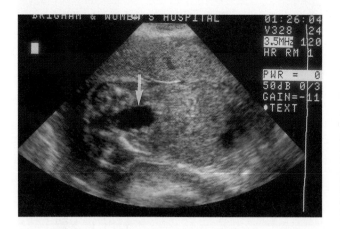

Figure 29–28   Bladder. Longitudinal view of the fetus demonstrating the fluid-filled bladder (**arrow**) in the pelvis.

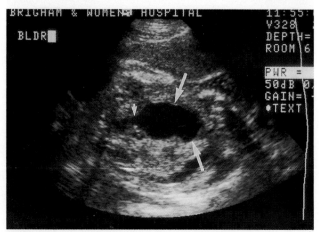

Figure 29–29   Posterior urethral valves. Sonogram of the pelvis of a fetus with posterior urethral valves. The bladder is dilated (**arrows**) and the dilated posterior urethra (**arrowhead**) is seen inferiorly.

cause this defect is not usually associated with other anomalies.[18]

Other Fetal Structures

Although other fetal anatomic structures, such as the extremities, are not listed specifically in the published standards, a thorough examination of the fetus should include scanning the fetus from head to toe. Partial evaluation of the fetal extremities is a standard part of the obstetrical sonogram, because the femur length is measured routinely to assess gestational age and growth of the long bones.[4,5] The other fetal extremities can be followed with real-time scanning to be certain they are present and normally formed. In particular, examination of the feet permits diagnosis of clubfoot when the bones of the feet lie in parallel with the bones of the lower leg (**Fig. 29–33**).

References

1. Moore KL, Persaud TVN. *The developing human*, 5th ed. Philadelphia: W.B. Saunders Co., 1993, p. 1–13.
2. Ewigman BG, Crane JP, Frigoletto RD, et al. Effect of prenatal ultrasound screening on perinatal outcome. *N Engl J Med* 1993;329:821—7.
3. Nyberg DA, Mahony BS, Pretorius DH. *Diagnostic ultrasound of fetal anomalies*. Chicago: Year Book Medical Publishers, Inc., 1990, p. 21—31.
4. ACR standard for antepartum obstetrical ultrasound. American College of Radiology Standards, 1995, p. 183—6.
5. Guidelines for performance of the antepartum obstetrical ultrasound examination. American Institute of Ultrasound in Medicine, 1994.
6. Nyberg DA, Mack LA, Hirsch J, Mahony BS. Abnormalities of fetal cranial contour in sonographic detection of spina bifida: evaluation of the "lemon" sign. *Radiology* 1988;167:387—392.
7. Cardoza JD, Goldstein RB, Filly RA. Exclusion of fetal ventriculomegaly with a single measurement: the width of lateral ventricular atrium. *Radiology* 1988;169:711—714.

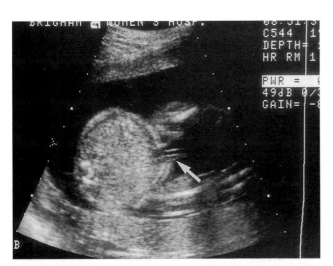

Figure 29–30 Normal umbilical cord insertion. Transverse view of the fetal abdomen at the umbilical cord insertion demonstrates the vessels of the umbilical cord (**arrow**) entering the abdomen.

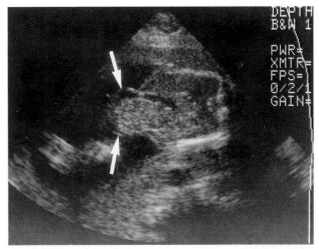

Figure 29–31 Omphalocele. Transverse sonogram of fetal abdomen at the level of the umbilical cord insertion, showing the omphalocele (**arrows**) extending anterior to the anterior abdominal wall.

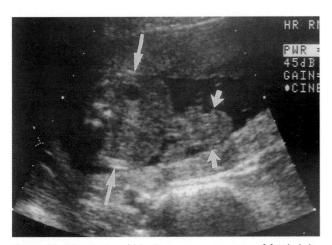

Figure 29–32 Gastroschisis. Transverse sonogram of fetal abdomen (**arrows**) demonstrating herniated loops of bowel freely floating in the amniotic cavity (**arrowheads**).

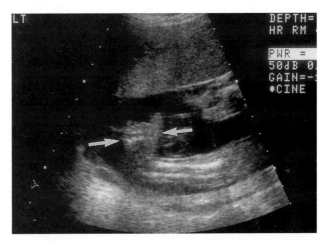

Figure 29–33 Clubfoot. Sonogram of the lower leg demonstrating the foot (**arrows**) turned such that the bones of the feet are in the same plane as the tibia and fibula in the lower leg.

8. Cardoza JD, Filly RA, Podrasky AE. The dangling choroid plexus: a sonographic observation of value in excluding ventriculomegaly. *AJR* 1988;151:767—770.

9. Nadel AS, Bromley BS, Frigoletto FD, Estroff JA, Benacerraf BR. Isolated choroid plexus cysts in the second-trimester fetus: is amniocentesis really indicated? *Radiology* 1992;185:545—548.

10. Benacerraf BR, Stryker J, Frigoletto FD. Abnormal US appearance of the cerebellum (banana sign): indirect sign of spina bifida. *Radiology* 1989;171:151—153.

11. Goldstein RB, Podrasky AE, Filly RA, Callen PW. Effacement of the fetal cisterna magna in association with myelomeningocele. *Radiology* 1989;172:409—413.

12. Bromley B, Parad R, Estroff JA, Benacerraf BR. Fetal lung masses: prenatal course and outcome. *J Ultrasound Med* 1995;14:927—936.

13. uibaud L, Filiatrault D, Garel L, et al. Fetal congenital diaphragmatic hernia: accuracy of sonography in diagnosis and prediction of the outcome after birth. *AJR* 1996;166:1195—1202.

14. Benacerraf BR, Pober BR, Sanders SP. Accuracy of fetal echocardiography. *Radiology* 1987;165:847—849.

15. Silverman NH, Schmidt KG. Ultrasound evaluation of the fetal heart. In: Callen PW, ed. *Ultrasonography in Obstetrics and Gynecology*, 3rd ed. Philadelphia: W.B. Saunders Company 1994; p. 291—332.

16. Benson CB, Doubilet PM. Fetal Genitourinary Anomalies. In: Fleischer AC, Manning FA, Jeanty P, Romero R, eds. *Sonography in Obstetrics and Gynecology, Principles and Practice*, 5th ed. Stamford: Appleton and Lange, 1996; p. 433—446.

17. Nyberg DA, Fitzsimmons J, Mack LA, et al. Chromosomal abnormalities in fetuses with omphalocele, significance of omphalocele contents. *J Ultrasound Med* 1989;8:299—308.

18. Langer JC, Khanna J, Caco C, Dykes EH, Nicolaides KH. Prenatal diagnosis of gastroschisis: development of objective sonographic criteria for predicting outcome. *Obstet Gynecol* 1993;81:53—56.

30 Family History of Congenital Heart Disease

Douglas L. Brown

Congenital heart disease (CHD) is estimated to occur in 0.4—0.8% of live births.[1,2] Because the majority of fetuses with CHD do not have a known risk factor,[3—5] it is important to evaluate the heart of every fetus who has a sonogram. However, there are maternal factors that increase the risk of CHD. These risk factors include metabolic disorders, teratogens, and a family history of CHD.[6] Diabetes mellitus and phenylketonuria are metabolic disorders that predispose to CHD. Teratogens that are associated with CHD include lithium, anticonvulsants (such as phenytoin, trimethadione, and valproic acid), ethanol, and retinoic acid.

While about 10—15% of CHD is considered to be due to chromosomal abnormalities (such as trisomy 21, 18, and 13, or Turner's syndrome), genetic syndromes (such as Noonan's or William's syndrome), or teratogens,[6] the cause of the majority of cases of CHD is not well understood and is believed to be multifactorial. When a previous child has CHD, the recurrence risk for most types of CHD in a subsequent pregnancy is estimated at about 2—4%,[1,7] representing a three to tenfold increase over the baseline population risk of CHD. If two siblings have had CHD, the risk is higher, estimated at 3–10%.[7] When cardiac anomalies are considered in terms of their developmental mechanism rather than by anatomy,[8] there seems to be a higher risk for lesions due to abnormal flow patterns, which includes hypoplastic left heart syndrome, coarctation of the aorta, aortic valve stenosis, pulmonary valve stenosis, and membranous ventricular septal defects.[1,2,9] However, when CHD does recur, it is not necessarily the same anatomic defect.[9] A full pregnancy history is important as a teratogen or maternal metabolic disease may be an etiologic factor in some cases, rather than having a true familial increased risk. A careful family history is also important as some families may have multiple individuals with CHD and an attendant higher risk of CHD.

The above risk estimates are based on a sibling having CHD. If a parent has CHD, the recurrence risk in the fetus seems to be higher, and estimated at 10—14%,[2,10] though not all studies have found this high a recurrence risk.[11] There is also some evidence that maternal CHD carries a higher risk of CHD in the fetus than paternal CHD,[11,12] but this also has not been confirmed in other studies.[10]

The association of cardiac anomalies with deletions in the long arm (q) of chromosome 22 has been increasingly recognized in the last several years. It is important to be aware of this particular association because other than trisomy 21, deletions in 22 q11 are believed to be the most important chromosomal cause of heart malformations.[13] The majority of patients with DiGeorge syndrome and velo-cardio-facial (Shprintzen) syndrome have deletions in chromosome 22 q11.[13] The clinical features of these two syndromes overlap, but the majority of patients with either syndrome have cardiac defects. While many types of CHD have been reported in patients with deletions in 22 q11, the most common cardiac defects associated with 22 q11 deletions include tetralogy of Fallot, pulmonary atresia, truncus arteriosus, and type B interrupted aortic arch.[14—16] Renal abnormalities, which may also be identified prenatally, have been reported in association with 22 q11 deletions.[16,17] About three-fourths of cases of 22 q11 deletions arise de novo, and the other one-fourth are inherited in an autosomal dominant manner.[13,16] An individual who has a 22 q11 deletion has a 50% risk of transmitting the deletion to his or her offspring.[13]

The pregnant patient with an increased risk for fetal cardiac anomalies such as a family history of congenital heart disease is understandably anxious. The parents level of anxiety will likely vary with their past experience. Parents whose child has had serious heart disease with numerous hospitalizations and surgery are likely to be more anxious than those whose child had a minor defect such as a small isolated ventricular septal defect. With a properly performed obstetric sonogram, one can identify the majority of fetuses with cardiac anomalies. In the following sections, we will discuss when and how to perform the sonographic exam, reasonable expectations of sonography for identifying CHD, and review the sonographic features of the more common structural cardiac anomalies.

Timing of the Ultrasound Exam of the Fetal Heart

At what gestational age should one examine the fetal heart by sonography? One wants to identify CHD as early as possible but also needs to perform the exam at a gestational age when the heart can be adequately evaluated. Not surprisingly, the ability to obtain the four-chamber (4 C) view in normal second-trimester fetuses increases with gestational age. In fetuses of 16—17 weeks gestational age, the 4 C view can be obtained in about 80% of normal fetuses, increasing to 95% or greater after 18 weeks.[17] Adequate views of the aortic and pulmonary outflow tracts can also be obtained in more than 95% of fetuses after 18 weeks.[18—20] While the fetal heart is most easily evaluated at about 20—24 weeks,[21] one generally wants to identify CHD somewhat earlier, if possible. In our practice, we try to evaluate the fetal heart, with 4 C and outflow tract views, in all fetuses starting at 16 weeks and can obtain these views in most 16- to 17-week fetuses. However, for the fetus with a known increased risk of CHD, 18 weeks gestational age seems a reasonable time to plan the sonogram as the 4 C and outflow tracts views can be obtained in the vast majority of fetuses at this age. There will be a small minority of patients at increased risk for fetal CHD who will need follow-up sonograms due to an inability to fully evaluate the heart for such technical reasons as maternal obesity or poor fetal position.

In some centers transvaginal sonography has been used to evaluate the fetal heart in the late first, or early second, trimester. The expertise to perform such exams is not widely available and this earlier examination is less reliable than the usual examination later in the second trimester.[22] The majority of anomalies diagnosed at this earlier gestational age are severe, complex anomalies.[22] With transvaginal sonography the 4 C and outflow tract views can be obtained in 70—100% of fetuses at 13—14 weeks gestational age.[22] Transvaginal sonography is limited by restricted angles of imaging, decreased penetration, and the small size of the fetal heart.[22] Additionally, some anomalies may not be evident until later in gestation.[22—24] Therefore, if one does obtain a normal transvaginal study of the fetal heart at 13—15 weeks, it should be followed by a more complete study later in the second trimester.

Expectations of Sonography for Identifying CHD

A wide range (4—96%) has been reported for the sensitivity of the 4 C view for identifying CHD.[5] While several factors may help explain the variable sensitivity in different studies, a large part of the variable sensitivity probably has to do with how well the heart is seen and what criteria are used to consider the 4 C view as normal. There is more to the 4 C view than just seeing four chambers. What constitutes an adequate 4 C view will be discussed in the next section. In the RADIUS study, the sensitivity for "complex" CHD using the 4 C view was 43%.[25] A reasonable estimate of the sensitivity of the 4 C view for CHD is probably around 50—60%, increasing to about 80—85% when the outflow tracts are also evaluated.[19, 26, 27] The variably reported sensitivity, however, should reinforce the notion that more consistent and complete sonographic examinations are needed to achieve optimal sensitivity.[5]

There are several cardiac anomalies which are particularly difficult to detect even with an optimal sonographic exam. These include patent ductus arteriosus (PDA), secundum atrial septal defect (ASD), small ventricular septal defect (VSD), mild degrees of aortic or pulmonary valve stenosis, total anomalous pulmonary venous return, and coarctation of the aorta. PDA and secundum ASD (the most frequent type of ASD) are rarely, if ever, diagnosed prenatally as the ductus arteriosus and foramen ovale are normally patent in the fetus. Small VSDs, mild degrees of aortic or pulmonary valve stenoses, total anomalous pulmonary venous return, and coarctation of the aorta are sometimes difficult to diagnose because the lesion is small or produces only minor changes in the appearance of the 4 C or outflow tract views. It is important for parents to be aware of these limitations of fetal cardiac sonography. Because ASDs and small VSDs are relatively common lesions, it is particularly important for parents who have a previous child with one of these lesions to understand the limitations of sonography.

Though the prenatal diagnosis of a specific cardiac lesion will not be always exactly correct, false-positive diagnoses of CHD are uncommon, that is, it is uncommon to diagnose fetal CHD and then the heart be normal postnatally. Small VSDs and coarctation of the aorta are probably the most frequent false-positive diagnoses and will be discussed subsequently.

General Aspects of the Ultrasound Exam of the Fetal Heart

The basic view for imaging the fetal heart is the four-chamber view, which is essentially a transverse view through the fetal thorax (**Fig. 30–1**). For the 4 C view to be considered normal, one should be able to determine that (1) the four chambers are normal in size, (2) the ventricular septum is intact, (3) the "crux" region of the heart is intact, and (4) the general appearance (i.e., size, position, and axis) of the heart is normal.[28—30] The two atria are generally of the same width, as are the two ventricles, though the right-sided chambers of the heart may be minimally larger than the left-sided chambers. The ventricular septum should be continuous, with no defect in it. The membranous portion of the ventricular septum is normally thin and, as will be discussed subsequently, may be difficult to image well. The "crux" of the heart refers to the area where the ventricular and atrial septa meet the atrioventricular valves.[28] At the crux, the septa should be intact, and the tricuspid valve should appear to attach to the septum just slightly more toward the apex of the heart than does the mitral valve. Overall assessment of the heart reveals that it normally occupies about one-third of the cross-sectional area of the thorax. The heart is basically midline but with cardiac apex to the left, and the ventricular septum is usually oriented at about a 45° angle to the midline sagittal plane.[31, 32] The normal range of cardiac axis is reported as 20—55 degrees in one study[31] and 22—75 degrees in another study.[32] While fetuses with CHD may have a normal cardiac axis, an abnormal cardiac axis is frequently associated with CHD.[31—33] Ideally, one should also determine if the abdominal situs (position of abdominal organs) is normal. The stomach of course should be on the left side of the fetus, and, particularly, if one suspects a situs abnormality, the inferior vena cava should be assessed for abnormal location or for interruption of its hepatic segment, which may occur with polysplenia or asplenia.

While imaging of the outflow tracts is not currently included in most standards for obstetric sonography, their evaluation does help identify abnormalities of the great arteries that are likely to be missed on the 4 C view

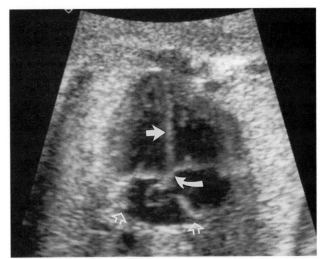

Figure 30–1   Four-chamber (4 C) view. The ventricles are approximately equal in size as are the atria in this normal 4 C view. The ventricular septum is intact (**arrow** is within left ventricle and points to ventricular septum). The crux region (**curved arrow** is within right atrium and points to crux where tricuspid valve is attached) is intact with the tricuspid valve slightly more toward the apex than the mitral valve at this level. Two of the pulmonary veins (**open arrows**) can be seen entering the left atrium.

alone.[20, 30] We find a long axis view most helpful for evaluating the left ventricular outflow tract (**Fig. 30–2**). It is attained by slight cranial angulation (with respect to the fetus) of the transducer from the 4 C view and slight rotation of the transducer (if the fetal spine is posterior, rotate the transducer clockwise on the maternal abdo-

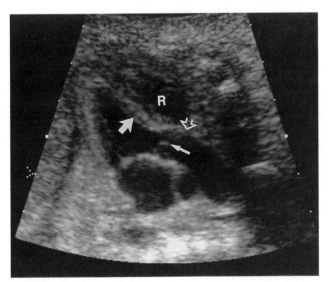

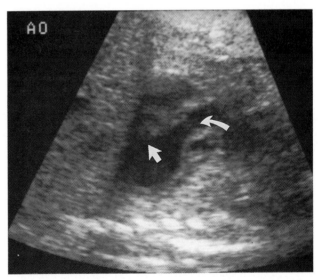

Figure 30–2   Left ventricular outflow tract views. (**A**) This view from a normal fetus demonstrates continuity of the ventricular septum (**solid arrow** within left ventricle and points to septum) and the wall of the aorta (**open arrow**). **Small arrow** in ascending aorta indicates aortic valve. A portion of the right ventricle (R) is seen on the other side of the ventricular septum. The view is used to assess for an overriding aorta and one may not recognize an overriding aorta if the view does not include at least a small portion of the right ventricle. Reprinted with permission from Problems and pitfalls in the sonographic diagnosis of fetal cardiac anomalies by DL Brown, LK Hornberger. **Ultrasound Q** 1995;13:221—227. (**B**) This view from a different fetus illustrates an inadequate left

ventricular outflow tract view. It may be tempting to accept a view like this as normal, but it is not adequate to exclude overriding of the aorta. While it does show the aorta (**curved arrow**) arising from the left ventricle, it does not adequately demonstrate continuity of the ventricular septum and aorta (**straight arrow** is within left ventricle and points to part of ventricular septum). Other views did show an overriding of the aorta in this fetus who had tetralogy of Fallot. One should be able to see a portion of the right ventricle (as in **A** above) on the other side of the ventricular septum before continuity of the ventricular septum and aorta can be adequately evaluated.

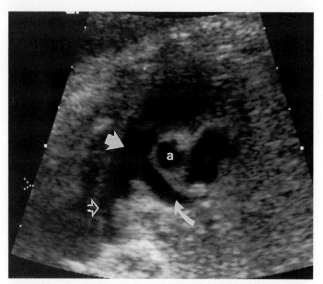

Figure 30–3 Right ventricular outflow tract view. The pulmonary artery appears to "wrap around" the aorta (a), seen in cross-section, in this normal fetus. The pulmonary artery (**solid arrows**) appears to bifurcate into the ductus arteriosus (**open arrow**) and the right pulmonary artery (**curved arrow**). The left pulmonary artery is not seen in this view. In the course of obtaining the two outflow tract views, one observes that the aorta and pulmonary artery criss-cross at right angles to one another as they exit the heart. This is shown indirectly in this view where one sees the aorta in cross-section and a longitudinal segment of the pulmonary artery. Reprinted with permission from Problems and pitfalls in the sonographic diagnosis of fetal cardiac anomalies by DL Brown, LK Hornberger. **Ultrasound Q** 1995;13:221—227.

Table 30–1 Summary of abnormalities to consider on each view

I. Four-chamber view
  A. Septal defect
    1. Ventricular septal defect
    2. Atrioventricular canal defect
  B. Left ventricle relatively smaller than right ventricle
    1. Hypoplastic left heart syndrome
    2. Coarctation
    3. Severe intrauterine growth restriction
    4. Total anomalous pulmonary venous return
  C. Right ventricle relatively smaller than left ventricle
    1. Pulmonary atresia/severe pulmonary stenosis
    2. Critical aortic stenosis
    3. Tricuspid atresia
  D. Enlarged right atrium
    1. Ebstein's anomaly
    2. Other tricuspid valve anomalies: dysplasia, absent leaflets, Uhl's anomaly
    3. Pulmonary atresia/severe pulmonary stenosis
  E. Mass within cardiac chamber
    1. Tumor
    2. Distinguish from echogenic foci, prominent moderator band

II. Outflow tract evaluation
  A. Overriding of the aorta
    1. Tetralogy of Fallot
    2. Truncus arteriosus
    3. Pulmonary atresia with VSD
  B. Absence of "criss-crossing" of aorta and pulmonary artery
    1. Complete transposition
    2. Double-outlet right ventricle
    3. Corrected transposition

men). More detailed discussion of how to obtain the outflow tract views is available elsewhere.[6] The key feature to note on this view is that the ventricular septum is continuous with the anterior wall of the aorta. The right ventricular outflow tract can be imaged with slightly more cranial angulation and rotation of the transducer in the opposite direction. This gives a short axis view which shows bifurcation of the main pulmonary artery (PA) into the right pulmonary artery and ductus arteriosus (**Fig. 30–3**). The left pulmonary artery is not seen in this plane. A key feature to note in obtaining the two outflow tract views is that the great arteries cross at right angles to each other as they exit the heart. The PA is usually slightly larger than the aorta.[34]

Color Doppler is sometimes helpful,[35–37] but is not generally needed for evaluation of the normal fetal heart.[35] Color Doppler is most helpful when an abnormality is suspected, particularly abnormalities of the great arteries or pulmonary veins and to assess for valvular regurgitation.

From the above discussion, there are six key features (four features on the 4 C view and two features on the two outflow tract views) that will allow one to decide if the fetal heart is normal or abnormal. The six features, posed as questions, are listed below. If all six questions can confidently be answered "yes," then the heart is very likely to be normal.

Regarding the 4 C view, the following is noteworthy:

1. Are 4 chambers present and symmetric in size?
2. Is the ventricular septum intact?
3. Is the crux region of the heart normal?
4. Is the size/position/axis of the heart in the chest normal?

On the 2 outflow tract views, the following is significant:

5. Is the wall of the aorta continuous with the ventricular septum?
6. Do the aorta and pulmonary artery criss-cross as they exit the heart?

In the following section we will consider the more common abnormalities of the fetal heart that one may identify, first on the 4 C view and then on the outflow tract views (**Table 30–1**). Possible abnormal findings that may be seen on each view will be reviewed and their differential diagnosis discussed. Further examples of abnormalities that can be seen on the 4 C view, outflow tract views, and also normal variants can be found in several sources.[20, 29, 30, 38—40]

The question is sometimes asked as to whether the pregnant patient with an increased risk of CHD should have a more detailed fetal echocardiogram performed by a pediatric cardiologist. This is perhaps a debatable issue and probably one without a clear, universal answer. The ability of obstetric sonographers and sonologists to evaluate the fetal heart varies considerably, and different approaches to evaluate the fetal heart are probably reasonable in different locales. The wide range of reported sensitivities of prenatal sonography for CHD suggests that to achieve high sensitivity, one should evaluate the heart in a careful and consistent manner. If the sonographer and sonologist performing the obstetric sonogram are adequately trained and capable of evaluating the heart as discussed in this chapter, it is unlikely that major CHD will be missed. If one is not comfortable evaluating the heart in such a manner, then the exam should be performed by someone who is, which in some locales may be the pediatric cardiologist. In our practice, we value the expertise of our pediatric cardiologists, who have experience in fetal cardiology, and we send patients to them for a more detailed study if we identify a cardiac anomaly or if we encounter an uncertain finding in the fetal heart. We feel that in such cases, it is important for the fetus to have a more detailed sonographic evaluation so that the most accurate diagnosis can be made. The patient can then receive appropriate counseling from the cardiologist about the prognosis.

The Four-Chamber View: Abnormal Findings

Defects in the Septum

A *ventricular septal defect* (VSD) is identified as a gap in the ventricular septum (**Fig. 30–4**). It is often seen on the 4 C view, but as a single 4 C image only evaluates part of the septum, one needs to sweep through the en-

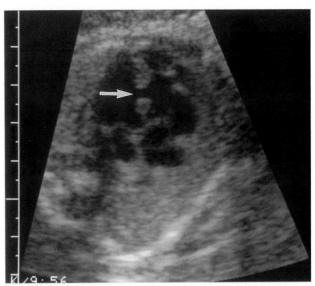

Figure 30–4   Ventricular septal defect. The 4 C view shows a distinct defect (**arrow**) in the muscular portion of the ventricular septum. Defects in this portion of the septum tend to be easier to recognize than those in the membranous septum, closer to the atrioventricular valves. Reprinted with permission from Problems and pitfalls in the sonographic diagnosis of fetal cardiac anomalies by DL Brown, LK Hornberger. **Ultrasound Q**   1995;13:221—227.

tire septum. A VSD can be both over- and under-diagnosed. A potential pitfall can occur with an apical 4 C view (where the sound beam is parallel to the septum); there may appear to be a defect in the membranous septum (**Fig. 30–5**). This is probably due to the limitations of lateral resolution and the relative thinness of the membranous portion of the septum. This artifact can

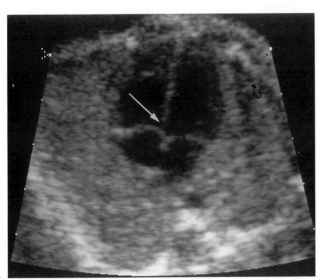

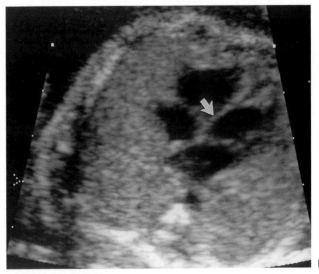

A   B

Figure 30–5   Pseudo-ventricular septal defect. (**A**) In this apical 4 C view (referred to as apical because cardiac apex points toward the transducer), the ventricular septum is essentially parallel to the ultrasound beam. In such a view, one may question if there is a small defect in the thin, membranous portion of the ventricular septum (**arrow**). This can be a difficult area in which to diagnoses small VSDs and both false-positive and false-negative sonographic diagnoses are possible. One should, however, be cautious about diagnosing an isolated VSD in this location, based just on one view such as this. (**B**) The most helpful feature before diagnosing such a small VSD is that one should be able to also see the VSD in a view where the ultrasound beam is more perpendicular to the septum. Further imaging in this patient, with such a view, showed an intact ventricular septum (**arrow**). Reprinted with permission from Problems and pitfalls in the sonographic diagnosis of fetal cardiac anomalies by DL Brown, LK Hornberger. **Ultrasound Q**   1995;13:221—227.

usually be recognized by its characteristic location, by a gradual fading of the septum as opposed to a more abrupt termination of the septum with a true VSD and (probably most importantly) by the absence of a defect when imaging more perpendicular to the septum.[28, 38]

While a VSD is the most frequent cardiac anomaly seen postnatally, it seems to be a difficult lesion to diagnose prenatally. The sensitivity of prenatal ultrasound for VSDs has been reported from 0—71% with most of these studies reporting well under 50% sensitivity.[19, 25, 41-46] Small isolated VSDs are most likely to escape detection. Such small isolated VSDs may not be important clinically as it has been reported that 74% of isolated VSDs in the fetus will close spontaneously, sometimes before birth.[47] One should look carefully for other cardiac anomalies as a VSD may just be one component of a more complex lesion.

Atrioventricular canal defect (AVCD) is identified as a defect in the lower portion of the atrial septum and upper portion of the ventricular septum and is an important reason to evaluate the "crux" of the heart (**Fig. 30–6**). The normal differential insertion of the atrioventricular (AV) valves is lost and a common AV valve may be present. AVCD is associated with Down's syndrome and also with polysplenia and asplenia. About 30—40% of patients with AVCD will have trisomy 21. Complete heart block may be present due to distortion of the conduction tissue. Heart block or atrioventricular valve regurgitation may lead to congestive heart failure and hydrops. One should be aware that the entrance of the coronary sinus into the right atrium can simulate a defect in the lower atrial septum, which might raise concern for an ostium primum atrial septal defect that may be a component of AVCD.[48]

Left Ventricle Smaller than Right Ventricle

We will consider ventricular size discrepancy in relative, rather than absolute, terms. The ventricles are normally the same size or the right ventricle may be slightly larger than the left ventricle. Care must be taken not to oblique the plane of imaging, thus falsely producing an image of one ventricle being small. When the left ventricle is very small, hypoplastic left heart syndrome (HLHS) is the most likely lesion. When the left ventricle is only slightly small, coarctation of the aorta is the main lesion to consider but the differential diagnosis also includes total anomalous pulmonary venous return, changes secondary to intrauterine growth restriction (IUGR), and some forms of pulmonary atresia.

In *HLHS*, the left ventricle is usually severely underdeveloped (**Fig. 30–7**) but there is a spectrum of severity. Typically, the mitral valve is hypoplastic while the aortic valve is an imperforate membrane. The ascending aorta and arch are usually very small. In utero there may be no hemodynamic consequence as the right ventricle supplies both the pulmonary and systemic circulations. The ascending aorta fills retrograde via the ductus arteriosus.[49]

Coarctation of the aorta produces a less marked decrease in LV size than does HLHS (**Fig. 30–8**). It is unlikely to cause significant hemodynamic disturbance in the fetus. The sonographic diagnosis is challenging but should be suspected when the left ventricle is relatively smaller than the right ventricle.[50-54] The sensitivity of prenatal sonography for coarctation remains only moderate however, around 50—62%.[46, 54] A relatively small left ventricle (LV) is usually first detected with subjective evaluation. Norms for ventricular size can be used for more objective evaluation.[55-59] However, not all fetuses

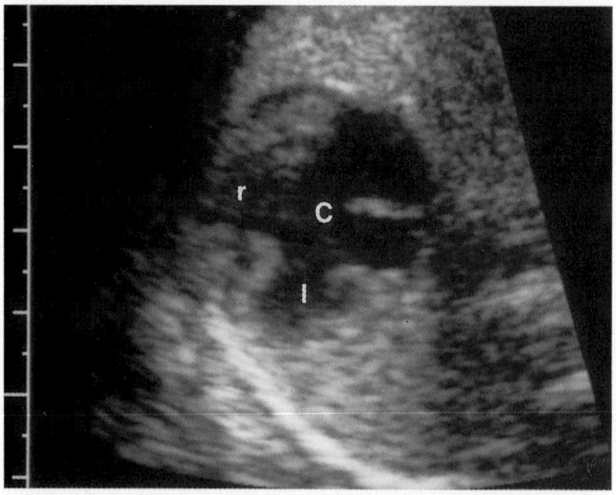

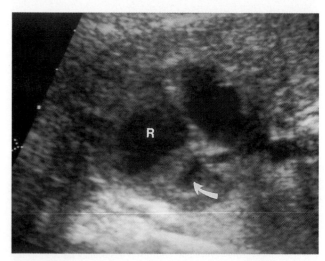

Figure 30–6 Atrioventricular canal defect. This 4 C view shows the characteristic defect at the crux (c) of the heart. The defect includes the upper portion of the ventricular septum and lower portion of atrial septum. (r, right ventricle and l, left ventricle).

Figure 30–7 Hypoplastic left heart syndrome (HLHS). The left ventricle (**curved arrow**) is very small relative to the right ventricle (R). In some cases of HLHS, the left ventricle is even smaller than this and may be difficult to identify. Other views in this fetus demonstrated a very small aorta.

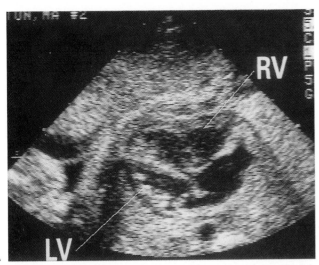

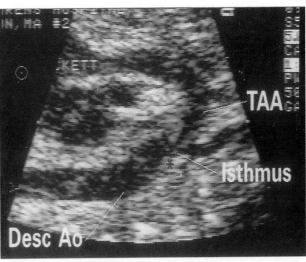

Figure 30–8   Coarctation of the aorta. (**A**) In this 4 C view, the left ventricle (LV) is slightly smaller than the right ventricle (RV). Such ventricular size discrepancy is an indirect finding that may be seen with coarctation, but can be problematic as some fetuses with mild discrepancy will have a normal heart. When we identify such a finding, we generally refer patients to our pediatric cardiology colleagues for more detailed assessment, particularly of the aortic arch. (**B**) An image of the aortic arch in this same fetus revealed a small transverse aortic arch (TAA) and isthmus, which is supportive evidence of a coarctation. (Desc Ao, descending aorta). Reprinted with permission from Problems and pitfalls in the sonographic diagnosis of fetal cardiac anomalies by DL Brown, LK Hornberger. **Ultrasound Q**   1995;13:221—227.

with a slightly small left ventricle will have coarctation and some will be normal at birth. The right ventricle (RV) normally becomes larger, relative to the left ventricle (LV), with increasing gestational age. Thus, the LV:RV ratio (ratio of left ventricular to right ventricular width) decreases with increasing gestational age and at term the mean LV:RV ratio is 0.78.[56] False-positive diagnoses of coarctation, based on ventricular disproportion, are more likely in the third trimester.[53, 54] Accurate prenatal diagnosis remains difficult in many cases. Evaluation of the size of the aortic arch (typically small with coarctation) may help improve the accuracy of prenatal diagnosis.[60, 61] The actual narrowing in the aortic arch is often difficult to image directly, and conversely, slight narrowing in the isthmus of the aorta can be seen in some normal fetuses.

Some fetuses with severe *intrauterine growth restriction* (IUGR) may have ventricular disproportion due to an enlarged right ventricle.[62, 63] This is postulated to be secondary to the increased placental vascular resistance which the right ventricle pumps against and/or to myocardial dysfunction related to hypoxemia.[62]

Total anomalous pulmonary venous return (TAPVR) may produce a slightly small left ventricle compared to the right ventricle.[28] One should suspect TAPVR if no pulmonary veins are seen to enter the left atrium, if there is a common pulmonary venous chamber posterior to the left atrium, and/or if the anomalous draining vein is seen. Though TAPVR is uncommon, it remains one of the more frequently missed cardiac anomalies by prenatal sonography.

Fetuses with *pulmonary atresia* can have variable right ventricular size. While the RV may be large, and thus be considered in this differential diagnosis, it more frequently is small and will be discussed in the next section.

Right Ventricle Smaller than Left Ventricle

Pulmonary atresia is considered in this section, although the RV can be either small, normal, or slightly large.[64] This variability may be related to two types of pulmonary atresia.[65] *Pulmonary atresia with an intact ventricular septum (PA-IVS)* may be an "acquired" congenital lesion. The valve typically has minimal to no abnormality. The pulmonary artery is often large and the right ventricle, while variable in size, is usually small (**Fig. 30–9**). *Pulmonary atresia with a VSD (PA-VSD)* is probably a severe form of tetralogy of Fallot. The valve is usually abnormally formed and the pulmonary artery is usually small. The right ventricle is usually normal in size.

Right atrial enlargement may be present, due to tricuspid regurgitation, and can be so severe that pulmonary hypoplasia results. Pulmonary atresia and severe pulmonic valvular stenosis may appear similar prenatally, and one may not be able to distinguish them unless antegrade flow through the pulmonic valve is detected by Doppler ultrasound (thereby excluding pulmonary atresia).[66] Obstructive lesions of the pulmonary (or aortic) valve may evolve in utero, sometimes progressing from valve stenosis to atresia (at least functional atresia).

Critical aortic stenosis generally causes an enlarged, poorly contractile left ventricle (**Fig. 30–10**). The endocardium may be very echogenic due to associated endocardial fibroelastosis. The aortic valve is often small. The left atrium may be enlarged due to mitral regurgitation. This lesion can progress in utero to what appears to be HLHS at birth.

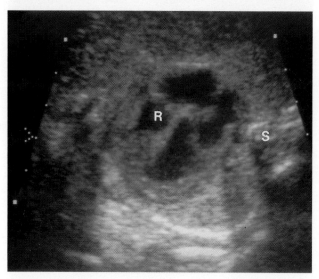

Figure 30–9 Pulmonary atresia, with intact ventricular septum. In this 4 C view, the right ventricle (R) has a small chamber size and a slightly thick wall. Other views demonstrated a relatively normal sized pulmonary artery and more detailed assessment showed no flow through the pulmonary valve. Severe pulmonary stenosis may have a similar appearance prenatally. This view also shows an abnormal cardiac axis. The ventricular septum is oriented at nearly 90 degrees to the midline sagittal plane (S, spine).

Tricuspid atresia is an uncommon lesion in which the RV may be small. The tricuspid valve is absent and one may see a thick band of tissue in its expected location. Doppler helps confirm absence of flow from the right atrium to right ventricle. Transposition of the great arteries coexists in some cases.

Enlarged Right Atrium

Abnormalities of both the pulmonic valve and tricuspid valve need to be considered when the right atrium is enlarged. Pulmonary atresia/severe stenosis has been discussed previously. We will mainly consider tricuspid valve abnormalities in this section.

Ebstein's anomaly is due to downward displacement, to varying degrees, of the septal and posterior leaflets of the tricuspid valve. The valve may also be dysplastic. The tricuspid valve is usually insufficient, leading to further right atrial enlargement. Ultrasound demonstrates variable degrees of downward displacement of the tricuspid valve into the right ventricle and variable degrees of right atrial enlargement[67–69] (**Fig. 30–11**). The resulting right ventricular cavity may be small, as may the pulmonary artery. There is a wide spectrum of clinical severity of Ebstein's anomaly. Other cardiac anomalies, such as pulmonary atresia/stenosis or transposition anomalies may coexist with Ebstein's anomaly. Ebstein's anomaly has been associated with maternal lithium use.

Ebstein's anomaly is part of a spectrum of malformations that has variable degrees of dysplasia of the tricuspid valve and/or right ventricle.[70] Any of the anoma-

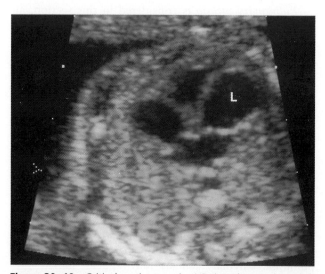

Figure 30–10 Critical aortic stenosis. 4 C view shows a large left ventricle (L) in this 21-week fetus. At real-time scanning, there was poor contractility of the left ventricle. Serial scans during pregnancy revealed no growth of the left ventricle, and, at term, the left ventricle was relatively small with an appearance suggesting hypoplastic left heart syndrome. Reprinted with permission from Problems and pitfalls in the sonographic diagnosis of fetal cardiac anomalies by DL Brown, LK Hornberger. **Ultrasound Q** 1995;13:221—227.

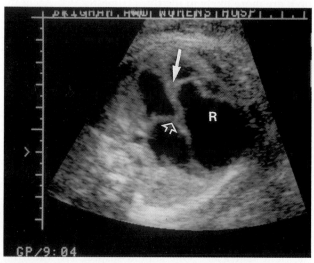

Figure 30–11 Ebstein's anomaly. In this 4 C view, the right atrium (R) is enlarged and part of the tricuspid valve inserts lower on the ventricular septum than normal (**solid arrow**). While the tricuspid valve attachment to the ventricular septum is normally slightly more toward the cardiac apex than is the mitral valve attachment (**open arrow**), the difference in insertion levels in this fetus is much more than normal.

lies in this spectrum may cause a large RA. Also in this spectrum is *dysplasia of the tricuspid valve*, where the valve is abnormally thickened but normally attached.[67–69] Other rare anomalies in this spectrum of malformations are Uhl's anomaly and congenital absence of tricuspid valve leaflets.

Masses within the Cardiac Chambers

Cardiac tumors are the primary consideration here. One should be aware that the apex of the RV is normally blunted, due to the moderator band, and should not be mistaken for a mass.

Rhabdomyomas are the most common type of fetal cardiac tumor.[71] Tuberous sclerosis is frequently present when a cardiac tumor is seen, although the diagnosis of tuberous sclerosis may not be made for several months, or sometimes years, after birth. Aside from this association, cardiac tumors are generally isolated anomalies. Size and location of tumors vary considerably. While most are benign, they should be followed during pregnancy as congestive heart failure may occur if the tumor is positioned such that there is obstruction of blood flow. Arrhythmias have been reported, most frequently supraventricular tachycardia,[28] but also bradycardia,[72] and can also cause congestive failure. Sonographically, one observes a hyperechoic mass within the heart (**Fig. 30–12**).

Most tumors can be distinguished from the more frequent echogenic foci within the ventricles by assessment of their echogenicity and size. The echogenic foci are generally due to papillary muscle mineralization[73] and are more brightly echogenic than tumors. These echogenic foci are small (generally less than 3 mm), whereas tumors are more variable, and often larger, in size. There does seem to be a slightly increased frequency of these echogenic foci in fetuses with trisomy 21 and trisomy 13.[74–77] The clinical significance of a ventricular echogenic focus, as an isolated finding, remains controversial.

Outflow Tract Views: Abnormal Findings

The most important points to note when evaluating the great arteries are that there normally is continuity between the ventricular septum and the anterior wall of the aorta and that the great arteries cross at right angles to each other as they initially exit the heart. The aorta crosses from left to right and the pulmonary artery from right to left. Demonstration of these two normal relationships helps exclude abnormalities of the great arteries such as tetralogy of Fallot, truncus arteriosus, and transposition anomalies.

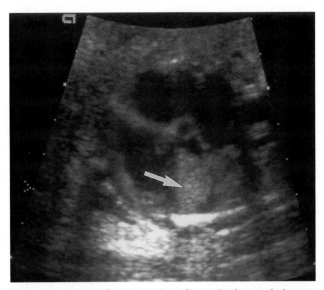

Figure 30–12 Cardiac tumor. A moderate size hyperechoic mass (**arrow**) fills much of the left ventricle in this 4 C view. Additional cardiac tumors were also seen in this fetus; however, the pregnancy progressed uneventfully, and no hydrops or arrhythmias occurred.

Overriding Aorta

While the aorta normally courses over the plane of the ventricular septum as it leaves the heart, the septum is intact. With an overriding aorta, one observes a VSD and the aorta displaced toward the right side. This disrupts the normal continuity of the ventricular septum and the wall of the aorta. It is possible, however, to falsely produce an image of aortic overriding. The origin of this artifact is uncertain, though it may be due to partial volume artifact of the more superior pulmonary artery or of a sinus of Valsalva. If overriding is seen, then it needs to be confirmed with slightly different angulation of the transducer.[38] At least in some cases of pseudo-overriding, close observation of the site of apparent discontinuity will show that it is actually distal to the aortic valve, whereas with true overriding, the discontinuity is proximal to the aortic valve.

Tetralogy of Fallot (TOF) is the primary diagnosis to consider when overriding of the aorta is seen (**Fig. 30–13**). The VSD and overriding of the aorta are the two features that generally suggest the diagnosis prenatally. The pulmonary artery may be small, but infundibular pulmonary stenosis may not be apparent, particularly early in pregnancy.[28] Right ventricular hypertrophy is not typically seen in the fetus.[78] If the pulmonary valve is absent, there is usually dilatation of the pulmonary artery and its more peripheral branches.

When one observes an overriding aorta, the pulmonary artery is a key structure to evaluate[28] to help distinguish TOF from other lesions that may have apparent overriding of the aorta. In TOF the pulmonary artery arises normally from the right ventricle. *Truncus arteriosus*, while a less common lesion, is the likely diagnosis if

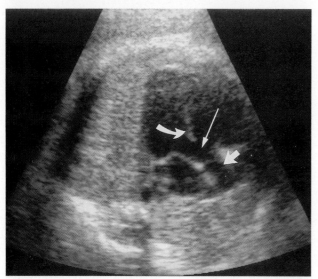

Figure 30–13 Tetralogy of Fallot. Left ventricular outflow tract views shows a ventricular septal defect (**thin arrow** is within right ventricle and points to the septal defect) and overriding of the aorta. The overriding appears as a lack of continuity between the ventricular septum (**curved arrow** is in left ventricle and points to septum) and wall of the aorta (**thick straight arrow**). The aorta is shifted toward the right ventricle and appears to "straddle" the ventricular septum. Additional views showed the pulmonary artery arising normally from the right ventricle, helping to confirm tetralogy of Fallot. If the pulmonary artery had not been found arising from the right ventricle, then truncus arteriosus or pulmonary atresia with ventricular septal defect would have been possible.

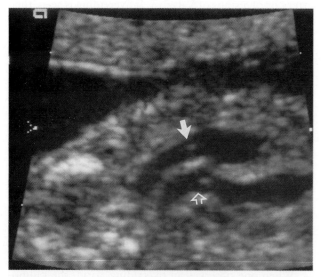

Figure 30–14 Transposition of the great arteries. A normal right and left ventricular outflow tract view could not be obtained in this fetus. Instead, the aorta (**solid arrow**) and the pulmonary artery (**open arrow**) are in a parallel orientation as they exit the heart. Additional views confirmed which great artery was the aorta by demonstrating the head and neck arteries arising from it. (Image courtesy of P. Doubilet, M.D., Ph.D; Boston, MA.)

the pulmonary artery (or arteries) arises from the aorta. The pulmonary artery may arise as a single vessel from the truncus arteriosus or the right and left pulmonary arteries may arise separately from the truncus arteriosus. If the pulmonary artery is not present or is very small, *pulmonary atresia with a VSD* (probably a severe form of TOF) should be considered.

Parallel Aorta and Pulmonary Artery

The normal "criss-crossing" of these two arteries occurs in their initial course, as they exit the heart. Slightly more distally in their course (e.g., near the aortic arch level) one normally observes a segment of parallel orientation of the aorta and pulmonary artery/ductus arteriosus. When the great arteries exit the ventricles in parallel, some type of transposition abnormality is probably present.

In *complete transposition* of the great arteries, the aorta arises from the right ventricle and the PA from the left ventricle. Usually there is no hemodynamic consequence in utero although if pulmonary stenosis is present, congestive heart failure can occur. Sonographically one observes parallel orientation of the aorta and the PA as they exit the heart (**Fig. 30–14**). The aorta can be correctly identified by noting the head and neck arteries originating from it.

Double-outlet right ventricle (DORV) is a type of transposition abnormality. It occurs when the pulmonary artery and most of the aorta arise from the right ventricle. As in complete transposition, the normal criss-crossing of the aorta and PA is lost, but one observes both great arteries arising predominantly from the right ventricle. A VSD is usually also present. Accurate diagnosis may be difficult at times, as the abnormality may appear similar to either complete transposition of the great arteries or tetralogy of Fallot. DOVR may coexist with other anomalies such as HLHS.

Corrected transposition is an uncommon anomaly but may also produce an initial parallel course of the great arteries. The blunted appearance of the apex, due to the moderator band, may help one identify the morphologic right ventricle which is now the more posterior ventricle and gives rise to the aorta. The morphologic left ventricle, with its pointed apex, is now the more anterior ventricle and gives rise to the pulmonary artery. This anomaly is frequently associated with situs abnormalities.[79] Other lesions such as pulmonic stenosis or a VSD may be present. Atrioventricular block may occur due to distortion of the conducting tissue.

Summary — Structural Abnormalities

While evaluation of the 4 C view is included in most guidelines for obstetric sonography, further evaluation of both outflow tracts will improve the sensitivity of obstetric ultrasound for CHD. If the sonographer and sonologist can adequately evaluate the six key features discussed above, four on the 4 C view and two on the outflow tract views, then the majority of congenital heart anomalies can be diagnosed before birth, both in patients at higher risk for CHD and those at lower risk.

References

1. Ardinger RH. Genetic counseling in congenital heart disease. *Ped Annals* 1997;26:99—104.
2. Boughman JA, Berg IA, Astemborski JA, et al. Familial risks of congenital heart defect assessed in a population-based epidemiologic study. *Am J Med Genetics* 1987;26:839—849.
3. Cooper MJ, Enderlein ME, Dyson DC, Roge CL, Tarnoff H. Fetal echocardiography: retrospective review of clinical experience and an evaluation of indications. *Obstet Gynecol* 1995;86:577—582.
4. Allan L. Fetal cardiology (Editorial). *Ultrasound Obstet Gynecol* 1994;4:441—444.
5. Spevak PJ. New developments in fetal echocardiography. *Current Opinion Cardiol* 1997;12:78—83.
6. Abuhamad A. *A Practical Guide to Fetal Echocardiography.* Philadelphia: Lippincott-Raven Publishers, 1997, p. 1—6;41.
7. Nora JJ, Nora AH. Update on counseling the family with a first-degree relative with a congenital heart defect. *Am J Med Genetics* 1988;29:137—142.
8. Clark EB. Pathogenetic mechanisms of congenital cardiovascular malformations revisited. *Semin Perinatol* 1996;20:465—472.
9. Thompson MW, McInnes RR, Willard HF. *Genetics in Medicine*, (5 th ed.) Philadelphia: W.B. Saunders Company, 1991, p. 351—358.
10. Whittemore R, Wells JA, Castellsague X. A second-generation study of 427 probands with congenital heart defects and their 837 children. *J Am Coll Cardiol* 1994;23:1459—1467.
11. Burn J, Brennan P, Little J, et al. Recurrence risks in offspring of adults with major heart defects: results from first cohort of British collaborative study. *Lancet* 1998;351:311—316.
12. Nora JJ, Nora AH. Maternal transmission of congenital heart diseases: new recurrence risk figures and question of cytoplasmic inheritance and vulnerability to teratogens. *Am J Cardiol* 1987;59:459—463.
13. Thomas JA, GrahAm JM. Chromosome 22 q11 deletion syndrome: an update and review for the primary pediatrician. *Clin Pediatrics* 1997;36:253—266.
14. Strauss AW, Johnson MC. The genetic basis of pediatric cardiovascular disease. *Semin Perinatol* 1996;20:564—576.
15. Johnson MC, Hing A, Wood MK, Watson MS. Chromosome abnormalities in congenital heart disease. *J Med Genet* 1997;70:292—298.
16. Ryan AK, Goodship JA, Wilson DI, et al. Spectrum of clinical features associated with interstitial chromosome 22 q11 deletions: a European collaborative study. *J Med Genet* 1997;34:798—804.
17. Shultz SM, Pretorious DH, Budorick NE. Four-chamber view of the fetal heart: demonstration related to menstrual age. *J Ultrasound Med* 1994;13:285—289.
18. DeVore GR. The aortic and pulmonary outflow tract screening examination in the human fetus. *J Ultrasound Med* 1992;11:345—348.
19. Bromley B, Estroff JA, Sanders SP, et al. Fetal echocardiography: accuracy and limitations in a population at high and low risk for heart defects. *Am J Obstet Gynecol* 1992;166:1473—1481.
20. Benacerraf BR. Sonographic detection of fetal anomalies of the aortic and pulmonary arteries: value of four-chamber view vs direct images. *AJR* 1994;163:1483—1489.
21. Jeanty P. A practical approach to the ultrasound investigation of the fetal heart. In: Wladimiroff JW, Pilu G, ed. *Ultrasound and the Fetal Heart.* New York: The Parthenon Publishing Group, 1996, p. 15—32.
22. Gembruch U, Baschat AA, Knopfle G, Hansmann M. First- and early second-trimester diagnosis of fetal cardiac anomalies. In: Wladimiroff JW, Pilu G, ed. *Ultrasound and the Fetal Heart.* New York: The Parthenon Publishing Group, 1996, p. 39—46.
23. Hornberger LK, Sanders SP, Sahn DJ, et al. In utero pulmonary artery and aortic growth and potential for progression of pulmonary outflow tract obstruction in tetralogy of Fallot. *J Am Coll Cardiol* 1995;25:739—745.
24. Hornberger LK, Sanders SP, Rein AJJT, et al. Left heart obstructive lesions and left ventricular growth in the midtrimester fetus: a longitudinal study. *Circulation* 1995;92:1531—1538.
25. Crane JP, LeFevre ML, Winborn RC, et al. A randomized trial of prenatal ultrasonographic screening: impact on the detection, management, and outcome of anomalous fetuses. *Am J Obstet Gynecol* 1994;171:392—399.
26. Kirk JS, Riggs TW, Comstock CH, Lee W, Yang SS, Weinhouse E. Prenatal screening for cardiac anomalies: the value of routine addition of the aortic root to the four-chamber view. *Obstet Gynecol* 1994;84:427—431.
27. Achiron R, Glaser J, Gelernter I, Hegesh J, Yagel S. Extended fetal echocardiographic examination for detecting cardiac malformations in low risk pregnancies. *Br Med J* 1992;304:671—674.
28. Allan LD. *Manual of Fetal Echocardiography.* Lancaster, England: MTP Press Limited, 1986, p. 11—48;98—99,167.
29. McGahan JP. Sonography of the fetal heart: findings on the four-chamber view. *AJR* 1991;156:547—553.
30. Brown DL, Emerson DS, Cartier MS, et al. Congenital cardiac anomalies: Prenatal sonographic diagnosis. *AJR* 1989;153:109—114.
31. Shipp TD, Bromley B, Hornberger LK, Nadel A, Benacerraf BR. Levorotation of the fetal cardiac axis: a clue for the presence of congenital heart disease. *Obstet Gynecol* 1995;85:97—102.
32. Comstock CH, Smith R, Lee W, Kirk JS. Right fetal cardiac axis: clinical significance and associated findings. *Obstet Gynecol* 1998;91:495—499.
33. Smith RS, Comstock CH, Kirk JS, Lee W. Ultrasonographic left cardiac axis deviation: a marker for fetal anomalies. *Obstet Gynecol* 1995;85:187—191.
34. Cartier MS, Davidoff A, Warneke LA, et al. The normal diameter of the fetal aorta and pulmonary artery: echocardiographic evaluation in utero. *AJR* 1987;149:1495—1003.
35. Copel JA, Morotti R, Hobbins JC, Kleinman CS. The antenatal diagnosis of congenital heart disease using fetal echocardiography: is color flow mapping necessary? *Obstet Gynecol* 1991;78:1—8.
36. Sharland GK, Chita SK, Allan LD. The use of colour Doppler in fetal echocardiography. *Int J Cardiol* 1990;28:229—236.
37. Rice MJ, McDonald RW, Sahn DJ. Contributions of color Doppler to the evaluation of cardiovascular abnormalities in the fetus. *Sem Ultrasound, CT MRI* 1993;14:277—285.
38. Brown DL, DiSalvo DN, Frates FC, et al. Sonography of the fetal heart: normal variants and pitfalls. *AJR* 1993;160:1251—1255.
39. Nyberg DA, Emerson DS. Cardiac malformations. In: Nyberg DA, Mahony BS, Pretorius DH, ed. *Diagnostic Ultrasound of*

Fetal Anomalies: Text and Atlas. Chicago: Year Book Medical Publishers, Inc., 1990, p. 300—341.

40. Silverman NH. *Pediatric Echocardiography*. Baltimore: Williams and Wilkins, 1993, p. 533—595.

41. Tegnander E, Eik-Nes SH, Johansen OJ, Linker DT. Prenatal detection of heart defects at the routine fetal examination at 18 weeks in a non-selected population. *Ultrasound Obstet Gynecol* 1995;5:372—380.

42. Stoll C, Alembik Y, Dott B, Roth PM, De Getter B. Evaluation of prenatal diagnosis of congenital heart disease. *Prenatal Diagnosis* 1993;13:453—461.

43. Wigton TR, Sabbagha RE, Tamura RK, et al. Sonographic diagnosis of congenital heart disease: comparison between the four-chamber view and multiple cardiac views. *Obstet Gynecol* 1993;82:219—224.

44. Benacerraf BR, Pober BR, Sanders SP. Accuracy of fetal echocardiography. *Radiology* 1987;165:847—849.

45. Copel JA, Pilu G, Green J, Hobbins JC, Kleinman CS. Fetal echocardiographic screening for congenital heart disease: the importance of the four-chamber view. *Am J Obstet Gynecol* 1987;157:648—655.

46. Kirk JS, Comstock CH, Lee W, et al. Sonographic screening to detect fetal cardiac anomalies: a 5-year experience with 111 abnormal cases. *Obstet Gynecol* 1997;89:227—232.

47. Orie J, Flotta D, Sherman FS. To be or not to be a VSD. *Am J Cardiol* 1994;74:1284—1285.

48. Brown DL, Hornberger LK. Problems and pitfalls in the sonographic diagnosis of fetal cardiac anomalies. *Ultrasound Q* 1995;13:221—227.

49. Cartier MS, Emerson DS, Plappert T, St. John Sutton M. Hypoplastic left heart with absence of the aortic valve: prenatal diagnosis using two-dimensional and pulsed Doppler echocardiography. *J Clin Ultrasound* 1987;15:463—468.

50. Allan LD, Chita SK, Anderson RH, et al. Coarctation of the aorta in prenatal life: an echocardiographic, anatomical, and functional study. *Br Heart J* 1988;59:356—360.

51. Benacerraf BR, Saltzman DH, Sanders SP. Sonographic sign suggesting the prenatal diagnosis of coarctation of the aorta. *J Ultrasound Med* 1989;8:65—69.

52. Emerson D, Cartier M, DiSessa T, Brown D, Felker R. Prenatal sonographic identification of coarctation of the aorta. *J Ultrasound Med* 1988;7:S271.

53. Sharland GK, Chan K, Allan LD. Coarctation of the aorta: difficulties in prenatal diagnosis. *Br Heart J* 1994;71:70—75.

54. Brown DL, Durfee SM, Hornberger LK. Ventricular discrepancy as a sonographic sign of coarctation of the fetal aorta: how reliable is it? *J Ultrasound Med* 1997;16:95—99.

55. Tan J, Silverman NH, Hoffman JIE, Villegas M, Schmidt KG. Cardiac dimensions determined by cross-sectional echocardiography in the normal human fetus from 18 weeks to term. *Am J Cardiol* 1992;70:1459—1467.

56. Sharland GK, Allan LD. Normal fetal cardiac measurements derived by cross-sectional echocardiography. *Ultrasound Obstet Gynecol* 1992;2:175—181.

57. Wladimiroff JW, Stewart PA, Vosters RPL. Fetal cardiac structure and function as studied by ultrasound. *Clin Cardiol* 1984;7:239—253.

58. DeVore GR, Siassi B, Platt LD. M-mode assessment of ventricular size and contractility during the second and third trimesters of pregnancy in the normal fetus. *Am J Obstet Gynecol* 1984;150:981—988.

59. Sahn DJ, Lange LW, Allen HD, et al. Quantitative real-time cross-sectional echocardiography in the developing normal human fetus and newborn. *Circulation* 1980;62:588—597.

60. Hornberger LK, Weintraub RG, Pesonen E, et al. Echocardiographic study of the morphology and growth of the aortic arch in the human fetus: observations related to the prenatal diagnosis of coarctation. *Circulation* 1992;86:741—747.

61. Hornberger LK, Sahn DJ, Kleinman CS, Copel J, Silverman NH. Antenatal diagnosis of coarctation of the aorta: a multicenter experience. *J Am Coll Cardiol* 1994;23:417—423.

62. Siassi B. Normal and abnormal transitional circulation in the IUGR infant. *Semin Perinatol* 1988;12:80—83.

63. DeVore GR. Examination of the fetal heart in the fetus with intrauterine growth retardation using M-mode echocardiography. *Semin Perinatol* 1988;12:66—79.

64. Allan LD, Crawford DC, Tynan MJ. Pulmonary atresia in prenatal life. J Am Coll Cardiol 1986;8:1131—1136.

65. Kutsche LM, Van Mierop LHS. Pulmonary atresia with and without ventricular septal defect: a different etiology and pathogenesis for the artesia in the 2 types. *Am J Cardiol* 1983;51:932—935.

66. Hornberger LK, Benacerraf BR, Bromley BS, Spevak PJ, Sanders SP. Prenatal detection of severe right ventricular outflow tract obstruction. *J Ultrasound Med* 1994;13:743—750.

67. Hornberger LK, Sahn DJ, Kleinman CS, Copel JA, Reed KL. Tricuspid valve disease with significant tricuspid insufficiency in the fetus: diagnosis and outcome. *J Am Coll Cardiol* 1991;17:167—173.

68. Roberson DA, Silverman NH. Ebstein's anomaly: echocardiographic and clinical features in the fetus and neonate. *J Am Coll Cardiol* 1989;14:1300—1307.

69. Sharland GK, Chita SK, Allan LD. Tricuspid valve dysplasia or displacement in intrauterine life. *J Am Coll Cardiol* 1991;17:944—949.

70. Kumar AE, Gilbert G, Aerichide N, Van Praagh R. Ebstein's anomaly, Uhl's disease and absence of tricuspid valve leaflets: a new spectrum (abstract). *Am J Cardiol* 1970;25:111—112.

71. Groves AMM, Fagg NLK, Cook AC, Allan LD. Cardiac tumors in intrauterine life. *Arch Dis Child* 1992;67:1189—1192.

72. Gresser CD, Shime J, Rakowski H, et al. Fetal cardiac tumor: a prenatal echocardiographic marker for tuberous sclerosis. *Am J Obstet Gynecol* 1987;156:689—690.

73. Brown DL, Roberts DJ, Miller WA. Left ventricular echogenic focus in the fetal heart: Pathologic correlation. *J Ultrasound Med* 1994;13:613—616.

74. Manning JE, Ragavendra N, Sayre J, et al. Significance of fetal intracardiac echogenic foci in relation to trisomy 21: a prospective sonographic study of high-risk pregnant women. *AJR* 1998;170:1083—1084.

75. Roberts DJ, Genest D. Cardiac histologic pathology characteristic of trisomies 13 and 21. *Human Pathol* 1992;23:1130—1140.

76. Bromley B, Lieberman E, Shipp TD, Richardson M, Benacerraf BR. Significance of an echogenic intracardiac focus in fetuses at high and low risk for aneuploidy. *J Ultrasound Med* 1998;17:127—131.

77. Lehman CD, Nyberg DA, Winter TC, et al. Trisomy 13 syndrome: prenatal US findings in a review of 33 cases. *Radiology* 1995;194:217—222.

78. Allan LD, Sharland GK. Prognosis in fetal tetralogy of Fallot. *Pediatr Cardiol* 1992;13:1—4.

79. Romero R, Pilu G, Jeanty P, Ghidini A, Hobbins JC. *Prenatal Diagnosis of Congenital Anomalies*. Norwalk: Appleton and Lange, 1988, p. 125—194.

31 The Role of Sonography in the Evaluation of Pregnant Women with High Maternal Serum α-Fetoprotein

Ruth B. Goldstein

Alpha-Fetoprotein Screening

α-Fetoprotein (AFP) screening was shown to be effective for detecting neural tube defects (NTDs) in the 1970s.[1] In 1991, the American College of Obstetrics and Gynecology (ACOG) endorsed offering maternal serum- (MS) AFP testing to all pregnant women. Since then, screening in the United States became more widespread and experience in this country and others has demonstrated considerable benefits from AFP screening, not only for the detection of NTDs, but also for a number of other fetal abnormalities (i.e., twins, ventral abdominal wall defects and chromosomal abnormalities). In one study, either high or low maternal serum AFP was associated with 34% of all major congenital defects.[2] Further, even in the absence of multiple gestations and discrete fetal defects, women with high MS-AFP have a much higher rate of adverse pregnancy outcome (i.e., fetal death, growth retardation, premature birth and preeclampsia).[3,4] It is estimated that as many as 20—38% of women with unexplained high MS-AFP will suffer adverse pregnancy outcomes,[5,6] and this information is another important benefit of MS-AFP screening.

The state of California implemented a statewide screening program in 1986. It is now required by California State law that women who begin prenatal care before 20 weeks be offered MS-AFP screening. Currently, over 300,000 pregnant women in California are tested annually. Among the first 1.1 million women screened through the California AFP Screening Program, 1390 fetal anomalies (morphologic and chromosomal) were detected (prevalence of 1.3/1000). These included 710 NTDs (417 anencephaly, 247 spina bifida, and 46 encephalocele), 286 ventral abdominal wall defects, 163 fetuses with Down syndrome, and 231 cases of other chromosomal anomalies. Impressively, of all anomalies detected in this program, nearly three-quarters involved two organ-systems: the neural axis (51%) and ventral abdominal wall (21%). This distribution of "likely" fetal anomalies is especially germane to the sonologist examining women with elevated MS-AFP. As discussed below, these two groups of fetal defects (and many others) can now be accurately detected on targeted prenatal sonograms performed by experienced examiners.

Alpha-Fetoprotein: Where it Comes From, How it Gets There

AFP is a glycoprotein produced initially by the yolk sac and fetal gut, and later predominantly by the fetal liver. At the end of the first trimester, it is present in the fetal serum in *milligram* quantities, in the amniotic fluid in *microgram* quantities, in the maternal serum in quantities measured in *nanograms*. In the fetus, serum AFP level increases until approximately 14—15 weeks, and then falls progressively. In normal pregnancies, AFP from fetal serum enters the amniotic fluid through fetal urination, fetal gastrointestinal secretions and transudation across fetal membranes (amnion and placenta) and immature epithelium. Detectable quantities of AFP in the maternal serum gradually increase during gestation, peaking at 30—32 weeks, and declining thereafter. Maternal serum levels are usually reported in multiples of the median (MoM) to standardize interpretation among laboratories.

There are a number of potential ways that fetal AFP can enter the maternal serum in abnormal quantities. Among fetal defects, the most common mechanism is through fetal cutaneous defects, such as anencephaly or myelomeningocele. These defects result in leakage of fetal serum proteins into the amniotic fluid, and secondarily into maternal serum. Other abnormalities, including intrinsic placental abnormalities and maternal-fetal hemorrhage, also allow fetal AFP to mix with maternal serum. In some cases, the precise mechanism for the feto-maternal transfer is not known (proximal gut obstruc-

---

[1] These fetal deaths occur mainly in the second trimester, and the risk appears to be directly related to the degree of maternal serum-AFP elevation.[4]

tion, renal agenesis), and may be secondary to diminished fetal gut degradation or elevated fetal serum concentrations of AFP.

It would be ideal if a single MS-AFP level could completely segregate normal from abnormal fetuses. Unfortunately, this is impossible owing to considerable overlap in MS-AFP levels between normal and abnormal pregnancies. Thus, the choice of a judicious cutoff value which maximizes detection of anomalies and minimizes the number of false-positive results is necessary for this screening program to be effective. Most screening programs in the United States have settled on a serum value of ≥ 2.5 MoM. Using this cutoff, approximately 90% of anencephalic fetuses, 75—80% of fetuses with an open spinal defect, 98% of fetuses with gastroschisis and approximately 70% of fetuses with omphaloceles will be detected.[7] Further, using 2.5 MoM as the cutoff has resulted in a reasonably low screen-positive rate (approximately 4—5%).

MS-AFP Screening Programs: How Patients are Triaged

It is optimal to test maternal serum between 16 and 18 weeks. If the MS-AFP is only marginally elevated (between 2.5 and 3.0 MoM) and the gestational age is below 17 weeks, then the maternal serum may be retested. Accurate dating is critical for AFP screening because serum AFP levels rise approximately 15% per week during the 16- to 18-week window. MS-AFP values are also corrected for maternal weight, race and the presence of diabetes (diabetes has a depressing effect on MS-AFP so lower levels may be found in association with NTDs).[8]

In California, approximately 2% of screened women have elevated MS-AFP levels (≥ 2.5 MoM), and approximately 3% have MS-AFP levels ≤ 0.5 MoM. The latter group will be discussed elsewhere. Roughly 6—15% of women with high MS-AFP have some type of major congenital defect,[2,9,10] and this risk increases with the magnitude of MS-AFP elevation.

If MS-AFP is elevated, then a nontargeted standard antepartum obstetrical sonogram ("level 1") is performed for the purpose of identifying easily recognized causes of "false-positives" (gestational age ≥ 2 weeks more advanced than estimated clinically, multiple gestations, fetal death, and obvious fetal defects). The intent of a standard antepartum obstetrical sonogram is to provide a general assessment of fetal/pregnancy health and it is performed according to the published guidelines endorsed by the AIUM and ACR.[11] The standard antepartum obstetrical sonogram is an important step in the triage of patients with high MS-AFP; impressively, approximately 20—50% of the elevated MS-AFP levels will be explained by findings on this preliminary sono-

gram (including the detection of a number of neural tube and abdominal wall defects).[12,13] If the elevated MS-AFP is not explained by findings of the standard antepartum obstetrical sonogram, traditionally, the next step has been to counsel patients and offer amniocentesis for measurement of amniotic fluid-(AF) AFP. Among women who choose to undergo amniocentesis following an "unrevealing" sonogram, > 90% will have normal AF-AFP (< 2.0 MoM), and no further diagnostic evaluation is done.[14] If the AF-AFP is elevated (≥ 2.0 MoM), then acetylcholinesterase (an isoenzyme important in neurotransmission) is tested on the amniotic fluid sample. Acetylcholinesterase is present in association with exposed neural tissue (and occasionally with abdominal wall defects). High AF-AFP plus positive acetylcholinesterase is quite specific for a fetal defect. In most screening programs, karyotype testing is also routinely performed on the amniotic fluid specimen.

If the AF-AFP is elevated (≥ 2.0 MoM), a targeted fetal sonogram ("level 2") is offered. Among women with elevated AF-AFP, approximately one-third of fetuses are anomalous.[14] Similar to MS-AFP, the likelihood of a neural tube or other defect increases proportionately with the degree of AF-AFP elevation, but clearly not all of these fetuses will be abnormal. The targeted sonogram is performed in these cases to determine (1) whether any fetal anomaly is present: (AF-AFP may be false-positive), (2) if the fetus is abnormal, what the nature of the anomaly is (i.e., NTD versus omphalocele), and (3) if present, the severity of the anomaly and presence/absence of associated malformations (i.e., spinal level of myelomeningocele).

AF-AFP testing is a highly sensitive method for detecting or excluding NTDs. The negative predictive value of a normal AF-AFP is approximately 97% and elevated AF-AFP plus acetylcholinesterase allows > 99% accurate detection of NTDs.[15] High-resolution, targeted ultrasonography performed in conjunction with abnormal AF-AFP is also highly accurate in identifying anomalous fetuses (i.e., > 99% accurate).[14,16] Nevertheless, there is a small but important procedural fetal loss rate associated with amniocentesis, generally quoted to be 1/200 (0.5%). As a result, women with elevated MS-AFP have, in increasing numbers, opted to go directly from the serum AFP test to a targeted fetal sonogram (i.e., to skip the amniocentesis). The latter approach has become more popular in the last few years for two major reasons. First, sonographic detection of the "likely" anomalies associated with high MS-AFP has improved over the last 10—15 years. Expected rates of sonographic detection for neural tube and abdominal wall defects are currently > 90% (several series report 100% sensitivity using ultrasound).[16—20] It is estimated that a complete, detailed, normal sonogram can now reduce the MS-AFP-based risk of a neural tube or ventral abdominal wall defect by 95%.[21,22] Second, going directly to a targeted sonogram circumvents the small but important procedural risk of fetal loss from amniocentesis. Indeed, the UK has adopted this paradigm and detailed, targeted sonograms are now routinely performed as the second diagnostic step in women with high MS-AFP.

Some have cautioned against adopting a routine policy of circumventing the amniocentesis[23] because (1) this approach will require a much larger number (i.e., ten times as many) of targeted sonograms, and the larger number of experienced examiners may not be available or patients may be required to travel a long distance for the targeted sonogram, (2) that even "experienced" examiners, especially as the prevalence of defects falls in the population scanned, may not detect as many defects as AF-AFP testing,[18] and (3) skipping amniocentesis will cause potentially detectable chromosomal abnormalities to be missed. The last issue remains controversial, and multicenter consensus has not been reached. Some favor a paradigm in which targeted sonography follows a high MS-AFP, arguing that there is only a very small risk of an abnormal karyotype in a fetus without morphologic defects. Recall that most of the unsuspected autosomal trisomies detected with AFP screening will occur in the *low* MS-AFP group, and that autosomal trisomies represent the minority of abnormal karyotypes found in women with high MS-AFP. For example, trisomies 13, 18, and 21 account for only 28% of abnormal karyotypes in women with high MS-AFP compared with 75% of abnormal karyotypes in women ≥ 35 years of age. Further, fetuses with autosomal trisomies,[13, 18, 21] detected as a result of high MS-AFP, often have sonographically detectable structural abnormalities.[19, 24] If the targeted sonographic fetal survey in a woman with elevated MS-AFP is normal, it has been estimated that the risk of a fetal chromosomal abnormality is only 0.6—1.1%,[21, 24—27] and sex chromosome aberrations (other than 45 X) account for many (30—50%) of the chromosomal abnormalities in these fetuses.[24]

There is no "right" choice but all women facing the choice of targeted sonography versus amniocentesis should be fully informed of these controversies during their counseling. Decisions to perform an amniocentesis versus a targeted sonogram will vary according to patient (maternal age, other serologic markers, i.e., HCG, estriol, and personal choice) and institution (depending on availability of experienced sonologists). Although many patients will elect to have a targeted sonogram instead of amniocentesis, amniotic fluid testing should still be strongly considered in the following patients: (1) fetal position or maternal body habitus precludes an adequate sonographic fetal anatomic survey, (2) equivocal sonographic findings (i.e., abnormal posterior fossa but spinal defect not seen), (3) experienced sonographic examiner not available, and (4) nonlethal anomaly detected on standard antepartum obstetrical sonogram for which karyotype testing is appropriate.

Increased MS-AFP: What Should You Look For?

Accurate sonographic diagnosis has become extremely important in light of AFP screening in pregnancy. If the preliminary, standard antepartum sonogram is unrevealing or an amniocentesis shows an elevated AF-AFP, a targeted fetal survey is performed. Because the most commonly encountered defects are those of the neural tube and ventral abdominal wall, the neural axis and ventral abdominal wall will be the most critical regions for scrutiny during the targeted sonogram.

A focused examination of the neural axis in each fetus should include an assessment of overall cranial size and contour, ventricular size (transaxial diameter of ventricular atrium > 10 mm is abnormal),[28] posterior fossa including cerebellar morphology and cisterna magna.[28—30] At UCSF, we also include images of the cavum septum pellucidum as a check for forebrain malformations. The spine should be carefully examined in each fetus, including segment by segment images in the transaxial and sagittal planes from the craniocervical junction through the sacrum. Sagittal and transaxial images of the spine should demonstrate an intact dorsal skin line. The normal curvature of the spine should be documented, and the ossified posterior elements examined for abnormal splaying. The ventral abdominal wall of the fetus is examined with focused attention on the umbilical cord insertion. The examiner should maintain a heightened sensitivity to the presence of bowel loops within the umbilical cord or floating in the amniotic fluid distant from the cord insertion/abdominal wall.

A number of other important fetal anomalies are associated with elevated AFP, and these potential defects should also be sought on the targeted sonogram. Less common defects include fetal teratoma (pharyngeal, sacral), defects caused by the amniotic band syndrome (asymmetric cephaloceles, gastropleuralschisis), cystic hygroma, lesions that alter the placentomaternal barrier (i.e., placental chorioangioma, lakes and abruption/hemorrhage), proximal fetal gut obstructions (i.e., esophageal and duodenal atresias), some renal abnormalities[31] [including multicystic dysplastic kidney, pelviectasis, congenital (Finnish) nephrosis] and oligohydramnios. Thus, careful examination of the face, posterior neck, oropharynx, thorax, abdomen (including a normally filled stomach) should be performed.[32] The limbs and digits should be assessed for abnormalities suggesting the amniotic band syndrome or the VACTERL (vertebral, anorectal, cardiac, tracheoesophageal fistula, renal and limb anomalies) association. Amniotic fluid volume should be qualitatively or semiquantitatively assessed in addition to careful examination of the placenta. The most commonly encountered individual defects are discussed below.

Anencephaly

Anencephaly accounts for approximately half of all NTDs (**Fig. 31–1**). On average, anencephaly is associated with the highest AF-AFP and MS-AFP values of all NTDs, and approximately 90% will be detected by an MS-AFP ≥ 2.5 MoM. This is a lethal anomaly in which the bony calvarium is absent above the orbits. Normal cerebral cortex is absent. Some dysplastic "brain tissue," histologically representing angiomatous stroma, may be observed above the orbits, apparently floating freely in the amniotic fluid. Owing to its irregular shape and absence of recognizable normal morphology, it is unlikely to be confused for normal brain. One should be cautious, however, not to confuse an engaged fetal head (in which the convexity may not be well visualized) for anencephaly. This distinction is accomplished by the observation of amniotic fluid above the orbits and the calvarial defect. It is critical that this be diagnosed accurately because most patients will electively terminate their pregnancies following this diagnosis. Anencephaly can be diagnosed in virtually all affected fetuses after 14 weeks gestation.[33]

Myelomeningocele

Myelomeningocele occurs in approximately 1:1000 live births in California (slightly higher in the southwestern USA). The myelomeningocele sac can be detected on sagittal or transverse views but the sensitivity for detection of the spinal dysraphism is especially important if a sac is not seen or has ruptured. A myelomeningocele is suggested by a defect in the normal smooth dorsal skin line and splayed posterior ossification centers on the transaxial image (**Fig. 31–2**). Widening of the posterior ossification centers can also be seen on coronal images of the spine. The majority of spinal dysraphisms occur in the lumbrosacral region, so this area should be scrutinized with extra care. Very abnormal spine curvature may be associated with the amniotic band syndrome or limb—body wall complex (**Fig. 31–3**). If the fetus is persistently in breech presentation and the distal spine is not well visualized with transabdominal imaging, then endovaginal scanning should be performed.

Spinal defects in some fetuses with spina bifida can be very difficult to observe owing to their small size, absence of a discrete myelomeningocele sac, and relatively inconspicuous bony defects. This is undoubtedly the reason that sonographic detection was only mediocre (50—80%) in reports from the early 1980 s.[9,34,35] Descriptions of several important cranial findings associated with "open" spinal bifida have been tremendously beneficial and have dramatically improved our ability not only to detect fetal myelomeningocele sensitively but also to confidently exclude it. Cranial findings as-

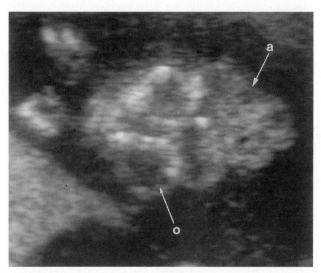

Figure 31–1 Anencephaly. The cranial bones are absent and angiomatous stroma is seen floating in the amniotic fluid (a) above the orbits (o).

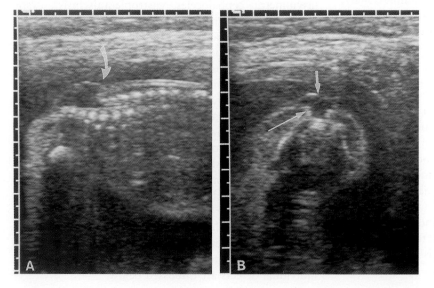

Figure 31–2 Myelomeningocele, **A:** Sagittal image demonstrates the break in the skin line (**curved arrow**). The top of the lesion is L5. **B:** Transaxial image shows the myelomeningocele sac (**short arrow**) and divergent posterior ossification centers (**long arrow**).

sociated with open (nonskin covered) fetal myelomeningoceles include the "lemon sign,"[21, 36—38] "banana sign,"[38] effaced cisterna magna,[29] ventriculomegaly[28, 39] and small biparietal diameter.[40] At least one of these findings is present in > 99% of affected fetuses.[21]

The *lemon sign* (**Fig. 31–4**) describes an inward scalloping of the frontal cranial bones seen in nearly all second-trimester fetuses with open spina bifida, but tends to disappear in affected fetuses in the third trimester. Importantly, the lemon sign may also be seen in as many as 1% of normal fetuses[37, 41] in addition to a number of other neural axis anomalies diminishing its positive predictive value for spina bifida.[42] Thus, sonographic diagnosis of spina bifida should never be based solely on the observation of a lemon sign.

The *banana sign* and the effaced cisterna magna occur secondary to the hindbrain malformation known as the Chiari II malformation, which is present in almost all (> 95%) fetuses who have open spinal lesions.[2] The posterior fossa is small in the Chiari II malformation and the developing cerebellum is cramped. As a result, the cerebellum often herniates superiorly through the tentorium or inferiorly through the foramen magnum. Neither of these potential herniations are seen sonographically but the deformation of the cerebellum can be easily recognized. The crowded cerebellum appears to wrap around the brain stem (creating a transaxial cerebellar configuration akin to the shape of a banana) or, at the minimum, the cisterna magna is completely or nearly obliterated. These are extremely important observations, and have enhanced the sensitivity of sonographic detection of fetal spinal bifida. The banana sign is highly specific for the Chiari II malformation but not quite as sensitive as effacement of the cisterna magna (some of the posterior fossa deformities of the Chiari II malformation are not severe enough to produce a banana cerebellum). Effacement of the cisterna is more sensitive for detection of the Chiari II malformation but less specific (and can be seen in association with hydrocephalus and also in normals). The cisterna magna (3—10 mm) can be visualized in 97% of normal fetuses at 15—25 weeks gestation. Because the Chiari II malformation (and myelomeningocele) is nearly always associated with an abnormal-appearing posterior fossa, a small or absent cisterna should raise suspicion for a spinal lesion. As a corollary, the presence of a normal-appearing cerebellum and cisterna magna has a negative predictive value for the Chiari II malformation of > 98%. Thus, especially if the distal spine is somewhat obscured, it should be reassuring to the examiner that a normal-appearing posterior fossa reduces the risk of an open spinal lesion by > 98%.

Other cranial findings associated with spina bifida include a biparietal diameter that is small for dates (second trimester) and ventricular enlargement. The degree of ventricular dilatation in fetuses with myelomeningoceles tends to increase with gestational age.[39] In a series of 51 fetuses with spina bifida aperta (nonskin-covered), we found ventriculomegaly (atrium >10 mm) present in only 44% of myelomeningocele fetuses examined before 24 weeks but present in 94% of fetuses scanned in the third trimester.[39] The degree of ventriculomegaly is also related to the degree of visualized posterior fossa deformity[39] but not to the spinal level of the lesion.[43] It should be emphasized that even though the cranial findings have so greatly improved the sensitivity with which we can detect myelomeningocele (currently reported to be > 90% and > 95% in many centers),[14, 22] the final diagnosis of a myelomeningocele should only be made after direct observation of the spinal defect.

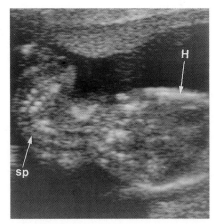

Figure 31–3 Limb—body wall complex. A ventral abdominal wall defect (not shown) was seen in association with a dramatic fixed angulation of the spine (sp). H, head.

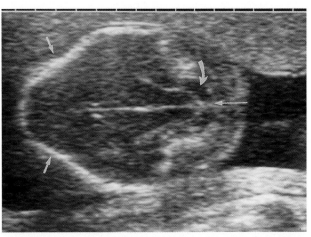

Figure 31–4 Cranial findings associated with "open" spina bifida and the Chiari II malformation: inward scalloping of the frontal bones (**short arrows**), also known as the "lemon sign," small posterior fossa and banana-shaped cerebellum ("banana sign") (**curved arrow**) and effaced cisterna magna (**long arrow**).

---

2 The Chiari II malformation usually is not associated with skincovered (closed) spinal abnormalities (skin-covered myelomeningocele, lipomeningocele, or midline spinal hematoma). Therefore, the banana sign and effaced cisterna magna will not appreciably improve sonographic detection of these fetal abnormalities.

If a Myelomeningocele Is Detected...

Outcome of fetuses with myelomeningocele is influenced by the presence of associated malformations, chromosomal abnormalities, the level of the spinal lesion (children with higher lesions have more severe motor handicaps), and childhood shunt infections.[44] Prenatal sonography has little to offer in estimating the number and severity of shunt infections but we can offer important and accurate information regarding the presence of ventriculomegaly, the level of the spinal lesion, and the presence of associated malformations. The bony level of the defect can be accurately estimated (± one spinal level), sonographically, in 79% of fetuses.[45] This is accomplished in most cases by "counting up" from the last sacral ossification center (assumed to be S4 in the second trimester and S5 in the third) (**Fig. 31–2**). Associated malformations in addition to the Chiari malformation and hydrocephalus are rare in childhood series but present in 13—24% of fetuses with myelomeningocele.[17,39,46] Multiple malformations increase the likelihood of fetal karyotype abnormalities[47—49] but chromosomal abnormalities are reported in 10—15%[48,50] of fetuses with *isolated* myelomeningocele. Thus, if the parents plan to carry the pregnancy, it is prudent not only to perform a complete, detailed, fetal anatomic survey but also to offer fetal karyotype testing.

Cephalocele

Cephaloceles are relatively rare (1.2/10,000 births) midline cranial defects which contain meninges, and cerebrospinal fluid (meningocele) ± neural tissue (encephalocele).[51] These lesions only account for approximately 3% of fetal anomalies detected with MS-AFP screening and 6% of detected NTDs.[23,52] In the United States, most (80—85%) of these occur in the occipital location,[53] a small percentage occur in the frontal (10—15%) or parietal (10—15%) area. Because encephaloceles occur in the midline, off-midline cranial defects should suggest the presence of the amniotic band syndrome. Occipital cephaloceles are usually easily recognized, particularly on images of the posterior fossa and cisterna magna (**Fig. 31–5**). Small frontal and parietal lesions, however, may be difficult to detect because these regions of the cranium do not usually receive focused attention. Most occipital lesions are associated with abnormalities of the posterior fossa and parietal lesions may also be associated with the Chiari malformation. The face and orbits should be carefully examined. The interorbital distance is usually widened in association with a frontal encephalocele.

Prognosis of fetuses with cephaloceles is generally poor (only 21% liveborn in our series)[53] and outcome is related to the presence of associated neural and nonneural malformations (common), as well as the size and content of the lesion; poorer outcome is associated with a large volume of herniated brain. Associated brain malformations include the Dandy-Walker malformation, agenesis of the corpus callosum, cerebellar hypoplasia and migrational abnormalities. Karyotype abnormalities are common, found in 44% of tested fetuses in one report.[53] It is important to remember that many encephaloceles are skin-covered (60% in one series)[52] and, therefore, may elude detection with MS-AFP screening.[1,54] Occipital cephaloceles may occur as part of the heritable (autosomal recessive) Meckel's syndrome (encephalocele, cystic dysplastic kidneys, and polydactyly).[55] Affected pregnancies may be terminated without adequate pathologic diagnosis. Therefore, prenatal recognition of this potential syndromic association is important for counseling regarding future pregnancies, because the 25% risk of recurrence associated with Meckel syndrome greatly exceeds the recurrence risk of other cephaloceles (3%).[15]

Ventral Abdominal Wall Defects

Ventral abdominal wall defects include omphalocele, gastroschisis, and those defects associated with the amniotic band syndrome or limb body wall complex. Scrutiny of the fetal umbilical cord insertion and ventral abdominal wall allows sonographic detection of omphalocele and gastroschisis in > 90% of fetuses.[14,22] Omphaloceles occur in approximately 1:4,000 livebirths, and include a spectrum of midline defects which range from large (usually containing liver and bowel) (**Fig. 31–6**) to small (which may contain only 1 or 2 bowel loops). The exteriorized viscera are contained by an amnioperitoneal membrane, and the umbilical cord inserts midline into the sac. Very large lesions can be difficult to repair postnatally, but features most predictive of prognosis are other serious malformations (expected in 50—75% of affected fetuses, including cardiac in

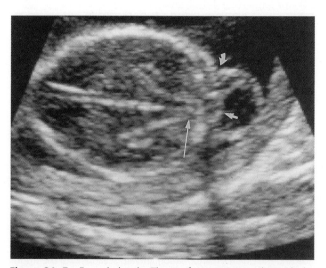

Figure 31–5 Encephalocele. The sac forms acute angles with the scalp (**curved arrow**). Cerebellar tissue is herniated into the sac (**short arrow**). Also note the beaked tectum (**long arrow**).

30—35%) and chromosomal abnormalities (approximately 10—20%), mainly trisomies 18 and 13. Although "bowel only" omphaloceles (**Fig. 31–7**) are generally smaller, sonographically less conspicuous, and often easier to repair postnatally, the rate of chromosomal abnormalities (perhaps 70—80%) is 8—10 times higher than that found in fetuses in whom the omphaloceles contain liver within herniated sac.[36,56] Be aware that small bowel-only omphaloceles may contain only one or two loops of bowel that have migrated into the cord so that the abnormality may not be recognized solely by examination of the cord *insertion* into the fetal abdomen. Thus, examination of the umbilical cord beyond the fetal abdomen for several centimeters is prudent.

Gastroschisis is a full-thickness, paramedian, abdominal wall defect, usually occurring to the right of the fetal umbilical cord insertion, through which bowel is exteri-

orized. Importantly, there is no covering membrane (**Fig. 31–8**). Associated malformations other than gut malrotation and atresia are rare, and the prevalence of chromosomal abnormalities is not increased. Fetal growth retardation is seen in up to 40%.[57] Bowel dilatation and mild thickening are common as gestation progresses. The degree of bowel dilation and wall thickening loosely correlate with seriously damaged bowel requiring resection postnatally.[57] Early in the second trimester (< 20 weeks), gastroschisis may be difficult to observe. The defect in the abdominal wall is small (1—3 cm) (**Fig. 31–8**) and, early on, the bowel is usually nondilated. As mentioned above, sensitivity to the presence of tubular structures other than cord floating in the amniotic fluid will allow detection of most cases.

A large population-based study involving 72,782 consecutively screened pregnancies was used to establish

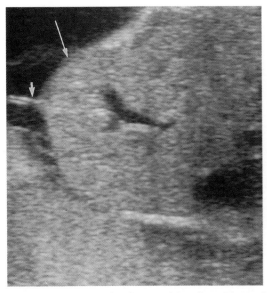

Figure 31–6 Omphalocele containing liver. The umbilical cord (**short arrow**) inserts centrally into the sac. (Covering amnioperitoneal membrane not shown.)

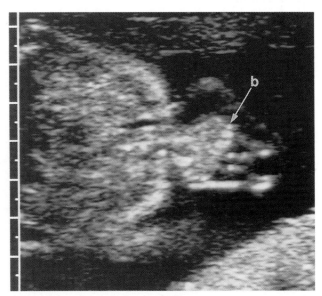

Figure 31–7 "Bowel only" omphalocele. A few loops of bowel are herniated into the base of the umbilical cord (**long arrow**). This type of omphalocele (liver not exteriorized) is associated with a higher rate of chromosomal anomalies. b, bowel loops.

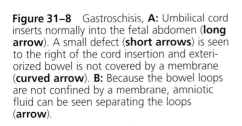
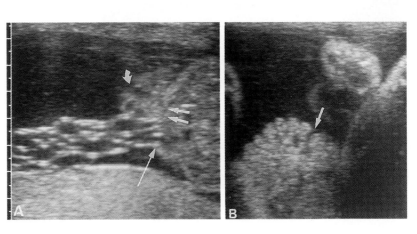

Figure 31–8 Gastroschisis, **A:** Umbilical cord inserts normally into the fetal abdomen (**long arrow**). A small defect (**short arrows**) is seen to the right of the cord insertion and exteriorized bowel is not covered by a membrane (**curved arrow**). **B:** Because the bowel loops are not confined by a membrane, amniotic fluid can be seen separating the loops (**arrow**).

distributions of AFP in pregnancies with gastroschisis and omphalocele.[7] Based on a cutoff of 2.5 MoM, all fetuses (20/20) with gastroschisis and approximately 70% (10/18) with omphaloceles were detected during MS-AFP screening.

Less Commonly Observed Fetal Defects Associated with Elevated MS-AFP

The AF- and MS-AFP may be elevated in fetuses with *cystic hygroma* (CH) (**Fig. 31–9**). Although the precise mechanism is not known, it is speculated that fetal serum proteins may leak through the membrane/integument covering the CH, or perhaps enter the maternal blood through an intrinsic, placental abnormality associated with an abnormal karyotype (present in 60—80% of second- and third-trimester fetuses with CH).

Teratomas (most commonly sacral (**Fig. 31–10**) but also oropharyngeal and lingual) can grow to a very large size in fetal life. These tumors often ulcerate, allowing leakage of fetal protein into the amniotic fluid and sec-

ondarily into maternal serum. In many cases, they are not completely skin-covered. Transverse axial views of the oropharynx, coronal and axial views of the face (to exclude oropharyngeal and lingual teratomas), and transverse and longitudinal views of the sacral area (sacrococcygeal teratomas are most common) should be obtained in patients referred for elevated MS-AFP. How sensitively teratomas are detected by MS-AFP screening is not known.

Esophageal atresia and *duodenal atresia* have been associated with elevated AFP. Some have speculated that a smaller than average degradation of swallowed AFP might account for the AFP elevation. A normally filled fetal stomach and the absence of a persistently filled or dilated duodenum should be sought. The normal fetal duodenum empties immediately and a persistently filled duodenum (even if it does not appear "over-distended") is always abnormal. The presence of a fetal "double bubble" (**Fig. 31–11**) suggests duodenal obstruction (usually atresia but can be due to stenosis, Ladd's bands, annular pancreas). Importantly, nearly one-third of fe-

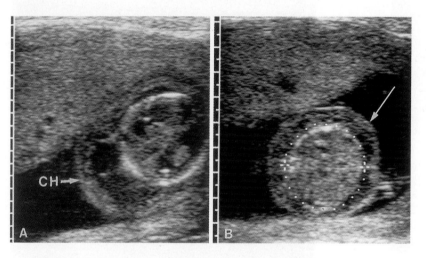

Figure 31–9 Cystic hygroma associated with diffuse lymphangiectasia at 15 weeks, **A:** Cystic hygroma (CH). Diffuse integumentary edema is seen around the abdomen (**long arrow**).

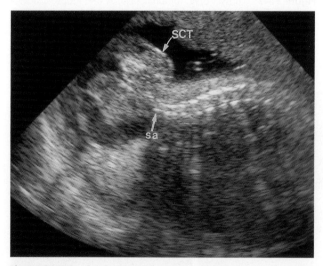

Figure 31–10 Sacrococcygeal teratoma (SCT) growing from the sacrum (sa).

Table 31–1 Defects Associated with High Maternal Serum Alpha-Fetoprotein

I. Common
- A. Neural tube defects
  - Anencephaly
  - Myelomeningocele (Chiari II)
  - Cephalocele
- B. Abdominal wall defects
  - Omphalocele
  - Gastroschisis
  - Gastropleuralschisis associated with abdominal band syndrome or limb-body wall

II. Uncommon
- A. Cystic hygroma
- B. Renal abnormalities
  - Finnish nephrosis (no defect observed sonographically)
  - Multicystic dysplastic kidney
  - Pelviectasis
- C. Chorioangioma
- D. Teratoma
- E. Esophageal/duodenal atresia

Figure 31–11 Duodenal atresia, **A:** Double bubble dilated stomach (s) and duodenum. **B:** Care should be taken to demonstrate that the stomach and duodenum are connected (**arrow**).

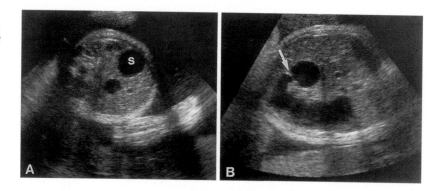

tuses with duodenal atresia have Down's syndrome. Thus, if a double bubble is detected, a focused examination of the fetal heart is performed and karyotype testing is offered to the parents.

Esophageal atresia is suggested by an absent/unfilled stomach (**Fig. 31–12**) and polyhydramnios but this constellation of observations is insensitive (< 50%) for the sonographic detection of fetal esophageal atresia before the third trimester. This is due to the fact that the proximal esophageal pouch is only rarely seen in fetuses, and a fistula exists between the lower esophagus and bronchial tree in > 90%, allowing passage of some fluid into the fetal stomach. A small, not absent stomach was observed in 5 of 12 fetuses with proven esophageal atresia by McKenna et al.[32] In addition, frank polyhydramnios is typically not seen before 20—24 weeks gestation.

Renal abnormalities including congenital (Finnish) nephrosis, multicystic dysplastic kidney, renal agenesis, and pelviectasis have been associated with elevated MS-AFP.[31, 58] In some cases the AFP is elevated secondary to abnormal leakage of proteins into fetal urine. *Congenital nephrosis* results in a dramatic fetal proteinuria in utero and, because there are no renal morphologic features, this is a very difficult diagnosis to make with certainty antenatally. The clue to the diagnosis is that both the MS- and AF-AFP levels are extremely high (i.e., typically ≥ 10 MoM!) with negative amniotic fluid acetylcholinesterase and without evidence of maternal-fetal hemorrhage or other fetal morphologic defects.[59] In cases of renal agenesis, the mechanism for MS-AFP elevation is not known but it is speculated that these fetuses may have higher serum protein levels owing to diminished excretion.

Finally, placental abnormalities including chorioangioma, placental abruption, periplacental hemorrhages (i.e., subchorionic hemorrhage), and placental lakes may result in elevated MS-AFP. A careful examination of the placenta should be performed.[60—62] Relatively minor placental abnormalities (i.e., placental lakes, large marginal veins) are seen commonly in pregnancy patients. Although the placenta should be carefully examined in all women referred for high AFP, a placental lesion should only be the diagnosis of exclusion (after

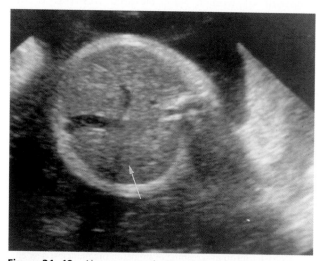

Figure 31–12 Absent stomach. No stomach bubble is observed (**arrow**). Diagnosis is esophageal atresia.

morphologic defects have been excluded), as the cause of increased MS-AFP.

Comment

Recall that amniocentesis performed following an elevated MS-AFP eliminates almost 90% of women with elevated MS-AFP from further testing. If we do not have AF-AFP levels to help us in triaging patients, 10 times as many targeted sonograms will be required to find the same number of fetal defects. Further, the likelihood of finding an anomaly during each targeted sonogram referred for high MS-AFP will be considerably lower than it is in the population scanned for high AF-AFP. Therefore, the examiner must "work harder" to remain vigilant while searching for fetal defects in this low prevalence population. The level of MS-AFP elevation may provide guiding information. The likelihood of finding a fetal defect increases with MS-AFP levels. Minor elevations of MS-AFP (i.e., 2.5—3 MoM), are associated with fetal defects in only 3—4%.[63] Whereas, if the MS-AFP is > 5 MoM, the prevalence of fetuses with defects may be as high as 20—30%,[5] and if the MS-AFP is > 7 MoM, the prevalence of abnormal fetuses may be as high as 30—40%.[63, 64] Thus the risk of a neural tube defect is almost ten times (13%) greater among women with MS-AFP > 7 MoM compared to those with elevations 2.5—2.9 MOM (1.4%).[63] This MS-AFP-related risk also parallels the rate of neural tube and ventral wall defects reported with increasing levels of AF-AFP.[14]

This information may be useful to the examiner and counselor of women with elevated MS-AFP. If she chooses to circumvent the amniocentesis, the degree to which her MS-AFP is elevated not only helps to adjust your index of suspicion for an anomaly but also helps to prepare and counsel the pregnant patient.

References

1. Wald NJ, Cuckle H, Brock JH, Peto R, Polani PE, Woodford FP. Maternal serum-alpha-fetoprotein measurement in antenatal screening for anencephaly and spina bifida in early pregnancy. Report of U.K. collaborative study on alpha-fetoprotein in relation to neural-tube defects. *Lancet* 1977;i:1323—1332.

2. Milunsky A, Jick SS, Bruell CL, et al. Predictive values, relative risks, and overall benefits of high and low maternal serum alpha-fetoprotein screening in singleton pregnancies: new epidemiologic data. *Am J Obstet Gynecol* 1989;161:291—297.

3. Davis RO, Goldenberg RL, Boots L, et al. Elevated levels of midtrimester maternal serum alpha-fetoprotein are associated with preterm delivery but not with fetal growth retardation. *Am J Obstet Gynecol* 1992;167:596—601.

4. Maher JE, Davis RO, Goldenberg RL, Boots LR, DuBard MB. Unexplained elevation in maternal serum alpha-fetoprotein and subsequent fetal loss. *Obstet Gynecol* 1994;83:138—141.

5. Crandall BF, Robinson L, Grau P. Risks associated with an elevated maternal serum alpha-fetoprotein. *Am J Obstet Gynecol* 1991;165:581—586.

6. Robinson L, Grau P, Crandall BF. Pregnancy outcomes after increasing maternal serum alpha-fetoprotein levels. *Obstet Gynecol* 1989;74:17—20.

7. Palomaki GE, Hill LE, Knight GJ, Haddow JE, Carpenter M. Second-trimester maternal serum alpha-fetoprotein levels in pregnancies associated with gastroschisis and omphalocele. *Obstet Gynecol* 1988;71:906—909.

8. Macri JN. Critical issues in prenatal maternal serum alpha-fetoprotein screening for genetic anomalies. *Am J Obstet Gynecol* 1986;155:240—246.

9. Robinson HP, Hood VD, Adam AH, Gibson AA, Ferguson-Smith MA. Diagnostic ultrasound: early detection of fetal neural tube defects. *Obstet Gynecol* 1980;56:705—710.

10. Haddow JE, Kloza EM, Smith DE, Knight GJ. Data from an alpha-fetoprotein pilot screening program in Maine. *Obstet Gynecol* 1983;62:556—560.

11. American Institute of Ultrasound in Medicine (AIUM). Guidelines for performance of the antepartum obstetrical ultrasound examination. *J Ultrasound Med* 1991;10:576—578.

12. Burton BK, Sowers SG, Nelson LH. Maternal serum alpha-fetoprotein screening in North Carolina: experience with more than twelve thousand pregnancies. *Am J Obstet Gynecol* 1983;146:439—444.

13. Lindfors KR, Gorczycz DP, Hanson FW, et al. The roles of ultrasonography and amniocentesis in evaluation of elevated maternal serum alpha-fetoprotein. *Am J Obstet Gynecol* 1991;164:1571—1576.

14. Robbin M, Filly RA, Fell S, et al. Elevated levels of amniotic fluid alpha-fetoprotein: sonographic evaluation. *Radiology* 1993;188:165—169.

15. Main DM, Mennuti MT. Neural tube defects: issues in prenatal diagnosis and counselling. *Obstet Gynecol* 1986;67:1—16.

16. Sepulveda W, Domalson A, Johnson RD, Davies G, Fisk NM. Are routine alpha-fetoprotein and acetylcholinesterase determinations still necessary at second-trimester amniocentesis? Impact of high-resolution ultrasonography. *Obstet Gynecol* 1995;85:107—112.

17. Hogge WA, Thiagarajah S, Ferguson JE II, Schnatterly PT, Harbert GM Jr. The role of ultrasonography and amniocentesis in the evaluation of pregnancies at risk for NTD. *Am J Obstet Gynecol* 1989;161:520—524.

18. Platt LD, Feuchtbaum L, Filly R, et al. The California maternal serum alpha-fetoprotein screening program: the role of ultrasonography in the detection of spina bifida. *Am J Obstet Gynecol* 1992;166 L:1328—1329.

19. Morrow RJ, McNay MB, Whittle MJ. Ultrasound detection of neural tube defects in patients with elevated maternal serum alpha-fetoprotein. *Obstet Gynecol* 1991;78:1055—1057.

20. Benacerraf BR. Should patients with elevated levels of maternal serum alpha-fetoprotein always undergo amniocentesis? *Radiology* 1993;188:17—18.

21. Watson WJ, Chescheir NC, Katz VL, Seeds JW. The role of ultrasound in evaluation of patients with elevated maternal serum alpha-fetoprotein: a review. *Obstet Gynecol* 1991;78:123—128.

22. Nadel AS, Green JK, Holmes LB, Frigoletto FD Jr, Benacerraf BR. Absence of need for amniocentesis in patients with elevated levels of maternal serum alpha-fetoprotein and normal ultrasonographic examinations. *New Engl J Med* 1990;323:557—561.

23. Filly RA, Callen PW, Goldstein RB. Alpha-fetoprotein screening programs: what every obstetric sonologist should know. *Radiology* 1993;188:1—9.

24. Megerian G, Godmilow L, Donnenfeld AE. Ultrasound-adjusted risk and spectrum of fetal chromosomal abnormality in women with elevated maternal serum alpha-fetoprotein. *Obstet Gynecol* 1995;85:952—956.

25. Feuchtbaum LB, Cunningham G, Waller DK, et al. Fetal karyotyping for chromosome abnormalities after an unexplained elevated maternal serum alpha-fetoprotein screening. *Obstet Gynecol* 1995;86:248—254.

26. Thiagarajah S, Stroud CB, Vavelidis F, et al. Elevated maternal serum alpha-fetoprotein levels: what is the risk of fetal aneuploidy? *Am J Obstet Gynecol* 1995;173:388—392.

27. Barth WH, Frigoletto FD Jr, Krauss CM, et al. Ultrasound detection of fetal aneuploidy in patients with elevated maternal serum alpha-fetoprotein. *Obstet Gynecol* 1991;77:897—900.

28. Filly RA, Goldstein RB, Callen PW. Fetal ventricle: Importance in routine obstetrical sonography. *Radiology* 1991;181:1—7.

29. Goldstein RB, Podrasky AE, Filly RA, Callen PW. Effacement of the fetal cisterna magna in association with myelomeningocele. *Radiology* 1989;172:409—413.

30. Cardoza JD, Goldstein RB, Filly RA. Exclusion of fetal ventriculomegaly with a single measurement: the width of the lateral ventricular atrium. *Radiology* 1988;169:711—714.

31. Townsend RR, Goldstein RB, Filly RA, et al. Sonographic identification of autosomal recessive polycystic kidney disease associated with increased maternal serum/amniotic fluid alpha-fetoprotein. *Obstet Gynecol* 1988;71:1008—1012.

32. McKenna KM, Goldstein RB, Stringer MD. Prognostic significance of a small or absent fetal stomach. *Radiology* 1995;197:729—733.

33. Goldstein RB, Filly RA, Callen PW. Sonography of anencephaly: pitfalls in early diagnosis. *J Clin Ultrasound* 1989;17:397—402.

34. Persson PH, Kullander S, Gennser G, Grennert L, Laurell CB. Screening for fetal malformations using ultrasound and measurements of alpha-fetoprotein in maternal serum. *BMJ* 1983;286:747—749.

35. Roberts CJ, Evans KT, Hibbard BM, et al. Diagnostic effectiveness of ultrasound in detection of neural tube defects. The South Wales experience of 2509 scans (1977—1982) in high-risk mothers. *Lancet* 1983;ii:1068—1069.

36. Nyberg DA, Mack LA, Hirsch J, Mahony BS. Abnormalities of fetal cranial contour in sonographic detection of spina bifida: evaluation of the "lemon" sign. *Radiology* 1988;167:387—392.

37. Van den Hof MC, Nicolaides KH, Campbell J, Campbell S. Evaluation of the lemon and banana signs in one hundred thirty fetuses with open spina bifida. *Am J Obstet Gynecol* 1990;162:322—327.

38. Nicolaides KH, Campbell S, Gabbe SG, Guidetti R. Ultrasound screening for spina bifida: cranial and cerebellar signs. *Lancet* 1986;ii:72—74.

39. Babcook CJ, Goldstein RB, Barth RA, et al. Prevalence of ventriculomegaly in association with myelomeningocele: correlation with gestational age and severity of posterior fossa deformity. *Radiology* 1994;190:703—707.

40. Wald N, Cuckle H, Boreham J, Stirrat G. Small biparietal diameter of fetuses with spina bifida: implications for antenatal screening. *Br J Obstet Gynaecol* 1980;87:219—221.

41. Campbell J, Gilbert WM, Nicolaides KH, Campbell S. Ultrasound screening for spina bifida: cranial and cerebellar signs in a high-risk population. *Obstet Gynecol* 1987;70:247—250.

42. Ball R, Filly RA, Goldstein RB. The "lemon sign": not a specific indicator of myelomeningoceles. *J Ultrasound Med* 1993;12:131—134.

43. Babcook CJ, Goldstein RB, Filly RA. Spinal level of fetal myelomeningocele: does it influence ventricular size or severity of the posterior fossa deformity? (Abstr) American Roentgen Ray Society, Boston, March

44. Sturgiss S, Robson S. Prognosis for fetuses with antenatally detected myelomeningocele. *Fetal Maternal Med Rev* 1995;7:235—249.

45. Kollias SS, Goldstein RB, Cogen PH, Filly RA. Prenatally detected myelomeningoceles: sonographic accuracy in estimation of the spinal level. *Radiology* 1992;185:109—112.

46. Luthy DA, Wardinsky T, Shurtleff DB, et al. Cesarean section before the onset of labor and subsequent motor function in infants with meningomyelocele diagnosed antenatally. *New Engl J Med* 1991;324:662—666.

47. Babcook CJ, Goldstein RB, Filly RA. Prenatally detected fetal myelomeningocele: is karyotype analysis warranted. *Radiology* 1995;194:491—494.

48. Drugan A, Johnson MP, Dvorin E, et al. Aneuploidy with neural tube defects: another reason for complete evaluation in patients with suspected ultrasound anomalies or elevated maternal serum alpha-fetoprotein. *Fetal Ther* 1989;4:88—92.

49. Lindfors KK, McGahan JP, Tennant FP, Hanson FW, Walter JP. Midtrimester screening for open neural tube defects: correlation of sonography with amniocentesis results. *AJR* 1987;149:141—145.

50. Harmon JP, Hiett AK, Palmer CG, Golichowski AM. Prenatal ultrasound detection of isolated neural tube defects: is cytogenetic evaluation warranted? *Obstet Gynecol* 1995;86:595—599.

51. Lorber J. The prognosis of occipital encephalocele. *Develop Med Child Neurol* 1967;Suppl 13:75—86.

52. Chan A, Robertson EF, Haan EA, Ranieri E, Keane RJ. The sensitivity of ultrasound and serum alpha-fetoprotein in population-based antenatal screening for neural tube defects, South Australia 1986—1991. *Br J Obstet Gynaecol* 1995;102:370—376.

53. Goldstein RB, LaPidus AS, Filly RA. Fetal cephaloceles: diagnosis with US. *Radiology* 1991;180:803—808.

54. Simpson JL, Palomaki GE, Mercer B, et al. Associations between adverse perinatal outcome and serially obtained second- and third-trimester maternal serum alpha-fetoprotein measurements. *Am J Obstet Gynecol* 1995;173:1742—1748.

55. Johnson VP, Holzwarth DR. Prenatal diagnosis of Meckel syndrome: case reports and literature review. *Am J Med Genet* 1984;18:699—711.

56. Getachew MM, Goldstein RB, Edge V, Goldberg JD, Filly RA. Correlation between omphalocele contents and karyotype abnormality: sonographic study in 37 cases. *AJR* 1992;158:133—136.

57. Babcook CJ, Hendrick MH, Goldstein RB, et al. Gastroschisis: can sonography of the fetal bowel accurately predict postnatal outcome? *J Ultrasound Med* 1994;13:701—706.

58. Petrikovsky BM, Nardi DA, Rodis JF, Hoegsberg B. Elevated maternal serum alpha-fetoprotein and mild fetal uropathy. *Obstet Gynecol* 1991;78:262—264.

59. Albright SG, Warner AA, Seeds JW, Burton BK. Congenital nephrosis as a cause of elevated alpha-fetoprotein. *Obstet Gynecol* 1990;76:969—971.

60. Williams MA, Hickok DE, Zingheim RW, et al. Elevated maternal serum alpha-fetoprotein levels and midtrimester placental abnormalities in relation to subsequent adverse pregnancy outcomes. *Am J Obstet Gynecol* 1992;167:1032—1037.

61. Salafia CM, Silberman L, Herrera NE, Mahoney MJ. Placental pathology at term associated with elevated midtrimester maternal serum alpha-fetoprotein concentration. *Am J Obstet Gynecol* 1988;158:1064—1066.

62. Fleischer AC, Kurtz AB, Wapner RJ, et al. Elevated alpha-fetoprotein and a normal fetal sonogram: Association with placental abnormalities. *AJR* 1988;150:881—883.

63. Reichler A, Hume RF Jr, Drugan A, et al. Risk of anomalies as a function of level of elevated maternal serum alpha-fetoprotein. *Am J Obstet Gynecol* 1994;171:1052—1055.

64. Killam Wm P, Miller RC, Seeds JW. Extremely high maternal serum alpha-fetoprotein levels at second-trimester screening. *Obstet Gynecol* 1991;78:257—260.

32 Triple Marker Screening Test Positive for Down Syndrome

Catherine J. Babcook

Introduction

Down syndrome (trisomy 21) is the most common chromosomal abnormality, occurring in the United States with a reported incidence of 1/700 to 1/1000 live births.[1] Women of advanced maternal age (≥ 35) have long been recognized as having an increased risk of conceiving a fetus with trisomy 21, and these women are traditionally offered amniocentesis for fetal karyotype assessment. However, only 20% of fetuses with Down syndrome are born to women in this advanced age group. Women under 35, therefore, carry 80% of trisomy 21 fetuses[2] and a method has been sought to identify women in this age group who are at risk. The Triple Marker screen can identify 60% of fetuses with Down syndrome.[3] Many women are, therefore, undergoing this prenatal testing, and approximately 6% of women test positive for Down syndrome. These women usually undergo genetic counseling to explain the implications of the test results and are then referred for prenatal sonography. Down syndrome occurs in all populations and is characterized by a number of physical characteristics such as short stature, epicanthal folds, flat nasal bridge, and simian creases. Everyone with Down syndrome is mentally disabled, but the severity of disability varies from mild to severe, with most being moderately affected. Approximately 40% have congenital heart defects. The life span of affected individuals is, in general, reduced, and the extent of the reduction is related to the presence or absence of congenital anomalies.

Triple Marker Screening Test

The Triple Marker screening test consists of maternal serum measurements of alpha-fetoprotein (AFP), human chorionic gonadotropin (HCG), and unconjugated estriol (uE3). Each is reported as multiples of the median (MoM). If the test is abnormal, then the patient is assigned to a risk category based on the pattern of the abnormal serum results (**Table 32–1**). AFP is a protein, primarily produced in the fetal liver, and released into the fetal circulation and amniotic fluid. A small amount crosses the placenta and is detectable in the maternal serum with levels increasing through the second

Table 32–1 Pattern of serum chemicals in positive screen tests

Risk Category	AFP	HCG	uE3
Neural tube defect/ abdominal wall defect	↑	Not applicable	Not applicable
Trisomy 21	↓	↑	↓
Trisomy 18	↓	↑	↑

AFP, alphafetoprotein; HCG, human chorionic gonadotropin; uE3, unconjugated estriol.

trimester. AFP levels are lower, on average, in Down syndrome pregnancies. The placenta synthesizes and secretes HCG. Levels of HCG rise quickly in the first 10 weeks of pregnancy and then decline between 10 and 20 weeks. Levels are higher, on average, in Down syndrome pregnancies. Unconjugated estriol is a hormone produced by the fetal adrenal glands and liver and the placenta, with levels that normally rise throughout gestation and that are lower, on average, in Down syndrome pregnancies. The profile in pregnancies at risk for Down syndrome is, therefore, low AFP, high HCG, and low uE3. If the levels of these chemicals result in a risk estimate of 1/250 or higher, the test is considered positive.

Differential Diagnosis

Pregnancies that are screen positive may have fetal trisomy 21, or they may be normal or have other chromosome abnormalities such as triploidy and Turner syndrome.[3] The screen may also be positive if the last menstrual period (LMP) dating is incorrect and the pregnancy is not as far along as originally thought.

Diagnostic Workup

When a triple marker screen is positive for trisomy 21, the patient usually undergoes genetic counseling to explain the implications of the positive screen and the diagnostic possibilities, and to outline the options. The patient is then referred for ultrasound evaluation.

Sonography has two primary roles in the setting of a positive triple marker screen for Down syndrome. The first is to date the pregnancy to ensure that the serum screen was performed at the appropriate time in gestation. Maternal blood must be drawn between 15 and 20 weeks gestation. If the patient's dating is inaccurate, and the blood was drawn too early or too late, the serum measurements will be inaccurate, and the risk assignment may be erroneous. In this situation, the serum test should be repeated if the gestational age is still within the 15- to 20-week window. If the menstrual dating is confirmed, amniocentesis is offered. The results of amniocentesis are available 10—14 days following the procedure. Occasionally, peripheral umbilical blood vein sampling instead of amniocentesis will be offered to assess fetal karyotype, when there is a need for more rapid evaluation. Results of this test are available in 48 h but the test is associated with a higher miscarriage rate (1 to 3%) than amniocentesis (approximately 1/300).

The second role of sonography is to identify fetal anomalies or sonographic findings that are associated with trisomy 21. Although amniocentesis for karyotype analysis is the only definitive way to detect abnormal fetal chromosomes, most women with a positive screen for Down syndrome undergo sonography for dating and this provides an opportunity to evaluate for the presence of additional sonographic information that could alter risk assignment. While some patients will choose to undergo amniocentesis regardless of the sonographic findings and will have made this decision (assuming dates are correct) before the ultrasound, others will base their decision on both the expanded AFP risk assessment and the sonographic findings. This is particularly true for couples who have had difficulty conceiving and are extremely reluctant to accept even the small risk of miscarriage associated with amniocentesis. For sonographic findings to be clinically useful they need to be reliably obtained, effective in discriminating between chromosomally abnormal fetuses and normals, and obtainable at a gestational age that is early enough to provide the parents with management options.

Sonographic Findings in Trisomy 21 (Down Syndrome)

General

Ultrasound to evaluate fetuses for the presence trisomy 21 was first described in 1985 by Benacerraf et al.[4] The goal of exploring the utility of sonographic evaluation in the setting of Down syndrome was to assist high-risk women in decision making regarding amniocentesis and to identify otherwise low-risk women carrying affected fetuses. Since that time, much has been written about the role of sonography in differentiating Down's fetuses from chromosomally normal fetuses. There are a number of sonographic signs that have been

suggested to have importance in this evaluation. An understanding of the significance of these signs is important not only for those specializing in prenatal diagnosis but also for those who perform general obstetrical sonography, so that appropriate interpretation and referral can be made. While some investigators suggest that it is possible to detect 87% of fetuses at risk for Down syndrome using ultrasound,[5] others have detected only 50% of affected fetuses sonographically.[6] Therefore, a normal sonogram does not exclude trisomy 21, as 13 to 50% of Down's fetuses will have no sonographic abnormality.

Major Structural Anatomic Abnormalities

The identification of a major structural abnormality always raises the possibility of a chromosomal abnormality. The most common major anatomic abnormality associated with trisomy 21 is a congenital cardiac defect (CHD). Forty to 50% of neonates with trisomy 21 have CHD. Atrioventricular canal defect is the abnormality often mentioned (**Fig. 32–1**) but ventricular septal defect (VSD) and atrial septal defect (ASD) are the most common. Unfortunately, sonography is fairly insensitive for detecting CHD prenatally in these fetuses. In one series, CHD were identified in only five (5.3%) of 94 fetuses with trisomy 21 and two of these were identified after 24 weeks.[7] Fourteen additional defects were identified postnatally or at postmortem (total of 20% of fetuses had CHD) and because follow-up was incomplete, this likely underestimates the total number of cardiac defects in this group. Nine of the 14 missed defects had been ex-

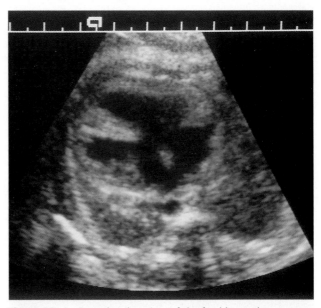

Figure 32–1   Four-chamber view of the fetal heart shows a central discontinuity in the ventricular and atrial septae resulting in a common ventricle and common atrium characteristic of an atrioventricular canal defect.

amined before 24 weeks. Other major anatomic abnormalities that have been reported in association with trisomy 21 include duodenal atresia (**Fig. 32–2**), hydrothorax (**Fig. 32–3**), hydrops, omphalocele (**Fig. 32–4**), and others (**Fig. 32–5**). Duodenal atresia is well known to occur in fetuses with Down syndrome. However, it rarely manifests sonographically before 24 weeks gestational age and is therefore not helpful at the time of triple marker screening. When any cardiac abnormality or other significant fetal anomaly is identified sonographically, including those described above, trisomy 21 as well as other chromosomal abnormalities should be considered.

Nuchal Thickness

In general, an increased fetal nuchal thickness is associated with an increased risk of a chromosomal abnormality. The pathophysiologic mechanism for this finding remains unclear but theories include transient overperfusion of the developing brain, lymph overproduction, and jugular lymphatic overdistention secondary to failure of communication with the internal jugular vein.[8] Fetal nuchal thickness increases with increasing gestational age so the criteria for diagnosing abnormally increased nuchal thickness change with gestational age. Most studies that have evaluated nuchal thickness and

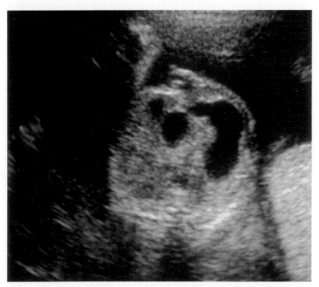

Figure 32–2 Transverse view of the fetal abdomen showing a fluid-filled stomach and duodenal bulb secondary to duodenal atresia.

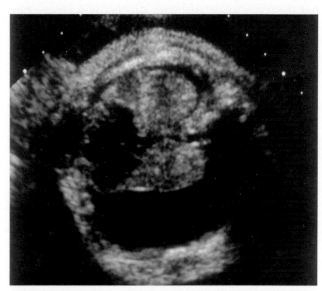

Figure 32–3 Transverse view of the fetal chest shows the lungs surrounded by bilateral pleural effusions (hydrothorax).

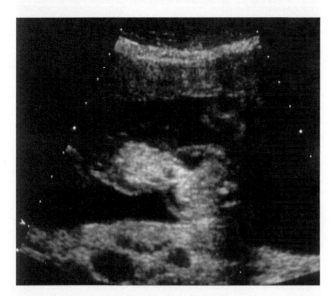

Figure 32–4 Transverse view of the fetal abdomen demonstrates increased soft tissue echogenicity extending from the fetal abdomen into the base of the umbilical cord consistent with a bowel-only omphalocele.

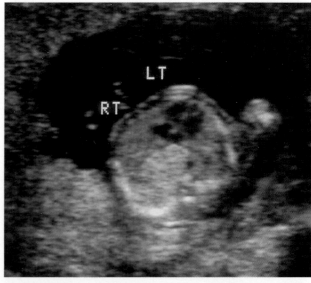

Figure 32–5 Transverse view of the fetal chest in a fetus with trisomy 21 shows an echogenic mass in the region of the posterior right lung due to a cystic adenomatoid malformation.

the risk of aneuploidy have studied fetuses between 14 to 21 weeks.[9—15] Nuchal thickness measuring ≥ 6 mm at 14 to 21 weeks is abnormal (**Fig. 32–6**). Accurate measurement of the nuchal thickness requires attention to the appropriate plane of section in which the measurement is made. Measurements at improper angles may lead to overestimation of nuchal thickness.[9, 16—19] The nuchal measurement should be made on a slightly angled axial view of the fetal head, which includes cavum septi pellucidi anteriorly, cerebral peduncles centrally, and the cerebellum and cisterna magna posteriorly. Careful utilization of these landmarks will prevent too coronal a plane from being used which overestimates nuchal thickness (**Fig. 32–7**).[12] Data from two large, early studies of women age 35 or older, or with low MSAFP found that 40% of fetuses with trisomy 21 had abnormal nuchal thickening and 29% of fetuses with trisomy 21 had this sign as an isolated finding. The positive predictive value (PPV) of nuchal thickening for Down Syndrome was 18%.[9, 10] Others have substantiated the utility of measuring nuchal thickness to identify the fetus with Down syndrome,[15, 19] although they have not shown positive predictive values as high as the early studies did.

Echogenic Bowel

Increased echogenicity of the fetal bowel has been associated with trisomy 21 (**Fig. 32–8**),[7, 20—22] other chromosomal abnormalities,[7, 21—23] cystic fibrosis[23,] intrauterine growth retardation (IUGR)[22] intraamniotic bleeding,[24] and normal fetuses.[25] The criteria for what constitutes echogenic bowel have varied in different studies. Some studies considered bowel to be echogenic if it

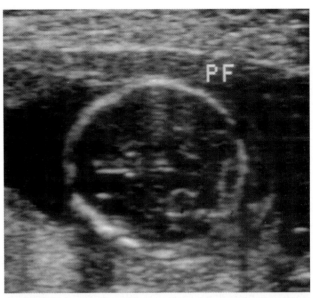

Figure 32–6   Transverse view of the fetal head shows a thickened nuchal fold extending posteriorly from the bony occiput (PF, posterior fossa).

were "more echogenic than normal."[21] Others considered it abnormal if it were of similar or greater echogenicity than surrounding bone.[22, 23] Nyberg et al.[7] compared the bowel echogenicity to that of the liver and graded it as 1 = mildly echogenic, 2 = moderately echogenic, or 3 = markedly echogenic (nearly as echogenic as bony structures). The latter two categories contained the majority of fetuses with adverse outcome. It is therefore probably best to consider bowel to be abnormally echogenic if it approaches or matches the echogenicity of ad-

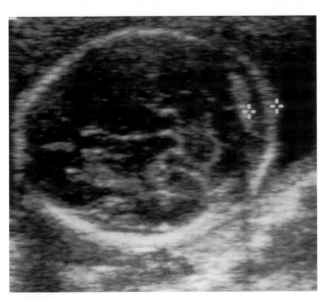

Figure 32–7   Transverse view of the fetal head, demonstrating the appropriate landmarks for measuring the nuchal thickness, shows a thickened nuchal fold in this fetus with trisomy 21.

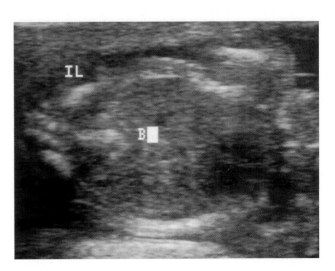

Figure 32–8   Coronal view of the fetal abdomen shows an echogenic bowel loop in the lower abdomen in this fetus with trisomy 21. (B, bowel, IL, iliac wing)

jacent bone and this appearance is consistent in all planes of visualization (transverse, coronal, and sagittal). Overall, studies have shown that 50 to75% of fetuses with echogenic bowel are normal, 16 to 27% have a chromosome abnormality, and 12 to 23% have trisomy 21.[7,21–23] One of the difficulties in interpreting the findings of these studies with respect to the positive triple marker screen is that some of the studies included only fetuses from a high-risk population while other studies used the general obstetrical population. While most studies showed an association between echogenic bowel and trisomy 21, one study of fetuses with echogenic bowel contained no fetuses with trisomy 21 and found a previously unidentified relationship with IUGR and neonatal death (Fig 32–9).[23] On balance, it appears that markedly echogenic bowel (approaching bone echogenicity) is associated with trisomy 21.

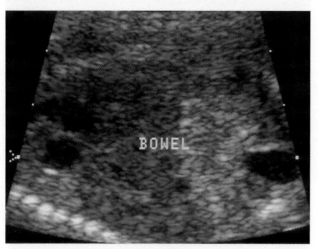

Figure 32–9   Coronal view of the fetal abdomen shows increased echogenicity of the fetal bowel surrounding the bladder. This fetus had a normal karyotype but was small for gestational age and died in utero.

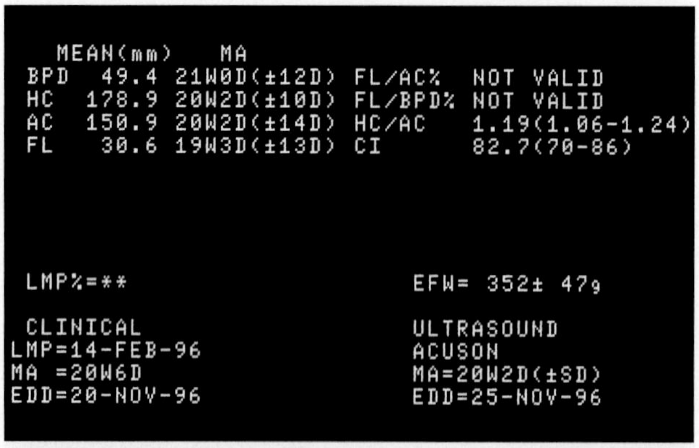

```
   MEAN(mm)     MA
BPD   49.4   21W0D(±12D)   FL/AC%    NOT VALID
HC   178.9   20W2D(±10D)   FL/BPD%   NOT VALID
AC   150.9   20W2D(±14D)   HC/AC     1.19(1.06-1.24)
FL    30.6   19W3D(±13D)   CI        82.7(70-86)



LMP%=**                     EFW=  352± 47g

CLINICAL                    ULTRASOUND
LMP=14-FEB-96               ACUSON
MA =20W6D                   MA=20W2D(±SD)
EDD=20-NOV-96               EDD=25-NOV-96
```

Figure 32–10   Biometric data in a fetus with trisomy 21 shows a relatively short femur compared to the other biometric measurements and the gestational age by LMP.

Biometric Measurements and Ratios

Cephalic Index

Despite the fact that brachycephaly is commonly present in infants with Down syndrome, the cephalic index in fetuses with Down syndrome does not differ significantly from normals.[26]

Femur Length and Ratios

Fetuses with Down syndrome have been shown to have shorter femur lengths (FL), relative to the expected length for their gestational age and relative to their biparietal diameter than do normal fetuses (**Fig. 32–10**). However, studies evaluating the utility of screening programs based on FL shortening associated with Down syndrome have shown marked discrepancies in the results from different centers. Variations in methods may account for some of this variability. In any case, the magnitude of femoral shortening in Down syndrome is probably insufficient to make it a useful and reproducible sonographic marker.

Decreased sonographic FL in Down syndrome was first described by Lockwood and coworkers in 1987 in a high-risk population (AMA, low MSAFP).[27] They reported that a BPD/FL ratio above 1.5 SD above the mean for their center had a PPV of 1/37, or 2.7% for women 35 or older, and a PPV of 1/103 or 0.97% for the general OB population. This group developed a regression equation to determine the measured versus expected FL for fetuses and reported that a ratio of measured to expected FL of 0.91 had a PPV of 12% for women 35 or older and 3.3% for the general OB population. Other investigators have agreed that the PPV of FL measurement for Down syndrome (3% for age ≥ 35) was better than the PPV of AMA and low MSAFP but have not been able to duplicate the very high positive predictive values of Lockwood's regression formula.[28] Still other investigators have not been able to substantiate that FL in Down syndrome fetuses differs significantly from normals.[29] A study of twins in which one twin had trisomy 21 showed no significant difference in femur length ratios between the affected twin and its cotwin, suggesting that it is not a useful differentiating sign.[30]

A postmortem study of FL in fetal specimens with trisomy 21, compared with normal controls, showed that only 3/37 femurs fell more than 2 S.D. below the mean, and that only 16% of trisomy 21 fetuses had actual to expected femur lengths below 0.91.[31] These data suggest that while FL in fetuses with trisomy 21 may be shorter than the norm, the magnitude of this difference may not be sufficient to be clinically useful for screening.

Humeral Length and Ratios

There is less data relating to the utility of humeral length as a screening tool for trisomy 21 but the issues remain the same as for femur length. A postmortem study of fetal specimens with trisomy 21 suggested that the differences between humeral lengths of trisomy 21 fetuses and normals are greater than the differences for femoral length between these groups.[31]

Benacerraf and coworkers showed a PPV of 4.6% for humeral length combined with nuchal thickness for identifying trisomy 21 among women 35 or older and a PPV of 1.2% for the general population.[32]

On balance, it appears that measurements of femur length and humerus length and their ratios with BPD may not be reliable indicators of increased risk of trisomy 21 when used alone. If any of these ratios are to be used, it appears prudent that each ultrasound lab develop its own normative data to be used in the calculations.

Fetal Pyelectasis

In 1990, Benacerraf and coworkers reviewed sonograms from 7400 pregnancies and found that 2.8% had pyelectasis.[33] They reported that the prevalence of Down syndrome among these fetuses with pyelectasis was 3.3% and, therefore, suggested that when pyelectasis was present, the risk of Down syndrome was substantially higher than that associated with advanced maternal age or a low serum AFP (**Fig. 32–11**). The criteria used for pyelectasis were an anteroposterior diameter of the renal pelvis of 4 mm or greater between 15 and 20 weeks, 5 mm or greater between 20 and 30 weeks, and 7 mm or greater between 30 and 40 weeks.

Using criteria of > 4 mm before 33 weeks gestation and 7 mm or more at 33 weeks and later, Wickstrom et al found that isolated pyelectasis resulted in a 3.9-fold increase in the risk of Down syndrome over the age-related a priori risk.[34] In contrast, Vintzileos et al. found that isolated pyelectasis was not associated with an increased risk for trisomy 21.[35] The increase in risk above the risk assigned by the triple marker screen (if any) is unknown.

Choroid Plexus Cysts

Recent evidence indicates that the frequency of choroid plexus cysts (CPC) among fetuses with trisomy 21 is not significantly different from normal fetuses and that the previous reports of a few fetuses with trisomy 21 having CPC is likely the result of coincidence(**Fig. 32–12**).[36]

Echogenic Intracardiac Focus

In a population at 1/250 risk for trisomy 21, Bromley and coworkers suggested that there is an increased incidence of trisomy 21 among fetuses with intracardiac echogenic foci (**Fig. 32–13**),[37] although most fetuses with this finding are normal (**Fig. 32–14**). Of 1334 fetuses, 66 had an echogenic intracardiac focus, most commonly in the LV but also in the RV and bilaterally, and four of these 66 fetuses had trisomy 21. Eighteen other fetuses identified with trisomy 21 during the study period did not have echogenic intracardiac foci. The

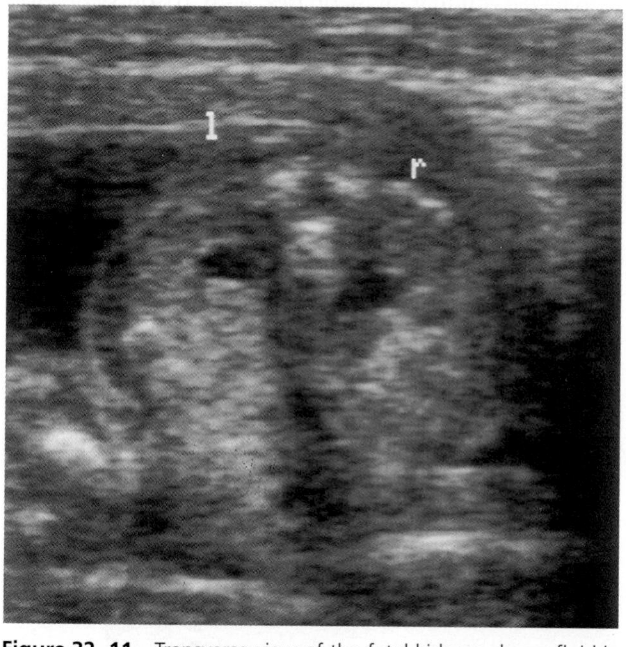

Figure 32–11 Transverse view of the fetal kidneys shows fluid in the renal pelves bilaterally consistent with mild fetal pyelectasis.

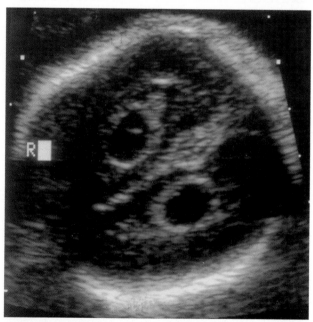

Figure 32–12 Semicoronal view of the fetal head shows bilateral cystic lesions in the choroid plexus of the lateral ventricles consistent with choroid plexus cysts. (R, right)

positive predictive value of an echogenic intracardiac focus for trisomy 21 was 6.1% in their population where the incidence of trisomy 21 was 1.6% (significantly higher than the standard quoted 1/250 or 0.4% for women ≥ 35 years). However, one of the six fetuses also had nuchal thickening and one was scanned at 14 weeks, making it difficult to determine whether this was truly an isolated finding. Thus, only two of their fetuses with isolated echogenic intracardiac foci had complete anatomical surveys. The risk ratio of trisomy 21 in this setting is not statistically significant.

A recent study by Manning et al. has also suggested a statistically significant association between intracardiac echogenic foci and trisomy 21.[38] Of 901 at-risk fetuses in their study, 24 had an echogenic focus. Of these 24, three (13%) had trisomy 21. Of the 877 fetuses without echogenic foci, 14 (2%) had trisomy 21. The sensitivity, specificity, and positive and negative predictive values of

echogenic intracardiac foci for trisomy 21 in their study were 18%, 98%, 13%, and 98% respectively. Therefore, in women with a positive triple marker screen, this sign should probably be interpreted as suggestive of Down syndrome in the fetus.

Iliac Wing Angle

It has long been known that infants with trisomy 21 have greater iliac wing angles than do normal infants.[39] Recently, Bork et al. found that this difference could be identified in fetuses.[40] They found that, using a cutoff of 90 degrees, they could detect 91% of fetuses with trisomy 21. Using this criterion, their positive predictive value for trisomy 21 was 33% and their negative predictive value was 99.7%. This study suggests that this may be an extremely valuable marker for trisomy 21. Further investigation with larger numbers of fetuses is needed.

Frontal Lobe Shortening

Children with Down syndrome have been shown to have brachycephaly related to decreased frontal lobe growth.[41] Winter et al. recently evaluated the difference between the frontothalamic distance in fetuses with trisomy 21 and normal fetuses.[42] They found that fetuses with trisomy 21 had statistically significantly smaller frontal lobes than normal and suggests that this may be a useful adjunctive screening marker with other signs in the sonographic evaluation for Down syndrome.

Separation of the Great Toe

Separation of the great toe from the second toe is a recognized finding in neonates with trisomy 21. Recently, this finding was reported in two fetuses who had trisomy 21 (**Fig. 32–15**).[43] This finding also occurs in

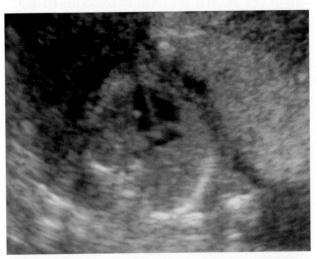

Figure 32–13 Four-chamber view of the fetal heart showing an echogenic intracardiac focus in the left ventricle in a fetus with trisomy 21.

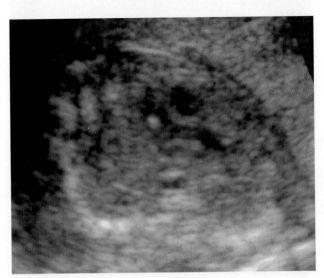

Figure 32–14 Left ventricular outflow tract view shows an echogenic intracardiac focus in the left ventricle of a normal fetus.

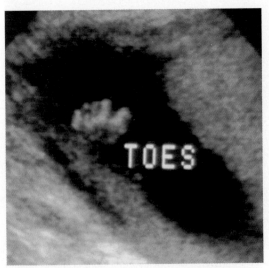

Figure 32–15 View of the fetal foot shows separation between the great toe and the second toe in a fetus with trisomy 21.

many normal babies (**Fig. 32–16**) and there are insufficient data to determine the PPV of this finding for trisomy 21 or guide management when this finding is made in low- or high-risk patients.

Hypoplasia of the Fifth Middle Phalanx and Clinodactyly

These anatomic findings are also recognized in neonates with trisomy 21 and, although their presence has been reported antenatally in fetuses with trisomy 21 (**Fig. 32–17**), there is too little information available to determine PPV or the utility of making these observations in utero.

Scoring Index Based on Combination of Sonographic Findings

It would seem logical that the identification of more than one of the aforementioned fetal sonographic markers for trisomy 21 would increase the likelihood that the fetus is affected. In 1992, Benacerraf and colleagues developed a scoring system using a combination of sonographic findings to assist in assigning a risk for trisomy 21 to a particular fetus.[13] This scoring index continues to undergo modification as additional information is obtained.[37,44] Other investigators have followed suit and these scoring indices are outlined in **Table 32–2** for comparison.[5,6] Nyberg et al. were the only group to look specifically and exclusively at women with positive triple marker screens. As shown in **Table 32–2**,

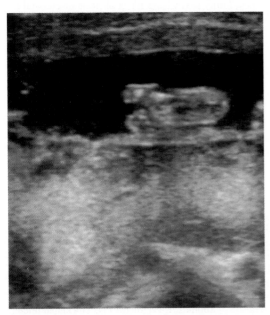

Figure 32–16 View of the fetal foot shows separation of the great toe and second toe in a normal fetus.

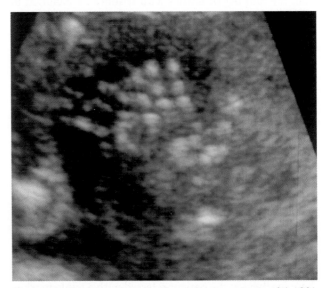

Figure 32–17 View of the fetal hand shows curving in of the fifth phalanx toward the fourth consistent with clinodactyly in a fetus with trisomy 21.

Table 32–2 Outcomes of scoring indices from three different authors utilizing different sonographic markers

Sonographic finding	Author scoring index		
	Benacerraf et al., 1994[a] Score ≥ 2	Nyberg et al., 1995[b] Score ≥ 1	Vintzilleos et al., 1997[c] Score ≥ 1
Cardiac defect or other major abnormalities	2	1	NA
Nuchal thickening	2	1	1
Echogenic bowel	1	1	NA
Short femur or short humerus	1	NA	NA
Short Femur	NA	1	1
Short humerus	NA	NA	NA
Mild pyelectasis	1	1	1
Cerebral ventricular dilatation	NA	1	NA
For scores:	Score ≥ 2	Score ≥ 1	Score ≥ 1
Sensitivity	73%	50%	87%
Specificity	96%	NA	NA
False-positive rate	3.8%	5.1%	6.7%
PPV	6.9%	NA	NA
NPV	NA	NA	NA

[a] Reference 44. [b] Reference 6. [c] Reference 5. NA, not available.

there is marked variability in the performance of the scoring indices reported by different authors, and they are difficult to compare as each utilizes different combinations of markers. A large multicenter trial with uniform scoring criteria is needed.

Risk Adjustment Based on Sonographic Findings

In theory, the risk of fetal trisomy 21 based on an abnormal triple marker can be modified based on the sonographic assessment. In particular, the risk of trisomy 21 will decrease if the fetal sonogram is normal.[6,45,46] Unfortunately, as yet the quantification of risk reduction is not possible, because the risks associated with various markers have varied among published studies. In addition, the number of fetuses with trisomy 21 included in these studies is often very small[6,46] making it impossible to quantify risk accurately. One meta-analysis of second-trimester sonographic assessment for Down syndrome suggested using the fetal sonographic finding to modify risk assessment in both high- and low-risk fetuses.[35] Others, however, have questioned their methods and suggested that using sonography in this way is premature.[47]

Summary

There are many sonographic markers that have been reported to be associated with trisomy 21. Along with the many markers is significant controversy regarding their individual and collective utility in accurately predicting the presence of Down syndrome. In utilizing these markers in the patient referred with a triple marker screen positive for Down syndrome, it should be remembered that their sensitivities, specificities, and positive and negative predictive values were often established in patient populations characterized by low AFP and advanced maternal age. How their individual or collective presence affects the risk assigned by the triple marker screen is not yet quantified, nor is how the triple marker screen and sonographic findings can be used jointly to define risk quantified. Multicenter studies including large numbers of trisomy 21 fetuses are needed to address these issues with sufficient statistical power to draw meaningful conclusions.

References

1. Adams MM, Erickson JD, Layde PM et al. Down syndrome: recent trends in the United States. *JAMA* 1981;246:758.
2. Youings S, Gregson N, Jacobx P. The efficacy of maternal age screening for Down syndrome in Wessex. *Prenat Diagn* 1991;11:419—425.
3. The California expanded alpha-fetoprotein screening program prenatal care provider handbook. California Department of Health Services, Genetic Disease Branch. 2151 Berkeley Way, Annex 4, Berkeley, CA 94704.
4. Benacerraf BR, Barss VA, Laboda LA. A sonographic sign for the detection in the second trimester of the fetus with Down's syndrome. *Am J Obstet Gynecol* 1985;151;1078—1079.
5. Vintzileos AM, Campbell WA, Guzman ER et al. Second-trimester ultrasound markers for detection of trisomy 21: which markers are best? *Obstet Gynecol* 1997;89:941—944.
6. Nyberg DA, Luthy DA, Cheng EY et al. Role of prenatal ultrasonography in women with positive screen for Down syndrome on the basis of maternal serum markers. *Am J Obstet Gynecol* 1995;173:1030—1035.
7. Nyberg DA, Dubinsky T, Resta RG et al. Echogenic fetal bowel during the second trimester: clinical importance. *Radiology* 1993;188:527—531.
8. Pajkrt E, Bilardo CM, Van Lith JMM et al. Nuchal translucency measurement in normal fetuses. *Obstet Gynecol* 1995;86:944—947.
9. Benacerraf BR, Frigoletto FD Jr, Cramer DW. Down syndrome: sonographic sign for diagnosis in the second-trimester fetus. *Radiology* 1987;163:811—813.
10. Benacerraf BR, Gelman R, Frigoletto FD. Sonographic identification of second-trimester fetuses with Down's syndrome. *N Eng J Med* 1987;317:1371—1376.
11. Benacerraf BR, Cnann A, Gelman R et al. Can sonographers reliably identify anatomic features associated with Down syndrome in fetuses? *Radiology* 1989;173:377—380.
12. Crane JP, Gray DL. Sonographically measured nuchal skinfold thickness as a screening tool for Down syndrome: results of a prospective clinical trial. *Obstet Gynecol* 1991;77:533—536.
13. Benacerraf BR, Laboda LA, Frigoletto FD. Thickened nuchal fold in fetuses not at risk for aneuploidy. *Radiology* 1992;184:239—242.
14. Donnenfeld AE, Carlson DE, Palomaki GE et al. Prospective multicenter study of second-trimester nuchal skinfold thickness in unaffected and Down syndrome pregnancies. *Obstet Gynecol* 1994;84:844—847.
15. Watson WJ, Miller RC, Menard MK et al. Ultrasonographic measurement of fetal nuchal skin to screen for chromosomal abnormalities. *Am J Obstet Gynecol* 1994;170:583—586.
16. Toi A, Simpson GF, Filly RA. Ultrasonically evident fetal nuchal skin thickening: is it specific for Down syndrome? *Am J Obstet Gynecol* 1987;156:150—153.
17. Hill LM, Guzick D, Belfar HL et al. The current role of sonography in the detection of Down syndrome. Obstet Gynecol 1989;74:620—623.
18. Ginsberg N, Cadkin A, Pergament et al. Ultrasonographic detection of the second-trimester fetus with trisomy 18 and trisomy 21. *Am J Obstet Gynecol* 1990;163:1186—1190.
19. Grandjean H, Sarramon M-F. Sonographic measurement of nuchal skinfold thickness for detection of Down syndrome in the second-trimester fetus: a multicenter prospective study. *Obstet Gynecol* 1995;85:103—106.
20. Nyberg DA, Resta TG, Luthy DA et al. Prenatal sonographic findings of Down syndrome: review of 94 cases. *Obstet Gynecol* 1990;76:370.

21. Scioscia AL, Pretorius DH, Budorick NE et al. Second-trimester echogenic bowel and chromosomal abnormalities. *Am J Obstet Gynecol* 1992;167:889—894.

22. Bromley B, Doubilet P, Frigoletto FD Jr et al. Is fetal hyperechoic bowel on second-trimester sonogram an indication for amniocentesis? *Obstet Gynecol* 1994;83:647—645.

23. Dicke JM, Crane JP. Sonographically detected hyperechoic fetal bowel: Significance and implications for pregnancy management. *Obstet Gynecol* 1992;80:778—782.

24. Sepulveda W, Hollingsworth J, Bower S et al. Fetal hyperechogenic bowel following intra-amniotic bleeding. *Obstet Gynecol* 1994;83:947—950.

25. Fakhry J, Reiser M, Shapiro LR et al. Increased echogenicity in the lower fetal abdomen: a common normal variant in the second trimester. *J Ultrasound Med* 1986;5:489—492.

26. Wald NJ, Smith D, Kennard A et al. Biparietal diameter and crown-rump length in fetuses with Down's syndrome: implications for antenatal serum screening for Down's syndrome. *Br J Obstet Gynecol* 1993;100:430—435.

27. Lockwood C, Benacerraf B, Krinsky A et al. A sonographic screening method for Down syndrome. *Am J Obstet Gynecol* 1987;157:803—808.

28. Perrela R, Duerinckx AJ, Grant EG et al. Second-trimester sonographic diagnosis of Down Syndrome: role of femur-length shortening and nuchal-fold thickening. *AJR* 1988;151:981—985.

29. LaFollette L, Filly RA, Anderson R et al. Fetal femur length to detect trisomy 21: a reappraisal. *J Ultrasound Med* 1989;8:657—660.

30. Lynch L, Berkowitz GS, Chitkara U et al. Ultrasound detection of Down syndrome: is it really possible? *Obstet Gynecol* 1989;73:267—270.

31. FitzSimmons J, Droste S, Shepard TH et al. Long-bone growth in fetuses with Down syndrome. *Am J Obstet Gynecol* 1989;161:1174—1177.

32. Benacerraf BR, Neuberg D, Frigoletto FD Jr. Humeral shortening in second-trimester fetuses with Down syndrome. *Obstet Gynecol* 1991;77:233—227.

33. Benacerraf BR, Mandell J, Estroff JA et al. Fetal pyelectasis: a possible association with Down syndrome. *Obstet Gynecol* 1990;76:58—60.

34. Wickstrom EA, Thangavelu M, Parilla BV et al. A prospective study of the association between isolated fetal pyelectasis and chromosomal abnormality. *Obstet Gynecol* 1996;88:379—382.

35. Vintzileos AM, Egan JFX. Adjusting the risk for trisomy 21 on the basis of secondrimester ultrasonography. *Am J Obstet Gynecol* 1995;172:837—844.

36. Bromley B, Lieberman E, Benacerraf BR. Choroid plexus cysts: not associated with Down syndrome. *Ultrasound Obstet Gynecol* 1996:8;232—235.

37. Bromley B, Lieberman E, Laboda L et al. Echogenic intracardiac focus: a sonographic sign for fetal Down syndrome. *Obstet Gynecol* 1995;86:998—1001.

38. Manning JE, Ragavendra N, Sayre J et al. Significance of fetal intracardiac echogenic foci in relation to trisomy 21: a prospective sonographic study of high-risk women. *AJR* 1998;170:1083—1084.

39. Caffey J, Ross S. Mongolism (mongloid deficiency) during early infancy: some newly recognized diagnostic changes in the pelvic bones. *Pediatrics* 1956;17:6442—6451.

40. Bork MD, Egan JFX, Cusick W et al. Iliac wing angle as a marker for trisomy 21 in the second trimester. *Obstet Gynecol* 1997;89:734—737.

41. Schmidt-Sidor B, Wisniewski K, Shepard T et al. Brain growth in Down syndrome subjects 15 to 22 weeks of gestational age and birth to 60 months. *Clin Neuropathol* 1990;9:181—190.

42. Winter TC, Reichman JA, Luna JA et al. Frontal lobe shortening in second-trimester fetuses with trisomy 21: usefulness as a US marker. *Radiology* 1998;207:215—222.

43. Wilkins I. Separation of the great toe in fetuses with Down syndrome. *J Ultrasound Med* 1994;13:229—231.

44. Benacerraf BR, Nadel A, Bromley B. Identification of second-trimester fetuses with autosomal trisomy by use of a sonographic scoring index. *Radiology* 1994;193:135—140.

45. Nadel AS, Bromley B, Frigoletto FD et al. Can the presumed risk of autosomal trisomy be decreased in fetuses of older women following a normal sonogram? *JUM* 1995;14:297—302.

46. Bahado-Singh RO, Goldstein I, Uerpairojkit B et al. Normal nuchal thickness in the midtrimester indicates reduced risk of Down syndrome in pregnancies with abnormal triple-screen results. *Am J Obstet Gynecol* 1995;173:1106—1110.

47. Palomaki GE, Haddow JE. Can the risk for Down syndrome be reliably modified by second-trimester ultrasonography? *Am J Obstet Gynecol* 1995;173(5):1639—1640.

33 Diabetes Mellitus and Pregnancy: The Role of Ultrasound

Peter W. Callen

It has been estimated that diabetes mellitus affects between one and two million women of childbearing age in the United States.[1] The management of this disease has evolved from an attempt to improve maternal survival in the 1900s and fetal survival in the middle part of the century to the prevention of fetal morbidity in the 1990s. The diagnosis and management of the maternal complications of diabetes mellitus are numerous and complex and will not be addressed in this discussion. Rather, the fetal complications, including fetal malformations, growth disturbances, including intrauterine growth restriction, and macrosomia, and prematurity will be discussed.[2, 3]

Pathophysiology and Classification

Pregnancy itself has often been referred to as diabetogenic. In fact, this is only partially true. In the first trimester, estrogen and progesterone induced pancreatic ß-cell hyperplasia result in increased insulin production and a lowering of fasting blood sugar in both diabetic and nondiabetic pregnancies. In the second and third trimesters, the levels of human placental lactogen, a polypeptide hormone which is an insulin antagonist, rise. In addition, prolactin, cortisol, estrogen, and progesterone also exert a contrainsulin effect.

Diabetes mellitus occurring during pregnancy has been traditionally categorized according to the White classification. The basis of this system relied upon the fact that the severity of diabetes can be quantified and is directly related to both maternal and perinatal outcomes. The White classification grouped patients into classes A through F on the basis of the type of therapy administered, the duration of maternal diabetes before pregnancy, and the presence or absence of maternal vascular complications. Class A refers to those patients with gestational diabetes, whereas classes B,C, and D include patients with diabetes mellitus predating their pregnancies. Classes F, R, and H represent those diabetic women with evidence of vascular disease. While the White classification has been useful for identifying women at risk for an adverse outcome, it has recently fallen into disuse. As our understanding of diabetes and pregnancy has improved it has become clear that most of the fetal risk is related to the time during pregnancy when diabetes is present, the degree of metabolic control achieved with therapy, the presence of maternal vascular complications and the presence of medical complications, such as hypertension and urinary tract infections.

A more modern classification divides patients into two large groups: those whose diabetes antedated pregnancy (pregestational diabetes) and those whose diabetes was first diagnosed during gestation (gestational diabetes).[4] Fetal risks in the former group include those derived from maternal metabolic abnormalities during the first trimester (birth defects and spontaneous abortion) as well as the second and third trimesters (i.e., macrosomia, hyperinsulinemia, and stillbirth). Fetal risks in women with gestational diabetes are primarily dervied from metabolic abnormalities in the second and third trimesters. In addition to the above classifications, diabetes mellitus may also be characterized as Type I, insulin-dependent diabetes mellitus (IDDM) and Type II, noninsulin-dependent diabetes mellitus. Type I diabetes is the ketotic-prone form of the disorder, while Type II is the so-called *maturity-onset*, nonketotic prone form of the disease.

Ultrasound in the Diabetic Pregnancy

Through the use of fetal biometry, ultrasound is able to determine fetal age, weight, and growth. The accurate determination of fetal gestational age is important in the diabetic patient to aid in the timing and interpretation of maternal serum AFP levels, aid in the timing of third trimester amniocentesis and delivery, and in the evaluation of fetal growth. In patients in whom the menstrual history is uncertain, first trimester ultrasound may be necessary to establish the gestational age to aid in the timing of either maternal serum AFP testing or amniocentesis. Accuracy within 4—7 days may be achieved in most cases. As will be discussed later, while the accuracy for estimating gestational age is excellent, the ability to detect many significant fetal malformations is poor in the first trimester. A sonogram performed between 18 and 20 weeks of gestation will still have an accuracy of +/- one week for defining gestational age and have a greater than 90% likelihood of detecting serious fetal malformations.

Fetal Malformations

Perhaps the most significant fetal complication of pregnancy encountered by pregestational diabetic women is a significantly increased risk of fetal congenital malformations. An association between diabetes mellitus and congenital malformations was suspected as early as 1885 when it was reported that infants of diabetic mothers had an increased incidence of congenital malformations.[5–7] In a study done between 1926 and 1963, 6.4% of infants of diabetic mothers had major congenital malformations compared to 2.1% in the control group.[8] Virtually all other studies done subsequently have verified the increased incidence of congenital malformations in this population to be three to four times that of controls.[5,9,10] Congenital malformations account for 35 to 40% of all perinatal deaths and are the leading cause of death among infants of diabetic mothers.[1]

The malformations most commonly observed are cardiac defects, neural tube defects, caudal regression syndrome (sacral agenesis), and renal abnormalities (**Fig. 33–1, 33–2**). Although the focus of many clinical centers is on the detection of neural tube disease in pregestational diabetics, cardiac abnormalities are by far the most common abnormalities in these patients. The

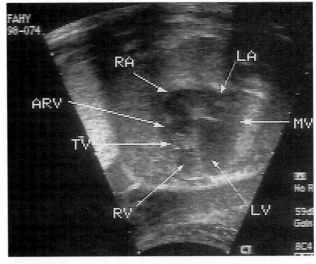

Figure 33–1 Four-chamber view from a fetal echocardiogram in a diabetic patient. Typical findings of inferior displacement of the triscuspid valve (TV) with an atrialized right ventricle (ARV) is seen. RA, right atrium; LA, left atrium; MV, mitral valve; RV, right ventricle; LV, left ventricle. (Case courtesy of Norman Silverman, M.D., San Francisco, CA, U.S.A.)

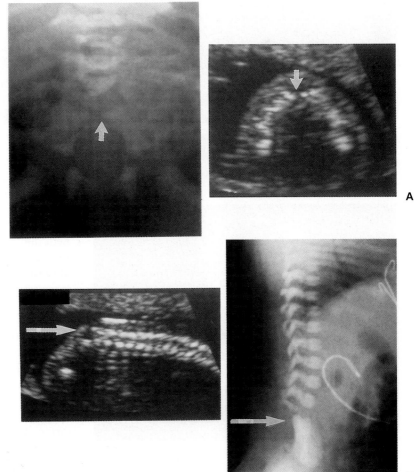

Figure 33–2 (A) AP radiograph and sonographic transverse axial plane of section of a fetus with sacral agenesis and preconceptional diabetes at 26 weeks gestation. Medial aspects of the iliac wings are in close proximation to one another (**arrow**). (**B**) Sagittal plane of section sonogram and lateral radiograph from the same patient as in **A**. Absence of the normal continuation of the spine into the sacrum is seen (**arrow**). (Case courtesy of Nancy Budorick, M.D., New York, NY, U.S.A.).

reported incidence of cardiac abnormalities is increased to between 2 and 4% in pregestational diabetics as compared to the incidence of 0.8% in the general nondiabetic population.[1,11] The abnormalities most commonly seen are conotruncal abnormalities such as transposition of the great vessels (**Fig. 33–3**), truncus arteriosis, (**Fig. 33–4**), tetralogy of Fallot (**Fig. 33–5**), and ventricular septal defects (**Fig. 33–6**). Many of the abnormalities will not be detected with just the standard four chamber view of the heart. In a recent study by Smith et al., the sensitivity of ultrasound for detecting an abnormal heart increased from 73% with the four-chamber view (**Fig. 33–7**) to 82% with the addition of the aortic outflow tract view (**Fig. 33–8**). There were two false-negative and no false-positive diagnoses. In their study, when the four-chamber view and outflow tracts appeared normal, additional views such as the ductal and aortic arches did not detect a cardiac defect. Additional cardiac abnormalities which may be seen in the diabetic patient include cardiomyopathy (**Fig. 33–9**) and aortic coarctation. Clearly, if a gravid diabetic patient is to have an ultrasound evaluation for the purpose of detecting morphologic abnormalities, it should include an evaluation of the fetal heart by an experienced fetal and/or pediatric echocardiographer.

Neural tube defects are increased in the diabetic population. The incidence of neural tube defects is said to be 19.5 per thousand in diabetic mothers compared to one to two per thousand in the general population.[12] Anencephaly (**Fig. 33–10**) as well as myelomeningoceles (**Fig. 33–11**) may be seen in this population. Caudal regression syndrome (sacral agenesis) is wrongly often assumed to be an abnormality seen only in the diabetic population. Caudal regression, in which there is hypo-

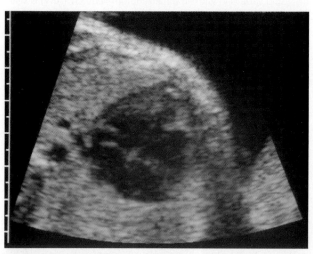

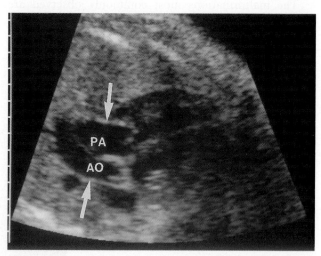

Figure 33–3 Transposition of the great vessels. (**A**) Normal four-chamber view of the fetal heart. (**B**) View of cardiac outflow tracts demonstrates the two great vessels arising from the heart in parallel to each other (**arrows**) with the aorta (AO) arising from the right ventricle and the pulmonary artery (PA) arising from the left ventricle. (Case courtesy of Carol B. Benson, M.D., Boston, MA, U.S.A.)

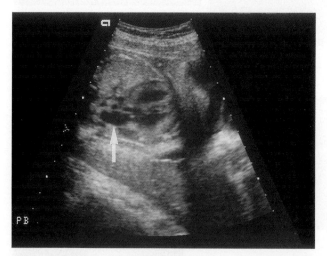

Figure 33–4 Truncus arteriosus. Long axis view of fetal heart demonstrating single large vessel (**arrow**) arising from both ventricles (Case courtesy of Carol B. Benson, M.D., Boston, MA, U.S.A.)

plasia of the sacrum and lower extremities was first described in 1964 as being more common in infants of diabetic mothers.[13] Associated anomalies which may be seen at birth are fusion of the lower limbs (sirenomelia), absence of the bladder, imperforate anus, absence of external genitalia, renal agenesis, and single umbilical artery. As was stated above, the abnormalities that form the basis of caudal regression syndrome may be seen in nondiabetics as well.

A number of other abnormalities may also be seen in pregestational diabetics including fetal hydronephrosis, skeletal abnormalities, and ocular and skin defects. A study by Petrikovsky et al. evaluated a group of 12 patients with a hypoplastic umbilical artery (**Fig. 33–12**) (artery to artery difference of greater than 50%).[14] They found that 1/3 of the patients were diabetic. Another study by Weissman et al. found that the umbilical cord was significantly larger in fetuses of mothers with ge-

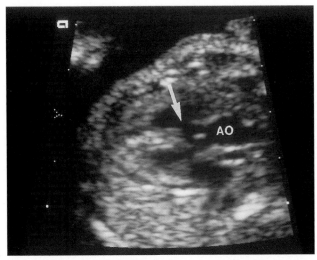

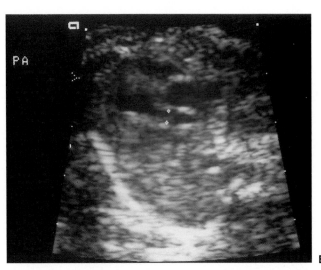

Figure 33–5 Tetralogy of Fallot (**A**) Long axis view of fetal aortic outflow tract demonstrating overriding aorta (AO) and ventricular septal defect (**arrow**). (**B**) The pulmonary artery (calipers) was small. (Case courtesy of Carol B. Benson, M.D., Boston, MA, U.S.A.)

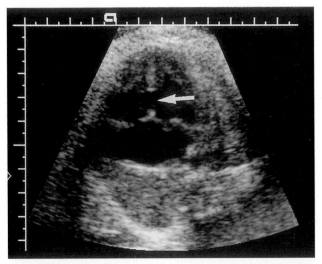

Figure 33–6 Ventricular septal defect. four-chamber view of fetal heart demonstrating defect in ventricular septum (**arrow**). (Case courtesy of Carol B. Benson, M.D., Boston, MA, U.S.A.)

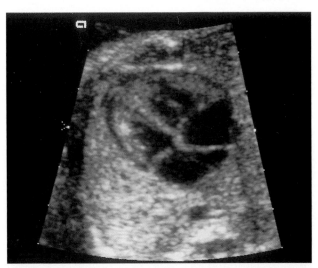

Figure 33–7 Normal four-chamber view of fetal heart. (Case courtesy of Carol B. Benson, M.D., Boston, MA, U.S.A.)

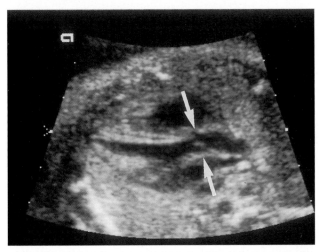

Figure 33–8 Normal aortic outflow tract (**arrows**) arising from left ventricle. (Case courtesy of Carol B. Benson, M.D., Boston, MA, U.S.A.)

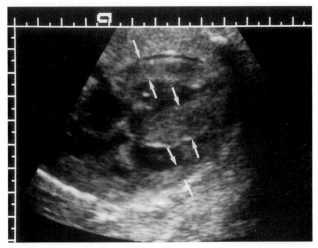

Figure 33–9 Cardiomyopathy. Four-chamber view of fetal heart demonstrating thickening of the walls of both ventricles (**arrows**) and the septum. (Case courtesy of Carol B. Benson, M.D., Boston, MA, U.S.A.)

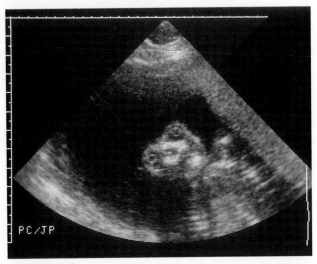

Figure 33–10 Ancencaphlic fetus. Sonogram demonstrates fetal face with absence of cranium. (Case courtesy of Carol B. Benson, M.D., Boston, MA, U.S.A.)

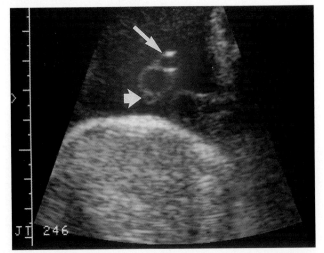

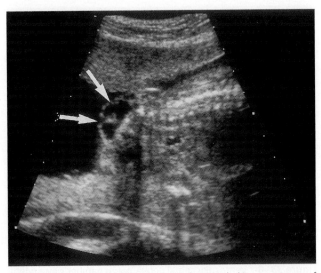

A

B

Figure 33–11 Meningomyelocele (**A**) Transverse sonogram of lower spine demonstrating spinal defect with cystic dorsal sac (**arrows**). (**B**) Longitudinal view of lower spine demonstrating disruption of spine and posterior cystic mass (**arrows**). (Case courtesy of Carol B. Benson, M.D., Boston, MA, U.S.A.)

Figure 33–12 Hypoplastic umbilical artery. Transverse image of three-vessel umbilical cord with one normal umbilical artery (**arrow**) and one hypoplastic (**arrowhead**). (Case courtesy of Carol B. Benson, M.D., Boston, MA, U.S.A.)

stational diabetes than in the normal population.[15] The main increase in width was attributed to an increase in Wharton jelly content.

The exact mechanism leading to an increased incidence of congenital malformations is controversial. Insulin is unlikely to be the cause of malfomations as it does not cross the placenta, and fetal insulin is not produced until after organogenesis. Hyperglycemia has been implicated as the main cause of malformations. Maternal glycosylated hemaglobin (Hb A1 c) is a reflection of average maternal glucose levels during the preceding 6 to 8 weeks. When these values are found to be elevated in the early second trimester, it raises the concern that the diabetes is poorly controlled and that hyperglycemia may have been present at the time of organogenesis. One study found a 22% incidence of congenital anomalies among infants of diabetic mothers if the Hb A1 c was greater than 8.5%, and a 3% incidence if the Hb A1 c was less than 8.5%.[16]

Although the above-stated risks and malformations apply to the pregestational insulin-dependent diabetic, they do not apply to the patient with gestational diabetes. Historically, the chance of fetal malformations in gestational diabetics has been reported as not being appreciably different from that of the general population. The Collaborative Perinatal Project, a prospective study of 48,437 subjects from 14 institutions, revealed that diabetic women with pregnancy-induced glucose intolerance were not at increased risk for producing infants with congenital malformations.[10] These facts strongly implicate a first-trimester metabolic teratogen contribution in the pregestational diabetic population and give further credance to the notion of attempting to achieve optimal preconceptional glucose control in an attempt to decrease the risk of fetal malformations. An interesting, recent study by Schaefer et al. attempted to determine the risk of congenital malformations based upon the degree of hyperglycemia in women with gestational diabetes.[17] In their study, one or more major congenital anomalies were present in 2.9% of the newborns and an additional 2.4% had only minor abnormalities. In this study the highest fasting serum glucose level at diagnosis was the best predictor of the likelihood of congenital anomalies. When the authors stratified women into subgroups based upon the fasting serum glucose level at diagnosis, the incidence of major anomalies was as follows: 2.1% with a fasting serum glucose < 120 mg/dl, 5.2% with a fasting serum glucose level of 121 to 260 mg/dL and 30.4% with a fasting serum glucose level > 260 mg/dL. Their conclusion was that a fasting glucose level below that of overt diabetes outside of pregnancy carries an important risk of major anomalies that should be considered in the counseling of gravid patients.

Growth Disturbances

Infants of diabetic mothers can be affected by major growth disturbances, most commonly macrosomia. The etiology of the macrosomia is thought to be due to excess levels of insulin resulting from maternal hyperglycemia. The accelerated fetal growth seen in macrosomia is likely due to the structural similarity of insulin to human growth hormone. It should be remembered that while diabetic women have a higher incidence of macrosomia than nondiabetics, only approximately 2% of macrosomic fetuses will be born to mothers with diabetes mellitus.[18,19]

Macrosomia has been traditionally defined as a birth weight greater than the 90th percentile for gestational age or a birth weight greater than 4000 g. Ultrasound is capable of estimating fetal weight utilizing measurements of the fetus, of which the fetal abdomen is the most important. While fetal weight estimates are fairly accurate throughout pregnancy, they tend to be less so in the macrosomic fetus. One possible explanation is the greater amount of adipose tissue (not accounted for in most formulas for fetal weight estimation) in these fetuses.[18] A second problem is that because one of the definitions of macrosomia relates the weight to the menstrual age, when the menstrual age is not known this relationship is no longer meaningful. It is for this reason that menstrual age-independent indicators, such as the absolute measurement of the fetal abdomen or the relationship of the fetal abdomen to the fetal femur, have been used as methods of detecting these fetuses. These methods are far from perfect, however.

As shoulder dystocia is a major problem in the macrosomic diabetic fetus, several investigators have recently evaluated the utility of ultrasound in predicting this condition. Studies have evaluated either fetal subcutaneous tissue around the extremities or abdomen or various combinations of relationships of the fetal abdomen to other fetal parts.[20–22] In several studies, humeral soft tissue thickness greater than 12 mm was predictive of macrosomia with sensitivities of 88 to 96%.[23,24] There are, however, a number of studies in which ultrasound is only marginally better than clinical evaluation for the prediction of macrosomia.[25]

While macrosomia is the most common growth disturbance in diabetic pregnancies, intrauterine growth retardation can be seen in these patients as well. It is likely that the etiology in this population is decreased uteroplacental perfusion secondary to vascular compromise. The commonly used definition of fetuses below the 10% weight for gestational age is also used in this population.

Polyhydramnios

Virtually every discussion concerning polyhydramnios will list diabetes mellitus as a common etiology. While it is true that polyhydramnios can be seen in patients with diabetes mellitus, it relates more to three factors than the actual disease itself: (1) Patients with poor glycemic control are more likely to have polyhydramnios than those whose blood glucose are normal, (2) those patients with macrosomic fetuses (either diabetic or nondiabetic) are more likely to have polyhydramnios, and (3) fetuses with morphologic abnormalities (which may be seen in the pregestational diabetic group) may have polyhydramnios.

Prematurity

Diabetic patients tend to have an increased incidence of premature deliveries, two to three times that of the general population.[2,26] Many of these deliveries are due to maternal complications including hypertension and preeclampsia. An additonal problem is that insulin-dependent diabetic pregnancies have delayed lung maturation. A recent series demonstrated that approximately 23% of patients with insulin-dependent diabetes were negative for amniotic fluid phosophatidylglycerol as late as 39 weeks.[4] Because of the risk for prematurity and respiratory distress syndrome, it is important that gestational age be established as accurately as possible. In general, the earlier in pregnancy that fetal biometry is performed using the ultrasound, the more accurate it is likely to be. While early first-trimester ultrasound examinations are quite accurate for establishing gestational age, they do not allow the accuracy in detection of fetal morphologic abnormalities. A reasonable compromise is to obtain a sonogram at 18 to 20 weeks of gestation, when the sonographic accuracy is still within 1 week.

References

1. 1. Reece EA. Diabetes-associated congenital anomalies:pathogenesis and prenatal diagnosis. *Ultrasound in Obstetrics and Gynecology.* In: F.C. Chervenak, G.C. Issacson, and S. Campbell, eds., Boston: Little, Brown and Co., 1993, p. 771—781.

2. Macones G, Silverman N. Diabetes during pregnancy. In: A.R. Spitzer, ed. *Intensive Care of the Fetus and Neonate,* St. Louis: Mosby-Year Book, Inc., 1996.

3. Costini NV, Kalkhott RK. Relative effects of pregnancy, estradiol and progesterone on plasma insulin and pancreatic islet insulin secretion. *J Clin Invest* 1971;50:992—999.

4. Buchanan TA and Coustan DR. Diabetes mellitus. In: G.N. Burrow and T.F. Ferris, eds. *Medical Complications During Pregnancy.* Philadelphia: WB Saunders and Co., 1995.

5. Shah, DM. Sonography in diabetic pregnancies. In: A.C. Fleischer et al., eds. *Sonography in Obstetrics and Gynecology,* Stamford: Appleton and Lange, 1996, p. 531–546.

6. Mills JL, Baker L, Goldman AS. Malformations in infants of diabetic mothers occur before the seventh gestational week: implications for treatment. *Diabetes* 1979;28:292.

7. Mills JL. Malformations in infants of diabetic mothers. *Teratology,* 1982;25:385.

8. Pedersen IM, Tygstrup I, Pedersen J. Congenital malformations in newborn infants of diabetic women. Correlation with maternal diabetic vascular complications. *Lancet* 1964;1:1124.

9. Kucera J. Rate and type of congenital anomalies among offspring of diabetic women. *J Reprod Med* 1971;7:61.

10. Chung CS, Myrianthopoulos NC. Factors affecting risks of congenital malformations: Report from the Collaborative Perinatal Project. *Birth Defects* 1975;11:23.

11. Rowland TW, Hubbell JP, Nadas AS. Congenital heart disease infants of diabetic mothers. *J Pediatr* 1973;83:815.

12. Milunsky A, et. al Prenatal diagnosis of neural tube defects VIII. The importance of serum alpha-fetoprotein screening in diabetic pregnant women. *Am J Obstet Gynecol* 1982;142:1030.

13. Lenz W, Maier W. Congenital malformations and maternal diabetes. *Lancet* 1964;2:1124.

14. Petrikovsky B, Schneider E. Prenatal diagnosis and clinical significance of hypoplastic umbilical artery. *Prenatal Diagn* 1996;16:938—940.

15. Weissman A, Jakobi P. Sonographic measurements of the umbilical cord in pregnancies complicated by gestational diabetes. *J Ultrasound Med* 1997;16:691—694.

16. Miller E, Hare JW, Cloherty JP, et al. Elevated maternal hemoglobin A1c in early pregnancy and major congenital anomalies in infants of diabetic mothers. *N Engl J Med* 1981;304:1331.

17. Schaefer UM, Songster G, Xiang A, et al. Congenital malformations in offspring of women with hyperglycemia first detected during pregnancy. *Am J Obstet Gynecol* 1997;177:1165—1171.

18. Hadlock FP. Ultrasound evaluation of fetal growth. In: P.W. Callen, ed. *Ultrasonography in Obstetrics and Gynecology,* Philadelphia: W.B. Saunders and Co., 1994, p. 129—143.

19. Boyd ME, Usher RH, McLean FH. Fetal macrosomia: Predictions, risks, proposed management. *Obstet Gynecol* 1983;61:715.

20. Santolaya-Forgas J, Meyer WJ, DW.,G, Kahn D. Intrapartum fetal subcutaneous tissue/femur length ratio: an ultrasonographic clue to fetal macrosomia. *Am J Obstet Gynecol* 1994;171:1072—1075.

21. Petrikovsky BM, Oleshuk C, Lesser M, Gelertner N, Gross B. Prediction of fetal macrosomia using sonographically measured abdominal subcutaneous tissue thickness. *J Clin Ultrasound* 1997;25:378—382.

22. Cohen B, Penning S, Major C,et al. Sonographic prediction of shoulder dystocia in infants of diabetic mothers. *Obstet Gynecol* 1996;88:10—13.

23. Sood A, Yancey M, Richards D. Prediction of fetal macrosomia using humeral soft tissue thickness. *Obstet Gynecol* 1995;85:937—940.

24. Mintz MC, Landon MB, Gabbe SG, et. al. Shoulder soft tissue width as a predictor of macrosomia in diabetic pregnancies. *Am J Perinatol* 1989;6:240.

25. Johnstone FD, Prescott RJ, Steel JM, et al. Clinical and ultrasound prediction of macrosomia in diabetic pregnancy. *Br J Obstet Gynaecol* 1996;103:747—754.

26. Greene MF, Hare JW, Krache M, et. al. Prematurity among insulin requiring diabetic women. *Am J Obstet Gynecol* 1986;154:44.

34 Sonographic Evaluation of Fetus Following Teratogen Exposure

Mark. A. Kliewer

The original meaning of the word teratology was the study of monsters. In the prescientific era, babies born with deformities or defects were sometimes thought to represent monsters, grostesqueries, portents, and expressions of divine judgment.[1] Today, science has transformed teratology into the study of the causality, mechanism, and pathogenesis of human birth defects and congenital malformations. Broadly understood, teratogenesis results from genetic and environmental factors that singly or in concert alter the normal development of the embryo. Genetic aberrations are determined before conception, or at least differentiation, and exert a preemptive governing effect on development. Every neonate has at least a 5% risk of having a serious congenital abnormality, be it a malformation, mental retardation, or a functional deficit that becomes apparent only later in life.[2] Excluding those human malformations that can be attributed primarily to genetic aberrations and those for which no identifiable cause can be found, environmental teratogens account for approximately 10% of observed human malformations.[3] Those environmental agents that can cause developmental abnormalities include drugs, chemicals, infection, procedures, radiation, and hyperthermia.

Clinical Principles

Teratogens are identified and characterized on the basis of case reports of individuals, epidemiological studies of populations, and controlled laboratory studies on animals. Observed effects can be organized into four basic categories: malformation, growth retardation, death, and functional impairment.[4] Of these, growth disturbances are the most common and sensitive signs of exposure.[5]

There are four cardinal principles of teratogenicity.

Teratogens Exert Their Effects Idiosyncratically Across Individuals of a Population and Between Species

The expression of teratogenic effects is determined by a multitude of factors that interact in complex and unpredictable ways. The genetic constitutions of mother and fetus interact to create a unique background of resilience and vulnerability to a teratogen. Teratogenic effects can be further modified by the size, metabolism, parity, age, social class, and nutritional state of the mother, as well as the ethnicity, race, and gender of the baby.[6] In addition, numerous environmental factors, such as season, temperature, and geography have been shown to potentially influence the incidence of malformations.[4]

Interspecies differences are commonplace.[7] Though animal studies are invaluable for the investigation of mechanism and pathogenesis, the results of these studies are not always directly transposable to the human case. This was tragically and pointedly demonstrated in the case of thalidomide, where tests on rodents indicated the benignity of the drug before its release, with devastating consequences for thousands of human babies.

Susceptibility of a Developing Fetus to a Teratogenic Agent Depends on the Developmental Stage of the Fetus at the Time of Exposure

Three important stages are usually distinguished (**Fig. 34–1**).[8] The first stage, encompassing the two weeks from fertilization to early implantation, is a period before cellular differentiation has occurred in the embryo and before the establishment of a placental connection to the blood supply of the mother. The embryo is relatively invulnerable to most teratogens during this period. Unless an agent can reach the embryo through the mucous blanket of the maternal genital tract or by other means independent of the maternal blood system, the embryo will not be affected. Those agents, such as radiation, which are not delivered by the maternal blood supply will result in embryonic death if significant cell loss or chromosomal defects are produced. Countervailing these effects is the plasticity of omnipotential embryonic cells which can mount a potent reparative response. If affected at all, the embryo will tend to either recover or die. This binary response has been referred to as the "all or none" phenomenon. This is not to say that malformations cannot occur in this period, only that there is a propensity toward embryolethality rather than surviving malformed embryos.

The second stage of development extends from roughly the third to the eighth week after fertilization.

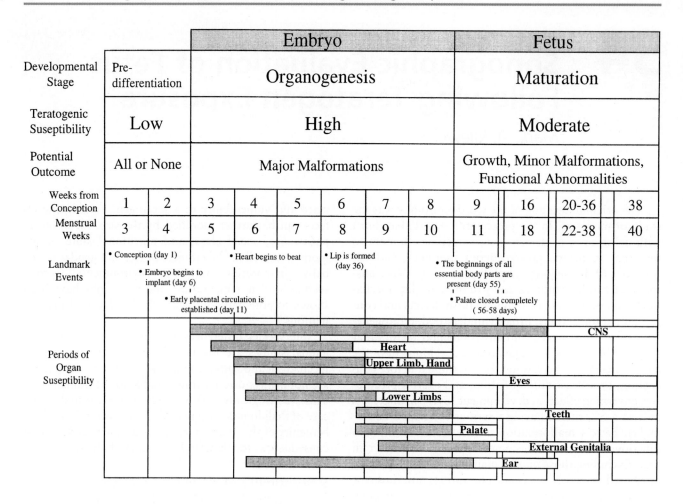

	Embryo								Fetus			
Developmental Stage	Pre-differentiation	Organogenesis							Maturation			
Teratogenic Susceptibility	Low	High							Moderate			
Potential Outcome	All or None	Major Malformations							Growth, Minor Malformations, Functional Abnormalities			
Weeks from Conception	1	2	3	4	5	6	7	8	9	16	20-36	38
Menstrual Weeks	3	4	5	6	7	8	9	10	11	18	22-38	40

Landmark Events:
- Conception (day 1)
- Embryo begins to implant (day 6)
- Early placental circulation is established (day 11)
- Heart begins to beat
- Lip is formed (day 36)
- The beginnings of all essential body parts are present (day 55)
- Palate closed completely (56-58 days)

Periods of Organ Susceptibility:
- CNS
- Heart
- Upper Limb, Hand
- Eyes
- Lower Limbs
- Teeth
- Palate
- External Genitalia
- Ear

Figure 34–1 Human embryonic development. Periods of greatest sensitivity (shaded) and lesser sensitivity to malformation are shown for individual organs. This chart is modified with permission from **Peace of Mind During Pregnancy** by C. Kelly-Bu- chanan, Philadelphia: Dell Publishers, 1989 and **The Developing Human — Clinically Oriented Embryology**, 4th ed., by K.L. Moore. Philadelphia: Publisher, 1988.

(Early developmental stages in this chapter are defined as weeks from the time of fertilization. The corresponding gestational age or menstrual age is calculated by adding two weeks.) This is the embryonic period when organogenesis occurs. During this stage, cells take on specific roles, grouping together to form organs at pre- scribed critical periods of formation.[9] Each organ, then, has a window of particular vulnerability to teratogenic insult. Unfortunately, this period of greatest teratogenic susceptibility begins before most women know them- selves to be pregnant, and sometimes even before the condition of pregnancy can be reliably ascertained.

The last stage of development, known as the fetal stage, begins after the ninth week after conception. With the important exceptions of the genitourinary system, the palate, and the brain, most organs have formed and thereafter proceed to mature, function, and grow. Tera- togenic insults during this period can lead to growth failure, and eventual disturbances of behavior or fertil- ity. Examples of behavioral teratogenicity include the hyperactivity, inattention, and tremulousness of children of narcotic addicted mothers; the mental retardation of children of women exposed to anticonvulsants, alcohol, and lead; and the abnormal reflexes of children of mothers exposed to methyl mercury.[10]

Teratogenic Induction is a Threshold Phenomenon

A dosage threshold must be exceeded for irreparable damage to be done. This can occur either as a single large dose or as repeated chronic exposure. The interaction of two or more drugs or chemicals may be synergistic. Equally important, especially for the parents, is the inverse formulation of this principle: there is a level below which no embryopathic effects can be measured.[11] The concept of a placental barrier has been debunked as specious: Most drugs and chemicals readily reach the fetus in significant concentration soon after administration.[12]

Typically, Teratogens Cause Characteristic Patterns of Malformations Rather Than Single Defects

The pattern of malformations represents not only the consequences of initial injury mediated through cell death and disruption of cell growth and metabolism, but also that of secondary reparative and regenerative processes. For example, the intraabdominal and intracranial calcifications characteristic of some viral infections represent a reparative response to initial injury.

Sonographic Approach

The sonologist evaluating a patient with teratogen exposure will need to assess first the developmental risks of the exposure. This requires interviewing the patient to determine the agent, the dose, and the timing of the exposure. Specific agents tend to produce specific patterns of abnormality. Both the incidence and severity of malformations tend to increase with the dose (Tables 34–1 and 34–2). As stated earlier, timing is crucial. Teratogenic exposures in the first two weeks following conception are less likely to result in malformation in embryos that survive. Exposures occurring during the embryonic stage should be placed as precisely as possible in those critical six weeks so that the examination can be concentrated on those organs most susceptible to injury **(Fig. 34–1)**.

Once risk is assessed, the sonologist will likely benefit from any of a number of informative or consultative resources. On-line data bases provide perhaps the most current and readily accessible summaries of the medical literature and estimates of risk. Such a particularly valuable service is the ReproTox system.[13] Other useful electronic resources that can be accessed on-line are the Teratogen Information System (TERIS),[14] ReproRisk, and Shepards Catalog of Teratogenic Agents.[15] If an unusual abnormality or pattern of abnormalities is found in a fetus, possible etiologies can be found in such data bases as POSSUM (Pictures Of Standard Syndromes and Undiagnosed Malformations), Platypus, and the London Dysmorphology Database. Finally, there are several excellent books and review articles that list teratogens and their described effects, though these will be variably current.[16—20] Though somewhat dated, the book, *Peace of Mind during Pregnancy* by Christine Keller-Buchanan, is particularly useful for counseling patients because it is

Table 34–1 Historical recognition of chemical teratogenesis in humans

Date discovered	Drug	Approximate number of malformed cases
1903	Antithyroid compounds	140
1950	Aminoglycoside antibiotics	60
1952	Anticancer agents	50
1953	Androgenic hormones	250
1956	Tetracyclines	Thousands
1961	Thalidomide	7700
1963	Phenytoin	Hundreds
1965	Hypervitaminosis A	20
1966	Coumarin anticoagulants	55
1967	Alcohol	Thousands
1970	Methadione anticonvulsants	40
1970	Lithium	25
1970	Diethylstilbestrol	Hundreds
1971	Penicallimine	5
1976	Primidone	25
1982	Valproic acid	100
1983	Vitamin A analogues	115
1987	Cocaine	Hundreds
1988	Carbamazepine	70

Reprinted with permission from *Chemically Induced Birth Defects,* 2nd ed. by James L. Schardein, New York: Marcel Dekker, Inc, 1993.

written in direct and clear language that will be accessible to most patients.[21]

Ultimately, the sonographic study of a pregnancy with a known teratogenic exposure will need to be more comprehensive and meticulous than routine studies. In addition to the routine fetal survey, scrutiny will need to be directed to the face, calvarium, spine, hear, limbs, hands, feet, and genitalia as well as the measures of fetal growth, amniotic fluid volume, and placental function. Knowing the probable effects of a teratogen will help focus this rather formidable and extensive survey (**Table 34–2**). This said, one small study of 126 pregnancies studied by ultrasound for teratogen exposure found only one structural abnormality.[22] This study, however, made no accounting of the magnitude or the timing of the exposures and included a broad miscellany of agents, most of which contribute five or less episodes of exposure each. Only the most virulent of teratogens is likely to demonstrate an effect in such a compilation of cases.

Craniofacial anomalies can generally be depicted with routine imaging, though more subtle abnormalities may require morphometric analysis.[23] Standardized linear measurements have been proposed to describe the growth of normal craniofacial structures, including the mandible. [24—26]

Even so, the morphometric approach has not been widely adopted in prenatal laboratories, partly due to the problem of obtaining reproducible planes of imaging, and partly due to the inherent imprecision of the relatively small measurements. Nonetheless, these techniques have been well established in infants and children,[27] and may yet prove to be transposable to the fetus.

Table 34–2   Sites of teratogenic abnormality   Sites routinely visited and documented

Agent		Central nervous system	Spine	Abdomen	Kidneys	Growth	Placenta, cervix
Thalidomide			Spine malformations	Duodenal atresia Esophageal atresia	Renal agenesis		
Antithyroid agents							
Anticonvulsant therapy	Hydantoins	Microcephaly					
	Valproic acid	Microcephaly, hydrocephaly	Neural tube defects				
	Trimethadione	Microcephaly[a]		Esophageal atresia	Renal malformation	IUGR[a]	
	Carbamazepine		Neural tube defect	Anal atresia, absent gallbladder		IUGR	
Coumarin		Microcephaly, hydrocephaly, Dandy Walker, Agenesis of the corpus callosum	Scoliosis			IUGR	
Retinoids		Hydrocephalus,[a] absent cereballar vermis, cerebellar hypoplasia, microcephaly					
Cyclophosphamide	(Alkylating agents)	Microcephaly		Imperforate anus		IUGR[a]	
Methotrexate	(Antimetabolic agents)	Skull malformation, hydrocephaly,[a] anencephaly, cerebral hypoplasia	Neural tube defect			IUGR[a]	
Lithium		Hydrocephalus	Neural tube defects				
Tetracycline						Depression of bone growth[a]	
Progestins, estrogens			Vertebral anomalies (?)	Anorectal atresia (?) TEF (?)	renal abnormalities(?)		
Ethanol		Microcephaly,[a] Holoprosencephaly, agenesis of the corpus callosum	Neural tube defect, scoliosis	Diaphragmatic hernia	Hydronephrosis, small kidneys	IURG[a]	
Cocaine		Cranial defects, encephalocele, cerebral infarction		Bowel obstruction,[a] intestinal perforation	Hydronephrosis,[a] renal agenesis, renal ectopica[a]	IUGR[a]	Abruption,[a] premature labor

[a] Dominant effects. CHD, congenital heart disease, tetralogy of Fallot; HLH, hypoplastic left heart; VSD, ventricular septal defect; ASD, atrial septal defect; TGV, transposition of the great vessels; TEF, tracheo-esophageal fistula; IUGR, intrauterine growth restriction.

Functional and neurobehavioral effects may be revealed in observations of fetal breathing, movement, behavior, and adaptability to stimulus. The agitated behavioral state of a cocaine-exposed fetus may be the only detectable abnormality. Choanal atresia in a coumarin-exposed fetus could theoretically be detected by an abnormal pattern of fetal breathing visible with color Doppler techniques. Such observations test the limits of the capabilities, skills, and patience of the examiner. The success of the enterprise, however, will finally depend on the ability of the sonologist to make subtle and careful observation.

Pharmaceuticals

The use of drugs is endemic in our society. An average of 1% of pregnant women are exposed to drugs sometime during their gestation, and the average number of drugs taken is approximately six.[28] Nonetheless, apart from exposures to established teratogens, the risk of a major fetal malformation following general maternal drug use is low: Case-control studies from large birth registries suggest an odds ratio of 1.2.[29]

The notion that the uterus is a privileged sanctuary for the fetus, largely impervious to the noxious agents of

B. Sites that require more scrutiny than usual

Face	Heart	Limbs, Hands, Feet	Genitalia
Malformed ear,	TOF	Limb reduction defects,	
facial hemangiomata	CHD	phocomelia, mesomelia	
Goiter			
Cleft lip-palate, hypertelorism, depressed nasal bridge, malformed ears, depressed nasal bridge,	CHD	Digital and nail hypoplasia	
	CHD, TOF	Radial ray defects	
Cleft lip-palate, malformed ears,	CHD, VSD	Malformed hands, feet	Ambiguous genitalia
Nasal hypoplasia, cleft lip-palate	CHD, ASD		Ambiguous genitalia
Nasal hypoplasia, depressed nasal bridge, choanal atresia, eye defects	CHD	Stippled epiphyses, brachydactyly, rhizomelia	
Midface hypoplasia, micrognathia, small malformed ears, hypertelorism, cleft palate	TGV, TF, VSD, truncus arteriosis, aortic arch abnormality		
Flattened nasal bridge, cleft palate	CHD(TOF), single coronary artery	Ectrodactyly (absence of one or more digits), syndactyly	
Micrognathia, hypertelorism, wide nasal bridge	Dextroposition of heart	Mesomelic shortening, syndactyly, talipes equinovarus	
	Ebstein's anomaly, tricuspid atresia, VSD, coarctation of the aorta		
		short bone lengths, especially the fibula, club foot	
	CHD, TGV(?)	Limb reduction defects (?)	Masculinization of female fetus
Midface hypoplasia, micrognathia, cleft lip-palate	VSD, ASD, TOF, great vessel anomalies	Upper limb synostosis, radial ray defects	Genital hypoplasia
Eye defects, Cleft lip-palate	TGV, hypoplastic right heart, VSD	Limb reduction defects	

the maternal world, was shattered by the thalidomide catastrophe. To be sure, an association had been reported between maternal rubella infection and severe fetal malformations as early as 1941, but the extreme vulnerability of the fetus to drugs and chemicals had not been widely suspected.[30–32] In subsequent years, a broad spectrum of drugs have come under closer scrutiny. Even so, only 19 drugs or drug groups have been established as human teratogens to date (Tab. 34–1).[28]

Thalidomide

Once a popular tranquilizer outside the United States, thalidomide damaged an estimated 7700 children before its teratogenic effects were discovered.[33, 34] These effects included limb reduction defects, esophageal and duodenal atresia, tetralogy of Fallot, renal agenesis, facial hemangiomata, and anomalies of the external ear (**Fig. 34–2**). Following the catastrophe, the use of thalidomide as a sedative ended in the 1960s, but currently the Food and Drug Administraiton (FDA) of the United States is considering thalidomide for the treatment for

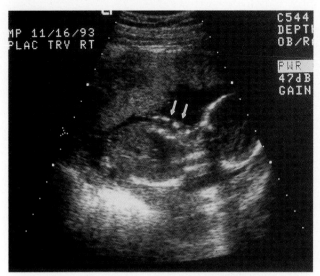

Figure 34–2 Phocomelia and micromelia. The upper limb of this fetus (**arrows**) is markedly short with complete or partial absence of individual bones. Such an abnormality was found in babies of mothers who had taken the sedative thalidomide. Though no longer used as a sedative, this drug is being reintroduced as a treatment for skin disease.

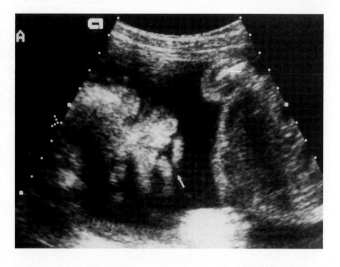

Figure 34–3 Cleft lip and palate. A complete unilateral defect (**arrow**) is seen in this modified coronal view. This finding can be found following exposure to hydantoins, valproic acid, trimethadione, retinoids, cyclophosphamide, ethanol, cocaine, and hyperthermia.

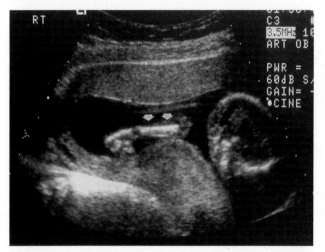

Figure 34–4 Radial ray defect. Only one long bone was found in the forearm of this fetus (**arrows**). Teratogens such as valproic acid and ethanol have been identified as causes of such abnormalities.

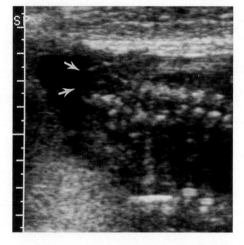

Figure 34–5 Neural tube defect. Spinal dysraphism and a meningomyelocele (**arrows**) is demonstrated in this fetus. This abnormality is a prominent feature of embryopathy resulting from valproic acid, carbamazepine, methotrexate, lithium, ethanol, and hyperthermia.

leprosy and other dermatological disorders. The drug is also being studied for other diseases such as AIDS, cancer, lupus, and rheumatoid arthritis.

Antithyroid Agents

Antithyroid agents, such as iodine-131, readily cross the placental membrane and are taken up by the fetal thyroid with an avidity that exceeds even that of the mother.[35] These agents are known to cause goiter and hypothyroidism when the fetal thyroid begins to concentrate iodide at 10—12 weeks of gestation, but there is no convincing evidence for induction of nonthyroid malformations.[36] Thyroid replacement agents, in distinction, are predominantly protein bound, and therefore, do not

readily cross the placenta.[37] These agents are considered to have a low teratogenic potential.

Anticonvulsants

The rate of congenital malformation is increased two to three times for epileptics receiving anticonvulsant therapy over nonepileptics or epileptics who were not medicated.[38,39] Anticonvulsant therapy has been particularly associated with the induction of cleft lip-cleft palate, and congenital heart disease (**Fig. 34–3**). More specific patterns of malformation have been attributed to five anticonvulsant drugs: phenytoin, trimethadione, valproic acid, primidone, and carbamazepine. The syndrome associated with hydantoins, such as Dilantin, is manifest by characteristic craniofacial features which include hypertelorism and depressed nasal bridge, limb anomalies such as digital and nail hypoplasia, and growth retardation. Many of these abnormalities are subtle, and at least one study indicated that sonograms ast 18—20 weeks are unlikely to reveal the structural defects associated with this drug.[40]

Those abnormalities associated with valproic acid, however, have been described in the ultrasound literature. Specifically, these include neural tube defects and radial ray limb defects (**Fig. 34–4 and 34–5**).[41—43] Similar phenotypic changes are seen with primidone, phenobarbital, and carbamazepine (Tegretol). Trimethadione is the most potent teratogen of the anticonvulsant group. The trimethadione syndrome is manifested by intrauterine growth retardation, microcephaly, cardiac anomalies, renal malformations, and mental retardation.[44] The increased teratogenic risk estimates for anticonvulsants are 80% for trimethadione exposure, 6% for phenobarbital—hydantoin exposure, and about 1% for valproic acid.

Anticoagulants

Coumarin anticoagulants, such as warfarin, produce characteristic teratological abnormalities of the skeleton in those fetuses exposed during the cirtical sixth to ninth week after fertilization. The most frequent abnormalities found in babies are stippled epiphyses and nasal hypoplasia. Stippled epiphyses are difficult to demonstrate prenatally by ultraound although one report does purport to depict this finding in a 22-week (gestational age) fetus with Conradi-Hünermann syndrom.[45] The nasal hypoplasia may be severe and associated with choanal atresia. Coumarin can cause intrauterine growth retardation and central nervous system (CN) abnormalities such as microcephaly, Dandy Walker malformation, eye defects, and agenesis of the corpus callosum.[46] Developmental retardation has been associated with second- and third-trimeter exposure . In a small number of cases, congenital heart disease has been described.

Both the nasal hypoplasia and the stippled epiphyses likely result from the interference by coumarin of chondrogenesis, rather than hemorrhage.[47] The CNS defects are probably caused by microhemorrhages in the developing tissues, although one case report does suggest a direct coeffect of warfarin on the developing CNS.[48] For the critical first-trimester period, many authorities recommend using heparin, which does not cross the placenta, as an alternative to warfarin.[49]

Vitamin A Congeners

Retinoids are among the most potent teratogens on the market. Used primarily in the treatment of severe acne and psoriasis, these vitamin A congeners carry an approximately 25% risk of malformation among fetuses who survive to 20 weeks gestational age following maternal exposure to therapeutic doses.[50] These malformations include craniofacial defects (small malformed ears, mandibular, and midfacial underdevelopment, and wide palatal clefts), cardiovascular malformations (especially conotruncal defects, transposition of the great vessels, tetralogy of Fallot, ventricular septal defects, and aortic arch abnormality), and central nervous defects (hydrocephalus and absence of the cerebellar vermis). One retinoid drug in particular, etretinate, is extrmely lipophilic and can be stored in body fat, and produce blood levels up to one year after cessation of treatment. Indeed, several cases of malformation have been reported in infants whose mothers discontinue treatment 7—12 months before their conceptions.[51] Vitamin A itself has much less teratogenic potential, though hydronephrosis, hemifacial micromelia, microhydrocephaly, and partial sirenomelia have been described after massive doses.[52, 53]

Anticancer Agents

Cyclophosphamide and other alkylating cancer thereapeutic agents carry an estimated risk of malformation of one in every six exposures. These malformations are typically skeletal and palate defects, as well as malformations of the limbs and eyes.[54] Exposure in the second and third trimesters is associated wih a much smaller risk of malformation, though growth retardation and pancytopenia have been described.[55] Other alkylating agents, such as busulfan and chlorambucil also produce malformations, but these more often cause abnormalities of the kidneys, ureters, and CNS closure.

Lithium

Lithium is the most controversial entry on the list of known teratogens. This drug has been associated with congenital heart disease, and, in particular, the rare Ebstein's anomaly (**Fig. 34–6**).[56—58] Though the true risk of congenital heart disease is unresolved, the repeated observation of heart defects appears to be more than coincidental. Though a 7 to 8% incidence has been cited, many believe a 1 to 5% range is more realistic.[13, 59—61] The issue is confounded by lack of a control population, the likely overreporting of abnormal cases, the prevalence of drug use and heavy smoking in this population, and a possible increased background risk of perinatal death and heart disease in the offspring of women with manic—depressive illness, regardless of drug therapy. Second-trimester sonographic screening has been recommended for any woman exposed to lithium in early pregnancy.[62, 63]

Tetracycline

Tetracycline has never been convincingly associated with major birth defects. Only minor defects have been

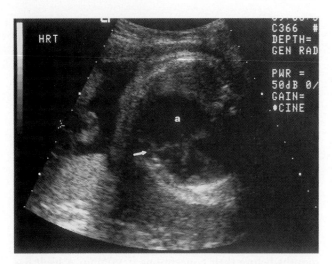

Figure 34–6   Ebstein's anomaly. This rare cardiovascular anomaly is characterized by displacement of the tricuspid valve into the right ventricle (**arrow**), creating a large right atrium (a) and right ventricular outflow obstruction. This anomaly has been reported in an unusually large number of lithium exposed fetuses.

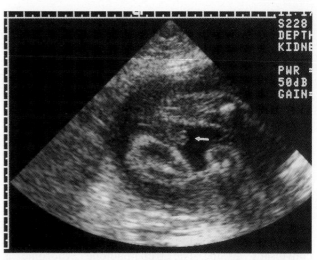

Figure 34–7   Ambiguous genitalia. Abnormalities of the genitalia (**arrow**) are features of trimethadione and carbamazepine, progestin, and ethanol exposures. Female fetuses exposed to natural progestin can demonstrate clitoral and labial enlargement, resulting in masculinization of the female genitalia.

described with consistency, the most common of these is a discoloration effect on developing teeth. At high doses, there has been depression of skeletal bone growth — particulary the fibula — and hypoplasia of tooth enamel.[64] Case reports of limb reduction defects have not been supported by epidemiologic or animal studies.

Hormones

Progestins and Estrogens

Fetal exposure to progestins and estrogens usually results from the continued use of birth control pills following conception by women unaware that they are pregnant.[65] Alternatively, women are sometimes exposed to these hormones as treatment for threatened abortion in the first trimester. Early retrospective studies proposed an association between exposure to female sex hormones and abnormalities such as cardiovascular defects (particularly, transposition of the great vessels), limb reduction defects, the VACTER syndrome, and malformations of the external genitalia.[66] These studies were, however, limited retrospective studies with small sample sizes. In many reported cases, exposure occurred outside of the critical period of organ formation. Most investigators now believe that progesterones and progesterone—estrogen combinations carry an extremely small teratogenic risk.[67] The risks that may be present seem to be limited to the increased incidence of hypospadias in male fetuses exposed to progestin, and clitoral and labial enlargement in female fetuses exposed to natural progestin (**Fig. 34–7**). Interestingly, the masculinization of female genitalia results from the converson of progestins to androgens in the mother and unborn baby.

Dietheylstilbestrol (DES)

Dietheylstilbestrol (DES) was at one time used to prevent miscarriage, premature delivery, and other pregnancy complications. In utero exposure to DES has been associated with subsequent development of vaginal adenosis and carcinoma in young women exposed to DES in utero. These daughters also have been found to have increased incidence of premature deliveries associated with increased perinatal mortality.[67] Abnormal morphology of the uterus, the "T-shaped appearance," as well as other uterine lesions have been described in this population. Detection of abnormalities in utero, however, has not been described. At least 25% of women with first-trimester DES exposure develop genital tract anomalies, inlcuding vaginal adenosis, cervical malformations, vaginal septae, uterine cavity anomalies, and fallopian tube anomalies.[68] A parallel increase in male urogenital abnormalities has not been substantiated, though microphallus, cryptorchidism, and hypoplastic testes have been reported.[69]

Substance Abuse

Alcohol and recreational drugs are the most significant developmental toxicants of the modern day.

Alcohol

Alcohol consumption during pregnancy is now the most frequent cause of mental retardation in the Western world, producing between 3000 and 6000 damaged babies in the United States alone.[70] And these numbers likely represent an underreporting of the true incidence.

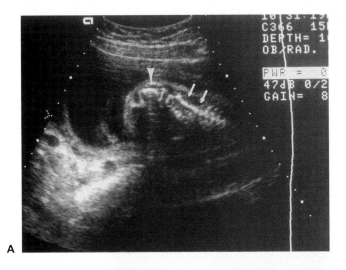

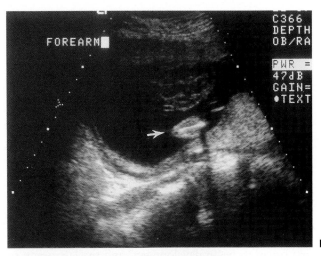

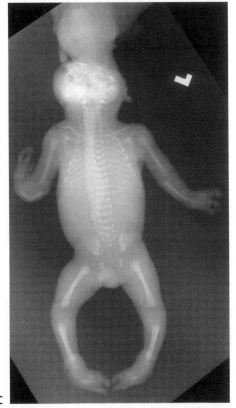

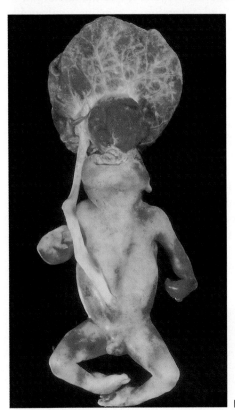

Figure 34–8   Ethanol exposure. The mother of this fetus was a chronic alcoholic who admitted to daily alcohol consumption. (**A**) Prenatal ultrasound demonstrated an intact cervical spine (**arrows**) and occiput (**arrowhead**), but absent anterior calvaria. Facial features could not be discerned. Disorganized neural tissue was seen arising above the expected level of the orbits. (**B**) Sonographic depictions of the forearms revealed only one bone (**arrow**) on each side. Abnormal hands and feet were seen on other views. (**C**) Postnatal radiography of the abortus demonstrates a large defect extending from the face to the cranium (faciocranioschisis), bilateral radial aplasia, ulnar bowing, bilateral ectrodactyly, bilateral club feet. (**D**) Photograph of the abortus shows that the extruded neural tissue from the head which adheres to the placenta. (Case courtesy of Martha Decker-Phillips, M.D.).

Alcohol teratogenicity produces central nervous system dysfunction, prenatal and postnatal growth retardation, characteristic craniofacial abnormalities, and a variable number of major and minor malformations.[71–73] Described CNS abnormalitiies include microcephaly, hydrocephaly, neural tube defects, and holoprosencephaly (**Fig. 34–8 A—D**). Facial features include midface hypoplasia, hypoplastic maxilla, micrognathia, cleft palate and lip, as well as short upturned nose, short palpebral fissures, thin upper lip, and flat philtrum. Other associated malformations include cardiac defects (VSD, ASD, great vessel anomalies, and tetralogy of Fallot), hydronephrosis, small kidneys, scoliosis, radial ulnar synostosis, polydactyly, and hernias of the diaphragm, umbilicus or groin, and hypoplastic external genitalia. Though the kidneys of ethanol-exposed infants are significantly smaller than normal controls, the prevalence of structural malformation may not be increased in the exposed group.[74]

Despite such pervasive abnormalities, prenatal detection of fetal alcohol syndrome is difficult, with subtle features appearing only late in pregnancy.[20] Quantitative characterization of the craniofacial dysmorphism has been reported in a nonblinded study of three fetuses at 16, 19, and 24 weeks gestational age.[75] Such results have not been corroborated in all laboratories. Gross abnormalities are most likely to be found in heavy drinkers: the risk for fetal alcohol syndrome is approximately 5.6% when alcohol is consumed at greater than 3 oz per day.[73] Even so, there is no clear dosage threshold or period of susceptibility yet defined: the brain is both the first organ to begin development, and the last organ to complete it, and therefore, remains vulnerable throughout gestation. The most critical period of exposure may be soon after conception.

Cocaine

Though it is clear that cocaine is a significant development toxicant, the teratogenic potential of the drug is difficult to characterize, in part, because fetuses of cocaine-abusing mothers are also exposed to the potentially deleterious effects of malnutrition, polydrug abuse, and inadequate prenatal care.[76] In addition, malformations resulting from cocaine abuse vary too widely among patients to constitute a recognized syndrom. Some studies have found a 15 to 20% incidence of congenital abnormalities in cocaine-abusing populations, and all such pregnancies are at increased risk of spontaneous abortion, stillbirth, premature rupture of membranes, placental abruption, premature labor and delivery, and intrauterine growth retardation.[77—79] In some large urban hospitals, cocaine abuse occurs during pregnancy in at least 16% of births.[80]

The teratogenic actions of cocaine likely stem from its physiologic effects, specifically, vasoconstriction, transient hypertension and vascular disruption.[81] Cocaine use has been associated with reduction or disruption of blood to the placenta, uterus, and fetus, making generalized intrauterine growth retardation a logical consequence. Specific malformations are multifarious and wide-ranging, but can be broadly categorized as cranial defects (exencephaly, encephalocele, parietal bone defects), cerebral infarction, limb reduction defects, urogenital abnormalities, and intestinal perforation, obstruction, and atresia (Fig 34–9).[13]

Neurosonographic studies on neonates have demonstrated subependymal germinal matrix cysts,[82, 83] and prenatal studies have demonstrated choroid plexus cysts.[81] These cysts may represent focal ischemia or hemorrhage. The incidence of abnormality on postnatal neurosonographic studies varies among studies and may be quite low.[84] Heart abnormalities include transposition of the great vessels and hypoplastic right heart syndrome. The increased incidence of malformations of the urinary tract is perhaps the most convincingly demonstrated manifestation of exposure: The estimated risk is approximately four times control.[85, 86] Such urologic abnormalities include hydronephrosis, renal infarction, crossed fused ectopic, prune belly syndrome, renal and ureteral agenesis, and hypospadius (Fig. 34–10). The developmental neurotoxicity of cocain, evident as ad-

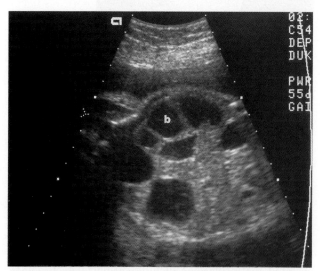

Figure 34–9   Dilated loops of bowel (b) in the fetal abdomen. Intestinal perforation, obstruction, and atresia are features found in the fetuses of cocaine-abusing mothers. Vascular disruption is presumed to cause ischemic and infarctive bowel injury in these fetuses.

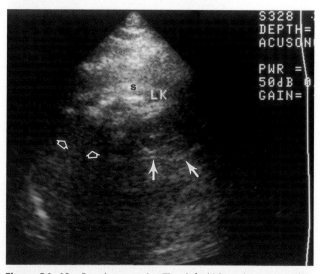

Figure 34–10   Renal agenesis. The left kidney is present (**arrows**), but the right is absent (**open arrows**) on this axial image with the spine (s) up. Malformations of the urinary tract, such as this, have been convincingly shown to have an increased incidence in fetuses exposed to cocaine. The urologic abnormalities, however, are wide ranging and include both malformation, infarction, and obstructon.

verse behavioral changes, has also been seen even on pre-natal ultrasound.[87]

Recreational Drugs

Teratogenicity has never been conclusively demonstrated for marijuana, heroin, opium, or lysergic acid diethylamide (LSD). To be sure, LSD use has been associated with limb defects, ocular defects, and CNS abnormalities. Heroin use has been associated with fetal growth retardation, but as yet no discernible pattern of defects has been identified.[88] Likeweise, impaired fetal growth has ben associated with marijuana, though this effect is difficult to substantiate when the confounding effects of social status and concurrent alcohol and drug use are considered.

Obstetrical Intervention and Procedures

Methotrexate

Though guidelines for the use of methotrexate for the medical treatment of ectopic pregnancy have been established, the misapplication of these guidelines is becoming more frequent as the treatment approach diffuses through general obstetrical practice. As a result, mothers carrying early intrauterine pregnancies, which may or may not have a discernible gestational sac by ultraosund, have been given methotrexate for the presumptive diagnosis of ectopic pregnancy. If the embryo survives, a broad orange of serious malformations can be found. These include malformations of the skull, such as sutural synostosis, defective ossification of the calvarium, micrognathia, brachycephaly, and a "clover leaf" configuration. Abnormalities of the CNS have included anencephaly, hydrocephaly, meningomyelocele, and cerebral hypoplasia. Ocular hypertelorism and a wide nasal bridge, and limb deformities, such as syndactyly, talipes equinovarus, and mesomelic shortening of the forearms have been seen in several infants (**Fig. 34–11**).[89, 90] Growth retardation was also a feature of the few cases that have been reported to date. Of note, however, several normal pregnancies have been reported after methotrexate and aminopterin exposure.

Much of what is known about the teratogenicity of methotrexate has been derived from case reports of mothers undergoing cancer treatment. A folic acid antagonist, methotrexate interferes with the replication of nucleic acid and consequently prevents the division and multiplication of cells. Aminopterin, a drug closely related to methotrexate, was used in the first trimester as a single dose for the purpose of inducing abortion. The anomalies identified in the abortuses and in the surviving babies represent one of the very few teratogenic experiments performed in humans.

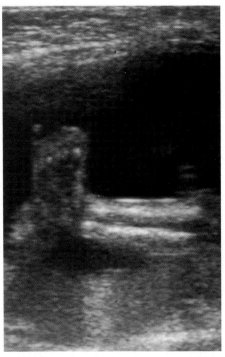

Figure 34–11   Talipes equinovarus or club foot. On this single scan plane, the tibia and fibula can be demonstrated in perpendicular relation to the metatarsals. This malformation can be produced by deformation of the foot in utero or after exposure to methotrexate and tetracycline.

Chorionic Villus Sampling

Chorionic villus sampling (CVS), a technique of first-trimester genetic diagnosis, has been implicated in the production of limb defects. This association was suggested by population studies and CVS registries in which an unexpected number of mothers who had had a CVS gave birth to babies with transverse limb reduction defects and oromandibular-limb reduciton hypogenesis syndrome, a syndrome characterized by limb deficiency, hypoglossia, and micrognathia.[91, 92] This association is controversial, and not corroborated by all studies.[93] Most investigators now believe that the risk, if real, is small (estimated at 1/3000 births), and may be related to the technique and timing of the procedure. There is no convincing evidence for an increase in limb reduction defects following CVS performed at 10 weeks gestational age or later, but there may be an increased risk for procedures performed earlier than 10 weeks gestational age.[94] Because CVS involves a biopsy of the developing placenta, the etiology of these malformations may be the embolization of trophoblastic tissue from the placenta to the fetus, resulting in ischemic or infarctive injury. Other proposed mechanisms suggest that the function of the placenta is compromised, or that the release of vasoactive placental angiotensin initiates the fetal injury.

Radiation and Heat

Radiation

More than any single issue in teratology, misunderstanding of the risks of radiation exposure to the developing embryo and fetus has caused excessive and unncessary anxiety.[21] Radiation is certainly one of the best known and earliest recognized teratogens, but the effects of radiation have been documented in pregnant women who have received large amounts of ionizing radiation either as therapy for cervical cancer or as atomic bomb survivors. The principle effects include microcephaly, intrauterine growth retardation, mental retardation, and eye malformations, but spina bifida cystica, cleft palate, and skeletal and visceral abnormalities have also been described. Studies indicate that microcephaly and mental retardation are associated with doses of 50 rads or greater, and no morphologic abnormality has been substantiated in a fetus that has not exhibited growth retardation or a CNS abnormality. Radiation effects are clearly dose related: radiation risks to the embryo are negligible at doses of 5 rads or less, which is well below the range of typical exposures from diagnostic X-ray studies.[95] There is no proof that human congenital malformations have ever been caused by diagnostic levels of radiation.[96,97]

Hyperthermia

Hyprthemia is defined as a body temperature of at least 102° F (38.9° C). Though hyperthermia is a demonstrated teratogen in laboratory animals, particularly guinea pigs, the risks to humans are less clear. Epidemiological studies of hyperthermia have suggested an increase in abdominal wall defects, cardiovascular malformations (atrial septal defects, hypoplastic left heart), and neural tube defects.[13] Exposures between 14 and 28 days after conception are thought to pose an increased risk for neural tube defects (spina bifida and anencephaly). From 4 to 14 weeks gestational age, there is an increased risk associated with hyperthermia of mental retardation, hypotonia, and facial defects (cleft lip and palate, external ear abnormalities, and midface hyopoplasia.[98] In most cases where birth defects have been reported, the mother had had a high fever that persisted for days. Theoretical risks exist for heat exposures in hot tubs and saunas. Though it has been suggested that a mother would become intolerably uncomfortable in a hot tub or sauna before her temperature reached 102° F, and would in all likelihood remove herself from the heat, there are conflicting reports of the reliability of subjective discomfort to prevent overheating.[99,100]

Infection

The collection of infectious agents into the TORCH acronym (toxoplasmosis — other — rubella — cytomegalovirus — herpes simplex virus) is convenient but misleading. Certainly, there is no recognizable "TORCH" syndrome per se, inasmuch as that implies a single entity, pattern of malformation, or clinical presentation. The types and frequencies of abnormalities vary from one agent to the next.[101]

Rubella

Rubella is a very efficient teratogen. The 1941 report that linked German measles to birth defects was the first to attribute congenital malformations in the human to an exogenous environmntal agent.[30] Rubella infection causes detectable defects in 85% of fetuses for exposures in the first eight weeks, 52% between nine and 12 weeks, and 16% betwen 13 and 20 weeks of pregnancy. The consequences of infection tend to be severe: death, cardiac malformation (pulmonary artery stenosis, patent ductus arteriosus), deafness, eye defects (particularly, cataracts), growth retardation, and mental retardation. Thankfully, with the advent of the rubella vaccination, the incidence of infection has decreased by more than 99%, and the fetal malformations from rubella virus have drastically decreased. Nonetheless, failure to be vaccinated has left 10 to 20% of the population susceptible to exposure, and this has not changed since the 1970 s. The principle aim of the vaccination program is the prevention of congenital rubella.

Cytomegalovirus

The most common viral infection of the human fetus is cytomegalovirus infection. Most such infections result in embryonic death, but those that survive can demonstrate intrauterine growth retardation, microphthalmia, microcephaly, ventriculomegaly, calcifications in the fetal abdomen and brain, hepatosplenomegaly, cardiac dysrhythmia, hydronephrosis, and hydrops (**Fig. 34–12 A—C**).[8,20,101] The findings of cerebral ventriculomegaly and decreased head circumference may be particularly ominous.[102]

Toxoplasmosis

Toxoplasmosis, caused by a protozoan parasite, is a common infection but a rare disease. Maternal infection is most often caused by eating poorly cooked meat, contact with infected cats, or from soil contaminated with cat feces. Transmission of the infection from the mother to the fetus occurs only with primary infection during pregnancy except when the mother has an immunosuppressive condition, such as AIDS. With maternal infec-

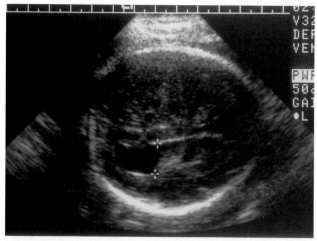

A

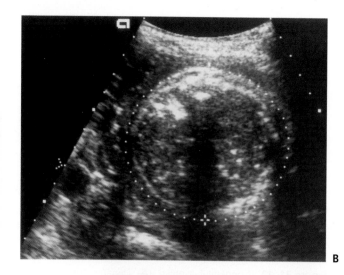

B

Figure 34–12 Fetal cytomegalovirus infection. This is the most common viral infection of the human fetus. In this case, the infection was evident by ventriculomegaly (**A**) and calcifications in the fetal abdomen (**B**). Postnatal CT examination (**C**) later demonstrated periventricular cerebral calcification (**arrow**) as well.

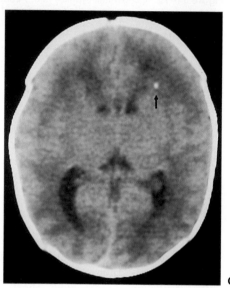

C

tion, the rate of transmission to the fetus is approximately 17 to 25% in the first and second trimester and 65% in the third trimester. The majority of the fetuses however, are asymptomatic, and the rate at which infection produces clinical illness is only 16% in the first and second trimesters and 5% in the third trimester. In the first trimester, the toxoplasma parasite can cause destructive changes of the brain and eyes, resulting in microcephaly, microphthalmia, and hydrocephalus.[8] Prematurity, growth retardation, cerebral calcification, hepatosplenomegaly, ascites, and pleural and pericardial fluid collection can also evolve.[20]

Varicella-Zoster

Varicella-zoster virus, which causes both chicken pox and shingles, is a neutotropic agent that causes abnormalities when acquired by the fetus in the first trimester of pregnancy. There is about a 25% chance of abnormality when infection occurs during this time, and these abnormalities include skin scarring, muscle atrophy, limb reduction defects, microcephaly, microphthalmia, ascites, liver calcifications, talipes equinovarus, hydrocephalus, and meningoceles.

Syphilis

The incidence of congenital syphilis has increased steadily since 1980. Treponema pallidum is an efficient teratogen causing infection of nearly 100% of fetuses born to women with untreated primary or secondary syphilis. Many pregnancies end in prenatal or perinatal fetal death, and the remaining fetuses demonstrate either congenital abnormalities or symptoms of infection.

Manifestations of congenital syphilis seen with prenatal ultrasound include hepatosplenomegaly, hydrops, bowel obstruction, bone changes, and abnormally large placental size (**Fig. 134–13 A, B**).[20, 103, 104] The bone changes are evident as surface irregularities and abnormal curvature and bowing of in the long bones of fetuses.[104] The classical stigmata of congenital syphilis infection, such as saddle nose, saber shin, and dental abnormalities, evolve from the destructive consequences of early childhood disease, and are seen only later in life.[13]

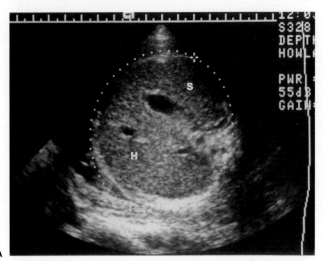

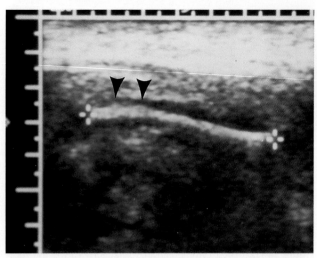

A

B

Figure 34–13 Congenital syphilis. (**A**) Hepatosplenomegaly is often the first, and sometimes the only finding of infection.[20] In this case, enlargement of the spleen causes displacement of the stomach (s) toward the midline. The liver (h) is also markedly enlarged. The measured abdominal circumference corresponds to approximately 35 menstrual weeks, though the fetus was only 22 weeks of age. (**B**) Views of the femurs showed surface irregularities of the bone (**arrowheads**) and abnormal bowing. These features have been described in a recent case report.[84] (Case courtesy of Sheryl Jordan, M.D.)

Herpes Simplex Virus

Infection of the fetus by herpes simplex virus usually occurs late in pregnancy. Described congenital abnormalities include microcephaly, microphthalmia, and mental retardation.

Parvovirus

Parvovirus is being increasingly recognized as the cause of previously unexplained nonimmune hydrops, spontaneous abortion, and stillbirth.[20] Infection typically results in spontaneous abortion in the first trimester, hydrops in the second trimeser, and stillbirth in the third trimester. This said, one study has indicated that parvovirus is a relatively common cause of second-trimester fetal death, and most such cases do not demonstrate hydrops.[105] Parvovirus may also cause isolated pleural or percardial effusion,[106] and possibly also structural malformations of the fetal brain and heart, mediated by vasculitis.[107] Only 39 to 60% of adults are seropositive to the virus, leaving approximately 40 to 70% of the population susceptible to disease. Parvovirus appears to be a relatively poor teratogen, causing congenital infection from an infected mother in only 10 to 20% of cases, and adverse outcome in only about 3% of pregnancies showing evidence of a recent maternal infection.[108]

Human Immunodeficiency Virus

The prenatal and perinatal transmission rate of the human immunodeficiency virus (HIV) is estimated to be at 40 to 50%. The effects of HIV infection on the outcome of pregnancy are controversial: some studies have noted premature rupture of membranes, premature birth, and growth retardation, but others find no such effects when the confounding factor of intravenous drug use is eliminated. Initial descriptions of an "AIDS embryopathy" have been disputed, and the diagnosis is now in disfavor. This syndrome was said to include growth failure, microcephaly, and a distinctive craniofacial dysmorphism (box-like forherad, hypertelorism, flat nasal bridge, obliquity to the axis of the eyes).[109] Reports of such a craniofacial dysmorphism have been severely criticized for failing to control for ethnic variation, maternal substance abuse, and other potentially teratogenic agents.[110] At present, there is no compelling evidence for an embryopathy that can be attributed to HIV alone.

Conclusion

Many embryos and fetuses exposed to teratogens will not have a demonstrable abnormality.[22] Even so, it is incumbent on the sonologist to be alert to potential teratogenic effects, so that a purposeful and orderly survey of the fetus can be made for the often subtle signs which may be the only indication of a teratogen. The use of ultrasound to establish the presence or abscence of discernible abnormality may be the best and only reassurance available to parents tormented by the fear that they have brought harm to their unborn child through a potentially preventable exposure.

Acknowledgments: Thanks to Barbara Hertzberg, M.D. and Martha Decker-Phillips, M.D. for case materials; Trisha Peters-Brown, C.G.C. for resource guidance; Eileen P. Ahearn, M.D., Ph.d. for editing suggestions; and Susan Murray for manuscript preparation.

References

1. Barrow MV. A brief history of teratology to the early 20th century. *Teratology* 1971;4:119—130.
2. Beckman DA, Brent RL. Mechanisms of teratogenesis. *Ann Rev Pharmacol Toxicol* 1984;24:483.
3. Brent RL, Beckman DA. Environmental teratogens. *Bull NY Acad Med* 1990;66:123—163.
4. Principles of teratogenesis applicable to drug and chemical exposure. In: Schardein JL, ed. *Chemically Induced Birth Defects*, 2nd ed. New York: Marcel Dekker, Inc, 1993, p. 1—62.
5. Risks. In: Kelly-Buchanan C, ed. *Peace of Mind During Pregnancy*. Philadelphia: Dell Pub., 1989, p. 7—26.
6. Kalter H. Experimental investigation of teratogenic action. *Ann NY Acad Sci* 1965;123:287—294.
7. Kalter H. Teratology of the central nervous system. Chicago, IL: University of Chicago Press, 1968, p. 3—20.
8. The causes of human congenital malformations. In: Moore KL, ed. *The Developing Human — Clinically Oriented Embryology*, 4th ed. Philadelphia: 1988, p. 131—158.
9. Wilson JG. Experimental studies on congenital malformations. *J Chronic Dis* 1959;10:111—130.
10. Tanimura T. Introductory remarks on behavioral teratology. *Congenital Anom* 1980;20:301—318.
11. Wilson JG. Mechanisms of abnormal development. In: Newburgh R, ed. *Proceedings, Conference on Toxicology: Implications to Teratology*. Washington, DC: NICHHD, 1971, p. 81—114.
12. Brent RL. (Editorial comment.) Definition of a teratogen and the relationship of teratogenicity to carcinogenicity. *Teratology* 1986a;34:359—360.
13. ReproTox (Database). Washington, DC: Columbia Women's Hospital.
14. TERIS (Data base). Seattle: Department of Pediatrics, University of Washington, Seattle.
15. Shepard TH, ed. *Catalog of Teratogenic Agents*. Baltimore: Johns Hopkins University Press, 1989.
16. Schardein JL, ed. *Chemically Induced Birth Defects*, 2nd ed. New York: Marcel Dekker, Inc, 1993.
17. Briggs GG, Freeman RK, Yaffe SJ, eds. *Drugs in Pregnancy and Lactation*, 5th ed. Baltimore: Williams & Wilkins, 1998.
18. Gilstrap III LC, Little BB, eds. *Drugs and Pregnancy*. New York: Elsevier Science Pub, 1992.
19. Koren G, Edwards MB, Miskin M. Antenatal sonography of fetal malformations associated with drugs and chemicals: a guide. *Am J Obstet Gynecol* 1987;156:79—85.
20. Sanders RC, ed. *Structural Fetal Abormaliities — The Total Picture*. St. Louis: Mosby-Year Book Inc, 1996.
21. Kelly-Buchanan, C, ed. *Peace of Mind During Pregnancy*. Philadelphia: Dell Publishers, 1989.
22. Levine D, Filly RA, Goldberg JD. Teratogen exposure: lack of morphological abnormalities by detailed fetal sonography. *Ultrasound Obstet Gynecol* 1994;4:452—456.
23. Turner GM, Twining P. The facial profile in the diagnosis of fetal abnormalities. *Clin Radiol* 1993;47:389—395.
24. Escobar LF, Bixler D, Padilla LM, Weaver DD. Fetal craniofacial morphometrics. In utero evaluation at 16 weeks gestation. *Obstet Gynecol* 1988;72:674—679.
25. Escobar LF, Bixler D, Padilla LM, Weaver DD, Williams CJ. A morphometric analysis of the fetal craniofacies by ultrasound: fetal cephalometry. *J Craniofacial Genet Develop Biol* 1990;10:19—27.
26. Watson WJ, Katz VA. Sonographic measurement of the fetal mandible: standards for normal pregnancy. *Am J Perinatol* 1993;10:226—228.

27. Garn SM, Smith RH, La Velle M. Applications of pattern profile analysis to malformations of the head and face. *Ped Radiol* 1984;150:683—690.
28. Drug use in pregnancy. In: Schardein JL, ed. *Chemically Induced Birth Defects*, 2nd ed. New York: Marcel Dekker, Inc, 1993; p. 63—78.
29. Queiber-Luft A, Eggers, I, Stolf G, Kieninger-Baum D, Schlaefer K. Serial examination of 20,248 newborn fetuses and infants: correlations betweeen drug exposure and major malformations. *Am J Med Genet* 1996;63:268—276.
30. Gregg NM. Congenital cataract following German measles in the mother. *Trans Opthalmol Soc Aus* 1941;3:35—46
31. Lenz W. Kindchemissbildungen nach Medikamenteneinnahme während der Gravidität? *Dtsch Med Wochenschr* 1961;86:2555—2556.
32. McBride WG. Thalidomide and congenital abnormalities. *Lancet* 1961;2:1358.
33. Thalidomide symposium: Papers presented at the 26th meeting of the Teratology Society, July 6—10, 1986, Boston, MA. *Teratology* 1988;38:201—251.
34. Gollop TR, Eigier A, Neto JG. Prenatal diagnosis of thalidomide syndrome. *Prenat Diag* 1987;7:295—298.
35. Speert H, Quimby EH, Werner SC. Radioiodine update by the fetal mouse thyroid and resultant effects in later life. *Surg Gynecol Obstet* 1951;93:230.
36. Bargman GJ, Gardner LI. The cloistered thyroidologist. *Lancet* 1969;2:562.
37. Fischer DA, Klein AH. Thyroid development and disorders of thyroid function in the newborn. *N Eng J Med* 1981;304:702—712.
38. Anticonvulsants. In: Schardein JL, ed. *Chemically Induced Birth Defects*, 2nd ed. New York: Marcel Dekker, Inc, 1993, p. 157—207.
39. Lindhout D, Omtzigt GC. Teratogenic effects of antiepileptic drugs: implications for the management of epilepsy in women of childbearing age. *Epilepsia* 1994;35:(Suppl 4):S19—S28.
40. Wladimiroff JW, Stewart PA, van Swaay RE, Lindhout D, Sachs ES. The role of ultrasound in the early diagnosis of fetal structural defects following maternal anticonvulsant therapy. *Ultrasound Med Biol* 1988;14:657—660.
41. Sharony R, Garber A, Viskochil D, et al. Preaxial ray reduction defects as part of valproci acid embryofetopathy. *Prenat Diag* 1993;13:909—918.
42. Langer B, Haddad J, Gasser B, Maubrt M, Schlaeder G. Isolated fetal bilateral radial ray reduction associated with valproic acid usage. *Fetal Diag Ther* 1994;9:155—158.
43. Ylagan LR, Burorick NE. Radial ray aplasia in utero: a prenatal finding associated with valproic acid exposure. *J Ultrasound Med* 1994;13:408—411.
44. Sharony, R, Graham Jr, JM. Identification of fetal problems associated with anticonvulsant usage and maternal epilepsy. *Obstet Gynecol Clin N Am* 1991;18:933—951.
45. Avni EF, Rypens F, Zappa M, et al. Antenatal diagnosis of short-limb dwarfism: sonographic approach. *Pediat Radiol* 1996,267:171—178.
46. Harrod MJE, Sherrod PS. Warfarin embryopathy in siblings. *Obstet Gynecol* 1981;57:673—676.
47. Howe AM, Webster WS. The warfarin embryopathy: a rat model showing maxillonasal hypoplasia and other skeletal disturbances. *Teratology* 1992;46:379—390.
48. Kaplan LC. Congenital Dandy Walker malformation associated with first trimester warfarin: a case report and literature reivew *Teratology* 1985;32:333.
49. Nageotte MP, Freeman RK, Garile, TJ et al. Anticoagulation in pregnancy. *Am J Obstet Gynecol* 1981;141:472.
50. Sulik KK, Alles AJ. Teratogenicity of the retinoids. In: Saurat JH, ed. *Retinoids: 10 Years On*. Basel, Switzerland: S. Karger, 1991, p. 282—295.

51. Verloes A, Dodinval P, Koulischer L, Lambotte R, Bonniver J. Etretinate embryotoxicity 7 months after discontinuation of treatment. *Am J Med Genet* 1990;37:437—438.

52. von Lennap E, El Khazen N, De Pierreux G, et al. A case of partial sirenomelia and possible vitamin A teratogenesis. *Prenat Diag* 1985;5:35—40.

53. Rosa FE, Wilk AL, Kelsey FO. Teratogen update: vitamin A congeners. *Teratology* 1986;33:355—364.

54. Greenberg LH, Tanaka KR. Congenital anomalies probably induced by cyclophosphamide. *JAMA* 1964;188:423—426.

55. Nicholson HO. Cytotoxic drugs in pregnancy: review of reported cases. *J Obstet Gynaecol Br Commonw* 1968;75:307—312.

56. Nora JJ, Nora AH, Toews WH. Lithium, Ebstain's anomaly and other congenital heart defects. *Lancet* 1974;Sept 7:594—595.

57. Källén B, Tandberg A. Lithium and pregnancy — a cohort study on manic-depressive women. *Acta Psychiatr Scand* 1983;68:134—139.

58. Källén B. Comments on teratogen update: lithium. *Teratology* 1988;38:597.

59. Cohen LAS, Friedman JM, Jefferson JW, Johnson M, Weiner ML. A reevaluation of risk of in utero exposure to lithium. *JAMA* 1994;271:146—150.

60. Jacobson SJ, Jones K, Johnson K, et al. Prospective multicentre study of pregnancy outcome after lithium exposure during first trimester. *Lancet* 1992;339:530—533.

61. Zalzstein E, Koren G, Einarson T, Freedom RM. A case-control study on the association between first trimester exposure to lithium and Ebstein's anomaly. *Am J Cardiol* 1990;65:817—818.

62. Allan LD, Desei G, Tynan MJ. Prenatal echocardiographic screening for Ebstein's anomaly for mothers on lithium therapy. *Lancet* 1982;2:875—876.

63. Loebstein R, Koren G. Pregnancy outcome and neurodevelopment of children exposed in utero to psychoactive drugs: the motherisk experience. *J Psychiatry Neurosci* 1997;22:192—196.

64. Rendle-short TJ. Tetracycline in teeth and bone. *Lancet* 1962;1:1188.

65. Jones KL. Effects of therapeutic, diagnostic, and environmental agents. In: Creasy R, Resnik R, eds. *Maternal-Fetal Medicine*, 3rd ed. 1994.

66. Katz Z, Lancet M, Skornik J, et al. Teratogenicitiy of progestogens given during the 1st trimester of pregnancy. *Obstet Gynecol* 1985;65:77—78.

67. Hormones and hormonal antagonists. In: Schardein JL, ed. *Chemically Induced Birth Defects*, 2nd ed. New York: Marcel Dekker, Inc, 1993, p. 271—339.

68. Senekjian EK, et al. Infertility among daughters either exposed or not exposed to diethylstilbestrol. *Am J Obstet Gynecol* 1988;158:493—498.

69. Stillmann RJ. In utero exposure to diethylstilbestrol: adverse effects on the reproductive tract and reproductive performance in male and female offspring. *Am J Obstet Gynecol* 1982;142:905.

70. Clarren SK, Smith DW. The fetal alcohol syndrome. *N Engl J Med* 1978;298:1063—1067.

71. Clarren SK, Recognition of fetal alcohol syndrome. *JAMA* 1981;245:2436—2439.

72. Day NL, et al. Prenatal exposure to alcohol: effect on infant growth and morphologic characteristics. *Pediatrics* 1989;84:536—541.

73. Ernhart CB, et al. Alcohol teratogenicity in the human: a detailed assessment of specificity, critical period and threshold. *Am J Obstet Gynecol* 1987;156:33—39.

74. Taylor CL, Jones KL, Jones MC, Kaplan GW. Incidence of renal anomalies in children prenatally exposed to ethanol. *Pediatrics* 1994;94:209—212.

75. Escobar LF, Bixler D, Padilla ■. Quantitation of craniofacial anomalies in utero: fetal alcohol and Crouzon syndromes and thanatophoric dysplasia. *Am J Med Genet* 1993;45:25—29.

76. Chasnoff I, Burns W, Schnoll S, Burns K. Cocaine use in pregnancy. **N Engl J Med** 1985;313:666—669.

77. MacGregor SN, Keith LG, Chasnoff IJ, et al. Cocain use in pregnancy: adverse perinatal outcome. *Am J Obstet Gynecol* 1987;157:686—690.

78. Viscarello RR, Ferguson DD, Nores J, Hobbins JC. Limbbody wall complex associated with cocaine abuse: further evidence of cocaine's teratogeniticity. *Obstet Gynecol* 1992;80:523—526.

79. Townsend RR, Laing FC, Jeffrey RB, Jr. Placental abruption associated with cocaine abuse. *AJR* 1988;150:1339—1340.

80. van Dyke DC, Fox AA. Fetal drug exposure and its possible implications for learning in the preschool-age population. *J Learn Disabil* 1990;23:160—163.

81. Hume RF, JR, Gingras JL, Martin LS, et al. Ultrasound diagnosis of fetal anomalies associated with in utero cocaine exposure: further support for cocaine-induced vascular disruption teratogenesis. *Fetal Diagn Ther* 1994;9:239—245.

82. Cohen HL, Sloves JH, Laungani S, Glass L, DeMarinis P. Neurosonographic findings in full-term infants born to maternal cocaine abusers: visualization of subependymal and periventricular cysts. *J Clin Ultrasound* 1994;22:327—333.

83. Dogra VS, Shyken JM, Menon PA, et al. Neurosonographic abnormalities associated with maternal history of cocaine use in neonates of appropriate size for their gestational age. *Am J Neuroradiol* 1994;15:697—702.

84. Bebnke M, Eyler FD, Conlon M, et al. Incidence and description of structural brain abnormalities in newborns exposed to cocaine. *J Pediatr* 1998;132:291—294.

85. Battin M, Albersheim S, Newman D. Congenital genitourinary tract abnormalities following cocaine exposure in utero. *Am J Perinatol* 1995;12:425—428.

86. Chavez GF, et al. Masternal cocaine use during early pregnancy as a risk factor for congenital urogenital anomalies. *JAMA* 1989;262:795—798.

87. Hume JR RF,, O'Donnell KJ, Stanger CL, Killam AP, Gingras JL. In utero cocaine exposure: observations of fetal behavioral state may predict neonatal outcome. *Am J Obstet Gynecol* 1989;161:685—690.

88. Schardein JL. Personal and social drugs. In: Schardein JL, ed. Chemically Induced Birth Defects, 2nd ed. New york: Marcel Dekker, Inc, 1993, p. 398—641.

89. Milunsky A, Graef JW, Gaynor MF. Methotrexate-induced congenital malformations with a review of the literature. *J Pediat* 1968;72:790—795.

90. Goodman RM, Gorlin RJ, eds. *The Malformed Infant and Child: An Illustrated Guide.* New York: Oxford University Press, 1983, p. 14—15.

91. Firth HV, Chamberlain P, MacKenzi IZ, Lindenbaum RH, Huson SM. Severe limb abnormalities after chorion villus sampling at 56—66 day's gestation. *Lancet* 1991;337:762—763.

92. Burton BK, Schulz CJ, Burd LI. Limb anomalies associated with chorionic villus samplnig. *Obstet Gynecol* 1992;79:726—730.

93. Olney RS, Khoury MJ, Alo CJ, et al. Increased risk for transverse digital deficiency after chorionic villus sampling: results of the United states multistate case-control study, 1988—1992. *Teratology* 1995;51:20—29.

94. Rodeck CH, Fetal development after chorionic villus sampling. *Lancet* 1993;341:468—469.

95. Brent RL. The effects of embryonic and fetal exposure to x-ray, microwaves, and ultrasound. *Clin Obstet Gynecol* 1983;26:484—510.

96. Berlin L. Radiation exposure and the pregnant patient. *AJR* 1996;167:1377—1379.

97. Taylor L. Lauriston Taylor reviews radiation risks. *J Nucl Med* 1985;26:118—121.

98. Pleet H, Graham JM, Smith DW. Central nervous system and facial defects associated with maternal hyperthermia at 4 to 14 weeks gestation. *Pediat* 1981;61:785—789.

99. Milunsky A, Ulcickas M, Rothman KJ, et al. Maternal heat exposure and neural tube defects. *JAMA* 1992;268:882—885.

100. Ridge BR, Budd GM. how long is too long in a spa pool? *N Engl J Med* 1990;323:835.

101. Drose JA, Dennis MA, Thickman D. Infecton in utero: US findings in 19 cases. *Radiology* 1991;178:369—374.

102. Twickler DM, Perlman J, Mabrry MC. Congenital cytomegalovirus infecton presenting as cerebral ventriculomegaly on antenatal sonography. *Am J Perinatol* 1993;10:404—406.

103. Nathan L, Twickler DM, Peters MT, Sánchez PJ, Wendel Jr GD. Fetal syphilis: correlation of sonographic findings and rabbit infectivity testing of amniotic fluid. *J Ultrasound Med* 1993;2:97—101.

104. Raafat NA Birch AA, Altieri LA, et al. Sonographic osseous manifestations of fetal syphilis: a case report. *J Ultrasound Med* 1993;12:783—785.

105. Wright C, Hinchcliffe SA, TAylor C. Fetal pathology in intrauterine death due to parvovirus B19 infection. *Br J Obstet Gynaecol* 1996;103:133—136.

106. Parilla BV, Tamura RK, Ginsberg NA. Association of parvovirus with isolated fetal effusions. *Am J Perinatol* 1997,14:357—358.

107. Katz VL, McCoy C, Kuller JA, Hansen WF. An association between fetal parvovirus B19 infection and fetal anomalies. a report of two cases. *Am J Perinatol* 1996;13:43—45.

108. Guidozzi F, Ballot D, Rothberg AD. Human B19 parvovirus infection in an obstetric population — a prospective study determining fetal outcome. *J Reprod Med* 1994;39:36—38.

109. Marion RW, Wiznia AA, Hucheon RG, Rubinstein A. Fetal AIDS syndrome score — correlation between severity of dysmorphism and age at diagnosis of immunodeficiency. *AJDC* 1987;141:429—431.

110. Qazi QH Sheikh TM, Fikrig S, Menikoff H. Lack of evidence for craniofacial dysmorphism in perinatal human immunodeficiency virus infection. *J Pediat* 1988;112:7—11.

35 Postpartum Hemorrhage

Jeanne A. Cullinan, Donna M. Kepple

Introduction

Hemorrhage and infection remain major causes of postpartum morbidity and mortality. Statistics issued by the United States Department of Health & Human Services report a perinatal mortality of 73.7 per 100 000 live births in 1950. This had decreased to under seven per 100 000 live births by the mid 1990 s.[1] Data from the Maternal Mortality Collaborative Project from 1980 through 1985 implicated hemorrhage in 11% of maternal deaths.[2] Statistics on morbidity are more difficult to ascertain due to reporting practices. Postpartum infection and/or hemorrhage may account for up to 5 to 10% of patients with morbidity following childbirth.[3] This article will outline etiologies of postpartum infection and bleeding. Although these entities are separated for the purposes of discussion, it should be recognized that patients with postpartum hemorrhage are prone to the subsequent development of postpartum infection. Significant overlap is seen in history, symptomatology, and imaging of these patients.

Clinical Diagnosis

Postpartum Hemorrhage

Postpartum hemorrhage is defined as a blood loss of greater than 500 mL after the completion of the third stage of labor.[4] This definition is imprecise because it is based on a subjective assessment. Blood loss at delivery is often underestimated or unrecognized, particularly if it occurs into the retroperitoneum. In certain clinical conditions, the bleeding may be concealed and not obvious to the clinician. Many investigators have advocated an objective definition. One such definition that has been proposed is a drop in the hematocrit from admission to the postpartum period of 10%, or the need for transfusion therapy. This correlates roughly with a blood loss of 1000 cc.[5]

The visual estimate of blood loss is notoriously inaccurate, particularly in difficult vaginal deliveries or cesarean sections. Physical signs, including blood pressure and pulse, are also often inaccurate in the immediate postpartum period. Care must be taken to prevent a normotensive blood pressure reading from creating a false sense of security, in the setting of obvious hemorrhage or signs of intravascular compromise.[6]

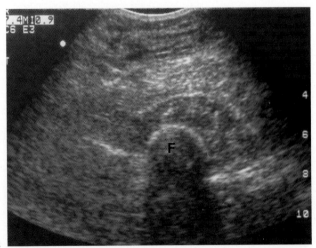

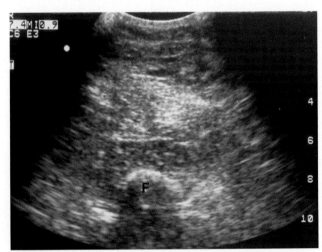

Figure 35–1 Postpartum hemorrhage: other etiologies. **A:** This patient presented with a significant drop in her hematocrit on day 4 postcesarean section for HELLP Syndrome. She had an enlarged tender left thigh. Imaging of the normal right thigh, demonstrates the normal muscular layers of the mid-thigh with posterior shadowing noted from the femur (F). **B:** In the left thigh, there is an increase in echogenicity, as well as an increase in thickness of the soft tissues of the left thigh. This represented intramuscular bleeding at an injection site.

The etiology of postpartum hemorrhage is complex. In a patient with diffuse coagulopathies due to pregnancy-related disorders, including abruption, fetal demise, or sepsis, hemorrhage may be quite severe. Other maternal etiologies of bleeding disorders include congenital coagulopathies or anticoagulation therapy. In these patients, the etiology of the bleeding is usually apparent from the history and abnormal laboratory data (**Fig. 35–1, 35–2**).

In the absence of a coagulation defect, hemorrhage often results from a physical cause, and the source of the bleeding should be established. The first area inspected should be the perineum. Visual inspection may show the presence of a vaginal or perineal hematoma. Perineal hematomas are seen in 1 and 300 to 1 and 1500 deliveries.[7] The incidence of hematomas among reported series varies significantly, probably due to differences in reporting, in definitions of significant hematomas, and in the rate of instrumentation at delivery. The true incidence is probably somewhere around 1 in 500 deliveries.[8] The hematoma results from bleeding into the surrounding tissues after a vascular injury. Causes for such hematomas include direct trauma, pressure necrosis, or inadequate hemostasis at the time of tissue repair. With operative vaginal deliveries, there is an increase in the incidence of this complication. Puerperal hematomas are often seen in patients with pudendal block, particularly if there is a coexisting clotting disorder. Vulvar and vaginal hematomas pose a risk of significant morbidity or even mortality if unrecognized.

The most commonly used classification of hematomas is based on the anatomic location. They are described as vulvar, vaginal, or subperitoneal.[8] Vaginal hematomas often involve the descending branch of the uterine artery.[7] Vulvar hematomas may involve branches of the pudendal artery. Vulvar hematomas may develop rapidly, producing excruciating pain, and a hematoma of moderate size may be seen bulging into the vagina or along the perineum. When the disrupted vessels extend above the pelvic fascia, the bleeding may dissect into the retroperitoneum. Of greatest clinical concern is the subperitoneal hematoma. When the bleeding extends into the retroperitoneal space, significant blood loss with hypovolemic shock may occur.

Inspection of the cervix may demonstrate lacerations, which may result from precipitous labor, obstructed labor, or intrapartum manipulations. Diagnosis is made by physical examination, rather than imaging modalities. If vaginal bleeding persists despite a firm uterus, then cervical lacerations should be suspected. These patients are prone to peritoneal bleeding if the laceration extends into cervical branches of the uterine artery.

After local causes for hemorrhage have been excluded by physical examination, the attention is turned to the uterus. Postpartum hemorrhage can be divided into two discrete diagnostic entities, primary and sec-

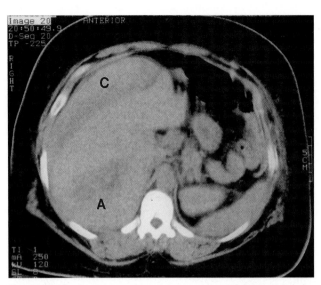

Figure 35–2 Postpartum hemorrhage: other etiologies. Vascular compromise was noted in this patient with a ruptured hepatic adenoma in the immediate postpartum period. A hypodense collection (C) is seen surrounding the liver representing clot. The adenoma (A) is seen as a hypodense area in the right posterior lobe of the liver.

ondary. Primary postpartum hemorrhage occurs during the first 24 h postpartum and is associated with acute clinical etiologies. This is the more common postpartum hemorrhage. Clinical circumstances at the time of delivery and physical examination will usually point to the diagnosis and aid in therapeutic interventions. Secondary postpartum hemorrhage occurs after 24 h. This is seen in fewer than 1% of patients.[3]

Postpartum hemorrhage accounts for more than 75% of serious postpartum complications within the first 24 h of delivery.[5] Uterine bleeding is responsible for up to 90% of cases of postpartum hemorrhage and is often severe. An immediate cause of hemorrhage is uterine atony. Uterine atony may be due to either an overdistended uterus or certain anesthetic agents. Clinically, the uterus is enlarged and boggy and fails to regress despite uterine massage or medical therapy.

Abnormal placentation sites also present with persistent vaginal bleeding. At the placental site, hemostasis is normally obtained by contraction and retraction of the myometrium to compress the small spiral arteries. Adherent placenta or large retained blood clots prevent effective myometrial contractions, which impairs hemostasis.[6] Abnormally adherent placenta remains the primary cause for emergency peripartum hysterectomies.

Uterine rupture may present as postpartum hemorrhage. *Uterine rupture* is defined as the disruption of all layers of the uterus, including the decidua, myometrium, and serosa. Predisposing conditions include previous uterine surgery or long difficult labor. In patients with vaginal deliveries after a previous cesarean section, uterine rupture can occur at the cesarean scar. Clinical presentation of uterine rupture includes significant bleeding postpartum and failure of the uterus to respond to uterine massage. In patients with cesarean sections, one must consider the postpartum scar and wound as other sources for the postpartum hemorrhage.

Secondary postpartum hemorrhage may be caused by retained placental tissue or subinvolution of the placental site. Retained placental fragments, as a result of either partial placental accreta or subinvolution of the placental bed, are common causes of such hemorrhage.[9] In many cases, however, the presence of tissue is not confirmed pathologically at the time of D&C.[10] Noninvoluted uteroplacental arteries are the cause of secondary postpartum hemorrhage in some cases.[11] The subinvolution may result from an aberrant interaction between the uterine cells and the trophoblast. Bleeding in these cases may be extensive and difficult to control, even in cases with retained fragments, because curettage may incite further hemorrhage at the site of abnormal placentation. Surgical intervention may also increase the probability of uterine adhesions with subsequent infertility.[12]

Infection

Postpartum infection is defined as a fever of 38 °C or higher that occurs on any two of the first 10 postpartum days exclusive of the first 24 h.[13] Postpartum infection occurs in 3 to 4% of vaginal deliveries and after 10 to 15% of cesarean deliveries, with the risk being higher in populations at risk.[14,15]

While the most common etiologies of persistent fever after childbirth are genital tract infections, it is important that patients be examined for extragenital causes before instituting therapy. As in the case of the patient with postpartum hemorrhage, thorough physical examination and laboratory assessment should be performed. Other possible causes for fever include respiratory complications, pyelonephritis, breast engorgement or infection, thrombophlebitis, and wound infections (**Fig. 35–3**). Clinical symptoms may include localized pain, continuous hemorrhaging, urine or bowel symptoms, vaginal discharge, or incisional drainage. Physical examination should include evaluation for genital and nongenital sources of infection. This includes assessment of the lungs, breast, abdomen, and pelvis, as well as the incision site. Chest X-ray, urine culture, as well as blood culture, may be obtained. In general, culture of the endometrial cavity is fraught with difficulties due to the potential for contamination. Occasionally, less common etiologies may account for fever in the postpartum period (**Fig. 35–4**).[16]

The route of delivery is the single most important risk factor for postpartum uterine infection. Infection occurs 10 to 20 times more frequently after cesarean section than vaginal delivery. Preoperative antibiotics have

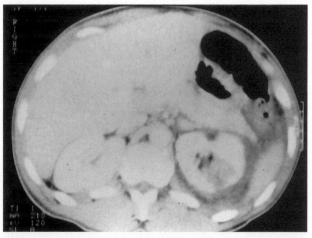

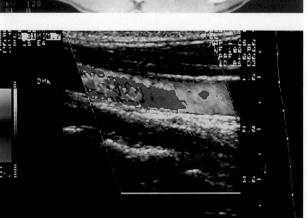

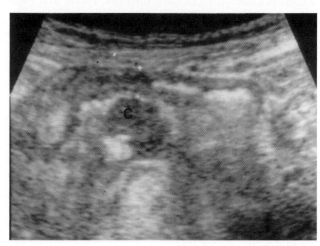

Figure 35–3 Postpartum fever: other etiologies. **A:** A hypodense area is noted in the interpolar region of the left kidney with stranding of the perinephritic fat. These findings were consistent with the clinical history of pyelonephritis. **B:** A noncompressible, blind-ending loop of bowel is seen. There is echogenic material in its distal tip with dirty "ringdown" shadowing. A small hypoechogenic collection is seen in the mesentery (C). Pathology confirmed a diagnosis of appendicitis. **C:** A noncompressible right common femoral vein was identified consistent with thrombophlebitis.

decreased the incidence of postpartum endometritis. After vaginal delivery, postpartum endometritis may be seen in patients following prolonged membrane rupture, multiple cervical examinations, or interpartum bacterosis.[17]

Postpartum endometritis following cesarean section is fairly common. The incidence is particularly high in patients who have multiple risk factors and do not receive antibiotic prophylaxis. Prophylactic antibiotics have decreased life-threatening complications to less than 2%.[18,19] Postpartum infection with pelvic cellulitis is another cause of postpartum infection. In patients with endometritis who fail to respond to antibiotics, a more extensive infection may ensue. Endometritis with cellulitis is typically a retroperitoneal infection. If cellulitis is extensive, then there may be areas of induration into the broad ligament with a resultant phlegmon. Symptoms of peritonitis, including an adynamic ileus, should raise concern for other etiologies, such as wound dehiscence or bowel injury.

Another important source of postpartum temperature elevation is the breast. In up to 15% of women, breast engorgement may cause a brief fever that rarely exceeds 39 °C.[20] This temperature elevation is usually transient and appears in the first 2—3 days postpartum. Postpartum mastitis is encountered in approximately 10% of women with breast engorgement. Infection of

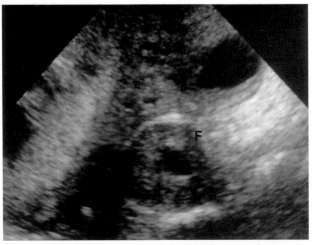

Figure 35–4   Postpartum fever: other etiologies. This patient presented with a postpartum fever due to necrosis of a fibroid of the broad ligament. Follow-up examination demonstrates a hypoechogenic center within the uterine fibroid (F) representing the area of necrosis.

the mammary glands can occasionally be seen as early as the first week postpartum, but, as a general rule, mastitis is not seen until later in the postpartum period. Approximately 10% of patients with postpartum mastitis may develop an abscess (**Fig. 35.5**), accompanied by constitutional symptoms.[21]

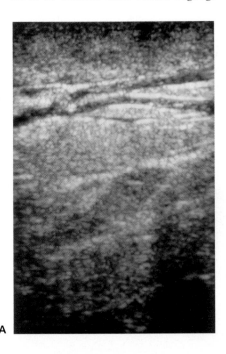

A

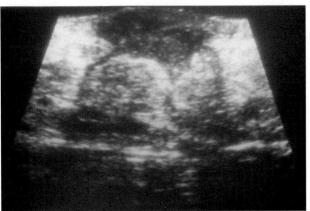

B

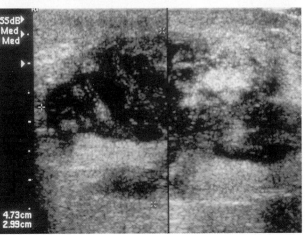

C

Figure 35–5   Postpartum fever: mastitis. **A:** Minimal dilatation of the mammary ducts is seen in the lactating patient. **B:** With mastitis, periareolar inflammation with focal abscess formation may be demonstrated. These often respond to conservative management. **C:** Deeper infections of the breast parenchyma may require surgical intervention if they fail to respond to antibiotic therapy. Sonogram illustrates a large complex collection deep to the right nipple in a patient who required surgical incision and drainage.

Postpartum thrombophlebitis or ovarian vein thrombosis typically presents with persistent fevers.[13] Ovarian vein thrombophlebitis is reported in 1 in 600 deliveries.[22] Clot in the ovarian veins may extend into the inferior vena cava. Clinical suspicion should be raised in patients who continue to have spiking fevers, despite antimicrobial therapy. Ovarian vein thrombosis is seen predominantly on the right. On the left, the ovarian vein flow is antegrade during pregnancy, while on the right ovarian vein flow is retrograde. Venous flow decreases sharply in the postpartum period, causing partial collapse and stasis within the veins. Valves in the right ovarian vein increase the risk of pooling and thrombosis.[23] Before using imaging modalities, patients often receive a therapeutic trial of anticoagulation. The patient usually responds within 48 to 72 h.

Imaging

Normal Anatomic Changes

The process of normal uterine involution following delivery occurs with rapid reversal of the growth changes seen during pregnancy. The most rapid involution takes place during the first week postpartum, with over a 50% reduction in the size of the uterus. Involution of the gravid uterus is usually complete by 6 to 8 weeks postpartum.[3] The uterus regresses during the postpartum period as a result of loss of fluid and protein and a reduction in cell size.[19] Typically, after 2 weeks the uterus is only mildly enlarged, and the endometrium is thin. Small amounts of blood or fluid are often seen in the uterine cavity (**Fig. 35–6**).[24] Excess fluid in the endometrial cavity, measuring more than 2 cm, may be a sign of postpartum atony or retained products of conception.

Postpartum Hemorrhage

Postpartum hemorrhage may result from retained products of conception, and ultrasound is often used to assess for the presence of retained products (**Fig. 35–7**). The most common sonographic finding with retained placental fragments is an echogenic mass in the uterine cavity.[25] If the cavity is distended more than 1.5 cm in the anteroposterior measurement with echogenic or heterogeneous material, then the probability of retained products increases. If hyperechoic foci are seen with no intraluminal mass, then products of conception are unlikely. Retained fragments are also unlikely in the presence of a normal endometrial stripe or fluid in the uterine cavity.[25,26] In cases of postpartum hemorrhage from suspected retained products, it is recommended that sonographic evaluation be performed before uterine instrumentation to avoid confusion from iatrogenically introduced air or bleeding.

Recently, sonohysterography has been reported to be of value in the evaluation of patients for residual trophoblastic tissue.[27] Sonohysterography will outline endometrial contents and provide added information to the transvaginal sonogram. Conservative management is preferred in patients in the absence of retained fragments, to reduce the risk of perforation or adhesion formation (**Fig. 35–8**).[12,27]

Another cause of postpartum hemorrhage that must be ruled out is uterine rupture. This is particularly important to consider in patients with previous cesarean section. Sonographic findings of uterine rupture include thinning of the uterine wall to less than 5 mm and a wedged-shaped myometrial defect.[28]

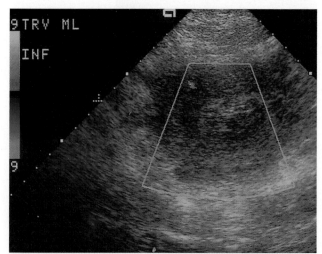

Figure 35–6 Normal postpartum uterus. **A:** A sagittal image of the uterus demonstrates a thin endometrial interface with a small amount of blood/debris (D) in the region of the lower uterine segment. **B:** A small amount of echogenic material is seen within the endometrial cavity with no significant flow seen.

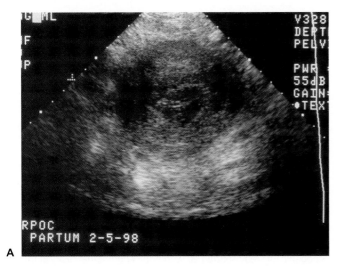

A

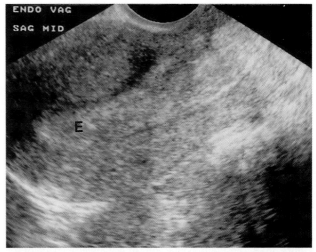

B

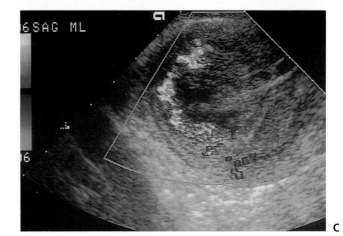

C

Figure 35–7   Postpartum hemorrhage. **A:** A midline image of the uterus demonstrates minimal debris within the cavity. **B:** A sagittal image of the uterus demonstrates a thick echogenic endometrial interface (E). Pathology confirmed retained products of conception. **C:** This patient presented with significant vaginal bleeding due to retained products of conception. A large amount of vascularity at the endometrial—myometrial interface is seen.

Postpartum Infection

Imaging studies in pelvic infection often are not helpful. Sonographic findings may be normal with uncomplicated endometritis. Gas within the endometrial cavity is a common finding, seen in 21% of patients in the first 3 days postpartum, and, therefore, is not diagnostic if a uterine infection.[29, 30] Seven percent of patients without infection have gas in the cavity up to 3 weeks postdelivery. Blood and fluid in the endometrial cavity are also a common finding in normal women.[31, 32] These fluid collections usually resolve within 1 week postpartum.

Endometritis is the most common cause of fever in the postpartum period. Retained products of conception may predispose patients to infection, as these serve as a nidus for bacterial overgrowth. Sonographic findings may be normal with uncomplicated endometritis, or endometrial fluid and/or gas or a localized abscess may be identified (**Fig. 35–9**). Abscesses appear sonographically as complex intrauterine masses which are primarily cys-

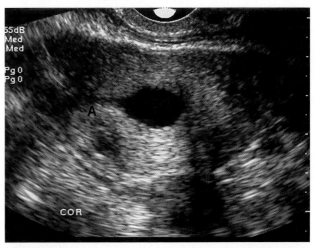

Figure 35–8   Intrauterine adhesions. This coronal image in the fundal region from a saline enhanced examination shows coapted walls representing adhesions (A) in the right cornu in a patient status-postinstrumentation.

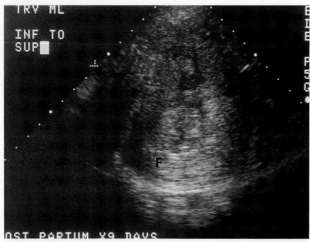

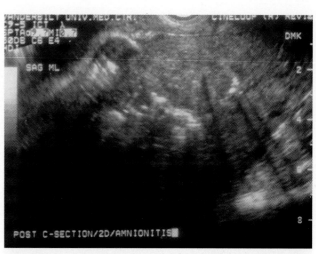

Figure 35–9 Postpartum infection. **A:** A transverse image of the uterus demonstrates echogenic material (F) within the cavity with small echogenic foci in the fundus consistent with either air and/or infection. **B:** A sagittal image demonstrates retained material with echogenic foci representing air within the endometrial cavity in this patient two days after surgery, now with an elevated temperature, white count, and uterine tenderness.

tic but may contain internal debris.[3] On computed tomography (CT), an endometrial abscess appears as a low density mass in the uterus. Such infections may require prolonged antibiotic therapy for resolution.

With prolonged infection, sonography may be useful in diagnosing the infection, as well as in assessing response to therapy.[33, 34]

Special considerations are needed for imaging patients with fever postcesarean section. In patients with possible uterine dehiscence, for example, the imaging must be correlated with the clinical symptoms (**Fig. 35–10**). Patients presenting with fever or significant blood loss after cesarean section are at risk for hematoma and abscess formation near the bladder or underneath the wound incision. These collections appear sonographically as complex masses at the site of the surgical inci-

sion or behind the bladder (**Fig. 35–11**).[35] Unfortunately, many patients without infection after cesarean section have parametrial fluid as a normal postoperative finding. This makes the diagnosis by imaging difficult. It is also common to see a small amount of fluid within the region of the bladder flap.[36] The presence of a large collection in this area, especially if it contains air, makes the diagnosis of infection or abscess more likely. The sonographic appearance of the collection depends on the degree of organization. When collections greater than 2 cm in diameter are identified, hematoma formation should be suspected. Bladder flap collections greater than 3.5 cm are associated with increased postpartum morbidity.[37]

Both transabdominal and transperineal ultrasound can be used to assess for complications of cesarean sec-

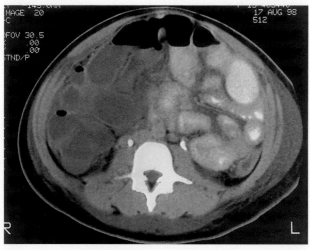

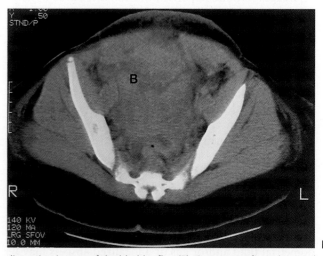

Figure 35–10 Postpartum hemorrhage: uterine dehiscence. **A:** A CT image of the mid abdomen demonstrates distended small bowel loops consistent with an ileus. **B:** In the pelvis, necrosis and disruption is seen of the bladder flap (B). Surgery confirmed wound dehiscence with necrosis.

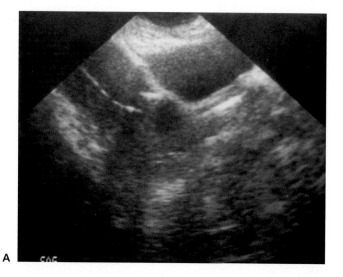

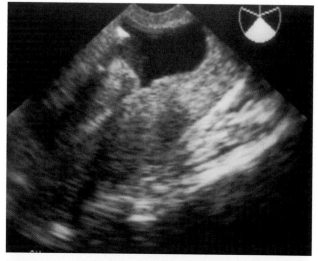

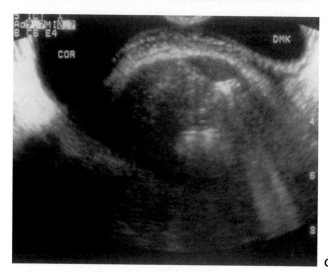

Figure 35–11 Postpartum endometritis: bladder flap collection. **A:** A sagittal transabdominal image of the uterus demonstrates an echogenic focus with ringdown shadowing in a small bladder flap collection. **B:** Transvaginal sonography confirmed this finding. **C:** A similar appearance is noted in a second patient with a postpartum fever after cesarean section. The bladder flap hematoma has echogenic material as well as air.

tion, although transabdominal scanning demonstrates a broader area.[38] The region of the uterine wound is usually well seen by either approach. Bladder flap hematomas and subfascial hematomas should be evaluated with transabdominal scanning.

Sonography is usually reserved for patients who present with significant vaginal bleeding or infection, to assess the uterus and parametrium, as well as abdominal or uterine incision (**Fig. 35–12**). Sonography is also useful for evaluating patients with vaginal or vulvar masses (**Fig. 35–13**), as well as patients with subperitoneal hematomas that dissect into the retroperitoneal space or along the pelvic side walls (**Fig. 35–14**).

Imaging may be useful in patients with refractory fevers from suspected ovarian vein thrombosis. Computed tomography, ultrasound, and magnetic resonance (MR) have all been utilized in the diagnosis of ovarian vein thrombosis. Computed tomography findings include distension of the ovarian vein with a nonenhancing mass within the lumen representing the thrombus. The vein appears as a tubular structure extending into the ret-

roperitoneal region with an enhancing vessel wall. On sonography, the abnormal vein may appear as an anechoic to hypoechoic structure extending superiorly from the adnexa. Magnetic resonance imaging is also useful for demonstrating thrombus.[33,39,40] Because the ovarian veins may be difficult to see due to overlying bowel gas, computed tomography and magnetic resonance imaging are the modalities of choice for diagnosing this disorder.

Arterial Embolization

Historically, control of postpartum hemorrhage has been accomplished via surgery. Bilateral hypogastric ligation significantly reduces pelvic blood flow and pulse pressure beyond the ligation.[41] Uterine artery ligation is also effective in controlling hemorrhage.[42] Failures of uterine artery ligation occur in patients with uterine atony or infection, placenta previa with extensive bleeding, or bleeding into the broad ligament. In these patients it may be necessary to ligate the ovarian or hypogastric arteries.

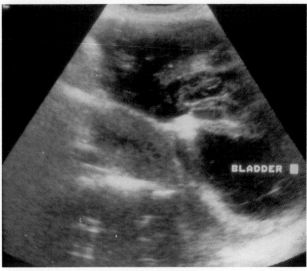

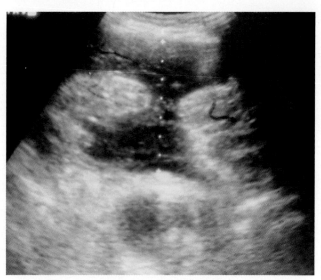

Figure 35–12 Postpartum hemorrhage: wound hematoma. **A:** An extensive wound hematoma was noted requiring surgical invention in this patient with HELLP Syndrome. A transverse image of the abdominal wall illustrates the collection. **B:** The collection has a ground glass appearance consistent with a hematoma and is seen splaying the bellies of the rectus muscles on this transverse image.

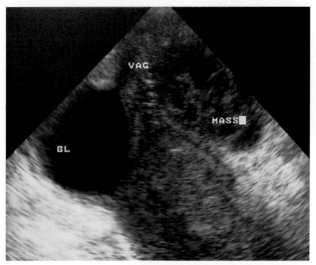

Figure 35–13 Postpartum hemorrhage: perineal hematoma. A large complex mass was noted posterior to the vagina in this patient status-postvaginal delivery with a mediolaterial episiotomy.

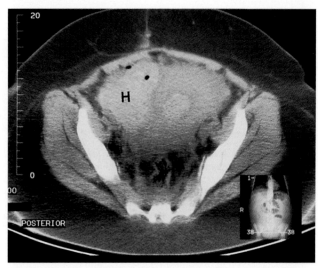

Figure 35–14 Postpartum hemorrhage: cervical laceration. A large hematoma containing air is noted to the right uterine body (H). This represented an intraperitoneal extension of a cervical laceration. The echogenic material seen within the uterus was in keeping with the patient's recent delivery.

Angiographic embolization is often useful in patients with postpartum hemorrhage. In capable hands, this is a safe and relatively rapid procedure. It should be considered before ligation of the hypogastric vessels, as ligation results in loss of access to the vessels. Success rates of angiographic embolization range from 40 to 100% in contemporary studies. [43–48] Complications from post-cesarean section embolotherapy are reported in approximately 6 to 7% of patients, with no deaths reported. The complications include abscess and fever.

Transcatheter arterioembolization has emerged as a highly effective technique for controlling acute genital bleeding. Transcatheter embolization of the hypogastric artery may be utilized as a nonsurgical method to man-age significant pelvic hemorrhage in patients in whom future fertility is a consideration (**Fig. 35–15**). After the procedure, normal menses returns and childbearing is not compromised.[49–51]

The standard for the treatment of serious obstetrical hemorrhage had been ligation of the hypogastric arteries or emergency hysterectomies. Angiographic embolization has proven effective in a high percentage of cases where even surgical intervention had been unsuccessful. Because patient at highest risk may be identified before delivery, some investigators have suggested the use of prophylactic placement of angiographic catheters before delivery.[47, 52, 53]

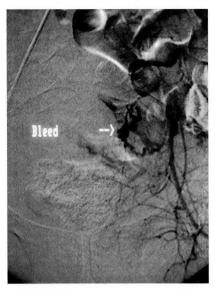

Figure 35–15 Postpartum hemorrhage: embolization. Interventional angiography successfully controlled bleeding in this patient with significant postpartum hemorrhage.

Conclusion

Postpartum hemorrhage and infection pose significant maternal risks. Imaging modalities provide useful clinical information in the diagnosis and subsequent follow-up of these patients. They allow for a timely diagnosis of potentially life threatening complications in the puerperal period.

References

1. Maternal mortality rates for complications of pregnancy, childbirth, and the puerperium according to race and age: United States, selected years 1950—93. Health United States, 1995. U.S. Department of Health and Human Services

2. Rochart RW, Koonin LM, Atrash HK, Jewett JF. (The Maternal Mortality Collaborative): Maternal mortality in the United States: Report from the Maternal Mortality Collaborative. *Obstet Gynecol* 1988;72:91

3. Fleischer AC, Manning FA, Jeanty P, Romero R. *Sonography In Obstetrics & Gynecology: Principles & Practice.* In: Lavery PJ, Gadwood KA. Postpartum Ultrasound, 5th ed. Appleton & Lange, 1995, p. 739—754.

4. Cunningham FG, MacDonald PC, Gant NF, Leveno KJ, Gilstrap LC III. Obstetrical Hemorrhage In: *Williams Obstetrics*, 19th ed. Norwalk, CT: Appleton & Lange, 1993, p. 819.

5. Roberts RE. Emergency obstetric management of postpartum hemorrhage. *Obstet Gynecol Clin North Am* 1995;22(2):283—302.

6. Cunningham FG, MacDonald PC, Gant NF, Leveno KJ, Gilstrap LC II.: Obstetrical Hemorrhage. In: *Williams Obstetrics*. 19th ed. Norwalk, CT: Appleton & Lange, 1993, p. 821.

7. Zahn CM, Yeomans ER. Postpartum hemorrhage: placental accreta, uterine inversion and puerperal hematomas. *Clin Obstet Gynecol* 1990;33:422.

8. Ridgway.LE: Puerperal emergency: vaginal and vulvar hematomas. *Obstet & Gynecol Clin North Am* 1995;22(2):357—367.

9. Khong TY, Khong TK. Delayed postparum hemorrhage: a morphologic study of causes and their relation to other pregnancy disorders. *Obstet Gynecol* 1993;82(1):17.

10. Dewhurst CJ. Secondary postpartum hemorrhage. *J Obstet Gynaecol Br Commonw* 1996;73:53.

11. Andrew AC, Bulmer JN, Wells M, Morrison L, Buckley CH. Subinvolution of the uteroplacental arteries in the human placental bed. *Histopathology* 1989;15:375.

12. Buttram VC. What sets the stage for IUA? *Contemp Ob-Gyn* 1978;11:33.

13. Cunningham FG, MacDonald PC, Gant NF, Leveno KJ, Gilstrap LC III. *Puerperal infection.* In: Williams Obstetrics, 19th ed. Norwalk, CT: Appleton & Lange, 1993, p. 627.

14. Gibbs RS, Rodgers PJ, Castaneda YS et al. Endometritis following vaginal delivery. *Obstet Gynecol* 1988;72:519.

15. Willison JR. The conquest of cesarean section related infections. *Obstet Gynecol* 1988;72:519.

16. Lee WL, Chiu LM, Wang PH, Chao HT, Yuan CC. Fever of unknown origin in the puerperium. A case report. *J Reprod Med* 1998;43(2):149—52.

17. Cunnningham FG, MacDonald PC, Gant NF, Leveno KJ, Gilstrap LC III. Puerperal Infection. 19th ed. Norwalk, CT: Appleton & Lange, 1993, p. 628.

18. Zuckman J, Levine D, McNicholas MJ, et al. Imaging of pelvic postpartum complications. *AJR* 1997;168(3):663—667.

19. Lavery JP, Shaw LA. Sonography of the puerperal uterus. *J Ultrasound Med* 1989;8:481—486.

20. Calhoun BC, Brost B. Emergency management of sudden puerperal fever. *Obstet Gynecol* 1995;22(2):357—367.

21. Cunningham FG, Macdonald PC, Gant NF. *Other Disorders of the Puerperium.* In: Williams Obstetrics, 19th ed., Norwalk, CT: Appleton & Lange, 1993, p. 647.

22. Thromboembolism in Pregnancy. ACOG Education Bulletin. Washington, D.C.: ACOG. March 1997.

23. Munsick R, Gillanders L. A review of the syndrome of puerperal ovarian vein thrombophlebitis. *Obstet Gynecol Surv* 1981;36:57—66.

24. Wachsberg RH, Kurtz AB, Levine CD et al. Real-time ultrasonographic analysis of the normal postpartum uterus. *J Ultrasound Med* 1994;13:215—221.

25. Wachsberg RH, Kurtz AB. Gas within the endometrial cavity after postpartum US: a normal finding after spontaneous vaginal delivery. *Radiology* 1992;183:431.

26. Garagiola D, Tarver R, Gibson L, Rogers R, Wass J. Anatomic changes in the pelvis after uncomplicated vaginal delivery: a CT study on 14 women. *AJR* 1989; 153:1239—1241.

27. Woo GM, Twickler DM, Stettler RW, Erdman WA, Brown, CEL. The pelvis after cesarean section and vaginal delivery: normal MR findings. *AJR* 1993;161(12):1249—1252.

28. Williams AB, Brown ED, Kettritzz UL, Kuller, JA, Semelka RC. Anatomic changes in the pelvis after uncomplicated vaginal delivery: Evaluation with serial MR imaging. *Radiology* 1995;195(4):91—94.

29. Hertzberg, BS, Bowie JD: Ultrasound of the postpartum uterus. *J Ultrasound Med* 1991;10:451—456.

30. Lee CY, Madrazo B, Drukker BH. Ultrasonic evaluation of the postpartum uterus in the managment of postpartum bleeding. *Obstet Gynecol* 1981;58:227.

31. Wolman I, Hartoov J, Pauzner D, et al. Transvaginal sonohysterography for the early diagnosis of residual trophoblastic tissue. *J Ultrasound Med* 1997;16:257—261.

32. Michaels WH, Thompson HO, Boutt A, et al. Ultrasound diagnosis in the scarred lower uterine segment during pregnancy. *Obstet Gynecol* 1988;71:112.

33. Brown CEL, Lowe TW, Cunningham FG, Weinreb J. Puerperal pelvic thrombophlebitis, impact on diagnosis and treatment using x-ray computed tomography and magentic resonance imaging. *Obstet Gynecol* 1986;68:789—794.

34. Lev-Toaff AS, Baka JJ, Toaff ME, et al. Diagnostic imaging in puerperal febrile morbidity. *Obstet Gynecol* 1991;78:50.

35. Twickler DM, Setiawan AT, Harrell RS, Brown CEL. CT appearance of the pelvis after cesarean section. *Am J Radiol* 1991;156:523.

36. Baker ME, Bowie JD, Killam AP. Sonography of post-cesarean-section bladder-flap hematoma *AJR* 1985;144(4):757.

37. Hertzberg BS, Bowie JD, Kliewer, MA. Complications of cesarean section: role of transperineal US. *Radiology* 1993;188(2):533.

38. Shaffer P, Johnson J, Bryan D, et al. Diagnosis of ovarian vein thrombophlebitis by computed tomography. *J Comput Assist Tomogr* 1981;5:436—439.

39. Savader SJ, Otero RR, Savader BL. Puerperal ovarian vein thrombosis: evaluation with CT, US and MR imaging. *Radiology* 1988;167:637—639.

40. Grant TH, Schoettle BW, Buchsbaum MS. Postpartmen ovarian vein thrombosis: diagnosis by clot protrusion into the inferior vena cava at sonography. *AJR* 1993;60:551—552.

41. Burchell RC. Physiology of internal iliac artery ligation. *J Obstet Gynaecol Br Commonw* 1968;75:642—651.

42. O'Leary JL, O'Leary JA. Uterine artery ligation for control of postcesarean section hemorrhage. *Obstet Gynecol* 1974;43:849—853.

43. Evans S, McShane P. The efficacy of internal iliac artery ligation in obstetric hemorrhage. *Surg Gynecol Obstet* 1985;160:250—253.

44. Clark SL, Phelan JP, Yeh S, Bruce SR, Paul RH. Hypogastric artery ligation for obstetric hemorrhage. *Obstet Gynecol* 1985;66:353—356.

45. Thavarasah AS, Sivalingam N, Almohdzar SA. Internal iliac and ovarian artery ligation in the control of pelvic haemorrhage. *Aust N Z J Obstet Gynaecol* 1989;29:22—25.

46. Chattopadhyay SK, Deb Roy B, Edress YB. Surgical control of obstetric hemorrhage: hypogastric artery ligation or hysterectomy? *Int J Gynaecol Obstet* 1991;32:345–351.

47. Mitty HA, Sterling KM, Alvarez M, Gendler R. Obstetric hemorrhage: prophylactic & emergency arterial catheterization and embolotherapy. *Radiology* 1993;88(1):183.

48. Vedantham S, Goodwin SC, McLucas B, Mohr G. Uterine artery embolization: an underused method of controlling pelvic hemorrhage. *AJ Obstet & Gynecol* 1997;176(4):938

49. Stancato-Pasik A, Mitty HA, Richard HM, Eshkar N. Obstetric embolotherapy: effect on menses and pregnancy. *Radiology* 1997;204:791.

50. Greenwood LH, Glickman MG, Schwartz PE, Morse SS, Denny DF. Obstetric and non-malignant gynecologic bleeding: treatment with angiographic embolization. *Radiology* 1987;164:155–159.

51. AbdRabbo SA. Stepwise uterine devascularization: a novel technique for management of uncontrolled postpartum hemorrhage with preservation of the uterus. *Am J Obstet Gynecol* 1994;171:694—700.

52. Alvarez M, Lockwood CJ, Ghidini A, et al. Prophylactic and emergent arterial catheterization for selective embolization in obstetric hemorrhage. *Am J Perinatol* 1992;9:441–444.

53. Likeman MA. The boldest procedure possible for checking the bleeding-a new look at an old operation, and a series of 13 cases from an Australian hospital. *Aust N Z J Obstet Gynaecol* 1992;32:256—62.

Pediatric Patient

36 Pediatric Abdominal Masses

Debra M. Lau and Marilyn J. Siegel

The role of diagnostic imaging in the evaluation of an abdominal mass in the neonate or older child is the determination of the origin, character, and extent of the lesion, with a minimum number of imaging procedures. Ultrasonography has gained widespread acceptance as a useful method to assess abdominal masses because of its widespread availability and relative ease of performance. This chapter addresses the clinical and sonographic features of selected common abdominal masses in infants and children. Advantages and limitations of other imaging procedures will also be described.

Differential Diagnosis

Neonatal Abdominal Masses

As many disease processes are age characteristic, this chapter is organized by age of presentation. Pediatric abdominal masses can be divided into two groups: those that present neonatally and those that present in the older infant and child.

Abdominal masses in neonates and infants under 2 months of age are predominantly retroperitoneal in location.[1,2] Fortunately, the majority of masses are benign and have an excellent prognosis. Most neonatal and infantile abdominal masses are renal in origin, and the most are hydronephrosis and multicystic dysplastic kidney. Together, these two entities account for approximately 70% of renal masses and 40% of all abdominal masses. Far less common entities that present in this age group include autosomal recessive polycystic disease, mesoblastic nephroma, renal vein thrombosis, and nephroblastomatosis.

Genital masses, such as hydrometrocolpos and ovarian cysts, and gastrointestinal masses including duplication cysts, volvulus, and mesenteric-omental cysts, each account for about 15% of neonatal masses.[1,2] The remainder of neonatal abdominal masses are extrarenal retroperitoneal masses (10%) and hepatobiliary masses (5%). The extrarenal retroperitoneal masses almost entirely comprise adrenal hemorrhages and rare neuroblastomas. The most frequently encountered hepatobiliary masses are hemangioendothelioma and choledochal cyst.

Abdominal Masses in the Older Infant and Child

The majority of abdominal masses occurring in the older infant (after 2 months of age) and child is still predominantly of retroperitoneal origin.[1,2] However, important differences in the specific types and incidence of lesions encountered exist. Although the overall frequency of renal masses is the same (55%), there is a significant increase in the incidence of Wilms' tumor and a decreased incidence of nonhydronephrotic cystic masses. Wilms' tumor account for 22% of renal masses in this older age group. Nonrenal retroperitoneal tumors also occur more frequently in this age group, and account for 23% of abdominal masses. This difference reflects both the increased prevalence of neuroblastoma and the concomitant decrease in adrenal hemorrhage. Hence, the percentage of malignant retroperitoneal neoplasms is significantly higher in older infants and children than in neonates.

Intraperitoneal masses are encountered less often in the older infant and child; this is primarily due to the decreased frequency of genital masses (4%).[1,2] Hepatobiliary masses and gastrointestinal lesions occur with similar overall frequencies to those seen in neonates (6% and 12%, respectively); however, there is a notably higher percentage of malignant hepatic neoplasms in this age group than in the neonate. Concurrently, there is a marked decrease in the frequency of congenital gastrointestinal masses and an increase in inflammatory masses (e.g., appendiceal abscess).

In the workup of a newborn with a clinically suspected abdominal mass, plain abdominal radiography is recommended as the initial imaging procedure. The primary role of radiography is to confirm the presence of the mass and suggest its size and position. If intestinal obstruction is suggested radiographically, then contrast examination of the gastrointestinal tract is the next most appropriate step. The decision of whether to perform an upper gastrointestinal series or barium enema is based on the suspected level of obstruction. Alternatively, if an extraintestinal mass is suggested, sonography should be performed as the next procedure.

Diagnostic Workup

Other Imaging Tests

The imaging techniques most frequently employed in the evaluation of suspected abdominal masses include plain radiography, scintigraphy, ultrasonography, and computed tomography (CT). Abdominal radiography is simple and readily available, but rarely diagnostic. Its utility lies in confirming the presence of an intraabdominal mass and in detecting the presence or absence of associated calcifications. Additional examinations are usually required for further characterization and specific diagnosis.

Similarly, radionuclide imaging has a limited diagnostic role in the evaluation of abdominal masses. The main limitations are its poor anatomic resolution and relative organ specificity; however, it is a valuable tool for the detection of functioning tissue in renal or hepatobiliary masses. Renal scintigraphy is superior to urography for identifying and quantifying functional renal tissue in cases of renal obstruction. In the case of a suspected biliary mass, hepatobiliary imaging is an excellent technique for confirming the diagnosis of a choledochal cyst. If a hepatic mass is present, radionuclide angiography is helpful in suggesting the presence of a hemangioendothelioma.

Ultrasonography has become an increasingly relied upon imaging modality in the workup of abdominal and pelvic masses in children.[3–7] It is especially useful in the neonate because of the lack of need for patient sedation. Other advantages include the ability to perform dynamic imaging in multiple planes and the lack of ionizing radiation. Sonography is useful for identifying the organ of origin, disease extent, and solid or cystic nature of a mass. Unfortunately, it cannot assess the function of a mass. Technically, sonographic interpretation may be hampered by intervening bowel gas or bone artifact. Additionally, compared with the other imaging modalities, sonography is more technically challenging to yield high-quality images and diagnostic information.

Computed tomography offers several advantages over the aforementioned radiologic techniques. First is its ability to identify small differences in attenuation values and, thus, reliably distinguish between blood, fat, and calcium. Second, CT is able to provide cross-sectional images that are unobscured by overlying structures such as bowel gas or bone; this is especially helpful in evaluating the retroperitoneum. Additionally, contrast-enhanced CT may provide information about the vascular anatomy and function of an abdominal mass. The disadvantages of CT in children include exposure to ionizing radiation, the necessity for sedation in most children under 5 years of age, and the need for oral contrast agents. The administration of oral contrast agents is especially important in pediatric imaging because, unlike adults, infants and children typically have little periviseral fat which serves to improve delineation of intraabdominal anatomy.

Approach to Imaging

Assuming technically adequacy, if the sonographic examination is normal, the need for further evaluation is generally eliminated. If renal sonography demonstrates hydronephrosis, renal scintigraphy may be employed to identify functional renal tissue in the hydronephrotic kidney and quantify the split renal function. A voiding cystourethrogram should also be included in the radiologic work up of hydronephrosis to differentiate obstructive causes of dilatation from nonobstructive causes, such as reflux. Computed tomography is usually unnecessary, but is sometimes performed if the level of obstruction is uncertain or a malignant neoplasm is suspected.

Similarly, if sonography shows benign cystic lesions in the adrenal glands, liver or ovaries, further imaging usually is not needed. However, if ultrasonography reveals a solid adrenal, hepatic or ovarian mass, CT is recommended. Contrast-enhanced CT can differentiate vascular lesions from other types of neoplasms, as well as define the extent of disease. When sonography suggests the presence of a choledochal cyst, confirmation by hepatobiliary scintigraphy is useful; hepatic excretion and accumulation within the sonographically detected mass is diagnostic of a choledochal cyst.

Sonographic Findings of Abdominal Masses

Kidneys

Neonates

The normal neonatal kidney demonstrates several unique sonographic features that are important to recognize (**Fig. 36–1**).[8] First, renal cortical echogenicity is increased and usually is equal to that of the liver or spleen, rather than being hypoechoic relative to those structures. The renal cortex becomes hypoechoic relative to liver or spleen in the majority of patients by 2 or 3 months, and nearly all infants demonstrate an adult echo pattern by the end of the first year. A second unique feature of the neonatal and infant kidney is that the medullary pyramids are hypoechoic and prominent. The pyramids attain an adult appearance by 1 year of age. Finally, the renal sinus in neonates, infants, and young children is not as echogenic as it is in adolescents and adults. The central sinus echogenicity increases with age, and the echogenic renal pelvis, characteristic of adults, is observed by adolescence. Other normal variations in anatomy include fetal lobulations, the junctional parenchymal defect and the interrenuncular septum (or junctional parenchymal line).[9]

Hydronephrosis

The goals of sonography in the evaluation of neonatal hydronephrosis are to evaluate kidney and bladder morphology, identify congenital anomalies which may be causative, and provide a baseline study for future reference.

Hydronephrosis is the most common cause of an abdominal mass in the neonate, accounting for approximately 25% of mass lesions.[1,2] Five disorders account for virtually all cases of hydronephrosis: ureteropelvic junction obstruction, 44%; ureterovesical junction obstruction, 21%; vesicoureteral reflux, 14%; duplication anomalies with an obstructed moiety, 12%; and posterior urethral valves, 9%.[4] Most cases of neonatal hydronephrosis are detected on in utero sonograms. If diagnosis is delayed beyond the neonatal period, then hydronephrosis is frequently complicated by superimposed infection and infants present with signs and symptoms of urinary tract infection.

The diagnosis of hydronephrosis is based on the presence of multiple communicating cysts of uniform size which connect to the central renal pelvis. The amount of renal parenchyma and degree of morphologic changes seen in hydronephrosis are dependent upon the severity and duration of the underlying lesion. In most cases of mild to moderate obstruction, renal scintigraphy and excretory urography is able to demonstrate some degree of preserved renal function on delayed images. However, in cases of severe hydronephrosis, there may be near complete absence of renal function; this can be scintigraphically and urographically indistinguishable from multicystic dysplastic kidney.

Ureteropelvic junction (UPJ) obstruction is the most common congenital urinary tract anomaly. The etiology of UPJ obstruction is controversial, but it has been postulated to be secondary to intrinsic stenosis, extrinsic compression from a fibrous band or aberrant vessel, or abnormal development of the muscle fibers at the ureteropelvic junction resulting in ineffective peristalsis and obstruction. Sonographically, the diagnosis is suggested by the presence of a dilated renal pelvis and calyces in the setting of a nondilated ureter and a normal bladder (**Fig. 36–2**).[10] The degree of pelvicaliectasis and parenchymal thinning is variable and bears no direct correlation with renal function. Other findings include increased parenchymal echogenicity and cortical cysts, reflecting renal dysplasia.[11] Renal scintigraphy is able to confirm an UPJ obstruction and can provide additional information regarding total and split renal function.

Ureterovesical junction obstruction may be divided into three types: (1) nonobstructive, nonrefluxing megaureter, (2) obstructive megaureter, and (3) refluxing megaureter. In primary megaureter, there is no juxtavesical obstruction or reflux. In obstructive megaureter, the most distal part of the ureter is narrowed and aperistaltic.[12] This segment is typically short, less than 4 cm, and

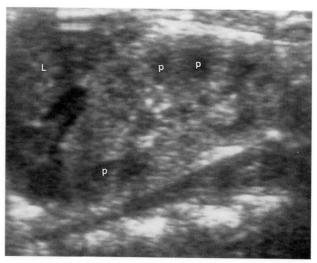

Figure 36–1   Normal renal anatomy. Neonatal kidney, longitudinal scan. Note the characteristic features of the neonatal kidney: similar echogenicity of the cortex and adjacent liver (**L**); prominent, hypoechoic medullary pyramids (**p**); and a paucity of central renal sinus echogenicity.

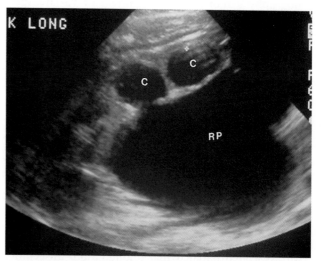

Figure 36–2   Ureteropelvic junction obstruction in a neonate. Longitudinal sonogram of the left kidney shows dilated calyces (C), a large renal pelvis (RP), and a thin rim of surrounding renal parenchyma. A distal ureter was not identified.

is located in the juxtavesical portion of the ureter. Sonography demonstrates unilateral or bilateral ureteral dilatation (**Fig. 36–3**).[12,13] The ureters are peristaltic proximal to the aperistaltic distal segment, which may or may not be identified as a short segment of fixed narrowing. The degree of hydronephrosis is variable. The diagnosis of primary megaureter may be confirmed by renal scintigraphy or excretory urography. In the neonate, the differential diagnosis of ureterectasis includes vesicoureteral reflux, ectopic ureter (isolated or associated with renal duplication), and infection-induced ureteral atony.

Ultrasonography is a poor predictor of primary vesicoureteral reflux (VUR) as variable degrees of urinary

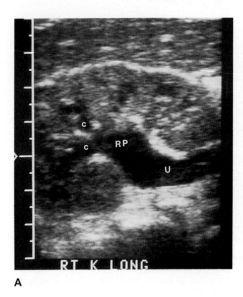

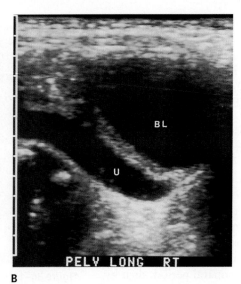

A   B

Figure 36–3 Megaureter. **A:** Longitudinal scan of the right flank reveals mild caliectasis (c) and dilatation of the renal pelvis (RP) and proximal right ureter (U). **B:** Longitudinal image through the lower pelvis of the same patient shows a dilated distal ureter (LU) which tapers just prior to entering the bladder (BL). At surgery, there was a stricture at the ureterovesical junction.

tract dilation may be present. However, because VUR is a dynamic process, the diagnosis may be suggested if sonography demonstrates intermittent or variable pelviectasis and ureterectasis. The presence of uroepithelial thickening, due to mucosal redundancy, is also suggestive of VUR. Voiding cystourethrography (VCUG) is the gold standard in the detection of VUR.[14] Vesicoureteral reflux may coexist with other forms of congenital obstruction, such as UPJ obstruction, UVJ obstruction, and duplex renal anomalies.

Renal duplication anomalies, due to complete or partial separation of the pelvicaliceal system and ureters, are present in about 1% of the population. According to the Weigert-Meyer rule, if the duplication is complete, the ectopic upper pole ureter inserts medially and inferiorly relative to the ureter from the lower pole moiety. The classic sonographic feature of a duplex system with an ectopic ureter is dilatation of the upper pole moiety with associated parenchymal thinning, and an ectatic, tortuous upper pole ureter.[15, 16] The ureter often terminates in the bladder as a ureterocele, but it may also terminate ectopically in the bladder base (**Fig. 36–4**), urethra, vagina or perineum. Concomitant hydronephrosis of the lower pole moiety may also be seen and is nearly always due to lower pole VUR. The ureterocele appears as a rounded, thin-walled, fluid-filled mass near or protruding into the bladder base.

Posterior urethral valves are the most common cause of urethral obstruction in infants and children. The valves are believed to result from anterior fusion of the normal plicae colliculolaris. Sonographic findings of posterior urethral valves include bilateral hydronephrosis and hydroureter, parenchymal thinning, bladder wall thickening, and posterior urethral dilatation.(**Fig. 36–5**).[17] The dilated prostatic urethra is best seen on longitudinal scanning directly over the perineum rather than by conventional transabdominal scanning using the urinary bladder as an acoustic window.[18] Complications of

posterior urethral valves include renal dysplasia (**Fig. 36–5 A**), urinary ascites, and urinomas. Urinary ascites and subcapsular or perinephric urinomas are the results of urine leakage secondary to forniceal rupture or a tear in the renal parenchyma. Hydronephrosis may be absent or minimal on sonography if there has been urine leakage or ascites, both of which allow decompression of the collecting systems.

The prune belly syndrome (also known as Eagle-Barrett syndrome) is characterized by a triad of deficient abdominal musculature, urinary tract dilatation, and cryptorchidism.[19] It usually is diagnosed in the neonatal period, affects boys almost exclusively, and has a prevalence between 1 and 35 000 and 1 in 50 000 live births. The diagnosis of prune-belly syndrome is established on the combination of clinical and radiologic findings. The sonographic features include a variable degree of hydronephrosis, ureteral dilatation, and bladder enlargement. Changes of renal dysplasia also may be seen, causing increased parenchymal echogenicity or small parenchymal cysts. Other findings include a patent urachus and posterior urethral dilatation secondary to hypoplasia or agenesis of the prostate.

In older children and adolescents, duplex Doppler sonography may be useful in detecting the presence or absence of obstruction. A resistive index (RI) of 0.7 or greater is suspicious for obstruction, whereas an RI of less than 0.7 favors nonobstructive dilatation. Resistive indices are less reliable in the neonate, because the normal values can be as high as 0.9.[20, 21]

Multicystic dysplastic kidney

Multicystic dysplastic kidney accounts for about 15% of abdominal masses identified in the neonatal period.[1, 2] Multicystic dysplastic kidney is usually unilateral and occurs with greater frequency on the left. Bilateral dysplastic kidneys are incompatible with survival past the newborn period; death is due to pulmonary hy

Figure 36–4 Ureteral duplication with an ectopic ureter in a 2-day-old boy. **A:** Longitudinal sonogram of the left kidney demonstrates marked dilatation of the upper pole (UP) moiety with associated parenchymal thinning. **B:** Longitudinal image more caudally again shows a dilated upper pole (UP) moiety along with a mildly dilated lower pole (LP) moiety and the dilated ureter (U) from the upper pole.

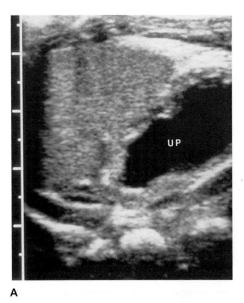
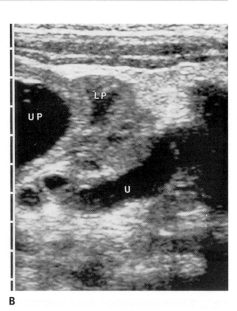

A   B

poplasia and renal failure. Thought to be the result of pelvic-infundibular atresia, the multicystic dysplastic kidney presents as a nonreniform mass comprising macrocysts and intervening dysplastic tissue with no recognizable renal pelvis.[22] The less common but more severe hydronephrotic type of multicystic dysplastic kidney results from localized atresia of the upper ureter without atresia of the renal pelvis and infundibulum. In the hydronephrotic type, the macrocysts are oriented radially around the central renal pelvis.[23,24]

Although multicystic dysplastic kidney may mimic the appearance of hydronephrosis, there are several sonographic features that distinguish these two entities. In contrast to hydronephrosis, the anechoic cysts seen in the multicystic dysplastic kidney are variable in size, randomly distributed, and noncommunicating. The renal pelvis is small or absent, and there is no definable renal parenchymal tissue (**Fig. 36–6**).[10,24—28] Doppler waveforms either are absent or show a low systolic peak frequency and absent diastolic flow.[29] Renal scintigraphy fails to demonstrate renal function on delayed images. The atretic ureter can be demonstrated by voiding cystourethrography as a blind-ending tube, which is of variable length. It is important to examine the contralateral kidney as the contralateral kidney is at increased risk for abnormalities such as UPJ obstruction, VUR, and dysplasia.[30,31]

Serial sonography has shown that the multicystic dysplastic kidney regresses in size or disappears entirely in the majority of patients.[27,32,33] Therefore, nonoperative management of multicystic dysplastic kidney has been recommended unless there are complications of infection or hypertension. In patients in whom the decision is made to leave a dysplastic kidney in place, serial imaging studies are needed because of a slightly increased incidence of Wilms' tumor.

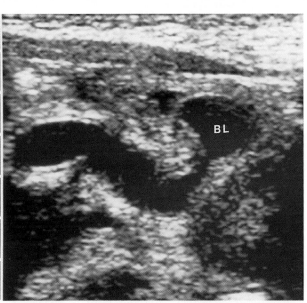

Figure 36–4 C Longitudinal sonogram of the lower pelvis shows the dilated upper pole ureter extending toward the bladder (BL) base. At surgery, the ureter entered the bladder at its junction with the posterior urethra.

Autosomal Recessive Polycystic Kidney Disease

Autosomal recessive polycystic disease (ARPD) results from growth disturbances along the branching of the ureteral bud. On gross examination, numerous small cysts, 1 to 2 mm in diameter, are seen involving both the cortex and medulla. Microdissection demonstrates cystic dilatation of the collecting tubules; the nephrons are normal.[34] Cystic changes in the liver and bile duct proliferation with periportal fibrosis are commonly associated features. In fact, ARPD constitutes a spectrum with the renal disease and hepatic fibrosis varying inversely. Neonates with ARPD present predominantly

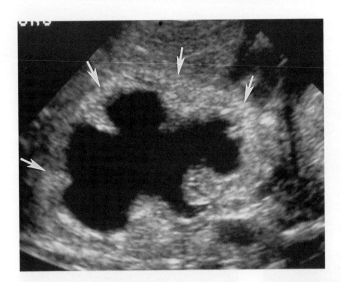

Figure 36–5 Posterior urethral valves, associated dysplasia. **A:** Longitudinal scan of the right kidney shows pelvocalyceal dilatation and diffusely echogenic parenchyma (**arrows**) secondary to dysplasia. **B:** The left intrarenal left collecting system and ureter (U) are also dilated. **C:** Longitudinal view of the pelvis shows a dilated urinary bladder (BL) and posterior urethra (Ur).

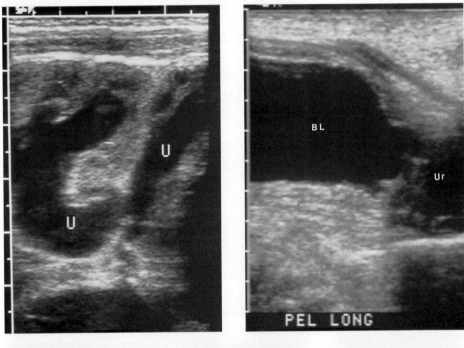

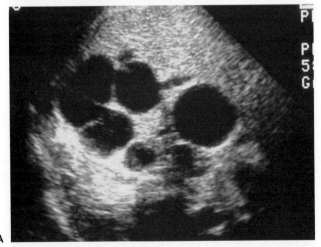

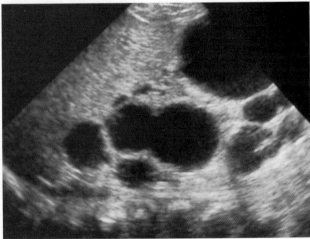

Figure 36–6 Multicystic dysplastic kidney in a 2-month-old boy. **A:** Transverse and **B:** longitudinal scans of the right kidney reveal multiple randomly distributed cysts of various size. There is no rec- ognizable renal parenchyma or central renal pelvis seen. The cysts completely involuted on a follow-up examination 1 year later.

with renal failure; the hepatic disease is clinically insignificant. Older children and adolescents typically present with complications of portal hypertension and esophageal varices, which are secondary to underlying hepatic fibrosis; the hepatic manifestations predominate over the renal disease in this form.

Sonography identifies bilateral renal enlargement with diffuse hyperechogenicity (**Fig. 36–7**). [25, 26, 35—37] The increased echogenicity is due to the innumerable fluid-tubular wall interfaces. In approximately 50% of kidneys, there is a sonolucent band, corresponding to compressed normal cortex, surrounding the central echogenic medulla.[38] Cysts that are sonographically discernible are usually small and located in the renal medulla. The portal triads within the liver may also appear hyperechoic secondary to periportal fibrosis and there may be bile duct ectasia. Excretory urography can confirm the diagnosis of ARPD by demonstrating bilateral nephromegaly, impaired renal function, and radiating "brush-like" striations extending from the renal papillae to the cortex; these striations represent stasis of contrast material within dilated tubules (**Fig. 36–8**).

Autosomal Dominant Polycystic Kidney Disease

Autosomal dominant polycystic disease (ADPD) involves both the collecting tubules and nephrons. On gross examination, small islands of normal renal parenchyma are seen interposed between numerous cysts in the cortex and medulla. Microdissection studies demonstrate the continuity of these cysts with both the collecting tubules and nephrons.[34] Despite progressively declining renal function, ADPD often remains clinically silent until late in the disease. Clinical manifestations do not usually become clinically apparent until early adulthood when hypertension or hematuria develops.

In the neonate, the sonographic findings in the autosomal dominant form of the disease may be similar to those seen in autosomal recessive polycystic disease. Bilaterally enlarged, echogenic kidneys similar to those seen in autosomal recessive disease are identified.[39] Unlike the autosomal recessive form, ADPD may present with asymmetric renal enlargement that can mimic the appearance of an unilateral cystic renal mass. Renal cysts in ADPD are more readily detectable than in ARPD (**Fig. 36–9**); however, the absence of detectable cysts does not exclude the diagnosis of autosomal dominant disease. The classic finding of multiple, variably sized cysts becomes increasingly apparent with advancing age. The presence of cysts in a subcapsular distribution also favors the diagnosis of autosomal dominant kidney disease. Cysts may also occur in the liver and pancreas, but unlike ARPD, no significant periportal hepatic fibrosis is present.

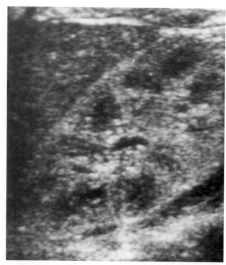

Figure 36–7 Autosomal recessive polycystic kidney disease in a 3-month-old boy. Longitudinal scan of the right flank shows an enlarged and diffusely hyperechoic right kidney. The left kidney had a similar appearance.

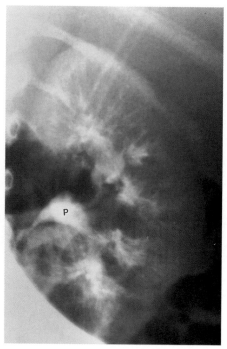

Figure 36–8 Autosomal recessive polycystic kidney disease. A coned-down image from an excretory urogram shows the classic "brush-like" striations radiating from the renal papillae into the cortex, representing contrast material in dilated renal tubules. P, renal pelvis.

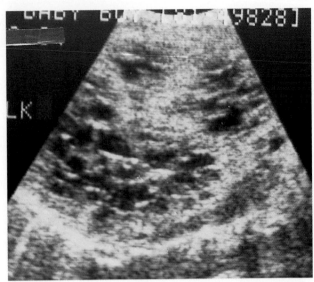

Figure 36-9 Autosomal dominant cystic disease in a newborn boy. Coronal sonogram of the left flank shows an enlarged, echogenic kidney with numerous small cysts. The right kidney had a similar appearance.

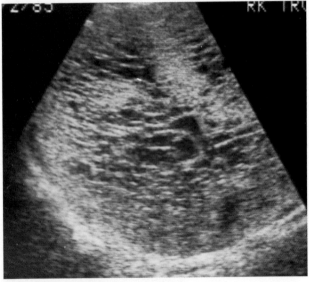

Figure 36-10 Glomerulocystic disease in a neonate. Transverse scan of the right flank demonstrates a markedly enlarged, echogenic kidney containing multiple small cysts.

Glomerulocystic Disease

Glomerulocystic disease is a rare, sporadic condition with no familial pattern, although it has been associated with other malformations, such as Zellweger's syndrome, oral-facial-digital syndrome, and renal-retinal dysplasia. Pathologic features include cystic dilatation of Bowman's space in the renal cortex, dilatation of the collecting tubules, periportal hepatic fibrosis, bile duct hyperplasia and dilatation, and hepatic cysts. Most patients present in the neonatal period with palpable abdominal masses and renal failure.[40,41] Sonography shows renal enlargement with generalized increased echogenicity, poorly defined renal margins, and loss of definition of the cortical medullary junction. Occasionally, discrete cortical cysts can be identified (**Fig. 36-10**).

Cystic Kidney Disease Associated with Syndromes

Among the more common syndromes in which cystic renal disease is present are tuberous sclerosis, Meckel-Grüber syndrome, von Hippel-Lindau syndrome, Zellweger's syndrome (cerebrohepatorenal syndrome),[42] and asphyxiating thoracic dystrophy. There is also an association with several chromosomal disorders, particularly trisomies 13, 18, and 21.

Tuberous sclerosis, or Bourneville's disease, is the most common malformation syndrome in which renal cysts can be demonstrated.[43,44] The cysts can mimic autosomal dominant polycystic kidney disease on sonography. Thus, careful physical examination to identify physical manifestations of tuberous sclerosis, such as cafe-au-lait spots and cranial imaging to detect subependymal nodules and cortical tubers, are indicated.

Meckel-Grüber syndrome is a less common malformation syndrome which can be detected on prenatal ultrasound. It is characterized by a the triad of cystic renal disease, encephalocele, and polydactyly.

Von Hippel-Lindau is a syndrome characterized by multiple cysts involving the kidneys, pancreas and liver. The greatest clinical significance in this condition is in the increased incidence of pheochromocytoma and renal cell carcinoma. Sonography is a very useful tool in screening for renal and adrenal masses.

Mesoblastic Nephroma

Solid renal tumors are rare in neonates and infants. Similar to cystic lesions, the presentation is usually that of a palpable mass or hematuria. Mesoblastic nephroma, also known as fetal renal hamartoma, is the most common solid renal mass in the neonate, typically replacing most or all of the kidney. However, mesoblastic nephroma is usually limited to the kidney and does not invade adjacent organs. It is composed of a monotonous sheet of uniform spindle-shaped cells with no cellular atypia. Occasionally, vascular channels and cartilage are present within the mass. Necrosis and hemorrhage, which are common features of Wilms' tumor, are rare.[44-46]

On sonography, a large, well-defined solid mass of variable echogenicity is seen (**Fig. 36–11**). Mesoblastic nephroma is typically homogeneous but can demonstrate a more heterogeneous appearance if cystic degeneration, necrosis or hemorrhage is present. Mesoblastic nephroma cannot reliably be differentiated from the rare neonatal Wilms' tumor by ultrasonography. The treatment of choice is nephrectomy, which is curative in the majority of cases.

Nephroblastomatosis

Nephroblastomatosis is an abnormality of nephrogenesis characterized by the persistence of fetal renal blastema beyond 36 weeks of gestation. Although not itself malignant, nephroblastomatosis is considered a precursor to Wilms' tumor.[47–51] Foci of nephroblastomatosis have been found in 25% of patients with unilateral Wilms' tumor and in virtually all patients with bilateral Wilms' tumors.

Nephroblastomatosis usually occurs before 2 years of age, with the majority of cases presenting before the age of 4 months. Two patterns of renal involvement are identified. Diffuse nephroblastomatosis presents clinically with bilateral flank masses. Sonographically, the diffuse form is seen as bilateral nephromegaly with poor corticomedullary differentiation (**Fig. 36–12**). In contrast, multifocal nephroblastomatosis may or may not result in renal enlargement. Foci of nephroblastomatosis are often found during nephrectomy for Wilms' tumor. Sonographically, multifocal nephroblastomatosis is seen as multiple subcapsular masses or nodules. Nephroblastomatosis is usually hypoechoic to the normal renal parenchyma but can be iso- or hyperechoic. Isoechoic masses are only detectable sonographically if contour deforming.[52, 53]

Renal Vein Thrombosis

Renal vein thrombosis in the pediatric population is primarily a disease of the newborn. It most frequently results from dehydration and secondary hemoconcentration; hemoconcentration can also occur secondary to blood loss, diarrhea, or sepsis. Infants of diabetic mothers are also at increased susceptibility for renal vein thrombosis due to water depletion.

Classically, the neonate presents with a palpable flank mass, hematuria, and transient hypertension. In the appropriate clinical setting, sonography is the imaging test of choice.[54] It is diagnostic in most cases and, thus, obviates the need for additional contrast studies. In the acute phase, the kidney enlarges and appears diffusely hyperechoic secondary to edema and hemorrhage. Loss of corticomedullary distinction and progressive decrease in echogenicity is seen over the next 1 to 2 weeks (**Fig. 36–13**). Then, as cellular infiltration and fibrosis develop, the variably sized kidney again becomes

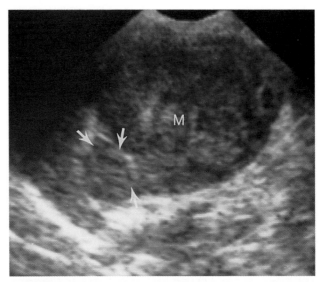

Figure 36–11 Mesoblastic nephroma. Transverse sonogram of the left kidney shows a homogeneous, echogenic mass (M) in the lower pole of the left kidney. A small amount of normal parenchyma (**arrows**) is noted posteriorly.

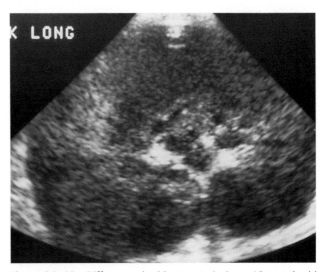

Figure 36–12 Diffuse nephroblastomatosis in a 13-month-old girl. Longitudinal scan of the right kidney shows marked enlargement, diffusely decreased echogenicity, and loss of corticomedullary differentiation.

more echogenic. At any stage, an echogenic intraluminal thrombus may be identified in the renal vein or inferior vena cava. Duplex and color Doppler can confirm the absence of venous signal.[55] Other findings supportive of renal vein thrombosis include loss of normal flow phasicity in the renal vein, diastolic arterial dampening, flow reversal, and an elevated resistive index (**Fig. 36–13 C**).

The fate of the kidney largely depends on the extent of thrombosis and on the rapidity of venous occlusion. The presence of collateral circulation or venous recanalization diminishes the degree of intrarenal edema, allow-

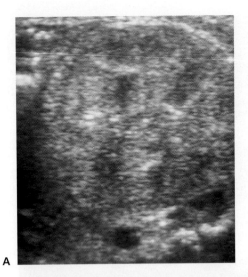

A

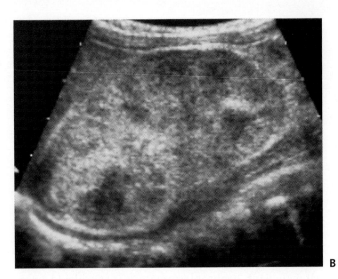

B

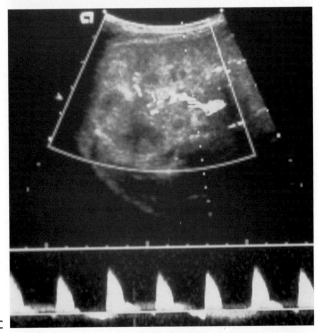

C

Figure 36–13   Renal vein thrombosis. **A:** Transverse sonogram of the left flank in a 1-day-old girl shows an enlarged, mildly echogenic left kidney with poor corticomedullary differentiation. **B:** Longitudinal sonogram 2 weeks later demonstrates a normal reniform kidney with heterogeneously echogenic parenchyma. The overall echogenicity of the renal cortex has decreased compared with the initial examination. **C:** Doppler interrogation of the kidney demonstrates increased vascular resistance in the main renal artery with systolic and diastolic arterial damping and flow reversal. Venous flow was absent.

ing continued arterial perfusion and a more favorable prognosis. The resultant parenchymal damage is, therefore, quite variable and ranges from near complete recovery to renal atrophy. Often, the end-stage hypoplastic kidney contains lace-like calcifications which extend outward from the pelvis into the parenchyma. These calcifications are readily apparent on both sonography and plain radiography, and reflect the distribution of the venous thrombi.

Older Children and Adolescents

Malignant Tumors

Wilms' Tumor

Wilms' tumor is the most common renal malignancy in children older than 1 year of age. It accounts for approximately 22% of all abdominal masses.[1,2] Charac-

teristically, Wilms' tumor is a large, bulky mass that nearly replaces the involved kidney. Pathologically, Wilms' tumor is a sharply circumscribed tumor which usually contains areas of necrosis, hemorrhage, and cystic degeneration, and is surrounded by a pseudocapsule composed of compressed renal parenchyma. Wilms' tumor spreads by either contiguous invasion of adjacent organs or extension into the renal vein and inferior vena cava. Because of the propensity for intravascular spread of tumor, there is also a tendency for systemic dissemination to the lung and liver.

Wilms' tumor usually presents in children under the age of 4 years; the mean age at presentation is 3 years. Over 90% of children present with an asymptomatic flank mass. Less frequent presentations include abdominal pain, fever, and hematuria. Despite the large size of the mass at presentation, metastatic disease at the time of diagnosis is rare. An increased incidence of Wilms' tumor is seen in association with several entities, which include Beckwith-Wiedemann syndrome, sporadic aniridia, hemihypertrophy, and the Drash syndrome (male pseudohermaphroditism and glomerular disease).

The diagnosis of Wilms' tumors must be considered whenever an intrarenal mass is identified in a young child on sonography. Common sonographic findings include an echogenic intrarenal mass with a heterogeneous or homogeneous appearance (**Fig. 36–14**), reflecting varying degrees of hemorrhage and necrosis; a hypo- or hyperechoic rim, corresponding to the pseudocapsule; and secondary characteristics, such as renal vein or inferior vena caval thrombosis, lymphadenopathy, and hepatic metastases.[56] Rarely, Wilms' tumor contains focal areas of fat[57] or calcifications. The tumor may also invade the collecting system producing a botryoid pelvicalyceal mass.[58] Increased vascularity it noted on color Doppler sonography.[59]

Renal Cell Carcinoma

Renal cell carcinoma accounts for less than 1% of pediatric renal tumors. The peak age incidence is approximately 9 years. Presenting signs and symptoms are nonspecific and include abdominal or flank pain (50 to 60%), a palpable abdominal mass (50 to 60%), and hematuria (30 to 60%).[60–62] Renal vascular invasion occurs in about 25% of cases.

On sonography, renal cell carcinoma may appear as a hypo-, iso-, or hyperechoic intrarenal mass (**Fig. 36–15**).[61, 62] The average diameter of the tumor at the time of diagnosis is 4 cm. Calcifications occur in approximately 25% of tumors. The tumor spreads by either direct extension into the retroperitoneum and lymph nodes or by invasion of the renal vein. Differentiation between renal cell carcinoma and Wilms' tumor is not possible and based only on the sonographic findings, but the age of the patient usually is helpful in suggesting the correct diagnosis.

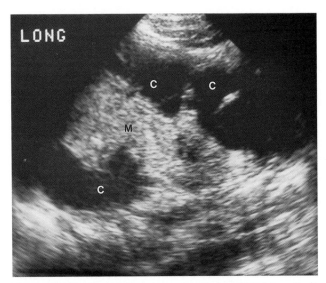

Figure 36–15 Renal cell carcinoma in a 7-year-old girl. Longitudinal scan of the left kidney demonstrates an echogenic mass (M) in the mid pole of the left kidney distorting moderately dilated calyces (C). The tumor had invaded the collecting the system causing hydronephrosis.

Rare Renal Tumors

Clear cell sarcoma and malignant rhabdoid tumor are rare renal masses. Malignant rhabdoid tumor usually affects young infants with a medium age of 13 months, whereas clear cell sarcoma favors children between 3 and 5 years of age. The presenting symptoms and signs are nonspecific and similar to those of Wilms' tumor. On sonography, both tumors may appear as homogeneously or heterogeneously echogenic masses. A thickened renal capsule and subcapsular fluid collections with tumor implants are frequent findings associated with rhabdoid tumor (**Fig. 36–16**).[63–65] Concomitant primary tumors of the posterior cranial fossa,

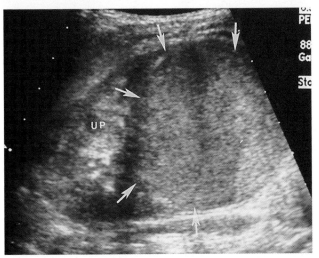

A

Figure 36–14 Wilms' tumor in a 18-month-old boy. **A:** Coronal image of the left kidney show a large, fairly well-defined and homogeneously echogenic mass (**arrows**) arising from the lower pole.

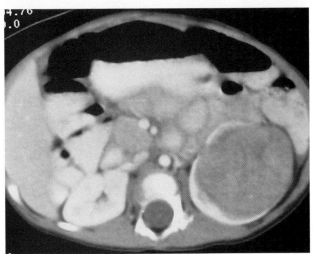

B

Normal parenchyma is seen in the upper pole (UP) of the kidney. **B:** Contrast-enhanced CT scan confirms a large, intrarenal soft-tissue mass surrounded by enhancing parenchyma.

soft tissues and thymus frequently occur in association with malignant rhabdoid tumor. Clear cell sarcoma may metastasize to bone.

Lymphoma

Renal involvement by lymphoma occurs late in the course of the disease and is usually asymptomatic and discovered only at autopsy. Renal involvement by lymphoma is more common with nonHodgkin's lymphoma than with Hodgkin's disease. Renal involvement may result from hematogenous spread or contiguous extension of retroperitoneal lymphoma.[66]

Four patterns of lymphomatous involvement have been reported. The most common pattern is multiple soft tissue masses (**Fig. 36–17**). Less frequent patterns include direct invasion from contiguous lymph nodes, solitary renal masses, and diffuse infiltration. On sonography, renal lymphoma is anechoic or hypoechoic relative to normal renal parenchyma.[67]

Benign Renal Masses

Multilocular Cystic Nephroma

Multilocular cystic nephroma, also known as multilocular cyst, benign cystic nephroma, and cystic hamartoma, is a nonhereditary, benign renal mass. It tends to affect young boys, usually younger than 4 years, and older women. In children, it presents as a painless abdominal mass; hematuria and hypertension are less common presenting signs. Pathologically, multilocular cystic nephroma is a well-circumscribed, encapsulated mass that contains multiple noncommunicating, fluid-filled cysts separated by fibrous stroma. The sonographic appearance varies with the size of the cysts and the amount of fibrous stroma present. When the cysts are large, ultrasonography will demonstrate a complex, renal mass with numerous anechoic or hypoechoic cysts separated by echogenic septae (**Fig. 36–18**).[68, 69] It is the cystic nature of this benign lesion which differentiates it from Wilms' tumor. However, the characteristic multiloculated appearance may not be appreciated if the cysts are too small to be resolved or if they contain mucoid material. In such instances, the appearance is nonspecific and similar to that of other solid renal tumors. Most multilocular nephromas are benign, although foci of Wilms' tumor have been reported in the cyst walls. The usual treatment is partial or total nephrectomy.

Angiomyolipoma

Angiomyolipoma is a benign renal tumor containing angiomatous, myomatous, and lipomatous elements.[70–73] It is rarely seen in the general pediatric population, but can be identified in as many as 80% of children with tuberous sclerosis. Also termed *renal hamartoma*, the lesions are usually small, asymptomatic, and discovered incidentally. However, due to the vascular nature of these lesions, angiomyolipomas may present with symptoms of intratumoral or retroperitoneal hemorrhage. The sonographic appearance ranges from uniformly increased renal echogenicity in cases of diffuse involvement to marked heterogeneity with multiple echogenic foci corresponding to fat. Rarely, a dominant mass is noted. Angiomyolipomas may coexist with small renal cysts (**Fig. 36–19**).[73] CT is useful to confirm the presence of fat.

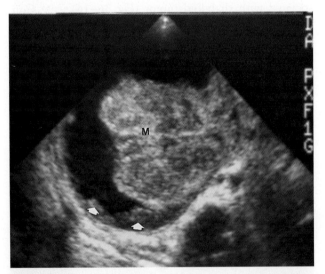

Figure 36–16   Malignant rhabdoid tumor in a 7-month-old boy. Transverse sonogram of the right kidney demonstrates a lobulated echogenic mass (M) replacing the renal parenchyma. Subcapsular fluid collection with tumor nodules (**arrows**) surrounds the parenchymal tumor.

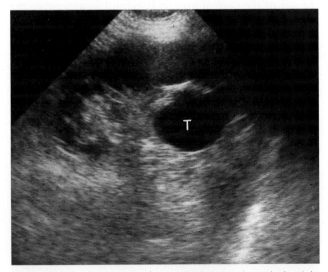

Figure 36–17   Lymphoma. Longitudinal image through the right flank demonstrates anechoic tumor (T) in the right kidney.

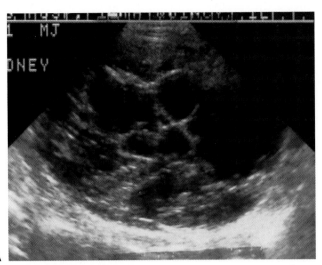
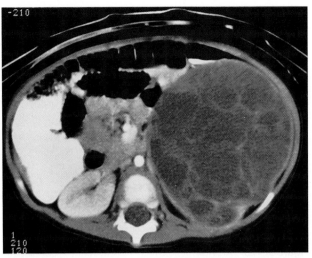

Figure 36–18 Multilocular cystic nephroma. **A:** Longitudinal scan of the left kidney shows numerous anechoic locules separated by echogenic septae. **B:** Contrast-enhanced CT confirms a multilocular mass with enhancing septations replacing the renal parenchyma.

Simple Renal Cyst

Although extremely common in the adult population, simple renal cysts are rarely seen in children.[74,75] Most are clinically asymptomatic, but they can present as a palpable abdominal mass. Typically unilocular and solitary, simple cysts demonstrate a single epithelial lining layer and a surrounding fibrous wall. The sonographic criteria for a simple cyst include round or ovoid shape, thin wall, acoustic enhancement, and the absence of internal echoes. Occasionally, simple cysts have a more complicated appearance, which likely reflects underlying hemorrhage, infection or calcification. In the older child, ultrasound-guided percutaneous aspiration may be both diagnostic and therapeutic.

Nonrenal Retroperitoneal Masses

Neonates

Adrenal Hemorrhage

Adrenal hemorrhage is a relatively common cause of an adrenal mass in neonates. Clinical features, in addition, to an abdominal mass, include jaundice and anemia. The exact etiology is unknown but birth trauma, anoxia, neonatal sepsis, and dehydration have all been implicated as possible causes. Renal vein thrombosis, usually left-sided, is a common associated lesion.[76]

The sonographic appearance of adrenal hemorrhage is dependent on the stage of the hemorrhage.[77–79] The characteristic sonographic finding in the acute stage is a hyperechoic suprarenal mass, which often displaces the ipsilateral kidney inferiorly. As the hemorrhage evolves, it acquires a more typical hypo- or anechoic appearance of a hematoma (**Fig. 36–20**). As clot forms and undergoes retraction, the mass again becomes more echoic.

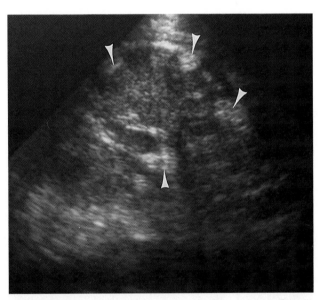

Figure 36–19 Angiomyolipomas. Longitudinal of a patient with tuberous sclerosis shows multiple echogenic fatty masses throughout the renal parenchyma.

Calcifications subsequently develop and become radiographically apparent within several weeks. Initially outlining the adrenal glands in a rim-like fashion, the calcifications become progressively more dense and eventually assume the triangular shape of the adrenal gland.

The primary differential diagnostic dilemma is the rare case of congenital neuroblastoma that presents as a dominant adrenal mass with little evidence of metastatic disease. Serial ultrasonography, however, can nearly always distinguish between these two disorders.[78,79] In general, masses due to adrenal hemorrhage generally demonstrate a rather rapid decrease in size and typically resolve within several weeks; neuroblastoma is unlikely to demonstrate any significant interval change in size on short-term follow-up sonography.

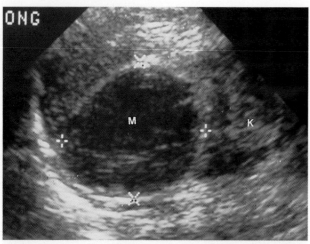

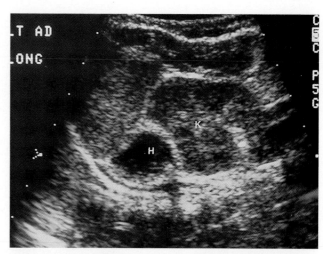

A

B

Figure 36–20 Adrenal hemorrhage in an infant of a diabetic mother. **A:** Two-day old infant girl. Longitudinal scan of the left flank reveals a predominantly hypoechoic mass (M) adjacent to the upper pole of the kidney (K). The interface between the mass and kidney is preserved. **B:** Three weeks later, the hematoma (H) has undergone marked involution. The adrenal gland is smaller, triangular in shape, and more hypoechoic. K, left kidney.

Neuroblastoma

Neonatal neuroblastoma is primarily a disease characterized by extensive metastatic disease, which usually involves the liver, skin, and bone marrow, and a small retroperitoneal or adrenal mass.[80] Rarely, the adrenal mass may be quite large. Destructive bony lesions are unusual in the neonatal period. Patients presenting in the neonatal period with disseminated disease usually have a good prognosis despite the extensive disease. On ultrasonography, the metastases and primary adrenal tumor are typically heterogeneously echogenic (**Fig. 36–21**). Echogenic foci, representing calcifications, also may be seen.[81] Rarely, large cystic areas are observed and may even predominate; they reflect the presence of necrosis, hemorrhage, or even cystic change.[82] MRI or CT usually are indicated to determine the full extent of disease.

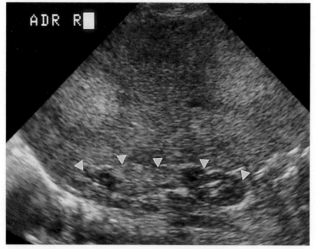

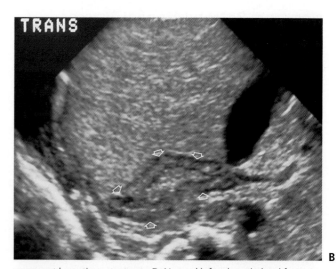

A

B

Figure 36–21 Disseminated neuroblastoma in a 1-day-old girl who presented with hepatomegaly. **A:** Longitudinal sonogram of the right upper quadrant shows a mildly enlarged, echogenic adrenal gland (**arrowheads**). The medulla and cortex of the gland cannot be separated. Also note the echogenic foci in the liver which represent hepatic metastases. **B:** Normal left adrenal gland for comparison. Transverse sonogram demonstrates the normal Y-shaped appearance of the adrenal gland. Corticomedullary differentiation is preserved with the echogenic medulla being surrounded by more hypoechoic cortex.

Older Children

Neuroblastoma

Neuroblastoma is the second most common cause of an abdominal mass in childhood and usually presents before 5 years of age with an age of peak incidence at 2 years; 75% of patients are under 4 years of age.[83, 84] Of neural crest tissue origin, neuroblastoma can arise anywhere along the sympathetic chain but the primary site is in the abdomen, with the vast majority arising in the adrenal medulla. Most patients present with a large, palpable abdominal mass. Approximately three-fourths of children will have metastases at the time of presentation, usually to bone marrow, skeleton, liver, and skin.[80] Symptoms and signs in these patients include skeletal pain, gastrointestinal complaints such as diarrhea or vomiting, and neurologic abnormalities such as opsoclo-cus-myoclonus, ataxia, nystagmus, and paraplegia. Elevated levels of serum or urinary catecholamine metabolites, particularly vanillylmandelic acid and homovanillic acid, are demonstrated in approximately 85% to 95% of cases.[80]

Important factors affecting prognosis are patient age at diagnosis, site of origin of the primary tumor, and tumor stage at diagnosis. With patients age under 1 year old, tumors arising in extraabdominal sites, and lower-stage tumors, a more favorable prognosis is indicated. Several biological tumors markers, such as the N-myc oncogene, have also been proven to have prognostic significance.

Neuroblastoma usually appears as a poorly defined, heterogeneously echogenic mass, reflecting the presence of calcification and high cellularity (**Fig. 36–22**). Small anechoic areas representing hemorrhage, necrosis, or cystic change may also be present. Although sonography is useful for detecting the primary tumor, it is of limited value in accurately defining tumor margins or in determining local extension because it is hampered by intervening bowel gas. Sonography is correct in the staging of neuroblastoma in about 55% of cases.[85] Patterns of intraabdominal extension of tumor include encasement of major vessels, spread to regional lymph nodes, intraspinal extension, and hepatic metastases.

Other Adrenal Neoplasms

Ganglioneuroblastoma and ganglioneuroma are also derived from neural crest tissue. The former comprises both primitive and differentiated cells, whereas the latter consists entirely of mature ganglion cells. Both may appear as heterogenous or homogenous echogenic masses with flecks of calcification. Differentiation of the various types of ganglion tumors requires tissue sampling.

Adrenocortical tumors are rare, accounting for less than 1% of all tumors in childhood. Of these adrenal carcinomas are the most frequent; pheochromocytomas are rarer. The mean age of presentation for carcinoma is approximately 6 years. Most adrenal carcinomas are

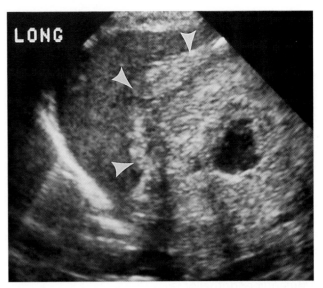

Figure 36–22 Neuroblastoma in a 1-year-old girl. Longitudinal sonogram of the left upper quadrant shows a large hyperechoic mass (**arrowheads**) containing a small cystic component which was shown to be necrosis at surgery.

hormonally active, secreting excessive amounts of androgen, and less frequently cortisol, estrogen, or aldosterone. Adrenal carcinomas are typically large, echogenic, or complex masses at the time of diagnosis, often greater than 4 cm in diameter. They have a sonographic appearance similar to that of neuroblastoma (**Fig. 36–23**).[84, 86]

Pheochromocytomas are catecholamine-secreting tumors arising from sympathetic ganglia. Approximately 75% are located in the adrenal medulla; the re-

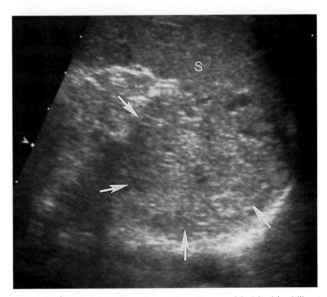

Figure 36–23 Adrenal carcinoma in a 4-year-old girl with virilization. Transverse sonogram of the left flank shows a round, nearly homogeneously echogenic mass (**arrows**) in the location of the adrenal gland. S, spleen.

mainder are extraadrenal in location, arising in the organ of Zuckerkandl, periaortic region, and wall of the urinary bladder. About 10% of pheochromocytomas in children are malignant and up to 70% are bilateral. Most children present with hypertension which is usually sustained. Sonography usually shows a relatively large, well-defined, predominantly echogenic tumor. Hypoechoic areas representing old blood or necrosis and hyperechoic areas representing acute hemorrhage or calcification may occasionally be seen.

Hepatic Masses

Neonates

Benign Tumors

Hemangioendothelioma

Primary hepatic tumors are uncommon, accounting for only 6% of neonatal abdominal tumors.[1,2] Benign hepatic tumors account for about one-third of all hepatic masses in children. The majority of benign hepatic neoplasms are of vascular origin. In the neonatal period, the most common is hemangioendothelioma.[87–90] More than 85% of hemangioendotheliomas are diagnosed in children under the age of 6 months. The clinical features depend on the rate of blood flow and the extent of arteriovenous shunting within the tumor. Hemangioendotheliomas with significant arteriovenous shunting present early in the neonatal period due to high-output cardiac failure. Tumors with little vascular shunting tend to present with a palpable abdominal mass or hepa-

tomegaly, acute abdominal symptoms from tumoral hemorrhage, thrombocytopenia secondary to platelet sequestration (Kasabach-Merritt syndrome), or as an incidental finding. Cutaneous hemangiomas are found in about 50% of neonates with hemangioendotheliomas.[87,88] On gross examination, hemangioendothelioma appears relatively avascular. Microscopically, however, the tumor is quite vascular, consisting of vascular channels of varying size lined by plump endothelium.

Like its clinical features, the sonographic features of hemangioendothelioma are variable. The appearance of hemangioendothelioma ranges from solitary to diffuse, from hypoechoic to hyperechoic, and from homogeneous to complex appearing (**Fig. 36–24**).[91–95] Increased blood flow is usually noted on color Doppler images (**Fig. 36–25**). On pulsed Doppler images, flow patterns include arterial and venous signals with high-frequency shifts and arteries with minimal systolic-diastolic flow variation.[95,96] Peak Doppler systolic shifts range from 0.8 to 5.5 kHz; by comparison the normal hepatic artery has a shift less than 0.7 kHz.[95,96] The diagnosis of hemangioendothelioma can be confirmed by CT, MRI, or technetium-labeled red blood cell scintigraphy.

Mesenchymal Hamartoma

Cystic mesenchymal hamartoma is the second most common benign liver mass in the neonate. Pathologically, it is a large, encapsulated mass composed of multiple cystic areas that contain mucoid material and are separated by fibrous stroma.[97–100] Although typically

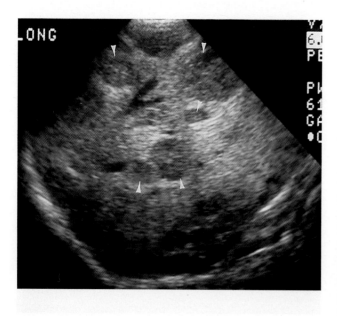

Figure 36–24 Diffuse hemangioendotheliomatosis in a 7-month-old girl. A transverse scan of the liver shows multiple hypoechoic masses (**arrows**) scattered throughout the liver.

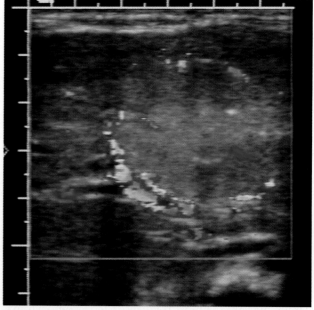

Figure 36–25 Solitary hemangioendothelioma. Color Doppler image shows a slightly echogenic mass with increased peripheral flow.

presenting as an abdominal mass, mesenchymal hamartoma may occasionally cause congestive heart failure secondary to arteriovenous shunting within the tumor. It is most commonly seen in children less than 2 years of age and is twice as frequent in boys than girls. Ultrasonography demonstrates a large, predominantly cystic mass containing anechoic spaces separated by echogenic septae.[97—100] If the cystic areas are small, the mass may appear relatively solid (**Fig. 36–26**). Aortic enlargement and large draining hepatic veins may be identified if significant arteriovenous shunting is present.

Malignant Tumors

Although congenital hepatoblastoma has been documented in this age group, malignant hepatic tumors in the neonatal period are rare. The vast majority of malignant liver neoplasms occur in the older infant and child (see below).

Older Children

Malignant Hepatic Tumors

Hepatic tumors are the third most frequent solid abdominal neoplasms, after Wilms' tumor and neuroblastoma and account for 6% of abdominal tumors in children.[1,2] In childhood, malignant liver tumors are twice as common as benign neoplasms. The most common are hepatoblastoma and hepatocellular carcinoma. Much less common are fibrolamellar hepatocellular carcinoma and embryonal cell sarcoma.[88,89,101,102]

The pathologic differentiation of hepatoblastoma from hepatocellular carcinoma depends on cellular maturity. Hepatoblastoma is composed of small primitive epithelial cells resembling fetal liver. Hepatocellular carcinoma contains large, pleomorphic, multinucleated

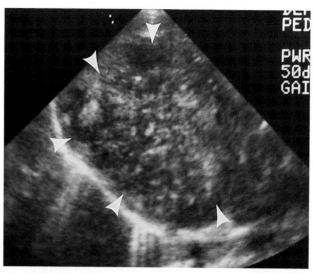

Figure 36–26 Mesenchymal hamartoma in a 2-year-old boy. Longitudinal sonogram of the liver demonstrates a complex, predominantly echogenic mass (**arrowheads**) with multiple hyperechoic areas representing debris and mucoid-filled cystic spaces.

cells with variable degrees of differentiation. The tumors are usually confined to a single lobe with the right lobe involved twice as often as the left lobe, but on occasion they may involve both lobes or there may be multicentric disease.[103,104]

Hepatoblastomas tends to occur in children under the age of 3 years; hepatocellular carcinomas occurs in slightly older children, usually after 5 years of age. Both tumors usually present as asymptomatic protuberant upper abdominal masses. They demonstrate similar sonographic features, typically appearing hyperechoic and heterogeneous relative to the adjacent hepatic parenchyma (**Fig. 36–27**).[92,103] Both tumors usually pre-

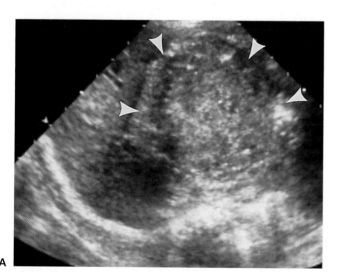

A

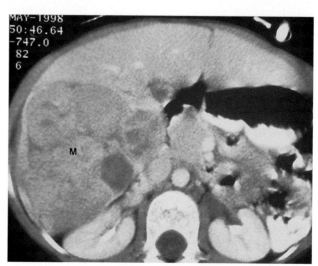

B

Figure 36–27 Hepatoblastoma in a 1-year-old girl. **A:** Transverse scan of the liver shows a heterogeneous, slightly hyperechoic mass (**arrowheads**) occupying the posterior segment of the right lobe. **B:** CT scan confirms a large soft-tissue mass (M) in the right lobe posteriorly.

sent as a solitary mass, a dominant mass with smaller satellite lesions, or multiple diffuse nodules; diffuse infiltration in rare. Blood flow within or around the tumor is commonly seen on color Doppler imaging. Vascular invasion is also common in both tumors. Vascular invasion appears as echogenic intraluminal thrombus. On pulsed Doppler sonography, primary hepatic malignancies demonstrate high peak systolic Doppler shifts (usually larger than 3 kHz).[105,106] Sites of distant metastases are the same for both neoplasms and include lungs, lymph nodes, brain, and skeleton.

Fibrolamellar carcinoma is a rare variant of hepatocellular carcinoma that is characterized by deeply eosinophilic hepatocytes and abundant fibrous bands arranged in a parallel pattern around the hepatocytes, hence, the term *fibrolamellar*.[107] The tumor tends to affect adolescents and young adults. The majority of patients present with abdominal pain or mass, weight loss, or fever. The fibrolamellar form of hepatocellular carcinoma has a better prognosis than does the conventional hepatocellular carcinoma. Sonographically, fibrolamellar carcinoma is usually seen as a well-defined solitary mass of variable echogenicity. Small central calcifications are present in about half of cases. Enlarged portal nodes also may be observed.

Embryonal sarcoma is a rare mesenchymal malignancy that occurs in older children and adolescents. On sonography, a heterogeneous mass with multiple cystic spaces is seen. The prognosis is poor, with a mean survival of less than 1 year.[108]

Benign Hepatic Tumors

In older children and adolescents, cavernous hemangioma is the most common benign primary hepatic tumor and is usually an incidental finding. Cavernous

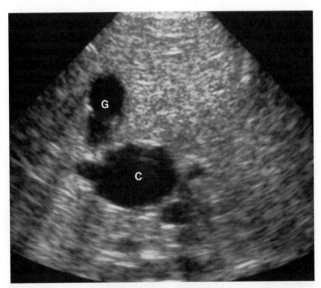

Figure 36–28 Choledochal cyst. Transverse sonogram through the liver of a 6-month-old girl shows a fluid-filled cyst (C), representing the dilated common bile duct, within the porta hepatis. The gallbladder (G) is identified separately from the choledochal cyst.

hemangiomas usually have a highly vascular appearance on gross pathology. Histologically, they are composed of dilated, blood-filled spaces lined by mature, flat endothelial cells and separated by fibrous septa. Most are sonographically homogeneous, hyperechoic, and have well-defined margins. Posterior acoustic enhancement is characteristic. They may, however, become more heterogeneous or hypoechoic secondary to degeneration, thrombosis, and fibrosis.[109] Doppler sonography often fails to show flow within cavernous hemangiomas. Doppler shifts when obtained are usually low, less than 1 kHz, reflecting the slow blood flow in these lesions.[110] On color Doppler imaging, there may be pulsatile peritumoral or mixed peritumoral and intratumoral flow.[111]

Biliary Masses

Choledochal Cysts

The most common biliary mass in children is choledochal cyst, which is a congenital dilatation of the biliary ductal system. The exact etiology of choledochal cysts is uncertain; although anomalous insertion of the distal common bile duct into the pancreatic duct permitting pancreatic-biliary reflux with resultant cyst formation has been proposed.[112,113] Three major types of choledochal cysts have been described. Type 1 refers to fusiform dilatation of the common bile duct with or without the hepatic duct dilatation; type 2 is an eccentric saccular diverticulum of the common bile duct; and type 3 is a dilatation of the intraluminal duodenal portion of the distal common bile duct, forming a choledochocele.

Nearly half of the patients with choledochal cysts are between 1 and 10 years of age at the time of diagnosis, although the lesion may present in neonates. Clinical findings include jaundice, abdominal mass and pain. Sonography reveals a cystic, fluid-filled mass in the region of the porta hepatis which is distinctly separate from the gallbladder (**Fig. 36–28**). The presence of proximal hepatic duct dilatation is variable; dilatation is usually limited to the right and left main hepatic ducts. Hepatobiliary imaging confirms the diagnosis by demonstrating hepatic uptake of tracer with excretion into the choledochal cyst and bowel on delayed images.

Pelvic Masses

Neonates

Gonadal Tumors

Pelvic masses in girls almost always arise from the genital tract and the majority comprises hydrometrocolpos and ovarian cysts.[114,115] Together, these two entities account for approximately 15% of all neonatal abdominal masses.[1,2] *Hydrocolpos* refers to dilatation of the vagina, and *hydrometrocolpos* to dilatation of both the uterus and vagina. In the neonate, vaginal obstruction may be the result of vaginal atresia or stenosis, a transverse septum, or a cloacal malformation.[116] Patients present with a palpable midline mass in the pelvis and/or abdomen resulting from the production and excess accumulation of vaginal secretions in utero secondary to maternal hormone stimulation. Urine may also be found in the vagina or uterus of neonates who have cloacal malformations. Associated congenital anomalies are common in neonates with cervical or vaginal stenosis or atresia; these include duplication anomalies of the uterus, fistula, urogenital sinus, imperforate anus, esophageal or duodenal atresia, and congenital heart disease.

The large dilated uterus and vagina are easily demonstrated on ultrasonography. The sonographic finding of hydrometrocolpos is a tubular, fluid-filled midline mass which is located midline between the bladder and rectum (**Fig. 36–29**). Internal echoes, reflecting cellular debris or blood, may be present. Like other pelvis masses, if large enough, hydrometrocolpos can cause hydronephrosis by displacing and obstructing the ureters.

Neonatal ovarian cysts resulting from maternal hormonal hyperstimulation of normal follicles are a common cause of abdominal and pelvis masses in the neonate.[117] The classic sonographic appearance of an ovarian cyst is an anechoic, thin-walled mass with increased through-transmission. A fluid—debris level (**Fig. 36–30**) or septations may be seen if there is associated adnexal torsion or hemorrhage into the cyst lumen. If large, then ovarian cysts can extend into the upper abdomen and be mistaken for a mesenteric or omental cyst.

Presacral Tumors

Presacral teratomas are congenital neoplasms that contain elements from all three germ layers. Although they may occur anywhere in the body, the most frequent site of occurrence is the sacrococcygeal region. Teratomas can be predominantly intrapelvic, extrapelvic, or both intra- and extrapelvic.[5,118] Over 90% of sacrococcygeal teratomas are diagnosed at birth, presenting as a large palpable gluteal mass, and the vast majority of these neonatal cases are histologically benign. In the remaining patients, the tumor is completely intrapelvic and presacral; in these cases, the patient may remain asymptomatic until older when urinary tract or bowel symptoms become apparent. Those lesions encountered beyond the neonatal period are more likely to contain malignant elements. Benign tumors are usually predominantly cystic (**Fig. 36–31**); the detection of a predominantly solid mass is suggestive of a malignant teratoma. Although sonography is helpful in tissue characterization, magnetic resonance imaging (MRI) is the preferred modality to assess the size and extent of the tumor. The differential diagnosis includes anterior meningocele, rectal duplication, and neural tumors.

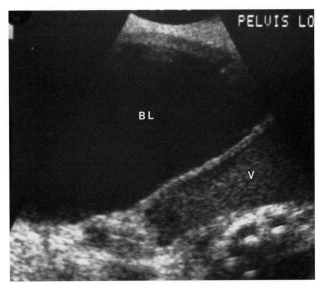

Figure 36–29 Hydrometrocolpos in a newborn girl. Longitudinal sonogram of the pelvis shows a dilated vagina (V) posterior to the urinary bladder (BL). The echogenic intravaginal contents reflect the presence of debris and blood.

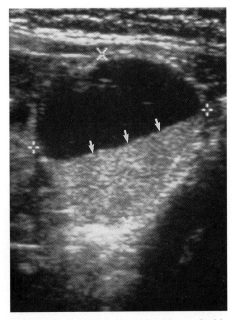

Figure 36–30 Torsed ovarian cyst in a neonate with a palpable lower abdominal mass. Transverse sonogram demonstrates a cystic mass (**calipers**) with a fluid—debris level (**arrows**) in the left lower quadrant. Exploratory laparotomy revealed a torsed follicular ovarian cyst containing blood.

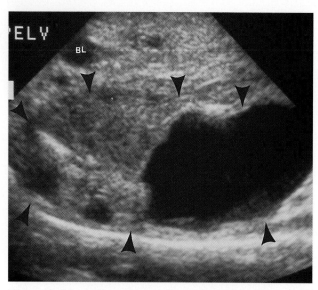

Figure 36–31 Benign sacrococcygeal teratoma in a neonate with a palpable gluteal mass. Longitudinal sonogram through the pelvis shows a complex mass (**arrowheads**) with a large cystic component. The bladder (BL) is displaced anteriorly and superiorly.

Older Children

Benign Masses

Ovarian Masses

Pelvic masses of genital origin in the older child are less frequent than in neonates. In the older child, genital masses account for only 3 to 4% of abdominal masses, and almost all of these are ovarian in origin.[1,2] The majority of ovarian tumors in children and adolescents are benign and usually cysts or teratomas.[114,115,119,120] Cystic teratomas account for more than 90% of all true benign ovarian neoplasms. Of the teratomas, approximately 90% are benign and 10% are malignant.[121] The remaining benign ovarian tumors are usually cystadenomas. Most benign lesions occur in girls between 10 and 15 years of age and present as asymptomatic pelvic and/or abdominal masses. However, acute abdominal pain may be the presenting symptom if the tumor undergoes torsion.

The most frequent appearance of teratoma, occurring in approximately 75% of patients, is a chiefly cystic mass containing an echogenic focus protruding from the inner wall, which represents the dermoid plug or Rokitansky nodule (**Fig. 36–32**).[122] These plugs contain hair, fat, teeth, bone, or any combination of these elements. The hypoechoic or anechoic components of the teratoma correspond to either sebum, which is liquid at body temperature, or serous fluid. Thin echogenic septations, floating masses, a fluid—debris level, and acoustic shadowing may also be observed.[122–124] Acoustic shadowing does not necessarily imply calcified material, such as teeth, but may instead represent a matted mixture of sebum and hair. The wall of the cyst is typically smooth and between 2- and 5-mm thick. On rare occa-

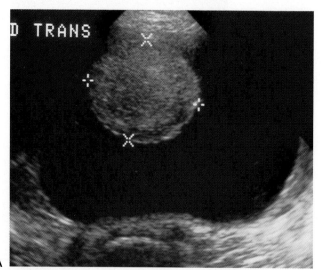

A

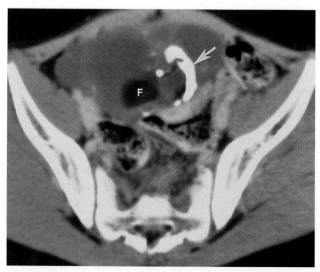

B

Figure 36–32 Ovarian teratoma in an 11-year-old girl. **A:** Transverse sonogram of the pelvis shows a cystic mass with a peripheral echogenic mural nodule (calipers). **B:** Contrast-enhanced CT scan shows the typical appearance of a teratoma—a predominantly low-attenuation mass with areas of fat (F) and calcification (**arrow**). At histopathologic examination, the cystic component of the teratoma contained a large amount of sebum; the mural nodule was composed of hair, fat and calcification.

sions, teratomas present as purely anechoic masses or echogenic masses.[122] Teratomas are bilateral in 20% of patients.

Vaginal/Uterine

Hydrometrocolpos or hydrocolpos can present in early adolescence with the initiation of menarche.[125] Vaginal obstruction in this age group is most often the result of a simple imperforate hymen or a transverse vaginal septum. Most patients present with an abdominal mass or recurrent lower abdominal pain, and absence of menses. In contradistinction to vaginal atresia in neonates, there is no increased association of congenital anomalies in the setting of an imperforate hymen. Ultrasonography is capable of confirming the presence of a midline mass arising from the pelvis and of documenting its fluid nature. Internal low-level echoes, representing cellular debris or blood, may be present within the mass.

Malignant Tumors
Ovarian

Malignant ovarian neoplasms account for only 2 to 3% of childhood cancers with germ cell tumors comprising 60 to 90% of these malignant neoplasms.[119,121] The malignant germ cell tumors in order of decreasing frequency are dysgerminoma, endodermal sinus tumor, teratoma, malignant mixed germ cell tumor, embryonal cell carcinoma, and choriocarcinoma.[121] Stromal neoplasms, either granulosa-theca tumors or Sertoli-Leydig cell tumors, account for nearly all the remaining malignant ovarian tumors in children. Malignant germ cell tumors are usually found in adolescent girls. The nongerm cell tumors usually affect girls under 10 years of age. Mucinous carcinoma is rare in childhood. Most malignant ovarian tumors present as large abdominal pelvic masses. Less frequent findings include abdominal pain or precocious puberty.

Sonographic findings of ovarian malignancy include an irregular solid mass or mixed solid-cystic mass with internal necrosis, thick septations, or papillary projections **(Fig. 36–33)**.[114,115,124] Cul-de-sac fluid is also frequently present. Findings of advanced disease include ascites, peritoneal implants, pelvic and retroperitoneal adenopathy, and hepatic metastases. Ovarian cancer may disseminate by lymphatic spread, direct local extension, or a hematogenous route. Variable degrees of central or peripheral flow may be seen on color Doppler sonography.[126] CT is superior to sonography in determining tumor extent.

Uterine and Vaginal Tumor

Rhabdomyosarcoma is the most common malignant tumor of the vagina and uterus in childhood, usually affecting girls under 4 years of age. It usually presents with vaginal discharge or bleeding.[7] On sonography, the

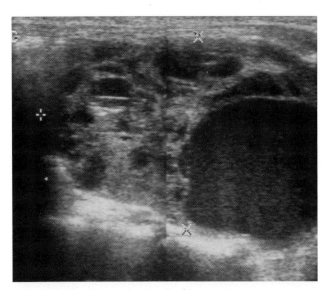

Figure 36–33 Dysgerminoma. Dual-image transverse sonogram of the right adnexal region shows a large complex mass (calipers) with solid and cystic areas.

tumor appears as a echogenic mass enlarging the vagina or uterus. Hypoechoic foci may be observed if the tumor undergoes necrosis or ulceration. Rhabdomyosarcoma metastasizes early by direct extension and hematogenous and lymphatic dissemination. Distant metastases are to liver, lymph nodes, lung, and bone.

Gastrointestinal Masses

Neonates

Duplication Cysts

Gastrointestinal masses account for 15% of neonatal abdominal masses.[1,2] Duplication cyst is the most common gastrointestinal cause of a mass in the neonate. An intestinal duplication is a spherical or tubular mass that contains an intestinal mucosal in the lining and smooth muscle in the wall.[127] Duplications are characteristically located along the mesenteric border of the bowel. Although they may occur anywhere along the gastrointestinal tract, the most common location is in the distal ileum near the ileocecal valve. They typically do not communicate with the bowel lumen and about 15% contain gastric mucosa.[127] Clinical features include a palpable abdominal mass, vomiting (secondary to bowel obstruction), and hemorrhage (secondary to peptic ulceration in those that contain gastric mucosa).

The sonographic appearance of a duplication cyst is that of a fluid-filled mass with increased through-transmission **(Fig. 36–34)**.[128,129] An inner echogenic mucosal layer surrounded by a hypoechoic muscular rim may be noted and is relatively specific for the diagnosis of duplication cyst. Occasionally, the cyst appears complex as a result of intraluminal hemorrhage or inspissated material.

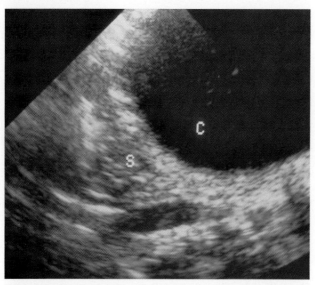

Figure 36–34   Gastric duplication cyst in a newborn girl. Transverse sonogram of the left upper quadrant shows an anechoic cystic mass (C) adjacent to the collapsed stomach (S).

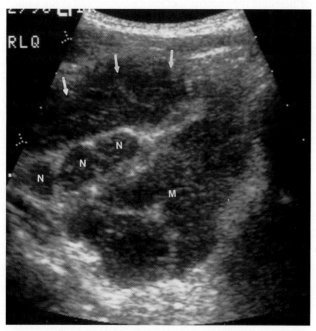

Figure 36–35   NonHodgkin's lymphoma. Transverse scan of the right lower quadrant demonstrates a thickened loop of distal ileum with hypoechoic walls (**arrows**). Also note several enlarged lymph nodes (N) and a large mesenteric mass (M).

Older Children

Lymphoma

In the older child, nonHodgkin's lymphoma is a common cause for an abdominal mass originating from the gastrointestinal tract. Gastrointestinal involvement by Hodgkin's disease almost never occurs. The distal ileum is the common site of lymphomatous involvement. The peak age of nonHodgkin's lymphoma in childhood is between 5 and 8 years. The most common clinical symptoms are abdominal mass and pain. The latter is the result of lymphomatous masses compressing adjacent structures or of small bowel obstruction secondary to acute intussusception. On sonography, lymphomatous involvement may appear as hypoechoic bowel thickening or as a lobulated, hypoechoic mesenteric mass (**Fig. 36–35**).[130,131] Associated lymph node enlargement is common.

Malignant intestinal tumors other than lymphoma are very rare in children. Leiomyosarcoma and adenocarcinoma have been reported and are often in advanced stages at the time of diagnosis.

Conclusion

The use of ultrasonography in the evaluation of pediatric abdominal masses has dramatically increased over the past decade Its increased use is due to its superb resolution, lack of invasiveness, and absence of ionizing radiation. Because of these features, it has become widely accepted as the initial imaging tool for evaluating an abdominal mass in the pediatric patient.

References

1. Kirks DR, Merten DR, Grossman H, et al. Diagnostic imaging of pediatric abdominal masses: an overview. *Radiol Clin North Am* 1981;19:527—545.
2. Merten DF, Kirks DR. Diagnostic imaging of pediatric abdominal masses. *Pediatr Clin North Am* 1985;32:1397—1425.
3. Brown T, Mandell J, Lebowitz RL. Neonatal hydronephrosis in the era of sonography. *AJR* 1987;148:959—963.
4. Preston A, Lebowitz RL. What's new in pediatric uroradiology. *Urol Radiol* 1989;11:217—220.
5. Shackelford GD. Adrenal glands, pancreas, and other retroperitoneal structures. In: Siegel MJ, ed. *Pediatric Sonography*. New York: Raven Press, 1995, p. 301—355.
6. Siegel MJ. Urinary tract. In: Siegel MJ, ed. *Pediatric Sonography*, 2nd ed. New York: Raven Press, 1995, p. 357—435.
7. Siegel MJ. Female pelvis. In: Siegel MJ, ed. *Pediatric Sonography*, 2nd ed. New York: Raven Press, 1995, p. 437—477.
8. Han BK, Babcock DS. Sonographic measurements and appearance of normal kidneys in children. *AJR* 1985;145:611—616.
9. Patriquin H, Lefaivre J-F, Lafortune M, Russo P, Boisvert J. Fetal lobation. An anatomo-ultrasonographic correlation. *J Ultrasound Med* 1990;9:191—197.

10. Sanders RC, Hartman DS. The sonographic distinction between neonatal multicystic kidney and hydronephrosis. *Radiology* 1984;151:621—625.

11. Sanders RC, Nussbaum AR, Solez K. Renal dysplasia: sonographic findings. *Radiology* 1988;167:623—626.

12. Meyer JS, Lebowitz RL. Primary megaureter in infants and children: a review. *Urol Radiol* 1992;14:296—305.

13. Wood BP, Ben-Ami T, Teele RL, Rabinowitz R. Ureterovesical obstruction and megaloureter: diagnosis by real-time US. *Radiology* 1985;156:79—81.

14. Lebowitz RL. The detection of vesicoureteral reflux in the child. *Invest Radiol* 1986;21:519—531.

15. Cremin BJ. A review of the ultrasonic appearances of posterior urethral valve and ureteroceles. *Pediatr Radiol* 1986;16:357—364.

16. Nussbaum AR, Dorst JP, Jeffs RD, Gearhart JP, Sanders RC. Ectopic ureter and ureterocele: their varied sonographic manifestations. *Radiology* 1986;159:227—235.

17. Macpherson RI, Leithiser RE, Gordon L, Turner WR. Posterior urethral valves: An update and review. *RadioGraphics* 1986;6:753—791.

18. Cohen, HL, Susman M, Haller JO, et al. Posterior urethral valves: transperineal US for imaging and diagnosis in male infants. *Radiology* 1994;192:261—264..

19. Berdon WE, Baker DH, Wigger HJ, Blanc WA. The radiologic and pathologic spectrum of the prune belly syndrome. *Radiol Clin North Am* 1977;15:83—92.

20. Patriquin H. Doppler examination of the kidney in infants and children. *Urol Radiol* 1991;12:220—227.

21. Platt JF, Rubin JM, Ellis JG, DePietro MA. Duplex Doppler US of the kidney: differentiation of obstructive from nonobstructive dilatation. *Radiology* 1989;171:515—517.

22. Griscom NT, Vawter GF, Fellers FX. Pelvoinfundibular atresia: the usual form of multicystic kidney: 44 unilateral and two bilateral cases. *Semin Roentgenol* 1975;10:125—131.

23. Felson B, Cussen LJ. The hydronephrotic type of unilateral congenital multicystic disease of the kidney. *Semin Roentgenol* 1975;10:113—123.

24. Kountz PD, Siegel MJ, Shapiro E. Flank mass in a newborn. *Urol Radiol* 1989;11:61—64.

25. Hayden CK Jr, Swischuk LE. Renal cystic disease. *Semin Ultrasound CT MR* 1991;12:361—373.

26. Hayden CK Jr, Swischuk LE, Smith TH, Armstrong EA. Renal cystic disease in childhood. *RadioGraphics* 1986;6:97—116.

27. Strife JL, Souza AS, Kirks DR, et al. Multicystic dysplastic kidney in children: US follow-up. *Radiology* 1993;186:785—788.

28. Wood BP. Renal cystic disease in infants and children. *Urol Radiol* 1992;14:284—295.

29. Hendry PL, Hendry GMA. Observations on the use of Doppler ultrasound in multicystic dysplastic kidney. *Pediatr Radiol* 1991;21:203—204.

30. Atiyeh B, Husmann D, Baum M. Contralateral renal abnormalities in multicystic-dysplastic kidney disease. *J Pediatr* 1992;121:65—67.

31. Nussbaum AR, Hartman DS, Whitley N, McCauley RGK, Sanders RC. Multicystic dysplasia and crossed renal ectopia. *AJR* 1987;149:407—410.

32. Pedicelli G, Jequier S, Bowen AD, Boisvert J. Multicystic dysplastic kidneys: spontaneous regression demonstrated with US. *Radiology* 1986;160:23—26.

33. Vinocur L, Slovis TL, Perlmutter AD, Watts FB Jr, Chang C-H. Follow-up studies of multicystic dysplastic kidneys. *Radiology* 1988;167:311—315.

34. Madewell JE, Hartman DS, Lichtenstein JR. Radiologic-pathologic correlation in cystic diseases of the kidney. *Radiol Clin North Am* 1979;17:261—279.

35. Melson GL, Shackelford GD, Cole BR, McClennan BL. The spectrum of sonographic findings in infantile polycystic kidney disease with urographic and clinical correlations. *J Clin Ultrasound* 1985;13:113—119.

36. Patriquin H. Stasis nephropathy. In: Siegel BA, Proto AV, eds. *Pediatric disease* (fourth series): *Test and Syllabus*. Reston, VA: American College of Radiology, 1993, p. 556—583.

37. Premkumar A, Berdon WE, Levy J, et al. The emergence of hepatic fibrosis and portal hypertension in infants and children with autosomal recessive polycystic kidney disease. Initial and follow-up sonographic and radiographic findings. *Pediatr Radiol* 1988;18:123—129.

38. Currarino G, Stannard MW, Rutledge JC. The sonolucent cortical rim in infantile polycystic kidneys. Histologic correlation. *J Ultrasound Med* 1989;8:571—574.

39. Pretorius DH, Lee ME, Manco-Johnson ML, et al. Diagnosis of autosomal dominant polycystic kidney disease in utero and in the young infant. *J Ultrasound Med* 1987;6:249—255.

40. Fitch SJ, Stapleton FB. Ultrasonographic features of glomerulocystic disease in infancy: similarity to infantile polycystic kidney disease. *Pediatr Radiol* 1986;16:400—402.

41. Fredericks BJ, de Campo M, Chow CW, Powell HR. Glomerulocystic renal disease: ultrasound appearances. *Pediatr Radiol* 1989;19:184—186.

42. Luisiri A, Sotelo-Avila C, Silberstein MJ, Graviss ER. Sonography of the Zellweger syndrome. *J Ultrasound Med* 1988;7:169—173.

43. Mitnick JS, Bosniak MA, Hilton S, et al. Cystic renal disease in tuberous sclerosis. *Radiology* 1983;147:85—87.

44. Narla LD, Slovis TL, Watts FB, Nigro M. The renal lesions of tuberosclerosis (cysts and angiomyolipoma)-screening with sonography and computerized tomography. *Pediatr Radiol* 1988;18:205—209.

45. Chan HSL, Cheng M-Y, Mancer K, et al. Congenital mesoblastic nephroma: a clinicoradiologic study of 17 cases representing the pathologic spectrum of the disease. *J Pediatr* 1987;111:64—70.

46. Hartman DS, Lesar MSL, Madewell JE, Lichtenstein JE, Davis CJ, Jr. Mesoblastic nephroma: radiologic—pathologic correlation of 20 cases. *AJR* 1981;136:69—74.

47. Bove KE, McAdams AJ. The nephroblastomatosis complex and its relationship to Wilms' tumor: a clinicopathologic treatise. *Perspect Pediatr Pathol* 1976;3:185—223.

48. Morello FP, Donaldson JS. Nephroblastomatosis. In: Siegel BA, Proto AV, eds. Pediatric disease (fourth series) test and syllabus. Reston, VA: American College of Radiology, 1993, p. 584—615.

49. Franken EA Jr., Yiu-Chiu V, Smith WL, Chiu LC. Nephroblastomatosis: clinicopathologic significance and imaging characteristics. *AJR* 1982;138:950—952.

50. Machin GA. Persistent renal blastema (nephroblastomatosis) as a frequent precursor of Wilms' tumor; a pathological and clinical review. Part 2. Significance of nephroblastomatosis in the genesis of Wilms' tumor. *Am J Pediatr Hematol Oncol* 1980;2:253—261.

51. Machin GA. Persistent renal blastema (nephroblastomatosis) as a frequent precursor of Wilms' tumor; a pathological and clinical review. Part 3. Clinical aspects of nephroblastomatosis. *Am J Pediatr Hematol Oncol* 1980;2:353—362.

52. Fernbach SK, Feinstein KA, Donaldson JS, Baum ES. Nephroblastomatosis: comparison of CT with US and urography. *Radiology* 1988;166:153—156.

53. White KS, Kirks, DR, Bove KE. Imaging of nephroblastomatosis: an overview. *Radiology* 1992;182:1—5.

54. Paling MR, Wakefield JA, Watson LR. Sonography of experimental acute renal vein occlusion. *JCU* 1985;13:647—653.

55. Laplante S, Patriquin HB, Robitaille P, et al. Renal vein

thrombosis in children: evidence of early flow recovery with Doppler US. *Radiology* 1993;189:37—42.

56. Reiman TH, Siegel MJ, Shackelford GD. Wilms' tumor in children: abdominal CT and US evaluation. *Radiology* 1986;160:501—505.

57. Fernbach SK, Donaldson JS, Gonzalez-Crussi F, Sherman JO. Fatty Wilms' tumor simulating teratoma; occurrence in a child with horseshoe kidney. *Pediatr Radiol* 1988;18:424—426.

58. Johnson KM, Horvath LJ, Gaisie G et al. Wilms' tumor occurring as a botryoid renal pelvicalyceal mass. *Radiology* 1987;163:385—386.

59. Van Campenhout I, Patriquin H. Malignant microvasculature in abdominal tumors in children: detection with Doppler US. *Radiology* 1992;183:445—448.

60. Dehner LP, Leestma JE, Price EB, Jr. Renal cell carcinoma in children: a clinicopathologic study of 15 cases and review of the literature. *J Pediatr* 1970;76:358—368.

61. Chan HSL, Daneman A, Gribbin M, Martin DJ. Renal cell carcinoma in the first two decades of life. *Pediatr Radiol* 1983;13:324—328.

62. Kabala JE, Shield J, Duncan A. Renal cell carcinoma in childhood. *Pediatr Radiol* 1992;22:203—205.

63. Eftekhari F, Erly WK, Jaffe N. Malignant rhabdoid tumor of the kidney: imaging features in two cases. *Pediatr Radiol* 1990;21:39—42.

64. Glass RBJ, Davidson AJ, Fernbach SK. Clear cell sarcoma of the kidney: CT, sonographic, and pathologic correlation. *Radiology* 1991;180:715—717..

65. Sisler CL, Siegel MJ. Malignant rhabdoid tumor of the kidney: Radiologic features. *Radiology* 1989;172:211—212.

66. Hartman DS, Davis CJ Jr, Goldman SM, Friedman AC, Fritzsche P. Renal lymphoma: radiologic—pathologic correlation of 21 cases. *Radiology* 1982;144:759—766.

67. Weinberger E, Rosenbaum DM, Pendergrass TW. Renal involvement in children with lymphoma: comparison of CT with sonography. *AJR* 1990;155:347—349.

68. Banner MP, Pollack HM, Chatten J, Witzleben C. Multilocular renal cysts: Radiologic—pathologic correlation. *AJR* 1981;136:239—247.

69. Madewell JE, Goldman SM, Davis CJ, Jr, et al. Multilocular cystic nephroma: a radiographic—pathologic correlation of 58 patients. *Radiology* 1983;146:309—321.

70. Bret PM, Bretagnolle M, Gaillard D, et al. Small, asymptomatic angiomyolipomas of the kidney. *Radiology* 1985;154:7—10.

71. Hartman DS, Goldman SM, Friedman AC, et al. Angiomyolipoma: ultrasonic—pathologic correlation. *Radiology* 1981;129:451—458.

72. Lemaitre L, Robert Y, Dubrelle F, et al. Renal angiomyolipoma: growth followed up with CT and/or US. *Radiology* 1995;197:598—602.

73. Narla LD, Slovis TL, Watts FB, Nigro M. The renal lesions of tuberosclerosis (cysts and angiomyolipoma)-screening with sonography and computerized tomography. *Pediatr Radiol* 1988;18:205—209.

74. McHugh K, Stringer DA, Hebert D, Babiak CA. Simple renal cysts in children: diagnosis and follow-up with US. *Radiology* 1991;178:383—385.

75. Steinhardt GF, Slovis TL, Perlmutter AD. Simple renal cysts in infants. *Radiology* 1985;155:349—350.

76. Brill PW, Jagannath A, Winchester P, Markisz JA, Zirinsky K. Adrenal hemorrhage and renal vein thrombosis in the newborn: MR imaging. *Radiology* 1989;170:95—98.

77. Cohen EK, Daneman A, Stringer DA, Soto G, Thorner P. Focal adrenal hemorrhage: a new US appearance. *Radiology* 1986;161:631—633.

78. Eklöf O, Mortensson W, Sandstedt B. Suprarenal hematoma versus neuroblastoma complicated by hemorrhage: a diagnostic dilemma in newborn. *Acta Radiol* 1986;27:3—10.

79. Heij HA, Taets van Amerongen AHM, Ekkelkamp S, Vos A. Diagnosis and management of neonatal adrenal haemorrhage. *Pediatr Radiol* 1989;19:391—394

80. Brodeur GM, Pritchard J, Berthold F, et al. Revisions of the international criteria for neuroblastoma diagnosis, staging, and response to treatment. *J Clin Oncol* 1993;11:1466—1477 x.

81. White SJ, Stuck KJ, Blane CE, Silver TM. Sonography of neuroblastoma. *AJR* 1983;141:465—468.

82. Atkinson GO JR, Zaatari GS, Lorenzo RI, Gay BB Jr, Gavin AJ. Cystic neuroblastoma in infants: radiographic and pathologic features. *AJR* 1986;146:113—117

83. Hayes FA, Smith EI. Neuroblastoma. In: Pizzo PA, Poplack DG, eds. *Principles and Practice of Pediatric Oncology.* Philadelphia: JB Lippincott; 1989, p. 607—622.

84. Daneman A. Adrenal neoplasms in children. *Semin Roentgenol* 1988;23:205—215.

85. Stark DD, Moss AA, Brasch RC, et al. Neuroblastoma: diagnostic imaging and staging. *Radiology* 1983;148:101—105.

86. Daneman A, Chan HSL, Martin J. Adrenal carcinoma and adenoma in children: a review of 17 patients. *Pediatr Radiol* 1983;13:11—18.

87. Dehner LP, Ishak KG. Vascular tumors of the liver in infants and children. A study of 30 cases and review of the literature. *Arch Pathol* 1971;92:101—111.

88. Dehner LP. Hepatic tumors in the pediatric age group: a distinctive clinicopathologic spectrum. *Perspect Pediatr Pathol* 1978;4:217—268.

89. Ein SH, Stephens CA. Benign liver tumors and cysts in childhood. *J Pediatr Surg* 1974;9:847—851.

90. Weinberg AG, Finegold MJ. Primary hepatic tumors of childhood. *Hum Pathol* 1983;14:512—537.

91. Dachman AH, Lichenstein JE, Friedman AC, Hartman DS. Infantile hemangioendothelioma of the liver: a radiologic—pathologic—clinical correlation. *AJR* 1983;140:1091—1096.

92. de Campo M, de Campo JF. Ultrasound of primary hepatic tumours in childhood. *Pediatr Radiol* 1988;19:19—24.

93. Fellows KE, Hoffer FA, Markowitz RI, O'Neill JA, Jr. Multiple collaterals to hepatic infantile hemangioendotheliomas and arteriovenous malformations: effect on embolization. *Radiology* 1991;181:813—818.

94. Keslar PJ, Buck JL, Selby DM. Infantile hemangioendothelioma of the liver revisited. *RadioGraphics* 1993;13:657—670.

95. Klein MA, Slovis TL, Chang CH, Jacobs IG. Sonographic and Doppler features of infantile hepatic hemangiomas with pathologic correlation. *J Ultrasound Med* 1990;9:619—624.

96. Paltiel HJ, Patriquin HB, Keller MS, Babcock DS, Leithiser RE, Jr. Infantile hepatic hemangioma: Doppler US. *Radiology* 1992;182:735—742.

97. Federici S, Galli G, Sciutti R, Cuoghi D. Cystic mesenchymal hamartoma of the liver. *Pediatr Radiol* 1992;22:307—308.

98. Giyanani VL, Meyers PC, Wolfson JJ. Mesenchymal hamartoma of the liver: computed tomography and ultrasonography. *J Comp Assist Tomogr* 1986;10:51—54.

99. Ros PR, Goodman ZD, Ishak KG, et al. Mesenchymal hamartoma of the liver: radiologic—pathologic correlation. *Radiology* 1986;158:619—624.

100. Stanley P, Hall TR, Woolley MM, et al. Mesenchymal hamartomas of the liver in childhood: sonographic and CT findings. *AJR* 1986;147:1035—1039.

101. Ein SH, Stephens CA. Malignant liver tumors in children. *J Pediatr Surg* 1974;9:491—494.

102. Exelby PR, Filler RM, Grosfeld JL. Liver tumors in children in the particular reference to hepatoblastoma and hepato-

cellular carcinoma: American Academy of Pediatrics Surgical Section Survey — 1974. *J Pediatr Surg* 1975;10:329—337.

103. Dachman AH, Pakter RL, Ros PR, et al. Hepatoblastoma: radiologic—pathologic correlation in 50 cases. *Radiology* 1987;164:15—19.

104. Lack EE, Neave C, Vawter GF. Hepatoblastoma a clinical and pathologic study of 54 cases. *Am J Surg Pathol* 1982;6:693—705.

105. Tanaka S, Kitamura T, Fujita M, Nakanishi K, Okuda S. Color Doppler flow imaging of liver tumors. *AJR* 1990;154:509—514.

106. Van Campenhout I, Patriquin H. Malignant microvasculature in abdominal tumors in children: detection with Doppler US. *Radiology* 1992;183:445—448.

107. Titelbaum DS, Burke DR, Meranze SG, Saul SH. Fibrolamellar hepatocellular carcinoma: pitfalls in nonoperative diagnosis. *Radiology* 1988;167:25—30.

108. Ros PR, Olmsted WW, Dachman AH, et al. Undifferentiated (Embryonal) sarcoma of the liver: radiologic—pathologic correlation. *Radiology* 1986;160:141—145.

109. Bree RL, Schwab RE, Glazer GM, Fink-Bennett D. The varied appearances of hepatic cavernous hemangiomas with sonography, computed tomography, magnetic resonance imaging and scintigraphy. *Radiographics* 1987;7:1153—1175.

110. Taylor KJW, Ramos I, Morse SS, et al. Focal liver masses: differential diagnosis with pulsed Doppler US. *Radiology* 1987;164:643—647.

111. Numata K, Tanaka K, Mitsui K, et al. Flow characteristics of hepatic tumors at color Doppler sonography: correlation with angiographic findings. *AJR* 1993;160:515—521.

112. Babbitt DP, Starshak RJ, Clemett AR. Choledochal cyst: a concept of etiology. *AJR* 1973;119:57—62.

113. Haller JO. Sonography of the biliary tract in infants and children. *AJR* 1991;157:1051—1058.

114. Siegel MJ. Pediatric gynecologic sonography. *Radiology* 1991: 179:593—600

115. States LJ, Bellah RD. Imaging of the pediatric female pelvis. *Semin Roentgenol* 1996;31:312—329.

116. Blask ARN, Sanders RC, Gearhart JP. Obstructed uterovaginal anomalies: demonstration with sonography. Part I neonates and infants. *Radiology* 1991;179:79—83.

117. Nussbaum AR, Sanders RC, Hartman DS, Dudgeon DL, Parmley TH. Neonatal ovarian cysts: sonographic—pathologic correlation. *Radiology* 1988;168:817—821.

118. Altman RP, Randolph JG, Lilly JR. Sacrococcygeal teratoma: American Academy of Pediatrics Surgical Section Survey —1973. *J Pediatr Surg* 1974;9:389—398.

119. Ehren IM, Mahour GH, Isaacs H. Benign and malignant ovarian tumors in children and adolescents. Am J Surg 1984;147:339—344.

120. Wu A, Siegel MJ. Sonography of pelvic masses in children: diagnostic predictability. *AJR* 1987;148:1199—1202.

121. Castleberry RP, Kelly DR, Joseph DB, Cain WS. Gonadal and extragonadal germ cell tumors. In: Fernbach DJ, Vietti TJ, eds. *Clinical Pediatric Oncology*. St. Louis: Mosby Year Book, 1991, p. 577—594.

122. Sisler CL, Siegel MJ. Ovarian teratomas: a comparison of the sonographic appearance in prepubertal and postpubertal girls. *AJR* 1990;154:139—141.

123. Sheth S, Fishman EK, Buck JL, Hamper UM, Sanders RC. The variable sonograhic appearances of ovarian teratomas: correlation with CT. *AJR* 1988;151:331—334.

124. Surratt JT, Siegel MJ. Imaging of pediatric ovarian masses. *RadioGraphics* 1991;11:533—548.

125. Blask ARN, Sanders RC, Rock JA. Obstructed uterovaginal anomalies: demonstration with sonography. Part II teenagers. *Radiology* 1991;179:84—88.

126. Fleischer AC, Rodgers WH, Kepple DM, et al. Color Doppler sonography of benign and malignant ovarian masses. *RadioGraphics* 1992;12:879—885.

127. Macpherson RI. Gastrointestinal tract duplications: clinical, pathologic, etiologic, and radiologic considerations. *RadioGraphics* 1993;13:1063—1080.

128. Barr LL, Hayden CK Jr, Stansberry SD, Swischuk LE. Enteric duplication cysts in children: are their ultrasonographic wall characteristics diagnostic? *Pediatr Radiol* 1990;20:326—328.

129. Teele RL, Henschke CI, Tapper D. The radiographic and ultrasonographic evaluation of enteric duplication cysts. *Pediatr Radiol* 1980;10:9—14.

130. Georg C, Schwerk WB, Goerg K. Gastrointestinal lymphoma: sonographic findings in 54 patients. *AJR* 1990;155:795—798.

131. Vade A, Blane CE. Imaging of Burkitt lymphoma in pediatric patients. *Pediatr Radiol* 1985;15:123—126.

37 Acute Abdominal Pain in Childhood

Carlos J. Sivit

Acute abdominal pain is a common complaint in childhood. It is associated with a large number of surgical and nonsurgical conditions. The initial evaluation begins with a careful history and physical examination. The differential diagnosis can usually be narrowed based on patient age, pain location, presence or absence of other signs and symptoms, and laboratory findings. However, it should be noted that many conditions resulting in acute abdominal pain in childhood may be seen across a wide age spectrum. Additionally, younger children may not be able to localize the site of pain well or verbalize other symptoms. Therefore, it may not always be easy for the clinician to narrow the number of differential diagnoses being considered on the basis of physical findings. The introduction of the graded-compression sonographic technique and continued improvement in gray scale and color Doppler technology have advanced the role of sonography in the initial evaluation of many conditions associated with acute abdominal pain in children. The principal challenge in the imaging evaluation of these children is to exclude conditions requiring emergency surgical intervention. When surgical disorders are present, an important secondary goal of sonography is to delineate the exact nature of these conditions.

Most children presenting with acute abdominal pain will have nonsurgical disease. The most frequent conditions requiring acute surgical intervention in children presenting with acute abdominal pain are acute appendicitis and intestinal intussusception. Among the other conditions commonly resulting in acute abdominal pain in the pediatric population are mesenteric lymphadenitis, acute pancreatitis, cholelithiasis, acute cholecystitis, and acute gynecologic conditions such as ovarian cyst, ovarian torsion, and pelvic inflammatory disease. An important contribution of sonography to the management of children with acute abdominal pain is in aiding in the diagnosis of a wide variety of conditions other than the principal ones being considered. Thus, consideration should be given to scanning the entire abdomen and pelvis, regardless of where the pain is localized.

In this chapter, the imaging evaluation of specific abdominal and pelvic conditions that result in acute abdominal pain in children are discussed, with emphasis on the sonographic assessment. This includes the clinical presentation of the condition, rationale for imaging, diagnostic workup of the condition including imaging tests other than sonography, techniques for optimal sonographic assessment, and findings at imaging assessment.

Intussusception

Intestinal intussusception results from a segment of bowel (intussusceptum) telescoping into a more distal segment (intussuscipiens) (**Fig. 37–1**). The most common type of intussusception is ileocolic, followed by ileoileocolic, ileoileal, and colocolic. Intussusception is the most common acute abdominal disorder of early childhood. The peak age incidence of the condition is between 5 and 9 months of age. It is rare under 3 months and over 3 years of age and this condition is more common in males than females. The majority of intussusceptions have no pathologic lead point. Such cases are called idiopathic and they are thought to result from hypertrophy of lymphoid tissues following a viral infection, resulting in increased intestinal peristalsis in an attempt to extrude the hypertrophied tissues. Recognizable lead points are found in 5—10% of children with intussusception. They should be strongly suspected in children who present under the age of 3 months, over the age of 3 years, or in cases of recurrent intussusception. The most common recognizable lead points include Meckel's diverticulum, intestinal polyp, enteric duplication, intramural hematoma, and lymphoma.

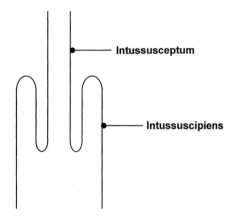

Figure 37–1 Diagram of an intussusceptum invaginating into an intussuscipiens.

The clinical presentation of intussusception is characterized by intermittent episodes of colicky abdominal pain, vomiting, and stool containing blood and mucus, described as "currant-jelly" stool. The child may initially appear comfortable between episodes of pain; however, the pain may become persistent over time. Somnolence and lethargy may also develop with prolonged duration of intussusception. Abdominal palpation demonstrates a sausage-shaped mass in approximately two-thirds of patients. Diffuse abdominal distension and tenderness may develop if the disorder is complicated by bowel obstruction.

The imaging evaluation of children with suspected intussusception has traditionally begun with abdominal radiographs. The principal role of conventional radiographs is to assess for possible complications of intussusception, including small bowel obstruction and perforation. Therefore, upright or lateral decubitus films should be included to assess for extraluminal air. Abdominal radiographs may detect the intussusception by demonstrating a rounded, soft tissue mass (**Fig. 37–2**). Abdominal radiographs are normal in nearly one-half of children with an intussusception. Thus, they are not a reliable measure for excluding the disorder.

Sonography has now gained acceptance as a reliable method for the diagnosis of intussusception and is being utilized with increasing frequency for the initial screening of children with such condition.[1–3] In various series, sonography has had a sensitivity of 100% for the diagnosis of intussusception.[1,2] The use of sonography as a screening examination allows for more selective use of contrast enema examinations, only for therapeutic purposes. A technique of graded-compression is utilized with pressure slowly applied with a linear, high-

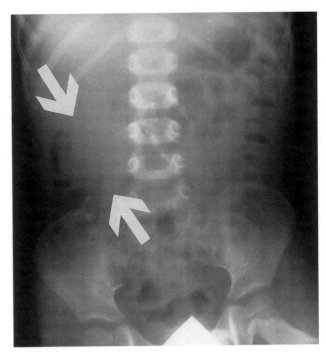

Figure 37–2 Intussusception. Abdominal radiograph shows a rounded, soft-tissue mass in the right mid-abdomen (**arrows**), representing an intussusception.

frequency transducer. The sonographic appearance of an intussusception is that of a mass lesion over 3 cm in maximal diameter. In the transverse plane, the appearance has been characterized as that of a "target" or "doughnut" due to its rounded appearance (**Fig. 37–3**), while in long axis it may have a more elongated or "pseudokidney" appearance (**Fig. 37–4**).[4]

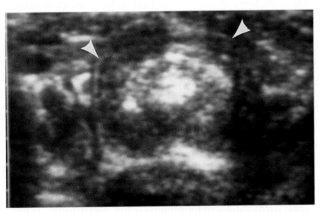

Figure 37–3 Intussusception with a target appearance. Transverse view through the right mid-abdomen demonstrates a rounded soft-tissue mass (**arrowheads**). Note the hypoechoic outer rim representing the receiver loop, or intussuscipiens. The central region is the intussusceptum.

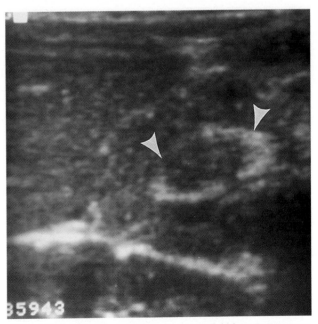

Figure 37–4 Intussusception with a pseudokidney appearance. Longitudinal view through the right upper quadrant demonstrates a soft-tissue mass (**arrowheads**) that resembles a kidney in shape.

A contrast enema examination is utilized for intussusception reduction. Intussusception reduction rates in most series range from 60% to 90%. Controversy exists as to the optimal choice of contrast material (air, water-soluble contrast (**Fig. 37–5**), or barium) for the treatment of intussusception. Proposed advantages of intussusception reduction with air include decreased cost, decreased fluoroscopy time, ability to monitor intraluminal pressure generated, and less fecal spillage and peritoneal contamination if perforation occurs. Proposed advantages of liquid reduction include improved visualization of the intussusception and of contrast refluxing into the small intestine and lower frequency and earlier visualization of perforation. There has been only one randomized, prospective study to date that has compared air and liquid contrast agents for reduction of intussusception. In that study, there was no statistically significant difference in the rate of intussusception reduction or complications with either contrast medium.

Various sonographic findings have been reported as predictive of the success of hydrostatic reduction. These include a thin external hypoechoic rim (< 8 mm in maximal diameter), absence of fluid trapped within the intussusception and presence of flow within the intussusception at color Doppler sonography.[1, 5—8] However, there are no sonographic findings that represent contraindications to attempted intussusception reduction. When evaluating flow within the intussusception, Doppler parameters should be set to maximize the detection of slow blood flow.

Sonography has also been utilized to guide the treatment of intussusception.[9, 10] The use of sonography to guide hydrostatic intussusception reduction has been reported with good results in several recent studies. A saline or tap water enema is administered while the patient is monitored by sonography until there is complete disappearance of the intussusception. This technique has been shown to be a safe treatment method, although its use in North America is currently limited.

Appendicitis

Acute appendicitis is the most common condition requiring emergency abdominal surgery in children. The incidence in the pediatric age group is estimated to be approximately 4 in every 1000 children. It is rare in children under the age of 2 years. The condition is felt to result from appendiceal luminal obstruction by hard concretions, fecal impaction, or appendiceal calculi. This is followed by luminal distension, ischemia, and secondary bacterial infection. Ultimately, if untreated, there is appendiceal wall necrosis, resulting in perforation and abscess formation.

The clinical presentation of appendicitis is characterized by abdominal pain that may originate in the periumbilical region and migrate to the right lower quadrant. Additional findings include focal tenderness over McBurney's point, fever, and leukocytosis. Diffuse abdominal distension and tenderness may develop if the disorder is complicated by bowel obstruction. Abdominal palpation may demonstrate a palpable mass following appendiceal rupture and development of a periappendiceal abscess. Unfortunately, the early clinical diagnosis of this condition remains difficult in children. Children who have the disease are likely to have signs and symptoms for a longer period of time than adults before a correct diagnosis is made, thus increasing the chance of perforation. Approximately one-third of children with appendicitis have an uncertain preoperative diagnosis based on clinical signs and symptoms. This is due to several factors, including the variable clinical manifestations of the disease, the inability of younger children to adequately communicate their complaints, and the large number of nonsurgical conditions, particularly acute gynecologic conditions, that may mimic appendicitis.

The consequences of missed or delayed diagnosis of appendicitis are serious. They include perforation, abscess formation, pylephlebitis, and peritonitis. These complications can result in prolonged hospitalization, an increased risk of infertility in females, and even death. At the other end of the spectrum, the percentage of appendectomies with false-positive findings is as high as 25% in some pediatric series.[11] False-positive diagnoses are associated with significant cost and morbidity, including later development of adhesions resulting in bowel obstruction. Therefore, the major challenges in the management of this condition are to establish an

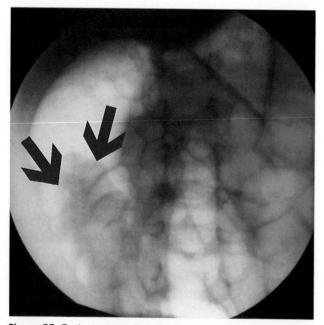

Figure 37–5 Intussusception. Spot-radiograph of the ascending colon during an air-contrast edema shows a soft-tissue mass (**arrows**) representing an intussusception.

early diagnosis in order to prevent progression to perforation and its associated complications and reduce the number of unnecessary appendectomies.

Sonography is the principal modality utilized in the assessment of children with suspected appendicitis,[12–14] and is particularly useful in the evaluation of children in whom the clinical findings are equivocal. In this group, sonography permits an earlier diagnosis and also minimizes the rate of unnecessary appendectomies due to false-positive sonographic findings.[13–15] The sonographic evaluation of appendicitis is based on the graded-compression technique. This method was first described by Puylaert in 1986 and is based on the observation that normal bowel loops and the normal appendix can be compressed with moderate pressure, but the inflamed appendix will not compress.[16] The use of graded compression with a linear 5.0- or 7.5-MHz transducer eliminates overlying bowel gas and reduces the distance from the transducer to the appendix. Compression is applied slowly to reduce patient discomfort. Adequate compression has been achieved if the iliac vessels and psoas muscle are visualized, as the appendix will always lie anterior to those structures. Sonography can be considered reliable for excluding appendicitis if the psoas muscle can be identified. Visualization of the appendix itself cannot be used as a criterion for a diagnostic examination, because the normal appendix is only visualized in one-quarter to one-half of patients. The examination in patients who have a normal graded-compression examination of the right lower quadrant should include a survey of the entire abdomen to assess potential abdominal and pelvic conditions that may mimic appendicitis.

The normal appendix is identified at sonography by its tubular appearance and blind end on long axis scans. It is usually curved and may be tortuous.[17] It is characterized at sonography by a thin, central, echogenic region corresponding to the submucosa, surrounded by a hypoechoic outer zone representing the muscularis propria (**Fig. 37–6**).[17] The normal appendix is compressible, and the maximum diameter does not exceed 6 mm. The appendix is differentiated from adjacent small bowel loops by the absence of peristalsis and the lack of change in configuration over time. It is differentiated from the ascending colon on the basis of its smaller size. The appendix can also be differentiated from bowel on the basis of its shape. The normal appendix will appear circular in the transverse plane while bowel has a flattened configuration.

The sonographic criteria for diagnosis of appendicitis includes visualization of an noncompressible appendix that has a maximum cross-sectional diameter of at least 6 mm (**Fig. 37–7**), identification of an appendicolith (an echogenic foci with acoustic shadowing) (**Fig. 37–8**), or demonstration of a complex mass or focal fluid collection, representing a periappendiceal abscess following appendiceal perforation (**Fig. 37–9**).[18,19] Color Doppler

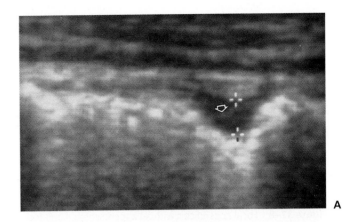

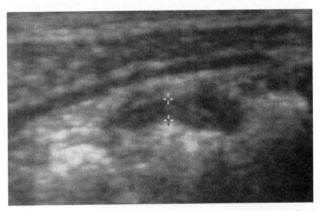

Figure 37–6 Normal appendix. Transverse (**A**) and longitudinal (**B**) views through the right lower quadrant demonstrate a normal appendix (between electronic calipers). Note the faint central echogenic mucosal and submucosal stripe (**open arrow**) and the outer hypoechoic muscularis.

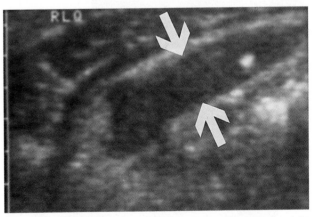

Figure 37–7 Appendicitis. Longitudinal view through the right lower quadrant demonstrates a noncompressible, enlarged appendix (**arrows**).

sonography is a useful adjunct in confirming the diagnosis of appendicitis by demonstrating blood flow in the appendiceal wall or in a right lower quadrant mass.[20] The normal appendix typically does not demonstrate any blood flow within its wall at color Doppler examination.

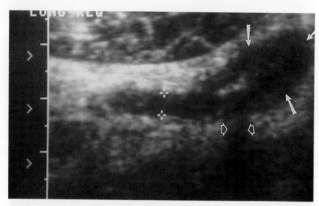

Figure 37–8 Focal appendicitis with an appendicolith. Longitudinal view through the right lower quadrant shows a normal-appearing proximal appendix measuring 4 mm in maximal diameter (calipers) with an enlarged bulbous distal appendix (**arrows**). Also note the echogenic appendicolith demonstrating acoustic shadowing (**open arrows**).

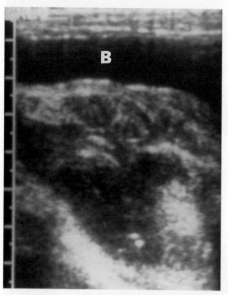

Figure 37–9 Perforated appendicitis. Longitudinal view through the pelvis demonstrates a complex mass behind the bladder (B), representing a periappendiceal abscess.

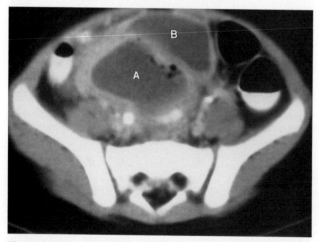

Figure 37–10 Perforated appendicitis. CT scan through the pelvis shows a thick-walled, low-attenuation collection behind the bladder (B), representing a periappendiceal abscess (A).

Another important contribution of sonography to the management of children with suspected appendicitis is in the diagnosis of other abdominal and pelvic conditions that can mimic appendicitis.[13—21] This is important as the majority of children referred for sonographic evaluation to rule out appendicitis will not have appendicitis. Appendicitis will be present in only approximately one-fourth to one-third of children referred for sonography with suspected appendicitis.[13—15,21] between one-third and one-half of these children will have resolution of abdominal pain without a specific diagnosis being established. However, approximately one-fourth to one-third of children assessed with sonography have a specific alternative diagnosis established by sonography.[13,21] Thus, the entire abdomen and pelvis should be scanned in children who have a normal graded-compression examination of the right lower quadrant.

The principal pitfalls associated with the sonographic diagnosis of appendicitis include focal appendicitis, retrocecal appendicitis, and perforated appendicitis. In focal appendicitis, inflammation is localized to the distal end (**Fig. 37–8**).[17] Therefore, it is important to image the entire length of the appendix to avoid a false-negative diagnosis, as the proximal appendix may appear normal in size. The appendiceal tip can be identified on the basis of its blind termination. A retrocecal appendix can be difficult to visualize, particularly if the ascending colon and distal small bowel contain large amounts of air that cannot be compressed. The appendix may also not be recognizable following perforation.[22,23] Additionally, even if a portion is identified, the diameter may be normal, as the intraluminal pressure has been relieved. Thus the principal finding in perforated appendicitis is a periappendiceal mass which may represent thickening of adjacent atonic bowel loops, interloop fluid pockets, phlegmon, or abscess (**Fig. 37–10**).

CT is also a useful modality for evaluating complications of appendicitis, such as perforation with phlegmon or abscess formation. It can delineate the location and extent of associated abdominal and pelvic abscess better than sonography (**Fig. 37–10**). Additionally, it can determine the relative size of liquefied and nonliquefied components. This is very useful in guiding management, as small collections, less than 3 cm in diameter, respond well to primary antibiotic therapy and no drainage. CT is also useful in the diagnosis of nonperforated appendicitis in children who are difficult to examine because of large girth or marked abdominal tenderness and when the sonographic findings are equivocal (**Fig. 37–11**).[24]

Mesenteric Adenitis/Mesenteric Lymphadenopathy

Mesenteric lymph node enlargement is associated with a variety of medical and surgical disorders in children that may result in acute right lower quadrant pain.[25–28] It is important to distinguish between the sonographic finding of mesenteric lymph node enlargement and the clinical syndrome of mesenteric lymphadenitis. Mesenteric lymph node enlargement at sonography is a nonspecific finding associated with a wide variety of abdominal and pelvic disorders, including appendicitis. The enlarged lymph nodes simply represent a marker for infectious, inflammatory, or neoplastic processes in the abdomen or pelvis. The precise origin of the primary condition is often not determined. The potential for coexistence of enlarged mesenteric lymph nodes and other associated conditions indicates that there should be a continued search for additional abdominal or pelvic abnormalities when enlarged mesenteric nodes are found at sonography. Sonography has been shown to be useful in establishing a specific diagnosis in approximately one-half of these cases.

Mesenteric lymphadenitis is a clinical entity where symptoms relate to benign inflammation of the lymph nodes by infectious or inflammatory processes. The clinical syndrome of mesenteric lymphadenitis can mimic an acute abdomen. Patients present with acute right lower quadrant pain, tenderness, fever, and leukocytosis. Although it is a nonsurgical condition, in several series mesenteric lymphadenitis was the most frequent diagnosis in children who went to surgery because of suspected appendicitis and had a normal appendix at surgery.[11] Histologic assessment of the lymph nodes typically demonstrates nonspecific, reactive lymphoid hyperplasia.[27]

Enlarged mesenteric lymph nodes are often identified in the right lower quadrant in children undergoing graded-compression sonography. Mesenteric lymph nodes have an oval shape, although they may appear somewhat flattened with graded compression (**Fig. 37–12**).[27-29] The shortest diameter of the lymph nodes is seen in the anteroposterior plane. Mesenteric lymph nodes are considered enlarged when the maximum anteroposterior diameter is at least 4 mm. The lymph nodes are iso- or hypoechoic relative to surrounding tissues and muscles.

Acute Gynecologic Conditions

Acute gynecologic conditions commonly result in acute right lower quadrant abdominal pain. The most common gynecologic causes of such pain include ovarian cyst, ovarian torsion, and pelvic inflammatory disease. Sonography is the principal imaging examination

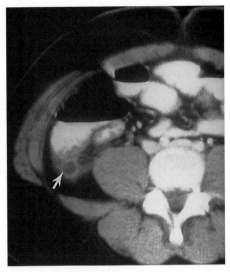

Figure 37–11 Nonperforated appendicitis. CT scan in a patient with an equivocal sonogram of the right lower quadrant demonstrates an enlarged, fluid-filled, retrocecal appendix (**arrow**). Note the associated stranding of the periappendiceal fat.

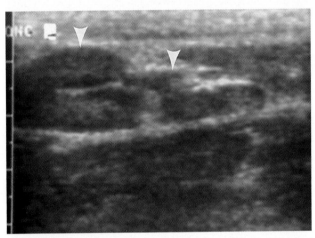

Figure 37–12 Enlarged mesenteric lymph nodes. Longitudinal view through the right lower quadrant at graded-compression sonography shows several enlarged, oval-shaped, mesenteric lymph nodes (**arrowheads**).

for the assessment of these conditions, serving as a useful complement to physical examination, cervical cultures, and, if indicated, a serum pregnancy test.

Sonographic assessment of pelvic pathology in children is based primarily on transabdominal sonography with a sector transducer. Adequate bladder distension is essential to evaluate the uterus and ovaries. The full bladder acts as an acoustic window for the pelvic structures. The lower abdomen should be scanned as well as the pelvis as the ovaries often have an intraabdominal location in prepubertal girls. Endovaginal sonography may provide additional diagnostic information in postpubertal females who are sexually active. It allows for a more precise characterization of ovarian and tubal pathology.

Ovarian cysts are a common cause of acute right lower quadrant or pelvic pain in postpubertal females. Symptoms result following cyst hemorrhage, rupture, or torsion. The majority of ovarian cysts are either follicular or corpus luteal cysts. Uncomplicated cysts typically have a thin rim and an anechoic appearance.[30–32] Peritoneal fluid may be noted if there has been prior cyst rupture. If there has been complicating hemorrhage, hypoechoic or echogenic internal contents, then a fluid debris level or septations may be noted within the cyst (**Fig. 37–13**). Distinction between a hemorrhagic ovarian cyst and other adnexal masses may not be possible on a single sonogram, and serial evaluation may be required once an acute signal emergency has been excluded.

Ovarian torsion results following rotation of the ovarian pedicle along its axis. It is seen more frequently

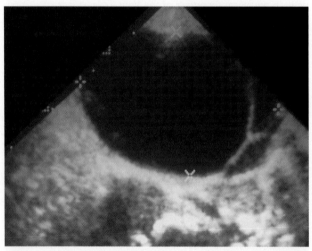

Figure 37–13 Ovarian cyst. Transverse view through the right adnexa shows a large cystic lesion (calipers) with several septa in the right ovary, representing an ovarian cyst.

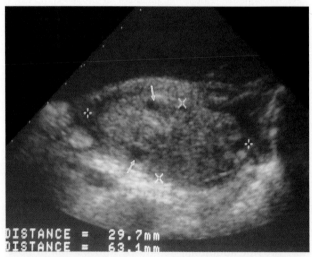

Figure 37–14 Ovarian torsion. Longitudinal view through the right adnexa demonstrates a solid mass (between the electronic calipers) with several peripheral follicles (**arrows**). Ovarian torsion was noted at surgery.

prior to puberty, owing to increased adnexal mobility prior to menarche. Torsion of a normal ovary may occur, although typically ovarian torsion is associated with a large ovarian cyst or ovarian neoplasm. Affected children usually present with acute right lower quadrant or pelvic pain. Anorexia, nausea, and vomiting are also common. Ovarian torsion is a surgical emergency as a compromise of the arterial blood supply to the ovary results in progressive congestion of ovarian parenchyma followed by hemorrhagic infarction and irreversible damage to the ovary. The gray scale sonographic findings of ovarian torsion are nonspecific and include a cystic or solid adnexal mass and enlargement of multiple ovarian follicles (**Fig. 37–14**).[32–34] Color Doppler sonography is essential in the evaluation of ovarian torsion by demonstrating absence of ovarian blood flow.[32] Caution should be utilized with this finding, however, because ovarian flow may not be observed in normal ovaries, particularly in younger children. Additionally, occasionally, some ovarian flow may be seen in ovarian torsion.

Pelvic inflammatory disease refers to infection of the upper genital tract. It is an ascending infection that originates in the cervix and may extend to the endometrium, fallopian tubes, ovaries, and peritoneal cavity. The infection is sexually transmitted. The most common organisms are *Chlamydia* and *Neisseria*. As the infection ascends, the fallopian tube is penetrated, causing cell destruction. The tubes become hyperemic, thickened, and filled with purulent exudate, resulting in a pyosalpinx. As the pressure increases, the tubal walls become thinned and convoluted. If the infection subsides at this stage, a hydrosalpinx may result. If inflammation progresses, then a tuboovarian complex may develop, as periovarian adhesions fuse the inflamed tube to the ovary. Further progression of infection results in the development of a tuboovarian abscess. The presenting signs and symptoms are variable, although right lower quadrant or pelvic pain and tenderness is common. Fever and leukocytosis may also be present, particularly following the development of a tuboovarian abscess.

Sonography may be normal in patients with mild tubal and ovarian inflammatory disease. Sonographic findings in patients with pelvic inflammatory disease include endometrial thickening, an enlarged uterus with indistinct margins, fallopian tube thickening, a fluid-distended fallopian tube representing a hydrosalpinx or pyosalpinx, and ovarian enlargement with indistinct borders.[35] A complex adnexal mass may be seen if a tuboovarian abscess develops (**Fig. 37–15**). Echogenic peritoneal fluid, representing pus, may also be seen. Once tuboovarian pathology has been diagnosed, follow-up sonography is useful to evaluate the efficacy of medical treatment.

Acute Pancreatitis

Acute pancreatitis in children most often results from blunt abdominal trauma. Nontraumatic causes in children include infection, drug toxicity, obstruction at the ampulla of Vater, pancreas divisum, and hereditary diseases including cystic fibrosis and hereditary pancreatitis. The most common infectious cause of pancreatitis is mumps. Obstruction at the ampulla of Vater most commonly occurs secondary to cholelithiasis. Pancreas divisum is a developmental anomaly of the pancreas in which the dorsal and ventral pancreatic ducts fail to fuse. The dorsal duct drains via the accessory duct of Santorini into the minor duodenal papilla, and the ventral duct drains via the common bile duct into the papilla of Vater. Pancreatitis is thought to result in these individuals if the duct of Santorini and the accessory papilla are too small to transmit the volume of pancreatic secretions that must flow through them, resulting in the pooling of pancreatic secretions. Pancreatitis develops in approximately 1% of children with cystic fibrosis. It is thought to result from ductal obstruction and leakage of pancreatic enzymes. Hereditary pancreatitis is an autosomal dominant disease characterized by recurrent attacks of acute pancreatitis.

Clinical findings of acute pancreatitis include upper abdominal pain that may localize to the epigastric region and radiate to the back, abdominal tenderness, vomiting, and fever. Pancreatic enzyme levels are elevated in blood and urine. Acute pancreatitis is classified as mild or severe on the basis of clinical and pathologic changes. Mild acute pancreatitis is characterized by minimal systemic signs and rapid response to medical therapy with improvement in physical signs and laboratory values within 48—72 h. It is characterized pathologically by interstitial edema. Rarely, microscopic foci of acinar cell necrosis may be noted. Severe acute pancreatitis is manifested by severe clinical findings including shock, renal failure, gastrointestinal tract bleeding, and pulmonary insufficiency. The development of pancreatic pseudocyst and abscess is common. It is characterized pathologically by pancreatic and peripancreatic fat necrosis. Patients who develop severe pancreatitis usually do so early in the course of their disease. Progression from mild to severe disease is rare.

Sonography is the principal modality utilized in the initial assessment of children with suspected pancreatitis. The pancreas may appear normal at sonography, particularly in cases of mild pancreatitis. Sonographic findings observed in pancreatitis include diffuse or focal gland enlargement (**Fig. 37–16**), pancreatic ductal dilatation (**Fig. 37–17**), increased or decreased pancreatic parenchymal echotexture, and extrapancreatic fluid collections.[36—41] Sonography has a low sensitivity and specificity in the diagnosis of pancreatitis. Its use should be limited to the assessment of complications of

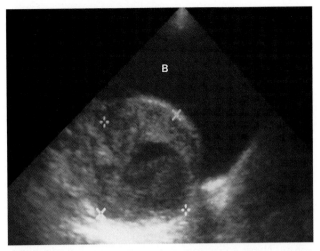

Figure 37–15 Tuboovarian abscess. Longitudinal view through the right adnexa demonstrates a complex mass (calipers) with a cystic center, representing a tubo-ovarian abscess. Note the mass effect on the bladder (B).

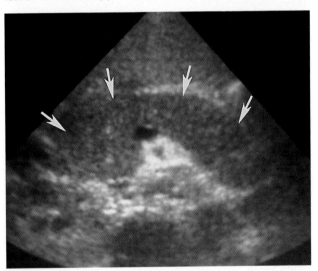

Figure 37–16 Pancreatitis with pancreatic enlargement. Transverse view through the pancreas in a child with pancreatitis demonstrates a diffusely enlarged pancreas (**arrows**).

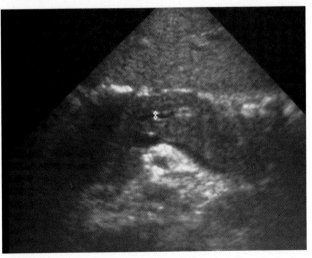

Figure 37–17 Pancreatitis with ductal dilatation. Transverse view through the pancreas in a child with pancreatitis shows dilatation of the main pancreatic duct (between electronic calipers).

pancreatitis, particularly extrapancreatic fluid collections. CT is a useful modality in children with pancreatitis for demonstrating the pancreas when it cannot be seen at sonography, usually because of overlying bowel gas and for assessing major complications of pancreatitis, including acute fluid collections, pseudocysts, pancreatic necrosis, and abscess.[42–44]

Acute fluid collections represent pancreatic juice that spreads throughout the connective tissue surrounding the pancreas, because the pancreas does not have a well-developed capsule.[41, 42] They are unencapsulated and take the shape of the peritoneal or retroperitoneal space in which they are located. The most common locations for these fluid collections are the anterior pararenal space, lesser sac, lesser omentum, and transverse mesocolon. These collections will appear anechoic or hypo-

echoic with increased through transmission at sonography (**Fig. 37–18**) and low attenuation at CT (**Fig. 37–19**). Most acute peripancreatic fluid collections resolve completely within a few weeks. A minority of these collections will evolve into pseudocysts. Formation of a pseudocyst requires at least 4 weeks following the onset of acute pancreatitis. Pseudocysts are round or oval in shape and are surrounded by a capsule containing fibrous tissue. They are typically found in close proximity to the pancreas. Although both sonography (**Fig. 37–18**) and CT (**Fig. 37–19**) can diagnose a pseudocyst, CT is superior for defining the extent of the lesion.[42] The treatment of choice for pancreatic pseudocysts is percutaneous catheter drainage. Pancreatic necrosis is defined as diffuse or focal zones of nonviable or devitalized pancreatic parenchyma, while pancreatic abscess is an intraabdominal collection of purulent material which is located in close proximity to the pancreas and contains little or no necrosis. CT is the preferred method for imaging both of these complications.[42–44] The CT appearance of pancreatic necrosis is a well-circumscribed, low-attenuation area that is larger than 3 cm in diameter or involves 30% or more of the area of the pancreas. A pancreatic abscess will appear at CT as a focal fluid collection with near-water attenuation and a relatively thick wall that may enhance. Differentiation between these two processes is important as pancreatic abscess can be drained percutaneously, while pancreatic necrosis may require surgical debridement.

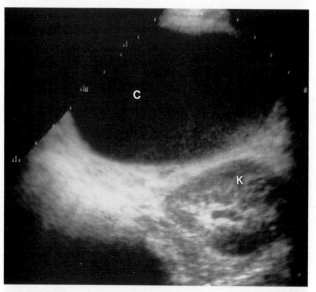

Figure 37–18   Pancreatic pseudocyst. Transverse view through the left upper abdomen demonstrates a large anechoic mass anterior to the left kidney (K), representing a pancreatic pseudocyst (C).

Cholethiasis

Gallstones may result from bile stasis, inflammation, infection, or abnormal hepatobiliary metabolism, either congenital or acquired. In children, associated conditions include cystic fibrosis, malabsorption, total parenteral nutrition, furosemide therapy, short gut syndrome, and hemolytic anemia. In many cases the cause is unknown. Clinical symptoms vary, depending on whether the stones are impacted in the gallbladder, cystic duct, or common bile duct. Gallbladder "colic" results in intermittent pain that is often localized to the right upper quadrant and that may radiate to the back. The episodes of pain typically last less than 4 h. Vomiting is also common. If a stone obstructs the common bile duct, then jaundice or pancreatitis may develop.

Sonography is the principal imaging modality utilized in the assessment of suspected cholelithiasis. Sonographic diagnosis of gallstones is dependent on three criteria: hyperechoic foci, acoustic shadowing, and mobility (**Fig. 37–20**).[45–47] If all three criteria are present, the sensitivity of sonography is greater than 95%. Stones generally respond to gravity and move to the most dependent position. Patients should be fasting to allow for maximal gallbladder distension. Abnormal distension of the gallbladder, a condition referred to as hydrops, may be caused by cystic duct obstruction.

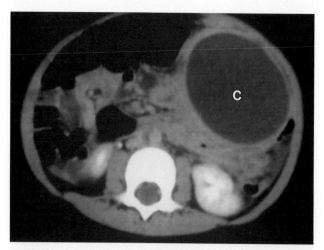

Figure 37–19   Pancreatic pseudocyst. Contrast enhanced CT scan through the upper abdomen demonstrates a low-attenuation lesion in the left anterior pararenal space, representing a pancreatic pseudocyst (C).

Pitfalls in the sonographic diagnosis of cholelithiasis include nonmobile hyperechoic foci, mobile hyperechoic foci without shadowing, impacted stones, and a nonvisible gallbladder. Nonmobile, hyperechoic foci may represent adherent stones, but they also may represent gallbladder septae, fibrous tissue, tumefactive sludge, and artifact. Acoustic shadowing is dependent on stone size, and small calculi may not shadow. Stones may impact in the gallbladder neck, and be difficult to image. Calculi in a contracted gallbladder are also easily missed at sonography. Additionally, when the gallbladder is filled with calculi it may be difficult to recognize.

Acute Cholecystitis

Acute cholecystitis can be seen in children, although less frequently than in adults. Cholecystitis may be due to bile stasis associated with persistent calculous obstruction of the cystic duct. This results in local damage to the gallbladder secondary to a change in bile concentration or its constituents. However, the majority of cases of acute cholecystitis in children are not due to calculi. Most cholecystitis in children is acalculous. Conditions associated with acalculous cholecystitis include recent surgery, fasting states, burns, hyperalimentation, dehydration, systemic illness, infection particularly due to streptococcal infection, Kawasaki disease, and generalized sepsis.

Acute cholecystitis is usually treated with cholecystectomy. Early surgical intervention is the most important factor in decreasing morbidity and mortality associated with this condition. Associated complications include gallbladder rupture, abscess, or peritonitis; however, the presenting signs and symptoms of acute

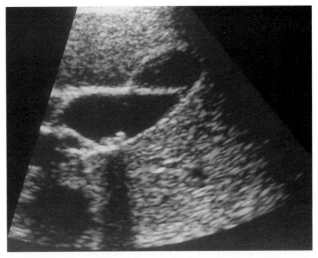

Figure 37–20 Cholelithiasis. Longitudinal view through the gallbladder shows a hyperechoic foci with acoustic shadowing, representing a gallstone.

cholecystitis vary widely, and the clinical diagnosis may be difficult. Thus, imaging assessment of this condition plays an important role in establishing an early diagnosis. Clinical findings include right upper quadrant pain, nausea, vomiting and low-grade fever. Focal tenderness over the gallbladder (Murphy's sign) may be present. There is usually elevation of liver enzymes, and jaundice may be occasionally present.

Sonography is commonly utilized in the assessment of children with suspected acute cholecystitis. Sonography is particularly useful in the evaluation of children with calculous cholecystitis by permitting assessment of associated biliary tract disease, including cholelithiasis, sludge, and biliary dilatation. However, the sonographic diagnosis of cholecystitis itself is insensitive and nonspecific. Sonographic findings associated with cholecys-

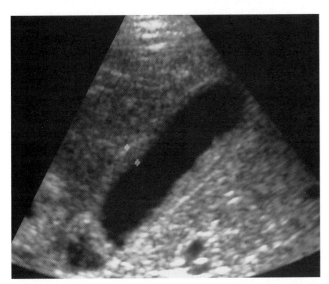

Figure 37–21 Acute cholecystitis. Longitudinal view through the gallbladder demonstrates gallbladder wall thickening (between electronic calipers).

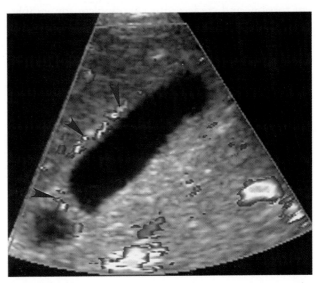

Figure 37–22 Acute cholecystitis. Longitudinal color Doppler sonogram through the gallbladder shows marked hyperemia (**arrowheads**) of the gallbladder wall.

titis include gallbladder wall thickening (> 3 mm) (**Fig. 37–21**), irregular anechoic areas and bands along the gallbladder wall, pericholecystic fluid, a positive sonographic Murphy's sign (localized tenderness over the gallbladder), gallbladder distension, and hypervascularity of the gallbladder wall at color Doppler imaging (**Fig. 37–22**).[48–52] Each of these features may be seen in the absence of cholecystitis. The best sonographic criteria for diagnosing acute cholecystitis are focal gallbladder tenderness in association with calculi.[53]

Hepatobiliary radionuclide imaging with the IDA group of compounds is also commonly used in the evaluation of children with suspected cholecystitis. Patients are evaluated in the fasting state to facilitate visualization of the gallbladder. Scintigraphic visualization of the gallbladder rules out the diagnosis of calculous cholecystitis with a high degree of accuracy because that condition is typically related to cystic duct obstruction. The hallmark finding of calculous cholecystitis at scintigraphy is visualization of radioisotope within the common bile duct and proximal small bowel with absence of gallbladder visualization due to cystic duct obstruction. However, the gallbladder may be visualized in the presence of acalculous cholecystitis.

Summary

In summary, sonography plays an important role in the evaluation of children with acute abdominal pain. The sonographic technique varies with the specific condition being assessed. The technique of graded-compression sonography is required for the assessment of intestinal intussusception, appendicitis, and mesenteric lymphadenopathy. Color Doppler sonography may be useful in the evaluation of intussusception, appendicitis, ovarian torsion, and cholecystitis. A complete sonographic assessment of the abdomen and pelvis should be performed when the clinical findings are equivocal as sonography often aids in the diagnosis of conditions other than the principal one being considered.

References

1. Pracros JP, Tran-Minh VA, et al. Acute intestinal intussusception in children: contribution of ultrasonography (145 cases). *Ann Radiol* 1987;30:525—530.
2. Verschelden P, Filiatrault D, Garel L, et al. Intussusception in children: reliability of US in diagnosis-a prospective study. *Radiology* 1992;184:741—744.
3. Weinberger E, Winters WD. Intussusception in children: the role of sonography. *Radiology* 1992;184:601—602.
4. Swischuk LE, Hayden CK, Boulden T. Intussusception: indications for ultrasonography and an explanation of the doughnut and pseudokidney signs. *Pediatr Radiol* 1985;15:388—391.
5. del-Pozo G, Albillos JC, Tejedor D. Intussusception: US findings with pathologic correlation-the crescent-in-doughnut sign. *Radiology* 1996;199:688—692.
6. del-Pozo G, Gonzalez-Spinola J, Gomez-Anson B, et al. Intussusception: trapped peritoneal fluid detected with US-relationship to reducibility and ischemia. *Radiology* 1996;201:379—383.
7. Lagalla R, Caruso G, Novara V, et al. Color doppler ultrasonography in pediatric intussusception. *J Ultrasound Med* 1994;13:171—174.
8. Lim HK, Bae SH, Lee KH, et al. Assessment of reducibility of ileocolic intussusception in children: usefulness of color doppler sonography. *Radiology* 1994;191:781—785.
9. Riebel TW, Nasir R, Weber K. US-guided hydrostatic reduction of intussusception in children. *Radiology* 1993;188:513—516.
10. Woo SK, Nim JS, Suh SJ, et al. Childhood intussusception: US-guided hydrostatic reduction. *Radiology* 1992;182:77—80.
11. Lau W, Fan S, Yiu T, et al. Negative findings at appendectomy. *Am J Surg* 1984;148:375—378.
12. Kao SCS, Smith WL, Abu-Yousef M, et al. Acute appendicitis in children: sonographic findings. *AJR* 1989;153:375—379.
13. Sivit CJ, Newman KD, Boenning DA, et al. Appendicitis: usefulness of US in a pediatric opulation. *Radiology* 1992;185:549—552.
14. Vignault F, Filiatrault D, Brandt ML, et al. Acute appendicitis in children: evaluation with US. *Radiology* 1990;176:501—504.
15. Ramachandran P, Sivit CJ, Newman KD, et al. Ultrasound as an adjunct in the diagnosis of acute appendicitis: a four year experience. *J Pediatr Surg* 1996;31:164—169.
16. Puylaert JCBM. Acute appendicitis: US evaluation using graded compression. *Radiology* 1986;158:355—360.
17. Sivit CJ. Diagnosis of acute appendicitis in children: spectrum of sonographic findings. AJR 1993;161:147—152.
18. Abu-Yousef MM, Bleicher JJ, James JW, et al. High resolution sonography of acute appendicitis. *AJR* 1987;149:53—58.
19. Jeffrey RB, Laing FC, Townsend RR. Acute appendicitis: sonographic criteria based on 250 cases. *Radiology* 1988;167:327—329.
20. Quillin SP, Siegel MJ. Appendicitis in children: color doppler sonography. *Radiology* 1992;184:745—747.
21. Siegel MJ, Carel C, Surratt S. Ultrasonography of acute abdominal pain in children. *JAMA* 1991;266:1987—1989.
22. Hayden CK, Kuchelmeister J, Lipscomb TS. Sonography of acute appendicitis in childhood: perforation versus nonperforation. *J Ultrasound Med* 1992;11:209—216.
23. Quillin SP, Siegel MJ, Coffin CM. Acute appendicitis in children: value of sonography in detecting perforation. *AJR* 1992;159:1265—1268.
24. Rao PM, Rhea JT, Novelline RA, et al. Helical CT technique for the diagnosis of appendicitis: prospective evaluation of a

focused appendix CT examination. *Radiology* 1997;202: 139—144.

25. Matsumoto T, Iida M, Sakai T, et al. Yersinia terminal ileitis: sonographic findings in eight patients. *AJR* 1991;156:965—967.

26. Rao PM, Rhea JT, Novelline RA. CT diagnosis of mesenteric adenitis. *Radiology* 1997;202:145—149.

27. Sivit CJ, Newman KD, Chandra RS. Visualization of enlarged mesenteric lymph nodes at US examination: Clinical significance. *Pediatr Radiol* 1993;23:471—475.

28. Puylaert JBCM. Mesenteric adenitis and terminal ileitis: US evaluation using graded compression. *Radiology* 1986;161:691—695.

29. Puylaert JCBM, Lalisang RI, van der Werf SDJ, et al. Campylobacter ileocolitis mimicking acute appendicitis: differentiation with graded-compression US. *Radiology* 1988;166:737—740.

30. Bass JS, Haller JO, Friedman AP, et al. The sonographic appearance of the hemorrhagic ovarian cyst in adolescents. *J Ultrasound Med* 1984;3:509—513.

31. Baltarovich OH, Kurtz AB, Pasto ME, et al. The spectrum of sonographic findings in hemorrhagic ovarian cysts. *AJR* 1987;148:53—58.

32. Siegel MJ. Pediatric gynecologic sonography. *Radiology* 1991;179:593—600.

33. Graif M, Itzchak Y. Sonographic evaluation of ovarian torsion in childhood and adolescence. *AJR* 1988;150:647—649.

34. Helvie MA, Silver TM. Ovarian torsion: sonographic evaluation. *J Clin Ultrasound* 1989;17:327—332.

35. Bulas DI, Ahlstrom P, Sivit CJ, et al. Comparison of transabdominal and transvaginal sonography in the evaluation of the adolescent patient with pelvic inflammatory disease. *Radiology* 1982;183:435—439.

36. Fleischer AC, Parker P, Kirchner SG, et al. Sonographic findings of pancreatitis in children. *Radiology* 1983;146:151—155.

37. Coleman BG, Arger PH, Rosenberg HK, et al. Gray-scale sonographic assessment of pancreatitis in children. *Radiology* 1983;146:145—150.

38. Jeffrey RB. Sonography in acute pancreatitis. *Radiol Clin North Am* 1989;27:5—17.

39. Siegel MJ, Sivit CJ. Pancreatic emergencies. *Radiol Clin North Am* 1997;35:815—830.

40. Siegel MJ, Martin KW, Worthington JL. Normal and abnormal pancreas in children: US studies. *Radiology* 1987;165:15—18.

41. Jeffrey RB, Laing FC, Wing VW. Extrapancreatic spread of acute pancreatitis: new observations with real-time US. *Radiology* 1986;159:707—711.

42. King LR, Siegel MJ, Balfe DM. Acute pancreatitis in children: CT findings of intra- and extrapancreatic fluid collections. *Radiology* 1995;195:196—200.

43. Balthazar EJ, Freeny PC, Van Sonnenberg E. Imaging and intervention in acute pancreatitis. *Radiology* 1994;193:297—306.

44. Balthazar EJ, Robinson DL, Megibow AJ, et al. Acute pancreatitis: value of CT in establishing prognosis. *Radiology* 1990;174:331—336.

45. Henschke CI, Teele RL. Cholelithiasis in children: recent observations. *J Ultrasound Med* 1983;2:481—484.

46. Franken EA, Kao SCS, Smith WL, et al. Imaging of the acute abdomen in infants and children. *AJR* 1989;153:921—928.

47. Cohen SM, Kurtz AB. Biliary sonography. *Radiol Clin North Am* 1991;29:1171—1198.

48. Wegener M, Borsch G, Schneider J, et al. Gallbladder wall thickening: a frequent finding in various nonbiliary disorders a prospective ultrasonographic study. *J Clin Ultrasound* 1987;15:307—312.

49. Ralls PW, Colletti PM, Lapin SA, et al. Real-time sonography in suspected acute cholecystitis: prospective evaluation of primary and secondary signs. *Radiology* 1985;155:767—771.

50. Simeone JF, Brink JA, Mueller PR, et al. The sonographic diagnosis of acute gangrenous cholecystitis: importance of the Murphy sign. *AJR* 1989;152:289—290.

51. Paulson EK, Kliewer MA, Hertzberg BS, et al. Diagnosis of acute cholecystitis with color doppler sonography: significance of arterial flow in thickened gallbladder wall. *AJR* 1994;162:1105—1108.

52. Uggowitzer M, Kugler C, Schramayer G, et al. Sonography of acute cholecystitis: comparison of color and power color doppler sonography in detecting hypervascularized gallbladder wall. *AJR* 1997;168:707—712.

53. Ralls PW, Colletti PM, Lapin SA, et al. Real-time sonography in suspected acute cholecystitis: prospective evaluation of primary and secondary signs. *Radiology* 1985;155:767—771.

38 Projectile Vomiting in an Infant

T. David Cox, Sam T. Auringer, and Thomas E. Sumner

The technical advances in ultrasound imaging have had a significant impact on the evaluation of an infant with projectile vomiting. In infants with a high clinical suspicion of hypertrophic pyloric stenosis, sonography has become the diagnostic tool of choice in many pediatric imaging centers. Other, less common, causes of vomiting in infancy may also be diagnosed with sonography.

Differential Diagnosis

Although pyloric stenosis is the most common cause of projectile vomiting in infancy,[1] the differential diagnostic considerations include both intestinal and extraintestinal disease processes. Other intrinsic lesions include pylorospasm, gastroesophageal reflux, malrotation with volvulus, duodenal atresia, congenital gastric outlet obstruction, and mural hematoma. Extrinsic causes of obstruction include Ladd bands, duplication cyst, and hematoma. Disease processes outside the gastrointestinal tract that may also cause vomiting in the neonate include infectious processes and diseases of the central nervous system.

Diagnostic Workup

Clinical Tests

The sensitivity of physical examination in the diagnosis of hypertrophic pyloric stenosis is as high as 70% when done by an experienced surgeon.[1] However, many clinicians lack the experience and confidence needed to make this diagnosis on the basis of palpation of the pyloric olive alone. Analysis of serum electrolytes is used primarily for supportive management of infants with projectile vomiting. In infants with prolonged vomiting secondary to gastric outlet obstruction (e.g., hypertrophic pyloric stenosis), a hypochloremic metabolic alkalosis is common.[2] Some investigators advocate placement of a nasogastric tube and quantification of the volume of aspirate. When the amount of aspirate is greater than 10 cc, more than 90% of infants with projectile vomiting are found to have hypertrophic pyloric stenosis.[3]

If gastroesophageal reflux is suspected, the gold standard for diagnosis is monitoring with a 24-h pH probe. However, the pH probe offers no information with regard to anatomic abnormalities or obstruction that may predispose to reflux, and does not detect nonacid reflux. Endoscopy is not typically used in evaluation of the vomiting infant, unless directed on findings of another modality.

Imaging Tests Other than Sonography

Selection of the appropriate imaging test in an infant with projectile vomiting is dependent on clinical findings. If bilious vomiting or abdominal distension is present, or if the vomiting occurs in the first few days of life, then conventional radiographs of the abdomen should be performed. If a distal obstruction is present, then a contrast enema is usually the imaging test of choice. If the obstruction is proximal or the bowel gas pattern is nonspecific, then an upper gastrointestinal series may be the most helpful examination. Bilious vomiting in an infant should be regarded as a surgical emergency, because of the possibility of malrotation with midgut volvulus.

If nonaccidental trauma is suspected in an infant with vomiting, then CT of the abdomen and pelvis may prove helpful in the evaluation of injuries to both solid and hollow viscera. Duodenal hematoma can also be diagnosed, as well as followed, with an upper gastrointestinal series. CT may also be helpful in evaluating a child with vomiting and a palpable abdominal mass, although determination of the organ of origin of the mass with sonography will help direct the imaging workup.

Gastroesophageal reflux, as well as disorders of gastric emptying, can be demonstrated with nuclear scintigraphy. Anatomic resolution is limited, and these tests are best used to quantify the severity of a functional abnormality at the pylorus or lower esophageal sphincter.

Sonography of Infants with Projectile Vomiting

Sonographic Technique

A linear, 5- to 10-MHz transducer should be used to evaluate infants with suspected pyloric stenosis; higher-frequency transducers provide superior near-field resolution. The pyloric region is best imaged from an anterior approach with the infant in a right posterior oblique position. This position allows fluid in the stomach to distend the antrum and pyloric region. A normal pylorus is shown in Fig. 38–1. Placement of a nasogastric tube may be helpful in some instances. In infants with a markedly distended stomach, aspiration of the gastric contents via a nasogastric tube can facilitate visualization of the pylorus (**Fig. 38–2**).[4] In other infants with an empty stomach, the introduction of a small volume of fluid into the stomach may be helpful in creating an acoustic window. Either glucose solution or water can be given orally or via a nasogastric tube.

Findings

Hypertrophic Pyloric Stenosis

Hypertrophic pyloric stenosis is the most common cause of projectile vomiting in infancy, with an incidence of between one in 300 and one in 400 infants. The condition is seen four times more often in boys than in girls.[5] There is an increased incidence of hypertrophic pyloric stenosis in infants of previously affected parents, particularly the mother, suggesting a genetic predisposition.[5] Patients with pyloric stenosis usually present between 2 and 6 weeks of age with nonbilious, projectile vomiting secondary to gastric outlet obstruction. With prolonged vomiting, the infant becomes dehydrated, with a meta-

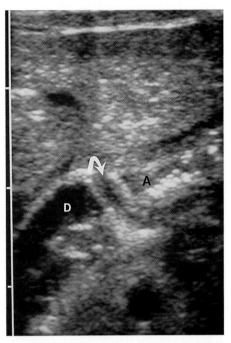

Figure 38–1 Normal pylorus. Transverse scan shows echogenic formula and gas in the distal antrum (A) and fluid in the duodenal bulb (D). Pyloric channel (**arrow**) is quite short.

bolic alkalosis caused by loss of gastric acid with the vomitus. In pyloric stenosis, the circular muscle at the pylorus becomes hypertrophic. The exact cause of the hypertrophy is unclear, although it may be due to a lack of innervation of the circular muscle fibers, as well as a diminished level of nitric oxide synthase, an enzyme that facilitates the relaxation of smooth muscle.[6]

The pylorus is most easily located by scanning in the transverse plane and locating the gallbladder and pancreatic head. Between these two structures, the duodenum and pylorus can then be located. Images of the pylorus are obtained in both longitudinal and cross-sectional planes.[7] On longitudinal scans, the findings of

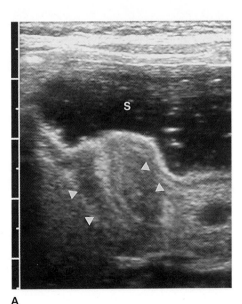
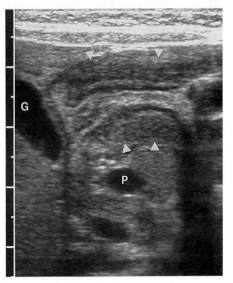

Figure 38–2 Hypertrophic pyloric stenosis. **A:** Sonogram oriented longitudinally to the pylorus reveals a thickened, but poorly seen pylorus (**arrowheads**) secondary to gastric distension (S) and posterior displacement of the pylorus. **B:** After emptying of the stomach, the thickend pyloric muscle on each side of the central echogenic mucosa is better seen, confirming the diagnosis of pyloric stenosis. G, gallbladder; P, portal vein.

pyloric stenosis are a thickened, elongated hypoechoic pyloric muscle impinging on the fluid-filled antrum (**Fig. 38–3**). On transverse images, the hypertrophied muscle has a bulls-eye appearance (**Fig. 38–4**). Other findings include the double-track sign created by the hyperechoic mucosa surrounded by the hypoechoic musculature, exaggerated peristaltic waves in the stomach, and poor gastric emptying.

Several measurements have been described for the diagnosis of hypertrophic pyloric stenosis.[8] These include the length of the pyloric channel, the length of the pyloric muscle, the diameter of the pylorus, and the thickness of the pyloric muscle (**Fig. 38–3**). Of these, pyloric muscle thickness is generally accepted as the most accurate and reproducible.[4,7,8] The exact thickness to be used for the threshold of diagnosis is controversial, with a range of 3—3.5 mm most commonly accepted. Pyloric channel lengths of 17 mm and greater are also considered abnormal. Early in the course of the disease, pyloric measurements may be equivocal; follow-up sonography in 2—3 days may be helpful in these cases (**Fig. 38–4**). Borderline thickness measurements are also not uncommon in malnourished infants secondary to prolonged vomiting, and in premature infants, even though pyloric stenosis is present. In these infants, the demonstration of mass effect on the distal antrum and elongation of the pyloric channel may be sufficient to confirm the diagnosis.

An increased incidence of genitourinary abnormalities has been reported with pyloric stenosis, and some investigators advocate surveying the kidneys in infants with pyloric stenosis.[9] However, results of a more recent study suggest that the incidence of renal abnormalities in infants with pyloric stenosis is just over 2%, a frequency seen in screened populations.[10]

Pylorospasm

Pylorospasm or antral dyskinesia is a common cause of nonbilious vomiting in infants and is an important consideration in the differential diagnosis of pyloric ste-

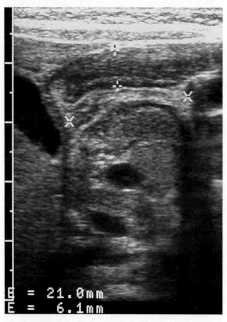

Figure 38–3 Hypertrophic pyloric stenosis. Sonogram oriented longitudinally to the pylorus shows abnormal thickening of the pyloric musculature (6.1 mm) and elongation of the echogenic pyloric channel (21 mm).

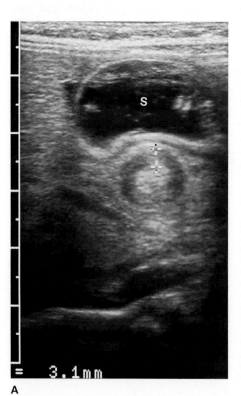

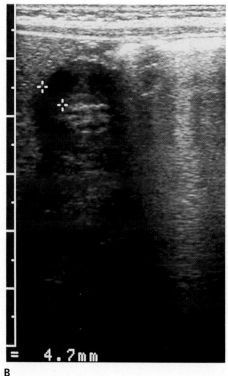

A   **B**

Figure 38–4 Hypertrophic pyloric stenosis. **A:** Sonogram oriented transversely to the long axis of the pylorus reveals the thickened muscle (3.1 mm) surrounding the echogenic mucosa. The pylorus is displaced posteriorly by the distended stomach (S). Although initially interpreted as consistent with pyloric stenosis, patient was followed clinically. **B:** Several days later, a repeat sonogram showed progressive thickening of the pyloric muscle (4.7 mm), confirming the initial diagnosis.

nosis. With pylorospasm, gastric emptying is delayed, and the pyloric channel may be mildly elongated. These findings can cause confusion between pylorospasm and hypertrophic pyloric stenosis at upper gastrointestinal series (UGI).[7]

In pylorospasm, the pyloric channel may be elongated at sonography, but there will be little, if any, thickening of the pyloric musculature. No mass effect on the gastric antrum will be seen, although the stomach may be fluid filled. Because pylorospasm is a self-limited, nonsurgical condition, accurate differentiation from the surgically managed pyloric stenosis is important.[7, 11]

Gastroesophageal Reflux

Gastroesophageal reflux is the most common cause of vomiting in children under 1 year of age.[1] Reflux is characterized by the low-pressure regurgitation of gastric contents, in contrast to vomiting, which is the forceful expulsion of gastric contents. The clinical differentiation can be difficult. Typically, vomiting secondary to gastroesophageal reflux is not projectile and not bilious. The clinical presentation of infants with gastroesophageal reflux is quite variable due to the wide range of severity of the condition.[1, 12] Reflux and regurgitation are seen in all infants to some degree, often until 6—9 months of age. The severity of reflux can be accentuated by overfeeding. With more severe reflux, infants may fail to thrive because of poor feeding or have respiratory symptoms secondary to aspiration pneumonitis or bronchospasm.[12] The role for diagnostic imaging in reflux is threefold: to assess for anatomic abnormalities that may predispose to reflux, quantify the severity, and assess for complications of reflux, such as strictures, esophagitis, and evidence of aspiration.

Sonography has been employed in Europe as a means of quantifying the severity of reflux.[12—14] The patient is scanned in the supine position with a curved 5-MHz transducer near the midline oriented in an oblique longitudinal scan plane over the distal thoracic esophagus and gastroesophageal junction.[13] The appearance of reflux depends on the ingested substance. Formula and milk are somewhat echogenic, while water and juice are nearly anechoic when seen filling the esophagus during a reflux episode. An advantage of sonography over pH probe monitoring is the detection of nonacid reflux.[13] However, because of technical considerations such as the relatively short duration of monitoring, this technique has not been embraced in the United States.

Intestinal Malrotation

Intestinal malrotation results from abnormal intestinal rotation and mesenteric fixation during embryologic development and causes a narrowed mesenteric pedicle and abnormally positioned duodenojejunal junction.[1, 15] The overall incidence of malrotation is unknown, as some individuals may be asymptomatic or the condition may not be detected until adulthood. Two-thirds of infants with symptomatic malrotation present in the first month of life with vomiting, typically bilious.[16] The two primary causes of vomiting in infants with malrotation are midgut volvulus and obstructing Ladd bands. In midgut volvulus, the small bowel twists around the superior mesenteric vasculature, resulting in a proximal bowel obstruction. The volvulus can result in vascular compromise to the small bowel as well. Ladd bands are peritoneal bands of tissue that arise secondary to abnormal mesenteric fixation.[16] They classically cross the second or third portion of the duodenum, resulting in vary-

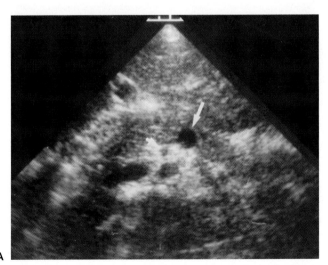

A

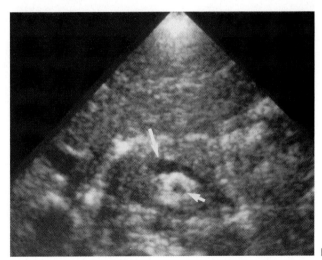

B

Figure 38–5 Malrotation. **A:** Transverse sonogram in the upper abdomen shows the superior mesenteric vein (**large arrow**) to the left of the superior mesenteric artery (**small arrow**), raising concern for malrotation. **B:** The normal anatomic relationship of the superior mesenteric artery and vein is seen in another patient. Reprinted with permission from Midgut malrotation by BA Siegel, AV Proto, eds. **Pediatric Disease** (Fourth series). **Test and Syllabus**. Reston, Virginia: American College of Radiology, 1993, p. 376—404.

ing degrees of obstruction. Infants with malrotation complicated by volvulus or Ladd bands are often asymptomatic except for bilious vomiting. The presence of peritoneal signs or hemodynamic instability suggests bowel infarction, and the infant requires urgent laparotomy.[1]

At sonography, the presence of malrotation may be inferred on the basis of an abnormal orientation of the superior mesenteric artery and vein (**Fig. 38–5**).[15,17,18] Care must be taken to scan directly anteriorly over these vessels in the transverse imaging plane. Normally, the superior mesenteric vein is to the right of the superior mesenteric artery, but with malrotation, the orientation is reversed. This sign is neither sufficiently sensitive nor specific to assess for malrotation, and an upper gastrointestinal series is necessary to confirm the presence or absence of malrotation. One small series demonstrated only a 67% sensitivity for this sign in patients with surgically proven malrotation.[17]

Findings secondary to midgut volvulus or obstructing Ladd bands may also be encountered at sonography of the vomiting neonate. Proximal duodenal obstruction may be seen, with a fluid-filled duodenum tapering into a beaked terminus at the point of obstruction (**Fig. 38–6**).[19] The whirlpool sign of intestine and mesentery coiling about the narrowed mesenteric root may be seen (**Fig. 38–7**).[16] In some patients, a nondescript mass may be present in the central abdomen; this mass represents the volved, and possibly ischemic bowel.[20] Coiling of the superior mesenteric vein about the artery may also be visible (**Fig. 38–8**). This finding is more evident with color Doppler interrogation. The presence of bowel wall thickening or ascites suggests vascular compromise of the small intestine.

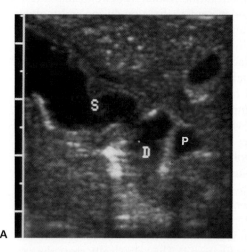
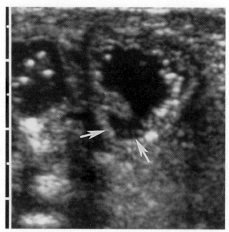

A   B

Figure 38–6   Malrotation with obstructing Ladd band. **A:** Transverse scan of the upper abdomen in a patient with situs inversus shows fluid distension of the stomach (S) and duodenum (D), as well as a preduodenal portal vein (P). **B:** More caudally in the abdomen, the distal duodenum tapers at the site of the obstructing Ladd band (**arrows**). Reprinted with permission from **Pediatric Sonography** by MJ Siegel. New York: Raven Press, 1995, p. 263—300.

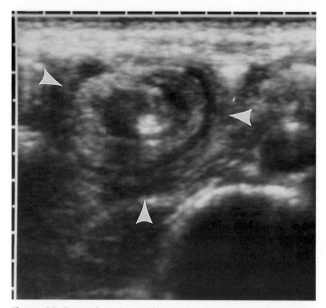

Figure 38–7   Malrotation with volvulus. Transverse sonogram of the mid-abdomen shows the "whirlpool" sign, concentric layered rings of mesentery and bowel forming a complex mass (**arrowheads**) in this patient with midgut volvulus. (Case courtesy of Dr. Marilyn J. Siegel, Mallinckrodt Institute of Radiology, St. Louis.)

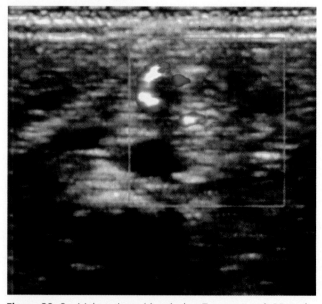

Figure 38–8   Malrotation with volvulus. Transverse color Doppler sonogram of the mid-abdomen reveals a poorly defined mass with the superior mesenteric vein coiling about the superior mesenteric artery, consistent with midgut volvulus.

Congenital Intrinsic Duodenal Obstruction

Patients with congenital duodenal obstruction typically present with vomiting. The site of obstruction is often in the periampullary region, and the vomiting is bilious if the obstruction is distal to the level of the ampulla of Vater.[1] Congenital duodenal obstruction is associated with Down's syndrome. The three major forms of congenital duodenal obstruction — duodenal atresia, stenosis and web, represent a spectrum of embryologic malformation. Duodenal atresia is uncommon, occurring in one in 8000 births.[1] This may be recognized in utero at prenatal sonography, manifesting as polyhydramnios as well as a double bubble sign. The double-bubble sign is caused by a fluid-filled, distended stomach and proximal duodenum. Infants with duodenal atresia present within hours of birth with vomiting, often bilious. Duodenal atresia may be accompanied by an annular pancreas.[1, 16] Neonates with complete duodenal obstruction secondary to duodenal atresia rarely undergo sonography as the diagnosis can almost always be made with conventional radiographs.[16] A sonogram demonstrating duodenal atresia is shown in Fig. 38–9.

Duodenal stenosis is a relatively uncommon congenital obstruction. The time to clinical presentation is dependent upon the degree of stenosis and obstruction. A duodenal web, like duodenal stenosis, may not present in the immediate postpartum period, depending on the size of the aperture in the web.[21] Only one-third of patients with duodenal web present in the first month of life. A thin diaphragm containing a small hole causes the obstruction. The diaphragm or web prolapses distally, yielding the characteristic windsock deformity seen at ultrasound and upper gastrointestinal examination.[21, 22]

In children with a duodenal web, a dilated proximal duodenum may be seen at sonography. A thin, echogenic web is outlined at the junction between the dilated, fluid-filled proximal duodenum and the distal collapsed duodenum (**Fig. 38–10**).[22] An upper gastrointestinal series is useful to confirm the diagnosis.

Enteric Duplication Cyst

Enteric duplication cysts are not common, but can occur anywhere in the gastrointestinal tract. Duplication cysts occur as a result of incomplete recanalization of the foregut during embryologic development.[1] Less than 4% of duplication cysts occur in the gastroduodenal region, where they often result in obstruction and vomiting.[1] Most gastroduodenal duplication cysts are diagnosed in the first year of life, with roughly one-third diagnosed in the newborn period. More distal duplications typically present with a mass or less often with obstruction secondary to volvulus or intussusception.[23]

Duplication cysts have a characteristic sonographic appearance. They are typically a unilocular, cystic mass with a wall comprising an inner echogenic layer repre-

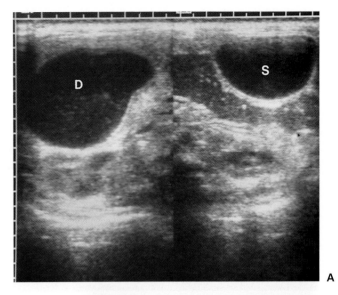

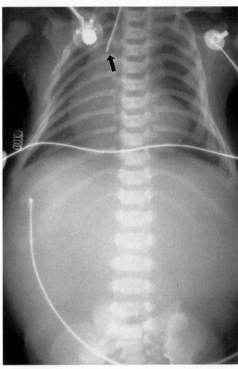

Figure 38–9 Duodenal atresia. **A:** Transverse sonogram of the upper abdomen demonstrates the dilated, fluid-filled stomach (S) and duodenum (D). Sonography was useful in this case, as the abdomen was gasless secondary to esophageal atresia without tracheoesophageal fistula. **B:** Conventional radiograph of the chest and abdomen shows the gasless abdomen and the nasogastric tube (**arrow**) in the esophageal pouch. (Case courtesy of Dr. Marilyn J. Siegel, Mallinckrodt Institute of Radiology, St. Louis.)

senting the mucosal lining and an outer hypoechoic layer of smooth muscle (**Fig. 38–11**).[23] This finding has been reported to be diagnostic of duplication cysts.[24] There is a potential artifactual pitfall that may mimic a double-layered wall. This artifact occurs only in the portion of the cystic mass that is deepest in the scan field and is seen only transiently, disappearing with slight movement of the transducer.[24]

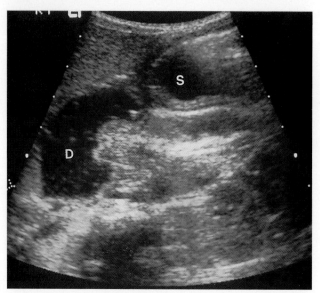

A

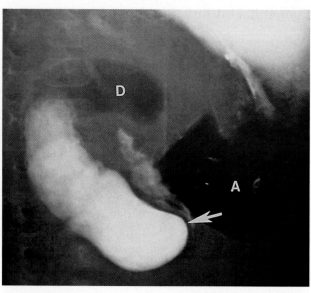

B

Figure 38–10 Duodenal web. **A:** Transverse sonogram of the upper abdomen reveals dilatation of the proximal duodenum (D), ending in a rounded pouch. The fluid-distended stomach (S) is also visible. **B:** Follow-up upper gastrointestinal series (B) confirmed the diagnosis of a duodenal web (**arrow**) causing partial obstruction of the duodenum. The gas-filled duodenal bulb (D) and gastric antrum (A) are identified.

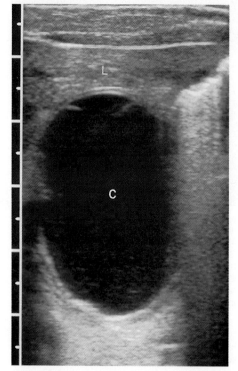

Figure 38–11 Enteric duplication cyst. Transverse sonogram of the upper abdomen in a 2-week-old infant with vomiting shows a cystic mass (C) caudal to the liver (L). The wall of the cystic mass has characteristic features of an enteric duplication cyst, with an inner echogenic layer (mucosa) and an outer hypoechoic layer (muscularis). The gallbladder and biliary tree were unremarkable.

Duodenal Trauma

There are 2.4 million cases of child abuse each year in the United States, and it is the most common cause of death in children from 6 to12 months of age.[1] With blunt trauma to the abdomen, both solid and hollow intestinal viscera are at risk for injury. The mechanism of injury is typically a blow with a closed fist or a kick. With blunt trauma, compression of the intestines over the spine can result in injuries to the bowel wall and mesentery ranging from mural hematoma to frank intestinal perforation. Duodenal hematoma in an infant or young child, in the absence of an appropriate history, is highly suggestive of nonaccidental trauma.[1] Infants and children with intestinal perforation may present with peritonitis or shock, but children with duodenal hematoma may present with vomiting and pain. The obstruction may not be clinically evident for 2 (or more) days after the injury, as the hematoma expands as it breaks down.

At sonography, the hematoma appears as a complex, hyperechoic or hypoechoic mass, which may contain septations or areas of liquefaction, depending on the age of the hematoma.[7] If it is large enough to cause obstructive symptoms, the stomach and proximal duodenum may be distended with fluid. Ultrasonography may be useful for follow-up to assess the size of the hematoma, as well as to monitor the patient for complications due to injuries of adjacent organs, particularly the pancreas.

Extraintestinal Causes of Vomiting

Vomiting may be a symptom of disease involving most organ systems in infancy. An infant with a urinary tract infection, otitis media, or pneumonia may present with vomiting. Vomiting is also caused by increased intracranial pressure, associated with central nervous system neoplasms and hydrocephalus.

Other Differential Considerations

Although infants with more distal causes of obstruction tend to present with abdominal distention, vomiting may also be present. Causes of distal obstruction in neonates include intestinal atresia, Hirschsprung disease, meconium ileus, and meconium plug syndrome.[16] Necrotizing enterocolitis, a potentially lethal condition seen in premature infants as well as in infants with congenital heart disease, may also cause vomiting. Later in infancy, intussusception is more commonly encountered and can result in vomiting. Sonograms of infants with a distal intestinal obstruction show multiple dilated loops of fluid-filled bowel throughout the abdomen. Determining the exact cause of obstruction is often not possible and better evaluated with conventional radiographs and a contrast enema. In meconium ileus, an echogenic mass representing the obstructing meconium may be seen at sonography in addition to dilated bowel loops.[25]

Although quite rare, other potential causes of projectile vomiting in an infant include congenital gastric outlet obstruction secondary to pyloric atresia or antral web, as well as congenital microgastria.[1, 7, 16, 26] Infants with these conditions present with feeding intolerance and nonbilious vomiting shortly after birth. Antral and pyloric webs may have a more delayed presentation, again depending on the degree of obstruction. Sonographic findings include a fluid-distended, hyperperistaltic stomach. Identification of an antral web at sonography is difficult and better assessed with an upper gastrointestinal series. Mesenchymal tumors of the stomach, including leiomyoma, leiomyosarcoma, and lipoma may cause vomiting in an infant secondary to obstruction but are extremely rare. The sonographic appearance of mesenchymal tumors is quite variable, ranging from a well-defined, echogenic lipoma to the more heterogeneous and poorly marginated leiomyosarcoma.[7, 16] An example of a gastric polyp is shown in Fig. 38–12.

Focal foveolar hyperplasia is a mucosal polypoid overgrowth that can result in gastric outlet obstruction and projectile vomiting. This condition typically occurs in adults but has been reported in children. It is believed to be secondary to mucosal hyperregeneration at a site of continuing injury.[27] The sonographic appearance is characterized by pronounced thickening of the echo-

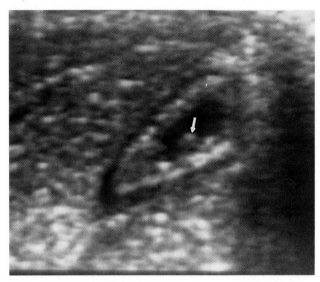

Figure 38–12 Gastric polyp. Oblique sonogram of the distal antrum demonstrates a small gastric polyp (**arrow**) arising from the antral mucosa. (Case courtesy of Dr. Marilyn J. Siegel, Mallinckrodt Institute of Radiology, St. Louis.)

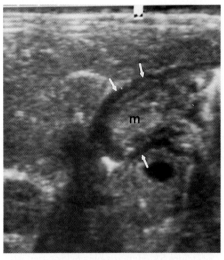

Figure 38–13 Focal foveolar hyperplasia. Longitudinal sonogram of the pyloric region demonstrates thickening of the echogenic mucosa (m), surrounded by a thin, normal muscularis (**arrows**). (Case courtesy of Dr. Marilyn J. Siegel, Mallinckrodt Institute of Radiology, St. Louis.)

genic mucosa in the antropyloric region (**Fig. 38–13**).[27] The surrounding muscular layer is of normal thickness, in contradistinction with pyloric stenosis. Mucosal hypertrophy in the distal antrum can also be caused by prostaglandin E.[28] Prostaglandin E is administered to newborn infants with some types of congenital heart disease, to maintain patency of the ductus arteriosus. Infants receiving prostaglandin E can develop projectile vomiting secondary to gastric outlet obstruction from the mucosal hypertrophy.[28] The condition is reversible with cessation of prostaglandin E therapy.

Benefits of Ultrasonography

The diagnostic accuracy of sonography in the evaluation of the vomiting infant has been most thoroughly investigated in patients with hypertrophic pyloric stenosis. Using a muscle thickness of 3 mm and a pyloric channel length of 17 mm as a threshold, both the sensitivity and specificity of ultrasound is greater than 98%.[4, 8] False-negative examinations may occur early in the course of the disease. In these infants, repeating the examination in a few days often yields a definitive diagnosis. False-positive results can be the result of improper scanning (e.g., tangentially scanning through the distal antrum and pylorus, creating pseudothickening of the muscle).[11] The cost-effectiveness of ultrasonography in the diagnosis of pyloric stenosis is debated. When reserved for infants with a clinical presentation consistent with hypertrophic pyloric stenosis, but without a palpable olive, sonography is an effective and inexpensive modality. In infants without a classic clinical presentation, those with bilious vomiting or in those who would require an upper gastrointestinal series if the sonogram were negative, sonography becomes less cost-effective.

References

1. Reyna TM, Reyna PA. Gastroduodenal disorders associated with emesis in infants. *Semin Pediatr Surg* 1995;4:190—197.
2. Van der Schouw YT, van der Velden MTW, Hitge-Boetes C, et al. Diagnosis of hypertrophic pyloric stenosis: value of sonography when used in conjunction with clinical findings and laboratory data. *Am J Roentgenol* 1994;163:905—909.
3. Finkelstein MS, Mandell GA, Tarbell KV. Hypertrophic pyloric stenosis: volumetric measurement of nasogastric aspirate to determine the imaging modality. *Radiology* 1990;177:759—761.
4. Neilson D, Hollman AS. The ultrasonic diagnosis of infantile hypertrophic pyloric stenosis: technique and accuracy. *Clin Radiol* 1994;49:246—247.
5. Deluca SA. Hypertrophic pyloric stenosis. *Am Fam Physician* 1993;47(8):1771—1773.
6. Vanderwinden J-M, Mailleux P, Schiffmann SN, et al. Nitric oxide synthase activity in infantile hypertrophic pyloric stenosis. *N Engl J Med* 1992;327:511—515.
7. Siegel MJ. Gastrointestinal tract. In Siegel MJ, ed: *Pediatric Sonography*. New York: Raven Press, 1995, p. 263—300.
8. Blumhagen JD, Maclin L, Krauter D, et al. Sonographic diagnosis of hypertrophic pyloric stenosis. *Am J Roentgenol* 1988;150:1367—1370.
9. Atwell JD, Levick P. Congenital hypertrophic pyloric stenosis and associated anomalies in the genitourinary tract. *J Pediatr Surg* 1981;16:1029—1035.
10. Fernbach SK, Morello FP. Renal abnormalities in children with hypertrophic pyloric stenosis—fact or fallacy? *Pediatr Radiol* 1993;23:286—288.
11. Swischuk LE, Hayden CK, Stansbury SD. Sonographic pitfalls in imaging of the antropyloric region in infants. *Radiographics* 1989;9:437—447.
12. Westra SJ, Derkx HHF, Taminiau JAJM. Symptomatic gastroesophageal reflux: diagnosis with ultrasound. *J Pediatr Gastroenterol Nutr* 1994;19:58—64.
13. Gomes H, Menanteau B. Gastro-esophageal reflux: comparative study between sonography and pH monitoring. *Pediatr Radiol* 1991;21:168—174.
14. Gomes H, Lallemand A, Lallemand P. Ultrasound of the gastroesophageal junction. *Pediatr Radiol* 1993;23:94—99.
15. Weinberger E, Winters WD, Liddell RM, et al. Sonographic diagnosis of intestinal malrotation in infants: importance of the relative positions of the superior mesenteric vein and artery. *Am J Roentgenol* 1992;159:825—828.
16. McAlister WH, Kronemer KA. Emergency gastrointestinal radiology of the newborn. *Radiol Clin North Am* 1996;34:819—844.
17. Zerin JM, DiPietro MA. Superior mesenteric vascular anatomy at US in patients with surgically proved malrotation of the midgut. *Radiology* 1992;183:693—694.
18. Kaminsky CK, Cleveland RH. Midgut malrotation. In Siegel BA, Proto AV, eds. *Pediatric Disease* (Fourth series). *Test and Syllabus*, Reston, VA: American College of Radiology, 1993, p. 376—404.
19. Hayden CK, Boulden TF, Swischuk LE, et al. Sonographic demonstration of duodenal obstruction with midgut volvulus. *Am J Roentgenol* 1984;143:9—10.
20. Pracos JP, Sann L, Genin G, et al. Ultrasound diagnosis of midgut volvulus: the "whirlpool" sign. *Pediatr Radiol* 1992;22:18—20.
21. Brown RA, Millar AJW, Linegar A, et al. Fenestrated duodenal membranes: an analysis of symptoms, signs, diagnosis, and treatment. *J Pediatr Surg* 1994;29:429—432.
22. Cremin BJ, Solomon DJ. Ultrasonic diagnosis of duodenal diaphragm. *Pediatr Radiol* 1987;17:489—490.
23. McAlister WH, Siegel MJ. Pediatric radiology case of the day. Duodenal duplication. *Am J Roentgenol* 1989;152:1328—1329.
24. Barr LL, Hayden CK, Stansbury SD, et al. Enteric duplication cysts in children: are their ultrasonographic wall characteristics diagnostic? *Pediatr Radiol* 1990;20:326—328.
25. Barki Y, Bar-Ziv J. Meconium ileus: ultrasonic diagnosis of intraluminal inspissated meconium. *J Clin Ultrasound* 1985;13:509—512.
26. Aintablian NH, Slim MS, Antoun BW. Congenital microgastria: case report and review of the literature. *Pediatr Surg Int* 1987;2:307—310.
27. McAlister WH, Katz ME, Perlman JM, et al. Sonography of focal foveolar hyperplasia causing gastric obstruction in an infant. *Pediatr Radiol* 1988;18:79—81.
28. Peled N, Dagan O, Babyn P, et al. Gastric-outlet obstruction induced by prostaglandin therapy in neonates. *N Engl J Med* 1992;327:505—510.

39 Sonography of Urinary Tract Infections in Children

Harriet J. Paltiel

Epidemiology

Urinary tract infection (UTI) is a common problem in childhood as well as an important cause of morbidity. Chronic or recurrent UTI can ultimately result in hypertension and renal failure, particularly when associated with obstructive uropathy or vesicoureteral reflux (VUR). Most UTIs are bacterial in origin. Diagnosis is made by documenting significant bacteriuria, defined as greater than 100,000 colony-forming units/mm^3 of a single organism, in one or more clean-voided specimens of urine. When the urine is obtained by suprapubic puncture or bladder catheterization, less than 100,000 colony-forming units/mm^3 can be considered significant.[1–3]

UTI in children can be asymptomatic or symptomatic. Symptomatic infections may be confined to the urethra (urethritis) or bladder (cystitis), or may involve the ureter (ureteritis), the collecting system (pyelitis), or renal parenchyma (pyelonephritis).

The prevalence of asymptomatic and symptomatic bacteriuria in children is determined by the age and sex of the patient, and by the method of diagnosis. The incidence of neonatal bacteriuria has been reported as ranging from 1% to 1.4%,[4–6] with a male-to-female ratio of between 2.8 and 5.4:1.[7,8] The sex ratio for bacteriuria in pre-school and school-age children is reversed from that seen in infancy, ranging from 0.7% to 1.9% of girls, and 0.2% to 0.4% of boys.[9–13] In a study of children living in Goteborg, Sweden published in 1974, Winberg et al. estimated that the aggregate risk for symptomatic UTI up to the age of 11 years was at least 3% for girls and 1.1% for boys.[14] In a more recent report from the same city, the prevalence of culture-documented, symptomatic UTIs in children up to the age of 7 years was higher than the previous estimate, with 8.4% of girls and 1.7% of boys affected.[15]

The majority of UTIs are caused by the family of gram-negative, aerobic bacilli known as Enterobacteriaceae that includes *Escherichia, Klebsiella, Enterobacter, Citrobacter, Proteus, Providencia, Morganella, Serratia,* and *Salmonella* species. Of these, *Escherichia coli* is by far the most frequently isolated organism, being responsible for approximately 80% of UTIs. *Pseudomonas* is a gram-negative, aerobic bacillus unrelated to the Enterobacteriaceae that may be isolated from the urine of patients with impaired immunologic defense mechanisms. The most common gram-positive organisms found in UTIs are *Staphylococcus* and *Enterococcus*. Gram-negative organisms usually infect the urinary tract by ascent from the perineum, while gram-positive organisms often reach the kidney hematogenously. Ascending infection occurs in approximately 97% of cases.

The true incidence of UTI is unknown because of the nonspecificity or absence of symptoms in young children. Poor feeding, failure to thrive, irritability, vomiting, or diarrhea may be the only signs indicative of an underlying problem. Fever occurs in most infants with symptomatic UTIs, but is often absent in neonates.[14] Once children develop speech and are toilet trained, symptoms of UTI are more readily detected. Disturbances of micturition often signal lower-tract UTI.[16] Symptoms and signs of lower urinary tract infection include dysuria, frequency, and cloudy, foul-smelling urine. Pyelonephritis often results in an acute, febrile illness associated with malaise, chills, vomiting, and flank pain. An infant with urosepsis may be critically ill, whereas in young children with less severe symptoms, it may be difficult to distinguish cystitis from pyelonephritis solely on the basis of clinical presentation.

Pathogenesis

Bacterial virulence

UTI occurs when bacterial virulence factors overwhelm host resistance.[17–19] Some of the most important bacterial virulence factors include adherence to uroepithelial cells, large amounts of K-antigen in the bacterial capsule, production of hemolysin and colicin, the ability to incorporate iron, and resistance to serum bacteriocidal activity.

Bacterial adherence is an essential step in the initiation of UTI. Uropathogenic bacteria attach both to specific receptor sites on the uroepithelium and in a nonspecific fashion by electrostatic hydrophobic means. As a consequence of this attachment, virulent bacteria may ascend into the upper urinary tract even in the absence of VUR or other structural abnormalities. Adhesion is mediated by antigens located on the bacterial cell surface known as pili or fimbriae. Clinical and experimental studies have shown that pyelonephritogenic *E. coli* often possess fimbriae that agglutinate erythrocytes of the P1 blood group. These pili are termed *P-fimbriae*. P-fimbriae attach to a specific carbohydrate receptor contained within the P blood group antigen, which is also present on human uroepithelial cells.[20, 21]

K-antigen is a capsular polysaccharide that has been shown to enhance the persistence of bacteria in the kidneys of experimental mice and shield bacteria from phagocytosis and complement lysis.[22, 23] It is isolated more often in children with pyelonephritis than in children with cystitis, asymptomatic bacteriuria, or healthy controls.[24] Hemolysins are cytotoxic proteins that damage renal tubular cells *in vitro*. Hemolytic strains of *E. coli* produce severe pyelonephritis in mice. Colicin is a protein produced by pyelonephritogenic bacteria that kills other bacteria in the vicinity. The colicin plasmid is believed to encode for an iron uptake system that promotes the survival and pathogenicity of colicin-producing organisms.[25] Most bacteria require iron for metabolism and optimal growth. Epidemiological studies have shown that the ability to bind iron is associated with enhanced virulence.[26, 27]

Host factors

Many host resistance factors protect the urinary tract from infection, including the presence of antibodies, male sex, a low density of bacterial receptor sites on host epithelial cells, lack of perineal colonization by virulent fecal bacteria, and unimpeded flow of urine.

Immunity to UTI is boosted in the neonatal period by the maternal transmission of antibodies through breastfeeding. The short urethra in girls appears to be the most obvious explanation for the increased relative incidence of UTIs in girls compared with boys, beyond the first year of life. There is a ten to 20-fold increase risk of UTIs in uncircumcised male infants in the first year of life, which is believed to be due to colonization of the prepuce by uropathogenic bacteria.[28—30]

Increased adherence of uropathogenic bacteria to periurethral and uroepithelial cells has been demonstrated in children prone to UTIs, implying a difference in host receptor affinity or density that influences the child's susceptibility to infection.[31, 32]

Anatomic/functional Abnormalities

Frequent and complete bladder emptying eliminates bacteria and prevents UTI. The predisposition to recurrent UTIs and VUR in children with dysfunctional voiding is related to overdistention from infrequent voiding, residual volume due to inadequate emptying, and increased intravesical pressure caused by uninhibited bladder contractions. Development of normal voiding pat-

terns in these children reduces the incidence of recurrent UTIs.[33, 34] A correlation had also been shown between constipation and recurrent UTIs in children.[35, 36] Improvement in bowel habits often results in a decrease in the incidence of recurrent UTIs.

Resistance to bacterial infection may be compromised by impedance to the unidirectional flow of urine out of the urinary tract, as may occur with VUR, obstruction, or both. Obstruction can occur at any site within the urinary tract. Children with obstruction of the distal end of the ureter [either primary ureterovesical junction (UVJ) obstruction or ectopic ureterocele] or the urethra (posterior urethral valves) often present with infection. Although the most common site of obstruction of the pediatric urinary tract occurs at the ureteropelvic junction (UPJ), children with this condition do not usually present with UTI.

Vesicoureteral Reflux

VUR is an abnormality that is frequently associated with UTI. With VUR, urine flows in a retrograde fashion into the ureter. VUR is almost always a primary phenomenon due to incompetence of the ureterovesical junction (UVJ) and is not secondary to infection or obstruction.[37, 38] VUR is especially common in neonates and infants. It occurs in families,[39] is less common in black children,[40, 41] and decreases in severity or resolves as the child gets older. Resolution is less likely to occur if the degree of VUR is severe, or is associated with other abnormalities such as voiding dysfunction.

VUR provides a pathway for bacteria within the bladder to reach the kidney. Due to the phenomenon of "aberrant micturition," part of the urine expelled from the bladder refluxes up the ureter and flows back into the bladder. The resulting stagnation of urine encourages bacterial overgrowth.[42] Secondary VUR is usually due either to an abnormality of micturition, such as dysfunctional voiding, a neurogenic bladder abnormality, or to the presence of a diverticulum at the UVJ.[34, 43] When VUR is present, it is the most significant host factor in the etiology of childhood pyelonephritis. The risk for acute pyelonephritis and subsequent renal scarring is related to the severity of VUR.[44, 45]

Pyelonephritis may result in the destruction of nephrons and their replacement by fibrous tissue. Once lost, these renal units are never regenerated or replaced. The destruction of renal parenchyma is directly proportional to the severity and frequency of episodes of infection. The increased burden placed on the remaining nephrons is thought to result in hyperfiltration injury and glomerulosclerosis.[46—48] The term *reflux nephropathy* is used to describe both the acute damage to the kidney as well as the long-term sequelae caused by reflux of infected urine.[49] Chronic pyelonephritis refers to the process of fibrosis and scar formation that follows bacterial infection.[50] The medulla is initially affected, but eventually the full thickness of renal parenchyma is involved. Scars are focal and frequently polar in location.

When VUR and ipsilateral obstruction coexist, infection is much more common and its clinical presentation and renal sequelae tend to be more severe. This is presumably due to the fact that pressure in the collecting system is elevated and drainage of infected urine is impeded.[51]

Clinical Outcome

Bacteria in the urinary tract may occur in an asymptomatic, healthy child or in association with an acute, severe febrile illness. The presence of bacteria requires prompt and adequate treatment because the sequelae of untreated infection or inadequate therapy are hypertension and/or chronic renal failure.

The significance of asymptomatic or covert bacteriuria is poorly understood. While some authorities believe such asymptomatic children should be treated, others have postulated that the bacteria may, in fact, be nonpathogenic and by blocking epithelial receptor sites may actually protect the patient from potentially more virulent organisms.[52, 53]

Diagnostic Workup

Nonimaging Tests

Evaluation of children with UTI begins with a history of voiding and bowel habits in those who are toilet trained. Family history should also be obtained, as heredity appears to be a factor in an individual's predisposition to bacteriuria and VUR.[39, 54] Physical examination includes abdominal palpation to detect bladder distention, bowel distention from fecal impaction, and flank masses. Circumcision status is important in male children because of the increased risk of UTIs in uncircumcised boys. Abnormal findings in girls include the presence of labial adhesions or vulvovaginitis, both of which may predispose to perineal colonization by bacteria.

In children with a significant history of voiding dysfunction associated with encopresis or constipation, an evaluation of perineal sensation, lower extremity reflexes, and an examination of the lower back for sacral dimpling or cutaneous abnormalities suggestive of underlying spinal abnormalities should be performed. Rectal examination for fecal impaction is indicated if there is a history of encopresis or severe constipation.

UTI can be diagnosed reliably only by urine culture. Thus, specimens for urine culture should be obtained in all patients in whom the clinical index of suspicion is high. In children who are not toilet trained, an initial urine specimen is often obtained by placing a collection bag on the perineum. Although this technique has been correctly criticized for producing a high rate of contaminated specimens, the method is reliable when the culture is negative. Contamination is directly related to the length of time the bag remains on the perineum. Confirmation of all positive urine specimens obtained in this fashion is advisable prior to treatment. Bladder catheterization or suprapubic aspiration should be performed whenever the clinical situation dictates immediate treatment or confirmation of a positive urine bag specimen. In older children who are toilet trained, significant bacteriuria in a single properly collected midstream, clean-catch urine specimen is reliable for diagnostic purposes.[55]

Imaging Tests Other than Ultrasonography

In most pediatric medical centers, children with UTI are treated as though they had pyelonephritis. This approach is due to the fact that, at present, no single imaging technique can reliably distinguish in all cases between a UTI limited to the bladder from one that involves the kidney, with its attendant risks of renal scarring, hypertension, and renal insufficiency. The outcome of this therapeutic approach has been successful in that renal scarring in patients with recurrent UTIs is very uncommon. Among patients treated according to current guidelines, recurrent chronic pyelonephritis accounts for less than 2% of end-stage renal disease among North American children.[56]

The purpose of imaging evaluation in the setting of UTI is to detect underlying anatomical or physiologic abnormalities that may predispose the child to infection, to identify renal structural damage, and to provide a baseline for subsequent evaluation of renal growth. It is widely agreed that all boys should be investigated after their first UTI. In girls, it has been recommended in the past that evaluation should only be done following a second UTI. However, significant renal scarring can occur after a single UTI.[57–62] The incidence of renal scarring is higher in children with VUR and recurrent UTI compared to those with VUR who have had only one infection.[61, 63] The signs and symptoms of UTI in infants and toddlers are often nonspecific, so that it may be impossible to ascertain whether or not a particular infection actually represents the first episode.[14] Therefore, in many centers, including our own, an imaging evaluation is performed in all boys and in all girls under 5 years of age who present after their first documented UTI.

Recommendations for particular radiologic studies in children with culture-documented UTI are, to a certain extent, based on the availability of various imaging modalities and the experience and expertise of the radiologist. Most children are not imaged during the acute phase of a UTI, although children hospitalized for febrile infections may be screened with ultrasonography (US) before discharge. US is the initial examination of choice for imaging children with UTI. The role of US is to rule out urinary tract obstruction. Voiding cystourethrography (VCUG) by bladder catheterization is also performed to detect the presence of VUR. VCUG is generally reserved for children under five years of age with their first documented UTI and for older children with febrile UTI or recurrent infections. Some radiologists prefer a conventional, fluoroscopically monitored VCUG, whereas others prefer nuclear cystography. Conventional contrast VCUG allows more precise determination of the severity of VUR and assessment of bladder and urethral anatomy. Nuclear cystography is associated with reduced gonadal radiation and permits continuous monitoring throughout the study, which increases its sensitivity to transient VUR.[64] Nuclear cystography is generally accepted to be the best examination for following children with known reflux, for documenting the result of antireflux surgery, and for screening children whose siblings have reflux.[65, 66] No further imaging is necessary in most cases if the cystogram and US of the kidneys and bladder are normal.

Additional imaging evaluation of the upper urinary tract in children with UTI varies from institution to institution. Planar scintigraphy or single photon emission computed tomography (SPECT) of the renal parenchyma with either technetium-(Tc) 99m-labeled dimercaptosuccinic acid (DMSA) or glucoheptonate (GH) have been used to detect acute pyelonephritis and renal scarring.[67] Tc-99m DMSA binds to the proximal renal tubules and provides excellent images of the parenchyma. Tc-99m GH also binds to tubular epithelial cells, but a large amount is filtered, allowing evaluation of the pelvicaliceal system, ureters, and bladder on early images, as well as the renal cortex on delayed images. Although both agents can show cortical involvement, Tc-99m DMSA is preferred over Tc-99m GH because of a lower gonadal dose. Renal cortical scanning may be of particular value when the diagnosis of pyelonephritis is unclear based on clinical and laboratory findings alone. For instance, neonates and young infants may present with nonspecific signs and symptoms. Urine cultures may not have been obtained in an appropriate fashion or before antibiotic treatment. Another example is of children with myelodysplasia who are managed by clean intermittent catheterization, where chronic asymptomatic bacteriuria is common. Thus, the diagnostic significance of a positive urine culture is limited when these patients present with unexplained fever.[65, 68]

When hydronephrosis and/or hydroureter are depicted by US and VUR is absent, a quantitative assessment of renal function and drainage of the dilated collecting system and ureter may be obtained with diuretic renography using either Tc-99m-labeled diethylenetriamine-pentaacetic acid (DTPA) or mercaptoacetyltriglycine (MAG-3).[69, 70] In most instances, nonobstructive dilatation can be reliably differentiated from true obstruction. Excretory urography (EU) has been largely sup-

planted by scintigraphic studies in the evaluation of acute pyelonephritis. EU depicts anatomy extremely well but provides only qualitative estimates of function. Computed tomography (CT) is not indicated in the child with uncomplicated UTI, but it may be of value in selected patients[71, 72] to determine the extent of the inflammatory process and the presence of abscess, ureteral or parenchymal calcifications, and gas. Urinary obstruction also can be confirmed.

The use of magnetic resonance imaging (MRI) has received little attention in the literature, to date. Lonergan et al. compared gadolinium-enhanced inversion-recovery MRI with renal cortical scintigraphy in the diagnosis of pyelonephritis in 37 children.[73] MRI detected more abnormalities than did renal cortical scintigraphy and had superior interobserver agreement.

Sonographic Imaging

The sonographic examination of the pediatric urinary tract includes images of the kidneys, ureters (if visible), and urinary bladder. The child may be given fluids to drink and cooperative children are asked not to void for several hours before the study. In a young child who is not toilet trained, the bladder must be checked first and often during the course of the examination, as it may fill and empty suddenly. The highest frequency transducer that will penetrate the area to be studied is used. For infants, 7- to 10-MHz transducers are optimal, while in children, 5-MHz transducers are usually employed. Routine examination includes longitudinal and transverse images of the kidneys and bladder. Scans are performed with the patient in both supine and prone positions. Supine images are best obtained with sector or convex transducers that can be positioned between the ribs, while prone images are performed with a convex or linear transducer. Images are recorded digitally or on hard-copy film.

Coronal images are obtained with the patient supine. The liver and spleen act as acoustic windows, thus permitting optimal visualization of the upper renal poles and comparison of the echogenicity of the renal parenchyma with that of the adjacent liver and spleen. Sagittal views obtained with the child prone are used to optimize visualization of the lower renal poles. Images of the bladder are obtained with the child supine and are optimally performed when the bladder is moderately distended, so that abnormalities such as bladder wall thickening can be appreciated but the patient is not uncomfortable. The proximal ureters are evaluated at the level of the renal pelvis as well as distally at the level of the bladder to detect dilatation and ureteroceles. Postvoid images of the kidneys and bladder are useful in children with hydronephrosis, hydroureter, and/or neurogenic bladder dysfunction to determine the effect of bladder distension on the degree of hydronephrosis.

Renal length measurements should be compared standards for patient age, height, weight, or body surface area.[74,75] Of interest are the recent papers by Carrico et al. and De Sanctis et al. in which sonographic measurements made with patients lying supine or in contralateral decubitus positions yielded slightly higher values than those made with the patient prone.[76,77]

Conventional color and pulsed Doppler US, as well as power Doppler imaging, are used in evaluating renal perfusion. Doppler settings are adjusted for depiction of slow flow by using the highest possible transducer frequency, the lowest wall filter and the lowest pulse repetition frequency and by restricting the color Doppler area of interest. A small sample volume and the lowest possible beam-to-vessel angle are used.

Cystitis

Acute cystitis in children is rarely associated with significant long-term morbidity. The recurrence rate of lower urinary tract UTI is relatively high.[78] Many of the children with recurrent UTI suffer from dysfunctional voiding. When inflamed, the bladder wall becomes thickened and irregular (**Fig. 39–1**). Blood clot or echogenic debris may be seen within the bladder lumen.[79,80]

Acute Pyelonephritis

The acutely infected kidney often appears normal on sonography.[81,82] However, in severe infections, gray-scale US can demonstrate diffuse renal enlargement; loss of corticomedullary differentiation; submucosal edema of the renal pelvis and/or ureter; and calyceal, pelvic, and/or ureteral dilatation (**Fig. 39–2**).[81–86] Occasionally, a localized area of hypo- or hyperechoic parenchymal abnormality may be identified, so-called "acute bacterial nephritis" or "lobar nephronia" (**Fig. 39–3**).[87] US can also be used to detect renal calculi which may predispose to infection (**Fig. 39–4**). There are few studies comparing the sensitivity and specificity of state-of-the-art US in the diagnosis of acute pyelonephritis to other imaging modalities. Conventional gray scale US has been shown to be superior to EU.[88,89] However, it fares poorly in comparison to CT and Tc-99m-DMSA scintigraphy, the current imaging standards.[89–94] A study of 91 children with culture-documented febrile UTI studied by DMSA scintigraphy and US showed changes consistent with pyelonephritis in 63% of the DMSA scans but in only 24% of the sonograms.[93]

With the advent of color and power Doppler imaging, the sensitivity and specificity of sonography in the diagnosis of acute pyelonephritis will probably be improved, due to better depiction of perfusion abnormalities.[95–98] To date, there have been no large studies comparing color and/or power Doppler imaging to state-of-the-art Tc-99m-DMSA SPECT or helical CT. Dacher et al. studied 30 children in whom acute pyelonephritis was clinically suspected using both power Doppler US and conventional incremental CT with intravenous contrast enhancement. With the CT findings as the reference standard, the sensitivity and specificity of power Doppler imaging were, respectively, 89% and 69%.[97] The recent development of Doppler contrast agents also holds promise for improving our ability to diagnose acute pyelonephritis with US technology.[99–101]

Complications of Acute Pyelonephritis

Complications of acute pyelonephritis include renal and perirenal abscesses and pyonephrosis.

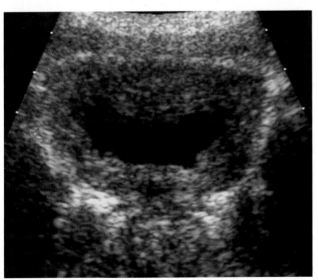
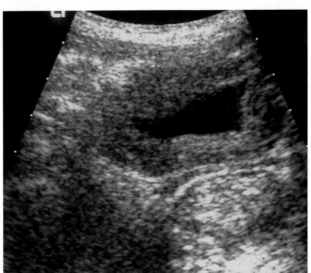

A   **B**

Figure 39–1 Cystitis in a patient with recurrent UTIs. Transverse (**A**) and sagittal (**B**) sonograms of the pelvis show a thick-walled bladder.

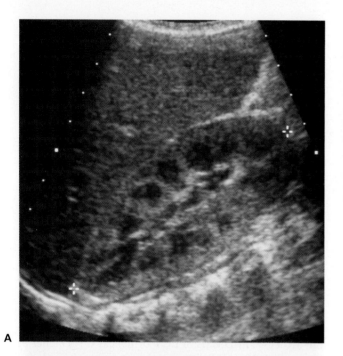

A

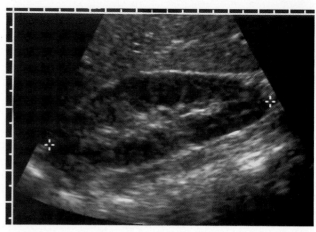

B

Figure 39–2 Acute pyelonephritis. (**A**) Longitudinal sonogram of the right flank demonstrates an echogenic kidney with prominent pyramids. (**B**) A repeat study obtained after antibiotic treatment shows a normal kidney with cortical echogenicity relatively hypoechoic to the adjacent liver.

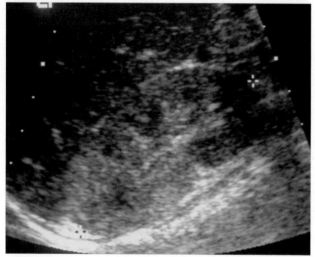

A

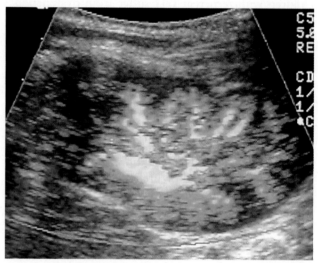

B

Figure 39–3 Acute focal bacterial nephritis. (**A**) Longitudinal sonogram of the right kidney reveals a swollen upper pole of increased echogenicity and loss of corticomedullary differentiation.

(**B**) Power Doppler image shows absent perfusion of the upper pole.

Abscess

When children with UTI do not respond rapidly to antibiotic treatment, repeat sonograms are warranted in order to detect complications that may require drainage. Renal abscesses are relatively uncommon in the pediatric population. They occur either from progression of acute pyelonephritis or as a result of hematogenous spread from a remote location. *Escherichia coli* and *Staphylococcus aureus* are the usual causative organisms. Renal abscesses tend to be multiple and bilateral when of hematogenous origin.

With US, a mature abscess appears as a well-circumscribed mass with an irregular, relatively echogenic wall and a hypoechoic or anechoic center due to liquified pus. Doppler US reveals absence of perfusion (**Fig. 39–5**).

Perinephric Abscess

Perinephric abscess is usually unilateral and results from inflammation of the soft tissues adjacent to the kidney. Infection of the perinephric space most often develops following rupture of a renal cortical abscess, but may follow seeding from blood-borne infections or

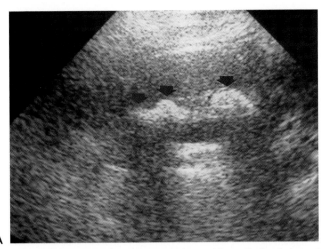

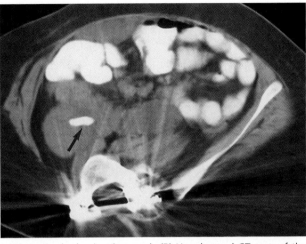

Figure 39–4 Staghorn calculus. Patient with myelodysplasia and UTI. (**A**) Longitudinal sonogram of the right kidney demonstrates foci of increased echogenicity in the renal sinus associated with dis- tal acoustic shadowing (**arrows**). (**B**) Unenhanced CT scan of the abdomen shows a calcified stone in the right renal pelvis (**arrow**).

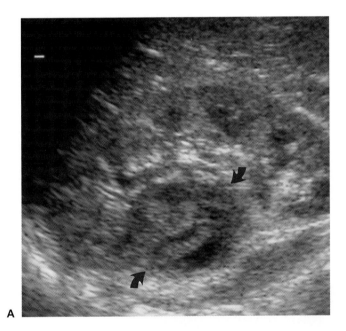

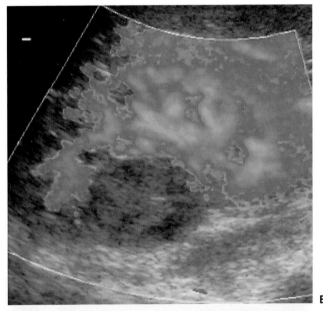

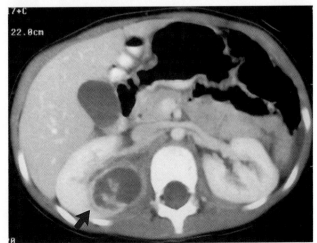

Figure 39–5 Renal abscess. (**A**) Sagittal sonogram of the right flank shows a heterogeneous, well-circumscribed mass (**arrows**). (**B**) Power Doppler image reveals no perfusion of the lesion. (**C**) Contrast-enhanced CT confirms the abscess (arrow) which contains irregular, thick septa.

after renal trauma (**Fig. 39–6**). US may be used to guide percutaneous aspiration and drainage in children with renal and perirenal abscesses.

Pyonephrosis

Pyonephrosis is a complication of pyelonephritis that consists of pus within a dilated renal collecting system. The diagnosis is suspected when fever and flank pain are associated with radiologic demonstration of urinary tract obstruction. The most common sonographic findings include hydronephrosis with a fluid/debris level (**Fig. 39–7**). However, the collecting system can be completely anechoic, contain only low-level echoes, or demonstrate very strong echoes due to the presence of gas-forming microorganisms. US may be used to guide aspiration and drainage of the collecting system. The sensitivity and specificity of US in the diagnosis of pyonephrosis have varied in different series from 25% to 67% and 96% to 100%, respectively. False-positive results occur with severe obstruction, where the collecting system is filled with proteinaceous material or debris.

False-negative results can occur when purulent material is not echogenic.[102—106]

Vesicoureteral Reflux

Conventional gray scale US is a poor screening method for the detection of VUR, because the study is frequently normal, particularly in patients with lesser degrees of reflux.[107—109] In the study of Alon et al., US was normal in 38 of 44 urinary systems with low-grade reflux (86%).[109] In the presence of long-standing, severe VUR, marked dilatation of the renal collecting system needs to be differentiated from obstructive hydronephrosis and hydroureter. In an effort to improve the sensitivity of US in the detection of VUR, air bubbles and, more recently, contrast agents have been instilled into the bladder (**Fig. 39–8**). Visualization of microbubbles or contrast material within the renal pelvis is indicative of VUR (**Fig. 39–9**).[110—113] These techniques, particularly the latter, hold promise, although they are currently somewhat difficult to perform.

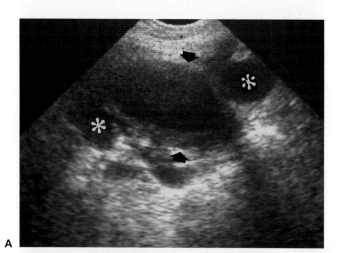

A

Figure 39–6 Renal abscess with perinephric inflammation. A patient with myelodysplasia and a history of extensive urinary tract reconstruction underwent dilatation of a stenotic jejunal ureter and placement of a nephrostomy tube. One month later, she developed fever and foul discharge from the catheter. (**A**) Sagittal sonogram of the right flank shows a hypoechoic fluid collection (**arrows**) along the lateral aspect of the kidney. Note the dilated upper and lower pole calyces (**asterisks**). (**B**) Contrast-enhanced CT obtained after placement of a drainage tube shows an abscess containing several gas bubbles within the superolateral portion of the right kidney. There is inflammatory change in the soft tissues posterolaterally and a small gas bubble is present (**arrow**). (**C**) Fluid is identified anterior and lateral to the right kidney. The drainage catheter lies within the abscess cavity.

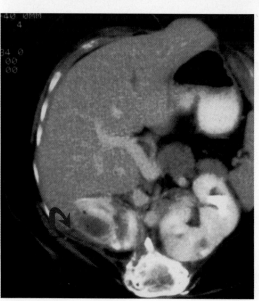

B

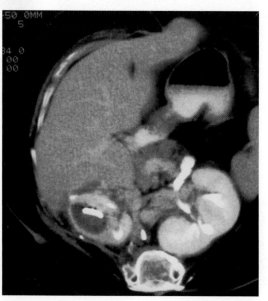

C

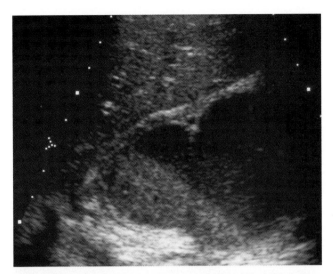

Figure 39–7   Pyonephrosis. A young girl with right UPJ obstruction developed a febrile UTI. Sagittal sonogram of the right flank shows massive hydronephrosis with a fluid-debris level. The renal parenchyma is markedly thinned. A nephrostomy tube placed in the renal pelvis drained a large amount of pus (not shown).

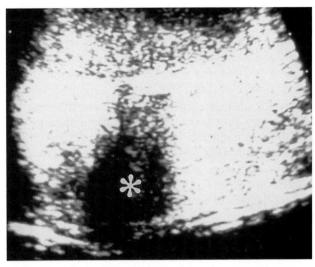

Figure 39–8   Sonicated albumin-enhanced sonography. Transverse image of the pelvis depicts the markedly hyperechoic, homogeneous contrast material within the bladder. Note the anechoic, saline-filled Foley catheter balloon (**asterisk**).

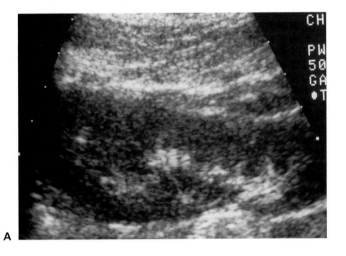

A

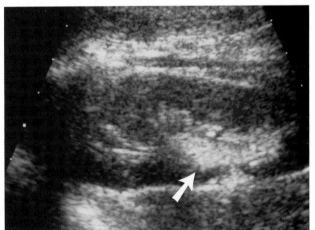

B

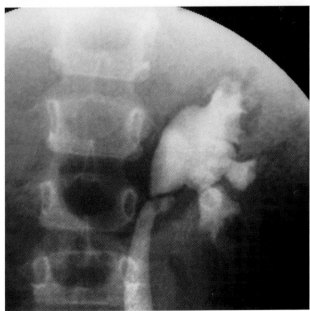

C

Figure 39–9   Documentation of VUR by sonicated albumin-enhanced sonography. (**A**) Sagittal sonogram of the left flank prior to contrast administration demonstrates a duplex kidney. (**B**) Following infusion of sonicated albumin into the bladder, sagittal sonogram of the left kidney reveals homogeneously increased echoes within the lower pole collecting system (**arrows**). (**C**) VCUG demonstrates left lower pole reflux.

Chronic Pyelonephritis

Chronic pyelonephritis results from repeated episodes of acute pyelonephritis. Sonographic findings include a small kidney with an irregular contour due to focal parenchymal loss (**Fig. 39–10**). Compensatory hypertrophy of the contralateral kidney can develop. The renal cortex may become more echogenic than normal and there is frequently loss of normal corticomedullary differentiation (**Fig. 39–11**). US can demonstrate renal atrophy and large scars, but it is not as sensitive or specific as 99m-Tc-DMSA scintigraphy in depicting milder degrees of scarring. In three recently published studies, the sensitivity and specificity of US to detect renal scarring varied respectively from 43% to 54%, and from 80% to 99%.[92,114,115]

Fungal Infection

Fungal infection of the urinary tract is most often due to *Candida albicans*. Immunodeficiency states, indwelling catheters, and prolonged antibiotic or immunosuppressive therapy are risk factors. Premature infants with diminished cellular immunity are especially susceptible to fungal infection. Seeding of the kidney is followed by the development of cortical abscesses and extension of inflammation into the interstitium and tubules. Complications include mycelial collections in the tubules, collecting system and urinary bladder, as well as necrotizing papillitis.

Sonographic abnormalities include renal enlargement and a generalized increase in parenchymal echogenicity with loss of normal corticomedullary differentiation (**Fig. 39–12**). Mycelial clumps (fungus balls) in

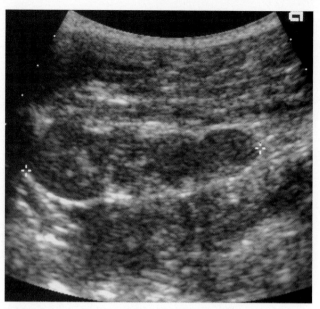

Figure 39–10 Chronic pyelonephritis. Longitudinal sonogram reveals a small right kidney (between cursors) with an irregular contour.

the collecting system and bladder appear as nonshadowing, echogenic masses and may cause obstruction (**Fig. 39–13**).[116—123]

Summary

US imaging in the child with a UTI is useful in depicting underlying anatomic abnormalities that may predispose to infection, identifying renal structural damage as a consequence of infection, and providing a baseline for subsequent evaluation of renal growth.

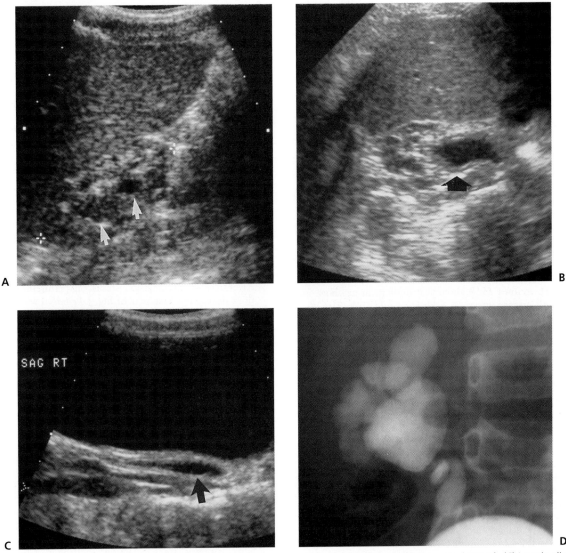

A

B

C

D

Figure 39–11   Chronic pyelonephritis. (**A**) Longitudinal sono-gram of the right flank demonstrates a small, echogenic right kid-ney (between cursors). The parenchyma is thin and there is poor corticomedullary differentiation. The calyces are mildly dilated (**ar-rows**). (**B**) Transverse sonogram reveals a moderately dilated right renal pelvis with thickened mucosa (**arrow**). (**C**) Longitudinal sono-gram of the pelvis depicts dilatation of the distal right ureter poste-rior to the bladder (**arrows**). (**D**) VCUG demonstrates right-sided grade 4 VUR.

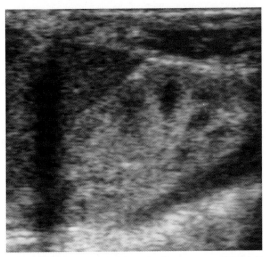

Figure 39–12   Neonatal candidiasis. Sagittal sonogram of the left flank demonstrates diffusely increased renal parenchymal echogen-icity. There is poor corticomedullary differentiation.

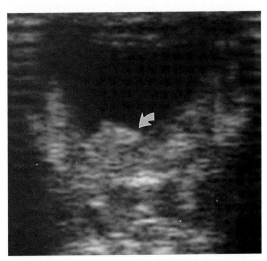

Figure 39–13   Neonatal candidiasis. Transverse sonogram of the bladder shows an intraluminal fungus ball (**arrow**).

References

1. Ginsburg CM, McCracken GH. Urinary tract infections in young infants. *Pediatrics* 1982;69:409—412.
2. Hoberman A, Wald ER, Reynolds EA, Penchansky L, Charron M. Is urine culture necessary to rule out urinary tract infection in young febrile children? *Pediatr Infect Dis J* 1996;15:304—309.
3. Nelson JD, Peters PC. Suprapubic aspiration of urine in premature and term infants. *Pediatrics* 1965;36:132—134.
4. Abbott GD. Neonatal bacteriuria: a prospective study in 1460 infants. *Br Med J* 1972;1:267—269.
5. Littlewood JM, Kite P, Kite BA. Incidence of neonatal urinary tract infection. *Arch Dis Child* 1969;44:617—620.
6. O'Doherty NJ. Urinary tract infection in the neonatal period and later infancy. In: O'Grady F, Brumfitt W, eds. *Urinary Tract Infection*, London: Oxford University Press, 1968, p. 113—122.
7. Bergström T, Larson H, Lincoln K, Winberg J. Studies of urinary tract infections in infancy and childhood. *J Pediatr* 1972;80:858—866.
8. Drew JH, Acton CM. Radiological findings in newborn infants with urinary infection. *Arch Dis Child* 1976;51:628—630.
9. Kunin CM, Deutscher R, Paquin A. Urinary tract infection in children: an epidemiologic, clinical and laboratory study. *Medicine* 1964;43:91—130.
10. Lindberg U, Claësson I, Hanson LÅ, Jodal U. Asymptomatic bacteriuria in schoolgirls. I. Clinical and laboratory findings. *Acta Paediatr Scand* 1975;64:425—431.
11. Newcastle symptomatic bacteriuria research group. Asymptomatic bacteriuria in schoolchildren in Newcastle upon Tyne. *Arch Dis Child* 1975;50:90—102.
12. Savage DC, Wilson MI, McHardy M, Dewar DA, Fee WM. Covert bacteriuria of childhood. a clinical and epidemiological study. *Arch Dis Child* 1973;48:8—20.
13. Saxena SR, Collis A, Laurance BM. Bacteriuria in preschool children (letter). *Lancet* 1974;2:517—518.
14. Winberg J, Andersen HJ, Bergström T, et al. Epidemiology of symptomatic urinary tract infection in childhood. *Acta Paediatr Scand* 1974;252 (Suppl):1—20.
15. Hellström A, Hanson E, Hansson S, Hjälmas K, Jodal U. Association between urinary symptoms at 7 years old and previous urinary tract infection. *Arch Dis Child* 1991;66:232—234.
16. Johnson CE, Shurin PA, Marchant CD, et al. Identification of children requiring radiologic evaluation for urinary infection. *Ped Infect Dis* 1985;4:656—663.
17. Torres VE, Kramer SA, Holley KE, et al. Interaction of multiple risk factors in the pathogenesis of experimental reflux nephropathy in the pig. *J Urol* 1985;133:131—135.
18. Roberts JA. Factors predisposing to urinary tract infections in children. *Pediatr Nephrol* 1996;10:517—522.
19. Ogata RT. Factors determining bacterial pathogenicity. *Clin Physiol Biochem* 1983;1:145—159.
20. Källenius G, Möllby R, Svenson SB, Winberg J, Hultberg H. Identification of a carbohydrate receptor recognized by uropathogenic *Escherichia coli*. *Infection* 1980;8(3):S288—S293.
21. Leffler H, Svanborg-Edén C. Glycolipid receptors for uropathogenic *Escherichia coli* on human erythrocytes and uroepithelial cells. *Infect Immun* 1981;34:920—929.
22. Horwitz MA, Silverstein SC. Influence of the *Escherichia coli* capsule on complement fixation and on phagocytosis and killing by human phagocytes. *J Clin Invest* 1980;65:82—94.
23. Svanborg-Edén C, Hagberg L, Hull R, et al. Bacterial virulence versus host resistance in the urinary tracts of mice. *Infect Immun* 1987;55:1224—1232.
24. Kaijser B, Hanson LÅ, Jodal U, Lidin-Janson G, Robbins JB. Frequency of *E. coli* K antigens in urinary-tract infections in children. *Lancet* 1977;1:663—664.
25. Williams PH. Novel iron uptake system specified by ColV plasmids: an important component in the virulence of invasive strains of *Escherichia coli*. *Infect Immun* 1979;26:925—932.
26. Carbonetti NH, Boonchai S, Parry SH, et al. Aerobactin-mediated iron uptake by *Escherichia coli* isolates from human extraintestinal infections. *Infect Immun* 1986;51:966—968.
27. Jacobson SH, Hammarlind M, Lidefeldt KJ, et al. Incidence of aerobactin-positive *Escherichia coli* strains in patients with symptomatic urinary tract infection. *Eur J Clin Microbiol Infect Dis* 1988;7:630—634.
28. Wiswell TE, Roscelli JD. Corroborative evidence for the decreased incidence of urinary tract infections in circumcised male infants. *Pediatrics* 1986;78:96—99.
29. Wiswell TE, Smith FR, Bass JW. Decreased incidence of urinary tract infection in circumcised male infants. *Pediatrics* 1985;75:901—903.
30. Wiswell TE, Miller GM, Gelston HM, Jones SK, Clemmings AF. Effect of circumcision status on periurethral bacterial flora during the first year of life. *J Pediatr* 1988;113:442—446.
31. Källenius G, Winberg J. Bacterial adherence to periurethral epithelial cells in girls prone to urinary tract infections. *Lancet* 1978;2:540—543.
32. Svanborg-Edén C, Jodal U. Attachment of *Escherichia coli* to urinary sediment epithelial cells from urinary tract infection-prone and healthy children. *Infect Immun* 1979;26:837—840.
33. Snodgrass W. Relationship of voiding dysfunction to urinary tract infection and vesicoureteral reflux in children. *Urology* 1991;38:341—344.
34. Koff SA, Murtagh DS. The uninhibited bladder in children: effect of treatment on recurrence of urinary infection and on vesicoureteral reflux resolution. *J Urol* 1983;130:1138—1141.
35. Neumann PZ, deDomenico IJ, Nogrady MB. Constipation and urinary tract infection. *Pediatrics* 1973;52:241—245.
36. O'Regan S, Yazbeck S, Schick E. Constipation, bladder instability, urinary tract infection syndrome. *Clin Nephrol* 1985;23:152—154.
37. Kiruluta HG, Fraser K, Owen L. The significance of the adrenergic nerves in the etiology of vesicoureteral reflux. *J Urol* 1986;136:232—235.
38. Gross GW, Lebowitz RL. Infection does not cause reflux. *AJR* 1981;137:929—932.
39. Noe HN, Wyatt RJ, Peeden JN, Rivas ML. The transmission of vesicoureteral reflux from parent to child. *J Urol* 1992;148:1869—1871.
40. Askari A, Belman AB. Vesicoureteral reflux in black girls. *J Urol* 1982;127:747—748.
41. Skoog SJ, Belman AB. Primary vesicoureteral reflux in the black child. *Pediatrics* 1991;87:538—543.
42. Hutch JA. Aberrant micturition. *J Urol* 1966;96:743—745.
43. Hernanz-Schulman M, Lebowitz RL. The elusiveness and importance of bladder diverticula in children. *Pediatr Radiol* 1985;15:399—402.
44. Majd M, Rushton HG, Jantausch B, Wiedermann BL. Relationship among vesicoureteral reflux, P-fimbriated *Escherichia coli*, and acute pyelonephritis in children with febrile urinary tract infection. *J Pediatr* 1991;119:578—585.
45. Bisset GS, Strife JL, Dunbar JS. Urography and voiding cystourethrography: findings in girls with urinary tract infection. *AJR* 1987;148:479—482.
46. Steinhardt GF. Reflux nephropathy. *J Urol* 1985;134:855—859.

47. Matsuoka H, Oshima K, Sakamoto K, Taguchi T, Takebayashi S. Renal pathology in patients with reflux nephropathy. The turning point in irreversible renal disease. *Eur Urol.* 1994;26:153—159.

48. Kincaid-Smith P. Glomerular lesions in atrophic pyelonephritis and reflux nephropathy. *Kidney Int* 1975;8:S81—S83.

49. Risdon RA. Reflux nephropathy. *Diagn Histopathol* 1981;4:61—70.

50. Hodson CJ. The radiological contribution toward the diagnosis of chronic pyelonephritis. *Radiology* 1967;88:857—871.

51. Hodson CJ. Reflux nephropathy: a personal historical review. *AJR* 1981;137:451—462.

52. Hansson S, Martinell J, Stokland E, Jodal U. The natural history of bacteriuria in childhood. *Infect Dis Clin North Am* 1997;11:499—512.

53. Chan RC, Reid G, Irvin RT, Bruce AW, Costeron JW. Competitive exclusion of uropathogens from human uroepithelial cells by *Lactobacillus* whole cells and cell wall fragments. *Infect Immun* 1985;47:84—89.

54. Fennell RS, Wilson SG, Garin EH, et al. Bacteriuria in families of girls with recurrent bacteriuria. A survey of 112 family members showed similar infections in 14 percent of the female siblings. *Clin Pediatr* 1977;16:1132—1135.

55. Hellerstein S. Urinary tract infections. Old and new concepts. *Pediatr Clin North Am* 1995;42:1433—1457.

56. North American pediatric renal transplant cooperative study. Annual Report, 1997.

57. Jakobsson B, Berg U, Svensson L. Renal scarring after acute pyelonephritis. *Arch Dis Child* 1994;70:111—115.

58. Ransley PG, Risdon RA. Reflux nephropathy: effects of antimicrobial therapy on the evolution of the early pyelonephritic scar. *Kidney Int* 1981;20:733—742.

59. Rushton HG, Majd M, Jantausch B, Wiedermann BL, Belman AB. Renal scarring following reflux and nonreflux pyelonephritis in children: evaluation with [99m]technetium-dimercaptosuccinic acid scintigraphy. *J Urol* 1992;147:1327—1332.

60. Smellie JM, Ransley PG, Normand IC, Prescod N, Edwards D. Development of new renal scars: a collaborative study. *Br Med J* 1985;290:1957—1960.

61. Winberg J, Bergström T, Jacobsson B. Morbidity, age and sex distribution, recurrences and renal scarring in symptomatic urinary tract infection in childhood. *Kidney Int* 1975;8:S101—S106.

62. Jodal U. Aspects of clinical trials of drug efficacy in children with uncomplicated infections. *Infection* 1994;22:S10—S11.

63. Smellie JM, Normand IC, Katz G. Children with urinary infection: a comparison of those with and those without vesicoureteric reflux. *Kidney Int* 1981;20:717—722.

64. Brendstrup L, Carlsen N, Nielsen SL, et al. Micturition cystourethrography using x-ray or scintigraphy in children with reflux. *Acta Paediatr Scand* 1983;72:559—562.

65. Rushton HG. Urinary tract infections in children. Epidemiology, evaluation, and management. *Pediatr Clin North Am* 1997;44:1133—1169.

66. Lebowitz RL, Mandell J. Urinary tract infection in children: putting radiology in its place. *Radiology* 1987;165:1—9.

67. Schlager TA, Dilks S, Trudell J, Whittam TS, Hendley JO. Bacteriuria in children with neurogenic bladder treated with intermittent catheterization: natural history. *J Pediatr* 1995;126:490—496.

68. Tarkington MA, Fildes RD, Levin K, et al. High resolution single photon emission computed tomography (SPECT) [99m]technetium-dimercaptosuccinic acid renal imaging: a state of the art technique. *J Urol* 1990;144:598—600.

69. Hauser W, Atkins HL, Nelson KG, Richards P. Technetium-99 m DTPA: a new radiopharmaceutical for brain and kidney scanning. *Radiology* 1970;94:679—684.

70. Bubeck B, Brandau W, Steinbächer M, et al. Technetium-99 m labeled renal function and imaging agents. II. Clinical evaluation of ^{99m}Tc MAG 3 (99m Tc mercaptoacetylglycylglycylglycine). *Nucl Med Biol* 1988;15:109—118.

71. Montgomery P, Kuhn JP, Afshani E. CT evaluation of severe inflammatory disease in children. *Pediatr Radiol* 1987;17:216—222.

72. Dacher JN, Boillot B, Eurin D, et al. Rational use of CT in acute pyelonephritis: findings and relationships with reflux. *Pediatr Radiol* 1993;23:281—285.

73. Lonergan GJ, Pennington DJ, Morrison JC, et al. Childhood pyelonephritis: comparison of gadolinium-enhanced MR imaging and renal cortical scintigraphy for diagnosis. *Radiology* 1998;207:377—384.

74. Rosenbaum DM, Korngold E, Teele RL. Sonographic assessment of renal length in normal children. *AJR* 1984;142:467—469.

75. Han BK, Babcock DS. Sonographic measurements and appearance of normal kidneys in children. *AJR* 1985;145:611—616.

76. Carrico CW, Zerin JM. Sonographic measurement of renal length in children: does the position of the patient matter? *Pediatr Radiol* 1996;26:553—555.

77. De Sanctis JT, Connolly SA, Bramson RT. Effect of patient position on sonographically measured renal length in neonates, infants, and children. *AJR* 1998;170:1381—1383.

78. Kunin CM. The natural history of recurrent bacteriuria in schoolgirls. *N Engl J Med* 1970;282:1443—1448.

79. Friedman EP, de Bruyn R, Mather S. Pseudotumoral cystitis in children: a review of the ultrasound features in four cases. *Br J Radiol* 1993;66:605—608.

80. Gooding GA. Varied sonographic manifestations of cystitis. *J Ultrasound Med* 1986;5:61—63.

81. Sty JR, Wells RG, Starshak RJ, Schroeder BA. Imaging in acute renal infection in children. *AJR* 1987;148:471—477.

82. Mackenzie JR, Fowler K, Hollman AS, et al. The value of ultrasound in the child with an acute urinary tract infection. *Br J Urol* 1994;74:240—244.

83. Dinkel E, Orth S, Dittrich M, Schulte-Wissermann H. Renal sonography in the differentiation of upper from lower urinary tract infection. *AJR* 1986;146:775—780.

84. Pickworth FE, Carlin JB, Ditchfield MR, et al. Sonographic measurement of renal enlargement in children with acute pyelonephritis and time needed for resolution: implications for renal growth assessment. *AJR* 1995;165:405—408.

85. Avni EF, Van Gansbeke D, Thoua Y, et al. US demonstration of pyelitis and ureteritis in children. *Pediatr Radiol* 1988;18:134—139.

86. Morehouse HT, Weiner SN, Hoffman JC. Imaging in inflammatory disease of the kidney. *AJR* 1984;143:135—141.

87. Klar A, Hurvitz H, Berkun Y, et al. Focal bacterial nephritis (lobar nephronia) in children. *J Pediatr* 1996;128:850—853.

88. Kangarloo H, Gold RH, Fine RN, Diament MJ, Boechat MI. Urinary tract infection in infants and children evaluated by ultrasound. *Radiology* 1985;154:367—373.

89. Monsour M, Azmy AF, MacKenzie JR. Renal scarring secondary to vesicoureteral reflux. Critical assessment and new grading. *Br J Urol* 1987;60:320—324.

90. Lavocat MP, Granjon D, Allard D, et al. Imaging of pyelonephritis. *Pediatr Radiol* 1997;27:159—165.

91. Mastin ST, Drane WE, Iravani A. Tc-99m DMSA SPECT imaging in patients with acute symptoms or history of UTI. Comparison with ultrasonography. *Clin Nucl Med* 1995;20:407—412.

92. Smellie JM, Rigden SP, Prescod NP. Urinary tract infection: a comparison of four methods of investigation. *Arch Dis Child* 1995;72:247—250.

93. Björgvinsson E, Majd M, Eggli KD. Diagnosis of acute pyelonephritis in children: comparison of sonography and ^{99m}Tc-DMSA scintigraphy. *AJR* 1991;157:539—543.

94. Verber IG, Strudley MR, Meller ST. ^{99m}Tc dimercaptosuccinic acid (DMSA) scan as first investigation of urinary tract infection. *Arch Dis Child* 1988;63:1320—1325.

95. Eggli KD, Eggli D. Color Doppler sonography in pyelonephritis. *Pediatr Radiol* 1992;22:422—425.

96. Winters WD. Power Doppler sonographic evaluation of acute pyelonephritis in children. *J Ultrasound Med* 1996;15:91—96.

97. Dacher J-N, Pfister C, Monroc M, Eurin D, Le Dosseur P. Power Doppler sonographic pattern of acute pyelonephritis in children: comparison with CT. *AJR* 1996;166:1451—1455.

98. Clautrice-Engle T, Jeffrey RB Jr. Renal hypoperfusion: value of power Doppler imaging. *AJR* 1997;168:1227—1231.

99. Pugh CR, Arger PH, Sehgal CM. Power, spectral, and color flow Doppler enhancement by a new ultrasonographic contrast agent. *J Ultrasound Med* 1996;15:843—852.

100. Brown JM, Quedens-Case C. Alderman JL, Greener Y, Taylor KJ. Contrast enhanced sonography of visceral perfusion defects in dogs. *J Ultrasound Med* 1997;16:493—499.

101. Taylor GA, Barnewolt CE, Adler BH, Dunning PS. Renal cortical ischemia in rabbits revealed by contrast-enhanced power Doppler sonography. *AJR* 1998;170:417—422.

102. Jeffrey RB Jr, Laing FC, Wing VW, Hoddick W. Sensitivity of sonography in pyonephrosis: a reevaluation. *AJR* 1985;144:71—73.

103. Schneider K, Helmig F-J, Eife R, et al. Pyonephrosis in children — is ultrasound sufficient for diagnosis? *Pediatr Radiol* 1989;19:302—307.

104. Wu TT, Lee YH, Tzeng WS, et al. The role of C-reactive protein and erythrocyte sedimentation rate in the diagnosis of infected hydronephrosis and pyonephrosis. *J Urol* 1994;152:26—28.

105. St. Lezin M, Hofmann R, Stoller ML. Pyonephrosis: diagnosis and treatment. *Br J Urol* 1992;70:360—363.

106. Coleman BG, Arger PH, Mulhern CB Jr., Pollack HM, Banner MP. Pyonephrosis: sonography in the diagnosis and management. *AJR* 1981;137:939—943.

107. Riccipetitoni G, Chierici R, Tamisari L, et al. Postnatal ultrasound screening of urinary malformations. *J Urol* 1992;148:604—605.

108. Jequier S, Forbes PA, Nogrady MB. The value of ultrasonography as a screening procedure in a first-documented urinary tract infection in children. *J Ultrasound Med* 1985;4:393—400.

109. Alon U, Berant M, Pery M. Intravenous pyelography in children with urinary tract infection and vesicoureteral reflux. *Pediatrics* 1989;83:332—336.

110. Schneider K, Jablonski C, Weissner M, Kohn M, Fendel H. Screening for vesicoureteral reflux in children using real-time sonography. *Pediatr Radiol* 1984;14:400—403.

111. Atala A, Wible JH, Share JC, et al. Sonography with sonicated albumin in the detection of vesicoureteral reflux. *J Urol* 1993;150:756—758.

112. Atala A, Ellsworth P, Share J, et al. Comparison of sonicated albumin enhanced sonography to fluoroscopic and radionuclide voiding cystography for detecting vesicoureteral reflux. *J urol* 1998;160:1820—1822.

113. Bosio M. Cystosonography with echocontrast: a new imaging modality to detect vesicoureteric reflux in children. *Pediatr Radiol* 1998;28:250—255.

114. Stokland E, Hellstrom M, Hansson S, et al. Reliability of ultrasonography in identification of reflux nephropathy in children. *Br Med J* 1994;309:235—239.

115. Rickwood AM, Carty HM, McKendrick T, et al. Current imaging of childhood urinary infections: prospective survey. *Br Med J* 1994;304:663—665.

116. Baetz-Greenwalt B, Debaz B, Kumar ML. Bladder fungus ball: a reversible cause of neonatal obstructive uropathy. *Pediatrics* 1988;81:826—829.

117. Cohen HL, Haller JO, Schechter S, et al. Renal candidiasis of the infant: ultrasound evaluation. *Urol Radiol* 1986;8:17—21.

118. Kintanar C, Cramer BC, Reid WD, Andrews WL. Neonatal renal candidiasis: sonographic diagnosis. *AJR* 1986;147:801—805.

119. Kirpekar M, Abiri MM, Hilfer C, Enerson R. Ultrasound in the diagnosis of systemic candidiasis (renal and cranial) in very low birth weight premature infants. *Pediatr Radiol* 1986;16: 17—20.

120. Patriquin H, Lebowitz R, Perreault G, Yousefzadeh D. Neonatal candidiasis: renal and pulmonary manifestations. *AJR* 1980;135:1205—1210.

121. Stuck KJ, Silver TM, Jaffe MH, Bowerman RA. Sonographic demonstration of renal fungus balls. *Radiology* 1981;142:473—474.

122. Pappu LD, Purohit DM, Bradford BF, Turner WR Jr., Levkoff AH. Primary renal candidiasis in two preterm neonates. Report of cases and review of literature on renal candidiasis in infancy. *Am J Dis Child* 1984;138:923—926.

123. Schmitt GH, Hsu AS. Renal fungus balls: diagnosis by ultrasound and percutaneous antegrade pyelography and brush biopsy in a premature infant. *J Ultrasound Med* 1985;4:155—156.

40 Amenorrhea in the Adolescent or Young Adult

Harry L. Zinn and Harris L. Cohen

Ultrasonography (US) of the pelvis and reproductive organs is indicated in a patient who presents with amenorrhea. *Primary amenorrhea* is defined as the lack of menses by age 16. Secondary amenorrhea is the cessation of menses at any point in time after menarche and before menopause.[1] In order to establish a diagnosis and cause of amenorrhea, the referring physician and radiologist need to understand the physiologic mechanisms regulating normal menses and the various abnormalities that may lead to its disruption. These abnormalities may be embryologic, genetic and/or endocrinologic.[2] An awareness of the patient's history, physical findings, and laboratory values and the spectrum of normal and abnormal imaging findings is also important in understanding the cause of amenorrhea.

The Normal Menstrual Cycle

Menstruation is the periodic vaginal bleeding that is the end result of the cyclical stimulation of ovarian follicles and the associated buildup and eventual shedding of uterine mucosa. In humans, the average time between one menses and the next is 28 days. The menstrual cycle is divided into follicular, ovulatory, and secretory phases. The first day of the cycle is arbitrarily defined as the first day of menstrual bleeding.[1, 3—5]

The follicular phase occurs between the 5th and 14th day of the menstrual cycle. During this phase, pulsatile release of gonadotropin releasing hormone from the hypothalamus stimulates the secretion of luteinizing hormone (LH) and follicle stimulating hormone (FSH) by the pituitary. These hormones stimulate several primordial ovarian follicles which enlarge and become surrounded by follicular fluid (**Fig. 40–1**). By the sixth day of the cycle, one follicle becomes dominant and the others become atretic. Under the influence of LH and FSH, this maturing ovarian (graafian) follicle continues to grow and eventually produces estrogen. Follicle stimulating hormone stimulates an increase in the number of granulosa cells of the graafian follicle as well as the number of FSH receptors on these cells. It also induces production of an enzyme necessary for the conversion of androgen precursors to estradiol. Under the influence of LH, the theca cells secrete androstenedione, testosterone, and estradiol into the bloodstream and into the follicle itself. Under the influence of estrogens (estradiol) from the developing follicles, the endometrium increases in thickness, reflecting a proliferation of glandular cells and stroma. By the midfollicular phase, FSH levels begin to decline. This is due to various mechanisms: feedback inhibition from the increasing levels of estrogen, direct blockage of FSH synthesis, and release of inhibit by the granulosa cells. The graafian follicle still responds to FSH despite decreasing FSH levels.

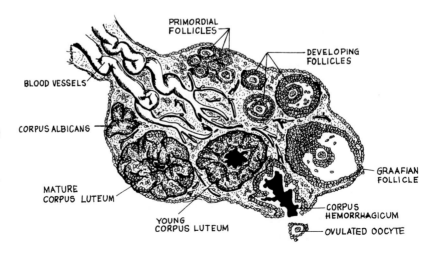

Figure 40–1 Cyclical changes in the postmenarchal ovary. Schematic drawing. The ovary undergoes various stages during the menstrual cycle. These include the follicular phase with formation of a dominant (graafian) follicle from among several stimulated primordial follicles; the ovulatory phase with formation of the corpus hemorrhagicum; and the secretory phase with formation of the corpus luteum, that produces estrogen and progesterone necessary for endometrial maturation. The corpus luteum degenerates, leaving scar tissue (corpus albicans), if no pregnancy occurs.

This is due to the earlier production of granulosa cells and FSH receptors, which amplify the effect of FSH. At the same time, the release intervals for LH increase.[2, 5]

At day 14 or midcycle, the increasing estrogen and progesterone levels result in a surge of LH. This LH surge causes the distended follicles to rupture and ovulation occurs (i.e., the ovulatory phase) (**Fig. 40–1**). The ovum enters the fallopian tube and either implants in the uterus after fertilization or passes through the uterus and out the body through the vagina. The start of the secretory cycle is remarkably constant, beginning at day 14.

The ruptured graafian follicle becomes hemorrhagic (corpus hemorrhagicum). The clotted blood is replaced by lipid-rich luteal cells which form the corpus luteum. The corpus luteum produces estrogen and progesterone which causes the endometrium to mature in preparation for possible implantation. This occurs within 8—9 days of ovulation. The endometrium becomes highly vascularized and slightly edematous with associated thickening of its mucosa and increase in glandular length. The production of prostaglandins by the endometrium also begins under the influence of progesterone.

If pregnancy occurs, the corpus luteum persists and no menses occurs until after delivery. If fertilization does not occur, the corpus luteum degenerates (**Fig. 40–1**) (starting at about 4 days prior to menses), eventually becoming an area of scar tissue (corpus albicans). With corpus luteal degeneration, the blood levels of estrogen and progesterone fall. With decreasing hormonal support, the endometrium thins. Foci of necrosis which soon coalesce appear in the endometrium. Lysosome breakdown in necrotic endometrial cells results in the release of prostaglandins. This subsequently causes vasoconstriction of the spiral arteries of the endometrium resulting in the initially spotty and then more confluent bleeding that is the menstrual flow. The superficial two-thirds of the endometrium, the stratum functionale, which is fed by the long coiled spiral arteries, is shed. The deepest third, the stratum basale, supplied by short straight basilar arteries, remains intact and serves as a regenerative layer for new endometrial proliferation in the next cycle.[1, 2, 4, 5]

Normal Physiology

Vaginal bleeding may be noted in the normal female in the immediate neonatal period. Newborns occasionally experience withdrawal bleeding after being exposed to high levels of maternal estrogen and progesterone in utero. The hormonal levels decrease after placental separation.[2, 7]

Ordinarily, menses does not begin until at least 8 years of age. An unknown "central restraining mechanism" that prevents the pulsatile release of gonadotropin releasing hormone from the arcuate nucleus of the hypothalamus is thought to prevent menses in younger children. The inhibition of gonadotropin releasing hormone production in patients with Turner syndrome who have no functioning gonadal tissue is evidence for this central control (rather than a negative feedback mechanism from ovarian hormone production).[8]

With the activation of gonadotropin releasing hormone at puberty, most girls undergo ovarian folliculogenesis without ovulation.[2, 9] Unopposed estrogen production leads to progressive uterine growth and endometrial proliferation. There is breast budding, physiologic leukorrhea, and accelerated linear growth. Axillary and pubic hair development are the result of androgen production by the ovaries and adrenal glands. The hypothalamic-pituitary-ovarian-uterine axis continues to mature. Over an approximately 2-year span, cycles with subnormal progesterone production and shortened intermenstrual intervals are replaced by normal menstrual cycles.[2]

The typical ovulatory cycle has a 24- to 35-day intermenstrual interval and usually a premenstrual molimina.[10] Longer intervals are often associated with anovulation, although when bleeding occurs it is often associated with some corpus luteal activity.[11] Menarche usually occurs 2—5 years after breast bud development.[2, 12] Improved nutrition and living conditions are thought responsible for the gradual decline in mean menarchal ages over the last century. In North America, it is currently 12.4 years with a range of 9—17 years.[13]

Genital Embryology

Differentiation of the primitive gonad into a testis begins at 7 weeks of fetal life in the presence of the HY antigen found on the Y chromosome. If there is no Y chromosome, ovarian differentiation begins at 17 weeks gestation in the presence of two X chromosomes.[14, 15]

Development of the urinary system and genital system are closely associated. Urogenital ridges develop from the intermediate mesoderm and are situated on each side of the primitive aorta. They gives rise to parts of the genital and urinary systems. The association of uterine and renal abnormalities are quite common, and when there is a gynecologic anomaly, one should evaluate the renal bed to rule out ectopia or agenesis (**Fig. 40–2**).[1, 14, 16, 17]

Both sexes develop two different pairs of genital ducts. In males, components of the wolffian (mesonephric) duct system develop into the epididymis, vas deferens, and seminal vesicles under the influence of testosterone. By 6 weeks, a mullerian (paramesonephric) duct develops lateral to each ipsilateral wolffian (mesonephric) duct. Male genital system development is "active," requiring the presence of testes and their production of testosterone and mullerian inhibition factor, which suppresses further development of the mullerian duct system. The production of dihydrotestosterone allows the wolffian duct system to develop into the epididymis, vas deferens, and seminal vesicles. The enzyme 5-alpha reductase converts testosterone intracellularly, within the target tissues, into the powerful dihydrotestosterone.[1, 15]

In the absence of androgens, the external genital development proceeds along female lines.[2, 14, 16] In females, the mullerian duct system develops into the fallopian tubes, uterus, and upper two-thirds of the vagina, and the wolffian system degenerates. If the mullerian duct system is dysgenetic, then the uterus or vagina may be absent or rudimentary as in the Mayer-Rokitansky-Kuster-Hauser syndrome. Such patients have normal karyotypes and normal secondary sex development, but have associated renal (50%) and skeletal (12%) anomalies.[2, 14, 17, 18]

By 11 weeks, a Y-shaped uterovaginal primordium has developed into the two fallopian tubes; subsequent fusion of a large portion of the bilateral mullerian duct systems results in a single uterus and upper two-thirds of the vagina. This occurs "passively," even if ovaries are not present, as long as there are no testes or high levels of androgens present.[1, 16]

The nonfusion or incomplete fusion of the mullerian duct system can lead to a wide spectrum of anomalies. Complete nonfusion results in a didelphys uterus, in which there are two vaginas, two cervices, and two uterine bodies. Various anomalies are associated with incomplete mullerian duct fusion. Partial fusion of only the caudal ends of the mullerian duct system results in a bicornuate uterus, characterized by variably separated uterine horns that communicate with a single uterine body, cervix, and vagina. The bicornuate uterus, which is wider than normal and has an anterior fundal depression, may be diagnosed on physical examination (usually when a patient is pregnant) or by sonography when two endometrial cavities are imaged. Optimally, the patient should be imaged either during the secretory phase of the menstrual cycle or during pregnancy (**Fig. 40–3**).[1, 14, 16]

The lower one-third of the vagina develops by elongation of the primitive vaginal plate into a core of tissue that canalizes by week 20.[1, 15, 19] The lumen of the vagina is separated from the vestibule of the vagina by a hymenal membrane until late in fetal life. The hymen usually ruptures in the perinatal period with only a thin fold of mucous membrane remaining around the vaginal entry.[16, 19]

Normal Pediatric Uterus

Ultrasonography helps in the evaluation of patients with amenorrhea by determining whether uterine shape and size is premenarchal (infantile) or postmenarchal (adult). The shape and size of the uterus changes during

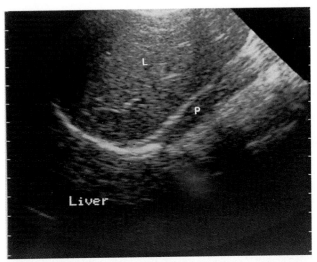

Figure 40–2 Renal agenesis associated with a congenital gynecologic anomaly. Right upper quadrant US. Longitudinal plane. The liver (L) and psoas muscle (P), but not the right kidney, are seen in the right upper quadrant of a 17-year-old with a mullerian duct system anomaly and right renal agenesis. If a kidney is not imaged in the renal bed it should be sought by nuclear medicine or other methods to rule out the possibility of an ectopic kidney rather than agenesis. Reprinted with permission from Pediatric and adolescent genital abnormalities by HL Cohen, J Haller. **Clin Diag Ultrasound** 1988;24:187—216.

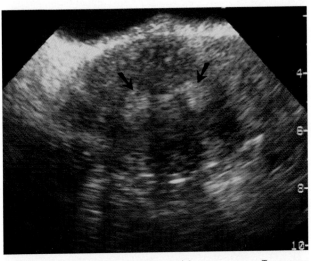

Figure 40–3 Bicornuate uterus. Pelvic sonogram. Transverse plane. Two echogenic endometrial cavity echoes (**arrows**) can be noted in this teenager whose uterus was imaged during the luteal phase of the menstrual cycle and whose diagnosis of a bicornuate uterus was an incidental finding. This image does not highlight the sometimes helpful associated finding of an anterior uterine depression where the uterine horns are separated.

pediatric life. During the first few months of life, uterine size, shape, and appearance are influenced by transiently high levels of gonadotropins levels that develop after placental separation. This hormonal stimulation results in some development of the neonatal uterus and sonographic findings which are typical of the adult uterus, including an echogenic central endometrial canal with a surrounding hypoechoic halo (seen in 29% of infant girls) and endometrial cavity fluid (seen in 23% of infant girls). These findings, when seen, suggest the potential for future estrogenization in adolescence.[1, 17]

The neonatal uterus has a mean length of 3.5 cm. The length decreases to 2.6—3 cm by the fourth month of life.[20, 21] In approximately 60% of newborns, the uterus is shaped like a spade with the anteroposterior (AP) measurement of the cervix greater than that of the fundus and the cervical length twice as long as the fundus (**Fig. 40–4**). In about 30% of newborns, the uterus is tube-shaped with the AP measurement of the cervix equal to that of fundus. Only 10% of premenarchal patients show the classic adult pear-shaped uterus with its fundus wider than the cervix (**Fig. 40–5**). After the first year of life, the uterus becomes tube-shaped (**Fig. 40–6**) and remains so through the next several years of childhood.[14, 17, 20]

The length of the uterus increases gradually between 3 and 8 years of age, reaching a measurement of 4.3 cm in the premenarchal child.[21, 22] The increase in uterine length, its change to a pear shape, and the reversal of the ratio of corpus to cervical length is not solely a matter of increasing estradiol levels. These changes are also believed to be a function of two other independent variables: patient age and size.[21] There is a moderate correlation between uterine length and weight (R = 0.69).[22]

After puberty, the typical uterus measures 5—8 cm in length. It descends deeper in the pelvis and no longer maintains the typical neutral position of the premenarchal years but may be anteverted or retroverted.[1, 23] Cyclic endometrial changes may be seen on US. A well-defined "triple line," representing the hypoechoic functional layers and the coapted echogenic canal are considered evidence of a proliferative endometrium. This triple line is replaced in the secretory phase of the cycle by a single echogenic stripe representing the conglomeration of the hyperechoic functional layers and the central echogenic canal. This echogenic stripe can increase in thickness with increasing endometrial thickness.[24]

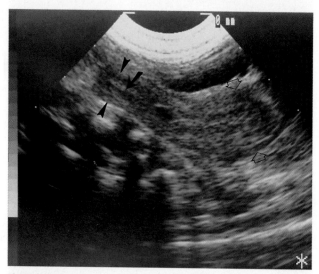

Figure 40–4 Neonatal uterus. Longitudinal midline plane. The typical uterus of a neonate has this spade shape. The cervix (**open arrows**) is thicker in anteroposterior dimension than is the fundus (**arrowheads**). An **arrow** points to the prominent echogenicity of the central endometrial cavity in the fundus. This is a consequence of the high gonadotropin levels in newborn girls.

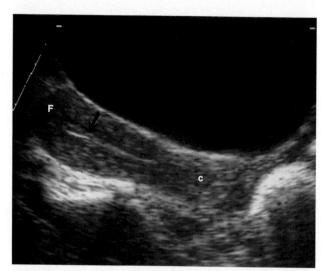

Figure 40–5 Normal postmenarchal adolescent uterus. Longitudinal midline plane. In the normal adult uterus, the AP dimension of the fundus is greater than that of the cervix (c). An **arrow** points to the central endometrial echogenicity which has a triple line appearance, typical of the follicular phase, rather than the single echogenic stripe typical of the secretory phase.

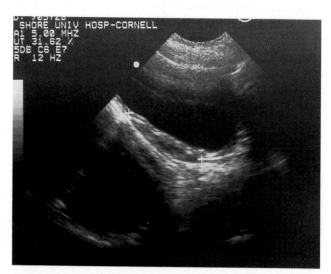

Figure 40–6 Tubular premenarchal uterus. Longitudinal midline plane. Cursors show the superior and inferior extent of a normal tubular, premenarchal uterus in a 5-year-old girl.

Imaging of Congenital Uterine Anomalies

The identification of the uterus and its size is the key piece of diagnostic information in the evaluation of several pediatric/adolescent gynecologic disorders.

Ultrasonography can aid in the diagnosis of anomalies of the mullerian duct system, particularly the bicornuate uterus and the uterus with partial or complete obstruction. Magnetic resonance imaging (MRI) with its multiplanar imaging also has been used successfully in the evaluation of several of these anomalies (**Fig. 40–7**). MRI can identify the tissue composition of an intrauterine septum, thereby helping differentiate between a bicornuate uterus whose septum contains myometrium and a septate uterus with a fibrous septum.[25, 26]

The Normal Pediatric Ovary

Pediatric and premenarchal ovaries can be imaged sonographically. The normal premenarchal ovaries are almond-shaped and often found posterior or lateral to the uterus. They are often seen lateral to the uterus on transverse sonographic images with the transducer angulated in a superior—inferior direction. On parasagittal scanning, they appear medial and anterior to the iliac vessels. Although usually at the level of the superior portion of the broad ligament, the ovaries may be present anywhere along their embryologic course from the inferior border of the kidneys to the broad ligament.[4] Although a rare occurrence, the absence of an ovary and its ipsilateral fallopian tube at surgery suggests an antenatal torsion with secondary necrosis.[1]

At one time, sonographic demonstration of pediatric ovaries was thought to be difficult, and normal mean ovarian volumes in patients under 10 years of age were reported to be as low as 0.7 cc.[27] However, we successfully imaged the ovaries in 64% of girls from birth to 2 years of age and in 78% of the ovaries of girls between 2 and 12 years.[7]

Concepts with regard to the sonographic analysis of the normal ovary for volume and echogenicity pattern have evolved over the last decade through the evaluation of both adults[28] and children.[7, 27] The once classic measurement of 3 x 2 x 1 cm (volume, 3 cc) is now recognized as underestimating the normal mean ovarian volume of 6—10 cc now reported in menstruating women. Mean volumes for premenarchal girls range between 0.75 and 4.18 cc.[21] Salardi et al. reported a statistically significant difference in ovarian size in children with Tanner 3 and higher stages of sexual development. These authors reported a volume of greater than 3 cc for Tanner 3; 4—4.6 cc for Tanner 4; and 5—7.5 cc for Tanner 5.[29] Golden and Cohen found the normal postpubertal ovarian volume to be 5.2 cc with a standard deviation

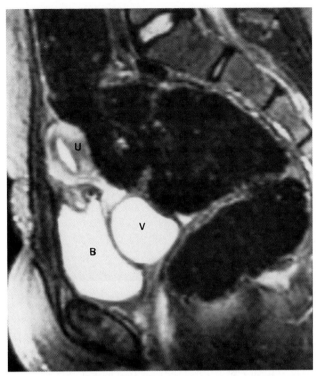

Figure 40–7 Vaginal obstruction as part of a mullerian duct anomaly. Sagittal T2-weighted MR image to the right of midline. The fluid-filled bladder (B) is noted anterior to the fluid-filled vagina (V) of a teenager with a didelphys uterus. This image shows only one of the two uteri (U) and vaginas; only one of the vaginas was obstructed.

of 2.7 cc.[30] Another study of women in their second decade found the mean ovarian volume to be 7.8 cc.[28]

At one time, the normal premenarchal ovary was typically described as homogeneously echogenic. The finding of follicles and/or cysts was thought to indicate menarche or near menarche. With improvements in sonographic resolution, normal premenarchal ovaries were found to usually be heterogeneous because of contained follicles and/or physiologic cysts (**Fig. 40–8**). Furthermore, it has been shown that follicle or cysts can be imaged throughout childhood.[17, 27] As a result, the presence of cysts does not help in differentiating between the normal child and the child with true isosexual precocious puberty. Microcysts (9 mm or less) can be demonstrated in as many as 72% of normal ovaries in children 2—6 years of age and in 68% of children 7—10 years of age. Even macrocysts (those greater than 9 mm) can be seen in premenarchal girls, although not as frequently as in postmenarchal girls.[27] These findings are consistent with reports in the pathology literature that have documented the presence of cystic follicles in the ovaries of fetuses, neonates, and children as well as adults.[31] One must conclude that ovarian follicles begin maturing at or before birth, and the pediatric ovary is a dynamic organ undergoing constant internal change.[17]

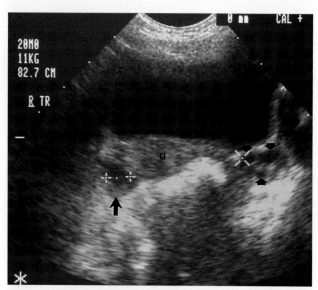

Figure 40–8 Normal premenarchal ovaries. Transverse plane. Follicles are seen in the ovaries of a normal 20-month-old girl. The largest follicle (**cursors**) in the right adnexa (**arrow**) measures 7 mm. Small arrows point to follicles in the left adnexa. Follicles are a normal finding, rather than a rarity, in premenarchal children. U, Uterus. Reprinted with permission from Imaging the pediatric pelvis: the normal and abnormal genital system and simulators of its diseases by HL Cohen, S Bober, S Bow. **Urol Radiol** 1992;14:273—283.

Table 40-1 Etiologies of Primary Amenorrhea (35)

Hypothalamus	Systemic illness
	Chronic disease
	Familial
	Stress
	Competitive athletics
	Eating disorders
	Obesity
	Drugs
Pituitary	Idiopathic hypopituitarism
	Tumor
	Hemochromatosis
Thyroid Gland	Hypothyroidism
	Hyperthyroidism
Adrenal Glands	Congenital adrenocortical hyperplasia
	Adrenal tumor
Ovaries	Gonadal dysgenesis
	Ovarian failure
	Polycystic ovary syndrome
	Ovarian tumor
Cervix	Agenesis
Vagina	Agenesis
	Transverse Septum
Hymen	Imperforate

Reprinted with permission from Pediatric Adolescent Gynecology by S. Emans, Goldstein D. Boston: Little Brown, 1990, p. 149—242.

Other Sonographic Techniques

Technologic advances in sonographic equipment over the last decade probably account for the more accurate imaging of premenarchal ovaries. The use of transvaginal (TV) imaging and, in virginal and other select patients, transperineal scanning, as well as the greater sensitivity of duplex and color Doppler imaging (CDI) have improved imaging of the female pelvis.[17] Transvaginal US has replaced the "water enema" technique in nonvirginal adults, although the latter technique is occasionally used for children. In the "water enema" technique, fluid is placed into the rectum by syringe injection through a foley catheter. This allows one to rule out a pseudomass (or pseudouterus) formed by air and stool within the bowel which can simulate a normal uterus. The "water enema" method can confirm the absence of a uterus, which is important information in the workup of patients with ambiguous genitalia and amenorrhea. In transvaginal US, a high-frequency transducer is placed into the upper vagina to evaluate adjacent pelvic structures. Transvaginal US has proven exceptionally valuable in the identification of early intrauterine and ectopic pregnancies and in the analysis of adnexal masses related to neoplasm or pelvic inflammatory disease (PID). Color Doppler imaging can be a useful adjunct in the evaluation of ectopic pregnancy, by showing the high-velocity, low-impedance color flow that can be seen at times in the wall of a viable ectopic gestational sac. It can also be used in the evaluation of ovarian and uterine flow.[17, 32]

Transperineal US or translabial sonography is performed by placing a transducer, covered by a glove or sheath containing gel, onto the introitus. This method has been used successfully to identify placenta previa in the late third trimester when transvaginal US may be less desirable.[33] In children and adolescents, transperineal US has been used to image vaginal outflow obstruction, usually caused by an intact hymen.[34]

Amenorrhea — Clinical and Laboratory Assessment

Sonographic evaluation of the adolescent pelvis is used for the diagnosis of both primary and secondary amenorrhea. It is also indicated if there is delayed or retarded sexual development, lower abdominal pain, and/or a pelvic mass.[1] There is an overlap in the clinical presentations and imaging findings among patients with amenorrhea. Most of the conditions that cause delay in pubertal development may cause primary or secondary amenorrhea.[35] Primary amenorrhea has many causes involving several organ systems (**Table 40-1**). It may be seen in adolescents with normal pubertal development as well as in those with delayed sexual development, delayed menarche, and some pubertal development, or delayed menarche, plus virilization.[2, 35]

Careful medical histories should be obtained from patients with amenorrhea and should include a neonatal history (e.g., maternal hormone ingestion or androgen-producing tumor may account for virilization; neonatal hypoglycemia may suggest hypopituitarism). Growth data during childhood and a history of prior surgery, irradiation, or chemotherapy, eating disorders or other psychological difficulty should be sought. The historical evaluation should also include a family history. Relevant information includes ages at menarche and a history of endocrine-related abnormalities, such as congenital adrenocortical hyperplasia, ovarian tumors, and thyroiditis.

Physical examination should rule out a visual field disturbance or neurologic findings that suggest pituitary or other CNS disease. A pelvic exam should include a vaginal smear and direct mucosal visualization. Red, thin vaginal mucosa is consistent with estrogen deficiency, while pink, moist vaginal mucosa is consistent with normal estrogenization. In pubertal patients, a pregnancy test should be done to rule out pregnancy as a cause of amenorrhea.[2, 35]

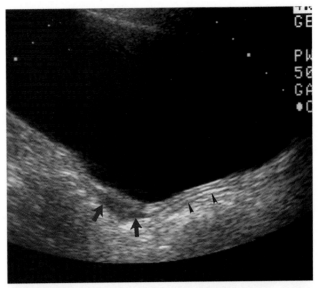

Figure 40–9 Infantile uterus in an 22-year-old woman with delayed puberty. Longitudinal midline plane. A small, premenarchal or infantile appearing uterus with a tubular shape (**arrows**) is noted posterior to a large fluid-filled bladder. Uterus length is 3.2 cm. **Arrowheads** outline the vagina.

Amenorrhea with Delayed Sexual Development

Sexual development is considered delayed if there is a lack of breast budding by age 13 years. Lack of pubertal development by 13 years is 2 standard deviations beyond normal and should be evaluated. Workup may be delayed for a year if there is a known debilitating illness or if the patient is involved in competitive or endurance sports such as running or ballet. Any interruption in sexual development is also a cause for concern and an endocrinologic workup should be performed. Only 0.03% of patients who do not undergo menarche by 15.5 years will develop it later.[35] Patients with primary amenorrhea typically have an infantile uterus with a small fundus, rather than an adult uterus (**Fig. 40–9**). These hypoestrogenic patients can be divided into two major groups, depending on their levels of gonadotropin (i.e., FSH, LH) production.[1, 2]

Hypogonadotropic Hypogonadism

Hypogonadotropic hypogonadism, characterized by low to normal LH, FSH levels, suggests pituitary or hypothalamic dysfunction as the cause of amenorrhea.[35] High prolactin levels suggest a pituitary cause of hypogonadotropic amenorrhea, while low prolactin levels suggest hypothalamic suppression of the pituitary.[2] Pituitary dysfunction may be the result of child abuse or head trauma leading to disruption of the pituitary stalk (usually with associated panhypopituitarism), tumors

such as craniopharyngiomas (often presenting with visual field disturbances, headaches, and behavioral changes), pituitary microadenomas, infiltrative diseases of the pituitary, or prolactinomas. Causes of hypothalamic dysfunction include hypothalamic tumors and Kallmann's disease (a lack of pulsatile release of gonadotropin-releasing hormone, associated with anosmia and, at times, midline craniofacial anomalies). Other "central" disorders, such as systemic illness or extreme physical, psychologic, or nutritional stress can also disrupt production of gonadotropin-releasing hormone. Systemic illnesses associated with such a disruption include chronic diseases, such as cystic fibrosis, sickle cell disease, and Crohn's disease (**Fig. 40–10**), endocrinopathies associated with pubertal delay include hypothyroidism, Cushing's disease and diabetes mellitus.[1, 2, 35, 36]

Anorexia nervosa, associated with the "fear of obesity," is also a central cause of amenorrhea. This condition is seen at a younger age than typical cases of anorexia. It can present as primary, but, more often presents as secondary amenorrhea after the development of secondary sexual characteristics. Amenorrhea associated with anorexia nervosa usually occurs when weight loss is greater than 20% of normal body weight. Sobanski et al. reported that anorexic patients had ovaries that were significantly smaller than expected for their age. Furthermore, those patients who recovered from anorexia had significantly greater ovarian volumes than those patients who did not recover. Sobanski suggested that sonographic measurements of ovarian volumes could be useful to determine the target weight required for recovery of ovarian function and a resumption of menses.[37]

Involvement in endurance sports is another central cause of amenorrhea. This form of amenorrhea may be due to alteration in diet or increased energy expenditures. Anomalies, injuries, or infections of the CNS including brain abscesses, tuberculosis, and prior cranial radiotherapy are associated with delayed sexual

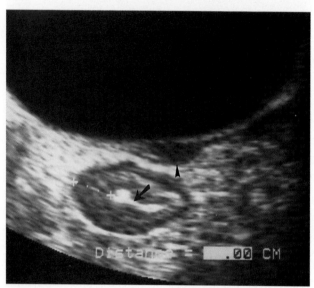

Figure 40–10 Amenorrhea in a patient with Crohn's disease. Transverse plane, right of midline. A thickened bowel wall (**calipers**), consistent with Crohn's disease, is seen posterior to the right adnexa (**arrowhead**). The bright area (arrow) noted eccentrically within the bowel is lumenal air. Amenorrhea or delayed puberty may be due to many chronic diseases.

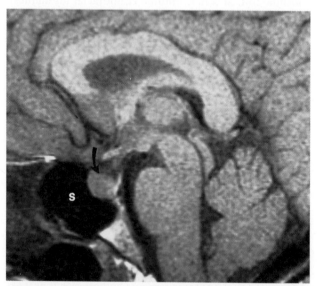

Figure 40–11 Pituitary adenoma. T1-weighted, midline sagittal image after gadolinium injection. A pituitary adenoma (**arrow**) is seen within the sella turcica of a young adult with headaches. The pituitary microadenoma is the most common pituitary tumor associated with amenorrhea. It is characteristically hypointense compared to the remainder of the pituitary on enhanced images. S, sphenoid sinus.

development. Evaluation of amenorrhea caused by central nervous system pathology (usually pituitary or hypothalamic) is best done by computed tomography (CT) or MRI (**Fig. 40–11**). The role of sonography in these patients is the determination of the size of the reproductive organs; this information provides support for the diagnosis of primary or secondary amenorrhea.

Hypergonadotropic Hypogonadism

Adolescents with hypergonadotropic hypogonadism, characterized by high FSH and high LH levels, have amenorrhea secondary to failure of the gonadal tissues to respond to endogenous gonadotropins. In pure forms, there will be failure of development of secondary sexual characteristics as well as amenorrhea. Hypergonadotropic amenorrhea also may be due to an abnormal karyotype such as Turner's syndrome or XY gonadal dysgenesis. Patients with normal karyotypes may have secondary ovarian failure due to radiation (usually 800 rads or greater to the pelvis), chemotherapy (transient amenorrhea occurs in 50% of women who undergo chemotherapy), or autoimmune oophoritis. Patients with these secondary causes of hypogonadotropic hypogonadism have varying degrees of pubertal development.[35, 38, 39]

Turner's syndrome, the most common human chromosomal abnormality, is also the most common example of gonadal dysgenesis associated with an abnormal karyotype. Half the patients are isochromatous, 45 X0. The remaining patients with Turner's syndrome may have a mosaic 45 X or 46 XX karyotype or have a structural abnormality of their second X chromosome. These patients present with a spectrum of clinical manifestations ranging from normal development to the classic stigmata of the pure 45 XO karyotype. Those patients who have an isochromosome of the short arm of one of the X chromosomes may have associated Hashimoto's thyroiditis.[2, 35]

Patients with classic Turner's Syndrome are short in stature and often have widely spaced nipples, a shield chest, low set ears, cubitus valgus, lymphedema, a high arched palette, a low hairline, short fourth and/or fifth metacarpals, large aortic roots, multiple pigmented nevi, and a webbed neck. One-fourth of patients have renal anomalies, usually horseshoe kidneys. Affected patients typically have a history of delayed onset of puberty and primary amenorrhea. In early adolescence, patients with Turner's syndrome have prepubertal genitalia, sparse axillary and pubic hair, and bilateral streak gonads. They have a normally formed uterus and vagina that will respond to exogenous hormones. In later adolescence, at around 15—16 years, many of these patients will develop pubic and axillary hair, but have no breast development or vaginal mucosal estrogenization.

Sonographic evaluation characteristically shows a prepubertal uterus (**Fig. 40–12**). The typical dysgenetic or streak gonads are difficult to image. The adnexa typically measure less than 1 cc, and, pathologically, there is oocyte depletion. Shawker et al. noted that some patients with Turner's syndrome, particularly those with mosaic karyotpyes, had normal ovaries. Such patients may have only partial ovarian failure and consequently the ovaries may be able to produce estrogen. Estrogen production in patients with Turner's syndrome also can be secondary to an associated theca lutein cyst or a germ cell tumor. If the karyotype of a patient with gonadal dysgenesis and ovaries includes a Y chromosome, there is an increased risk for the development of gonadoblastoma within the dysgenetic ovary. Evidence of asymmetrically sized, solid adnexa on sonography should arouse suspicion of a malignancy.[1, 2, 35, 40]

Pseudohermaphroditism

Sonography has been shown to be helpful in the evaluation of children whose karyotype, gonadal anatomy, and genital development are not in accord. This group of patients includes true hermaphrodites (a rare phenomenon), pseudohermaphrodites (also known as male and female intersex), and patients with mixed gonadal dysgenesis and testicular feminization syndrome.[1] Female pseudohermaphroditism (intersex) is a condition in which chromosomally normal females (46 XX) have masculinized external genitalia. It is usually diagnosed in the neonatal period and is most often due to adrenal hyperplasia, which is often congenital. Occasionally, however, it results from maternal ingestion of androgens in early pregnancy or less frequently from endogenous production of androgens by a masculinizing ovarian tumor in the mother. Sonography can depict the enlarged adrenal glands as well the presence of a normal uterus. These patients are potentially fertile after satisfactory genital reconstruction.[1, 19]

Male pseudohermaphrodites (male intersex) may present with findings of hypergonadotropic amenorrhea. Some patients may have incomplete testosterone production, while others with early destruction or dysgenesis of the testes will have no production of testosterone. Decreased testosterone levels and a lack of production of mullerian inhibition factor result in a karyotypically normal male with a female phenotype (except for partial masculinization of the external genitalia). There is variable development of the mullerian elements, such as the uterus, vagina, and fallopian tubes. These patients have no secondary sexual development at puberty and may have an infantile uterus on sonography.[1, 14]

An unusual form of intersex is the testicular feminization syndrome in which patients have 46 XY karyotypes and well-formed testes (usually undescended within the abdomen or inguinal region) that produce androgens and mullerian inhibition factor, but they lack an end organ response to androgens. Mullerian system development is inhibited, and, therefore, affected patients do not develop a uterus, fallopian tubes, or upper two-thirds of the vagina. Patients are phenotypically normal females, although they may have inguinal or labial masses due to the undescended testes. They have normal breast development (i.e., secondary female sexual characteristics) due to circulating estrogens (produced by the testes and adrenal gland) and a peculiar lack of body hair. Typically, patients present with amenorrhea. Ultrasonography fails to show the presence of either a uterus (**Fig. 40–13**) or ovaries.[1, 41]

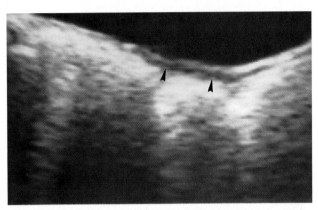

Figure 40–12 Turner's Syndrome in a teenager with delayed puberty. Midline longitudinal plane. An infantile uterus (**arrowheads**) is seen in this 15.5-year-old girl with a 45 X0 karyotype. Her ovaries could not be definitively imaged.

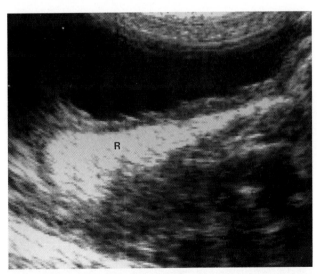

Figure 40–13 Testicular feminization syndrome. Midline longitudinal view. No uterus could be imaged in a phenotypically normal 17-year-old female who was raised as such and presented with amenorrhea. She proved to have a 45 XY karyotype with complete androgen insensitivity (i.e., testicular feminization syndrome). Echogenic air in the rectosigmoid region (R) facilitates demonstration of the absence of a uterus which normally should be seen between the bowel and the bladder wall (B). Reprinted with permission from Imaging the pediatric pelvis: the normal and abnormal genital system and simulators of its diseases by HL Cohen, S Bober, S Bow. **Urol Radiol** 1992;14:273.-283.

Female Adolescence with Virilization

Testosterone is the most potent of the circulating androgens. It is produced in normal females by the adrenal gland (25%), the ovaries (25%) and peripheral conversion of delta-4-androstenedione (50%). Only 1% is typically free and biologically active. Virilization from excess androgens produces voice deepening, clitorimegaly, increased muscle mass, and temporal balding. Testosterone-producing adrenal tumors rarely result in amenorrhea in adolescent patients.

Amenorrhea and virilization can occur in a patient with a hormonally active androgen-producing tumor. Increased free testosterone may be seen in virilizing tumors of the adolescent ovary. These are usually Sertoli-Leydig cell tumors (once known as androblastomas or arrhenoblastomas) or hilar cell tumors. The marked androgen production of these rare rapidly growing tumors results in amenorrhea, vaginal mucosal atrophy, decreased breast size, and virilization. Sonography will show a unilaterally enlarged solid ovary with abnormal echogenicity.[1,2,35,42]

Only one in 20 ovarian tumors have functional endocrine activity. The most common hormonally active malignant tumor of the ovary is the estrogen-producing granulosa cell tumor. These tumors grow rapidly and often disrupt the normal menstrual cycle, producing either amenorrhea or menorrhagia. Thecomas can also result in significant estrogen production.[2]

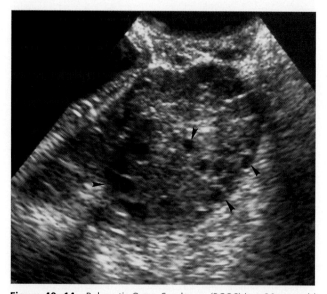

Figure 40–14 Polycystic Ovary Syndrome (PCOS) in a 20-year-old woman with hirsutism, obesity, and oligomenorrhea. Transvaginal US. Transverse oblique plane. This right ovary is enlarged and contains more than 10 follicles which measure less than 8 mm in diameter. The left ovary had a similar appearance. Arrowheads point to a few of the follicles. The area of bright echogenicity (**arrowhead**) in the middle of the ovary may represent increased ovarian stroma found in patients with PCOS.

Polycystic Ovary Syndrome

Androgen excess may result from causes unrelated to tumors. It may occur in association with idiopathic hirsutism, late-onset congenital adrenal hyperplasia, exaggerated adrenarche, Cushing's disease, hyperprolactinemia, and acromegaly. However, most hyperandrogenic adolescents will have polycystic ovary syndrome (PCOS), also known as Stein Leventhal syndrome.[43] Polycystic ovary syndrome is the most common cause of secondary amenorrhea associated with a hyperandrogenic state. Patients with this syndrome are usually 15—30 years of age and present with hirsutism (62%) and obesity (31%).[1] In a study of 466 women with PCOS, only 80% had menstrual irregularities.[2,43]

Laboratory confirmation of PCOS is based on the demonstration of an increased ratio of LS to FSH and elevated androstenedione levels.[45] The sonographic criteria for diagnosing PCOS are variable, irrespective of whether patients are examined by transabdominal or transvaginal ultrasonography.[46] Patients with PCOS often have an increased number of subcapsular follicles as well as enlarged, hyperechoic ovaries. (**Fig. 40–14**).

Herter et al. reported that ovarian volumes of greater than 10 cc in adolescent girls with menstrual disorders and/or hirsutism are suggestive of PCOS.[48] Takahashi et al. noted mean ovarian volumes of 10.3 cc in 47 affected patients, a volume significantly greater than those of a control group. In their study, 94% of the patients with PCOS had either an ovarian volume greater than 6.2 cc or had more than 10 follicles ranging between 2 and 8 mm in diameter. Only 6% of patients had a normal number of follicles and ovarian volume.[46] Increased ovarian echogenicity has been attributed to ovarian stromal hypertrophy, which is thought to be secondary to hyperandrogenism. Compared with normal ovaries, ovaries with stromal hypertrophy have larger volumes and lower vascular resistance in their arteries, resulting in low-resistive indices.[45] High-resistive indices are noted in the uterine arteries due to high androstenedione levels.[47]

Not all polycystic ovaries are due to hyperandrogenism. Unopposed estrogen stimulation from any source can result in polycystic ovaries. Genetic deficiencies of the enzymes 21-hydroxylase, 3-beta-hydroxysteroid dehydrogenase, or 11-beta hydroxylase are also associated with the development of polycystic ovaries.[1]

Eugonadism Estrogenization: Vaginal Obstruction

The absence of menses after development of secondary sexual characteristics suggests late disruption of the hypothalamic-pituitary-ovarian-uterine axis or outflow (uterine or vaginal) obstruction.[2] When a solid midline mass is discovered in an adolescent girl with amenorrhea, one must consider the possibility of a distended uterus (metra) or vagina (colpos) or combination of the two. Hematometrocolpos occurs in 1 in 1000—2000 teenagers.

Postmenarchal females with vaginal or uterine obstruction can present with a history of intermittent monthly abdominal or pelvic pain and no history of menses or with an abdominal mass. The degree of distention of the uterus/vagina is related to the degree of obstruction and the time that has elapsed between menarche and the diagnosis. The hematometrocolpos may be large enough to obstruct venous or lymphatic flow in the lower extremities or cause hydronephrosis due to obstruction of the ureters or bladder. Occasionally, patients have a history of difficulty with micturition.

Sonographic or MRI imaging of the vagina, cervix, and uterus helps provide important presurgical anatomical information.[1,6,14,17] On sonographic examination, hematometrocolpos (Fig. 40–15) appears as a distended midline tubular structure between the bladder and the rectum, containing fluid with variable echogenicity. The wall of the uterus is thicker than that of the ovary (due to normally thick myometrial layer). The scattered echoes in the fluid are due to cellular debris, mucoid material, and/or blood.

Hematometrocolpos is caused by an imperforate hymen in two-thirds of patients with otherwise normal pelvic anatomy. In the remaining patients, the obstruction may be due to a complete vaginal membrane, vaginal stenosis, or vaginal atresia. Transverse perineal US may define the thickness of the imperforate hymen (Fig. 40–16).[34] Vaginal outlet obstruction from causes

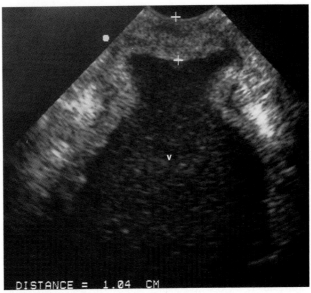

Figure 40–16 Hematometrocolpos. Transperineal technique. A transducer placed on the perineum of a teenager with imperforate hymen and hematometrocolpos shows a membrane (**cursors**) measuring 1.04 cm in thickness superficial to the distended, fluid-filled vagina. The vagina contains echogenic (hemorrhagic) debris. v, vagina.

other than an imperforate hymen have been associated with anomalies of the gastrointestinal tract, genitourinary tract, and cardiovascular and skeletal systems.[1,17]

When only hematometra is present, one must consider a more unusual abnormality such as cervical dysgenesis or obstruction of one horn in a bicornuate system. It can be more difficult to make a diagnosis when there is obstruction of only one uterine horn or one

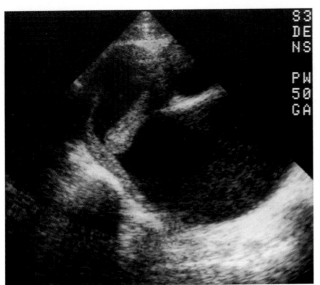

A

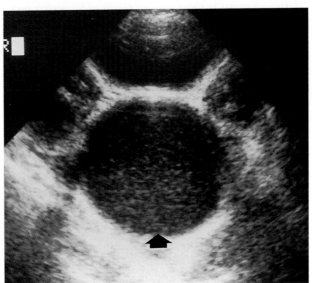

B

Figure 40–15 Hematometrocolpos. **A:** Longitudinal midline plane. There is echogenic (hemorrhagic) debris within the fluid-filled and dilated vagina (V) and uterus (U) of this 14-year-old girl with hematometrocolpos due to an imperforate hymen. An open arrow points to the thick uterine wall; by comparison, the wall of the distended vagina is thin. Reprinted with permission from Imag-

ing the pediatric pelvis: the normal and abnormal genital system and simulators of its diseases by HL Cohen, S Bober, S Bow. **Urol Radiol** 1992;14:273—283. **B:** Pelvic US. Transverse plane. An **arrow** points to the distended, debris-filled vagina of another teenager with hematometrocolpos due to an imperforate hymen.

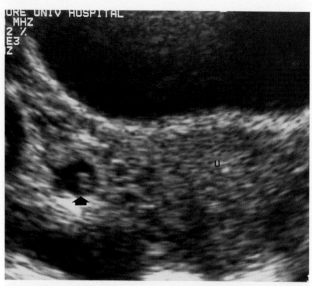

Figure 40–17 Ectopic pregnancy. Transverse plane. An arrow points to the ectopic gestational sac in the right adnexa of a 16-year-old girl with amenorrhea. No intrauterine pregnancy was noted. u, uterus.

vagina in a duplicated genital system (**Fig. 40–7**). Urometrocolpos has been reported in patients with ectopic ureters implanting in the vagina proximal to the site of obstruction.[1, 6, 14, 17]

Amenorrhea due to Uterine Aplasia or Hypoplasia

Fifteen percent of primary amenorrhea cases are thought to be due to absence or hypoplasia of the uterus. Uterine agenesis is most often a result of testicular feminization or the Mayer-Rokitansky-Kuster-Hauser syndrome. Mayer-Rokitansky-Kuster-Hauser syndrome patients have amenorrhea due to vaginal atresia with variable uterine abnormalities. They have a normal female karyotype and normal secondary sexual characteristics. Despite an absent or severely atretic uterus and vagina, the ovaries and the fallopian tubes are normal. Approximately 50% of patients have unilateral renal anomalies, and one-eighth have skeletal abnormalities.[1, 17, 49]

Secondary Amenorrhea

Secondary amenorrhea is amenorrhea that occurs after menses has been established. The conditions that cause delayed puberty and primary amenorrhea also may cause secondary amenorrhea.

Pregnancy is the most common cause of secondary amenorrhea in girls older than 9 years of age. As little as a 2- to 3-week delay in menses should raise a clinical concern for pregnancy and the need to perform a pregnancy test.[35] Ultrasonography is most effective in the diagnosis of suspected pregnancy. Transvaginal sonography allows an earlier and more accurate diagnosis of pregnancy, whether intrauterine or extrauterine (ectopic) in location (**Fig. 40–17**).

To be complete, another cause of secondary amenorrhea is Asherman's syndrome. This disorder, which is unusual in adolescence, follows intrauterine instrumentation, such as endometrial curettage. Deep curettage with denudation of the basalis layer of the endometrium is thought to interfere with normal endometrial regeneration. The inability to regenerate endometrium allows the formation of adhesions in the endometrial cavity. Not only is Asherman's syndrome a cause of amenorrhea, but it can also cause hypomenorrhea, sterility, or habitual abortions.[50]

Conclusion

The normal menstrual cycle and female reproductive physiology are marvels of complexity that depend on the integrated actions of several body systems. The intricacies of menses are not completely understood. Multiple factors have a role in menarche and in regulating the menstrual cycle; these include embryologic, genetic (karyotype), anatomic and endocrinologic factors, along with psychological and other, as of yet, not clearly understood factors. Imaging is only one part of the workup of patients with amenorrhea, but the information provided by imaging is vital. Ultrasonography is the key tool for screening patients with amenorrhea and is often the only imaging tool necessary for the pelvic evaluation of such patients.

References

1. Cohen HL, Haller JO. Pediatric and adolescent genital abnormalities. *Clin Diag Ultrasound* 1988;24:187—216.
2. Reid R. Amenorrhea. In: Copeland L, ed. *Textbook of Gynecology*. Philadelphia, Pa: WB Saunders, 1993, p. 367—387.
3. Emans S, Goldstein D. The physiology of puberty. In: Emans S, Goldstein D, eds. *Pediatric & Adolescent Gynecology*, 3rd ed. Boston, Ma: Little Brown, 1990, p. 95—124.
4. Haller J, Fellows R. The pelvis. *Clin Diag Ultrasound* 1983;8:65—185.
5. Ganong W. The gonads: development and function of the reproductive system. In: Ganong W. *Review of Medical Physiology*, 17th ed. Norwalk, CT: Appleton & Lange, 1995, p. 399—402.
6. Eldering J, Nay M, Hoberg L, Longcope C, McKracken J. Hormonal regulation of prostaglandin production by rhesus monkey endometrium. *J Clin Endocrinol Metab* 1990, 71:596—604.
7. Cohen HL, Shapiro M, Mandel F, Shapiro M. Normal ovaries in neonates and infants: a sonographic study of 77 patients 1 day to 24 months old. *AJR* 1993;160:583—586.
8. Conte F, Grumbach M, Kaplan S. A diphasic pattern of gonadotropin secretion in patients with the syndrome of

gonadal dysgenesis. *J Clin Endocrinol Metab* 1975;40:670—674.

9. Doring G. The incidence of anovular cycles in women. *J Reprod Fertil (Suppl)* 1967;6:77—81.

10. Rosenfeld R, Garcia C. A comparison of endometrial histology with simultaneous plasma progesterone determinations in infertile women. *Fertil Steril* 1976;27:1256—1266.

11. Sherman B, Korenman S. Hormonal characteristics of the human menstrual cycle throughout reproductive life. *J Clin Invest* 1975;55:699—706.

12. Tanner J, Davies P. Reply: pubertal data for growth velocity charts. *J Pediatr* 1986;109:564—565.

13. Bullough V. Age at menarche. A misunderstanding. *Science* 1981;213:365—366.

14. Cohen HL, Bober S, Bow S. Imaging the pediatric pelvis: the normal and abnormal genital system and simulators of its diseases. *Urol Radiol* 1992;14:273—283.

15. Grimes C, Rosenbaum D, Kirkpatrick J Jr. *Sem Roentgenol* 1982;17:284—301.

16. Moore K. *Before We Are Born. Basic Embryology and Birth Defects*, 3rd ed. Philadelphia, PA: WB Saunders 1989, p. 180.

17. Cohen HL. The female pelvis. In: Siebert J, ed. *Syllabus: Current Concepts: A Categorical Course in Pediatric Radiology.* Chicago, IL: RSNA Publications 1994, p. 65—72.

18. Rosenberg H, Sherman N, Tarry W, Duckett J, Snyder H. Mayer-Rokitansky-Kuster-Hauser Syndrome: US aid to diagnosis. *Radiology* 1986;161:815—819.

19. Goldman H, Eaton D. Pediatric uroradiology. In: Elkin M, ed. *Radiology of the Urinary System.* Boston, Ma: Little Brown, 1980, p. 1034—1109.

20. Nussbaum AR, Sanders RC, Jones MD. Neonatal uterine morphology as seen on real-time US. *Radiology* 1986;160:641—643.

21. Orsini L, Salardi S, Pilu G, Bovicelli L, Cacciari E. Pelvic organs in premenarchal girls: real-time ultrasonography. *Radiology* 1984;153: 113—116.

22. Eisenberg P, Cohen HL, Mandel F, et al. US analysis of premenarchal gynecologic structures. *J Ultrasound Med* 1991;10:S30.

23. Deutsch A, Gosink B. Normal female pelvic anatomy. *Sem Roentgenol* 1982;17:241—250.

24. Forrest T, Elyaderani M, Muilenburg M, et al. Cyclic endometrial changes: US assessment with histologic correlation. *Radiology* 1988;167:233—237.

25. Carrington B, Hricak H, Nuruddin R, et al. Mullerian duct anomalies: MR imaging evaluation. *Radiology* 1990;176:715—720.

26. Popovich M, Hricak H. Magnetic resonance imaging in the evaluation of gynecologic disease. In: Callen P, ed. *Ultrasonography in Obstetrics and Gynecology,* 3rd ed. Philadelphia, PA: WB Saunders, 1994, p. 660—688.

27. Cohen HL, Eisenberg P, Mandel F, Haller J. Ovarian cysts are common in premenarchal girls: a sonographic study of 101 children 2—12 years old. *AJR* 1992;159:89—91.

28. Cohen HL, Tice H, Mandel F. Ovarian volumes measured by US: bigger than we think. *Radiology* 1990;177:189—92.

29. Salardi S, Orsini L, Cacciari E, et al. Pelvic ultrasonography in premenarchal girls: relation to puberty and sex hormone concentrations. *Arch Dis Child* 1985;60:120—125.

30. Golden N, Cohen H, Gennari G, Neuhoff S. The use of ultrasonography in the evaluation of adolescents with pelvic inflammatory disease. *Am J Dis Child* 1987;141:1235—1238.

31. Polhemus D. Ovarian maturation and cyst formation in children. *Pediatrics* 1953;11:588—594.

32. Pellerito J, Taylor K, Quedens-Case C, et al. Ectopic pregnancy: evaluation with endovaginal color imaging. *Radiology* 1992;183:407—411.

33. Hertzberg BS, Bowie J, Carroll BA, Kliewer M, Weber T. Diagnosis of placenta previa during the third trimester: role of transperineal sonography. *AJR* 1992;159:83—87.

34. Scanlan K Pozniak M, Fagerholm M, Shapiro S. Value of transperineal sonography in the assessment of vaginal atresia. *AJR* 1990;154:545—548

35. Emans S, Goldstein D. Delayed puberty and menstrual irregularities. In: Emans S, Goldstein D, eds. *Pediatric & Adolescent Gynecology.* 3rd ed. Boston, MD: Little Brown, 1990, p. 149—242.

36. Falsetti L, Pasinetti E, Mazzani M, Gastaldi A. Weight loss and menstrual cycle: clinical and endocrinological evaluation. *Gynecol Endocrinol* 1992;6:49—56.

37. Sobanski E, Hiltmann WD, Blanz B, Klein M, Schmidt MH. Pelvic ultrasound scanning of the ovaries in adolescent anorectic patients at low weight and after weight recovery. *Eur Child Adolesc Psych* 1997;6:207—211.

38. Stillman R, Schinfeld J, Schiff I, et al. Ovarian failure in long-term survivors of childhood malignancy. *Am J Obstet Gynecol* 1981;139:62—66.

39. Bookman M, Longo D, Young R. Late complications of curative treatment in Hodgkin's disease. *JAMA* 1988;260:680—683.

40. Shawker T, Garra B, Loriaux, Cutler G, Ross J. Ultrasonography of Turner's syndrome. *J Ultrasound Med* 1986;5:125—129.

41. Shah R, Woolley M, Costin G. Testicular feminization syndrome: the androgen insensitivity syndrome. *J Ped Surg* 1992;27:757—760.

42. Larsen W, Felmar E, Wallace M, Frieder R. Sertoli-Leydig cell tumor of the ovary: a rare cause of amenorrhea. *Obstet Gynecol* 1992;79:831—833.

43. Rosenfield R. Hyperandrogenism in peripubertal girls. *Pediatr Clin North Am* 1990;37:1333—1358.

44. Goldzieher J, Green J. The polycystic ovary: I. Clinical and histologic features. *J Cin Endocrinol Metab* 1962;22:325—338.

45. Battaglia C, Artini P, D'Ambrogio G, Genazzani AN, Genazzani AR. The role of color Doppler imaging in the diagnosis of polycystic ovary syndrome. *Am J Obstet Gynecol* 1995;172:108—113.

46. Takahashi K, Okada M, Ozaki T, et al. Transvaginal ultrasonographic morphology in polycystic ovarian syndrome. *Gyn Obstetr Invest* 1995;39:201—206.

47. Battaglia C, Artini PG, Genazzani AD, et al. Color Doppler analysis in olig- and amenorrheic women with polycystic ovary syndrome. *Gynecol Endocrinol* 1997;11:105—110.

48. Herter L, Magalnaes J, Spritzer P. Relevance of the determination of ovarian volumes in adolescent girls with menstrual disorders. *J Clin Ultrasound* 1996;24:243—248.

49. Rosenblatt M, Rosenblatt R, Kutcher R, Coupey S, Kleinhaus S. Utero-vaginal hypoplasia. sonographic, embryologic and clinical considerations. *Pediatr Radiol* 1991;21:536—537.

50. Daya S. Habitual abortion. In: Copeland L, ed. *Textbook of Gynecology.* Philadelphia, PA: WB Saunders, 1993, p. 204—230.

51. Cohen HL. Evaluation of the adolescent and young adult with amenorrhea: Role of US. *RSNA Special Course Ultrasound* 1996;171—183.

41 Neonatal Hip Dislocation

Henrietta Kotlus Rosenberg

Clinical Features

Congenital dislocation of the hip is now referred to as developmental dysplasia of the hip (DDH), a broader term which encompasses all the variants of the disorder including dislocation, subluxation, and dysplasia, whether they occur prenatally (congenitally) or postnatally.[1] DDH requires early diagnosis in order to institute appropriate treatment and ensure normal development.

The incidence of DDH is approximately 1.5 per 1000. The condition is four times more common in females than males, and there is a 6% incidence in newborns with a family history of DDH.[1—3] DDH is suspected clinically when physical examination reveals asymmetrical skin folds, a shortened thigh due to superior dislocation of the femur, limited abduction of less than 70 degrees with the hips in flexion, loss of the normal mild hip and knee flexion with the patient in a supine position, instability of the hip, a palpable "clunk" during the Ortolani reduction test (**Fig. 41–1**) (performed by flexing the hip 90 degrees and gently abducting), or by an abnormal Barlow dislocation test (**Fig. 41–2**) (performed by grasping the thigh, adducting

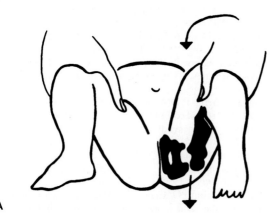
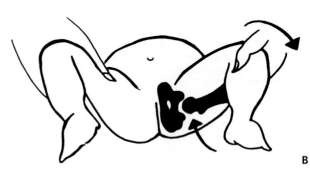

Figure 41–1 Physical examination: Ortolani's maneuver. **A,B:** Ortolani's maneuver attempts to reduce a dislocated hip. When the dislocated femoral head posses over the posterior labrum, it results in a palpable "clunk." (From Wenger DR. Developmental dysplasia of the hip. In: Wenger DR, Rang M, eds. **The Art and Practice of Children's Orthopedics**. New York: Raven Press, 1993, pp. 256—296.

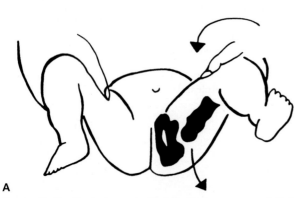
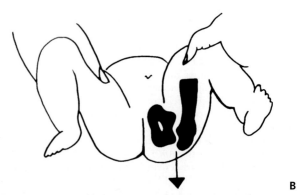

Figure 41–2 Physical examination: Barlow's maneuver. **A,B:** Barlow's maneuver attempts to dislocate an unstable hip. When the dislocatable femoral head passes over the posterior labrum, it results in a palpable "clunk." (From Wenger DR. Developmental dysplasia of the hip. In: Wenger DR, Rang M, eds. **The Art and Practice of Children's Orthopedics**. New York: Raven Press, 1993, pp. 256—296.

and exerting gentle downward pressure on the hip by pushing the knee posteriorly and superiorly, as in the functioning of a "piston"). Palpatory "clunks" have a low pitch which may be barely audible. "Clunks" should not be confused with "clicks" which have a high pitch and generally have no pathological significance. "Clicks" result from joint capsule and tendon stretching. Even in the best of hands, physical examination may be inaccurate, especially when the infant is not relaxed and crying. In infants with nonreducible dislocations due to muscle contraction and pseudoacetabulum formation, the Ortolani reduction test will be negative.[4]

DDH is thought to be due to abnormal laxity of the hip joint capsule, rather than a structural abnormality. Several mechanical and physiological factors predispose infants to DDH. Faulty intrauterine position of the fetus is an important risk factor in DDH. There is a 25% risk of DDH in babies with a breech presentation. The extension of the hips during birth tends to promote dislocation. The route of delivery (vaginal or Cesarean section) does not increase the risk of DDH.[5] Because fetuses tend to lie with their back to the maternal left side with the left thigh against the maternal sacrum, DDH tends to occur more frequently on the left. Oligohydramnios, which restricts the in-utero space, torticollis, foot deformities (metatarsus adductus or calcaneovalgus), and neuromuscular problems (spina bifida, arthrogryposis) also predispose to DDH (**Table 41–1**).[6] Excessive levels of circulating maternal estrogens are also thought to be important in DDH. Many newborns with DDH have elevated urine levels of estrogen and estradiol 17B, supporting the importance of maternal estrogens as a factor in DDH. The presence of excess estrogen blocks the maturation of collagen by impairing the cross-linkage of fibrils.[7]

Imaging Workup

Before the discovery of X rays in 1895 by the German physicist Wilhelm Konrad Roentgen, the diagnosis and follow-up of patients with congenital dislocation of the hip (CDH) depended solely on the clinical judgment of the attending physician.[8,9] Plain film radiography made a tremendous impact on the management of these patients by providing, for the first time, a means of imaging the relevant bony structures. Although the hips can be positioned in several different ways during filming, including neutral, frog lateral, and stressed positions [e.g., Andrew von Rosen view (internal rotation, 45 degrees thigh abduction)], false negatives may result because of the inability to image the cartilaginous portions of the infant hip joint (**Fig. 41–3**). On the other hand, false positives may result from improper positioning and rotation of the pelvis. Nevertheless, there are several classic landmarks, lines, and measurements for the plain film diagnosis of CDH. These include the contour of the

Table 41–1 Risk factors for DDH

Abnormal clinical examination (hips instability, click, limited range of motion)
Family history of DDH (parent, sibling)
Breech presentation at birth
Postural deformities (firstborn, oligohydramnios, torticollis)
Foot deformities (metatarsus adductus, calcaneovalgus)
Neuromuscular problems (spina bifida, arthrogryposis)
Sacral dimple

acetabulae (rounded, shallow, steep) and the presence and symmetry of the ossification centers. However, the capital femoral epiphyses ossify between 3 and 6 months in females and between 4 and 7 months in males, limiting the usefulness of this criterion for the diagnosis of DDH in young infants. On older infants, delayed ossification can be an indication of hip dysplasia. The acetabular index (AI), which is an indication of the slope of the acetabular roof, is another indicator of dysplasia. The AI is normally less than 30 degrees, measuring 28 degrees in male, and 26 degrees in female newborns, 23 degrees in male and 20 degrees in female infants under 6 months of age, and 21 degrees in males and 19.8 degrees in female infants 1 year of age. Disruption of the normally curved Shenton's line, which courses from the superior aspect of the obturator foramen and the medial femoral neck to the lesser trochanter, also suggests hip dislocation. The position of the femoral head can be surmised by evaluating the intersection of Hilgenreiner's line (YY line drawn through comparable points of the triradiate cartilage) and its intersection with Perkin's line (line drawn through superior/lateral aspect of acetabulum perpendicular to the YY line). In the normally positioned hip, the femoral capital epiphysis primarily occupies the medial inferior quadrant formed by these two lines.

In the late 1960 s, contrast arthrography became part of the imaging armamentarium for suspected hip dysplasia and provided a means of more completely evaluating the femoral head and acetabular contours. Hip instability and the success of reduction following treatment could be shown as well as soft tissue abnormalities such as a thickened ligamentum teres, acetabular labrum inversion, fibrofatty tissue (pulvinar) in the dysplastic acetabulum, and "hourglass" constriction of the joint by the iliopsoas tendon. The problem with arthrography, especially in the pediatric population, is that it is an invasive technique that utilizes ionizing radiation and carries a degree of risk, including not only complications of the procedure such as infection or hemorrhage, but also those of anesthesia and heavy sedation. In addition, it is impractical for children who require serial or frequent investigations.

The advent of computed tomography (CT) in the 1970 s provided, for the first time, a means of obtaining

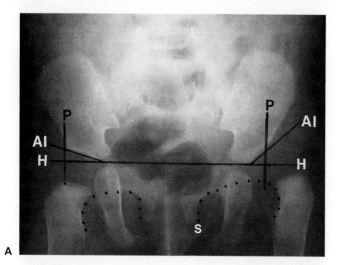

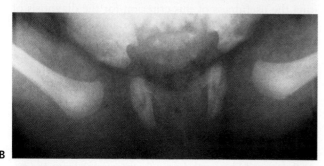

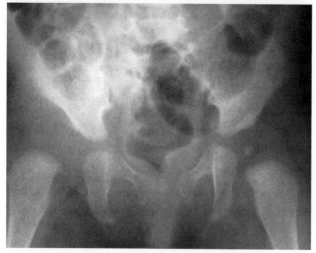

Figure 41–3   Plain film radiography of the hip. **A:** AP neutral view of infant hips and pelvis. The right hip is normally positioned in a nicely rounded acetabulum. The left hip is dislocated superolaterally; the acetabulum is dysplastic with a steep slope; and there is a hint of early pseudoacetabular formation superior to the upper lateral margin of the bony acetabulum. Note the disruption of Shenton's line (s). (H, Hilgenreiner's line, P, Perkin's line, AI, acetabular index). **B:** Frog lateral view of infant hips. In this infant with no evidence of DDH, the hips are normally articulated in abduction and external rotation with the cartilaginous femoral heads directed toward the triradiate cartilage. **C:** AP neutral view of hips and pelvis in 3-month old with asymmetric skin folds and clinical examination indicating dislocation of the right hip. The left hip is normally articulated with the developing ossification normally seated in a rounded acetabulum. The right femoral capital epiphysis is unossified and the right hip is dislocated superolaterally. The steep right acetabulum is poorly formed. A pseudoacetabulum is evident, and Shenton's line is disrupted.

cross-sectional images that could demonstrate the detailed anatomy of the hip joints in a noninvasive manner. However, the position of the cartilaginous portions of the femoral head and neck could only be inferred.[10] CT proved to be very useful to the orthopedic surgeon in planning the management of children with congenital hip dislocation in whom treatment was not instituted promptly and those in whom the result of treatment was not satisfactory. It is unnecessary in the management of the neonate or young infant with easily reducible congenital dislocation of the hip. CT requires the use of ionizing radiation and often requires sedation during the performance of the examination in young infants and children. It is, however, quite useful for the evaluation of concentricity of reduction after closed reduction, the detection of iliopsoas muscle deformity as a cause of failed closed reduction, the determination of the optimal time to perform surgery and the type of procedure, and the assessment of femoral torsion and acetabular configuration. Moreover, it can be performed even when the patient is in a cast.

The mid 1970s heralded the use of ultrasonography (US) as a practical tool for the evaluation of a wide gamut of pediatric abnormalities. Its potential for the evaluation of CDH was recognized by 1980 when the Austrian pediatric orthopedic surgeon Graf described an articulated arm scanning technique for the evaluation of the infant hip.[11–13] The 1980s heralded the arrival of high-resolution multiplanar real-time US, which proved to be reliable and accurate for the early diagnosis of congenital hip dislocation in the young infant.[14, 15] Both the cartilaginous femoral head and the acetabulum can be clearly seen without the use of ionizing radiation or the injection of contrast material and, in most patients, sedation is not necessary. Not only can detailed anatomy be demonstrated, but the hips can be observed as they are being maneuvered into neutral, flexed, stressed, and abducted positions. US is less useful once the secondary center of ossification exceeds 1 cm, as this bony structure can cause impedance of the ultrasound beam and the resultant shadowing of the US beam may mimic the triradiate cartilage and create confusing and possible spurious findings. It can be used in the operating room to guide hip reduction and postreduction, it can be used to examine the hip in a Pavlik harness, in traction, a brace, or a cast.[16, 17] A disadvantage of US that cannot be overemphasized is the fact that it is extremely operator-dependent.

In the mid-1980s, magnetic resonance imaging (MRI) was introduced as a nonionizing, noninvasive means of demonstrating exquisite anatomic detail of the clinically important soft-tissue and cartilaginous structures of the hip, even in casted patients.[18, 19] In addition, specific techniques have been developed to create an "arthrographic effect" by showing the synovial fluid. Sedation is generally necessary for the younger children, and it is not uncommon for older pediatric patients to complain of severe claustrophobia. In the mid-1990s, the alternative of "open" MRI has provided a more comfortable, although a slightly less detailed MRI examination.

Sonographic Techniques

Graf Technique

There are two major techniques available for examining the neonatal hip: the Graf technique and the dynamic technique. The Graf technique is based on a single direct coronal sonogram of the hip obtained with a linear-array transducer and the infant in the lateral decubitus position. The normal proximal femoral head appears as a round, hypoechoic speckled structure centered in the acetabulum.[11, 12] With this technique, three lines (A, B, and C) and two angles are drawn around the acetabulum and objective measurements of the depth of the acetabulum are made (**Fig. 41–4**).[13] The A line, the baseline of the "osseous convexity," connects the edge of the bony acetabulum to the point of insertion of the joint capsule to the periosteum. The B line, the "inclination line," connects the osseous convexity to the acetabular labrum. The C line, the "acetabular roof line," connects the lower edge of the acetabular roof medially to the osseous convexity.

The degree of acetabular convexity is determined by measuring the alpha angle which is formed by the intersection of lines A and C. In the normal hip, the alpha angle does not exceed 60 degrees; a small alpha angle indicates a shallow bony acetabulum. The angle of acetabular inclination is determined by measuring the beta angle which is formed by the intersection of line B and line A. This angle defines the position of the fibrocartilaginous labrum and also assesses how well the cartilaginous rim of the acetabulum covers the femoral head. It is considered normal when it is less than 55 degrees. An abnormally large beta angle indicates a laterally displaced femoral head.

Four basic hip types have been described based on the alpha and beta angles, the contour of the roof and the position of the femoral epiphysis relative to the acetabulum (concentric, subluxation, and/or dislocation (**Table 41–2**). Regardless of the type of hip pathology, the pathological process is always situated in the superior or in the superoposterior part of the acetabular roof.[20] The acetabulum is normal with a well-formed bony roof contour in types 1-A and I-B which are con-

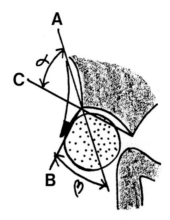

Figure 41–4 Graf technique: A, basic line; B, inclination line; C, line of acetabular roof (a angle characterizes osseous convexity, b angle characterizes the bone supplementing additional roofing by cartilaginous convexity).

sidered mature hips. In type I-A, the cartilaginous roof triangle is narrow extending far over the femoral head with the α angle > 60 degrees and the β angle < 55 degrees. In type I-B, the cartilaginous roof triangle is somewhat stubby, extending a short distance over the crown of the femoral head with the α angle > 60 degrees and the β angle > 55 degrees. Therapy is not required for types I-A and I-B. In II-A, the bony modeling of the acetabulum is normal, and the broad cartilaginous roof triangle covers the crown of the femoral head, but the α angle is smaller than normal (50—59 degrees), and the β angle is larger than normal (> 55 degrees). Although therapy is not required for type II-A, follow-up is necessary. Types II-B and II-C do require treatment with an abduction device. Types II-B and II-C are characterized by deficient bony modeling of the acetabulum with the broad cartilage roof triangle still covering the femoral head. The α angle varies from 50 to 59 degrees in type II-B and 43 to 49 degrees in type II-C, while the β angle is > 55 degrees and < 77 degrees respectively. The bony modeling of the acetabulum is highly deficient in type II-D with the cartilage roof triangle displaced, the α angle 43—49 degrees, the β angle >77 degrees, and the treatment is usually a reduction—abduction splint and eventually a plaster cast. This type of treatment is also necessary for the eccentric hips typed by Dr. Graf as III-A, III-B, and IV, all of which have poor bony modeling of the acetabulum, a angles < 43 and b angles > 77 degrees. In type III-A, the cartilage roof triangle is displaced and devoid of echoes, in III-B it is displaced and echogenic, and in type IV, it is trapped between the femoral head and the ilium.

Table 41–2 Sonographic acetabular morphology

Hip type	Alpha angle (degrees)	Beta angle (degrees)	Bony roof contour	Cartilaginous Rim
Type 1 A	60 or more	55 or less	Good	Narrow
Type 1 B	60 or more	55—77	Good	Covers head
Type 2	43—60	55—77	Satisfactory to deficient	Wide, covers head
Types 3/4	43 or less	77 or more	Poor	Wide, cranially displaced

The main points to be abstracted from Graf's work are that an angle > 60 degrees is normal at any age, an angle between 50 and 59 degrees can be normal in an infant younger than 3 months but requires follow-up, an angle between 50 and 59 degrees is abnormal in infants older than that, and an angle < 50 degrees is abnormal at any age.

Dynamic Technique

In 1984, Harcke et al.[15] demonstrated that a dynamic technique, which is now the most widely used technique, provides a reliable and accurate demonstration of the anatomic structures of the hip joint.[21] The dynamic technique allows classification of the relationship of the proximal femur with the acetabulum at rest and under stress.

Dynamic hip sonography should be performed with the highest possible frequency probe that permits penetration of the soft tissues. Usually a 7.5-MHz frequency transducer is adequate for infants under 3 months of age, a 5.0-MHz transducer for babies 3—7 months of age and a 3.0-MHz transducer for infants older than 7 months. Broadband linear-array probes are preferable. Because the examiner uses both hands for dynamic hip sonography, the ultrasound unit should be equipped with a foot pedal so that the examiner has personal control of which image will be frozen and then captured on hard or soft copy. For the left hip, it is recommended that the transducer be held in the right hand while the maneuvering of the hip is done with the left hand. The transducer is held with the left hand and the hip is positioned by the right hand when the right hip is examined. Although a linear transducer which covers a larger field of view and produces a rectangular image is preferable, the examination can be performed with a sector or curvilinear scanhead. Feeding the infant during the examination can increase patient comfort and cooperation.

With the dynamic Harcke approach, images are obtained with the child in a supine position and the transducer positioned over the lateral aspect of the hip. Both coronal and transverse images of the hips are essential components of the dynamic examination. The specific details, namely whether views need to be obtained in extension, flexion or both positions, is still somewhat controversial, and, in large part, depends on the preference of the examiner.[22, 23]. However, the minimal images include a coronal neutral view at rest, a coronal flexion view at rest, and transverse flexion view with stress (**Fig. 41–5** through **41–6**) (**Table 41–3**). At our institution, we believe that flexion views in both the transverse and coronal planes in three positions (neutral, adduction and abduction) are essential. Additionally, we obtain a coronal longitudinal view over the posterior lip of the acetabulum during stress maneuvers (**Table 41–4**). However, as noted above, the specific planes are variable and will depend on examiner experience and preference.

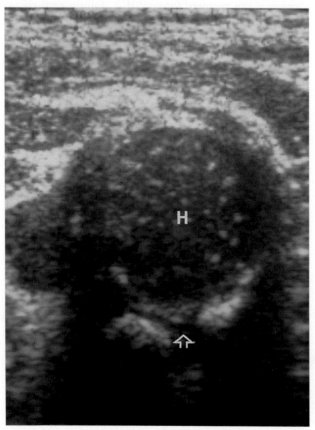

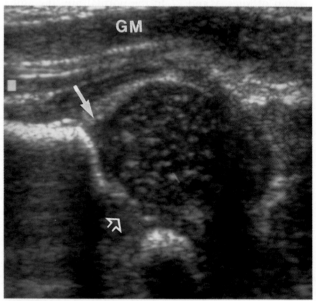

Figure 41–5   A: Transverse/neutral view of normal newborn hip: The well-rounded cartilaginous femoral head (H) is centered symmetrically above the triradiate cartilage (**open arrow**), through which there is increased sound transmission. **B:** Coronal/flexion view of normal newborn hip: The femoral head is well-seated in a nicely rounded acetabulum. The triradiate cartilage is noted by the **open arrow**. The cartilaginous labrum (**closed arrow**) and gluteal muscles (GM) appear normal (**open arrow)** joint capsule.

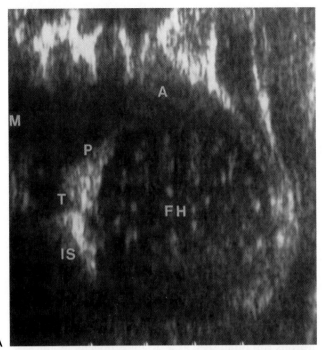

A

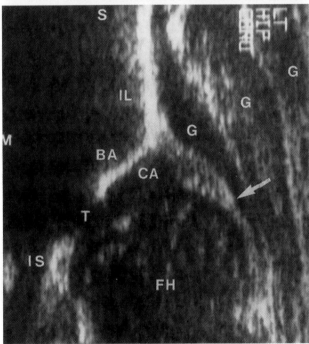

C

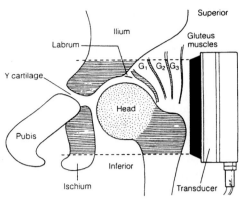

B

Figure 41–6 Sonogram of left hip in a newborn boy. **A:** Coronal view reoriented to be in anatomic position to match diagram in 6 b. (Reprinted with permission from Gerscovich EO. A radiologist's guide to the imaging in the diagnosis and treatment of developmental dysplasia of the hip. II. Ultrasonography: anatomy, technique, acetabular angle measurements, acetabular coverage of femoral head, acetabular cartilage thickness, three-dimensional technique, screening of newborns, study of older children. **Skel Radiol** 1997;26:447—456.) **B:** Coronal view, diagram. (From Leonidas JC. A sound way to identify congenital hip dislocation. **Contemp Pediatr** 1989;6:105—120.) **C:** Axial view reoriented to be in anatomic position to match diagram in 6 d. (Reprinted with permission from Gerscovich EO. A radiologist's guide to the imaging in the diagnosis and treatment of developmental dysplasia of the hip. II. Ultrasonography: anatomy, technique, acetabular angle measurements, acetabular coverage of femoral head, acetabular cartilage thickness, three-dimensional technique, screening of newborns, study of older children. **Skel Radiol** 1997;26:447—456.) **D:** Axial view, corresponding diagram. IL, ilium; BA, bony acetabulum; CA, cartilaginous acetabulum; t, triradiate cartilage; P, pubis; FH, femoral head; G, gluteus muscles; IS, ischium; **arrow**, labrum; S, superior; M, medial; A, anterior. (From Leonidas JC. A sound way to identify congenital hip dislocation. **Contemp Pediatr** 1989;6:105—120.)

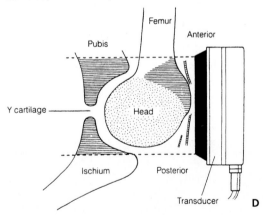

D

Table 41–3 Dynamic standard minimum

Hip examined at rest and when stressed
Views in orthogonal planes
Description of stability and morphology
Real-time linear-array transducer
Infant in supine or lateral position

Components
1. Either A or B:
  A. Coronal/neutral view in standard plane at rest
    Additional stress view optional
    Validation by line/angle measurement optional
  B. Coronal/flexion view in standard plane at rest
    Additional stress view optional
    Validation by line/angle measurement optional
2. Transverse flexion view with stress

Table 41–4 Protocol for US evaluation of infant hip for DDH (Albert Einstein Medical Center)

1. Transverse/flexion
  a. Neutral
  b. Adduction push
  c. Abduction

2. Coronal/flexion
  a. Neutral
  b. Adduction push over depth of acetabulum
  c. Adduction push over posterior lip
  d. Abduction

Note: For babies in harness, omit stress maneuvers until hip is stable and weaning process can begin.

Views in the transverse plane are mandatory. A view at rest is important to assess acetabular development (**Fig. 41–7**). Stress views are essential to evaluate motion. For the transverse views, the transducer is positioned over the lateral aspect of the hip in a plane that is perpendicular to the long axis of the body. The femoral head is easily identified by moving the transducer along the femoral shaft in a cephalad direction. In this view, the femoral head, the acetabulum, and the triradiate cartilage should be observed on one image. Harcke has compared the sonographic appearance of the cartilaginous head centered over the triradiate cartilage to a lollipop; the sound transmission through the triradiate cartilage represents the "stick" of the lollipop (**Fig. 41–5 a**). The bony acetabulum is highly echogenic, except at the triradiate cartilage which allows transmission of the ultrasound beam. Stress views are obtained with the hip in 90 degrees of flexion. Mandatory stress maneuvers are a push maneuver of the adducted hip and a pull maneuver of the abducted hip.

A coronal view in neutral position or in flexion is obtained at rest in the standard midacetabular plane to assess acetabular bone (**Fig. 41–8** through **41–9**). Stress views in the coronal plane are mandatory to evaluate stability (**Fig. 41–10**). For coronal views, the transducer is positioned along the lateral aspect of the hip and oriented in a coronal plane with respect to the acetabulum. The image obtained is orthogonal to the transverse plane. The femoral head is located by moving the transducer in an anterior/posterior direction. The iliac bone which is strongly echogenic and the bony acetabular roof can be identified and the coverage of the femoral head can be assessed (**Fig. 41–5 b**). The added value of the coronal/flexion view is that it reflects the position in which the physician places the hips during the dynamic physical examination.[24] For stress views, the hip is flexed 90 degrees and is abducted and adducted.

Normal Anatomy

On coronal views, the femoral capital epiphysis is contained within the cuplike acetabulum below the echogenic bony ilium (**Fig. 41–8, 41–9**). Normally, half of the diameter of the femoral head lies on either side of the ilium ("the equator sign") (**Fig. 41–10**).[25] If the acetabulum accommodates less than one-half but more than one-third of the femoral head, then acetabular dysplasia should be suspected. When one-third or less of the femoral head is accommodated, the presence of acetabular dysplasia is almost certain (**Fig. 41–11**). The joint capsule is seen as an echogenic linear structure surrounding the cartilaginous head and extending to the periosteum of the ilium. The acetabular labrum, often referred to as limbus or limbus cartilage, is composed of hyaline cartilage with a small fibrous cartilage rim. The limbus cartilage is normally superolateral to the femoral head. It is identifiable at the edge of the bony acetabulum beneath the joint capsule as an elongated, triangular, speckled, hypoechoic structure, with the fibrous rim often seen as a bright echogenic point.[26,27]

On transverse images, the femoral head is seated in the acetabulum formed by the ischium posteriorly, the pubic bone anteriorly and the triradiate cartilage centrally. The ossified portions of the acetabulum appear echogenic and produce an acoustic shadow (**Fig. 41–12**), while the triradiate cartilage is hypoechoic and permits sound transmission.

It is important to be aware that a certain amount of instability in the hips of newborns is normal. The pattern of laxity appears to be the same in both males and females; the laxity diminishes in most infants between the first and second days of life.[28,29] On the first day of life, the proximal left femur can usually be displaced between 2 and 4 mm with a mean of 3.2 mm; however, the extent of displacement can range from as little as 1 to as much as 6 mm. The extent of displacement of the proxi-

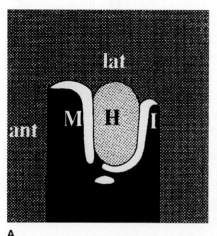

A

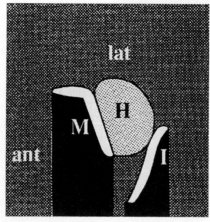

B

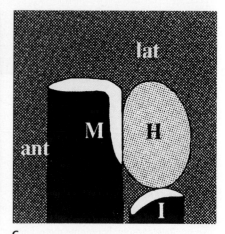

C

Figure 41–7 Transverse flexion views. **A—C:** Sonographic relationships in normal hip (**Fig. 41–10 a**) and in hips with subluxation (**Fig. 41–10 b**) and dislocation (**Fig. 41–10 c**). (H, femoral head; I, ischium; M, femoral metaphysis; ant, anterior; lat, lateral.) Reprinted with permission from Harcke HT. Hip and musculoskeletal US. In: Seibert JJ, ed. **Syllabus: Current Concepts: A Categorical Course in Pediatric Radiology.** Oak Brook: RSNA Publications, 1994

Figure 41–8 **A:** Coronal neutral view showing standard landmarks of the acetabulum. The standard plane through the midacetabulum. The ilium appears as a straight echogenic line extending to the lip of the acetabulum. The tip of the labrum (**arrowhead**) must be identified in this plane. This echogenic structure is composed of fibrocartilage and represents the outer edge of the acetabular cartilage. (H, femoral head; I, ischium; IL, ilium; M, femoral metaphysis; sup, superior; lat, lateral.) **B:** Type 1 hip. **C:** Type 2. **D:** Type 3 a. **E:** Type 4. Reprinted with permission from Harcke HT. Hip and musculoskeletal US. In: Seibert JJ, ed. **Syllabus: Current Concepts: A Categorical Course in Pediatric Radiology.** Oak Brook: RSNA Publications, 1994, p. 119—124.

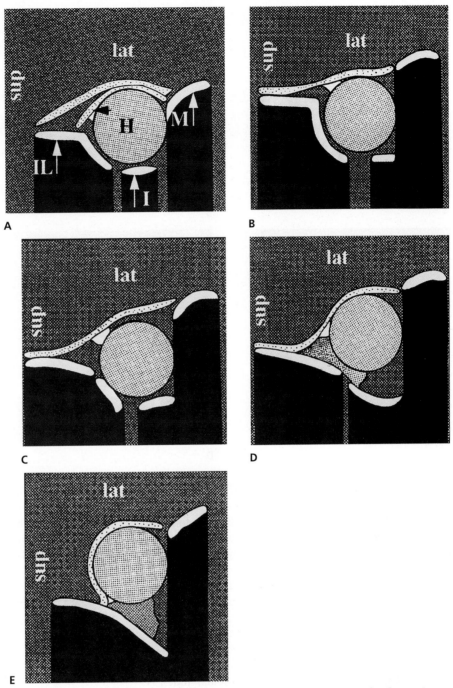

mal right femur ranges from 0 to 4 mm, with a mean of 2.3 mm. The laxity usually resolves in the first month of life without treatment.[21] Therefore, to avoid unnecessary treatment and/or follow-up sonography, US of the hips should be delayed until 4—6 weeks of life, unless there is clinical evidence of frank dislocation. By the fourth week of life, the hips are normal in approximately 78% of infants and by the ninth week, 90% of hips are normal.[30]

Pathologic Conditions

The diagnosis of hip dysplasia is based on abnormal position or abnormal mobility of the femoral head or insufficient acetabular depth to accommodate the femoral head, or both. The role of imaging using the dynamic approach is to determine if a hip is normal, lax with stress, subluxated (**Fig. 41–13**), or dislocated or dislocatable (**Fig. 41–14**) and whether or not an abnormal hip is reducible (**Table 41–5**) (**Fig. 41–13** through **41–14**).[31—34]

With subluxation, the femoral head is typically covered by a thickened stretched joint capsule, and the posterior portion of the bony acetabulum is flattened and underdeveloped. In frank dislocation, the joint capsule is frequently very thick and the bony acetabulum is abnormally small. The femoral head is not seated within the acetabulum but is displaced laterally and most often posteriorly and superiorly in relation to the acetabulum. The relationship of the limbus to the femoral head is im-

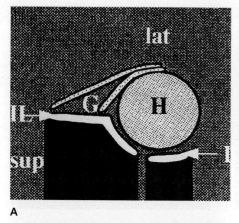

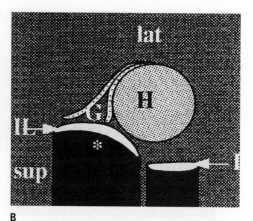

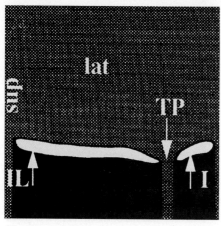

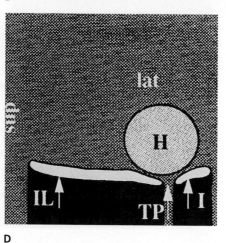

Figure 41–9 Coronal flexion views. **A,B:** Standard plane views, at rest, of the normal hip **(Fig. 41–9 A)** and a hip with subluxation and dysplasia **(Fig. 41–9 B)**. (*, iliac contour; G, gluteal muscle; H, femoral head, I, ischium; IL, ilium; sup, superior; lat, lateral.) **C,D:** Posterior lip view (coronal flexion), with stress: No part of the femoral head is seen over the posterior lip in the normal hip **(Fig. 41–9 C)**. The head projects over the posterior lip when there is posterior displacement **(Fig. 41–9 D)**. The femoral head is seen in the imaging plane. (H, femoral head; I, ischium; IL, ilium; TP, posterior lip of triradiate cartilage; sup, superior; lat, lateral.) Reprinted with permission from Harcke HT. Hip and musculoskeletal US. In: Seibert JJ, ed. **Syllabus: Current Concepts: A Categorical Course in Pediatric Radiology.** Oak Brook: RSNA Publications, 1994.

portant in the management of DDH. In the unstable, but reducible subluxed (partially dislocated) hip, the limbus is inverted. In the completely dislocated hip, the femoral head lies superolateral to the limbus and the limbus is interposed between the dislocated head and the acetabulum. Other abnormalities may be present including capsular adhesions, a taut iliopsoas tendon, and synovial hyperplasia, which often require operative reduction.

Insufficient acetabular depth is another feature of hip dysplasia. Uncoverage of the femoral head increases as the acetabular index increases. The mean area covered is 59.3% (range 37—89%) when the acetabular index is

normal, 46.2% (33—58%) when it is borderline, and 40.4% (range 8—58%) when it is abnormal. As a general rule, acetabuli with indices exceeding the normal range for the subject's age show head coverage of less than 33% **(Fig. 41–11)**.[35]

Table 41–5 Dynamic sonography classification

View and maneuver	Classification			
	Normal	**Laxity with stress**	**Subluxated**	**Disable/dislocated**
Coronal-neutral	N	N	A	A
Coronal-flexion	N	N to A	A	A
No stress-stress				
Transverse-flexion	N	N to A	N to A	A
Abduction-adduction				

N, = Normal
A, Abnormal
N to A, becomes abnormal with stress.

Reprinted with permission from **Syllabus: Current Concepts: A Categorical Course in Pediatric Radiology** by JJ Seibert, ed. Oak Brook: RSNA Publications, 1994, p. 119—124.

Figure 41–10   Normal newborn hip. **A:** Coronal/flexion view: The nicely rounded cartilaginous femoral head is well seated within a well-formed acetabulum with at least 50% coverage of the head, shown by a line drawn along the lateral aspect of the ilium in a horizontal plane. **B:** Coronal transverse/flexion view: the femoral head is well seated within the U-shaped cup formed by the bony femoral metaphysis (m) and the acetabulum (a). **C:** Coronal/flexion view of posterior lip of the acetabulum during the adduction push maneuver: The posterior lip (**arrow**) is well defined and there is no evidence of a subluxed or dislocated femoral head.

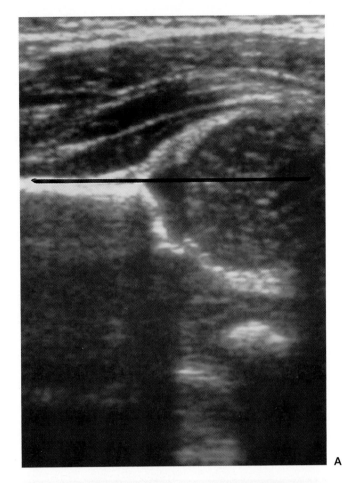

A

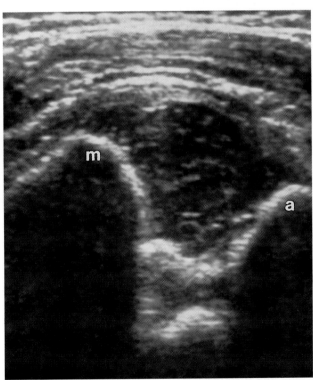

B

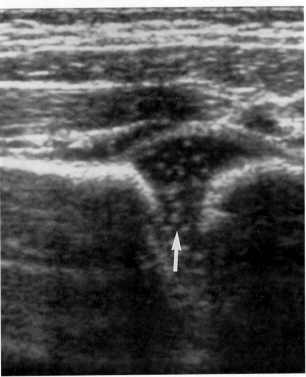

C

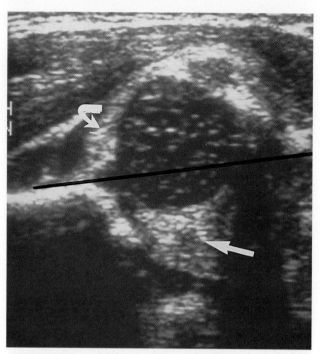

Figure 41–11 Coronal/flexion view of subluxated hip demonstrating increased echogenicity in the cartilaginous labrum due to increased fibrocartilage: There is a large amount of pulvinar (**arrow**) deep in the dysplastic acetabulum. The cartilaginous femoral head is supero-laterally subluxed with less than 33% coverage by the bony acetabulum and the cartilaginous labrum is hyperechoic consistent with fibrous deposition.

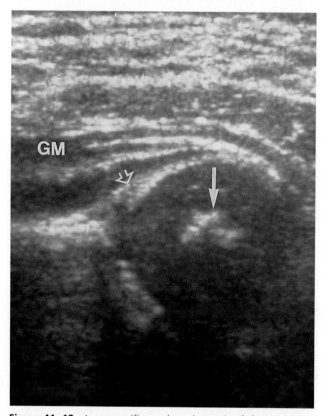

Figure 41–12 Large ossific nucleus (**arrow**) of femoral head causes shadowing of the ultrasound beam, mimicking the appearance of the triradiate cartilage.

Sonographic Accuracy

The sensitivity and specificity of sonography for the diagnosis of hip dysplasia is virtually 100%.[16] The acoustic shadowing from the ossific nucleus in the femoral capital epiphysis creates a defect in the bone medially which should not be mistaken for the triradiate cartilage (**Fig. 41–12**). The ability to visualize the acetabulum has been correlated with the size of the ossific nucleus. In general, when the size of the nucleus is less than 0.5 cm, the acetabulum should be visible.[36] Sonographic hip evaluation usually ceases to be reliable in children over 1 year because of the acoustic shadowing created by a large ossific nucleus which impairs visualization of the acetabulum.

Treatment and Follow-up Sonography

In addition to using US for the initial diagnosis of DDH, sonography can be used to follow infants during treatment.[32, 37] US provides a noninvasive accurate means of obtaining serial evaluations of the position of the femoral head, the acetabular contour and the development of the ossific nucleus (usually occurring between 6 weeks to 6 months of age) during the time of treatment. Congruent concentric reduction performed before 4 years of age results in a normal relationship of the acetabulum and the femur in more than 95% of patients. Follow-up US is not performed on hips that appear sonographically normal.

An infant with hip dysplasia and subluxation is treated with a Pavlik harness. In this device, the hips are held in flexion and abduction with the femoral heads directed toward the triradiate cartilage, thus promoting acetabular development. Although some movement is possible, the degree of restriction prevents subluxation or dislocation. After 6 weeks, US usually is performed with the infant in the harness to assess the position of the femoral head with respect to the acetabulum. A properly seated hip should be in the center of the acetabulum. If the hip is satisfactorily reduced, a 10-week weaning process is carried out, at the end of which time an anterior/posterior radiograph of the hips and pelvis is obtained to assess the bony acetabular configuration. This also serves as a baseline for comparison with follow-up radiographs should they be necessary.

An infant with frank dislocation is also treated with a Pavlik harness. In this condition, US is performed weekly until the femoral head is properly located. Once reduction is confirmed, US is repeated 3 weeks later to ensure that proper positioning has been maintained. A final sonogram is performed after an additional 3 weeks. If the hip is located and stable, the weaning program is begun and then the same ultrasound protocol is used as described for a subluxed hip (**Table 41–6**).

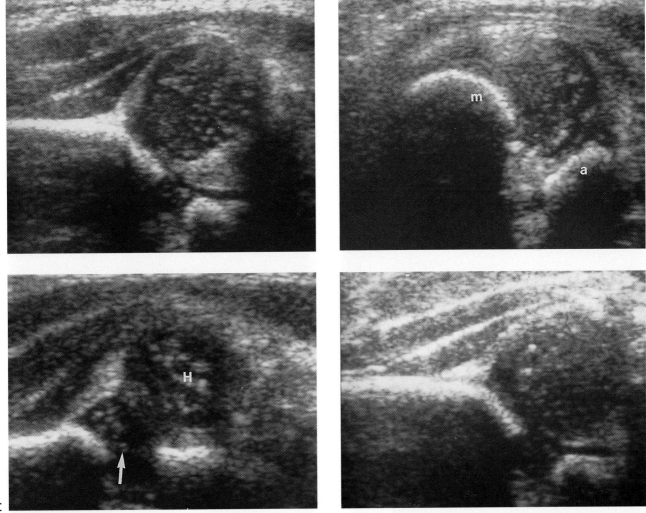

Figure 41–13 Subluxed hip. **A:** Coronal/flexion view of hip during the adduction push (stress) maneuver: The femoral head is subluxated superolaterally but it maintains contact with the upper lateral border of the steep bony acetabulum and the cartilaginous labrum. Note the large amount of pulvinar deep to the femoral head. **B:** Coronal transverse/flexion view of hip during stress maneuver: There is distortion of the normally U-shaped cup formed by the proximal femoral metaphysis (m) and the acetabulum (a) with a large amount of pulvinar seen deep to the subluxed femoral head. **C:** Coronal/flexion view of posterior lip of the acetabulum during stress maneuver: The femoral head (H) is subluxed posteriorly in relation to the posterior lip (arrow). **D:** Coronal/ flexion view of hip during abduction during treatment with a Pavlik harness: The head is better seated within the acetabulum indicating response to treatment.

Table 41–6 Recommendations for imaging after treatment initiated

Monitor hip position with US (dislocated hip tx successfully with harness reseats within 3 weeks)
If subluxed:
- Pavlik harness full-time 6 weeks
- US after 6 weeks (gentle stress)
- If stable, wean over 10 weeks (x-ray AP pelvis)

If dislocated:
- Pavlik harness (US weekly until head located)
- Repeat US in 3 weeks
- Repeat US 3 weeks later
- If located and stable, begin weaning program and follow protocol for subluxated hip

The transverse/flexion and coronal/flexion views are particularly useful for infants receiving treatment for DDH, such as with traction or a Pavlik harness. The transverse/neutral view should be eliminated, since the traction device or harness would need to be removed to place the hip into a neutral position.[32, 38]

When a spica cast is used for treatment, assessment of the position of the femoral head in the acetabulum by US requires that a window be cut in the side of the cast. However, this process can increase the risk of redislocation or subluxation. If a window is cut, it should be no larger than necessary for adequate examination and there should be no delay in repositioning the window and repairing the spica cast with additional plaster. CT is an alternative method (and in many institutions the preferred method) of evaluating the status of reduction if there is a cast in place.

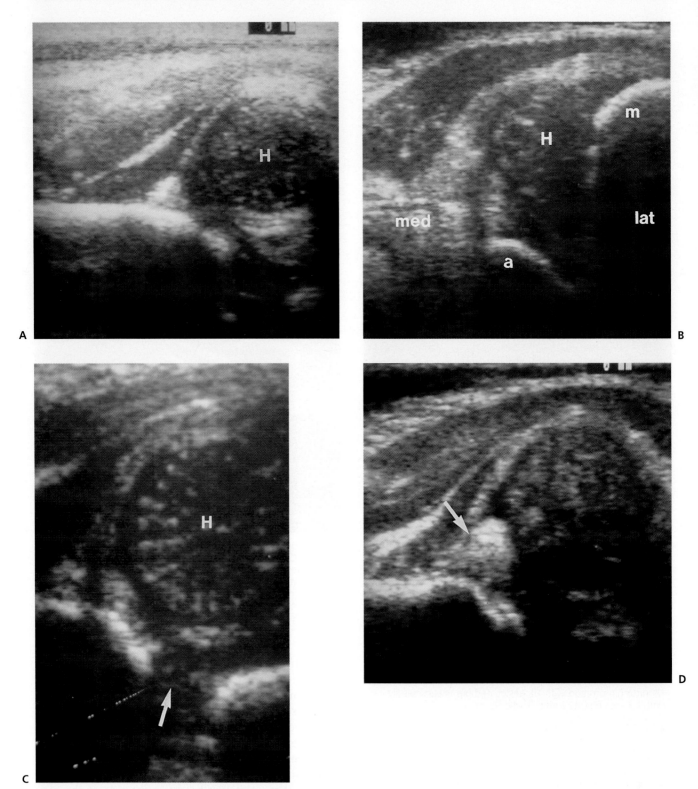

Figure 41–14 Dislocated hip. **A:** Coronal/flexion view: The femoral head (H) is dislocated superolaterally in relationship to the shallow acetabulum. Note the lack of contact with the femoral head and the bony acetabulum. **B:** Coronal transverse/flexion view: The femoral head (H) is dislocated superolaterally. There is total dis-tortion of the U-shaped cup formed by the metaphysis (m) of the femur and the acetabulum (a). **C:** Coronal/flexion view of posterior lip of acetabulum: The femoral head (H) is well seen indicating pos-terior dislocation. (**arrow**) posterior lip. **D:** Coronal/flexion view de-monstrating inverted limbus (**arrow**).

Screening

Clinical screening has been shown to decrease the incidence of late (missed) DDH by 50%.[39] Sonographic screening detects one-third more abnormalities than does the clinical examination.[40] The incidence of DDH found at screening US on newborns with a normal clinical examination at birth is 0.6 per thousand.[30] Infants with normal hip sonography at birth are unlikely to develop DDH. Of babies noted to have abnormal hip sonography on the first examination within the first 3 weeks of age, only 2.6% had clinically abnormal hips (subluxation or dislocation) noted on physical examination. Although it would be ideal to screen all newborn hips with ultrasound, it would require tremendous resources that are not readily available and there could be a tendency to overtreat. Thus, the approach in the United States is to limit ultrasound screening to infants with an abnormal physical examination or risk factors. The following guidelines for US screening have been established.[22]

1. Newborns with normal physical examination and no risk factors do not require sonography or follow-up.
2. Newborns with risk factors (see **Table 41–1**) are screened with sonography at 4—6 weeks.
3. Newborns with abnormal physical findings but with a stable hip that does not subluxate or dislocate; sonography is performed at 4—6 weeks.
4. Newborns with an abnormal physical examination and an unstable hip; sonography should be performed at 2 weeks.

Summary

The dynamic approach is now accepted as the primary imaging study for suspected DDH. Dynamic imaging allows evaluation of femoral head position and stability during stress maneuvers, as well as an evaluation of the labrum, pulvinar, and limbus. Based on the sonographic findings, four classes of hip pathology can be defined: normal, laxity with stress, subluxated, and dislocated. Knowledge of the type of dysplasia and its severity is critical in optimizing treatment.

References

1. Kilsic PJ. Congenital dislocation of the hip: a misleading term. *J Bone Joint Surg* 1984;71 B:136.
2. Phillips WE II, Burton EM. Ultrasonography of developmental displacement of the infant hip. *Appl Radiol* (May) 1995;25—30.
3. Staheli LT. Management of congenital hip dysplasia. *Pediatr Ann* 1989;18:24–32.
4. Gerscovich EO. A radiologist's guide to the imaging in the diagnosis and treatment of developmental dysplasia of the hip. I. General considerations, physical examination as applied to real-time sonography and radiography. *Skel Radiol* 1997;26:386—397.
5. Clausen I. Breech position, delivery route and congenital hip dislocation. *Acta Obstet Gynecol Scand* 1988;67:595—597.
6. Hensinger RN. Congenital dislocation of the hip. *Clin Sympos* 1979;31:3—31.
7. Ogden JA, Moss HL. Pathologic anatomy of congenital hip disease. In: Weil UH, ed. *Skeletal Dysplasias in Childhood. Progress in Orthopedic Surgery*, Vol. 2. New York: Springer-Verlag, Inc., 1978, p. 3–45.
8. Barlow TG. Early diagnosis and treatment of congenital dislocation of the hip. *J Bone Joint* 1962;44 B:292—301.
9. Ramsey PL. Congenital hip dislocation before and after walking age. *Postgraduate Med* 1976;60:114—120.
10. Hernandez RJ. Concentric reduction of the dislocated hip: computed-tomographic evaluation. *Radiology* 1984;150:266—268.
11. Graf R. The diagnosis of congenital hip-joint dislocation by the ultrasonic combound treatment. *Arch Orthop Traumat Surg* 1980;97:117—133.
12. Graf R. New possibilities for the diagnosis of congenital hip joint dislocation by ultrasonography. *J Pediatr Orthop* 1983;3:354—359.
13. Graf R. Classification of hip joint dysplasia by means of sonography. *Arch Orthop Trauma Surg* 1984;102:248—255.
14. Novick G, Ghelman B, Schneider M. Sonography of the neonatal and infant hip. *AJR* 1983;141:639—645.
15. Harcke HT, Clarke NMP, Lee MS, Borns PF, MacEwen GD. Examination of the infant hip with real-time ultrasonography. *J Ultrasound Med* 1984;3:131—137.
16. Boal DKB, Schwenkter EP. The infant hip: assessment with real-time US. *Radiology* 1985;157:667—672.
17. Clarke NMP, Harcke HT, McHugh P, et al. Real-time ultrasound in the diagnosis of congenital dislocation and dysplasia of the hip. *J Bone Joint Surg* 1985;67 B:406—412.
18. Fisher R, O'Brien TS, Davis KM. Magnetic resonance imaging in congenital dysplasia of the hip. *J Pediatr Orthop* 1991;11:617—622.
19. Johnson ND, Wood BP, Jackman KV. Complex infantile and congenital hip dislocation: assessed with MR imaging. *Radiology* 1988;168:151—156.
20. Graf R. Advantages and disadvantages of various access routes in sonographic diagnosis of dysplasia and luxation in the infant hip. *J Pediatr Orthop* 1997;6:248—252.
21. Harcke HT, Grissom LE. Performing dynamic sonography of the infant hip. *AJR* 1990;155: 837—844.
22. Harcke HT. Screening newborns for developmental dysplasia of the hip: The role of sonography. *AJR* 1994;162:395—397.
23. Harcke HT. Hip and musculoskeletal US. In: Seibert JJ, ed. *Syllabus: Current Concepts: A Categorical Course in Pediatric Radiology*. Oak Brook: RSNA Publications, 1994; 119—124.
24. Gerscovich EO. A radiologist's guide to the imaging in the diagnosis and treatment of developmental dysplasia of the hip. II. Ultrasonography: anatomy, technique, acetabular angle

measurements, acetabular coverage of femoral head, acetabular cartilage thickness, three-dimensional technique, screening of newborns, study of older children. *Skel Radiol* 1997;26:447—456.

25. Keller MS, Chawla HS, Weiss AA. Real-time sonography of infant hip dislocation. *RadioGraphics* 1986;6:447—456.
26. Keller MS, Chawla HS. Sonographic delineation of the neonatal acetabular labrum. *J Ultrasound Med* 1985;4:501—502.
27. Yousefzadeh DK, Ramilo JL. Normal hip in children: correlation of US with anatomic and cryomicrotome sections. *Radiology* 1987;165:647—655.
28. Novick GS. Sonography in pediatric hip disorders. *Radiol Clin North Am* 1988; 26:29—53.
29. Keller MS, Weltin GC, Rattner Z, Taylor KJW, Rosenfield NS. Normal instability of the hip in the neonate: US standards. *Radiology* 1988;169: 733—736.
30. Marks DS, Clegg J, Al-Chalabi AN. Routine ultrasound screening for neonatal hip instability. *J Bone Joint Surg Br* 1994;76:534—538.
31. Boal DKB, Schwenkter EP. Assessment of congenital hip dislocation with real-time ultrasound: a pictorial essay. *Clin Imaging* 1991;15:77—90.
32. Harcke HT, Kumar SJ. The role of ultrasound in the diagnosis and management of congenital dislocation and dysplasia of the hip. *J Bone Joint Surg* 1991;73 A:622—628.
33. Harcke HT, Grissom LE. Infant hip sonography: current concepts. *Semin US CT MR* 1994;15:256—263.
34. Millis MB, Share JC. Use of ultrasonography in dysplasia of the immature hip. *Clin Orthop Relat Res* 1992;274:160—171.
35. Morin C, Harcke HT, MacEwen GD. The infant hip: real-time US assessment of acetabular development. *Radiology* 1985; 157: 673—677.
36. Harcke HT, Lee MS, Sinning L, et al. Ossification center of the infant hip: Sonographic and radiographic correlation. *AJR* 1986;147:317—321.
37. Grissom LE, Harcke T, Kumar SJ, Bassett GS, MacEwen GD. Ultrasound evaluation of hip position in the Pavlik harness. *J Ultrasound Med* 1988;7:1—6.
38. Harcke HT, Grissom LE. Use of ultrasound in the evaluation of the infant hip. *Jefferson Orthopedic J* 1988;18:12—16.
39. Tredwell SJ, Davis L. A prospective study of congenital dislocation of the hip. *J Pediatr Orthop* 1989;9:386—390.
40. Boeree NR, Clarke NM. Ultrasound imaging and secondary screening for congenital dislocation of the hip. *J Bone Joint Surg Br* 1994;76:525—533.

42 Intracranial Hemorrhage and Ischemia in the Premature Infant

Richard D. Bellah

Intracranial Hemorrhage

Every year, approximately 50,000 infants are born who are less than 32 weeks gestation and who weigh less than 1500 g. Intracranial hemorrhage (ICH) and ischemia are major sources of morbidity and mortality in low birth weight (LBW) premature infants. Refinements in the patient management, prenatally and postnatally, have reduced the incidence of ICH in LBW infants to approximately 15 to 20 percent, almost one-half of what it was several years ago.[1–3] These refinements have also increased the survivability of very premature infants, or *micropremies*, with birth weight < 800 g. More than a decade ago, only a small percentage of infants born less than 26 to 27 weeks gestation survived. Neonatologists now readily resuscitate and provide life support for very LBW infants, with the caveat that the more premature the infant, the greater the likelihood of ICH.[4–6] A large number of preterm infants, therefore, continue to be affected by ICH, particularly those who are very LBW. ICH in these very premature infants can be severe, occur very early, and be associated with a fatal outcome.[5,6]

Since the early 1980s, transfontanelle (cranial) ultrasonography (US) has proven to be the modality of choice for the evaluation of the premature infant with possible ICH.[7–10] In many ways, cranial computed tomography (CT) and magnetic resonance imaging (MRI) are more sensitive for detecting ICH and its complications,[11] but US continues to have an invaluable advantage over these other modalities, that is, portability.

This chapter will review (1) risk factors for developing ICH in the premature infant, (2) optimal timing of the US examination to screen for ICH, (3) grading of ICH by US and how that information is utilized by clinicians, (4) pitfalls and limitations of US in the diagnosis of ICH and periventricular leukomalacia (PVL); and, (5) circumstances in which other neuroimaging modalities, such as CT or MR, may provide more clinically useful information.

Risk Factors for Developing ICH in the Premature Infant

Intracranial hemorrhage is a term that refers to a variety of hemorrhagic lesions. These include periventricular hemorrhage (PVH), intraventricular hemorrhage (IVH), intracerebellar hemorrhage, subdural hemorrhage, and/or subarachnoid hemorrhage. PVH-IVH occurs with greatest frequency in the premature infant, and the germinal matrix hemorrhage is the most common form.

The germinal matrix is the site of origin for migrating cerebral neuroblasts. Between 10 to 20 weeks gestation, these neuroblasts form basal ganglia and cerebral cortex.[12] The germinal matrix is highly cellular, gelatinous in texture, and richly vascularized. The vascular integrity is tenuous, however, because vessels within its capillary bed are immature, large in caliber, and thin-walled. From the middle of the second to the middle of the third trimester, the germinal matrix, lying along the subependymal surface of the lateral ventricles, gradually involutes. At 28 to 30 weeks gestation, the portion of germinal matrix that has not yet completely involuted is most prominent in the thalamostriate groove at the head of the caudate nucleus. This is the most common site for PVH-IVH in the premature infant. Before 28 weeks gestation, hemorrhage may occur in the germinal matrix that persists anywhere along the subependymal surface of the lateral ventricles, but this is not common.

One explanation for the increased frequency of bleeding in the germinal matrix is that the vascular border between end fields of the striate and the thalamic arteries within the germinal matrix contains a fragile capillary bed that is susceptible to injury caused by fluctuations in cerebral blood flow.[13] Fluctuations in cerebral blood flow, caused by cerebral ischemia and reperfusion, combined with the lack of a mature autoregulatory mechanism, are factors that could be largely responsible for the development of PVH-IVH in premature infants.[14] The other theory is that hemorrhage is venous in origin with perivenous extension of the extravasated blood.[15] Factors that predispose to fluctuations in perfusion and increased cerebral blood flow include aggressive resuscitation efforts, (tracheal suctioning, rapid intravenous bolus of fluid, mechanical ventilation), systemic abnormalities (pneumothorax, hypercarbia, hypoglycemia, patent ductus arteriosus), and neurologic disorders (seizures).[14–17] Decreased cerebral blood flow may be caused by perinatal asphyxia, hypotension, or perinatal myocardial depression. Decreased frequency of intracranial hemorrhage has been reported with the use of paralytic muscle agents (indomethacin, phenobarbital ethamsylate).

Timing of Cranial Sonography

Changes in the premature infant's clinical status do not necessarily accompany the occurrence of ICH or correlate with the extent of sonographic findings. Rarely, ICH in the preterm infant is accompanied by a catastrophic clinical event, such as seizure, unstable vital signs, decreased consciousness, or altered neurologic exam, but, in the majority of cases, ICH is a "clinically silent syndrome."[18, 19] Occasionally, an unexplained drop in hematocrit is the only clue. Cranial US, therefore, has an important role in screening the preterm infant for ICH.

In premature infants less than 1500 g, approximately 50% of ICH occur in the first postnatal day, 25% in the second postnatal day, and 15% by day 3 to 4 of life.[20] By approximately 72 to 96 h, at least 90% of ICH has occurred (and is detectable with US). ICH rarely occurs beyond the first week of life.

The timing for screening cranial US varies from institution to institution, but most examiners would agree that routine screening cranial US should be performed initially between days 3 and 7. An earlier sonogram may be indicated if there has been clinical deterioration.[21, 22] Because progression of hemorrhage occurs in about 20 to 40% of cases and typically reaches its maximal extent by 3 to 5 days of life,[2] a follow-up screening sonogram is usually recommended 7 to 10 days after birth. If an abnormality is found, weekly follow-up studies are often obtained to assess for stability or resolution of the findings. Based on a retrospective study, several investigators have suggested that the initial screening examinations be delayed to the second week of life. Such an approach would not appear to compromise patient care, but it could significantly decrease the cost of health care.[23]

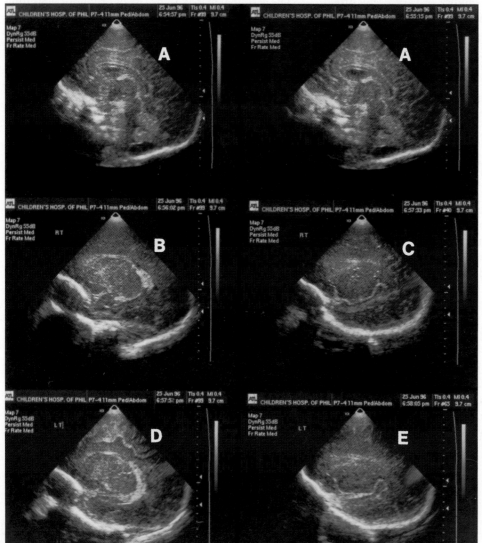

Figure 42–1 A: Sagittal views at the following levels. **A:** Corpus callosum, third and fourth ventricles; **B:** right lateral ventricle; **C:** right Sylvian fissure/periventricular white matter; **D:** left lateral ventricle; **E:** left caudothalamic groove. **F:** Left Sylvian fissure/periventricular white matter.

A

Following detection of IVH, serial US studies are important, as hydrocephalus develops in about three-fourths of patients. Hydrocephalus develops as a result of extension of germinal matrix or choroid plexus hemorrhage into the ventricular system. Choroid plexus hemorrhage by itself occurs more commonly in term than in pre-term infants. Ventricular dilatation usually occurs within the first 2 weeks following IVH. The degree of dilatation is generally related to the quantity of blood within the ventricular system. Serial sonography is needed to ensure resolution or arrest of dilatation; fortunately, this occurs spontaneously in more than two-thirds of patients.[24–27] Ventriculomegaly in preterm infants is not necessarily the result of previous IVH; it also may result from white matter loss (*ex vacuo*) due to PVL. Sonographically, it can be difficult to distinguish ventricular dilatation due to hemorrhage from that due to PVL. Moreover, both PVL and posthemorrhagic ventriculomegaly may coexist.

Neurosonographic Techniques: General Principles

Cranial sonography of the premature infant typically requires the use of a high-frequency transducer, usually 5- to 7.5-mHz, that has a footprint small enough to fit over the anterior fontanelle. Important technical details that must be attended to include (1) appropriate labeling, (2) appropriate depth, and (3) proper gain settings. The optimal depth allows visualization of the calvarium deep to the cerebellum. This is important to ensure detection of cerebellar bleeds. The overall gain needs to be adjusted to compensate for the ambient lights in most nurseries. If the ambient light in the room cannot be decreased, the overall gain needs to be increased. If gain is not optimized, then images that appear satisfactory on the monitor may transfer to bright or "gainy" images on hard copy or soft copy viewing.

Attention must be given to producing optimal hard or soft copy images. Inadequate hard or soft copy image can create problems with interpretation and follow-up

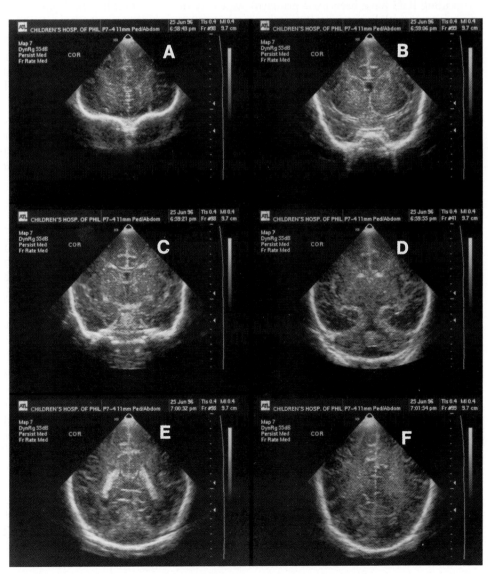

Figure 42–1 B: Sequences of normal images. Coronal views at the following levels.
A: Anterior to lateral ventricles; **B:** frontal horns; **C:** third ventricle; **D:** quadrigeminal cistern and cerebellar hemispheres; **E:** trigones of lateral ventricle; **F:** corona radiata just above lateral ventricles.

B

studies. A standard protocol also needs to be established and followed so that serial studies can be compared. At our institution, we perform a standard set of six coronal images followed by six parasagittal images for each infant (**Fig. 42–1**). Additional images or views may be acquired to confirm or exclude abnormalities. Finally, attention must be given to symmetry, especially in obtaining images in the coronal plane. Comparison of right and left cerebral hemispheres is a reliable technique for judging symmetry. The ventricles can normally be asymmetric, but structures such as the sylvian fissures, temporal-hippocampus lobes, and each side of the skull base are typically similar in appearance bilaterally.

Grading of ICH

Acute ICH appears as echogenic material and may be graded according to whether it lies within the subependymal region, within the ventricular system, or within the brain parenchyma. Since 1978, the systems for grading ICH have been used primarily as a way of communicating the appearance and degree of ICH.[22] With time, it has become apparent that the grade of ICH may serve as a predictor of neurodevelopmental outcome.[24]

The most widely used classification described by Papile[22] grades ICH as follows: grade 1, subependymal (germinal matrix) hemorrhage (SEH); grade 2, SEH with IVH in a nondilated lateral ventricle; grade 3, SEH with IVH and ventricular dilatation; and grade 4, SEH with IVH and intraparenchymal hemorrhage (IPH). Some investigators believe that this grading system has limitations and prefer to describe ICH rather than to grade it. Their objections to a grading scheme are that (1) ICH is

a dynamic, not static, event, and (2) grading does not necessarily allow for a detailed description of parenchymal abnormalities, such as extension of hemorrhage into cerebellum or thalamus.[28] Volpe, for example, refers to grade 1 as subependymal hemorrhage, grade 2 as IVH with less than 50% of ventricular area involved, and grade 3 as IVH with greater than 50% of ventricular area involved. Intraparenchymal hemorrhage is considered as a separate lesion (see below).[3,5]

PVH-IVH: Diagnosis, Pitfalls, and Neurosequelae

Grade 1 ICH

On coronal and sagittal views, acute grade 1 hemorrhage appears as an ovoid, unilateral or bilateral, echogenic mass anterior to the caudothalamic groove (**Fig. 42–2**), the site where the germinal matrix has yet to completely involute.

Besides the body of the lateral ventricle, SEH can occur in other areas where there is germinal matrix, although this is a rare occurrence. Potential pitfalls in diagnosis of subependymal germinal matrix hemorrhage include the normal specular reflection of the ventricular floor and the echogenic choroid plexus traversing the foramen of Monro. Over a period of weeks, grade 1 hemorrhage liquefies and eventually disappears or evolves into a subependymal cyst. The incidence of long-term major neurologic sequelae resulting from an uncomplicated grade 1 hemorrhage is small (< 15%).[24,29]

Grade 2 ICH

Intraventricular hemorrhage occurs in the majority of neonates with subependymal germinal matrix hemorrhage. The germinal matrix ruptures through the ependymal wall, allowing blood to enter the lateral ventricles. Rarely, IVH originates in the choroid plexus alone. This phenomenon occurs more commonly in acutely ill term infants than in preterm infants.[7,30] Grade 2 IVH appears as echogenic material within a nondilated ventricle (**Fig. 42–3**). It is distinguishable from the echogenic choroid plexus by the fact that it extends into the frontal horns anterior to the foramen of Monro and into the occipital horns beyond the trigones of the lateral ventricles. The associated SEH may be difficult to detect if there is substantial IVH. At times, it may be difficult to identify small amounts of hemorrhage in a nondilated ventricle, particularly if the echogenic choroid plexus is large, such as can be seen normally in very premature infants or in infants with Chiari II malformations. An enlarged, asymmetrically echogenic, or "lumpy" choroid plexus is suspicious for IVH adherent to the surface of the choroid plexus. The third ventricle can appear as an echogenic vertical line when blood extends into it. In-

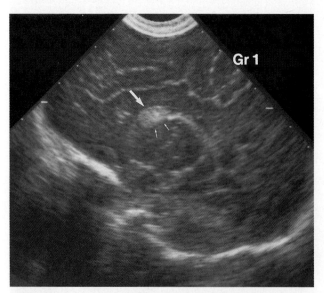

Gr 1

Figure 42–2 Grade 1 intracranial hemorrhage. Sagittal view shows an ovoid, echogenic hemorrhage (**large arrow**) anterior to the caudothalamic groove (**small arrows**).

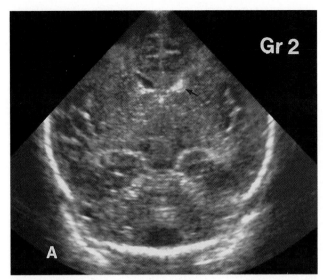

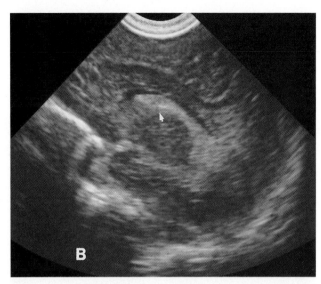

Figure 42–3 Grade 2 intraventricular hemorrhage (IVH). **A:** Coronal US view shows echogenic blood in nondilated left frontal horn (**arrow**). **B:** Sagittal US view shows echogenic blood within the left frontal horn, body, and occipital horn of a non-dilated lateral ventricle. **Arrow**, caudothalamic groove.

creased echogenicity of the ventricular wall, probably secondary to siderosis and glial response to IVH, is another finding of IVH (**Fig. 42–4**).[31] In cases where there is a question of blood in the occipital horn, insonation through the posterior fontanelle may be helpful to determine if blood clot is actually present (**Fig. 42–5**).[32] Power Doppler imaging may also prove useful in distinguishing normal vascularized choroid plexus from non-vascularized hemorrhage (**Fig. 42–6**).

One potential pitfall in diagnosis that can simulate IVH is a rounded, echogenic area occasionally detected in the trigone of the lateral ventricle.[33] This finding represents the *calcar avis*, a normal invagination of a portion of the occipital lobe into the trigone of the lateral ventricle (**Fig. 42–7**).

Like grade 1 ICH, grade 2 IVH (in the absence of PVL) has little to no major neurologic sequelae. Therefore, failure to recognize grade 2 IVH with US or differentiate between grade 2 IVH and SEH is not usually clinically important. Grade 2 IVH usually resolves completely over several weeks and rarely produces ventriculomegaly of any significant degree. Although usually benign, if detected, grade 2 IVH should be followed to resolution.[29] Marked ventriculomegaly has been described as a rare sequela. Because the long-term neurologic outcome depends in large part on the parenchymal injury that can accompany IVH, only an approximate relationship exists between the quantity of IVH and outcome. Major cognitive deficiencies and spastic deficits occur, therefore, in only a small percentage of patients with grade 2 IVH, probably between 5 and 15%.[34]

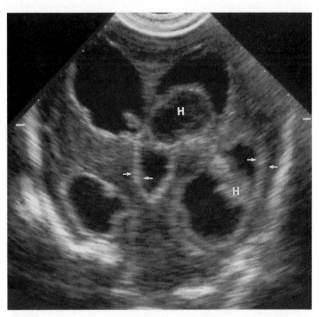

Figure 42–4 Post-hemorrhagic hydrocephalus. Coronal view shows lateral and third ventricular dilatation, hemorrhage (H) and thickened, echogenic ependymal lining (**arrows**).

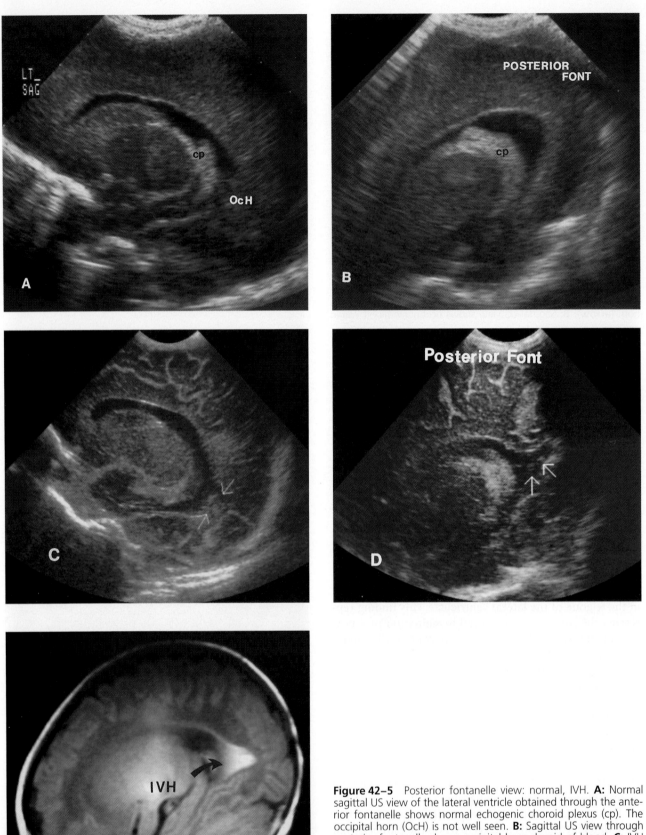

Figure 42–5   Posterior fontanelle view: normal, IVH. **A:** Normal sagittal US view of the lateral ventricle obtained through the anterior fontanelle shows normal echogenic choroid plexus (cp). The occipital horn (OcH) is not well seen. **B:** Sagittal US view through posterior fontanelle shows occipital horn devoid of blood. **C:** IVH sagittal view through anterior fontanelle shows questionable echogenic clot (**arrows**) in occipital horn. **D:** IVH sagittal view through the posterior fontanelle shows low level echoes (**arrows**) in the occipital horn consistent with IVH. **E:** IVH MRI (T_1-sagittal) in same patient also demonstrates high signal intensity of blood in occipital horn (**arrow**).

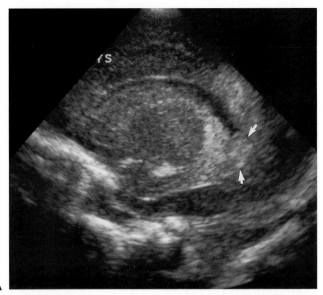

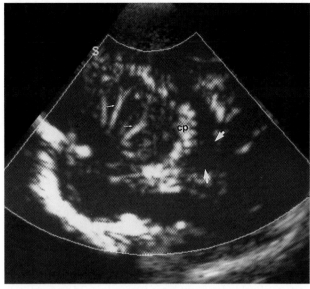

Figure 42–6   IVH – Power Doppler US. **A:** Sagittal view of a non-dilated lateral ventricle shows echogenic material, representing hemorrhage, in the trigone and occipital horn (**arrows**). **B:** Power Doppler US shows normal vascular flow within choroid plexus (cp) and thalamostriate vessels (**small arrows**), and absent flow (**arrows**) at the site of the echogenic material, consistent with IVH.

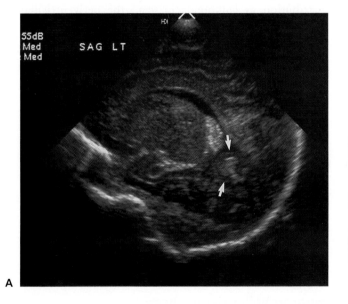

Figure 42–7   Calcar avis — simulating intraventricular hemorrhage. **A:** Sagittal view of the lateral ventricle shows echogenic material in the occipital horn (**arrows**). **B:** Power Doppler US (**sagittal view**) excludes hemorrhage by demonstrating intense vascular signal (**arrows**) at the site of echogenicity. **C:** Coronal view shows that the vascularized area represents a portion of occipital lobe, the **calcar avis**, invaginating into the trigone of the left lateral ventricle (**arrows**).

Grade 3 IVH

Hemorrhage that not only fills but enlarges one or both lateral ventricles is classified as grade 3 IVH (**Fig. 42–8**). Grade 3 IVH is recognized more easily than grade 2 IVH because the ventricles are dilated so blood (and clot) is more readily apparent. The blood may have a cast-like appearance, filling the ventricle. Occasionally, a blood-cerebrospinal fluid level may be noted in the occipital horn.

Over a period of weeks, clot within the ventricle retracts and may produce a "ventricle-within-a-ventricle" appearance; the ventricle itself usually remains dilated. Posthemorrhagic hydrocephalus develops in more than two-thirds of patients with grade 3 IVH (see Fig. 42–4). In 65 to 75% of patients, the dilatation will arrest or resolves spontaneously; in the remainder of patients, the ventricles increase in size, either slowly or rapidly, over 4 to 6 weeks. Hydrocephalus is typically mild or moderate with grade 3 ICH, and diversionary shunt placement is infrequently indicated.[35] In recent years, decline in incidence of grade 3 IVH has been attributed to improvement in clinical management.[4, 25] Grade 3 IVH still accounts for a large proportion (> 60%) of ICHs seen in very premature infants (< 700 g). Neurologic sequelae occur in 15 to 40% of premature infants with grade 3 hemorrhage.[34] Neurologic sequelae, mortality rates, incidence of hydrocephalus are higher if periventricular hemorrhagic infarction coexists with grade 3 IVH.

Grade 4 ICH

Intraparenchymal hemorrhage occurs in about 15% of infants with IVH. In the grading system of Papille, grade 4 hemorrhage is considered an extension of bleeding from IVH into brain tissue.[36] At sonography, parenchymal hemorrhage most often appears as an irregular area of increased echogenicity in the frontal or parietal lobe adjacent to the lateral ventricle. With large hemorrhages, there may be mass effect with midline shift.

Over 1 to 2 months, areas of increased parenchymal echogenicity (IPE) can liquefy and become hypoechoic. Cavitation eventually ensues that may or may not communicate with the adjacent lateral ventricle (**Fig. 42–9A,B,C**)]. Areas of IPE that do not cavitate may become smaller and persist as small foci of gliosis (**Fig. 42–9D**).

Controversy regarding the grading of ICH stems from work of Volpe and others who suggest that grade 4 IPH is not always an extension of IVH but rather can be due to hemorrhagic (venous) infarction. They observed that intraparenchymal hemorrhage occurs in the same distribution as leukomalacia (e.g., the periventricular frontal white matter). On this basis, they postulated that GMH-IVH obstructs the confluence of veins at the external angle of the lateral ventricle (**Fig. 42–10**). The resultant periventricular venous congestion and ischemia can lead to hemorrhagic infarction. Furthermore, in term infants as well, most examples of "grade 4" ICH are probably due to hemorrhagic infarction.[37—40] The neurodevelopmental outcome in grade 4 ICH is a function of the severity or extent of intraparenchymal echodensity. In infants with extensive IPE involving fronto-parietal-occipital origins, major deficits occur in 85 to 100%, while in infants with localized IPE, major deficits occur in 53 to 80%.[34]

Other Sites of Intracranial Hemorrhage

Intracerebellar Hemorrhage

Intracerebellar hemorrhage is more common in the premature infant than in the full-term infant. Based on the results of autopsy series, it has an incidence of 15 to 25% in neonates less than 32 weeks gestation. The likely cause of cerebellar hemorrhage in premature infants is bleeding in the subependymal germinal matrix of the fourth ventricle and subsequent extension of blood into the substance of the cerebellum; it occurs for the same reason that PVH-IVH occurs.[41—43]

Traumatic delivery with the use of forceps or straps for facemask ventilation and hypoxia are likely causes of cerebellar hemorrhage in term infants.[44] The cerebellar vermis is the initial site of hemorrhage in the majority of the term infants with intracerebellar hemorrhage. At US, cerebellar hemorrhage produces either a focal mass

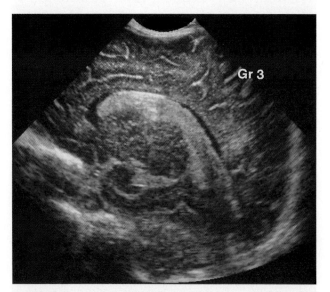

Figure 42–8   Grade 3 IVH. **A:** Sagittal view shows a mildly lateral ventricle filled with echogenic blood, extending into frontal and occipital horn.

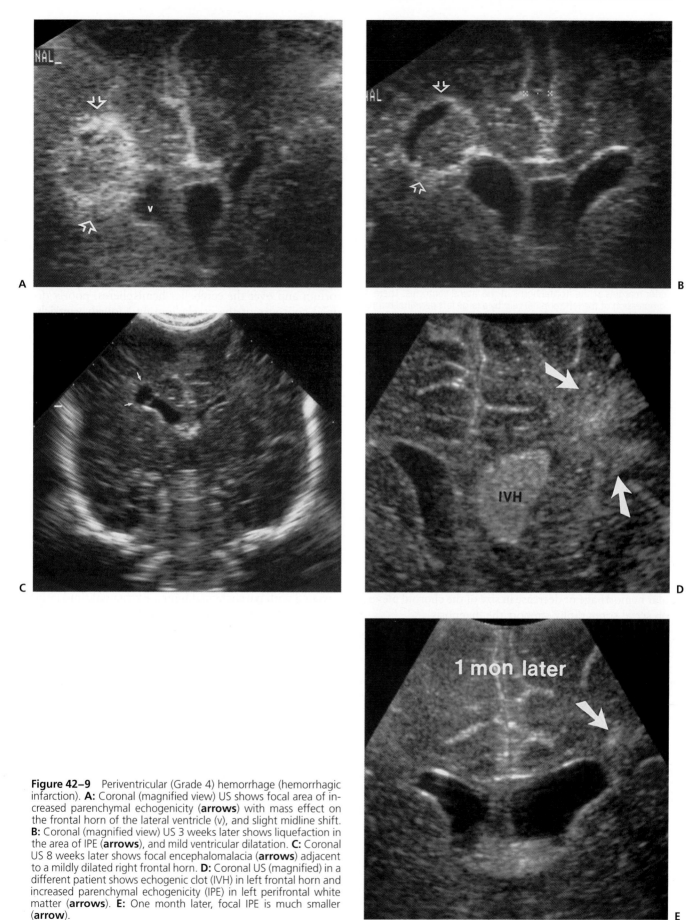

Figure 42–9   Periventricular (Grade 4) hemorrhage (hemorrhagic infarction). **A:** Coronal (magnified view) US shows focal area of increased parenchymal echogenicity (**arrows**) with mass effect on the frontal horn of the lateral ventricle (v), and slight midline shift. **B:** Coronal (magnified view) US 3 weeks later shows liquefaction in the area of IPE (**arrows**), and mild ventricular dilatation. **C:** Coronal US 8 weeks later shows focal encephalomalacia (**arrows**) adjacent to a mildly dilated right frontal horn. **D:** Coronal US (magnified) in a different patient shows echogenic clot (IVH) in left frontal horn and increased parenchymal echogenicity (IPE) in left perifrontal white matter (**arrows**). **E:** One month later, focal IPE is much smaller (**arrow**).

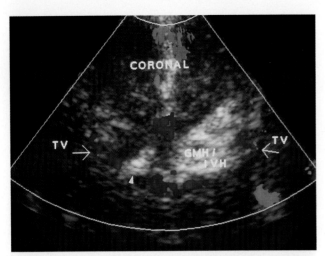

Figure 42–10 Color Doppler US (magnified coronal view of the frontal horns) shows terminal veins (TV-**arrows**) coursing along inferior margins of the frontal horns of the lateral ventricles. There is compression of the left terminal vein by a large left germinal matrix intraventricular hemorrhage (GMH-IVH) in dilated left frontal horn. Partial compression of right TV (**arrow**) by smaller right GMH (**arrowhead**).

within the cerebellar hemisphere or asymmetric cerebellar echogenicity.[43] Cerebellar hemorrhage may resolve completely or produce an area of encephalomalacia.

Choroid Plexus Hemorrhage

Choroid plexus hemorrhage occurs more often in term than in premature infants. Sonographically, it produces an enlarged echogenic plexus with an irregular contour. The diagnosis of choroid plexus hematoma often is difficult on sonography because the normal choroid plexus may be bulbous. Coexistent intraventricular hemorrhage or decrease in size of the choroid plexus on serial sonography support the diagnosis.

Extraaxial Hemorrhage

Subarachnoid hemorrhage can primarily result from disruption of bridging meningeal vessels, or secondarily occurs from extension of subdural, intraventricular, or intracerebral hemorrhage. Approximately 25% of infants with periventricular—intraventricular hemorrhage have subarachnoid hemorrhage.[45] Subarachnoid hemorrhage is more frequent in premature than term infants. Subarachnoid hemorrhage in prematures is usually due to asphyxia that leads to vascular engorgement and small vessel rupture; traumatic delivery is more often the cause in term infants. Sonography is relatively insensitive for detection of this form of hemorrhage because the echogenicity of the blood and gyral interfaces is similar. Large subarachnoid hemorrhages may be visible as fluid over the cerebral convexities or as a widened, echogenic Sylvian fissure. Subarachnoid hemorrhage is usually

clinically silent and of little prognostic importance. A rare complication of major primary subarachnoid hemorrhage is communicating hydrocephalus.

Subdural hemorrhage is the least common of major varieties of neonatal ICH. Subdural hemorrhage is more common in the full-term infant than in the preterm infant.[46] It usually is the result of traumatic delivery and resultant falcine or tentorial (more common) laceration. Laceration of the falx leads to supratentorial subdural hemorrhage. Tentorial laceration can result in rupture of vein of Galen, straight sinus, or transverse sinus, and produce infratentorial subdural hematoma.[47] Sonographic findings of supratentorial subdural hemorrhage include elliptical fluid collections over the surface of the brain, a widened intrahemisphere fissure, flattened gyri, and compressed ventricles. Infratentorial subdural hematoma appears as echogenic fluid beneath the tentorium and over the cerebellar hemispheres, poorly defined contours of the cerebellum and fourth ventricle, and compression of the cerebellum, fourth ventricle and aqueduct. Detection of subdural hematoma by US generally is difficult. Supratentorial subdural hemorrhages are more easily recognized than are infratentorial subdural hemorrhages. Extraaxial collections are initially echogenic but become hypoechoic with time.

One pitfall in the diagnosis of subdural hemorrhage is infantile (external) hydrocephalus which is a cause of enlarged extraaxial cerebral spinal fluid spaces. Infants with this condition present with macrocephaly, usually between 2 and 7 months of age. The precise location of the fluid — subdural or subarachnoid — is not clear. Sonography in benign external hydrocephalus typically shows bilateral symmetrical, extraaxial fluid collections. The brain parenchyma is normal, and the ventricles are normal to prominent. By comparison, traumatic subdural collections are asymmetric in size and may be associated with parenchymal injury. Extraaxial fluid in infantile hydrocephalus usually resolves by the second year of life.

Cortical Hemorrhage

Cortical hemorrhage, with or without periventricular/intraventricular hemorrhage, occurs more commonly in term than preterm infants. Major unusual and miscellaneous examples of ICH are associated with trauma[48] and hemorrhagic infarction.[49] As mentioned previously, most examples of "grade 4" ICH in term infants probably represent hemorrhagic infarction (**Fig. 42–11**).[46] Other causes include coagulation defects,[50] hypertension, emboli, and extracorpeal membrane oxygenation (ECMO). Infants on ECMO are at increased risk for cortical hemorrhage because of continuous heparinization.[51, 52] Acute hematoma appears as focal or diffuse increased gyral echogenicity. Multiple hematomas may occur in patients on ECMO.[53] As cortical hematomas evolve, they undergo clot lysis and retraction, becoming

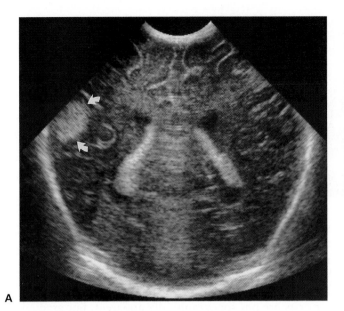

A

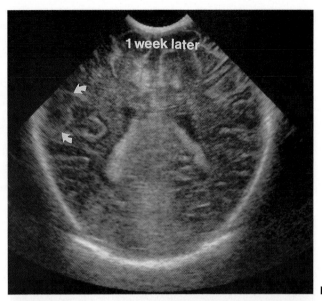

B

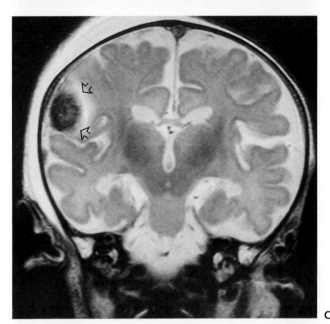

C

Figure 42–11 Cortical hemorrhage (probable hemorrhagic infarction, term infant). **A:** Coronal US shows focal area of increased parenchymal echogenicity on right (**arrows**). **B:** Coronal US (1 week later) shows the cortical hemorrhage (**arrows**) is isoechoic to brain. **C:** Coronal MR (T$_2$-weighted) 2 weeks later shows low signal intensity of hemosiderin in clot with high signal surrounding edema.

hypoechoic. Similar to parenchymal hematomas elsewhere, encephalomalacia may be a sequela.

Ischemic Brain Injury

Periventricular Leukomalacia

PVL is another manifestation of hypoxic-ischemic injury in the premature infant. The incidence ranges from 4 to 15% in very LBW infants. The most vulnerable time for white matter injury in the preterm infant is 28 to 32 weeks gestation during the period of myelinogenesis.[54] Anatomically, PVL, unlike periventricular hemorrhage, is usually bilateral and symmetric. Early sonographic findings are increased echogenicity at the arterial border zones, which include the optic radiations near the

trigones of the lateral ventricles, the periventricular white matter just lateral to the anterior horns, and corona radiata. The echodensities associated with PVL can be coarse, asymmetric, punctate, or patchy (**Fig. 42–12**). In some cases, periventricular hyperechogenicity may appear only transiently.[55]

The sensitivity of US for the diagnosis of acute PVL is low, about 25 to 30%.[56] The echogenicity associated with PVL can be mistaken for the normal periventricular echogenic halo or "blush." This finding is due to the anisotropic effect of the sound beam as it angles through the anterior fontanelle into the radiating neurofilaments.[57] The normal peritrigonal echogenicity should become less apparent when scans are obtained through the posterior fontanelle (**Fig. 42–13**).

Over a period of 2 to 3 weeks, abnormal areas of echogenicity due to PVL regress. Histopathologic data

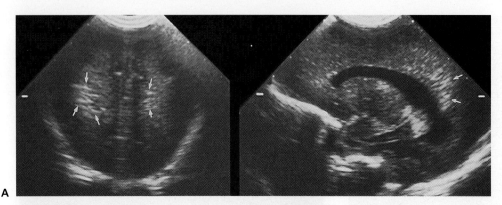

Figure 42–12 Early periventricular leukomalacia (PVL). **A:** Coronal and sagittal US views show patchy foci of hyperechogenicity (**arrows**) within the normally echogenic periventricular white matter (**arrows**). **B:** Coronal view 2 weeks later shows development of cysts (**arrows**) (cystic PVL).

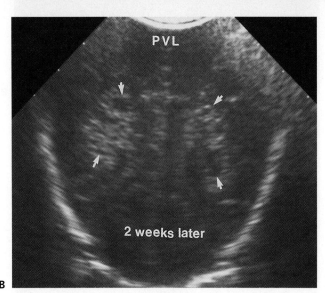

suggest that phagocytosis of necrotic tissue leads to cavitation and development of small cysts (cystic PVL) in 15 to 20% of affected infants (**Fig. 42–14**). These cysts are fine, multiple, septated, and rarely communicate with the ventricular system.[54, 56] In some cases, periventricular cysts are not sonographically apparent, but gradual loss of periventricular WM volume occurs with a concomitant increase in ventricular size. In this later stage of PVL, the diagnosis (of PVL) is more confidently made with MR (**Fig. 42–15**).

Recognizing increased parenchymal echogenicity, no matter whether it is due to periventricular venous infarction or PVL, is probably more important than identifying IVH. The reason is that long-term neurodevelopmental outcome is a function of parenchymal damage. The size or extent of hemorrhagic or ischemic change corresponds with the degree of patient morbidity

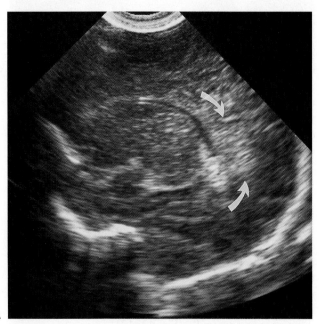

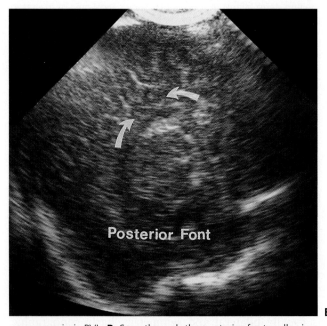

Figure 42–13 Normal peritrigonal "blush." **A:** Sagittal scan through lateral ventricle via anterior fontanelle approach shows normal periventricular hyperechogenicity (**arrows**). This appearance can mimic PVL. **B:** Scan through the posterior fontanelle view shows that the peritrigonal "blush" (**arrows**) disappears with this approach.

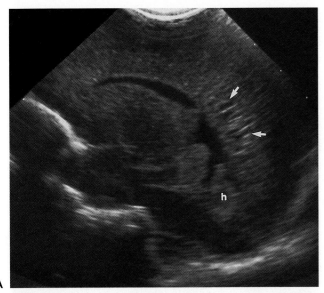

A

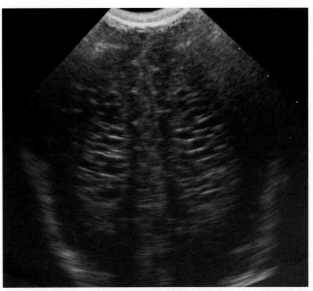

B

Figure 42–14 Cystic periventricular leukomalacia (PVL). **A:** Sagittal view shows mild dilatation of the lateral ventricle with echogenic hemorrhage (h) in the occipital horn, and small, cystic areas (**arrows**) in the peritrigonal white matter. **B:** One month later, coronal view through the corona radiata shows extensive bilateral cystic PVL. Widening of the interhemispheric fissure may be due to atrophy.

and mortality. Compared to IVH, the presence of intraparenchymal echogenicity more than doubles the likelihood of neurologic sequelae.[58] This information is critical for parental counseling and for overall prognostication. Furthermore, in the critically ill premature infant, the presence of intraparenchymal echogenicity may also be factored into the decision-making for determining the overall level of life support (conservative versus aggressive).

Depending on the extent and topography of the injury, PVL in infancy and childhood becomes clinically manifest as spastic hemiparesis or asymmetric spastic quadriparesis. Because of the arrangement of axons in the corticospinal tract, the lower extremities are affected more often than are the upper extremities. Unilateral localized frontal white matter damage due to hemorrhagic infarction usually has a better neurodevelopmental outcome than PVL, as PVL more often involves the posterior periventricular white matter, and, hence, cognitive (visual, auditory) development.[59] If possible, the radiologist should attempt to distinguish localized parenchymal echogenicity due to hemorrhagic infarction from the more extensive echogenicity due to PVL.

Limitations of Cranial Sonography

The major limitations of cranial sonography in the preterm infant are the inability to determine the presence and full extent of periventricular white matter damage, subarachnoid and subdural hemorrhage, and posterior fossa hemorrhage.

Increased parenchymal echogenicity may be due to hemorrhage, edema, infarction, or a combination of these. Some investigators have attempted to distinguish these by suggesting that intense hyperechogenicity in the periventricular area is more likely due to hemorrhage than to edema. This distinction is probably less important clinically, however, than determining the full extent of parenchymal injury.

MR is superior to US for assessing white matter once myelination is complete, and is the preferred modality for determining the nature and extent of white matter injury due to ischemic disease. MR is better at depicting the enlargement of cortical sulci and irregularity of the ventricular contour that can accompany PVL in its later stages. MR and CT are both limited, however, in their ability to identify early phases of PVL due to the normal high water content in the periventricular white matter of the unmyelinated brain. The sensitivity of MR for detecting ischemic damage increases directly with the degree of myelination. MRI is best performed between 8 months of age, when T1 myelination is nearly complete, and 18 months of age, when T2 myelination is nearly complete.[58–60]

Extraaxial (subarachnoid, subdural) hemorrhage occurs less frequently in premature infants than in term infants. CT is far more sensitive for detecting extraaxial hemorrhage than is US, especially with small bleeds. Whereas large convexity subdural hematomas may be recognized adjacent to the frontoparietal lobes, small hematomas or hematomas over the high convexities are more difficult to recognize by US, because of the inability to image the curved surfaces of the brain. Subarachnoid hemorrhage is extremely difficult to diagnose with US. It may cause the basilar cisterns or sylvian fissures to appear unusually echogenic and widened. Such a determination is difficult, however, because widening

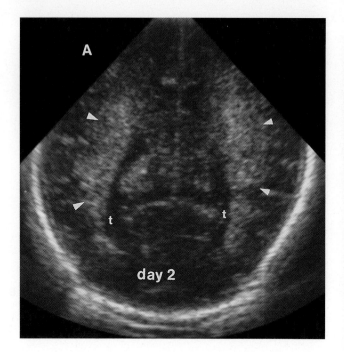

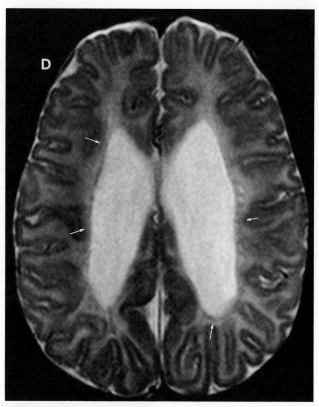

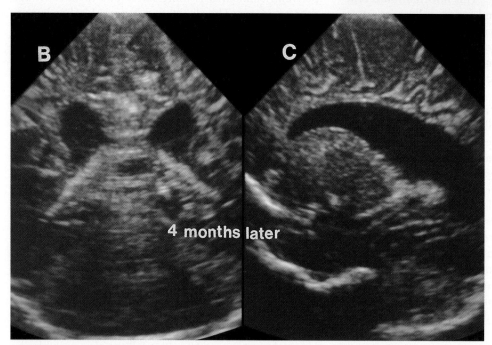

Figure 42–15   Periventricular leukomalacia (PVL). **A:** Coronal US view in a 2-day old at level of trigones (+) shows subtle symmetric periventricular hyperechogenicity, suspicious, but not diagnostic, for PVL (**arrows**). **B:** (coronal) and **C:** (sagittal) 4 months later show only ventriculomegaly (no cysts seen). This patient's clinical (neuro) exam was compatible with PVL. **D:** T₂-weighted axial MR in a similar older infant shows moderate ventricular enlargement secondary to diffuse white matter loss, or PVL (**arrows**). The medium signal intensity white matter is thin (**arrows**). The margins of the lateral ventricles are slightly wavy and irregular. The lower signal of cortical gray matter (and sulci) almost reach the margins of the ventricles. US at the time (not shown) revealed only ventriculomegaly.

and underoperculization of the sylvian fissures is a common finding in the immature brain.[61, 62]

While large cerebellar hemorrhages may be visualized sonographically using the anterior fontanelle as a window, small cerebellar hemorrhages may perhaps be seen better through a posterior approach (via the foramen magnum or occipito- or parieto-mastoid sutures) (**Fig. 42–16**). The ability to recognize blood in the poste-

rior fossa with US depends to some degree on the amount of blood present. Large posterior fossa hemorrhage usually distort the cerebellar hemispheres, as well as the fourth ventricle and cisterna magna, and are easier to recognize than small hemorrhages (**Fig. 42–17**). CT is the preferred method to confirm posterior fossa bleeding.[63]

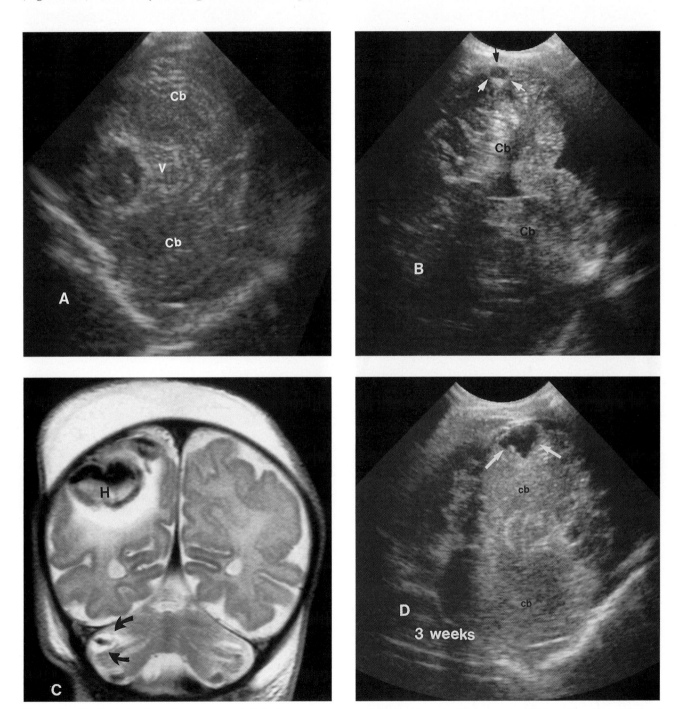

Figure 42–16 Posterior fossa (transverse-occipital) view — normal cerebellum and focal cerebellar hemorrhage. **A:** Normal high-resolution US through the occipitomastoid suture shows normal cerebellar hemispheres (cb) and vermis (v). **B, C, D:** Focal cerebellar hemorrhage. Posterior fossa (US) view (B) shows smalls complex cystic area (**arrows**) in right cerebellar hemisphere. MRI (coronal T$_1$- weighted) at 2 weeks (**C**) shows mixed high and low signal of blood at site of cerebellar hemorrhage (**arrows**). Patient also had right cortical hemorrhage (H). (**D**) Follow-up US (posterior fossa view) at 3 weeks shows area of encephalomalacia (**arrows**) in right cerebellar hemisphere.

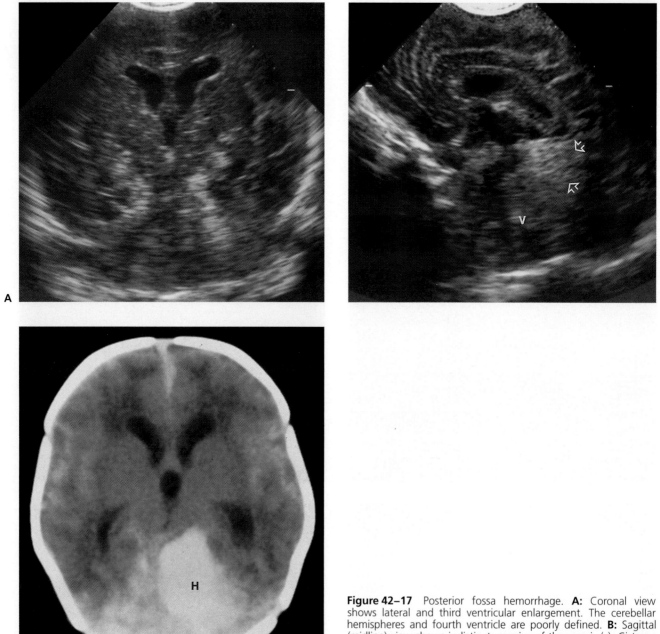

Figure 42–17 Posterior fossa hemorrhage. **A:** Coronal view shows lateral and third ventricular enlargement. The cerebellar hemispheres and fourth ventricle are poorly defined. **B:** Sagittal (midline) view shows indistinct margins of the vermis (v). Cisterna magna is obscured, and ill-defined hyperechogenicity (**arrows**) is seen in the supracerebellar cistern **C:** Unenhanced CT shows large posterior fossa hemorrhage (H), associated with supratentorial subarachnoid hemorrhage.

Recommendations

Sonography is the modality of choice for evaluating the brain of the preterm infant who is at risk for ICH. Because clinical signs are not often manifest with the onset of ICH, US should be performed routinely as a screen for infants with BWs less than 1500 g.

Limitations of cranial US for the preterm infant result mainly from an inability to distinguish hemorrhage from ischemia, evaluate the full extent of white matter injury, visualize hemorrhage in the extraaxial spaces, and diagnose early or small degrees of posterior fossa hemorrhage.

CT and MR are more informative than US in assessing the premature brain when there is suspicion of a mass lesion, congenital malformation, or infection. CT and MR are rarely performed in the acute setting for management of the sick premature infant. Difficulties with performing CT and MR are chiefly due to a reluctance to remove the fragile preterm infant from the intensive care environment for a prolonged period of time. CT or MR may be necessary acutely, however, if sonographic findings do not fully explain the clinical picture, if there is clinical suspicion of a life-threatening extraaxial hemorrhage, or if additional information is needed in determining the level of life support for a critically ill neonate. CT is excellent for detecting ICH and distinguishing hemorrhage in the periventricular region from nonhemorrhagic PVL; however, like MR, CT has limitations in detecting early changes of PVL. MR is more sensitive for detecting and estimating the age of hemorrhage, but, more importantly, for determining the effects of hypoxia/ischemia and extent of white matter injury.

References

1. Philip AG, Allan WC, Tito AM, et al. Intraventricular hemorrhage in preterm infants: declining incidence in the 1980 s. *Pediatrics* 1989;84:797—801.
2. Volpe JJ. Intraventricular hemorrhage in the premature infant — current concepts: part I. *Ann Neurol* 1989;25:3—11.
3. Cohen HL, Haller J. Review: advances in perinatal neurosonography. *AJR* 1994;163:801—810.
4. Strand C, Laptook A, Dowling S, et al. Neonatal intracranial hemorrhage: changing pattern in inborn low-birth-weight infants. *Early Human Dev* 1990;23:117—128.
5. Perlman JM, Volpe JJ. Intraventricular hemorrhage in the extremely small premature infants. *Am J Dis Child* 1986;140:1122—1124.
6. Bada H, Green R, Pourcyrous M, et al. Indomethecin reduces the risks of severe intraventricular hemorrhage. *J Pediatr* 1989;115:631—637.
7. Babcock DS, Bove KE, Han BK. Intracranial hemorrhage in premature infants: sonographic—pathologic correlation. *AJNR* 1982;3:309—317.
8. Grant EG. Sonography of the premature brain: intracranial hemorrhage and periventricular leukomalacia. *Neuroradiology* 1986;28:476—490.
9. Peterson CM, Smith WL, Franken EA. Neonatal intracerebellar hemorrhage detection by real-time ultrasound. *Radiology* 1984;150:391—392.
10. Kirks DR, Bowie JD. Cranial ultrasonography of neonatal perventricular/intraventricular hemorrhage: who, how, why, and when. *Ped Radiol* 1986;16:114—119.
11. Quisling RG, Reeder JD, Setzer ES, Kaude JV. Temporal comparative analysis of computed tomography with ultrasound for intracranial hemorrhage in premature infants. *Neuroradiology* 1983;24:205—211.
12. Szymonowilz W, Schatler K, Cussen L, et al. Ultrasound and necropsy study of periventricular hemorrhage in preterm infants. *Arch Dis Child* 1984;59:637—642.
13. Pape K, Wigglesworth J. In: Ischemia and the perinatal brain. Philadelphia: JB Lippincott, 1979.
14. Perlman JM, McMenamin J, Volpe J. Fluctuating cerebral blood flow velocity in respiratory distress syndrome. Relation to the development of intraventricular hemorrhage. *N Engl J Med* 1983;309:204—209.
15. Ghazi-Birry H, Moody D, Brown W, Challa V, Block S. Germinal matrix hemorrhage in the very low birth weight neonate is primarily venous in origin. Program abstract, ASNR, 1996.
16. Hill A, Perlman JM, Volpe JJ. Relationship of pneumothorax to occurrence of intraventricular hemorrhage in the premature newborn. *Pediatrics* 1982;69:144—149.
17. Funato M, Tamai H, Noma K, et al. Clinical events in association with timing of intraventricular hemorrhage in preterm infants. *J Pediatr* 1992;121:614—619.
18. Lazzara A, Ahmann P, Dykes F, et al. Clinical predictability of intraventricular hemorrhage in preterm infants. *Pediatrics* 1980;65:30—34.
19. Dubowitz L, Levene M, Movante A, et al. Neurologic signs in neonatal intraventricular hemorrhage: a correlation with real-time ultrasound. *J Pediatr* 1981;99:127—133.
20. Partridge C, Babcock DS, Han BK, Steichen J. Optimal timing for diagnostic cranial ultrasound in low birth weight infants: detection of intracranial hemorrhage and ventricular dilatation. *J Pediatr* 1983;102:281—287.
21. Rumack CM, Manco-Johnson ML, Manco-Johnson MJ, et al. Timing and course of neonatal intracranial hemorrhage using real-time ultrasound. *Radiology* 1985;154:101—110.
22. Papile L, Burstein J, Burstein R, Koffler H. Incidence and evolution of subependymal and intraventricular hemorrhage: a study of infants with birth weights less than 1500 gm. *J Pediatr* 1978;92:529—534.
23. Boal DK, Watterberg KL, Miles S, Gifford KL. Optimal cost-effective timing of cranial ultrasound screening in low-birth weight infants. *Pediatr Radiol* 1995;25:425—428.
24. Shankaran S, Slovis TL, Bedard MP, Poland RL. Sonographic classification of intracranial hemorrhage. A prognostic indicator of mortality, morbidity, and short-term neurologic outcome. *J Pediatr* 1982;100:469—475.
25. Dykes F, Dunbar B, Lazarra A. Post-hemorrhagic hydrocephalus in high-risk preterm infants. National history, management, and long-term outcome. *J Pediatr* 1989;114:611—618.
26. Volpe JJ. Intraventricular hemorrhage and brain injury in the premature infant. *Clin Perinatol* 1989;16:381—411.
27. Hill A. Ventricular dilatation following intraventricular hemorrhage in the premature infant. *Can J Neurol Sc* 1983;10:81—85.
28. Kuban K, Teele RL. Rationale for grading intracranial hemorrhage in premature infants. *Pediatrics* 1984;74:358—363.
29. Bowerman RA, Donn SM, Silver TM, Jaffe MH. Natural history of neonatal periventricular/intraventricular hemorrhage and its complications. *AJNR* 1984;5:527—538.

30. Reeder JD, Karede JV, Setzer ES. Choroid plexus hemorrhage in premature neonates: recognition by sonography. *AJNR* 1982;3:619—622.

31. Rypens F, Avri EF, Dussaussois L, et al. Hyperechoic thickened ependyma: sonographic demonstration and significance in neonates. *Pediatr Radiol* 1994;24:550—553.

32. Anderson N, Allan R, Darlow B, Malpas T. Diagnosis of intraventricular hemorrhage in the newborn: value of sonography via the posterior fontanelle. *AJR* 1994;163:893—896.

33. DiPietro MA, Brody BA, Teele RL. The calcar avis: demonstration with cranial ultrasound. *Radiology* 1985;156:363—364.

34. Volpe JJ. Intracranial hemorrhage: germinal matrix-intraventricular hemorrhage of the premature infant. In: Volpe JJ, ed. *Neurology of the Newborn*, 2nd ed. Philadelphia: WB Saunders, 1987, p. 403—463.

35. Volpe JJ. Current concepts of brain injury in the premature infant. Edward B. Neuhauser lecture. *AJR* 1989;153:243—251.

36. Babcock DS. Sonography of the brain in infants: role in evaluating neurologic abnormalities. *AJR* 1995;165:417—423.

37. Perlman J, Rollins N, Burns D, et al. Relationship between periventricular echodensities and germinal matrix — intraventricular hemorrhage in the very low birth weight neonate. *Pediatrics* 1993;91:474—480.

38. Nakamura Y, Okudera T, Fukuda S, et al. Germinal matrix hemorrhage of venous origin in preterm neonates. *Hum Pathol* 1990;21:1059—1062.

39. Guzzeta F, Shackelford G, Volpe S, Perlman JM, Volpe JJ. Periventricular intraparenchymal echodensities in the premature newborn: critical determinant of neurologic outcome. *Pediatrics* 1986;78:995—1006.

40. Takashima S, Mito T, Ando Y. Pathogenesis of periventricular white matter hemorrhage in preterm infants. *Brain Dev* 1986;8:25—30.

41. Martin CG, Snider AR, Katz SM, et al. Abnormal cerebral blood flow patterns in preterm infants with large patent ductus arteriosus. *J Pediatr* 1982;101:587—593.

42. Grunnet ML, Shilelds WD. Cerebellar hemorrhage in the premature infant. *J Pediatr* 1976;88:605—608.

43. Reeder JD, Setzer ES, Kaude JV. Ultrasonographic detection of perinatal intracerebellar hemorrhage. *Pediatrics* 1982;70:385—386.

44. Pape K, Armstrong D, Fitzhardinge P. Central nervous system pathology associated with mask ventilation in the very low birth weight infant: a new etiology for intracerebellar hemorrhage. *Pediatrics* 1976;58:473—483.

45. Govaert P, Van De Velde E, Vanhaesebrouck P, et al. CT diagnosis of neonatal subarachnoid hemorrhage. *Pediatr Radiol* 1990;20:139—142.

46. Volpe JJ. Intracranial hemorrhage: subdural, primary subarachnoid, intracerebellar, intraventricular (term infant), and miscellaneous. In: Volpe JJ, ed. *Neurology of the Newborn*, 2nd ed. Philadelpia: WB Saunders, 1987, p. 282—310.

47. Tanaka Y, Sakamoto K, Kobayashi S, et al. Biphasic ventricular dilatation following posterior fossa subdural hemorrhage in the full-term neonates. *J Neurosurg* 1988;68:211—216.

48. Lindenburg R, Freytag E. Morphology of brain lesion from blunt trauma in early infancy. *Arch Pathol* 1969;89:298.

49. Bergmann I, Bauer RE, Barmada MA, et al. Intracerebral hemorrhage in the full-term neonatal infant. *Pediatrics* 1985;75:488—496.

50. Burrows RF, Caco CC, Kelton JG. Neonatal alloimmune thrombocytopenia: spontaneous in utero intracranial hemorrhage. *Am J Hematol* 1988;28:98—102.

51. Babcock DA, Han BK, Weiss RG, Ryckman FC. Brain abnormalities in infants on extracorporeal membrane oxygenation: sonographic and CT findings. *AJR* 1989;153:571—576.

52. Taylor GA Fitz CR, Kapur S, Short BL. Cerebrovascular accidents in neonates treated with extracorporeal membrane oxygenation: sonographic-pathologic correlation. *AJR* 1989;153:355—361.

53. Bulas DI, Taylor GA, Fitz CR, et al. Posterior fossa intracranial hemorrhage in infants treated with extracorporeal membrane oxygenation: sonographic findings. *AJR* 1991;156:571—575.

54. Flodmark O, Lupton B, Li D, et al. MR imaging of periventricular leukomalacia in childhood. *AJR* 1989;152:583—590.

55. Appleton R, Lee R, Hey E. Neurodevelopmental outcome of transient neonatal intracerebral echodensities. *Arch Dis Child* 1990;65:27—29.

56. Schellinger D, Grant EG, Richardson JD. Cystic periventricular leukomalacia: sonographic and CT findings. *AJNR* 1984;5:439—445.

57. DiPietro MA, Brody BA, Teele RL. Peritrigonal echogenic "blush" on cranial sonography: pathologic correlates. *AJR* 1986;146:1067—1072.

58. Guit GL, van de Bor N, der Ouden L, et al. Prediction of neurodevelopmental outcome in the preterm infant: MR staged myelination compared with cranial US. *Radiology* 1990;175:107—109.

59. Dietrich RB, Bradley WG, Zavagoza EJ, et al. MR evaluation of early myelination patterns in normal and developmentally delayed infants. *AJR* 1988;150:889—896.

60. van de Bor M, der Ouden L, Gujit GL. Value of cranial ultrasound and magnetic resonance imaging in predicting neurodevelopmental outcome in preterm infants. *Pediatrics* 1992;90:196—199.

61. Huang CC. Sonographic cerebral sulcal development in premature newborns. *Brain Dev* 1991;13:27—31.

62. Winkler P. Pediatric Neurosonography. International Pediatric Radiology Conference. Neuroradiology Course. Boston, MA, 1996.

63. Carson SC, Hertzberg BS, Bowie JD, Burger PC. Value of sonography in the diagnosis of intracranial hemorrhage and periventricular leukomalacia: a postmortem study of 35 cases. *AJNR* 1990;11:677—683.

Vascular System

43 Sonographic Evaluation of the Carotid Arteries in Patients with TIA, Stroke, or Carotid Bruits

Joseph F. Polak

Introduction

The benefit of surgical interventions for patients with carotid artery stenoses is now well accepted. It has been shown for symptomatic[1,2] as well as asymptomatic[3] patients with significant internal carotid artery stenoses. The determination of what represents a significant carotid lesion has recently been determined to be a stenosis of 50% diameter narrowing, or more, graded according to the method used in the NASCET study.[4]

Understanding the role played by sonography in identifying patients who may benefit from surgery requires an appreciation of the incidence of ischemic stroke and the linkage to carotid artery disease. In order to better understand this linkage, the relationships between the pathologic aspects of atherosclerotic plaque growth and the diagnostic performance of carotid sonography must first be examined.

Stroke and TIA: Link to Carotid Artery Disease

Strokes and parenthetically transient ischemic attacks have many different etiologies. Two broad categories are hemorrhagic and ischemic. Events occurring in young subjects include primary brain hemorrhage associated with aneurysm rupture. In older individuals, brain hemorrhage can also occur in association with hypertensive episodes. In the broad category of ischemic insults, embolic phenomena account for most cases of stroke in the USA. Cardioembolic events tend to be associated with atrial fibrillation, with embolization of thrombi forming in the left atrium, to prosthetic valves with embolization of thrombi forming on the replacement valves or to left ventricular dysfunction with embolization of thrombi forming in the left ventricle. This linkage is supported by the detection of presumed embolic events with transcranial sonography: event rates are much greater for patients with prosthetic valves and atrial fibrillation than patients without.[5] Atheroembolism is the likely etiology of most strokes in patients with large carotid artery plaque deposits. This linkage is supported by transcranial Doppler signal detection of high intensity transitory signals (HITS) that increase in numbers as the severity of carotid plaques increase.[6] This does not exclude the possibility that carotid stenoses can progress and cause significant enough narrowing of the artery to cause an ischemic stroke because of a significant enough reduction in blood flow to cause underperfusion of the brain. This hypoperfusion syndrome affects the watershed area between the middle and the posterior and anterior circulations of the brain and is a much less common source of symptoms than embolic events from atherosclerotic plaque. Another major cause of ischemic events is lacunar strokes. These are believed to be caused by small vessel disease with lesions affecting the penetrating lenticulostriate branches of the middle cerebral arteries.

Differential Diagnosis

In the patient presenting with stroke, the clinical decision algorithm seeks, first of all, to distinguish ischemic from hemorrhagic strokes. The therapeutic options seem broader in the group of ischemic stroke because the inciting event often has an extracranial origin. Hemorrhagic strokes are often linked to intracranial pathologies, aneurysms or tumors, or to hypertensive episodes and small vessel rupture. Once a neurologic event has been classified as being ischemic, the role of sonography appears better defined: can sonography identify lesions that are directly associated with the presenting symptoms of an ischemic stroke? Arriving at an answer to this question requires three steps: (1) identifying the type of lesion that causes ischemic stroke and defining its appearance at sonography, (2) establishing the diagnostic accuracy of sonography in patients with and without neurological symptoms or carotid bruits and, (3) linking the results of sonographic examinations with outcomes.

Carotid Plaque: Appearance and Association with Ischemic Stroke

Examination of pathological specimens removed during carotid endarterectomy has shown that plaque hemorrhage is associated with the presence of transient ischemic attacks and with stroke.[7] Subsequent studies have suggested that areas of intraplaque hemorrhage correspond to hypoechoic zones seen with B-mode sonography.[8,9] Based on these observations, it would seem possible that sonography might be used to identify specific plaque characteristics that are indicative of an increased risk for subsequent stroke.

Studies have shown that the baseline appearance of carotid plaque is linked to the severity of carotid stenosis.[10,11] The sonographic appearance of carotid artery plaque changes as the severity of disease progresses: large plaques (causing greater degrees of stenosis) are more likely to be heterogeneous, with hypoechoic areas.[10] The hypoechoic areas seen with sonography need not correspond to zones of intraplaque hemorrhage. In fact, there is much overlap in the sonographic appearance of smooth muscle cells, lipid, and thrombus.[12] Pathologic studies have also shown that the presence of intra-plaque hemorrhage need not be associated with any symptoms.[13,14]

Surface irregularities in the atherosclerotic plaque are believed to serve as the nidus for the formation of platelet aggregates that then embolize. Carotid plaque ulceration seen during arteriography seems to be associated with a high likelihood for stroke.[15] This observation may be relevant to symptomatic individuals with high grade ($\geq 70\%$) stenoses. By itself, however, the arteriographic appearance of carotid plaque does not appear to predict the pathologic appearance.[8,15,16] Similarly, sonographic detection of carotid ulceration is poor when compared to pathologic specimens.[17,18]

The one characteristic of atherosclerotic plaque that consistently correlates with the risk of incident stroke is the severity of the internal carotid artery narrowing. The more the internal carotid artery is narrowed, the higher the likelihood for incident stroke.[1] The positive relationship between incident stroke and internal carotid artery disease has also been shown in patients where carotid artery stenosis severity has been measured with Doppler waveform analysis.[3,19] The ACAS, ECST, and NASCET studies did not, however, offer any evaluation of plaque characteristics. A prospective international multicenter natural history study of asymptomatic carotid stenosis (ACSRS), including plaque characterization, is now in progress. It does appear that hypoechoic plaque is associated with the risk of incident stroke in adults aged 65 years or more.[20]

Technique

A high-frequency transducer (7.5- to 10-MHz) is used to visualize the vascular structures because the carotid vessels are superficial. Evaluation of the vessels to characterize plaque is made in both the transverse and sagittal projections by high resolution gray scale alone, without CFDI (**Fig. 43–1**). After plaque characterization, CFDI is used to look for areas of turbulence, aliasing, or mosaic patterns. This helps identify the area of greatest stenosis. Doppler spectral analysis is used to determine the peak systolic velocity and the end diastolic velocity of the ICA by sampling at the area of turbulence. Measurements are made also of the peak systolic velocity and end diastolic velocity of the unobstructed CCA usually 2 cm proximal to the bulb. Ratios can be measured of peak systolic and end diastolic velocities.

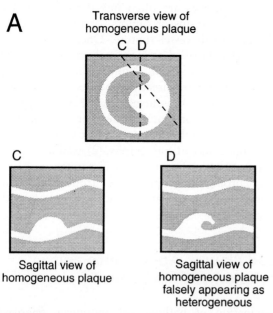

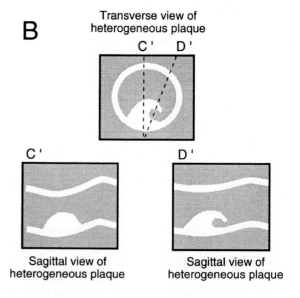

Figure 43–1 Line diagram showing the value of obtaining both transverse and sagittal images when characterizing plaque. In the sagittal plane, images can be obtained which would falsely simulate (**A**) homogeneous plaque (line C′) or (**B**) heterogeneous plaque (D).

Correlation in both planes is necessary to be certain that the plaque is characterized correctly. Reprinted with permission from Bluth E. Evaluation and characterization of carotid plaque. *Sem in US, CT, MRI* 1997;18:58.

Plaque Characterization

Several different classification schemes exist to characterize plaque. The homogeneous and heterogeneous descriptions have been popularized in the United States,[9,21-23] while in Europe a grading system has been used.[12] Both classification systems describe similar findings and, as a result, can be translated and in some cases interchanged.

Homogeneous plaque is relatively uniform in texture compared with the soft tissues surrounding the vessel wall. It has a smooth surface. Heterogeneous plaque has a complex echo pattern that contains at least one well-defined focal sonolucent area (**Fig. 43-2**). The intimal surface of the plaque can be smooth or irregular. In order to characterize plaque successfully, scanning must be performed in the sagittal and transverse planes. Alternatively, plaque can be classified into types I, II, III, and IV with type I the most echolucent and type IV the most echogenic. Several studies have linked the presence of heterogeneous or type I or II plaques with developing new neurologic events as well as ipsilateral CT brain infarcts.[20,24-26]

In order to develop a more reproducible and standardized method of plaque characterization and avoid the pitfalls of operator dependence, a new method has been developed to "normalize" different images by performing digital image processing. This has been successful in reducing the coefficient of variation from 47% to less than 5%.[27]

Diagnostic Accuracy of Sonography for Evaluating Carotid Artery Disease

Hemodynamically significant stenoses are, by definition, associated with a pressure drop as blood flows across the stenosis proper. This will typically take place when a plaque causes at least a 50% narrowing of the lumen diameter. The velocity of blood flow increases as the lumen narrows and is the greatest at the point of maximal stenotic narrowing. This phenomenon can be used to determine stenosis severity with continuous-wave Doppler waveform analysis (nonimaging),[28] pulsed-Doppler waveform analysis[29] and color flow imaging.[30] The zone of increased velocity that is established at the point of maximal stenosis can continue as a stenotic jet, typically extending 1 to 2 cm distal to the stenosis.[31]

Most imaging laboratories rely on color flow imaging in combination with pulsed Doppler waveform analysis to detect and grade the severity of internal carotid artery stenoses.[32] Stenosis severity can also be estimated directly from the color flow image: (1) by measuring the size of the color channel (**Fig. 43-3**) which corresponds to the residual lumen of the artery[30,33] or (2) by obtaining a mean blood flow velocity value from the frequency shift information on the color flow image. Direct measurements of residual lumen require that the color PRF (pulse repetition frequency) be set high enough to minimize bleeding of the color flow information outside of the artery walls or into the plaque. Mean velocity estimates can be made from the color map by determining the point where the color signals alias[34] or by selecting a velocity "tag".[30,35] These direct measurements are not possible when the calcified portions of plaque are sufficiently large to mask any Doppler information from the artery lumen.[33] However, because the flow disturbances associated with a stenosis

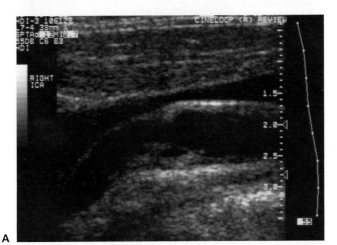

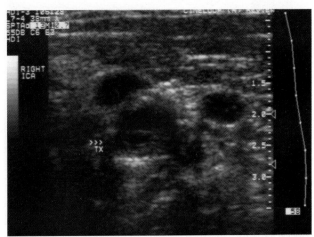

Figure 43–2 Sagittal (**A**) and transverse (**B**) images of heterogeneous or type II plaque. Note the presence of a well-defined focal hypo-echoic area within the plaque.

extend at least for at least one, and possibly two, centimeters downstream to the lesion,[29, 31, 36] the stenotic jet can still be sampled and graded with Doppler waveform analysis (**Fig. 43–4**). There is, therefore, a strong reliance on Doppler velocity estimates made with pulsed Doppler sonography when detecting the presence of lesions causing at least 50% diameter narrowing. Reported accuracies are close to 90%[32] or higher. Power Doppler (PD) sonography has been shown to help in distinguishing stenoses in the range of 50 to 70%.[37] Recently, it has been suggested that PD can be used as an accurate screening test.[38]

Blood flow velocity measurements are made by sampling the Doppler waveform at the site of stenosis and by correcting the frequency shift caused by moving blood with the aid of the Doppler equation. This requires that the sonographer estimate the direction of motion of blood. Errors made in determining the angle between Doppler ultrasound beam and the direction of flowing blood increase at angles above 60 degrees. The angle-corrected velocity measurements, therefore, become progressively less reliable as the angle between blood flow and the ultrasound beam increases above 60 degrees. Ambiguity in determining this angle is a source of intersonographer variability.

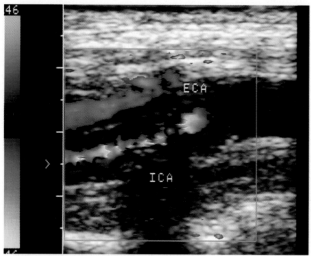

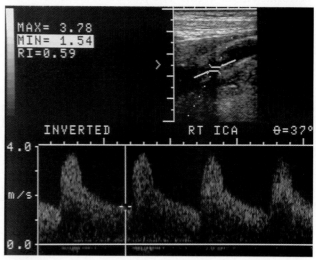

Figure 43–3 A: This color flow image shows a long stenosis of the internal carotid artery. The actual size of the color flow lumen cannot be used to grade the severity of the lesion as some of the color signals likely "bleed" into the diseased carotid wall. **B:** The high-grade lesion is confirmed by analysis of the Doppler waveform. Marked elevations of the peak systolic and end-diastolic velocities are consistent with a greater than 80% stenosis.

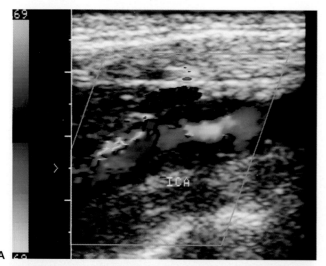

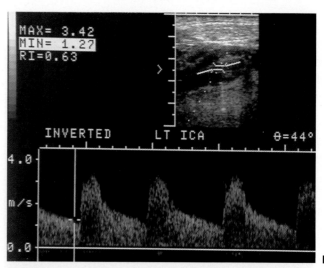

Figure 43–4 A: This color flow image shows aliasing of the color flow signals. Beyond the stenosis, the jet impacts on the outer wall of the internal carotid artery while a zone of flow reversal (**blue**) forms to the side and below. **B:** The high-grade stenosis is confirmed by Doppler waveform analysis showing marked elevations in the peak-systolic and end-diastolic velocities.

Stenosis grading

Grading stenosis has become an important issue as several randomized controlled trials involving more than 500 patients have demonstrated net benefits of carotid endarterectomy. The first NASCET[1] report has shown an absolute reduction in risk of 16.5% over a 2-year period for symptomatic patients with at least a 70% stenosis. A more recent NASCET report[39] of symptomatic patients with a 50 to 69% stenosis found an absolute risk reduction of 10.1% at 5 years, but no benefit for those with less than 50% stenosis. The ECST trial report documented an absolute risk reduction of 11.6% at 3 years in symptomatic patients with stenosis of 60% or greater as measured by the NASCET method.[40] The ECST Trial also showed that patients who had less than a 40% stenosis (by the NASCET Method) who underwent surgery had significantly poorer outcomes at 2 or 3 years than those treated medically.[41] Lastly, the ACAS[3] study showed an absolute reduction of 5.9% in the 5-year risk of ipsilateral stroke or any perioperative stroke or death for surgical intervention of asymptomatic patients who had a greater than 60% stenosis. These studies have now reemphasized the importance of identifying accurate noninvasive ways to identify flow limiting stenoses.

The second issue regarding grading stenosis has been the method to measure the angiographic correlations in the studies looking at surgical outcome of carotid endarterectomy. In the past, lumen diameter narrowing has often been measured by comparing the residual lumen of the internal carotid artery with a "best guess" of the diameter of the internal carotid artery[2, 29] (**Fig. 43–5**). This is the ECST technique and presently is still being used for the ACSRS study. The approach adopted by the NASCET and ACAS studies is to compare the residual diameter of the artery with that of the distal internal carotid artery beyond the stenosis (**Fig. 43–6**).

The differences of measuring techniques can and have been reconciled in order to compare results. A stenosis of 80% as measured in ECST is equivalent to a 60% NASCET or ACAS stenosis.[39-41] NASCET measurements of 30, 40, 50, 60, 70, 80, and 90% stenosis correspond to ECST stenosis grades of 65, 70, 75, 80, 85, 91, and 97% respectively.[39] As a result the Bluth, Stavros, Marich et al.[29] velocity criteria, which are based on ECST angiographic measurements, can still be used but the categories need to be adjusted upward to reflect NASCET technique for measuring angiograms. For example, the Bluth et al. > 80% stenosis categories of peak systolic velocity (PSV) of > 250 cm/sec, end diastolic velocity (EDV) > 100 cm/sec, systolic velocity ratio (SVR) > 3.7, and end diastolic velocity ratio (> 5.5) correspond with the 60% Moneta et al. criteria[42] (which use the NASCET methodology) of PSV > 260 cm/sec, EDV >70 cm/sec, and SVR > 3.5.

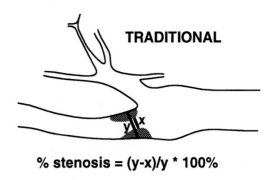

% stenosis = (y-x)/y * 100%

Figure 43–5 This diagram depicts the method of measuring stenosis severity as it has traditionally been performed.

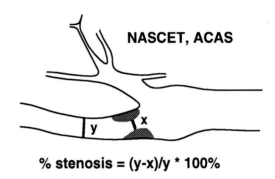

% stenosis = (y-x)/y * 100%

Figure 43–6 This diagram shows the current approach for determining stenosis severity based on the appearance of the distal internal carotid artery.

A diagnostic cut-point of 125 cm/sec in the peak-systolic velocity detects ≥ 50% stenosis when stenosis severity is graded with respect to the distal internal carotid artery.[32] Values for 70% diameter stenosis include a PSV of 230 cm/sec,[44] PSV ≥ 210 cm/sec,[45] PSV ≥ 130 cm/sec,[46] a PSV ratio of 4.0[45] or an end-diastolic velocity of 100 cm/sec[46] Moneta et al.[42] have described a PSV of ≥ 260 cm/sec corresponding to a 60% stenosis, while Carpenter et al.[43] suggests a cutoff of ≥ 170 cm/sec corresponds to the same degree of stenosis. All of these measurements of stenosis severity are made by relating the severity of carotid lumen diameter at the lesion to the internal carotid artery distal to the lesion (**Table 43–1**), at a presumed normal diameter.[47] How can we explain and reconcile all these differences? The values chosen to determine flow-limiting stenosis depend on the level of sensitivity and specificity the examiner hopes to achieve through the study. Increasing PSV and SVR increases specificity but decreases sensitivity and vice versa. Each laboratory must choose the velocity measurements that correspond with their ability to identify the correct degree of stenosis as compared with angiography or surgery and what degree of sensitivity and specificity they wish to achieve.[48]

Table 43–1   Current velocity cut-points for determining 70% or more stenosis of the internal carotid artery

Author	Parameter(s)	Accuracy
Hunink et al. [44]	ICA peak systolic velocity 230 cm/sec	sens .80, spec .90
Moneta et al. [42]	ICA/CCA peak systolic velocity ratio ≥ 4.0	sens .91, spec .87
Faught et al. [46]	ICA peak systolic velocity ≥ 130 cm/sec and ICA end diastolic velocity of ≥ 100 cm/sec	sens .81, spec .98
Neale et al. [73]	ICA peak systolic velocity ≥ 270 cm/sec and ICA end diastolic ≥ 110 cm/sec	sens .96, spec .91
Hood et al. [74].	ICA peak systolic velocity ≥ 130 cm/sec and ICA end diastolic velocity ≥ 100 cm/sec	sens .87, spec .97
Carpenter et al. [45]	ICA peak systolic velocity ≥ 210 cm/sec or ICA/CCA velocity ratio ≥ 3.0	sens .94, spec .77. sens .91, spec .78
Chen et al. [75]	ICA peak systolic velocity ≥ 125 cm/sec and ICA end diastolic velocity ≥ 135 cm/sec	sens .76, spec .93

Table 43–2   Current velocity cut-points for determining 60% or greater stenosis of the internal carotid artery

Author	Parameter(s)	Accuracy
Moneta et al. [76]	ICA peak systolic velocity ≥ 260 cm/sec and ICA end diastolic velocity ≥ 70 cm/sec	sens .84, spec .94
Carpenter et al.[43].	ICA peak systolic velocity ≥ 170 cm/sec	sens .98, spec .87
Fillinger et al. [77]	ICA/CCA peak systolic velocity ratio ≥ 2.6	sens .93, spec .97
	ICA peak systolic velocity ≥ 200 cm/sec	sens .95, spec, 93
	ICA peak systolic velocity ≥ 190 cm/sec	sens .87, spec 1.0
	ICA/CCA peak systolic velocity ratio ≥ 3.3	sens .95, spec .90
Jackson et al. [78]	ICA peak systolic velocity ≥ 245 cm/sec and ICA end diastolic velocity ≥ 65 cm/sec	sens .89, spec .92

Determining the relation between sonographic measurements of stenosis severity and outcomes is different than simply correlating the degree of stenosis on ultrasound with estimates made by arteriography. The ACAS study included sonographic evaluations of disease severity as part of the enrollment process.[3] At the early phases of the project, qualifying laboratories showed dismal performance in their ability to grade the severity of carotid artery disease.[49] Final outcome of the carotid ultrasound examination showed a specificity of 97%. The experimental design does not permit the determination of the diagnostic sensitivity of the sonographic examination.[3] However, review of the performance of different laboratories has shown that estimates of stenosis severity made by peak-systolic velocity measurements are less subject to interlaboratory differences.[50, 51] The diagnostic performance of sonography for detecting significant carotid artery disease in the NASCET study is very poor with a sensitivity of 68% and specificity of 67%.[52] There are many reasons why such estimates are biased towards poor performance: (1) no standard protocol, (2) lack of color flow imaging, (3) a process that averaged all of the velocity measurements from all laboratories involved without taking into consideration critical stenoses of ≥ 95%.[52]

Total versus Subtotal Occlusions

Very high-grade internal carotid artery lesions may be associated with a decrease in blood flow velocity rather than an increase.[28] The stenosis reaches such a level of severity that volume blood flow decreases thereby causing the velocities measured at the stenosis to decrease. This type of lesion can be difficult to evaluate with duplex sonography alone. The Doppler gate must be positioned over the very small residual lumen in the internal carotid artery. The hypoechoic elements of the stenosing plaque can obscure the normal residual lumen and mimic a stenosis of lesser severity. Alternatively, the residual lumen may be so small that it can be missed by duplex sonography alone. Color flow images, alternatively acquired in the longitudinal and the transverse planes, may help detect this very narrow residual lumen (**Fig. 43–4**). Once a patent lumen is identified, it can be directly interrogated with pulsed Doppler and waveform analysis is then possible. The color flow map can also be used to follow the course of the internal carotid to the point just downstream to the stenosis where blood flow signals are often distorted and of low amplitude. Doppler waveform analysis can then confirm patency of the internal carotid distal to the subtotal occlusion (**Fig. 43–7**). The accuracy of duplex sonography alone for distinguishing total from sub-total occlusions has been poor: approximately 50% in the early days of carotid Doppler sonography.[53] Color flow imaging may be more accurate than duplex ultrasound.[32, 54, 55] The total number of cases studied in the literature is too small to reach a firm

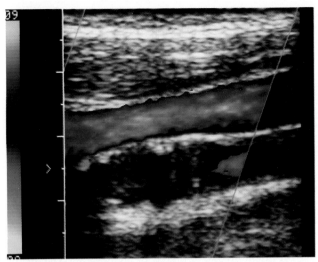
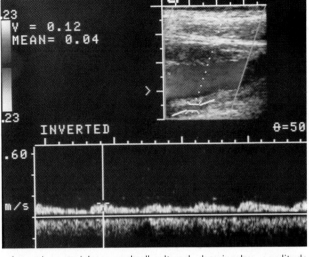

Figure 43–7 A This subtotal occlusion is difficult to appreciate on a longitudinal image of the internal carotid artery. Only faint color flow signals are seen proximal to the portion of the internal carotid artery that contains echogenic material. **B** Flow signals beyond the echogenic material are markedly altered, showing low amplitude and a low resistive index. This pattern is seen in the segment beyond the subtotally occluded internal carotid artery.

conclusion on the accuracy of the technique. Additionally, with the recent advent of PD, it is expected that the acccuracy has significantly improved.

Contralateral Stenosis

A critical stenosis on one side of the neck has a variable effect on the contralateral carotid system. There is a statistically significant increase in the measured velocity on the side contralateral to a high grade stenosis or total occlusion.[56] This may lead to overestimation of the severity of stenosis on the side contralateral to a high-grade stenosis.[57] There is no reliable way of predicting which patient will manifest this artifactual increase in blood flow velocity in the contralateral carotid artery. However, by paying careful attention to the correlation of the color or power image on transverse and sagittal sections, and correlating with the velocity measurements obtained, errors of overestimation can be avoided.

Hypoechoic Plaque

Color flow imaging is useful in evaluating lesions causing less than 50% diameter narrowing. Hypoechoic plaque that is not easily perceived on gray scale image can be quite readily depicted with color flow imaging[30,53] and, more recently, with PD.

Ulcerated Plaque

Gray scale imaging performs poorly in detecting ulcerated carotid plaque.[17,18] A localized zone of flow reversal or stagnation of blood flow can be seen in the ulcer crater.[58,59] This sign is specific, but not sensitive for detecting the presence of ulceration in lesions that cause a stenosis of less than 50% of the normal lumen diameter.[30] However, the presence of smaller irregularities in the contour of the plaque surface on color flow images appears to correlate with the presence of symptoms.[58]

Is Carotid Ultrasound Indicated in Patients with Stroke or Transient Ischemic Attacks?

Should carotid sonography be done in patients presenting with stroke or TIA? The current recommendations from an American Heart Association task force view carotid sonography as a secondary modality: "diagnostic studies aimed at establishing a likely etiology of acute ischemic stroke, including ultrasound or other imaging of intracranial or extracranial vessels, can, in some circumstances, be helpful in making decisions about treatment."[60]

A broader view suggests that ultrasound is an atraumatic way of determining whether a carotid lesion is possibly responsible for the patient's symptoms. The examination, conducted in the early stages of patient presentation, is done at a time when a TIA cannot be distinguished from a stroke. Operative intervention, in the early stages of a TIA or stroke, does not seem to carry a higher risk of morbidity than interventions done later.[61]

Once a carotid stenosis of clinical significance has been identified with sonography, additional evaluations have traditionally been done before the patient would be subjected to carotid artery surgery. Additional preoperative imaging with arteriography is considered the "gold standard." This strategy carries, however, a higher risk of stroke (1.2% in the ACAS study) than previously thought. One way to overcome this morbidity is to supplement sonography with Magnetic Resonance Angiography (MRA) of the carotid arteries.[62] Cases with conflicting results between MRA and sonography can then be sent to arteriography. Such a strategy is the more cost-effective than arteriography for symptomatic patients with ≥ 70% diameter stenosis of the internal carotid artery.[63] This strategy assumes a complete MRA examination consisting of 2 D Time-of-Flight as well as 3 D Time-of-Flight sequences. The accuracy of sonography is slightly greater than 2 D Time-of-Flight MRA while it may be slightly less than 3 D Time-of-Flight techniques.[64] For asymptomatic patients, the lower cut-point of 60% stenosis would favor the sole use of carotid ultrasound as a cost-effective strategy.[65] These strategic approaches are very dependent on the morbidity of the surgical procedure and assume rates of less than 5%.[63,65]

MRA evaluation of the carotid and innominate artery origin increases imaging time and cost. The frequency of unrecognized origin stenoses is estimated at 0.6%, and the more significant ones likely cause perturbations in the downstream Doppler waveform in the carotid branches.[66] The intracranial vessels can also be evaluated if there is a need. However, the diagnostic performance of Time-of-flight MRA does not seem to be very high.[63] The presence of tandem lesions that could possibly be missed with this diagnostic strategy likely does not affect outcome of subsequent carotid endarterectomy.[67] It appears, in fact, that the number of clinical risk factors might be a better predictor of a negative perioperative outcome.[68]

Is Carotid Ultrasound Useful in Patients with Carotid Bruits?

Patient selection based on carotid bruits is an interesting strategy. The presence of a carotid bruit is an insensitive and nonspecific indicator of carotid artery disease. In addition, the presence of a carotid bruit, although it is associated with an increased incidence of neurological events, need not predict an event on the same side as the bruit. The carotid bruit serves as a nonspecific marker of atherosclerotic disease.[69] Often, the bruit may be due to a lesion in the external carotid artery or be transmitted from a more proximal lesion. As a screening strategy, carotid ultrasound has much better sensitivity and specificity than the detection of a carotid bruit by physical examination.[70]

The finding of an internal carotid artery stenosis in an asymptomatic patient with a carotid bruit can lead to an interesting dilemma. If the findings from the ACAS study are to be believed, then an individual should undergo carotid endarterectomy if the stenosis causes a ≥ 60% narrowing in the diameter of the proximal internal carotid artery. With this apparent indication for carotid surgery, the patient may well be managed cost-effectively with carotid sonography as the sole preoperative diagnostic test.[65] However, reticence to believe that the ACAS results apply to both men and women or to individuals 68 years or less has lead to a conservative approach. A stenosis of ≥ 80% is still considered by many surgeons as the best cut-point for surgery in the asymptomatic patient. Further study of this important issue is necessary.

Estimating the Risk of Atheroembolism Based on the Findings of the Carotid Examination

Prevalent stroke is linked to stenosis severity in the internal carotid artery, but the stroke need not be on the same side as the more severely diseased carotid artery.[71] The relationship between carotid artery lesions and incident stroke is a bit clearer: the greater the severity of internal carotid artery stenosis measured by arteriography, the larger the risk of an incident stroke. In NASCET, for example, there is a positive dose—response curve between stenosis severity and the likelihood of incident stroke in symptomatic patients with ≥ 70% diameter stenosis. Sonographic estimates of disease severity do not appear to relate as nicely with incident strokes, at least in the NASCET study.[52] There are many possible explanations for the poor association between estimated carotid artery stenosis severity by Doppler ultrasound and incident stroke in the NASCET study. One likely explanation is the lack of a standardized carotid ultrasound imaging protocol. The lack of a standardized protocol has been shown to affect overall accuracy of the velocity estimates made with Doppler sonography.[49] Correcting these deficiencies dramatically improves the diagnostic performance of carotid sonography.[3]

As discussed previously, the morphology of internal carotid artery plaque also appears to be associated with stroke and TIA. The sonographic appearance of the carotid lesion correlates with symptoms and may be a predictor of subsequent stroke. This area remains somewhat controversial. The situation has, in fact, become less clear with the conclusion of the NASCET and ACAS studies. Most of the emphasis has now shifted to estimating internal carotid artery stenosis as lumen diameter narrowing. Presence or absence of ulceration or areas of plausible intraplaque hemorrhage has taken less importance. New studies looking at the impact of plaque characteristics on subsequent neurological events are therefore needed. A recent study has in fact shown that hypoechoic plaque seen on a carotid artery ultrasound can predict subsequent strokes.[20] A new international multicenter natural history study[27] is now in progress and may add new additional information.

Summary

Although Magnetic Resonance Angiography is increasingly being considered as a possible screening test for carotid artery disease, it is unlikely to replace duplex sonography. MRA complements duplex sonography and both techniques serve as a substitute for traditional contrast arteriography.

Color flow imaging and duplex sonography are cost-effective screening techniques. Use as the sole preoperative examination preceding carotid endarterectomy in a symptomatic population is increasing.[3] Adoption of a strategy where carotid sonography is the sole preoperative test requires careful attention to the technical aspects of the examination with quality control procedures taking on a great importance.[72]

References

1. North American Symptomatic Carotid Endarterectomy Trial Collaborators. Beneficial effect of carotid endarterectomy in symptomatic patients with high-grade stenosis. *New Engl J Med* 1991;325:445—453.

2. European Carotid Surgery Trialists' collaborative group. MRC European Carotid Surgery Trial: interim results for symptomatic patients with severe (70—99%) or with mild (0—29%) carotid stenosis. *Lancet* 1991;337:1235—1243.

3. Executive committee for the Asymptomatic Carotid Atherosclerosis Study. Endarterectomy for asymptomatic carotid artery stenosis. *JAMA* 1995;273:1421—1428.

4. Barnett HJM, for the NASCET Collaborators. Final results for the North American Symptomatic Carotid Endarterectomy Trial (NASCET). *Stroke* 1998;29:286.

5. Georgiadis D, Grosset DG, Kelman A, Faichney A, Lees KR. Prevalence and characteristics of intracranial microemboli signals in patients with different types of prosthetic cardiac valves. *Stroke* 1994;25:587—592.

6. Markus H, Droste D, Brown M. Detection of asymptomatic circulating cerebral emboli signals in patients with potential emboli sources. *Lancet* 1994;343:1011—1012.

7. Lusby RJ, Ferrell LD, Ehrenfeld WK, Stoney RJ, Wylie EJ. Carotid plaque hemorrhage: its role in production of cerebral ischemia. *Arch Surg* 1982;117:1479—1488.

8. O'Donnell TF, Erdoes L, Mackey WC, et al. Correlation of B-mode ultrasound imaging and arteriography with pathologic findings at carotid endarterectomy. *Arch Surg* 1985;120:443—449.

9. Bluth E, Kay D, Merritt C, et al. Sonographic characterization of carotid plaque: detection of hemorrhage. *AJR* 1986;146:1061—1065.

10. Polak JF, O'Leary DH, Kronmal RA, et al. Sonographic evaluation of carotid artery atherosclerosis in the elderly: relationship of disease severity to stroke and transient ischemic attack. *Radiology* 1993;188:363—370.

11. Lennihan L, Kupsky W, Mohr J, et al. Lack of association between carotid plaque hematoma and ischemic cerebral symptoms. *Stroke* 1987;18:879—881.

12. Widder B, Paulat K, Hackspacher J, et al. Morphological characterization of carotid artery stenoses by ultrasound duplex scanning. *Ultrasound Med Biol* 1990;16:349—354.

13. Svindland A, Torvik A. Atherosclerotic carotid disease in asymptomatic individuals: a histological study of 53 cases. *Acta Neurol Scand* 1988;1988:506—517.

14. Bassiouny HS, Davis H, Massawa N, et al. Critical carotid stenoses: morphologic and chemical similarity between symptomatic and asymptomatic plaques. *J Vasc Surg* 1989;9:202—212.

15. Eliasziw M, Streifler J, Fox A, et al. Significance of plaque ulceration in symptomatic patients with high-grade carotid stenosis. North American Symptomatic Carotid Endarterectomy Trial. *Stroke* 1994;25:304—308.

16. Imparato AM, Riles TS, Mintzer R, Baumann FG. The importance of hemorrhage in the relationship between gross morphologic characteristics and cerebral symptoms in 376 carotid artery plaques. *Ann Surg* 1983;197:195—203.

17. O'Leary DH, Holen J, Ricotta JJ, Roe S, Schenk EA. Carotid bifurcation disease: prediction of ulceration with B-mode US. *Radiology* 1987;162:523—525.

18. Bluth EI, McVay LV, Merritt CRB et al. The identification of ulcerative plaque with high resolution duplex carotid screening. *J Ultrasound Med* 1988;1:73—76.

19. Chambers BR, Norris JW. Outcome in patients with asymptomatic neck bruits. *N Engl J Med* 1986;315:860—865.

20. Polak JF, Shemanski L, O'Leary DH, et al. Hypoechoic plaque at US of the carotid artery: an independent risk factor for incident stroke in adults aged 65 years or older. *Radiology* 1998;208:649—654.

21. Bluth E. Evaluation and characterization of carotid plaque. *Sem in US, CT, MRI* 1997;18:57—65.

22. Reilly LM, Lusby RJ, Jeffrey RB et al. Carotid plaque histology using real time ultrasonography. Clinical and therapeutic implications. *Am J Surg* 1983;146:188—193.

23. Gray-Weale AC, Graham JC, Burnett JR et al. Carotid atheroma. Comparison of preoperative B-mode ultrasound appearance with carotid endarterectomy pathology. *J Cardiovasc Surg* 1988;26:676—681.

24. Geroulakos G, Domjan J, Nicolaides A, et al. Ultrasonic carotid artery plaque structure and the risk of cerebral infarction on computed tomography. *J Vasc Surg* 1994;20:263—266.

25. Sterpetti AV, Schultz RD, Feldhouse RJ. Ultrasonographic features of plaque and the risk of subsequent neurologic deficits. *Surgery* 1988;104:652—660.

26. Nicolaides AN. The value of computer analysis of ultrasonic plaque echolucency in identifying high risk carotid bifurcation lesions. *JEMU* 1996;17:404.

27. Nicolaides AN, Sabetai MM, Tegos TJ et al. The Echomorphology of the Atherosclerotic Carotid Plaque — the ACSRS Study. The World Congress on Cerebral Embolism New Orlean, La. Nov 1988 (Abs).

28. Spencer MP, Reid JM. Quantitation of carotid stenosis with Continuous-Wave (C-W) Doppler ultrasound. *Stroke* 1979;10:326—330.

29. Bluth EI, Stavros AT, Marich KW, et al. Carotid duplex sonography: a multicenter recommendation for standardized imaging and Doppler criteria. *RadioGraphics* 1988;8:487—506.

30. Steinke W, Kloetzsch C, Hennerici M. Carotid artery disease assessed by color Doppler flow imaging: correlation with standard Doppler sonography and angiography. *AJR* 1990;154:1061—1068.

31. Baxter GM, Polak J. Variance mapping in colour flow imaging: what does it measure? *Clin Radiol* 1994;49:262—265.

32. Polak JF, Dobkin GR, O'Leary DH, Wang AM, Cutler AS. Internal carotid artery stenosis: accuracy and reproducibility of color-Doppler-assisted duplex imaging. *Radiology* 1989;173:793—798.

33. Erickson SJ, Newissen MW, Foley WD, et al. Stenosis of the internal carotid artery: assessment using color Doppler imaging compared with angiography. *AJR* 1989;152:1299—1305.

34. Hallam MJ, Reid JM, Cooperberg PL. Color-flow Doppler

and conventional duplex scanning of the carotid bifurcation: prospective, double-blind, correlative study. *AJR* 1989; 152:1101—1105.

35. Landwehr P, Schindler R, Heinrich U, et al. Quantification of vascular stenosis with color Doppler flow imaging: in vitro investigations. *Radiology* 1991;178:701—704.

36. Vattyam HM, Shu MC, Rittgers SE. Quantification of Doppler color flow images from a stenosed carotid artery model. *Ultrasound Med Biol* 1992;18:195—203.

37. Griewing B, Morgenstern C, Driesner F, et al. Cerebrovascular disease assessed by color-flow and power Doppler ultrasonography. Comparison with digital subtraction angiography in internal carotid artery stenosis. *Stroke* 1996;27:95—100.

38. Bluth EI, Merritt C, Sullivan MA, et al. A screening test for carotid stenosis: a preliminary feasibility study. *Radiology Supplement* 1997;205:545.

39. Barnett HJ, Taylor DW, Eliasziw M et al. Benefit of carotid endarterectomy in patients with symptomatic moderate or severe stenosis. *N Engl J Med* 1998;339:1415—1425.

40. The European Carotid Surgery Trialists Collaborative Group. Randomized trial of endarterectomy for recently symptomatic carotid stenosis; final results of the MRC European Carotid Surgery Trial (ECST) *Lancet* 1998;351:1379—1387.

41. Chassin MR. Appropriate use of carotid endarterectomy. *NEJM*:1998;337:1468—1471.

42. Moneta GL, Edwards JM, Chitwood RW, et al. Correlation with North American Symptomatic Carotid Endarterectomy Trial (NASCET) angiographic definition of 70% to 99% internal carotid artery stenosis with duplex scanning. *J Vasc Surg* 1993;17:152—157.

43. Carpenter JP, Lexa FJ, Davis JT. Determination of sixty percent or greater carotid artery stenosis by duplex Doppler ultrasonography. *J Vasc Surg* 1995;22:697—705.

44. Hunink MGM, Polak JF, Barlan MM, O'Leary DH. Detection and quantification of carotid artery stenosis: efficacy of various Doppler velocity parameters. *AJR* 1993;160:619—625.

45. Carpenter JP, Lexa FJ, Davis JT. Determination of duplex Doppler ultrasound criteria appropriate to the North American Symptomatic Carotid Endarterectomy Trial. *Stroke* 1996;27:695—699.

46. Faught WE, Mattos MA, van Bemmelen PS, et al. Color-flow duplex scanning of carotid arteries: new velocity criteria based on receiver operator characteristic analysis for threshold stenoses used in the symptomatic and asymptomatic carotid trials. *J Vasc Surg* 1994;1994:818—828.

47. North American Symptomatic Carotid Endarterectomy Trial (NASCET) Steering Committee. North American Symptomatic Carotid Endarterectomy Trial. Methods, patient characteristics, and progress. *Stroke* 1991;22:711—720.

48. Zweibel WJ. New Doppler parameters for carotid stenosis. *Sem in US, CT MRI* 1997;18:66—71.

49. Howard G, Chambless LE, Baker WH, et al. A multicenter study of Doppler ultrasound versus angiography. *J Stroke Cerebrovasc Dis* 1991;1:166—173.

50. Howard G, Baker WH, Chambless LE, et al. An approach for the use of Doppler ultrasound as a screening tool for hemodynamically significant stenosis (despite heterogeneity of Doppler performance). A multicenter experience. Asymptomatic Carotid Atherosclerosis Study Investigators. *Stroke* 1996;27:1951—1957.

51. Kuntz KM, Polak JF, Whittemore AD, Skillman JJ, Kent KC. Duplex ultrasound criteria for the identification of carotid stenosis should be laboratory specific. *Stroke* 1997;28:597—602.

52. Eliasziw M, Rankin RN, Fox AJ, et al. Accuracy and prognos-

tic consequences of ultrasonography in identifying severe carotid artery stenosis. *Stroke* 1995;26:1747—1752.

53. Zwiebel WJ, Austin CW, Sackett JF, Strother CM. Correlation of high resolution, B-mode and continuous-wave Doppler sonography with arteriography in the diagnosis of carotid stenosis. *Radiology* 1983;149:523—532.

54. Hetzel A, Eckenweber B, Trummer B, Wernz M, von Reutern GM. Color-coded duplex ultrasound in pre-occlusive stenoses of the internal carotid artery (published erratum). *Ultraschall Med* 1993;14:240—246.

55. Berman S, Devine J, Erdoes L, Hunter G. Distinguishing carotid artery pseudoocclusion with color-flow Doppler. *Stroke* 1995;26:434—438.

56. Hayes AC, Johnston W, Baker WH, et al. The effect of contralateral disease on carotid Doppler frequency. *Surgery* 1988;103:19—23.

57. Spadone DP, Barkmeier LD, Hodgson KJ, Ramsey DE, Sumner DS. Contralateral internal carotid artery stenosis or occlusion: pitfall of correct ipsilateral classification — a study performed with color flow imaging. *J Vasc Surg* 1990;11:642—649.

58. Steinke W, Hennerici M, Rautenberg W, Mohr JP. Symptomatic and asymptomatic high-grade carotid stenoses in Doppler color-flow imaging. *Neurology* 1992;42:131—138.

59. Furst H, Hartl WH, Jansen I, et al. Color-flow Doppler sonography in the identification of ulcerative plaques in patients with high-grade carotid artery stenosis. *AJNR* 1992;13:1581—1587.

60. Adams H, Brott T, Crowell R, et al. Guideines for the management of patients with acute ischemic stroke. A statement for healthcare professionals, from a special writing group of the Stroke Council, American Heart Association. *Circulation* 1994;90:1588—1601.

61. Gasecki AP, Ferguson GG, Eliasziw M, et al. Early endarterectomy for severe carotid artery stenosis after a nondisabling stroke: results from the North American Symptomatic Carotid Endarterectomy Trial. *J Vasc Surg* 1994a;20:288—295.

62. Polak JF, Kalina P, Donaldson MC, et al. Carotid endarterectomy: preoperative evaluation of candidates with combined Doppler sonography and MR angiography. *Radiology* 1993;186:333—338.

63. Kent KC, Kuntz KM, Patel MR, et al. Perioperative strategies for carotid endarterectomy: an analysis of morbidity and cost-effectiveness in symptomatic patients. *JAMA* 1995;274:888—893.

64. Patel MR, Kuntz KM, Klufas RA, et al. Preoperative assessment of the carotid bifurcation. Can magnetic resonance angiography and duplex ultrasonography replace contrast arteriography? *Stroke* 1995b;26:1753—1758.

65. Kuntz KM, Skillman JJ, Whittemore AD, Kent KC. Carotid endarterectomy in asymptomatic patients — Is contrast angiography necessary? A morbidity analysis. *J Vasc Surg* 1995c;22:706—716.

66. Akers DL, Markowitz IA, Kerstein MD. The value of aortic arch study in the evaluation of cerebrovascular insufficiency. *Am J Surg* 1987;154:230—232.

67. Mattos MA, van Bemmelen PS, Hodgson KJ, et al. The influence of carotid siphon stenosis on short- and long-term outcome after carotid endarterectomy. *J Vasc Surg* 1993;17:902—910.

68. McCrory DC, Goldstein LB, Samsa GP, et al. Predicting complications of carotid endarterectomy. *Stroke* 1993;24:1285—1291.

69. Heyman A, Wilkinson WE, Heyden S, et al. Risk of stroke in asymptomatic persons with cervical arterial bruits. A population study in Evans County, Georgia. *N Engl J Med* 1980;302:838—841.

70. Ingall TJ, Homer D, Whisnant JP, Baker HL, O'Fallon WN. Predictive value of carotid bruit for carotid atherosclerosis. *Arch Neurol* 1989;46:418—422.

71. Norris JW, Zhu CZ. Silent stroke and carotid stenosis. *Stroke* 1992;23:483—485.

72. Chervu A, Moore WS. Carotid endarterectomy without arteriography. *Ann Vasc Surg* 1994;8:296—302.

73. Neale ML, Chambers JL, Kelly AT, et al. Reappraisal of duplex criteria to assess significant carotid stenosis with special reference to reports from the North American Symptomatic Carotid Endarterectomy Trial and the European Carotid Surgery Trial. *Stroke* 1994;20:642—649.

74. Hood DB, Mattos MA, Mansour A, et al. Prospective evaluation of new duplex criteria to identify 70% internal carotid artery stenosis. *J Vasc Surg* 1996;23:254—61;discussion 261—262.

75. Chen JC, Salvian AJ, Taylor DC, et al. Predictive ability of duplex ultrasonography for internal carotid artery stenosis of 70%—99%: a comparative study. *Ann Vasc Surg* 1998;12:244—247.

76. Moneta GL, Edwards JM, Papanicolaou G, et al. Screening for asymptomatic internal carotid artery stenosis: duplex criteria for discriminating 60% to 99% stenosis. *J Vasc Surg* 1995;21:989—994.

77. Fillinger MF, Baker RJ, Jr., Zwolak RM, et al. Carotid duplex criteria for a 60% or greater angiographic stenosis: variation according to equipment. *J Vasc Surg* 1996;24:856—864.

78. Jackson MR, Chang AS, Robles HA, et al. Determination of 60% or greater carotid stenosis: a prospective comparison of magnetic resonance angiography and duplex ultrasound with conventional angiography. *Ann Vasc Surg* 1998;12:236—243.

44 Leg Swelling with Pain or Edema

Edward I. Bluth

Introduction

Because they are at risk for having acute deep venous thrombosis (DVT), patients who present with leg swelling with pain or edema are of great clinical concern. Acute DVT is an important public health problem because it affects over twenty million individuals yearly in the United States. It occurs in both sedimentary outpatients as well as hospital inpatients although rarely in children. Among the predisposing factors are prolonged congestive heart failure, pelvic and lower extremity surgery, pregnancy, obesity, inactivity, coagulopathy, and paraplegia.[1]

The diagnosis of DVT has other significant implications as well. It has been known for more than a century that DVT may be a presenting feature of an occult neoplasm. Recently, a definite association between DVT and a subsequent clinically occult cancer has been shown, particularly in the first 6—12 months of follow-up.[2] However, in the study by Sorensen et al. 40% of the patients diagnosed with cancer within 1 year of the diagnosis of DVT had distant metastases. As a result, it is uncertain whether an extensive search for an occult neoplasm would be cost effective or warranted as early diagnosis may not change outcomes. The types of cancers most strongly associated with DVT in this Swedish study of more than 15 000 patients were cancer of the pancreas, ovary, liver (primary hepatic cancer) and brain.[2]

Presently, it is important to diagnose acute DVT because of its relationship with acute pulmonary embolism. The presence of DVT does not equate with pulmonary embolism, but detecting DVT may prevent pulmonary embolism from developing. It is reported that when significant acute venous thrombosis is diagnosed but not treated, pulmonary embolism is likely to occur in up to 50% of the cases.[3] More importantly, it is believed that in up to 30% of the episodes of pulmonary embolism the outcome is death.[3] Mortality can be significantly reduced when acute DVT is treated with anticoagulation. Because an estimated 90% of pulmonary emboli arise from the lower extremities, there is a great clinical need to accurately assess the venous system of the lower extremities when there is clinical suspicion of acute DVT.

Accuracy of Clinical Presentation

Patients who present with the clinical symptomatology of leg swelling with pain or edema certainly are at risk for acute DVT. However, the clinical accuracy of diagnosing this entity is known to be very poor. Every clinical sign attributed to DVT has been statistically analyzed and found to be of no value in reliably determining the presence or absence of DVT.[4] The location of signs and symptoms of pain or swelling is usually unrelated to the extent or location of clot within the veins. Symptoms localized to the calf may have an etiology in the femoral veins, and thigh pain may be related to occlusion of calf veins.[5] The specificity for clinical diagnosis is low as the symptomatology associated with acute DVT can have, among other causes, a musculoskeletal or lymphatic basis. Furthermore, asymptomatic DVT can commonly occur, and the sequelae can even be severe enough to cause death by pulmonary embolism.

In patients who present with bilateral leg symptoms, in the absence of significant risk factors (such as malignancy, paralysis, bed rest of more than 3 days, major surgery, strong family history of DVT, or leg, thigh, or calf swelling)[6] the first assumption should be that the etiology is cardiac disease or chronic peripheral vascular disease.[7] However, in patients with risk factors, the possibility of bilateral clot must be seriously considered, and a bilateral ultrasound (US) examination is warranted.

Differential Diagnosis

The differential diagnosis for the symptoms of leg swelling with pain or edema includes acute DVT, Baker's (popliteal) cyst, cellulitis, lymphadema, chronic venous insufficiency, superficial thrombophlebitis, popliteal venous aneurysm, popliteal artery aneurysm, femoral artery pseudoaneurysm, enlarged lymph nodes extrinsically compressing the veins, heterotopic ossification, hematoma and muscular tears.[5, 8—15] The appropriate use of imaging studies, and, in particular, the appropriate use of US, enables us to distinguish which of these clinical entities is present.

Baker's cysts appear as sonolucent or complex masses more commonly medial than lateral. When they rupture, the surface margins become irregular (**Fig. 44–1**). They appear separate and distinct from the popliteal artery or vein. The normal popliteal artery measures less than 1 cm. Veins and arteries should taper normally, and an outpouching would suggest aneurysmal dilatation. Frequently, thrombus may surround the residual lumen of an arterial aneurysm (**Fig. 44–2**). Aneurysms or pseudoaneurysms, owing to their expanded size, can compress the venous stuctures that surround them, resulting in swelling or edema of the distal extremity. The visualization of a concomitant vascular abnormality should, therefore, not preclude further evaluation of the more distal venous structures as the resultant stasis may be a predisposing factor to the development of DVT (**Fig. 44–3**). Patients with superficial thrombophlebitis have an increased risk of progressing to DVT. In one report, 11% of patients who initially had isolated superficial venous thrombus progressed to DVT.[16] In another study, 23% of patients with superficial thrombophlebitis had occult DVT of the lower extremities.[17] As a result, if superficial venous thrombosis is noted, then the deep venous system should be carefully studied. Similarly, enlarged lymph nodes can also extrinsically compress adjacent venous structures resulting in lower extremity symptoms (**Fig. 44–4**). On rare occasions, pain or swelling of the lower extremity may be the presenting symptom of lymphoma. Lymph nodes appear separate from the vascular structures and are easily distinguished using color flow Doppler imaging (CFDI). Hematoma are also separate and distinct from the arteries and veins and, depending on their age, appear as either complex or sonolucent masses.

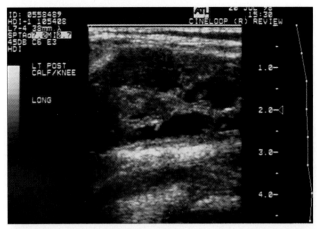

Figure 44–1   Oblique image of a complex mass in the popliteal space separate and medial to the artery and vein. This is characteristic of a ruptured Baker's cyst.

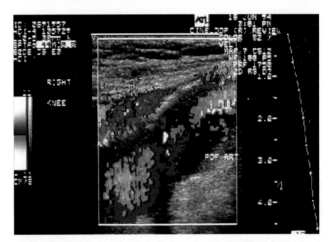

Figure 44–2   Sagittal color flow Doppler imaging (CFDI) image of a 2-cm popliteal artery aneurysm. Note large amount of thrombus present within the aneurysm.

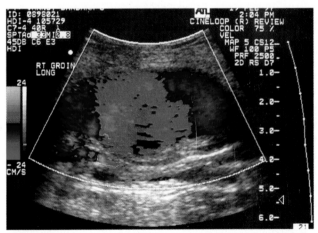

A

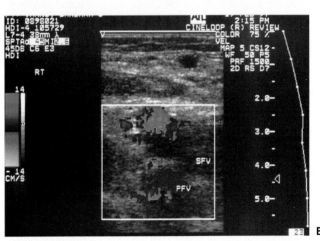

B

Figure 44–3   A: Large pseudoaneurysm of the right common femoral artery (CFA) post cardiac catheterization compressing the common femoral vein (CFV). **B**: Transverse image showing the more expanded hypoechoic noncompressible proximal superficial femoral vein (SFV) consistent with acute thrombus.

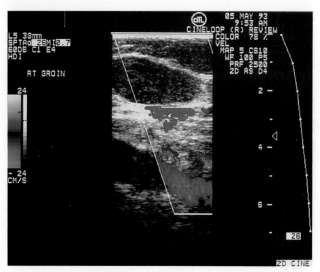

Figure 44–4 Solid mass density in the right inguinal area separate and apart from the CFA and CFV. On biopsy this mass of nodes was diagnosed as nonHodgkin's lymphoma.

Diagnostic Workup

Tests to evaluate the lower extremities include contrast venography, venous ultrasound including CFDI and Doppler spectral analysis, impedance plethysmography (IPG), various radionuclide approaches, magnetic resonance (MR) venography, computed tomography, nonimaging continuous wave Doppler, and thermography. All evaluation methods were studied by the Cardiovascular Appropriateness Panel of the American College of Radiology (ACR), and each of these methods was rated for appropriateness in 1995 (**Table 44–1**).[18]

Table 44–1 American College of Radiology Appropriateness Criteria for Clinical Condition: Suspected Deep Vein Thrombosis (DVT)

Radiologic exam procedure	Appropriateness rating
Duplex Doppler compression ultrasound (US)	9
Leg venography	6
Pelvic venography	5
IPG	5
MR venography	5
Color Doppler ultrasound (US) without compression	4
CT pelvis with contrast	4
Radionuclide venography	4
CW Doppler (nonimaging)	2
Plain film	1

Apropriateness Criteria Scale 1 2 3 4 5 6 7 8 9. 1 = least appropriate, 9 = most appropriate Reproduced with permission from the M American College of Radiology. Appropriate Criteria for suspected DVT. American College of Radiology 1993,3, Reston, Virginia.

Contrast venography has been the "gold standard" by which other examination methods have been rated, however, in 5—10% of patients it may not give a reliable result, and because it also requires the use of intravenous contrast with the associated risks of renal failure, extravasation, chemical-induced thrombophlebitis, and idiopathic contrast reactions, its appropriateness rating was only intermediate. In contrast, duplex Doppler compression ultrasound received the highest possible rating and, therefore, now should be used as the study of choice to evaluate symptomatic patients.

The panel reported also that thermography and nonimaging continuous wave Doppler analysis were inappropriate and should not be performed. IPG was given an intermediate appropriateness rating as was MR venography. The accuracy of IPG is reported to be close to 90% for DVT above the knees but it requires meticulous technique. Heijboer et al. reported that serial ultrasonography is a more accurate means of detecting DVT than is IPG. An abnormal IPG had a positive predictive value of 83% for DVT compared with a 94% rate for an ultrasound abnormality in patients with DVT.[19] Recently introduced MR venography appears to be promising, particularly to detect thrombi above the inguinal ligament or when extrinsic compression of the iliac veins mimicks DVT.[20, 21] However, larger-scale studies need to demonstrate MR's efficacy before it should be widely used for these applications. Radionuclide venography was given a lower intermediate rating. The accuracy of detecting large obstructive thrombi is reported to be close to 90%. Another approach which can be used and appears best to diagnose DVT below the knee or in the lower thigh is the active uptake of radionuclide-labeled fibrinogen, platelets, peptides, fibrin, and plasmin by thrombi. New imaging agents may also be helpful in differentiating acute recurrent from chronic DVT. Computed tomography is most useful for imaging thrombosis related to the iliac veins and is not particularly suitable for studying the femoro-popliteal veins.

Ultrasound Imaging

Evaluating patients with symptoms of leg swelling with pain or edema should involve using all the capabilities of US when available including Doppler spectral analysis, CFDI, transducer compression, and high-resolution B-mode imaging. The examination should integrate all these methodologies into the complete study of the venous structures of the lower extremity. Extended field of view sonography, a new option of some machines, may be useful in demonstrating more easily the full extent of disease. The use of contrast agents and harmonic imaging may be helpful, in the future, in cases in which the complete occlusion of vessels is uncertain.

Normal Sonographic Findings

With Doppler spectral analysis and CFDI, three parameters of normal lower extremity veins can be identified: respiratory phasicity, spontaneous flow, and augmentation. During the respiratory cycle, the change in venous flow is termed *respiratory phasicity* (**Fig. 44–5**). During inspiration (Fig 44–6 A), an increase in intraabdominal pressure causes compression of the inferior vena cava and a decease in the Doppler signal. In expiration, there is an increase in visualized flow and in the Doppler spectral analysis signal (**Fig. 44–6 B**). The Valsalva maneuver leads to stasis and venous dilatation. The normal physiologic response of the femoral vein is a 50—200% increase in diameter. At the end of the Valsalva maneuver, augmented venous flow normally occurs (**Fig. 44–7**). In a normal venous system, augmentation also occurs with distal mechanical compression (**Fig. 44–8**). Spontaneous venous flow is easily detected

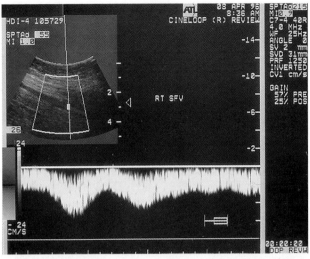

Figure 44–5 Normal phasic respiratory pattern of the superficial femoral vein (SFV) seen with Doppler spectral analysis.

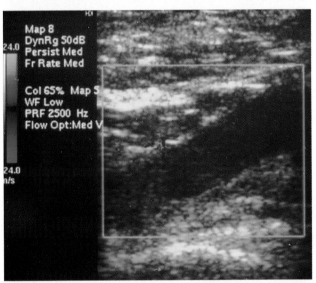

A

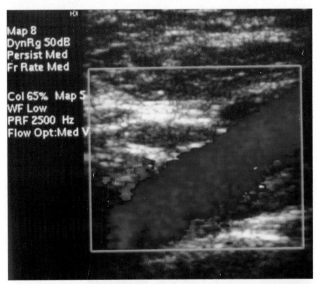

B

Figure 44–6 CFDI image of a normal common femoral vein demonstrating normal physiologic phasic respiratory changes. On deep inspiration (**A**), flow appears to be absent or decreased. On expiration (**B**), flow is increased (augmented).

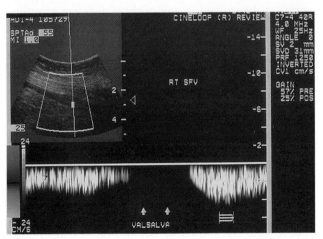

Figure 44–7 A normal superficial femoral vein demonstrating initially normal venous flow, then absence of flow during the Valsalva maneuver and then slight augmentation of flow following the maneuver.

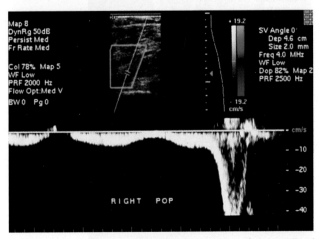

Figure 44–8 A normal augmentation response of the popliteal vein following distal compression.

in the large leg vessels but is frequently not seen in some of the smaller calf vessels. Augmentation will frequently be required to prove patency.

A normal vein also demonstrates compressibility, has unidirectional flow, and is free of internal echoes. Compressibility is best demonstrated when the transducer is held in the transverse position relative to the vein because the transducer will not roll off the vessel (**Fig. 44–9**). An adequate amount of pressure sufficient to dimple the overlying skin should be applied with the transducer in order to visualize the normal sonographic finding of a collapsed venous lumen. Unidirectional flow is best identified with CFDI.

Ultrasound Technique

The choice of tranducers for studying the lower extremities depends on the patient's body habitus and the depth of the vessel being studied. For the average patient, a 5-MHz transducer is most appropriate. Vessels ranging in size from 1 mm to slightly over 1 cm can be clearly visualized over a depth of 6 cm. For large-body habitus patients, transducers of 2.5 or 3.75 MHz can be used. Linear array transducers permit long segments of vessels to be imaged more rapidly and are therefore preferred. Transducers will frequently need to

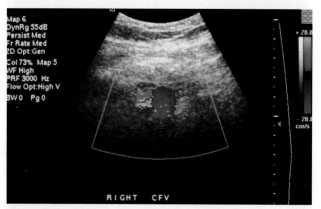

A

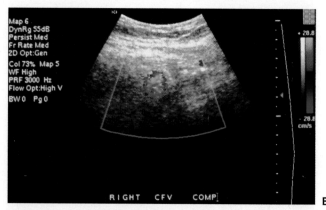

B

Figure 44–9 Transverse CFDI images demonstrating the normal common femoral vein (CFV — blue) and the common femoral artery (CFA — red) without (**A**) and with (**B**) compression. Note the collapse of the normal vein.

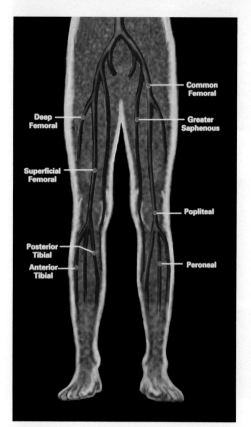

Figure 44–10 Vessels commonly visualized when evaluating the veins of the lower extremities.

be switched when the examiner moves from the inguinal region to the thicker thigh or the calf veins.

Vessels that can be studied include the common femoral veins; saphenous veins; superficial femoral veins; popliteal veins; calf veins including the anterior tibial, posterior tibial and peroneal veins; and if possible, the iliac veins (**Fig. 44–10**). The external iliac, common femoral, saphenous and superficial femoral veins are best evaluated with the patient supine. The popliteal veins can be studied in any of three different positions: with the patient prone and the leg flexed 20—30 degrees, with the patient decubitus and the study side up, and by elevating the foot and leg and scanning from below (**Fig. 44–11**). At times, a combination of these techniques is necessary. Flow augmentation of the calf veins can be achieved by having the patient plantar flex the foot. This self-augmentation technique helps in better visualization of these vessels. Some have advocated studying the calf veins by having the patient sitting up and dangling the legs over the side of the examining table.

Sonographers and sonologists should carefully scan the femoral veins to look for duplicated vessels. In a recent report, Screaton et al. demonstrated that multiple femoral veins were present in 177 (46%) of 381 venograms.[22] This is much more than the generally accepted frequency of duplication of 20—25%.[23] However, even with this high frequency of duplication, Screatin et al demonstrated only a 6% false-negative rate, which was not statistically significant compared to the 1% (four of 402 patients) false-negative rate found in patients with single femoral veins. However, for the inexperienced, it is important to realize that the incidence of duplication for femoral veins is significant and, therefore, special attention must be directed to insure that a duplicated thrombosed vessel is not ignored.

Examination Protocol

Recently, there has been considerable debate about what constitutes an adequate and appropriate examination. The traditional protocol described in the ACR Standard for Performance of The Peripheral Venous Ultrasound Examination adopted in 1993 calls for the careful examination of the full length of the common femoral vein, superficial femoral vein and popliteal vein.[18] Images with and without compression should be recorded at the common femoral, mid-superficial femoral and mid-popliteal veins. We use CFDI as an adjunct in nearly all our examinations as it helps speed identification of vessels. Power Doppler imaging can sometimes be useful in identifying early recanalization, but because there is no directionality of flow, it is not as useful as CFDI alone. Doppler spectral analysis is useful in assessing phasicity and augmentation responses and is particularly helpful as a secondary means of evaluating the patency of the iliac veins. Some centers also include the study of the greater saphenous vein where it enters the common femoral vein as part of the routine examination because of the risk of superficial thrombophlebitis extending into the deep system.

Limited Compression Examinations

Pezzullo, Perkins, and Cronan recently reported in a prospective study of 53 symptomatic patients and a retrospective study of 155 symptomatic patients that a limited compression examination of the common femoral (from the inguinal ligament to the takeoff of the profunda femoral vein) and of the popliteal vein (above and below the knee) depicted each case of DVT that was detected with the traditional more complete examination.[24] Additionally, they found a 54% reduction in examination time (9.7 min) with the limited study. As a result, they recommended studying just the common femoral and popliteal veins and repeating the study in 2—5 days if the patient was still symptomatic. In reaction, Frederick et al. prospectively studied 721 symptomatic patients and determined after 755 examinations that DVT limited to a single vein occurs with sufficient frequency that the study could not be abbreviated without loss of diagnostic accuracy.[25] They found that DVT was limited to the common femoral vein in eight studies (6.1%), to the superficial femoral vein in six

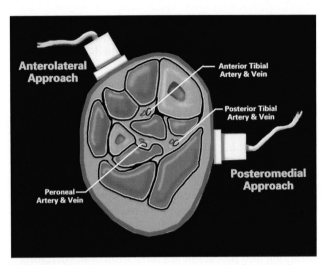

Figure 44–11 Diagram demonstrating practical anatomic approaches used to study the calf veins.

studies (4.6%), and to the popliteal vein in 14 studies (10.7%). They found no statistically significant difference between the frequency of isolated thrombus in any of these three veins. As a result, it appears that all these three major veins must still be carefully studied.

Calf Veins

The issue of what to do about studying the calf veins is also controversial. The ACR Standard does not require the study of calf veins because of the generally accepted principle that it is safe to withhold anticoagulation treatment for isolated calf vein thrombosis as no significant thrombi arise from these veins. However, while most calf vein thromboses resolve spontaneously, approximately 20% extend to the proximal venous system.[24] This suggests that if symptoms persist or worsen, a repeat study should be performed even if an initial study was negative. In 2% of patients who had an initial normal examination, abnormalities were evident on serial testing due to extension of calf vein thrombosis.[6] Even in the most careful and detailed examination of the calf veins, it is difficult to be certain that all of the possibly duplicated vessels are free of thrombus. It has been suggested, however, that a negative US combined with a normal plasma D-dimer value or low pretest risk factor probability can exclude DVT without further tests.[6] With the more recent aggressive interventional approaches to thrombolytic therapy for treating DVT, the accurate identification of calf vein thrombosis which might propagate proximally is becoming increasingly important, and including the calf veins in the assessment of the lower extremity is advisable.

How to Scan Carefully

How carefully the vessels are studied depends on the history and symptomatology. Usually, it is adequate to scan every 1—2 cm of the veins. In most symptomatic patients, the clot usually involves multiple or whole venous segments. However, orthopedic patients, particularly those who had hip fractures and joint replacements, have short and focal segments of thrombus above the knee and extensive thrombus in the calf veins. As a result, if the calf veins are not studied, the examiner should study the veins above the knee in shorter intervals than they might otherwise plan to do. Additionally, absent flow augmentation tells the examiner that there should be an obstruction between the site of Doppler sampling and the site of augmentation and, therefore, a detailed study of this area should be performed.

Unilateral or Bilateral?

Another controversial issue regarding technique is whether to study both lower extremities, which has traditionally been done. However, in a recent article, Naidich et al.[26] showed that in only 1% of patients was the thrombus found in the asymptomatic leg when evaluation of the symptomatic leg was negative. Cronan[7] described that the likelihood of finding clots solely in the asymptomatic leg as between 0% and 1% and therefore questioned the routine evaluation of the asymptomatic leg. However, the status of the venous structures is important, particularly in differentiating acute recurrent thrombus from chronic venous thrombus. Therefore, routine bilateral studies are probably worthwhile, if for no other reason than as a baseline for future comparison.

Benefits of Ultrasound

Classic Findings of Acute DVT

When classic findings are present, acute venous thrombosis appears to be hypoechoic. On CFDI it can be demonstrated as an intraluminal defect or color void. Acute DVT expands the venous lumen; it is noncompressible, does not demonstrate augmentation, and as an indirect sign, the distal vein demonstrates nonvariable venous signals or loss of phasicity (**Figs. 44–12—44–14**). The latter finding is particularly important when the iliac veins are not well visualized and they can only be secondarily evaluated by interrogating the common femoral veins.

Accuracy

Loss of compressibility of the veins is the most important of the criteria and is the most universally accepted as being highly accurate (**Fig. 44–7**). Cronan pooled the results of several series which totaled 1619 lower extremities and compared compression ultrasonography with ascending venography. This pooling resulted in a 95% sensitivity and a 98% specificity for compression ultrasound.[4] Many studies have similarly shown the high accuracy of compression sonography in diagnosing acute DVT. The sensitivities range from 88% to 100% and the specificities from 92% to 100%.[19,27—39] Additionally, in several outcome studies, patients who had negative compression ultrasounds and therefore were followed but not treated with anticoagulation did not have any evidence of developing pulmonary emboli.[40,41] This adds further credence to the accuracy of this technique. With CFDI, the normal vessels are usually completely filled in with color indicating patency. Additionally, compression, phasicity, and augmentation responses can be studied. Several studies have reported

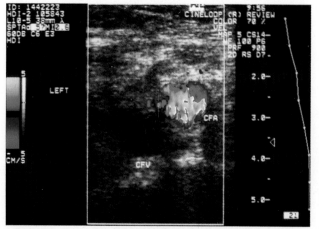
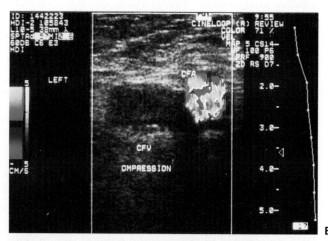

Figure 44–12 Transverse images of the left common femoral vein (CFV). In (**A**) the CFV is expanded, hypoechoic, and demonstrates no color. With compression (**B**) the vein remains expanded and does not compress. This is diagnostic of acute DVT.

that CFDI was comparable to compression sonography.[42, 43] Lewis et al. reported a sensitivity of 95%, a specificity of 99%, an accuracy of 98%, a positive predictive value of 95%, and a negative predictive value of 99%.[44] For isolated calf vein thrombosis, the sensitivity is significantly lower, ranging between 60% and 80%. Lewis et al. also reported that the rate for indeterminate results in their patients was 6% with CFDI, which was comparable to the rate of indeterminate examinations reported for compression sonography.

Complications

There are very few complications attributed to US. Although no complications are generally assumed to be the result of compression US, a few case reports have described documented cases of a pulmonary embolism developing as a result of a compression study of a superficial femoral vein.[45] Gentle compression is therefore advised particularly when acute thrombus is present.

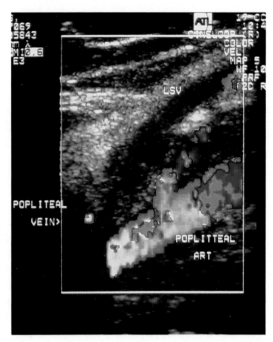

Figure 44–13 Sagittal CFDI image of an acutely occluded popliteal vein (PV) and lesser saphenous vein (LSV). Note that the thrombosed veins appear expanded and hypoechoic.

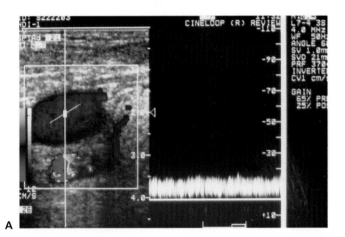

A

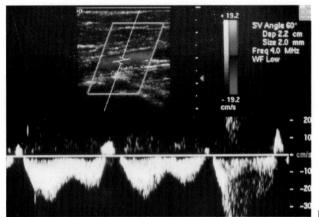

B

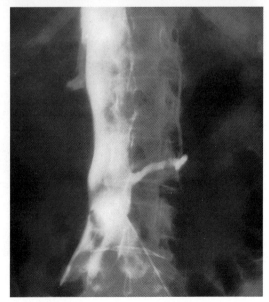

C

Figure 44–14 Duplex images of the right (**A**) and left (**B**) CFV showing flow in both vessels but loss of respiratory phasicity demonstrated by the flattened right Doppler spectral analysis pattern compared to the left. This suggests a proximal obstruction of either the more proximal femoral or iliac veins. The venogram (**C**), indicated extensive thrombus in the right iliac vein.

Limitations

The limitations of this technique include proximal obstruction by an extrinsic mass such as adenopathy, hematoma, or tumor, which may, therefore, limit compressibility of the venous structures and suggest a false-positive diagnosis. Additionally, congestive heart failure with secondary venous distension may also lead to an inaccurate assessment and false-positive diagnosis.

Other significant problems relate to differentiating chronic thrombus from an acute exacerbation. This is particularly difficult in patients with chronic DVT who have residual changes of a thickened venous wall and who have decreased compliance. When recurrent thrombus occurs in these patients, the venous wall cannot acutely expand and diagnostic certainty decreases.

False-negative examinations can occur in obese patients and patients with edematous extremities, which are therefore difficult to examine. Small nonocclusive thrombi less than 3 cm in length in the profunda femoral vein and the distal popliteal vein in particular are prone to being missed.[42, 43] The adductor canal is a particularly difficult site to produce a technically adequate examination, but luckily isolated thrombus in this location is rare.[29] Another pitfall is to mistake a patent lessor saphenous vein at the saphenopopliteal junction for a distal popliteal vein which is thrombosed (**Fig. 44–13**). Usually, the saphenous vein is more superficial and is smaller than the 3—4 mm popliteal vein.

Frequently, iliac veins are difficult to visualize, but if careful attention is paid to the spectral analysis patterns of the visualized portions of the distal iliac and femoral veins and loss of phasicity is noted, a secondary sign of proximal thrombosis will not be missed and the correct diagnosis will be suggested (**Fig 44–14**) . Collateral vessels can also be mistaken for occluded vessels. Collaterals can be differentiated by appreciating the fact that the true venous structure is adjacent to the artery while collateral veins have a more random relationship (**Fig. 44–15**). Lastly, the venous structures are frequently duplicated, and this duplication cannot always be visualized even with CFDI. Thrombosis in one of these duplicated vessels may go undetected.

Chronic Venous Thrombosis

Cronan has reported that after 6 months of acute DVT, 48% of veins will still have demonstrable abnormalities on US examination. In this study, 14% of the abnormal veins remained completely occluded.[4] A larger number of veins recanalized to some extent but remained with residual clot as organized thrombus material along the vein wall. This organized fibrous intimal venous thickening results from an ingrowth of inflammatory cells which begins to occur soon after acute thrombus adheres to the venous endothelium. This thickened vein will now resist compression, causing confusion with nonocclusive thrombosis, and can lead to the incorrect diagnosis of acute recurrent thrombosis.

Some findings that can help distinguish chronic from acute thrombosis include the fact that chronic thrombus does not expand the venous lumen, that chronic thrombus is generally more echogenic than acute thrombus, that collateral vessels when seen particularly with CFDI suggest a chronic etiology, and that flow is seen within the central venous lumen with CFDI and the wall changes may be better appreciated (**Fig. 44–16, 44–17**). However, in many cases, distinguishing recurrent acute venous thrombosis from chronic thrombosis is a very difficult diagnostic dilemma. Perhaps there may be a role for radionuclide imaging or MR in some of these indeterminate cases.

Chronic Venous Insufficiency Syndrome

The chronic venous insufficiency syndrome occurs as a result of destruction of venous valves secondary to acute DVT, allowing blood to flow from the deep to the superficial venous system. The resulting volume overload and distension or obstruction of these veins produces a clinical picture of pain, swelling, skin changes, necrosis, and superficial ulcerations. This syndrome can be identified by seeing reverse flow with CFDI for more than 1 s when the patient performs the Valsalva maneuver (**Fig. 44–18 A,B**). Other methods to test for reflux include applying compression to the limb above the area being evaluated and producing augmentation by squeezing the calf with the patient standing and then observing the venous response.[46] Johnson et al. reported that after an episode of DVT, 41% of patients developed features of the chronic venous insufficiency synrome although only 13% of patients

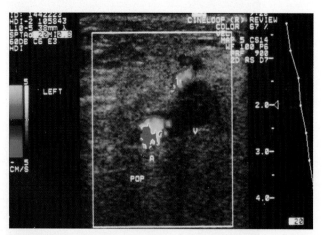

Figure 44–15 Large collateral vessel adjacent to an occluded popliteal vein. Note that the collateral vein is not immediately adjacent to the artery.

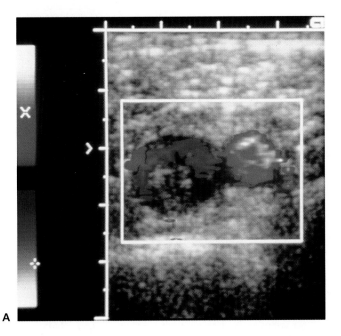

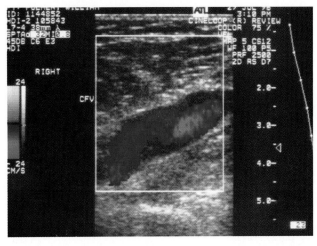

Figure 44–16 Transverse (**A**) and sagittal (**B**) images demonstrating recanalized flow around chronic thrombus in two different patients. The vein is not expanded and the thrombus is echogenic.

developed skin complications.[47] The magnitude of the reflux detected by US appears to be related to the likelihood of developing ulcerations.[46]

Summary

Ultrasound is now recognized as the first and most appropriate study to perform when a patient presents with symptomatic lower extremities suggesting acute venous thrombosis. There are numerous advantages to performing a sonographic study of the lower extremities. These evaluations can be performed portably, generally cause no complications, and do not involve the use of contrast media or radiation. In approximately 10% of patients, other abnormalities such as Baker's cysts, arterial aneurysms, or hematomas can be detected and can explain the symptoms (**Fig. 44–2—44–4**). The limitations of ultrasound are that it requires experienced

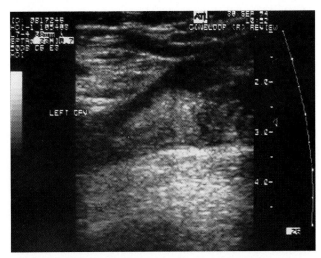

Figure 44–17 Sagittal image of a left CFV which contains chronic residual thrombus from a previous episode of DVT but now has superimposed acute recurrent thrombosis as evidenced by the expanded noncompressible CFV.

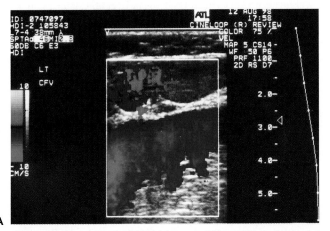

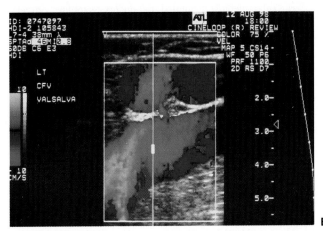

Figure 44–18 A: Sagittal CFDI image of the CFV during quiet breathing. **B:** Same vessel imaged after Valsalva maneuver. Note reversed flow which lasted for several seconds and was consistent with reflux.

operators, it is frequently hard to define the iliac and calf veins, it is difficult to distinguish chronic from acute recurrent thrombosis, and the presence of duplicated vessels can be a significant challenge to achieving an accurate study. Nonetheless, because it is the study of choice, it is important for all those who involved in diagnostic ultrasound to be comfortable in performing and interpreting these examinations.

References

1. Foley WD. Extremity venous disease. In: Foley WD, ed. *Color Doppler Flow Imaging.* Reading MA: Andover Press, 1991, p. 129—151.
2. Sorensen HT, Mellemkjaer L, Steffensen FH, Olsen JH, Nielsen GL. The risk of a diagnosis of cancer after primary deep venous thrombosis or pulmonary embolism. *N Engl J Med* 1998;338:1169—1173.
3. Needleman L, Polak J. Suspected lower extremity deep vein thrombosis. In: *American College of Radiology Appropriateness Criteria for Imaging and Treatment Decisions.* Reston VA: ACR 1995; CV-8.1—8.6.
4. Cronan JJ. Venous thromboembolic disease: the role of US. Radiology 1993;186:619—630.
5. Hirsh J, Hull RD. Venous thromboembolism: natural history, diagnosis and management. In: *Diagnosis of Venous Thrombosis.* Boca Raton, FL: CRC Press, 1987, p. 23—28.
6. Ginsberg JS. Management of venous thromboembolism. *N Eng J Med* 1996;335:1816—1828.
7. Cronan JJ. Controversies in venous ultrasound. *Sem US, CT, MR* 1997;18:33—38.
8. Bluth EI, Merritt CR, Sullivan MA. Gray-scale evaluation of the lower extremities. *JAMA* 1982;247:3127—3129.
9. Borgstede JP, Clagett GE. Types, frequency, and significance of alternative diagnoses found during duplex Doppler venous examinations of the lower extremities. *J Ultrasound Med* 1992;11:85—89.
10. Sandler DA, Mitchell JR. How do we know who has had deep venous thrombosis? *Postgrad Med J* 1989;65:16—19.
11. Grice GD, Smith RB III, Robinson PH, Rheudasil JM. Primary popliteal venous aneurysm with recurrent pulmonary emboli. *J Vasc Surg* 1990;12:316—318.
12. Ross GJ, Violi L, Barber LW, Vujic I. Popliteal venous aneurysm. *Radiology* 1988;168:721—722.
13. Lutter KS, Kerr TM, Roedersheimer LR, et al. Superficial thrombophlebitis diagnosed by duplex scanning. *Surgery* 1991;110:42—46.
14. Ikeda M, Fujimori Y, Tankawa H, Iwata H. Compression syndrome of the popliteal vein and artery caused by popliteal cyst. *Angiology* 1984;35:245—251.
15. Swett HA, Jaffe RB, McIff EB. Popliteal cysts: presentation as thrombophlebitis. *Radiology* 1975;115:613—615.
16. Chengelis DL, Bendick PJ, Glover JL, Brown OW, Ranjal TJ. Progression of superficial venous thrombosis to deep vein thrombosis. *J Vasc Surg* 1996;24:745—749.
17. Jorgensen JO, Hanel KC, Morgan AM, Hunt JM. The incidence of deep venous thrombosis in patients with superficial thrombophlebitis of the lower limbs. *J Vasc Surg* 1993;18:70—73.
18. American College of Radiology (1993). *ACR Standards for Performance of the Peripheral Venous Ultrasound Examination.* Reston, VA.
19. Heijboer H, Buller HR, Lensing AW, et al. A comparison of real-time compression ultrasonography with impedance plethysmography for the diagnosis of deep venous thrombosis in symptomatic outpatients. *N Engl J Med* 1993;329:1365—1369.
20. Evans AJ, Sostman HD, Knelson MH, et al. Detection of deep venous thrombosis: prospective comparison of MR imaging with contrast venography. *AJR* 1993;161:131—139.
21. Spritzer CE, Norconk JJ Jr, Sostman HD, Coleman RE. Detection of deep venous thrombosis by magnetic resonance imaging. *Chest* 1993;104:54—60.
22. Screaton NJ, Gillard JH, Berman LH, Kemp PM. Duplicated superficial femoral veins: a source of error in the sonographic investigation of deep vein thrombosis. *Radiology* 1998; 206:397—401.
23. Cronan JJ. Venous duplex US of the lower extremities: effect of duplicated femoral veins. *Radiology* 1998;206:308—309.
24. Pezzullo JA, Perkins AB, Cronan JJ. Symptomatic deep venous thrombosis: diagnosis with limited compression US. *Radiology* 1996;198:67—70.
25. Frederick MG, Hertzberg BS, Kliewer MA, et al. Can the US examination for lower extremity deep venous thrombosis be abbreviated? A prospective study of 755 examinations. *Radiology* 1996;199:45—47.
26. Naidich JB, Torre JR, Pellerito JS, et al. Suspected deep venous thrombosis; is US of both legs necessary? *Radiology* 1996;200:429—431.
27. Rosner NH, Doris PE. Diagnosis of femoropopliteal venous thrombosis: comparison of duplex sonography and plethysmography. *AJR* 1988;150:623—627.
28. White RH, McGahan JP, Daschbach MM, Hartling RP. Diagnosis of deep-vein thrombosis using duplex ultrasound. *Ann Intern Med* 1989;111:297—304.
29. Vogel P, Laing FC, Jeffrey RB Jr, Wing VW. Deep venous thrombosis of the lower extremity: US evaluation. *Radiology* 1987;163:747—751.
30. Cronan JJ, Dorfman GS, Scola FH, Schepps B, Alexander J. Deep venous thrombosis: US assessment using vein compression. Radiology 1987; 162:191—194.
31. Cronan JJ, Dorfman GS, Grusmark J. Lower-extremity deep venous thrombosis: further experience with and refinements of US assessment. *Radiology* 1988;168:101—107.
32. George JE, Smith MO, Berry RE. Duplex scanning for the detection of deep venous thrombosis of lower extremities in a community hospital. *Curr Surg* 1987;44:202—204.
33. Appelman PT, De Jong TE, Lampmann LE. Deep venous thrombosis of the leg: US findings. *Radiology* 1987; 163:743—746.
34. Lensing AWA, Prandoni P, Brandjes D, et al. Detection of deep venous thrombosis by real-time B-mode ultrasonography. *N Engl J Med* 1989;320:342—345.
35. Froehlich JA, Dorfman GS, Cronan JJ, et al. Compression ultrasonography for the detection of deep venous thrombosis in patients who have a fracture of the hip. A prospective study. *J Bone Joint Surg (Am)* 1989;71:249—256.
36. O'Leary DH, Kane RA, Chase BM. A prospective study of the efficacy of B-scan sonography in the detection of deep venous thrombosis in the lower extremities. *J Clin Ultrasound* 1988;16:1—8.
37. Aitken AGF, Godden DJ. Real-time ultrasound diagnosis of deep vein thrombosis: a comparison with venography. *Clin Radiol* 1987;38:309—313.
38. Killewich LA, Bedford GR, Beach KW, Strandness DE, Jr. Diagnosis of deep venous thrombosis: a prospective study comparing duplex scanning to contrast venography. *Circulation* 1989;79:810—814.
39. Becker DM, Philbrick JT, Abbitt PL. Real-time ultrasonography for the diagnosis of lower extremity deep venous thrombosis: the wave of the future? *Arch Intern Med* 1989;149:1731—1734.

40. Vaccaro JP, Cronan JJ, Dorfman GS. Outcome analysis of patients with normal compression US examinations. *Radiology* 1990;175:645—649.

41. Sarpa MS, Messina LM, Smith M, et al. Significance of a negative duplex scan in patients suspected of having acute deep venous thrombosis of the lower extremity. *J Vasc Tech* 1989;13:222—226.

42. Rose SC, Zweibel WJ, Nelson BD, et al. Symptomatic lower extremity deep venous thrombosis: accuracy, limitations, and role of color duplex flow imaging in diagnosis. *Radiology* 1990;175:639—644.

43. Foley WD, Middleton WD, Lawson TL, et al. Color Doppler ultrasound imaging of lower extremity venous disease. *AJR* 1989;152:371—376.

44. Lewis BD, James EM, Welch TJ, et al. Diagnosis of acute deep venous thrombosis of the lower extremities: prospective evaluation of color flow Doppler imaging versus venography. *Radiology* 1994;192:651—655.

45. Perlin SJ. Pulmonary embolism during compression US of the lower extremity. *Radiology* 1992;184:165—166.

46. Polak JA. Peripheral artery and veins: Contributions of CFDI. In Bluth EI, Divon MY, Laurel, MD eds. Update in duplex, power and color flow imaging. American Institute of Ultrasound in Medicine. 1996;51—62.

47. Johnson BF, Manzo RA, Bergelin RO, Strandness DE, Jr. Relationship between changes in the deep venous system and the development of the postthrombotic syndrome after an acute episode of lower limb deep venous thrombosis: a one- to six-year follow-up. *J Vasc Surg* 1995;21:307—312.

45 Pulsatile Groin Mass in the Postcatheterization Patient

Barbara A. Carroll

Introduction

Percutaneous catheterization of femoral vessels is a rapidly increasing method for performing diagnostic and therapeutic procedures as an alternative to more invasive surgical interventions. As the number of procedures and their complexity, utilizing larger vascular sheaths, lytic agents and anticoagulants, increases, the number of postcatheterization groin complications has also grown. While the majority of groin interventional procedures are followed by little more than a relatively small bruise, significant complications including large hematomas, pseudoaneurysms (PSA), and arteriovenous fistulas (AVF) can occur. The frequency of postcatheterization complications varies depending upon the nature of the intervention, whether diagnostic or therapeutic, and relative meticulousness of post-sheath removal techniques utilized. Complication frequencies reportedly range from less than 1% for diagnostic catheterizations, up to 9% for coronary angioplasty, and as high as 16% following placement of an intracoronary stent.[1] Color Doppler ultrasound is now the preferred technique for evaluating potential groin complications related to femoral artery catheterization.[2–5] The color Doppler findings characteristic of these complications will be presented, including unusual complications, potential diagnostic pitfalls, and an approach to ultrasound-guided compression pseudoaneurysm repair.

Diagnostic Workup

The majority of patients referred for a groin ultrasound examination after femoral artery catheterization have a palpable mass. These masses may be pulsatile and/or associated with a new bruit or palpable thrill. Color Doppler ultrasound provides a rapid, relatively pain free, portable imaging technique which can readily discern the cause of these auscultary and palpable abnormalities. The examination is usually performed using a 5-MHz linear array transducer; however, a 7.5-MHz may be used for thin patients or for superficial lesions, whereas in cases of obese patients or those with large hematomas overlying the vascular structures, a 3.5-MHz transducer may be required.

The examination consists of color and pulsed Doppler evaluation of the groin vessels beginning at the region of the inguinal ligament above the puncture site, at, and below the puncture site. Color Doppler should be used to confirm the patency of the femoral artery and vein and search the extravascular soft tissues for evidence of large hematomas, PSAs, or AVFs. The color Doppler gain threshold and flow detection parameters should be adjusted so that color fills the artery and vein but does not "bleed over" into the adjacent soft tissues. It may be necessary to decrease the gain or increase the pulse repetition frequency (PRF) in order to visualize the artery and vein if a significant color Doppler bruit secondary to an AVF is present. Similarly, gain and threshold adjustments may be necessary to eliminate color noise artificially written into soft tissues such as hematomas which may be confused with PSAs (**Fig. 45–1 A,B**). A complete ultrasound evaluation of the postcatheterization groin rarely takes more than 15—20 min. Alternative imaging tests are rarely needed, however, occasionally CT will be obtained to evaluate the extent of a retroperitoneal hematoma related to postcatheterization complications, and arteriography may occasionally be needed before surgical or percutaneous interventions.

Hematomas

Virtually all patients who have undergone a groin catheterization have a small localized hematoma or bruise. However, when the ecchymosis is extensive or there is a palpable mass, which may be pulsatile, patients are usually referred for color Doppler sonography. Localized hematomas present as discrete hypo to anechoic masses that do not contain blood flow. Color Doppler noise may appear in a hematoma if gain settings are not optimized; pulsed Doppler interrogation will show the absence of a characteristic signal (**Fig. 45–2**). Large hematomas may compress and displace femoral vessels posteriorly such that they are beyond the penetration range of higher-frequency range transducers (**Fig. 45–3**). A localized hematoma and a thrombosed PSA are indistinguishable in appearance. Occasionally a hypoechoic tract leading from the vessel to the thrombosed PSA will be seen. While hematomas and thrombosed PSAs are

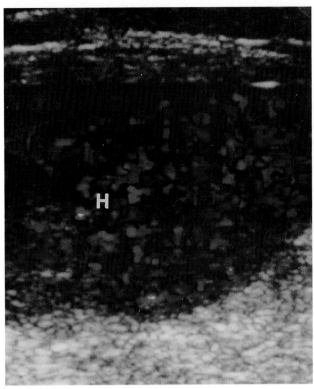

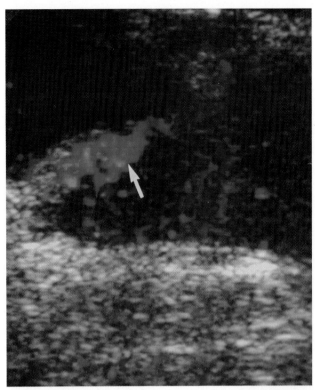

A

B

Figure 45–1 A: A large right thigh hematoma (H) is filled with red and blue color Doppler "noise" related to transmitted motion created by intermittent venous leakage into the large mass. **B:** The area of the intermittent vascular leak (**arrow**) is seen. The area of the low-velocity venous leak vanished by the end of the examination.

both avascular, inflammatory hypervascularity may be seen surrounding hematomas. Additionally, actively bleeding jets may be seen into a rapidly expanding hematoma (**Fig. 45–1 B**). Many clinically obvious hematomas are difficult to recognize on ultrasound because the hemorrhage has infiltrated diffusely into the soft tissues of the thigh or retroperitoneum, resulting in diffuse distortion of architecture and often suboptimal ultrasound penetration, but no discrete mass. Sonography is relatively insensitive for the evaluation of pelvic side wall or retroperitoneal hematomas. If a patient experiences a significant hematocrit drop or severe back pain following catheterization, computed tomography is usually indicated as a means of evaluating the presence and extent of a retroperitoneal hematoma.

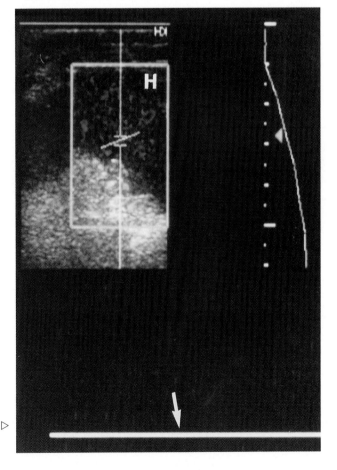

Figure 45–2 Pulsed Doppler analysis of color Doppler noise ▷ transmitted into a soft-tissue hematoma (H) shows absence of flow (**arrow**).

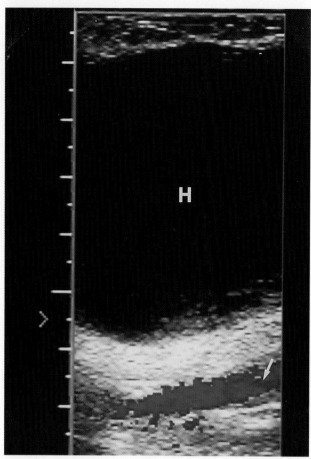

Figure 45–3 Large-groin hematoma (H) displaces the common femoral vein (arrow) posteriorly and compresses it.

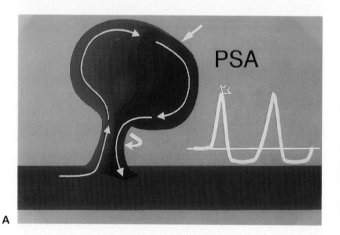

A

Figure 45–4 A: Diagrammatic representation of a pseudoaneurysm demonstrates the characteristic "Yin-Yang" color Doppler pattern within the pseudoaneurysm (**arrow**) and the characteristic to-and-fro waveform (**open arrow**) obtained from the region of the pseudoaneurysm neck (**curved arrow**). **B:** Duplex color Doppler image of a pseudoaneurysm (P). Note the characteristic red and blue flow pattern within the pseudoaneurysm. The pulsed Doppler waveform obtained from the neck (**arrow**) demonstrates the characteristic to-and-fro (**open arrows**) waveform.

Pseudoaneurysms (PSAs)

Following femoral arterial sheath removal, the artery is manually compressed to assure hemostasis at the puncture site. Typically, 15 min of manual compression are required following diagnostic procedures, however, therapeutic procedures may require longer periods of compression, particularly if anticoagulation is continued. A recent study showed that the incidence of PSA development following arterial catheterization was related to the type of intervention, with therapeutic procedures having a higher incidence of PSAs.[5] However, the greatest risk factor for developing a PSA, regardless of the type of intervention, was too brief a period of manual compression following sheath removal. If the arterial wall defect fails to seal, then pulsatile blood jets from the artery into the adjacent perivascular soft tissues. This hematoma connects with the artery via a neck or tract and is largely contained within the soft tissues. While these contained hematomas are referred to as PSAs, they do not have the characteristic fibrous wall of a true PSA; thus some feel it is more accurate to refer to these masses as "pulsatile hematomas."[2]

Color Doppler examination readily distinguishes PSAs from other pulsatile masses in the postcatheterization groin. Sonographic features of a PSA include the detection of a vascular mass connected to the artery by a neck or tract. During systole there is antegrade flow into the PSA through the neck (**Fig. 45–4 A—B**). During diastole, the increased pressure in the PSA, vis-a-vis underly-

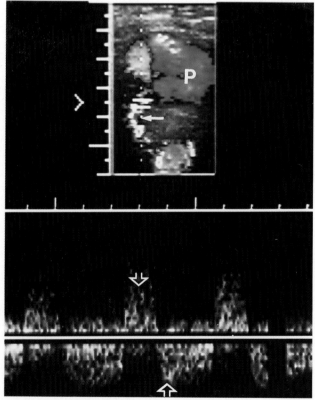

B

ing artery results in a retrograde flow out of the PSA through the neck and back into the artery. This results in a characteristic "to-and-fro" pulsed Doppler waveform in the PSA neck and produces a characteristic "Yin Yang" swirling color flow pattern within the body of the PSA. Some PSAs may be multilobed, producing a "string-of-beads" appearance (**Fig. 45–5**). These probably result from more extensive dissection of blood along fascial planes. Although two separate PSAs can occur following multiple punctures, multilobulated PSAs usually arise from a single puncture and interconnect between the artery and the multiple lobes. PSAs may also coexist with AVFs. In such cases, the Doppler features of either or both of the complications may be seen (**Fig. 45–6 A–C**). These patients may present with a bruit and a pulsatile mass. Some patients may demonstrate a linear track of blood flow that follows the expected track of the needle or sheath from the artery toward the actual puncture site.[6] These tracks may represent an abortive form of a PSA. However, these are very narrow, with varying waveforms not characteristic for a PSA. These tracks do not seem to be clinically important, nor do they appear to require further imaging or treatment if they are observed as isolated findings.

Complications of PSAs including pain, infection, compressive neuropathy, and most critically, rupture, can occur. Fortunately, this dire consequence is rare, but because this complication has such a potentially disastrous outcome, PSAs had been considered surgical emergencies. Recent studies have shown that PSAs are more benign and self-limited complications than previously thought.[7–9] Indeed, the majority of PSAs reported in many series have spontaneously thrombosed, suggesting that close monitoring and no further treatment may be sufficient. The majority of PSAs thrombose spontaneously within a week, and if imaged serially will demonstrate progressive thrombus of the PSA. PSAs with relatively small volumes of pulsatile flow and those with long necks are more likely to thrombose than will those with larger-flow volumes and short or wide necks.

Pseudoaneurysm Compression

Ultrasound guided compression therapy has been enthusiastically welcomed as an alternative to surgery.[10–12] This time-consuming, relatively noninvasive procedure obviates the need for surgical groin incisions which tend to heal poorly in these patients. Another attractive aspect of this procedure is that there is no need for the expense of operating room time. Although this procedure is less invasive, it is potentially painful and intravenous sedation is frequently needed.

The procedure consists of obtaining informed consent and administering pain medications and sedation as needed. The ultrasound transducer is then used to locate the PSA neck. Vigorous manual compression is applied

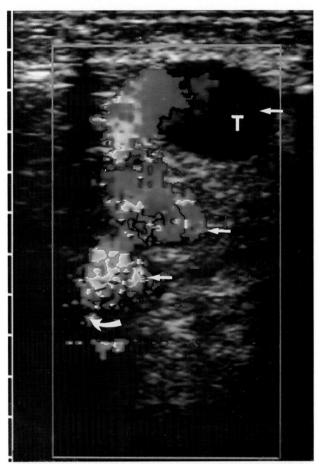

Figure 45–5 Tri-lobed pseudoaneurysm. The three lobes of the pseudoaneurysm (**arrows**) are seen arising from a single neck (**curved arrow**). Thrombus (T) is seen obliterating part of the lumen of the most superficial lobe.

directly to the PSA neck to determine if blood flow into the PSA can be completely obliterated (**Fig. 45–7 A—C**). Distal arterial pulses are checked to determine that arterial blood flow is maintained during this compression. If the PSA flow is obliterated and the arterial flow distally is maintained, then compression is continued for cycles of 20 min followed by a brief check of the status of the PSA. Arterial blood flow can be monitored either with color Doppler or by checking the dorsalis pedis or posterior tibial pulses manually or with a handheld Doppler during the procedure. We have found it helpful to approach this procedure as a "tag team" with the switching of operators following each 20-min period. We continue compressing the PSA for 20-min intervals, stopping for as brief a period as possible in between intervals until the PSA completely thromboses. Usually PSAs are completely obliterated within 1 h. However, in some cases compression fails. If after 60 min of compression there is no evidence of thrombus formation and no change, or even a slight increase, in size of the PSA, the procedure is terminated. If, however, the PSA has demonstrated significant thrombus, but remains patent at 1 h, we will continue compressing at 20-min intervals until

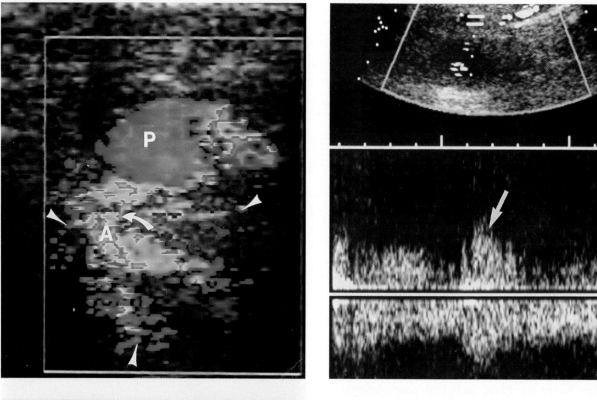

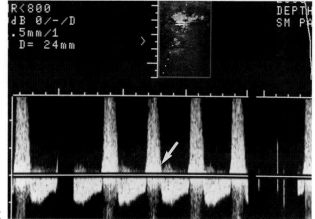

Figure 45–6 A: A color Doppler image of a pseudoaneurysm-AV fistula combination demonstrates the pseudoaneurysm (P) with its neck (**curved arrow**) and a large amount of soft tissue speckling (**arrowheads**). Common femoral artery (A). **B:** The neck of the pseudoaneurysm demonstrates characteristic to-and-fro waveforms (**arrow**). **C:** Pulsed Doppler waveforms obtained from a small fistulous track arising from the pseudoaneurysm and connecting with the greater saphenous vein demonstrates low-resistance "turbulent" arterial waveforms (**arrow**).

such time as the PSA is completely obliterated or further observations demonstrate no further progress.

Routine 24- to 48-h follow-up to document persistent thrombosis of PSAs is advocated by some; however, we do not do this routinely unless the patient has recurrence of symptoms or an enlarging hematoma in the region of the thrombosed PSA. Successful ultrasound-guided compression repair is reported to range from 66% to 100%. The incidence of success is related to many factors, including the size, multiplicity, and neck length of the PSA, the presence or absence of significant hematoma, the presence of an associated AVF, and most importantly, the presence of concurrent anticoagulation. If PSA compression is desired, we request that the referring physicians discontinue anticoagulation at least

4 h before the procedure. If the referring physicians believe that the risk of discontinuing anticoagulation outweighs the risk of either PSA rupture or failure to thrombose the PSA, we will attempt compression repair even though the patient is anticoagulated. In such cases, prolonged compression is frequently required and it is possible that mechanical clamp devices may be useful. Multilobed PSAs can be effectively compressed. While the success rate is slightly less than that for unilobular PSAs, that for multilobed PSAs exceeds 81%. The most important factor enabling success in these multilobulated PSAs is to clarify the course of the blood flow from the native artery. Applying compression to the most proximal neck nearest the artery usually results in obliteration of blood flow to all of the string of PSAs.

Figure 45–7 A: A diagrammatic representation of pseudoaneurysm compression demonstrates how transducer (T) is used to apply pressure over the neck of the pseudoaneurysm (**curved arrow**) to obliterate flow within the pseudoaneurysm. **B:** Pseudoaneurysm (P) with a long neck (**curved arrow**) prior to compression. **C:** Obtained following a successful thrombosis of the pseudoaneurysm demonstrates the patent common femoral artery (A) and the thrombosed hypoechoic neck (**curved arrow**) and body (**arrows**) of the pseudoaneurysm.

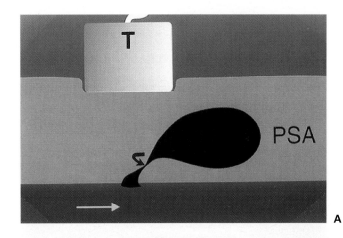

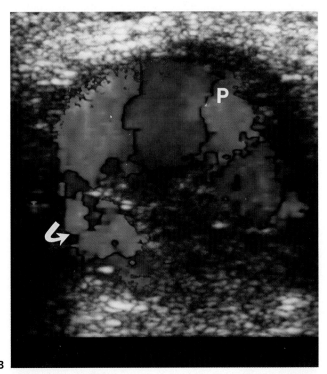

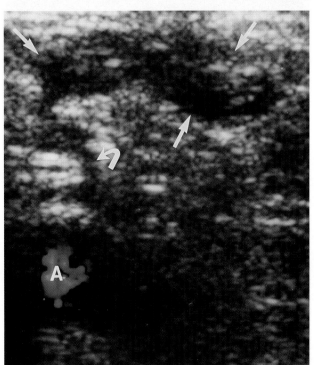

Ultrasound-guided compression repair complications are unusual. Reported complications include femoral artery thrombosis, embolization of plaque from compression, deep venous thrombosis, and PSA rupture. Although ultrasound-guided compression therapy has become a very desirable and widely utilized procedure, there are contraindications. Lower-limb ischemia, the possibility of groin infection (**Fig. 45–8**), skin ischemia overlying the PSA, and active pulsatile bleeding into the groin are contraindications. Although some have suggested that chronic PSAs are difficult to thrombose, success occurs in many cases, and this is not considered an absolute contraindication. Similarly, compression of PSAs associated with AVFs are less likely to be effective. AVFs are not effectively obliterated using this technique, however, the associated PSA may be thrombosed. Percutaneous transcatheter embolization of PSA or AVF with coils has been done when compression has failed, as a less invasive alternative to surgery.[13] Recent work supports the use of bovine thrombin or human thrombin injections to obliterate pseudoaneurysm.

Duplex sonography has promise for the evaluation of arterial trauma in patients with occult vascular injuries. For many years arterial injury has been perceived as a life- or limb-threatening event requiring immediate angiographic evaluation. Traumatic PSAs caused by knife, bullet, or other penetrating wounds (**Fig. 45–9 A,B**) do not seem to have the same propensity to spontaneous thrombosis as does iatrogenic injury. However, ultrasound could provide noninvasive useful information that would allow at least temporary nonoperative observation in a significant number of patients.[14, 15] These PSAs are probably best handled by surgical repair, particularly as there is greater vascular injury, significant soft tissue disruption surrounding the PSA, and a greater propensity for infection.

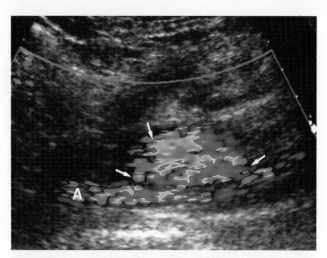

Figure 45–8 A patient several days postcardiac catheterization presents with increasing erythema and pain in the groin as well as a purulent discharge along the puncture site. There is a focal aneurysmal mass (**arrows**) arising from the common femoral artery (**A**). The mass has no discernible neck and the distinction cannot be made between a mycotic aneurysm versus a pseudoaneurysm. This mass required surgical intervention.

Arteriovenous Fistula

Simultaneous puncture of the femoral artery and vein can produce an AVF. AVFs most commonly result from the simultaneous catheterization of the left and right heart, however, inadvertent venous puncture associated with an arterial study can also result in an AVF. These are less frequently encountered than PSA following groin catheterization. Most AVFs are small and not hemodynamically significant. The majority resolve spontaneously and surgical repair is rarely required except in cases of high-output congestive heart failure, threatened limb ischemia, or severe varicosity. Physical findings of an AVF are most commonly the discovery of a new thrill or bruit at the puncture site. Although a "new" AVF may be discovered, many bruits at the puncture site may be due to preexisting atherosclerotic disease and/or the inadvertent production of an arterial dissection in the region of the puncture site.

The sonographic features of an AVF mirror the hemodynamic effects of an abnormal communication between a very high-resistance artery and a low-resistance vein without an intervening capillary bed (**Fig. 45–10**).[16, 17] Blood flow direction is always toward the region of lower pressures such that arterial blood flow preferentially shunts into the vein. Because the venous pressure is lower, this results in the loss of the high-resistance triphasic waveform in the artery proximal to the fistulous communication (**Fig. 45–11**). If a

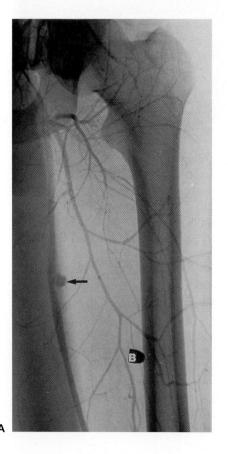

A

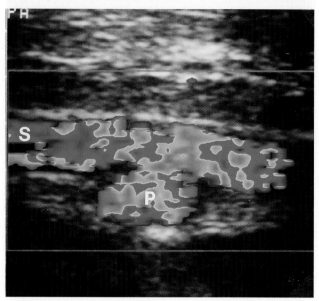

B

Figure 45–9 A: A lower-extremity arteriogram demonstrates a traumatic pseudoaneurysm (**arrow**) and associated vascular spasm involving the superficial femoral artery. The offending projectile (**B**) lies adjacent to the femur. **B:** Longitudinal image of the superficial femoral artery (S) demonstrates a broad-based pseudoaneurysm (P) arising from the vessel's posterior aspect. Because of its deep location, as well as significant soft tissue injury, it was decided to observe this patient and perform a follow-up ultrasound.

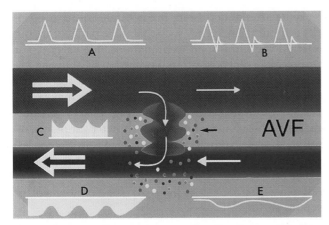

Figure 45–10 A diagram demonstrating the characteristic flow waveform changes seen with arteriovenous fistulas (AVFs). The low-resistance waveform (**A**) seen proximal to the AVF, the more normal triphasic waveform seen distal to the AVF (**B**), the disturbed low-resistance arterial flow seen within the AVF (**C**), the high-velocity pulsatile venous flow seen in the vein proximal to the AVF (**D**), and the more normal undulating low-velocity venous flow seen in the vein distal to the AVF (**E**), are diagrammed. Note also the soft tissue color Doppler speckling in the region of the AV communication (**arrow**).

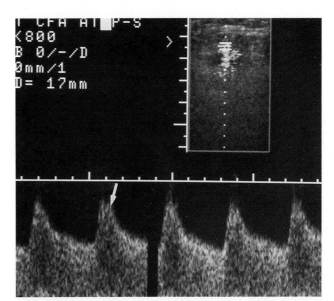

Figure 45–11 Characteristic low-resistance arterial waveforms (**arrow**) in the artery just proximal to the AV communication. Typically, resistive indices (RI) are 0.50 or less in the region of the AV communication.

large enough component of the blood flow is diverted into the fistula, there may be decreased blood flow in the distal artery, as well as increased pulsatile blood flow in the vein proximal to the communication (**Fig. 45–12 A,B**). The blood flow disturbance across the fistulous communication can be transmitted into the adjacent soft tissues resulting in a striking color Doppler soft-tissue bruit manifested by extensive heterogeneous color

speckling surrounding the AVF (**Fig. 45–13**). This soft tissue color collection contains high-velocity pulsatile flow with extensive spectral broadening and may be so extensive that it actually obscures the site of the AV communication. Appropriate alteration of gain, PRF, wall filter, and persistance settings can decrease or eliminate the soft tissue speckling, allowing one to visualize the AV communication.

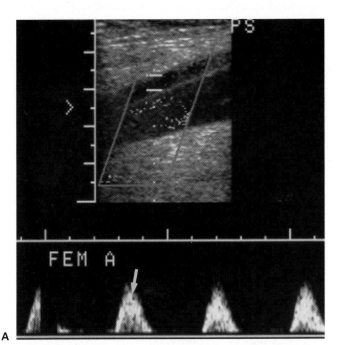

Figure 45–12 A: Demonstration of arterial waveforms distal to a significant AVF in a patient with unilateral decreased dorsalis pedis pulsus. The superficial artery waveform (**arrow**) demonstrates decreased velocities with loss of the normal triphasic waveform.

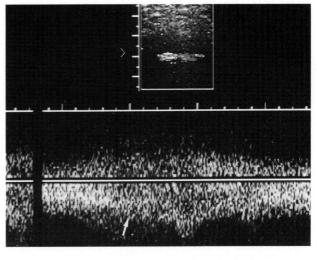

B: Interrogation of the superficial femoral vein proximal to a more distal AVF demonstrates high-velocity disturbed venous flow (**arrow**). Pulsed Doppler flow waveform inverted.

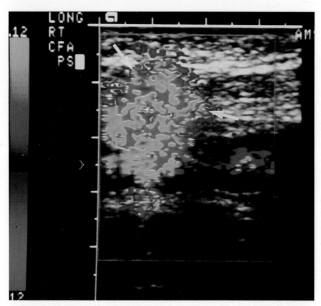

Figure 45–13 A longitudinal color Doppler of the right groin demonstrates a striking heterogeneous ball of color (**arrows**) produced by the transmitted soft tissue vibrations in the region of the AVF.

AVFs that involve small branch vessels or which have a long circuitous communication between the artery and vein may not produce the proximal and distal changes characteristic of an AVF. In such cases, the color Doppler bruit may be localized to the area of the communication with characteristic pulsatile low-resistance disturbed flow localized to the area of the tract (**Fig. 45–14 A—E**). The proximal artery and vein may demonstrate relatively normal waveforms.

Because patients with peripheral atherosclerotic disease may have bruits and loss of the normal triphasic waveform associated with significant stenosis or postcatheterization dissection, isolated findings of disturbed, low-resistance arterial flow waveforms and soft tissue speckling should not be considered diagnostic of an AVF (**Fig. 45–15 A,B**). The absence of corresponding venous changes and the presence of visible plaque or thrombus within the artery distinguishes such arterial disease from an AVF. High-velocity venous flow can also be seen in cases of venous stenosis. Venous compression by hematoma and transmitted pulsations from the adjacent artery can also mimic the venous flow changes seen in AVFs. However, the characteristic AVF communication and corresponding arterial waveform changes are not seen in these situations. Pulsatile venous flow is a frequent manifestation of increased right heart pressure; however, these waveforms manifest significant flow reversal and do not resemble the arterialized pulsatile flow associated with AVFs. Femoral artery dissections may be created by catheterization; however, they may be difficult to distinguish from plaque or thrombus unless arterial flow is seen within the false lumen. Rarely, these dissections may result in arterial occlusions. In the case of

an acute arterial occlusion, the ischemic cold leg is usually a surgical emergency such that these patients are not referred for ultrasound examinations. However, color Doppler can diagnose arterial occlusion by showing absence of flow as well as identifying collateral reconstitution. Occasionally, deep venous thromboses may be detected postgroin catheterization (**Fig. 45–16**). Hemorrhage and bleeding into the site of catheterization can result in large hematomas that produce extrinsic compression on the vein. In addition to that, the groin holding which takes place following the puncture as well as bed rest place the patient at high risk for development of venous thrombosis.

Potential Pitfalls

Color Doppler accurately diagnoses postcatheterization vascular complications in the groin; however, pitfalls do exist. Hyperemic lymph nodes can produce a pulsatile tender mass that may simulate a PSA on palpation.[18] These hyperemic lymph nodes may be extremely hypoechoic on gray scale and contain extensive internal vascularity with striking increased flow on color or power Doppler (**Fig. 45–17 A,B**). Although these inflamed lymph nodes might be mistaken for a partially thrombosed PSA, they do not demonstrate characteristic to-and-fro waveforms. The internal arterial waveforms are characteristically those of a normal arterial waveform (**Fig. 45–17 B**). Furthermore, the gray scale appearance of these lymph nodes usually shows the characteristic echogenic central hilum of the node with the radial distribution of blood vessels out into the parenchyma. While many hyperemic lymph nodes have relatively low-resistance waveforms, others may have high-resistance arterial waveforms. At least one case report of an inguinal hernia filled with fluid simulating a PSA exists.[19] In this case the swirling fluid within the hernia sac was shown to have flow that was in synchrony with respiratory motion rather than with the cardiac cycle. We have also seen venous aneurysms (giant varices) of the greater saphenous vein that contained the so-called "Yin-Yang" internal blood flow appearance. However, flow on pulsed Doppler was clearly venous in nature and showed a clearcut response to a valsalva maneuver.

True aneurysms may also present as a pulsatile groin mass. Furthermore, the flow within these aneurysms may have a swirling pattern reminiscent of a PSA. However, it is usually easy to determine that the aneurysm lies within the arterial lumen rather than outside of the wall of the vessel. If there is any question that a traumatic PSA exists, then further evaluation with angiography may be necessary.

The inferior epigastric artery arises from the distal external iliac artery in the region of the inguinal ligament and ascends to provide arterial blood supply to the ante-

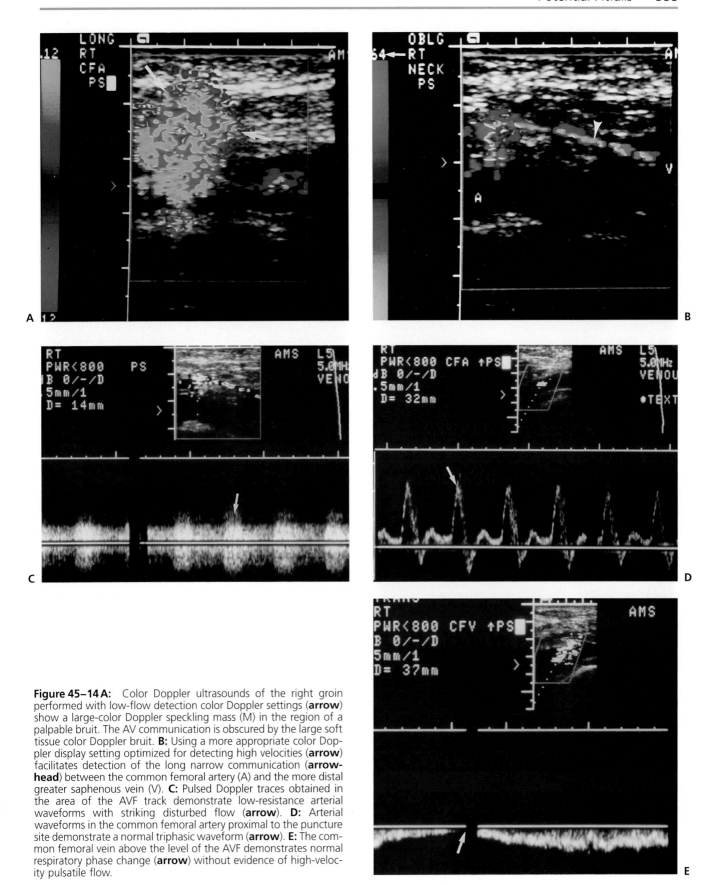

Figure 45–14 A: Color Doppler ultrasounds of the right groin performed with low-flow detection color Doppler settings (**arrow**) show a large-color Doppler speckling mass (M) in the region of a palpable bruit. The AV communication is obscured by the large soft tissue color Doppler bruit. **B:** Using a more appropriate color Doppler display setting optimized for detecting high velocities (**arrow**) facilitates detection of the long narrow communication (**arrowhead**) between the common femoral artery (A) and the more distal greater saphenous vein (V). **C:** Pulsed Doppler traces obtained in the area of the AVF track demonstrate low-resistance arterial waveforms with striking disturbed flow (**arrow**). **D:** Arterial waveforms in the common femoral artery proximal to the puncture site demonstrate a normal triphasic waveform (**arrow**). **E:** The common femoral vein above the level of the AVF demonstrates normal respiratory phase change (**arrow**) without evidence of high-velocity pulsatile flow.

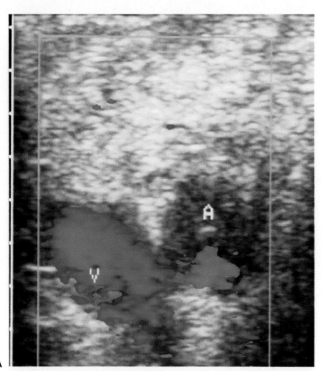

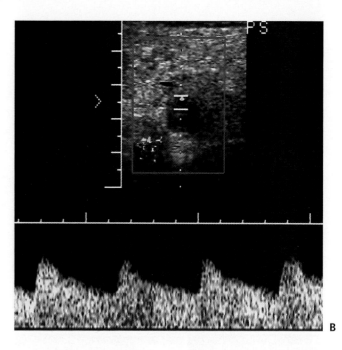

Figure 45–15 A: A transverse color Doppler ultrasound of the left groin in a patient with a new bruit status postcatheterization demonstrates a hypoechoic mass in the common femoral artery (**A**) which obliterates roughly two-thirds of the vascular lumen. Com-

mon femoral vein (V). **B:** Flow waveforms obtained from the region of this iatrogenic aortic dissection with thrombus demonstrate low-resistance disturbed flow waveforms similar to those that can be seen in the region proximal to an AVF.

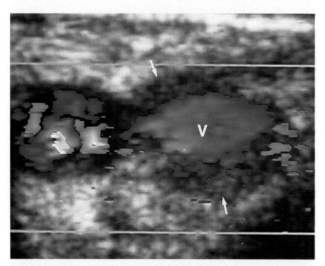

Figure 45–16 A transverse scan of the right groin in a postcatheterization patient demonstrates partial thrombosis (**arrows**) of the right common femoral vein (V).

rior abdominal wall musculature. Occasionally, this branch will be visualized in the upper thigh and should not be confused with a PSA neck, a patent needle track, or the arterial limb of an AVF. This vessel does have a relatively low-resistance waveform somewhat atypical of the femoral arterial system (**Fig. 45–18**). However, its course is different from that anticipated for a needle track or PSA neck, and corresponding venous changes are not present to suggest an AVF. Furthermore, no characteristic PSA to-and-fro flow will be observed along the course of this branch vessel.

Color Doppler imaging has made a significant contribution to the management of the postcatheterization groin. It has become the primary imaging modality for assessing complications and offers an elegant noninvasive method of treatment of PSAs.

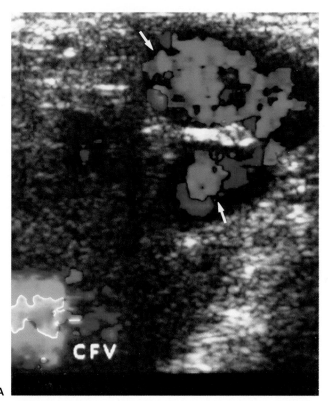

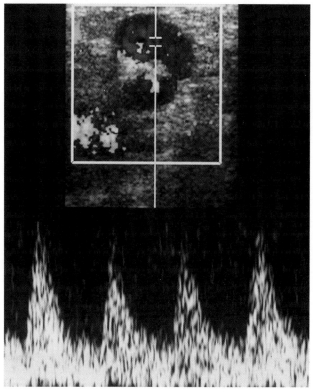

Figure 45–17 A: Hyperemic lymph nodes simulating a pseudo-aneurysm (**arrows**). **B:** Pulsed Doppler waveforms obtained within these masses demonstrate relatively low-resistance waveforms such as those commonly seen in hyperemic lymph nodes.

Figure 45–18 A longitudinal color Doppler ultrasound of the groin shows a branch vessel running cranially in the anticipated location of the inferior epigastric artery (**arrow**). Pulsed Doppler waveforms (**open arrow**) demonstrate an uncharacteristic waveform with more end diastolic blood flow than typical for a peripheral artery. The course of this vessel and its waveforms help distinguish it from a pseudoaneurysm neck or an AVF.

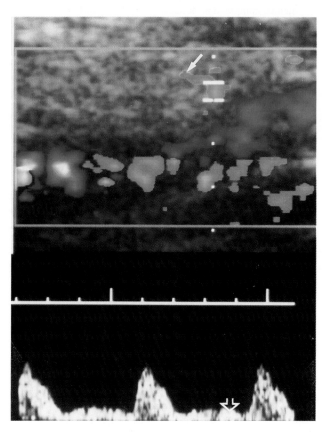

References

1. Lumsden AB, Miller JM, Kosinski AS, et al. A prospective evaluation of surgically treated groin complications following percutaneous cardiac procedures. *Am Surg* 1994;60:132—137.
2. Paulson EK, Kliewer MA, Hertzberg BS, et al. Color Doppler sonography of groin complications following femoral artery catheterization. *AJR* 1995;165:439—444.
3. Abu-Yousef MM, Wiese JA, Shamma AR. The "to-and-from" sign: duplex Doppler evidence of femoral artery pseudoaneurysm. *AJR* 1988;150:632—634.
4. Helvie MA, Rubin JM, Silver TM, Kresowik TF. The distinction between femoral artery pseudoaneurysms and other causes of groin masses: value of duplex Doppler sonography. *AJR* 1988;150:1177—1180.
5. Katzenschlager R, Ugurluoglu A, Ahmadi A, et al. Incidence of pseudoaneurysm after diagnostic and therapeutic angiography. *Radiology* 1995;195:463—466.
6. O'Malley CM, Paulson EK, Kliewer MA, et al. Color Doppler sonographic appearance of patent needle tracts after femoral arterial catheterization. *Radiology* 1995;197:163—165.
7. Johns JP, Pupa Jr LE, Bailey SR. Spontaneous thrombosis of iatrogenic femoral artery pseudoaneurysms: documentation with color Doppler and two-dimensional ultrasonography. *J Vasc Surg* 1991;14:24—29.
8. Allen BT, Munn JS, Stevens SL, et al. Selective non-operative management of pseudoaneurysms and arteriovenous fistulae complicating femoral artery catheterization. *J Cardiovasc Surg* 1992;33:440—447.
9. Paulson EK, Hertzberg BS, Paine SS, Carroll BA. Femoral artery pseudoaneurysms: value of color Doppler sonography in predicting which ones will thrombose without treatment. *AJR* 1992;159:1077—1081.
10. Fellmeth BD, Roberts AC, Bookstein JJ, et al. Postangiographic femoral artery injuries: nonsurgical repair with US-guided compression. Radiology 1991;178:671—675.
11. Coley BD, Roberts AC, Fellmeth BD, et al. Postangiographic femoral artery pseudoaneurysms: further experience with US-guided compression repair. *Radiology* 1995;194:307—311.
12. Paulson EK, Kliewer MA, Hertzberg BS, et al. Ultrasonographically guided manual compression of femoral artery injuries. *J Ultrasound Med* 1995;14:653—659.
13. Lemaire J-M, Dondelinger RF. Percutaneous coil embolization of iatrogenic femoral arteriovenous fistula or pseudoaneurysm. *Eur J Radiol* 1994;18:96—100.
14. Meissner M, Paun M, Johansen K. Duplex scanning for arterial trauma. *Am J Surg* 1991;161:552—555.
15. Frykbert ER, Crump JM, Dennis JW, Vines FS, Alexander RH. Nonoperative observation of clinically occult arterial injuries: a prospective evaluation. *Surgery* 1991;109:85—96.
16. Roubidoux MA, Hertzberg BS, Carroll BA, Hedgepeth CA. Color flow and image-directed Doppler ultrasound evaluation of iatrogenic arteriovenous fistulas in the groin. *J Clin Ultrasound* 1990;18:463—469.
17. Igidbashian VN, Mitchell DG, Middleton WD, Schwartz RA, Goldberg BB. Iatrogenic femoral arteriovenous fistula: diagnosis with color Doppler imaging. *Radiology* 1989;170:749—752.
18. Morton M, Charboneau JW, Banks PM, Internal lymphadenopathy simulating a false aneurysm on color flow Doppler sonography. *Am J Radiol* 1988;151:115—116.
19. Middleton MA, Middleton WD. Femoral hernia simulating a pseudoaneurysm on color Doppler sonography. *Am J Radiol* 1993;160:1291—1292.

46 Painful Legs After Walking

William J. Zwiebel

Leg pain after walking immediately brings to mind thoughts of intermittent claudication resulting from arterial insufficiency, but it is important to recognize that other disorders also may cause leg pain after walking, including neurogenic pain, acute venous thrombosis, chronic venous insufficiency, rupture of a popliteal cyst, and muscular hematoma.[1—3] In differentiating among these and other possible causes, the history and physical examination (PE) are the starting point. For certain diagnoses, such as arterial insufficiency, the history and PE generally are quite specific and are quite useful. For other causes of leg pain, however, the history and physical findings are nonspecific and do not permit definitive diagnosis. Furthermore, the history and PE may be nondiagnostic when two conditions coexist both of which might cause leg pain (e.g., arterial insufficiency and peripheral neuropathy). In such circumstances, it is difficult to determine which condition is causing the symptoms.

This chapter focuses on common causes of leg pain with walking — arterial insufficiency. We will review the clinical diagnosis of arterial insufficiency and the role played by ultrasound and other noninvasive diagnostic procedures. The other causes of leg pain listed above will not be covered in detail in this presentation, but several of these are included elsewhere in this text.

Arterial Insufficiency: Clinical Presentation

The term *claudication* is derived from a Latin word for limping or lameness.[4] Intermittent claudication refers to leg pain, weakness, or other discomfort that is absent at rest, commences after a period of ambulation, and subsides promptly when the patient stops walking.[1—3] In most instances, intermittent claudication is a sign of arterial insufficiency. At rest, the circulation is sufficient to meet the metabolic demands of the leg muscles and other tissues, but blood flow is insufficient to keep up with the metabolic demands of exercise. Lactic acid and other metabolites accumulate in the ischemic muscles, causing cramping pain.

History and Physical Examination

Intermittent claudication[1,2] occurs specifically in areas of muscle ischemia; therefore, the location of symptoms is a pretty good indication of the level of arterial obstruction. The most common location for intermittent claudication is in the calf, but claudication also may occur in the thigh, implying external iliac or common femoral artery obstruction, or in the buttock, implying aortic or common iliac artery blockage. Atypical claudication symptoms also occur, including foot pain or burning, and these atypical symptoms are particularly confusing from a diagnostic perspective. The severity of arterial insufficiency is implied by the amount of exercise that results in claudication. Therefore, intermittent claudication is commonly graded according to the distance the patient can ambulate before symptoms begin or limit ambulation (e.g., One- or two-block claudication).

The clinical diagnosis of arterial insufficiency[1—3] is based on a history of claudication symptoms and on diminished or absent arterial pulses. With severe arterial insufficiency, rubor (redness of the skin) may be evident in the leg and foot with the limb dependent, coupled with pallor of the skin when the leg is elevated. Moderate or severe arterial insufficiency is generally easy to diagnose solely on the basis of the history and physical findings. Mild arterial insufficiency, however, may not be detected with physical examination alone. Furthermore, the symptoms of other conditions may mimic those of arterial insufficiency, as discussed previously. These problems limit the accuracy of the history and PE. In addition, the history and PE are further limited because they are qualitative, not quantitative. Because they are qualitative, one clinician's assessment may vary from another, and it is difficult to compare one patient's symptoms with another, and the history and PE are relatively insensitive to changes in the patient's condition.

Diagnostic Workup

Physiological Tests

The deficiencies of the history and PE cited above led to the use of physiological tests for the assessment of lower-extremity arterial insufficiency.[2–6] The commonly used physiologic studies are segmental pressure measurements (thigh, calf, ankle, toe), plethysmography (which measures changes in limb volume with each arterial pulse), and Doppler waveform analysis (**Fig. 46–1, 46–2**). Treadmill ambulation is incorporated with these examinations to determine whether the arterial system can respond to increased metabolic demand. Together the physiological tests serve well to answer several important questions that are not adequately addressed by the history and PE.

1. *Are the patient's symptoms truly due to arterial insufficiency or should another cause be sought?* Post-treadmill pressure measurements are exquisitely sensitive for arterial insufficiency. Therefore, a normal segmental pressure examination or ankle—brachial index, coupled with a normal postexercise response, effectively excludes arterial insufficiency as a cause of ambulation-related symptoms.

2. *How severe is arterial insufficiency?* Pressure measurements provide a reliable way of quantifying arterial insufficiency and a fairly precise way for comparing one patient's condition with another. For example, an ankle—brachial index of 0.7 or 0.8 generally corresponds to mild arterial insufficiency and relatively mild claudication. An ankle—brachial index of 0.4 or less corresponds to severe arterial insufficiency, consistent with rest pain.

3. *Is arterial insufficiency stable or progressing?* Physiologic studies provide quantitative data that are more reliable than changes in symptomatology. In some cases the patient describes a lessening of symptoms, yet physiologic tests show worsening of arterial insufficiency, and vice versa.

4. *Has the patient responded to therapy?* The effects of medical or surgical therapy can be gauged quantitatively with physiologic tests.

The principal disadvantage of physiological studies, including segmental pressure measurements and Doppler waveform analysis is that these tests provide only limited information about the extent and location of arterial obstruction. This information, furthermore, is particularly unreliable with diffuse disease. Physiological studies also do not differentiate between arterial stenosis and occlusion. These failings prompted the use of duplex ultrasound as a means to enhance the noninvasive evaluation of arterial insufficiency.

Other Diagnostic Modalities

Magnetic resonance angiography (MRA) and computed tomographic angiography (CTA) are two imaging modalities that have great promise for noninvasive arteriography. Of these, MRA appears to have greater potential for lower-extremity arterial diagnosis as large areas can be covered and contrast material is not always necessary.[7, 8] Although MRA is not fully developed technically, it is reasonable to make a few educated guesses about its role in arterial diagnosis. First, it is not likely, in my opinion, that MRA will displace noninvasive physiological studies, as the latter are convenient, technically

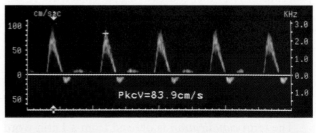

A

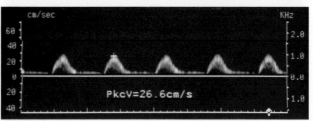

B

Figure 46–1 Physiological study. Segmental pressure and plethysmographic examination reveals left lower-extremity arterial insufficiency resulting from inflow (iliac) obstruction. At all levels on the left, systolic blood pressure is significantly reduced and pulse volume waveforms are damped. The left ankle—brachial index is 0.70, consistent with mild claudication. There is no evidence of arterial insufficiency on the right.

Figure 46–2 Doppler extremity arterial evaluation. **A:** A normal, triphasic arterial signal in this common femoral artery suggests absence of arterial insufficiency. Peak systolic velocity (PkcV) is within normal range (**Table 46–1**) **B:** A damped resting arterial waveform in this popliteal artery indicates arterial obstruction proximal to the examination site. Note the broad systolic peaks, slow upstroke in systole, low peak systolic velocity (PkcV), and forward flow in diastole.

simple, and inexpensive, and provide valuable clinical information. Second, MRA may replace duplex ultrasound for some lower-extremity arterial applications, but duplex will continue to be used for other applications as it is convenient and relatively inexpensive. Duplex certainly will continue to be used for graft surveillance, but MRA may well displace ultrasound for localizing obstructive lesions in native arteries. Finally, I believe that most diagnostic angiography in the lower extremities ultimately will be performed with MRA.

Duplex Ultrasound

The clinical utility of duplex ultrasound for lower-extremity arterial diagnosis[9—13] was advanced significantly by the development of color Doppler flow imaging, and more recently by the development of power Doppler flow imaging. In spite of these advancements, however, duplex examination of extremity arteries is arduous and time consuming. Only the femoral and popliteal arteries are relatively easy to examine, and even here difficulties may arise if there are multiple areas of obstruction and if the vessels are heavily calcified. Duplex examination of the iliac arteries is limited by interference from bowel contents, as well as vessel tortuosity. Duplex examination of calf vessels is limited by the small size of the vessels as well as acoustic shadows from calcification.

Considering these limitations, what is the utility of lower-extremity arterial sonography? It is possible to map out the entire arterial system, from the aorta to the calf, with ultrasound, but even the advocates of this procedure admit that this is difficult and may take as long as 2 h.[9,13] I believe that mapping the entire arterial tree with ultrasound generally is not an effective procedure and that the duplex ultrasound examination should be focused on specific questions raised by the history, physical examination, physiologic studies, or arteriography. Here are some questions that can be answered in a reasonable amount of time and with a reasonable amount of effort using duplex ultrasound.

1. *Is there a localized obstruction in the iliac system that is amenable to angioplasty or stent placement?* This information might be used, for instance, to separate patients treatable as outpatients from those requiring admission for surgery.
2. *Is an abnormal thigh pressure due to inflow obstruction or superficial femoral artery occlusion?* This important distinction often cannot be made with plethysmography, and duplex ultrasound usually can answer the question fairly quickly.
3. *Is an arteriographically identified stenosis hemodynamically significant?* Even when carefully performed, arteriography may reveal stenotic lesions of indeterminate importance from a hemodynamic perspective. Duplex ultrasound may be used for assessing the hemodynamic significance of such stenoses, facilitating surgical planning.
4. *Is there a stenosis in an arterial graft?* This is perhaps the most promising use of duplex arterial ultrasound, as there is evidence that timely detection of stenoses with ultrasound improves primary graft patency, as compared with surveillance by physical examination or pressure measurements.[14,15]

Ultrasound Imaging

Normal Duplex Ultrasound Values

Normal values for arterial diameter and velocity have been determined in adults, as listed in **Table 46–1**.[16]

Table 46–1   Normal arterial diameters and peak systolic velocities in adults

Artery	Diameter (mm)	Peak Systole (cm/s)
Ext. iliac/com. femoral	6.6—9.6	89—141
Sup. femoral	4.3—7.2	77—108
Popliteal	4.1—6.3	55—82

Reprinted with permission from **Noninvasive Diagnostic Techniques in Vascular Disease** by EF Bernstein, ed. St. Louis: Mosby, 1985, p. 876—892.
Modified from Jager KA, et al. [6]

Examination Method

The duplex ultrasound examination of extremity arteries should be conducted in a warm room so that the extremity is not vasoconstricted. The patient should be comfortable, as the examination may take some time. Although reactive hyperemia and exercise can enhance the detectability of hemodynamically significant lesions, the diagnostic criteria that are used for grading stenoses have been described for resting, nonhyperemic patients.

The examination should be focused on an area of clinical concern, as discussed previously. Start with color Doppler imaging and get oriented. Find the artery of interest and trace its course. Look for focal high velocities, disturbed flow, and occluded segments (absence of flow). Get an idea where the obstructive lesions are located and then go back and obtain Doppler information. The peak systolic velocity and spectral waveforms should be obtained proximal, within, and distal to areas of stenosis. Also obtain an end diastolic velocity in high-grade stenoses, in which flow is present throughout diastole. Get a sense of how severe the poststenotic flow disturbance is from the color Doppler image or the Doppler spectrum.

Doppler Criteria for Grading Stenoses

Lower-extremity arterial stenoses generally reach hemodynamic significance when the lumen diameter is reduced by 50%. Diagnostic criteria have been derived for this degree of stenosis as well as severe stenosis of 70% or greater diameter reduction.[9, 12] Absolute velocity criteria such as those used for carotid artery stenoses do not work in extremity arteries for reasons of hemodynamic variability. Therefore, extremity arterial stenoses

Table 46–2 Criteria for lower-extremity arterial stenosis

Minor stenosis (< 50% diameter reduction)

Pre/poststenosis
1. Waveforms and flow velocity normal prestenosis
2. Disturbed flow immediately beyond stenosis. Normal waveforms farther distal to stenosis

Within stenosis
1. Biphasic or triphasic waveform
2. Peak systolic velocity < 100% higher than prestenosis velocity
3. Reverse flow waveform component present

Severe stenosis (50—75% diameter reduction)

Pre/poststenosis
1. Possible low-velocity pre- and poststenosis
2. Highly disturbed flow immediately poststenosis
3. Damped waveforms farther distal to stenosis

Within stenosis
1. Peak systole 100% or greater than prestenotic velocity
2. Reverse component absent
3. End diastole < prestenotic peak systole

Very severe stenosis (> 75% diameter reduction)
1. Same as 50—75% stenosis, but
2. end diastole in stenosis > peak systole prestenosis

are principally graded using a ratio of peak systole in the stenosis divided by peak systole *proximal* to the stenosis. A ratio of 2 or greater generally indicates 50% or greater stenosis, and a ratio of 3—3.5 generally indicates 70% or greater stenosis.[9–12] Other criteria for grading stenoses are the shape of the Doppler waveform in and distal to the stenosis, and the degree of poststenotic flow disturbance. The Doppler criteria are outlined in **Table 46–2**, which the reader should review before proceeding to the examples of minor, moderate, and severe stenosis illustrated in **Fig. 46–3—46–5**.

In the author's experience, localized stenoses are most easily and accurately evaluated. The presence of multisegment occlusive disease makes it harder to assess the severity of individual lesions. Stenoses at vessel origins also are problems as no prestenotic velocity is available. If the corresponding contralateral artery is relatively disease free, then the velocity at the origin of that vessel may be used to formulate the ratio. This is not an option, however, if the contralateral vessel is seriously diseased.

Arterial occlusion (**Fig. 46–6**) is diagnosed on the basis of absent blood flow and damped distal arterial flow. The diagnosis of occlusion generally is straightforward, but a few words of caution are in order. First, be sure that your instrument is set to detect low-velocity flow. Otherwise, you may miss a "trickle" of flow in a highly stenosed vessel and make a false-positive diagnosis of occlusion. Second, doublecheck with spectral Doppler to confirm a color Doppler impression of arterial occlusion. Spectral Doppler may be more sensitive to low-flow states than color Doppler.

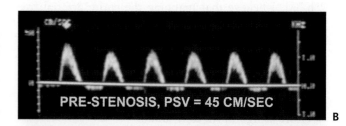
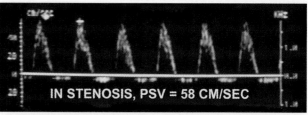
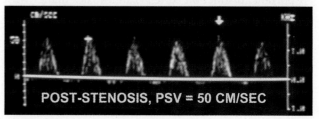

Figure 46–3 Mild arterial stenosis that is not hemodynamically significant. **A:** Color Doppler image shows plaque (P) in the superficial femoral artery that generates a region of increased velocity (**arrow**), but no appreciable poststenotic flow disturbance. **B:** Prestenotic peak systolic velocity is 45 cm/s. **C:** In the stenotic region, the Doppler waveform is biphasic and the peak systolic velocity is 58 cm/s. Systolic velocity ratio is 1.3. **D:** Poststenotic Doppler waveforms are biphasic and **not** damped, with peak systolic velocity similar to the prestenotic velocity. This constellation of findings indicates that lumenal diameter reduction is less than 50%, and the stenosis is not hemodynamically significant.

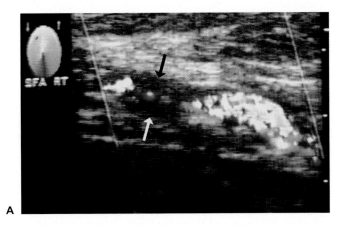

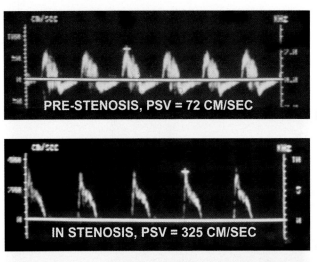

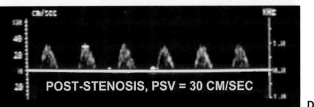

Figure 46–4 Moderate arterial stenosis. **A:** A color Doppler image shows substantial obstruction of the superficial femoral artery accompanied by moderate poststenotic flow disturbance. **B:** In the prestenotic region, the peak systolic velocity is 72 cm/s, and the Doppler waveforms are biphasic. **C:** In the stenosis, the peak systolic velocity is 325 cm/s, and the systolic velocity ratio is 4.5. The Doppler waveforms are monophasic, but without diastolic flow. **D:** In the poststenotic region, Doppler waveforms are monophasic and slightly damped, and peak systolic velocity is low.

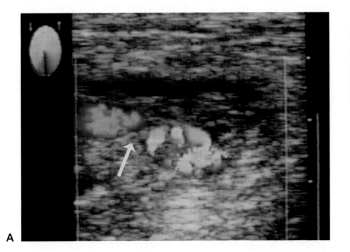

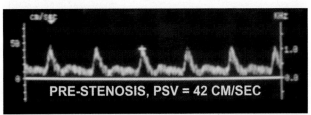

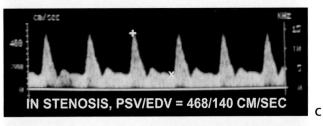

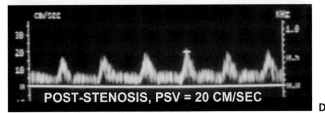

Figure 46–5 Severe arterial stenosis. **A:** Color Doppler examination of this reversed vein graft shows an eccentric, focal area of narrowing (**arrow**) accompanied by severe poststenotic flow disturbance. **B:** The prestenotic peak systolic velocity is 42 cm/s. **C:** Within the stenosis, peak systolic velocity is 468 cm/s, there is a large amount of diastolic flow, and end diastolic velocity is 140 cm/s. The systolic velocity ratio is 11.2, and **the end diastolic velocity exceeds the prestenotic peak systolic velocity.** **D:** Poststenotic Doppler waveforms are damped, peak systolic velocity is very low, and there is a large amount of flow throughout diastole.

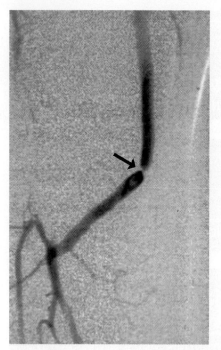

Figure 46–5 E Digital subtraction arteriogram confirming the ultrasound findings. The combination of very high velocity (and ratio) in the stenotic zone, a large amount of diastolic flow in the stenosis, and poststenotic damping with diastolic flow clearly indicates a very severe stenosis. We currently would not obtain arteriographic confirmation in a case such as this, but as this patient was seen early in our duplex arterial experience, arteriographic confirmation was obtained.

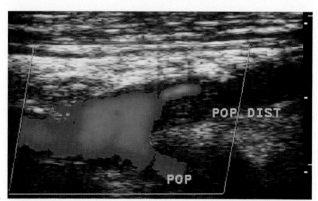

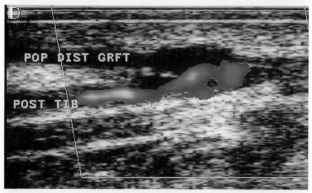

Figure 46–6 Occluded graft. Views of the proximal (**A**) and distal (**B**) anastomoses demonstrate absence of flow and echogenic intraluminal thrombus in this occluded popliteal-to-posterior tibial artery graft (POP DIST GRFT). POP, popliteal artery; POST TIB, posterior tibial artery.

Bypass Graft Examination

The examination principles described above and in **Table 46–2** apply to arterial bypass grafts as well as native arteries. It generally is much easier to examine grafts than native arteries, nonetheless, you can save a lot of time and aggravation, and you can avoid errors, if you know the surgical anatomy before setting out on a duplex graft examination. Begin the duplex examination by becoming oriented. It is extremely important to identify the proximal and distal anastomoses of arterial bypass grafts, as these are common locations for complications, including stenosis and aneurysm formation. Focal velocity elevation and flow disturbances are common at the anastomoses, and these should not be overdiagnosed as significant stenoses. Once the graft anatomy has been sorted out, obtain a Doppler spectral waveform and measure the peak systolic velocity in the inflow artery proximal to the graft and at the proximal anastomosis. Survey the graft with color Doppler and obtain velocity information in areas of stenosis, as described above for native arteries. If there are no flow disturbances, obtain a representative spectral waveform and systolic velocities in the vessel that feeds the graft, in the proximal, mid, and distal portions of the graft, and in the outflow vessel. *Compare the current study to a postsurgery baseline*, if available. If focal flow disturbance and high velocity are present on color Doppler examination (indicating stenosis), then use the criteria described in **Table 46–2** to evaluate the stenosis (**Fig. 46–5**).[14, 15] Graft stenoses with peak systolic velocity exceeding 300 cm/s and with a systolic velocity ratio exceeding 3.5 generally benefit from repair, whereas those with values lower than this generally can be followed.[17] When a severe stenosis is identified, the skin is marked over the narrowed area, facilitating surgical repair. In clearcut, uncomplicated cases surgical repair is performed on the basis of ultrasound findings, and arteriography is not needed.

A mid-graft peak systolic velocity of less than 40 cm/s is worrisome with respect to potential graft failure, but low levels of flow have not proven to be accurate predictors of graft failure.[9, 18] Flow velocity within the graft varies somewhat from one location to another because of inconsistencies in the graft diameter. The waveform shape in normally functioning grafts is usually biphasic but in some cases may be monophasic or triphasic. Comparison with a baseline study is necessary for evaluating waveform shape and flow velocity within the graft.

Accuracy

It appears that duplex assessment of lower extremity arteries is quite accurate in experienced hands. For native lower-extremity arterial occlusion, sensitivity exceeds 90%, and for stenosis of 50% or greater, sensitivity is at least 82% and is higher in some studies.[11] Duplex suffers, however, by overestimating stenosis severity in up to 18% of cases (78% specificity),[11] but one study reported specificity exceeding 90%.[19]

Practice Makes Perfect

The author has found that confidence with duplex ultrasound extremity arterial diagnosis increases with experience. It is advisable, therefore, to practice on the patient's postangiography until one gets the "feel" of the examination.

Summary

Walking-associated leg pain, in the form of intermittent claudication, classically is caused by arterial insufficiency; however, other conditions may cause walking-associated leg pain, including peripheral neuropathy, acute venous thrombosis, chronic venous thrombosis, muscular hematoma, and rupture of a popliteal cyst.

Diagnostic measures commonly used for assessing walking-related leg pain include history and physical examination, arterial pressure measurement, plethysmography, Doppler and duplex ultrasound, and angiography. The history and physical examination are accurate for diagnosis of arterial insufficiency that is moderate or severe, but physical examination is qualitative and subjective. Furthermore, mild arterial insufficiency cannot always be detected with physical examination. Arterial pressure measurement and plethysmography are highly sensitive for arterial insufficiency, especially when conducted postexercise, and serve well to differentiate between arterial insufficiency and other causes of leg pain, such as peripheral neuropathy. In addition, arterial pressure measurements are quantitative and are moderately accurate for localizing arterial obstruction. Duplex sonography is accurate for localizing and grading arterial occlusive lesions in the lower extremities, both in native arteries and arterial grafts. Although an adequate examination can be obtained in most patients, duplex ultrasound of native arteries is tedious and time consuming. Arterial graft examination is considerably easier, in most cases.

Normal duplex arterial parameters and criteria for stenosis grading are reviewed in **Table 46–2**. Duplex ultrasound is well established as an effective method for arterial bypass graft assessment. The role of duplex sonography in the assessment of native arterial lesions is less clear. This author feels that native artery duplex ultrasound is most effective when used to answer focused questions about localized areas of arterial disease.

References

1. Carter SA. Clinical problems in peripheral arterial disease: is the clinical diagnosis adequate? In: Bernstein EF, ed. *Noninvasive Diagnosis Diagnostic Techniques in Vascular Disease*. St. Louis: Mosby, 1985, p. 471—480.
2. Carter SA. Role of pressure measurements. In: Bernstein EF, ed. *Noninvasive Diagnosis Diagnostic Techniques in Vascular Disease*. St. Louis: Mosby 1985, p. 486—512.
3. Nicolaides AN. Basic and practical aspects of peripheral arterial testing. In: Bernstein EF, ed. *Noninvasive Diagnosis Diagnostic Techniques in Vascular Disease*. St. Louis: Mosby, 1985, p. 481—485.
4. Dorland Medical Dictionary, W. B. Sanders; Philadelphia PA, p. 343.
5. DeMasi RJ, Gregory RT, Wheeler JR, et al. Exercise testing: diagnosis and follow-up. *J Vasc Tech* 1994;18:257—261.
6. Macdonald NR. Pulse volume plethysmography. *J Vasc Tech* 1994;18:241—248.
7. McCauley TR, Monib A, Dickey KW, et al. Peripheral vascular occlusive disease: accuracy and reliability of time-of-flight MR angiography. *Radiology* 1994;192:351—357.
8. Rubin GD, Walker PJ, Drake MD, et al. Three-dimensional spiral computed tomographic angiography: an alternative imaging modality for the abdominal aorta and its branches. *J Vasc Surg* 1993;18:656—665.
9. Zierler RE. Duplex sonography of lower extremity arteries. In: Zwiebel WJ, ed. *Introduction to Vascular Ultrasonography*. Philadelphia: Saunders, 1992; p. 237—251.
10. Kohler TR. Duplex scanning for the evaluation of lower limb arterial disease. In: Bernstein EF, ed. *Noninvasive Diagnosis Diagnostic Techniques in Vascular Disease*. St. Louis: Mosby, 1985, p. 481—485.
11. Polak JF. Arterial sonography: efficacy for the diagnosis of arterial disease of the lower extremity. *AJR* 1993;161:235—243.
12. Kerr TM, Bandyk DF. Color duplex imaging of peripheral arterial disease before angioplasty or surgical intervention. In: Bernstein EF, ed. *Noninvasive Diagnosis Diagnostic Techniques in Vascular Disease*. St. Louis: Mosby, 1985, p. 481—485.
13. Burnham CB, Cummings C. Should arterial duplex imaging replace segmental pressures? *J Vasc Tech* 1993;17:49—51.
14. Beidle TR, Brom-Ferral R, Letourneau JG. Surveillance of infrainguinal vein grafts with duplex sonography. *AJR* 1994;162:443—448.
15. Berry SM, Dardik H, Ibrahim IM, Ragno I, Sussman BC. Comparative role of duplex imaging and ABI for surveillance of in situ and autologous vein grafts of the lower extremity.
16. Jager KA, Ricketts HI, Strandness DE. Duplex scanning for the evaluation of lower limb arterial disease. In: Bernstein EF, ed. *Noninvasive Diagnostic Techniques in Vascular Disease*. St. Louis: Mosby, 1985, p. 876—892.
17. Gahtan V, Payne LP, Roper LD, et al. Duplex criteria for predicting progression of vein graft lesions: which stenoses can be followed? *J Vasc Tech* 1995;19:211—215.
18. Dalsing MC, Cikrit DF, Lalka SG, Sawchuk AP, Schulz C. Femoro-distal vein grafts: the utility of graft surveillance criteria. *J Vasc Surg* 1995;21:127—134.
19. Kohler TR, et al. Duplex scanning for diagnosis of aortoiliac and femoro-popliteal disease. *Circulation* 1987;5:1074—1080.

47   Arm Swelling

Thomas R. Beidle and Janis Gissel Letourneau

Introduction

In the upper extremity, several mechanisms can produce swelling, a general term used to indicate the accumulation of extracellular fluids.[1] Increased capillary permeability, decreased oncotic pressure, increased intracapillary hydrostatic pressure, and increased lymphatic pressure are basic mechanisms that lead to swelling. A complete history and physical examination should help identify generalized edema, which is commonly caused by congestive heart failure, renal insufficiency, or nephrotic syndrome.[1] Swelling isolated to the arm implies a localized process, such as venous stasis, lymphatic obstruction, cellulitis, or angioneurotic edema. The patient's history will often indicate which conditions are the most likely causes of arm swelling.

Differential Diagnosis

Cellulitis is often caused by a penetrating injury or by the use of nonsterilized needles by intravenous drug abusers. The swelling of cellulitis is often localized, but it can involve the entire arm. If a focal area of the arm is particularly swollen, then an abcess should be considered and ultrasound (US) can be used to determine whether a fluid collection is present (**Fig. 47–1**). These collections can be aspirated and drained under US guidance. It is important to note that intravenous drug abuse can lead to thrombophlebitis, which can produce swelling and also coexist with cellulitis.

Treatment of breast cancer with axillary dissection and radiation therapy causes arm swelling in as many as 25% of patients.[2] The pathophysiology of swelling in these patients is controversial. In 1938, Veal[3] stated that 90% of instances of postmastectomy arm swelling were due to venous obstruction. Subsequently, however, Lobb and Harkins[4] showed that axillary vein resection did not increase the incidence of arm swelling. Lymphangiographic studies have shown anatomic abnormalities of the lymphatic channels after surgery and radiotherapy,[5] but these abnormalities were also seen in patients without arm swelling.[6] By using color and duplex Doppler sonography, Svensson et al.[7] showed that 57% of women with arm swelling after breast cancer treatment had evidence of venous outflow obstruction. Furthermore, venous thrombosis has been shown to occur after radiation therapy alone.[8] Thus, venous thrombosis, as well as lymphatic obstruction, should be considered as a possible cause of arm swelling in these patients (**Fig. 47–2**), particularly since, as described below, venous thrombosis can lead to significant complications: venous thrombosis is often directly treatable, whereas lymphatic obstruction is not. Other causes of lymphatic obstruction would include trauma or diseases such as elephantiasis, which is more common in the legs and is rarely seen in the Western world.[1]

Another cause of extremity swelling, angioneurotic edema, is usually well demarcated and localized. It involves only the deep layers of the skin and adjacent subcutaneous tissue. During physical examination, it can be distinguished from other causes of swelling because it is nonpitting; venous stasis and lymphatic obstruction tend to result in pitting edema.[9] Angioneurotic edema is frequently caused by an allergic reaction and is often self-limiting.

Venous stasis in the upper extremity is almost always caused by a venous outflow obstruction that results from partial or complete thrombosis of the axillary, subclavian, or innominate veins, or superior vena cava. Venous outflow obstruction can also be precipitated by extrinsic compression from an adjacent node, mass, or hypertrophied muscle; such extrinsic conditions can also lead to venous thrombosis, one example being effort thrombosis (Paget-Schroetter syndrome),[10]

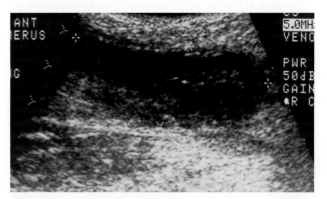

Figure 47–1   Single gray scale US image of upper arm of patient with cellulitis and history of intravenous drug abuse shows a cystic structure that contains debris and septations. Purulent material was aspirated, confirming the diagnosis of abcess.

caused by external compression of the subclavian vein by hypertrophied scalene muscles. Venous thrombosis resulting from prolonged erect posture is limited to the lower extremities. Current or previous placement of a central venous catheter through the subclavian vein or internal jugular vein (IJV) is the most common predisposing factor for thrombosis.[11, 12] Because the incidence of thrombosis in patients with indwelling catheters is so high, [13] the diagnosis of venous thrombosis should be ruled out in any of these patients who develop arm swelling. Bilateral findings raise the possibility of an obstruction of the superior vena cava (SVC) caused by either luminal caval stenosis or extrinsic compression from an adjacent tumor, such as lung carcinoma or lymphoma.

Arm swelling is only one of a number of symptoms that can occur as a result of venous outflow obstruction. Other signs include a poorly functioning catheter, local hyperemia, fever, pain, elevated white blood cell count, appearance of superficial varicosities in the arm, neck, and chest, and facial and neck swelling. However, these clinical signs and symptoms (including arm swelling) are nonspecific. The sensitivity of clinical diagnosis is also very low; thrombosis has been shown to be asymptomatic in 50% of patients with indwelling catheters.[14] Prompt diagnosis is important, as thrombosis can lead to permanent venous insufficiency, thrombophlebitis, and pulmonary embolism. Venous thrombosis of the upper extremity is associated with pulmonary embolism in up to 16% of cases.[15, 16]

Diagnostic Workup

History and physical examination obviously play an important role in determining the cause of arm swelling. Diagnostic tests are used to identify or exclude venous outflow obstruction, as it is potentially treatable and can lead to complications. Nonimaging studies such as plethysmography are now rarely performed in the lower extremities and were never proven to be accurate in the evaluation of the upper extremities. Therefore, imaging procedures are necessary when there is a question of venous obstruction.

Contrast venography has been the "gold-standard" for making this determination. However, venography is an invasive procedure that can cause pain, a phlebitic reaction, or skin necrosis, particularly in patients with thrombosis.[17] In addition, the potential for allergic or nephrotoxic reactions exists, and the procedure may be contraindicated in patients with renal failure.

Contrast material-enhanced computed tomography (CT) of the chest is accurate for detection of intrinsic and extrinsic obstruction of the SVC. Although accuracy has not been documented, subclavian venous obstruction can be identified using spiral CT.[18] However, CT has the same drawbacks as venography, because ipsilateral

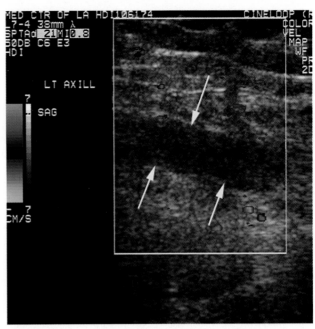

Figure 47–2 Color Doppler flow image demonstrates low-level echogenic material filling lumen of left axillary vein (**arrows**) of patient who had undergone left axillary dissection for breast carcinoma. Image shows that no flow is present within the vein. Note that pulse repetition frequency (PRF) has been lowered to detect any slow flow that may be present.

venous contrast material injection is needed to identify thrombosis.

Radionuclide venography has been used to assess patency of the upper extremity veins and indwelling catheters. False-positive and false-negative results can result from poor venous access, indwelling catheter, or collateral veins being mistaken for the subclavian vein.[19,20] Advantages of nuclear imaging are its low cost, relative noninvasiveness, and ability to assess catheter patency.

All of these imaging techniques focus on the subclavian vein but are inherently unable to evaluate the internal jugular vein. Kroger et al.[21] demonstrated that there is a high incidence of IJV thrombosis in patients with subclavian vein thrombosis. Extensive thrombosis of the IJV can lead to dural sinus thrombosis and possible cerebral venous infarction. Magnetic Resonance (MR) angiography is capable of imaging the IJV as well as the subclavian vein, innominate vein, and SVC. Two dimensional time-of-flight MR angiography is accurate and can image the extent of thrombus more completely than venography.[22,23] However, this test is expensive, not universally available, and difficult to perform in uncooperative patients or in patients in intensive care. MR angiography has also been used to evaluate occlusion of the subclavian vein in patients with thoracic outlet syndrome.[24]

Ultrasound Imaging

Ultrasound is an attractive alternative to other imaging modalities because it is noninvasive, portable, inexpensive, and capable of fully evaluating the IJV. However, the test can be challenging to perform and interpret.

Sonography of the thoracic inlet veins requires knowledge of the regional anatomy. The basilic and brachial veins merge at the lateral margin of the pectoralis minor muscle to form the axillary vein, which lies medial and inferior to the axillary artery (**Fig. 47–3**).[25] As it courses medially past the lateral margin of the first rib, the axillary vein becomes the subclavian vein, which

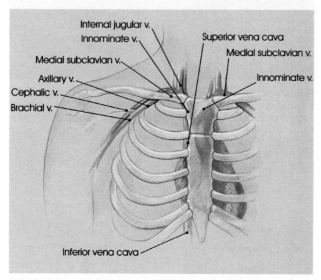

Figure 47–3 Anatomic drawing of the upper extremity and thoracic inlet veins shows normal relationships of the IJVs, innominate veins, subclavian veins, axillary veins, brachial veins, and cephalic veins.

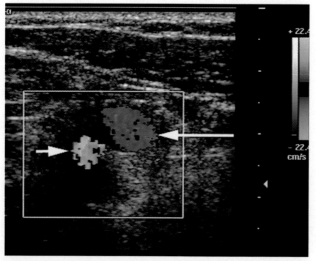

Figure 47–4 Color Doppler image obtained with a linear transducer in a plane axial to the vessel lumina. Note the normal relationship of the axillary vein (**long arrow**) anterior to the axillary artery (**short arrow**). Color PRF is set low in order to visualize flow in the vein. As a result, higher velocity in the artery causes aliasing.

lies anterior and inferior to the subclavian artery. If a vein becomes occluded, collateral veins enlarge and are often oriented parallel to the subclavian and axillary veins. Part of the sonographic examination involves following the artery and vein in a plane axial to the vessel lumina to ensure that a constant normal anatomic relationship between artery and vein is maintained (**Fig. 47–4**). This will help to ensure that a patent collateral vein is not mistaken for the axillary or subclavian vein. The subclavian vein courses over the first rib and posterior to the clavicle before turning inferiorly and merging with the IJV to form the innominate vein. The right innominate vein is shorter and more vertically oriented than the left innominate vein, and the junction of these veins behind the sternal manubrium forms the SVC. In dehydrated patients, visualization of the thoracic inlet veins may be difficult due to lack of venous distention. This situation can be remedied by placing the patient in the supine position with the head flat on the examining table, and elevating the legs if necessary.

A complete US examination of the upper extremity and the thoracic inlet veins includes bilateral evaluation of the IJVs, innominate veins, subclavian veins, and axillary veins. The cephalad portion of the SVC can be visualized in some patients (**Fig. 47–5**). If thrombosis of the axillary vein is present, the distal extent of thrombus can be documented by examining the brachial vein and its tributaries. Unless the patient is an IV drug abuser, has had trauma or surgery in the arm, or has a dialysis fistula, isolated thrombosis of an arm vein is rare. In addition, unless a dialysis fistula is present, isolated thrombosis of an arm vein is usually not symptomatic and is of less importance than a more proximal thrombosis, because of the presence of a large number of potential collateral veins.

Gray scale US, color Doppler imaging, and pulsed Doppler imaging are all essential for sonographic evaluation of the upper-extremity veins. A-high frequency (7—10 MHz) linear transducer is usually optimal for visualizing the peripherally located portions of the subclavian veins and IJVs, as well as the axillary vein and veins of the upper arm (**Figs. 47–6, 47–7**). Overlying osseous structures render visualization of the more centrally located veins more difficult.

Because of the greater ease with which the sonographer can angle the scan plane, a small footprint phased-array or sector transducer aids in visualization of the inferior IJV, the medial half of the subclavian vein, the innominate vein, and the SVC. Proper positioning of the probe is essential for imaging these vessels. The junction of the subclavian and jugular veins is best visualized with the probe positioned in the supraclavicular fossa, angling medially, inferiorly, and slightly anteriorly (**Figs. 47–6, 47–8, 47–9**). Note that the veins in this region are located anterior to the arteries. A small footprint 7-MHz transducer can be used in thin patients to view the superior portion of the innominate veins. A 5-MHz small

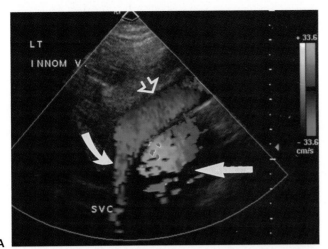

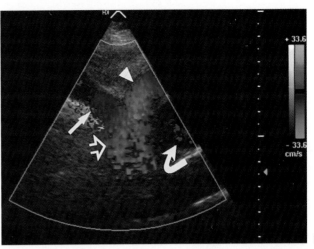

A

B

Figure 47–5   Color Doppler images of the central thoracic veins in a normal patient. **A:** Coronal image obtained through the left supraclavicular fossa with a phased array 7- to 4-MHz transducer shows the central portion of the left innominate vein (**open arrow**) turning into the SVC (**curved arrow**) over the aortic arch (**arrow**).

B: Coronal image with the transducer angled more to the right and slightly twisted in order to visualize the SVC bifurcation. The right innominate vein (**arrow**) joins the left innominate vein (**arrowhead**) to form the SVC (**open arrow**). The edge of the aortic arch (**curved arrow**) is also visualized.

Figure 47–6   Drawing demonstrates probe positioning for sonographic evaluation of thoracic inlet veins. The linear transducer can be used peripherally in the axillary vein and IJV. A small-footprint phased-array transducer is placed in the supraclavicular notch and angled medially to visualize the innominate veins and SVC. The probe is angled more laterally to visualize the remaining portion of the subclavian vein.

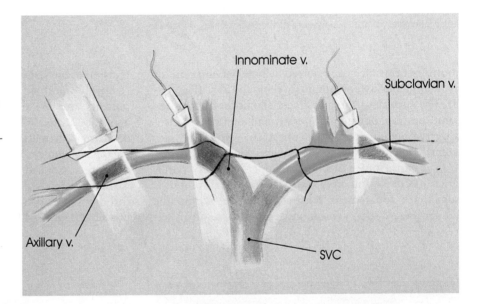

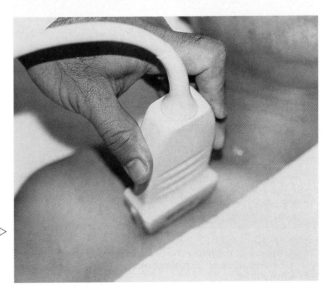

Figure 47–7   A 7-MHz linear transducer is used to visualize the ▷ axillary vein, inferior to the clavicle. The transducer should be turned 90 degrees to perform compression and confirm a normal relationship of the axillary vein to the axillary artery, in order to avoid mistaking a collateral vein for the axillary vein.

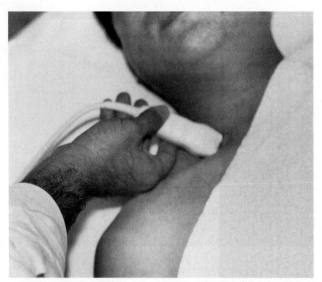

Figure 47–8 Positioning of small-footprint probe to visualize right innominate vein and SVC. Anterior view shows that the probe should be positioned in the supraclavicular fossa and angled medially. On the left side, greater medial angulation may be required, and, in some patients, sliding the probe toward the suprasternal notch may allow better visualization of the SVC (see Fig. 47–5).

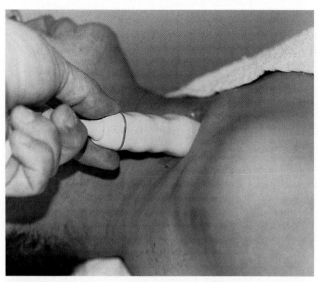

Figure 47–9 Lateral photograph shows probe in a coronal plane positioned to visualize the right innominate vein and SVC. In some patients more anterior angulation may be required.

footprint transducer is preferred in large patients and for evaluating the lower innominate veins and SVC (**Fig. 47–5**). The surface of the transducer should be kept in the same location, but angled laterally and inferiorly to visualize the midportion of the subclavian vein, which lies immediately posterior to the clavicle (**Fig. 47–6**).

The entire lumen of a normal upper-extremity vein is often anechoic. With gray scale sonography, thrombus is sometimes apparent as echogenic material within the lumen (**Fig. 47–10**). Thrombosis can also result in ex-

pansion of the venous lumen. However, thrombus can be relatively anechoic or difficult to appreciate in obese patients due to decreased resolution and increased acoustic scatter. The normal subclavian vein will decrease in diameter during a sniffing maneuver and increase in diameter during the Valsalva maneuver.[26] If pressure is applied with the transducer, a normal vein will completely collapse if no thrombus is present; any thrombosed segment of vein will not be completely compressible (**Fig. 47–11**). This technique should be applied

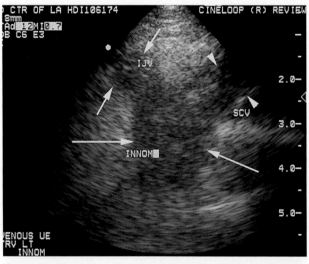

Figure 47–10 Gray scale coronal US image of left thoracic inlet shows material of midlevel echogenicity filling lumens of innominate vein (**long arrows**), IJV (**short arrows**), and medial subclavian vein (**arrowheads**).

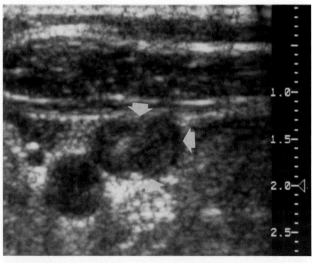

Figure 47–11 Axial gray scale US image shows thrombus within left IJV (**arrows**) that is not compressible.

in the more peripherally located veins, wherever a linear transducer is used. Because of the overlying clavicle, first rib, and sternum, compression is not possible in the medial half of the subclavian vein, the inferior IJV, the innominate vein, or the SVC.

Color Doppler sonography is an important part of the examination of the upper-extremity veins. It can aid in the identification of any major vessels that may be difficult to identify with standard sonography. The direction of flow can be quickly and easily ascertained. Color Doppler sonography is crucial for evaluation of the more centrally located veins that are not amendable to compression.[14] Although pulsed Doppler imaging findings can confirm the presence of flow, a nonocclusive thrombus can still be present. Therefore, color Doppler flow imaging is used to confirm that the vessel completely fills with color. Any portion that does not fill may contain a thrombus that may not have been visible at gray scale sonography. Because color Doppler imaging can help identify small channels of flow through a thrombus that appears to completely fill the venous lumen, it aids in distinguishing between an occlusive and a nonocclusive thrombus (**Fig. 47–12**). Color Doppler sonography can also facilitate identification of venous stenosis, which is characterized by luminal narrowing and color aliasing, indicating high velocity (**Fig. 47–13**). In addition, color Doppler imaging allows easy identification of collateral venous channels that arise as a result of venous obstruction (**Fig. 47–14**).[27] These collaterals may occur in the thoracic inlet region, in the axilla, or in the neck.

Even if optimal sonographic technique is employed, the innominate vein and medial subclavian vein can be difficult to evaluate in some patients, and the junction of the innominate veins is sometimes not visualized.[28] Therefore, the analysis of venous waveforms obtained with duplex sonography is geared toward identification of a centrally located venous obstruction that may not be directly visualized. Normally, waveforms within centrally located veins demonstrate respiratory phasicity resulting from decreased intrathoracic pressure that occurs during inspiration (**Fig. 47–15**). Cardiac pulsatility is also present and results from retrograde transmission of the changing right-atrial pressure during the cardiac cycle. A small retrograde component is often present, making the waveform biphasic. Waveforms are less phasic and pulsatile when obtained further away from the thoracic inlet. If a similar degree of phasicity and pulsatility is not present in waveforms obtained from a corresponding location on the opposite side, then venous obstruction should be suspected (**Figs. 47–16, 47–17**).[29] Therefore, even if symptoms are unilateral, Doppler interrogation should always be performed bilaterally.[30] A complete bilateral examination is needed because a disparity in peripheral waveforms can help identify a central obstructing lesion that may be overlooked initially using gray scale or color Doppler sonog-

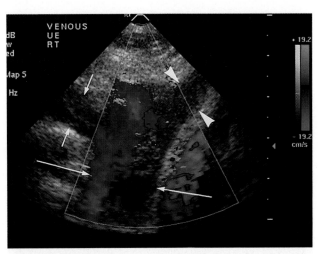

Figure 47–12 Thrombus is present throughout the right subclavian vein (**short arrows**), IJV (**arrowheads**), and innominate vein (**long arrows**). Blue color indicates a patent channel within the lateral portion of the innominate vein. The medially located vessel with red color is the caudal portion of the right common carotid artery.

raphy. In addition, although a collateral vein can be mistaken for a patent subclavian vein (**Fig. 47–17**),[27] the waveform obtained from a collateral vein will often differ from the unaffected subclavian vein on the opposite side, prompting a search for the ipsilateral thrombosed subclavian vein. Abnormally elevated venous velocities can occur at a site of narrowing. Narrowing may be caused by a nonocclusive thrombus or a stenosis resulting from a previous thrombosis or cannulation related trauma (**Fig. 47–13**).[31]

Additional maneuvers may be needed if thoracic outlet compression of the subclavian vein is suspected. In the majority of cases, thoracic outlet syndrome is caused by compression of the brachial plexus, and arm swelling from vascular compromise is not usually present.[32] However, the subclavian vein can be compressed at the thoracic outlet between the scalene muscles and the first rib. Compression of this vein can result in intermittent arm swelling and other symptoms of thoracic outlet syndrome. Repeated compression of the subclavian vein, often during strenuous exercise, can lead to the Paget-Schroetter syndrome (also known as *effort thrombosis*).[33, 34] If thrombosis is present, it should be detectable sonographically, employing the technique described above. If thrombosis is not identified, then a more extensive US examination may help to determine whether compression of the subclavian vein occurs during arm abduction. Color Doppler and pulsed Doppler imaging should be used to evaluate the subclavian vein with the arm abducted at 90, 135, and 180 degrees, as well as in any position that reproduces symptoms. Thoracic outlet compression may be present if cessation of flow or dampening of the venous waveform occurs.[35] However, some dampening has been shown to occur in a small percentage of asymptomatic individuals.[35]

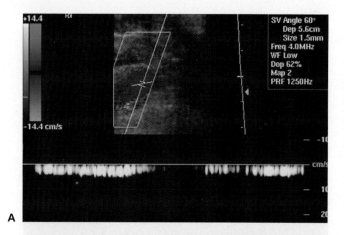

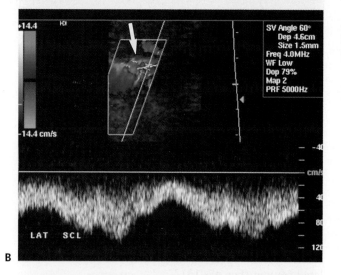

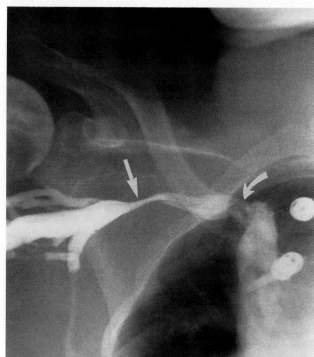

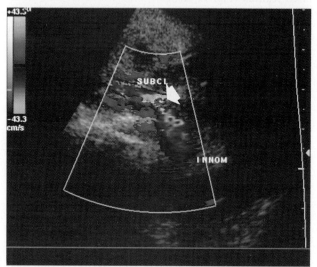

Figure 47–13 Patient had previous angioplasty for stenosis of the medial right subclavian vein, but arm swelling continued. Arm swelling worsened soon after surgical axillary to jugular venous bypass graft was placed. Color duplex sonography was performed followed by right arm venography. The surgical graft could not be identified and was occluded. **A:** Color duplex image of the axillary vein shows phasic flow with low velocity (5 cm/s). **B:** Near the axillary/subclavian junction, narrowing of the vessel lumen and color aliasing are identified (**arrow**). Velocity is elevated (110 cm/s). **C:** A second site of color aliasing (**arrow**) is identified at the junction of the right subclavian vein with the innominate vein. **D:** Venogram confirms stenosis of the medial axillary vein (**arrow**). CT and US findings indicated postoperative hematoma as the cause of extrinsic narrowing. Stenosis of the medial subclavian vein is also present (**curved arrow**).

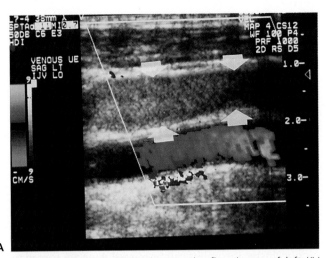

A

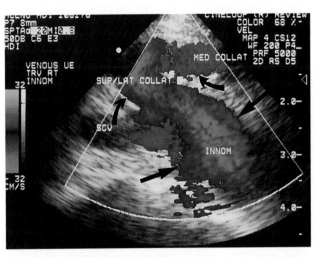

B

Figure 47–14 A: Sagittal color Doppler flow image of left IJV demonstrates thrombus filling the lumen (**arrows**). No color signal is present in the IJV, indicating a complete occlusion. **B:** Color Dop-pler flow image from right supraclavicular region in same patient shows large collateral veins (**curved arrows**) connecting to the innominate vein (**straight arrows**).

Figure 47–15 Color duplex US image of right innominate vein ▷ shows normal central vein waveform. Note respiratory phasicity (**long arrows**), cardiac pulsatility (**short arrows**), and small retro-grade component of flow (**arrowheads**).

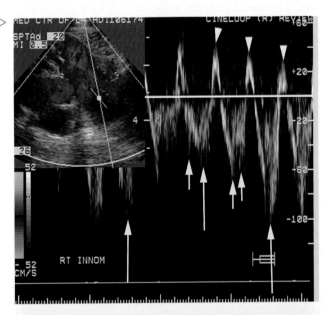

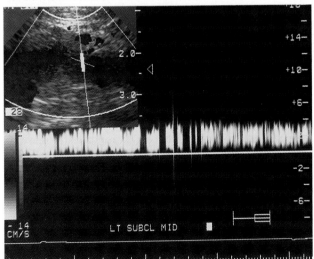

A

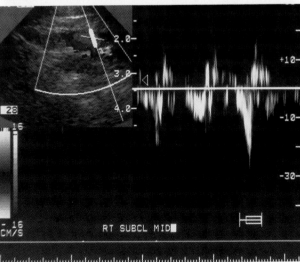

B

Figure 47–16 A: Duplex US image of left subclavian vein shows severely dampened waveform with low velocity (4 cm/s). **B:** Duplex US waveform of right subclavian vein shows respiratory phasicity and pulsatility. Thrombosis of IJV extending into left innominate vein was identified as the cause of subclavian venous obstruction.

Benefits of Ultrasound

Accuracy of Ultrasound

Determination of the accuracy of US of the thoracic inlet and upper extremity veins is complicated because of the variety of sonographic methods used to diagnose venous obstruction. Koksoy et al.[14] used color and duplex US and contrast venography to study 44 patients with subclavian venous catheters. They concluded that the most useful combination of parameters included visualization of thrombus, absence of spontaneous flow, and absence of respiratory phasicity. In their study, sonography had a sensitivity of 94% and a specificity of 96% for depiction of thrombus; its positive predictive value was 94%, and its negative predictive value was 96%. One potential weakness of this study is that it was limited to patients with subclavian venous catheters, a group of patients recognized to have a high incidence of venous complications. However, this study does demonstrate the accuracy of ultrasound in patients with a history of indwelling catheter, a group that comprises the vast majority of cases of upper extremity venous thrombosis in a hospital setting. Knudson et al.[28] reported a larger study with a more diverse population of 91 patients, but imaging correlation was available for only 22 of these patients. Sensitivity of US was 78%, and specificity was 92%. All four of the false-negative color Doppler examinations involved the innominate vein or SVC. This result is not unexpected as analysis of pulsed Doppler waveforms was not included as part of the sonographic technique. Baxter et al.[36] compared color Doppler sonography with venography in 19 patients and found a sensitivity of 89% and a specificity of 100%. The accuracy of US for detecting innominate or SVC obstruction was not documented. Although large studies comparing sonography with contrast venography are unavailable, most investigators have concluded that US is a useful test for detection of venous obstruction of the upper extremity veins.[10, 14, 17, 27, 28, 30, 36]

Limitations of Ultrasound

Because of the overlying osseous structures, upper-extremity venous US is a technically demanding study and can be difficult to interpret. Most of the inaccurate results in the above-mentioned studies involved the innominate veins and SVC, which are not visualized in a number of patients. Therefore, reliance on waveform analysis is often necessary to suggest a centrally located obstruction. The central portion of the subclavian vein, located posterior to the clavicle, can also be difficult to visualize. A nonocclusive thrombus in this region can be overlooked.[37] In addition, the entire subclavian vein and adjacent artery cannot be followed continuously with the probe oriented axially to the vessel lumina, which increases the likelihood of mistaking a collateral vein for the subclavian vein.[27] Bilateral waveform analysis may help prevent this potential pitfall, because flow within a collateral vein may be dampened when compared with the normal subclavian vein on the opposite side (**Fig. 4–17**).

Because the study is technically demanding, experience performing and interpreting these examinations probably increases accuracy. In addition, updated equipment with modern color Doppler technology probably improves accuracy by improving visualization of venous flow. This is particularly important for direct visualization of the lower innominate veins and SVC. A 5-MHz sector-type probe with a small footprint is essential for visualization of the SVC in a number of patients. Nonocclusive thrombus can be missed if we are forced to rely solely on waveform analysis. Although CT is more accurate for evaluation of the SVC, many patients are in an intensive care unit (ICU) setting where portable examinations are preferred.

Several other pitfalls must be avoided when obtaining and interpreting pulsed Doppler waveforms. Excessive pressure applied to the US transducer can narrow the vessel lumen and lead to increased velocity, decreased velocity, or dampening of the waveform. Large-bore indwelling catheters may cause turbulent flow or dampening of the Doppler waveform, although small-caliber catheters do not cause this phenomena.[38] The presence of a hemodialysis fistula may lead to increased flow and spectral broadening in the thoracic inlet veins of the ipsilateral arm (**Fig. 47–18**).[27] Dialysis patients are at risk for central venous obstruction as many have had central lines previously.

As mentioned previously, lymphadenopathy can cause extrinsic compression of a thoracic inlet vein (**Fig. 47–19**), resulting in high velocity and peripheral waveform dampening. Evaluation for thrombosis may be more difficult in these patients. Occasionally, an enlarged node can simulate an intraluminal thrombus (**Fig. 47–20**).

Role of Ultrasound

Color duplex sonography should be used as the initial imaging modality for detection of venous outflow obstruction in patients with arm swelling. Although large studies with complete correlation are still unavailable, multiple investigators have concluded that US is sufficiently accurate to be used as an initial screening test.[14, 27, 28, 30, 36] US is also noninvasive, inexpensive, often readily available, and portable. It can even be performed in an intensive care unit. US is most sensitive for the depiction of thrombosis of the axillary, subclavian, and jugular veins. It is less useful for the identification of obstruction of the innominate veins and SVC, but the presence of this condition is often suggested by waveform analysis, prompting further evaluation with

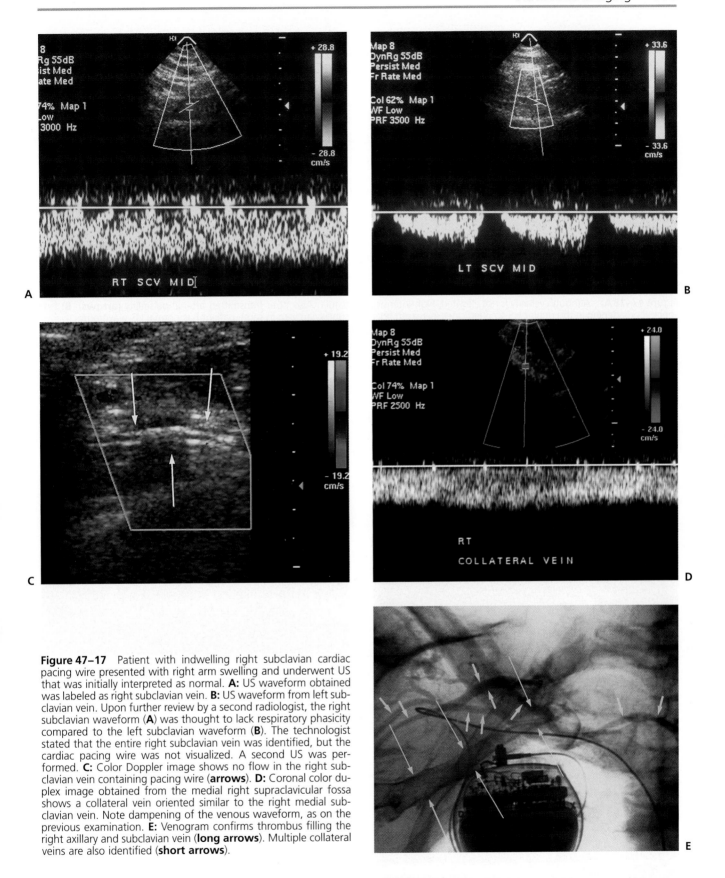

Figure 47–17 Patient with indwelling right subclavian cardiac pacing wire presented with right arm swelling and underwent US that was initially interpreted as normal. **A:** US waveform obtained was labeled as right subclavian vein. **B:** US waveform from left subclavian vein. Upon further review by a second radiologist, the right subclavian waveform (**A**) was thought to lack respiratory phasicity compared to the left subclavian waveform (**B**). The technologist stated that the entire right subclavian vein was identified, but the cardiac pacing wire was not visualized. A second US was performed. **C:** Color Doppler image shows no flow in the right subclavian vein containing pacing wire (**arrows**). **D:** Coronal color duplex image obtained from the medial right supraclavicular fossa shows a collateral vein oriented similar to the right medial subclavian vein. Note dampening of the venous waveform, as on the previous examination. **E:** Venogram confirms thrombus filling the right axillary and subclavian vein (**long arrows**). Multiple collateral veins are also identified (**short arrows**).

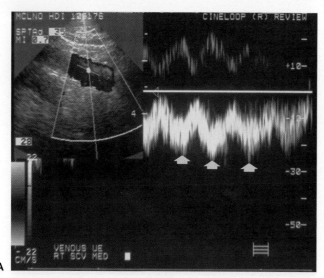

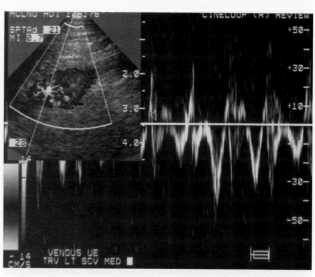

Figure 47–18 A: Although velocity is not elevated, high-intensity spectral broadening in this duplex US scan indicates increased flow in right subclavian vein of this patient with an ipsilateral dialysis fistula. Also note transmitted arterial pulsatility (**arrows**). **B:** Left subclavian vein in same patient has normal US waveform.

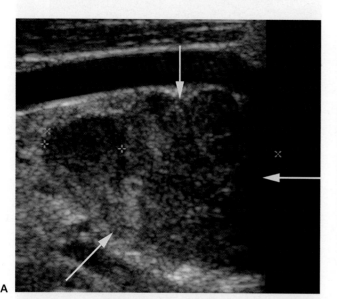

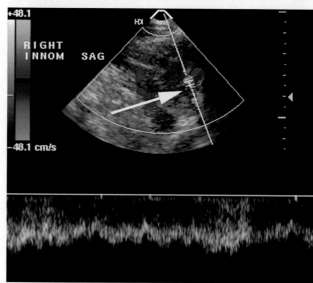

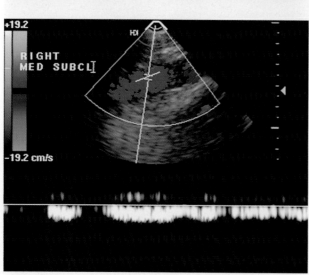

Figure 47–19 A: Gray scale US scan shows conglomerate of enlarged lymph nodes posterior to right clavicle in patient with lymphoma (**arrows**). **B:** Color duplex US image of right innominate vein shows region of color aliasing (**arrow**), indicating a site of high velocity. Pulsed Doppler imaging at this site helps confirm that velocity is elevated (120 cm/s), and spectral broadening is present. This narrowing is a result of extrinsic compression from adjacent nodes. **C:** US waveform in ipsilateral subclavian vein is dampened as a result of more centrally located narrowing.

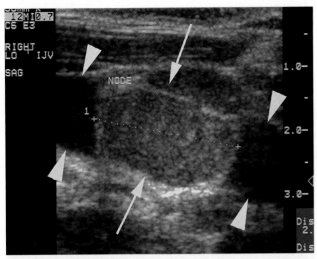

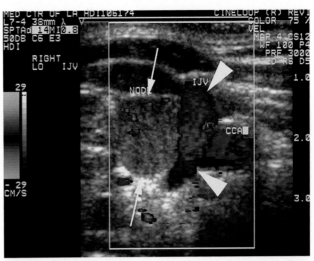

Figure 47–20 A: Sagittal gray scale US image shows enlarged lymph node (**arrows**) that appears to be a thrombus expanding the right IJV (**arrowheads**). **B:** Axial color Doppler flow image shows that the node (**arrows**) is compressing the IJV (**arrowheads**) medially. No color filling defects are present in the IJV lumen.

other imaging modalities. As mentioned previously, optimal technique and modern probe technology will allow sonographic evaluation of the SVC bifurcation in some patients. However, if an obstruction of the SVC is clinically suspected, CT or MR imaging may be used as the initial imaging test. Otherwise, CT, MR angiography, and contrast venography can be used as secondary imaging modalities in a few groups of patients. These groups would include patients without evidence of thrombus at gray scale or color Doppler sonography, but with abnormal duplex findings that suggest a centrally located obstruction, patients with normal US findings in whom thrombosis still seems likely on the basis of clinical information, and patients in whom surgical or radiological intervention is planned.

There are several treatment options for patients with upper extremity venous thrombosis. If a central venous catheter is present, removal of the catheter combined with anticoagulant therapy may relieve symptoms and prevent pulmonary embolism.[39] However, persistent morbidity including pain and swelling persists in a significant number of patients; morbidity rates vary depending on etiology of thrombosis and study population.[40,41] Percutaneous thrombolysis is more invasive but produces long-term symptomatic relief.[42] Success of therapy and follow-up can be evaluated with sonography (**Fig. 47–21**). Percutaneous recanaliztion and thrombolysis is also effective in reestablishing central venous access for parenteral therapy or nutrition.[43] Surgical decompression of the subclavian vein with first rib resection is usually reserved for patients with Paget-Schroetter syndrome who are shown to have thoracic outlet compression of the subclavian vein.[44] Sonography can also be used to follow these patients.

Summary

Venous outflow obstruction involving the thoracic inlet veins is a common and treatable cause of arm swelling that can lead to life-threatening complications. US can be used as the primary imaging modality for identifying patients with thrombosis, venous stenosis, or extrinsic venous compression. Sonography is noninvasive and accurate; frequently, it can help specifically confirm the existance of thrombosis. The US examination of the upper extremity veins requires knowledge of regional vascular anatomy and use of linear, as well as phased-array or sector, transducers to visualize vessels behind the sternum and clavicle. With modern ultrasound technology, it is possible to visualize the SVC in some patients. Maximum sensitivity and specificity are attained with combined use of gray scale, color Doppler, and pulsed Doppler modalities.

Frequently, US is able to help confirm or rule out the existence of thrombosis, and no further evaluation is needed. Even if the innominate veins are not completely visualized, central venous outflow obstruction can still be suggested on the basis of pulsed Doppler waveform analysis. Additional imaging with CT, MR imaging, or contrast venography can be used to help confirm the diagnosis.

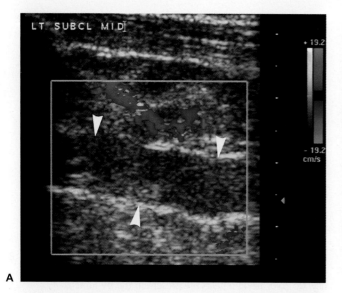

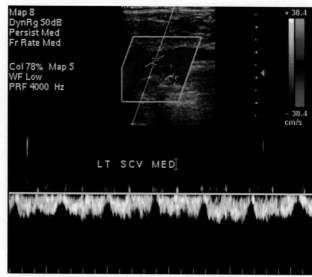

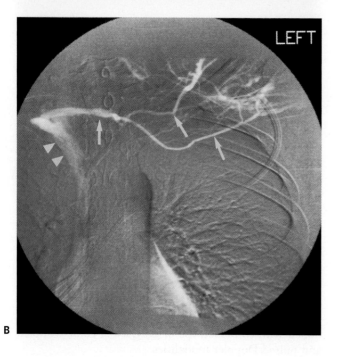

Figure 47–21 A: Color Doppler US image shows no flow in thrombosed left axillary vein (**arrowheads**). Red color indicates flow in a collateral vein. **B:** Left arm venogram show no opacification of left subclavian and axillary veins. Collateral veins (**arrows**) extend from the left arm to the right innominate vein (arrowheads). **C:** Color Doppler US 3 weeks later shows complete color filling of left subclavian vein with waveform that show pulsatility and phasicity.

References

1. Whalen RE. Cardiovascular problems. In: Samiy AH, Douglas RG, Barondess JA, eds. *Textbook of Diagnostic Medicine*. Philadelphia, PA: Lea & Febiger, 1987, p. 199—200.
2. Kissin MW, Quercidella Rovere G, Easton D, Westbury G. Risk of lymphoedema following the treatment of breast cancer. *Br J Surg* 1986;73:580—584.
3. Veal JR. The pathological basis for swelling of the arm following radical amputation of the breast. *Surg Gynaecol Obstet* 1938;67:752—760.
4. Lobb AW, Harkins HN. Postmastectomy swelling of the arm with a note on the effect of segmental resection of the axillary vein at the time of radical mastectomy. *Western J Surg Obstet Gynaecol* 1949;57:550—557.
5. McIvor J, O'Connell D. The investigation of postmastectomy oedema of the arm by lymphography and venography. *Clin Radiol* 1978;29:457—462.
6. Danese C, Howard JM. Postmastectomy lymphedema. *Surg Gynecol Obstet* 1965;120:797—802.
7. Svensson WE, Mortimer PS, Tohno E, Cosgrove DO. Colour Doppler demonstrates venous flow abnormalities in breast cancer patients with chronic arm swelling. *Eur J Cancer* 1994;30:675—660.
8. Wilson CB, Lambert HE, Scott RD. Subclavian and axillary vein thrombosis following radiotherapy for carcinoma of the breast. *Clin Radiol* 1987;38(1):95—96.
9. Austen KF. Diseases of immediate type hypersensitivity. In: Petersdorf RG, Adams RD, Braunwald E, Isselbacher KJ, Martin JB, Wilson JD, eds. *Harrison's Principles of Internal Medicine*, 10th ed. New York, NY: McGraw-Hill, 1983, p. 372—377.
10. Grassi CJ, Polak JF. Axillary and subclavian venous thrombosis: follow-up evaluation with color Doppler flow US and venography. *Radiology* 1990;175:651—654.

11. Drury EM, Trout HH, Giordano MD, Hix WR. Lytic therapy in the treatment of axillary and subclavian vein thrombosis. *J Vasc Surg* 1985;2:821—827.

12. Warden GD, Wilmore DW, Pruitt BA. Central venous thrombosis: a hazard of medical progress. *J Trauma* 1973;13:620—625.

13. Balestreri L, DeCicco M, Matovic M, Coran F, Morassut S. Central venous catheter-related thrombosis in clinically asymptomatic oncologic patients: a phlebographic study. *Eur J Radiol* 1995;20:108—111.

14. Koksoy C, Kuzu A, Kutlay J, et al. The diagnostic value of color Doppler ultrasound in central venous catheter related thrombosis. *Clin Radiol* 1995;50:687—689.

15. Horattas MC, Wright DJ, Fenton AH, et al. Changing concepts of deep venous thrombosis of the upper extremity: report of a series and review of the literature. *Surgery* 1988;104:561—567.

16. Monreal M, Raventos A, Lerma R, et al. Pulmonary embolism in patients with upper extremity DVT associated to venous central lines — a prospective study. *Thromb Haemostas* 1994;72(4):548—550.

17. Svensson WE, Mortimer PS, Tohno E, et al. The use of colour Doppler to define venous abnormalities in the swollen arm following therapy of breast carcinoma. *Clin Radiol* 1991;44:249—252.

18. Tello R, Scholz E, Finn JP, Costello P. Subclavian vein thrombosis detected with spiral CT and three-dimensional reconstruction. *AJR* 1993;160:33—34.

19. Fielding JR, Nagel JS, Pomeroy O. Upper extremity DVT correlation of MR and nuclear medicine flow imaging. *Clin Imag* 1997;21:260—263.

20. Podoloff DA, Kim EE. Evaluation of sensitivity and specificity of upper extremity radionuclide venography in cancer patients with indwelling central venous catheters. *Clin Nucl Med* 1992;17:457—462.

21. Kroger K, Gocke C, Schelo C, Hinrichs A, Rudofsky G. Association of subclavian and jugular vein thrombosis: color Doppler sonographic evaluation. *Angiology* 1998;49:189—191.

22. Finn JP, Zisk JH, Edelman RR, et al. Central venous occlusion: MR angiography. *Radiology* 1993;187:245—251.

23. Chang YC, Dai MH, Wang TC, Su CT, Chiu LC. 2-D Time-of-flight (TOF) MRA of thrombophlebitis of upper extremity and subclavian veins. *Angiology* 1996;47:1019—1022.

24. Esposito MD, Arrington JA, Blackshear MN, Murtagh FR, Silbiger ML. Thoracic outlet syndrome in a throwing athlete diagnosed with MRI and MRA. *JMRI* 1997;17:598—599.

25. Woodburne RT. *Essentials of Human Anatomy,* 7th ed. New York, NY: Oxford University Press, 1983.

26. Hightower DR, Gooding GW. Sonographic evaluation of the normal response of subclavian veins to respiratory maneuvers. *Invest Radiol* 1985;20:517—520.

27. Nazarian GK, Foshager MC. Color Doppler sonography of the thoracic inlet veins. *RadioGraphics* 1995;15:1357—1371.

28. Knudson GJ, Wiedmeyer DA, Erickson SJ, et al. Color Doppler sonographic imaging in the assessment of upper-extremity deep venous thrombosis. *AJR* 1990;154:399—403.

29. Pucheu A, Evans J, Thomas D, Scheuble C, Pucheu M. Doppler ultrasonography of normal neck veins. *JCU* 1994;22:367—373.

30. Longley DG, Finlay DE, Letourneau JG. Sonography of the upper extremity and jugular veins. *AJR* 1993;160:957—962.

31. Criado E, Marston WA, Jaques PF, Mauro MA, Keagy BA. Proximal venous outflow obstruction in patients with upper extremity arteriovenous dialysis access. *Ann Vasc Surg* 1994;8:530—535.

32. Pollak W. *Thoracic Outlet Syndrome: Diagnosis and Treatment.* Mount Kisko, NY: Futura, 1986.

33. Smith-Behn J, Althar R, Katz W. Primary thrombosis of the axillary/subclavian vein. *South Med J* 1986;79(9):1176—1178.

34. Thompson RW, Schneider PA, Nelken NA, Skioldebrand CG, Stoney RJ. Circumferential venolysis and paraclavicular thoracic outlet decompression for effort thrombosis of the subclavian vein. *J Vasc Surg* 1992;16:723—732.

35. Longley DG, Yedlicka JW, Monila EJ, et al. Thoracic outlet syndrome: evaluation of the subclavian vessels by color duplex sonography. *AJR* 1992;158:623—630.

36. Baxter GM, Kincaid W, Jeffrey RF, et al. Comparison of colour Doppler ultrasound with venography in the diagnosis of axillary and subclavian vein thrombosis. *Br J Radiol* 1991;64:777—781.

37. Haire WD, Lynch TG, Lund GB, Lieberman RP, Edney JA. Limitations of magnetic resonance imaging and ultrasound-directed (duplex) scanning in the diagnosis of subclavian vein thrombosis. *J Vasc Surg* 1991;13:391—397.

38. Burbidge SJ, Finlay DE, Letourneau JG, Longley DG. Effects of central venous catheter placement on upper extremity duplex US findings. *JVIR* 1993;4:399—404.

39. Haire WD. Arm vein thrombosis. *Clin Chest Med* 1995;16(2):341—351.

40. AbuRahma AF, Short YS, White JF. Treatment alternatives for axillary-subclavian vein thrombosis: long-term follow-up. *Cardiovasc Surg* 1996;4(6):783—787.

41. Becker DM, Philbrick JT, Walker FB. Axillary and subclavian venous thrombosis. *Arch Intern Med* 1991;151:1934—1943.

42. Beygui RE, Olcott C, Dalman RL. Subclavian vein thrombosis: outcome analysis based on etiology and modality of treatment. *Ann Vasc Surg* 1997;11:247—255.

43. Ferral H, Bjarnason H, Wholey M, et al. Recanalization of occluded veins to provide access for central catheter placement. *J Vasc Interv. Radial* 1996;7:681—685.

44. Adelman MA, Stone DH, Riles TS, et al. A multidisciplinary approach to the treatment of Paget-Schroetter syndrome. *Ann Vasc Surg* 1997;11:149—54.

Musculoskeletal System

48 Shoulder Pain

William D. Middleton, Sharlene A. Teefey, and Ken Yamaguchi

Introduction

The shoulder is recognized as a primary and common source of functional disability. It ranks second only to knee pain as the most common joint-related complaint prompting a patient to seek physician referral.[1] Shoulder pain may arise from a number of different sources including dysfunction or inflammation of local structures, abnormalities of more remote structures, or systemic illness. Accurate clinical evaluation will not only include a careful history and physical examination but also employ appropriate imaging modalities to help characterize any anatomic structures responsible for pain. By far the most common anatomic etiology for shoulder pain is rotator cuff disease. Multiple imaging modalities can be employed to provide useful information on the status of the rotator cuff. This chapter will focus primarily on evaluation of shoulder pain and illustrate the potential contributions that can be made with ultrasound.

Differential Diagnosis

Shoulder pain can arise from either primary or secondary etiologies.[1] Primary sources include various abnormalities of the local anatomy about the shoulder. Secondary sources include remote or systemic abnormalities which refer pain to the shoulder area. In an evaluation of a patient with shoulder pain, it is important to differentiate primary from secondary etiologies. Secondary sources of shoulder pain include cervical spine disease, thoracic outlet disorders, brachial plexus lesions, heart disease and certain infectious diseases such as Herpes zoster. Among the secondary causes for shoulder pain, the most common by far is cervical spine disease. Pain from this etiology can be differentiated from primary shoulder sources with a careful history and physical exam. In these patients, pain often extends below the elbow and into the hand and is associated with paresthesias in the fingers. The neurologic deficits follow radicular patterns rather than peripheral nerve patterns. Additionally, passive motion about the shoulder generally does not cause pain in those patients with cervical spine disease. Thoracic outlet disorders are primarily a diagnosis of exclusion when other primary or secondary sources do not appear to be significant. Medical dis-

orders such as heart disease, lung disease, or upper abdominal disorders should also be considered when the diagnosis is unclear.[1] Although these conditions are uncommonly seen in people who present with only shoulder pain, correct early diagnosis can be very important in the prognosis and treatment.

Primary shoulder pain can come from multiple intrinsic causes. These disorders include rotator cuff and biceps tendon disease, primary biceps tendon disease, glenohumeral instability, degenerative arthritis, and frozen shoulder.[2] It should be noted that some overlap usually exists between these entities. As stated earlier, rotator cuff disorders are by far the most common source of shoulder pain and dysfunction. The etiology of rotator cuff disorders is largely unknown. The two most common theories for the development of rotator cuff disease include intrinsic age-related changes and extrinsic sources such as mechanical abutment from degenerative spurs or repetitive overuse and microtrauma.[2,3] The more commonly accepted etiology for rotator cuff disorders is mechanical abutment. Mechanical abutment generally occurs when the rotator cuff is "pinched" between the humeral head below and the coracoacromial arch above. This mechanical abutment of the rotator cuff against the anterior acromion and coracoacromial ligament can be caused from either an osteophyte above the cuff or superior migration of the humeral head. The occurrence of an osteophyte at the anterior leading edge of the acromion is thought to increase the likelihood of mechanical abutment. The etiologies of these osteophytes is still largely unknown but is thought to occur secondary to degenerative changes in the coracoacromial ligament. Superior head migration occurs in the context of repetitive overuse and fatigue of the rotator cuff.

The importance of intrinsic, age-related degenerative changes to the rotator cuff is becoming increasingly apparent in the pathophysiology of rotator cuff disease. Multiple studies have shown an age-related incidence of rotator cuff tears. In a classic study by DePalma and colleagues, it was shown that 30% of individuals between the age of 50 and 70 had rotator cuff tears while approximately 90% above the age of 70 had tears.[4] Interestingly, 40% of these patients had no shoulder symptoms at the time of their death. An MRI study looking at the incidence of rotator cuff tears in documented asymptomatic people showed a 28% incidence of full-thickness rotator cuff tears in those people above the age of 65. Very few people below this age had full-thickness tears.[5] Using ultrasound, Milgrom and colleagues showed similar findings in asymptomatic volunteers. In this study, the cumulative percentage of partial-and full-thickness tears was 33% for those between the ages of 50 and 60, 55% for those between the ages of 60 and 70, and 70% between the ages of 70 and 80.[6] In addition to an age-related increasing incidence of rotator cuff tears, these studies also showed a high incidence of bilateral disease supporting the fact that this is a more intrinsic age-related process.

Diagnostic Workup

As with any other medical evaluation, obtaining an accurate history and physical examination is essential in the overall clinical assessment of shoulder pain and dysfunction. A thorough history and physical examination, in conjunction with appropriate diagnostic tests, will allow for the accurate diagnosis of the majority of patients with shoulder pain. Patients with rotator cuff disorders present with complaints of pain, both with activities and at times resting, especially at night. The pain is usually anterior and lateral and can radiate to the deltoid insertion. It is not uncommon for the pain to radiate to the level of the elbow, but, generally, it does not radiate further distally. With full-thickness rotator cuff tears, the pain can often be quite significant at night. Often, the patient has difficulty sleeping on the affected side. With further progression, the pain can be symptomatic in any position when lying flat. The patients can sometimes get symptomatic relief by sleeping in a recliner or some other position in which the back is elevated. Additionally, patients can present with complaints associated with limited motion and weakness. They often have difficulty reaching behind, for instance, to place their arm in a sleeve or obtain something from a back pocket.

Physical findings in patients with rotator cuff disease can be variable. Generally, patients without full-thickness rotator cuff tears can achieve full active elevation of their shoulder. Those with full-thickness tears have variable limits to their active motion, but passive elevation is generally preserved. While passive elevation can be maintained, it is nearly universal that impassive, internal rotation and extension is reduced on the affected side in comparison to the contralateral side. Generally, external rotation is preserved. Specific rotator cuff testing can also be performed for the teres minor, infra and supraspinatus muscles as well as the subscapularis. These include the "lift-off" exam, thumb-down abduction or "Jobe's" test, external rotation at the side, and external rotation and abduction. With large chronic tears, atrophy of the supra and infraspinatus muscles can be seen on inspection. Impingement signs are generally present in those patients with rotator cuff disorders. All im-

pingement signs rely on positioning of the arm in such a way that motion will produce compression of the rotator cuff against the anterior inferior acromion and coracoacromial ligament. An impingement *test* can be conducted in which the previous pain elicited during an impingement *sign* is reduced or completely relieved by an injection of local anesthetic into the subacromial space.[1–3,7]

After a careful history and physical examination, shoulder radiographs are the initial imaging tests obtained for most patients presenting with shoulder pain. For rotator cuff disease, plain radiographs are often normal. Superior migration of the humeral head and sclerosis of the anterior—inferior surface of the acromion can occasionally be seen but are only present in the presence of chronic and massive rotator cuff tears. An anterior—inferior acromial spur can also be detected by plain radiographs. These spurs suggest an increased likelihood of rotator cuff tears but are not diagnostic. Calcific tendinitis of the rotator cuff can also be seen infrequently on radiographs.

Additional imaging modalities for the rotator cuff include arthrography, MRI, and ultrasound. Historically, shoulder arthrography was the primary test used to confirm or exclude a clinical diagnostic of full-thickness rotator cuff tear. Arthrographic documentation of a communication between the glenohumeral joint and the subacromial bursa indicates a full-thickness rotator cuff tear. Identification of contrast only within the substance of the rotator cuff is the diagnostic criteriom for a partial-thickness tear. The sensitivity of arthrography for the detection of full-thickness rotator cuff tears has ranged from 93 to 100%.[8,9] Results for detection of partial-thickness tears have been less reliable and limited to tears only on the deep (articular) surface of the cuff. Although arthrography is sensitive for diagnosing full-thickness cuff tears, it has recently become less popular because it is an invasive and sometimes painful procedure. In most current practices, it is used as a problem-solving tool, rather than a primary diagnostic test.

Magnetic resonance imaging (MRI) is now widely used in diagnosis of rotator cuff tears. Multiple studies have shown high accuracy for the detection of full-thickness tears with reported sensitivities ranging from 80 to 100% and specificities similarly high, from 77 to 99%.[10–13] The detection of partial tears has been less reliable with MRI, with reported sensitivities ranging from 25 to 89% and specificities from 83 to 99%.[10–12,14] MR arthrography can improve the detection of partial-thickness tears but the sensitivity remains limited with a reported sensitivity in one series of only 46%.[14] In addition, MRI arthrography converts a noninvasive test into an invasive test.

In addition to its noninvasive nature and overall accuracy, an advantage of MRI is the ease and consistency with which images can be acquired. If established protocols are used, then the quality of the images are dependent more on the patient compliance than on the operator. However, during the course of an exam, the patients need to remain motionless in a tightly confined space. This can be uncomfortable, and in those patients with claustrophobia, poorly tolerated. In addition, as with other sophisticated imaging tests, interpretation of images requires knowledge of relevant soft tissue anatomy and an understanding of the relative strengths and weaknesses of individual MR signs for rotator cuff tears.[15]

Ultrasound

Like other musculoskeletal ultrasound exams, shoulder sonograms should be performed with high-frequency linear array transducers. For most patients, the operating frequency of the probe should be between 7 and 10 MHz. The exact choice of transducer will vary depending on the patient and the type of equipment used.

At our institution, patients are examined while seated on a stool that rotates. This allows the patient to be positioned so that both shoulders can be examined conveniently. The examiner stands behind and to the side of the patient. Initially, transverse and longitudinal views of the biceps tendon are obtained with the shoulder in a neutral position. Transverse and longitudinal views of the subscapularis are then obtained with the shoulder externally rotated. Finally, the supraspinatus and infraspinatus tendons are examined in long and short axis orientations with the shoulder extended and the patient's hand placed on the ipsilateral posterior hip. During the examination of the shoulder, the rotator cuff is compressed in a manner similar to lower-extremity venous studies. The criteria for rotator cuff tears will be discussed in more detail later.

Like MRI, ultrasound is a noninvasive means of imaging the rotator cuff. The normal sonographic appearance of the rotator cuff is well described[16, 17] and is illustrated in **Fig. 48–1**. The primary indication for shoulder sonography is to detect, localize, and quantify the width and degree of retraction of rotator cuff tears. There are a number of sonographic criteria for full-thickness tears.[18, 19] As with MRI, all of these findings should be understood and should be recognized to maintain high sensitivity.

When there is a tear of the rotator cuff the defect is often filled with fluid, which interrupts the normal echo-

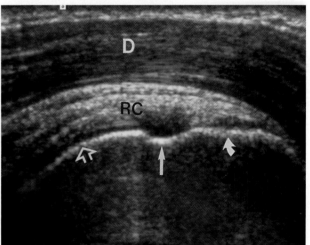

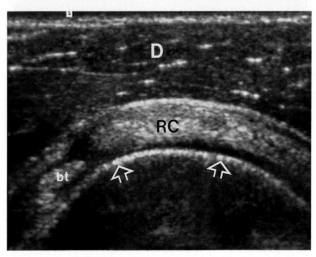

Figure 48–1 Normal rotator cuff **A:** Magnified transverse view of the rotator cuff demonstrates the different layers that are visualized sonographically. The bright curvilinear reflection in the deep aspect of the image arises from the cortex of the humeral head (**open arrows**). The overlying hypo/anechoic layer represents articular cartilage (c). The next hyperechoic layer is the rotator cuff (RC). Superficial to the rotator cuff is a thin hypoechoic layer corresponding to the subdeltoid bursa (b). The thin hyperechoic layer superficial to the bursa represents a small amount of peribursal fat (**arrows**). The most superficial hypoechoic tissue is the overlying deltoid muscle (D). Note the outwardly convex contour of the peribursal fat. This is an important normal finding. **B:** Long axis view of the supraspinatus insertion showing the greater tuberosity (**curved arrow**), the anatomic neck of the humerus (**arrow**), the humeral head (**open arrow**), the rotator cuff (RC), and the deltoid muscle (D). **C:** Short axis view of the rotator cuff shows the reflection from the humeral head (**open arrows**), the rotator cuff (RC), the intraarticular portion of the biceps tendon (bt), and the overlying deltoid muscle (D).

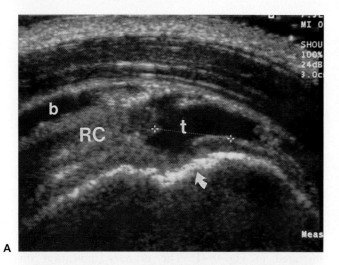

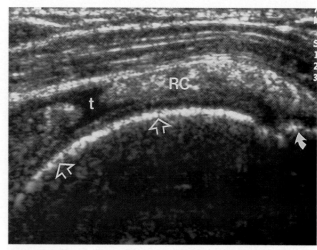

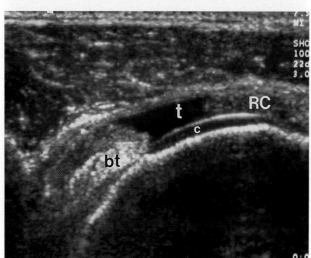

Figure 48–2   Full-thickness rotator cuff tears identified as fluid-filled defects. **A:** Long axis view of the rotator cuff (RC) demonstrates a tear (t) at the site of attachment to the greater tuberosity (**curved arrow**). A small amount of fluid is also seen in the subdeltoid bursa (b). Reprinted with permission from **Sonography of the Shoulder** by WD Middleton, SA Teefey, and K Yamaguchi. **Sem Musculoskel Rad** 1998;2:211—221. **B:** Long axis view of the rotator cuff (RC) demonstrates a small tear (t). In this case, the tear is located over the humeral head (**open arrows**) and is removed from the greater tuberosity (**curved arrow**). **C:** Short axis view of the rotator cuff (RC) demonstrates a tear (t) located immediately adjacent to the intraarticular portion of the biceps tendon (bt). In this case, fluid in the tear accentuates the reflection from the articular cartilage (c) producing an uncovered cartilage sign. Reprinted with permission from **Sonography of the Shoulder** by WD Middleton, SA Teefey, and K Yamaguchi. **Sem Musculoskel Rad** 1998;2:211—221.

genicity of the cuff and produces an anechoic or hypoechoic defect. This appearance is easy to understand and recognize. This is illustrated in **Fig. 48–2**.

If fluid does not fill the space created by the tear, then the deltoid muscle and the peribursal fat drop into the defect. This produces a change in the normal outwardly convex contour of the peribursal fat. The difference in appearance of a "wet" and a "dry" tear is illustrated in **Fig. 48–3**. Depending on the size of the tear and the shape of the underlying humerus, the contour of the peribursal fat may become concave (**Fig. 48–4**) or straight (**Fig. 48–5**).

In the majority of cases, the contour abnormality described above is easily detected with routine scanning. However, if the tear is filled with hypertrophied bursal synovial tissue or if there is no separation of the torn tendon ends, there may be no detectable defect and no visible contour abnormality. In these cases, when pressure is applied with the transducer, the synovial tissue will compress or the tendon ends will separate, and a contour abnormality will become visible (**Fig. 48–6**).

Massive tears of the rotator cuff are associated with a marked tendon retraction, often beneath the acromion process. In such cases, no normal rotator cuff will be visible covering the humeral head. Rather, the deltoid muscle and bursal tissue will come into direct contact with the humeral head and its cartilage. This appearance is referred to as nonvisualization of the rotator cuff (**Fig. 48–7**).

Irregularity of the greater tuberosity is also a common finding in patients with rotator cuff tears. In one study, all of the full-thickness tears were associated with tuberosity irregularities, while only 11% of shoulders without a cuff tear had tuberosity irregularity.[20]

Partial-thickness tears are seen as hypoechoic or mixed hypo and hyperechoic defects of the rotator cuff.[21,22] They usually occur on the deep surface of the cuff and are usually associated with irregular reactive changes in the underlying greater tuberosity (**Fig. 48–8**). Unlike full-thickness tears, most partial tears do not compress with transducer pressure.

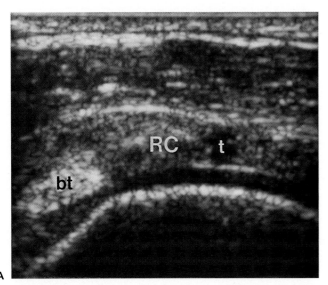

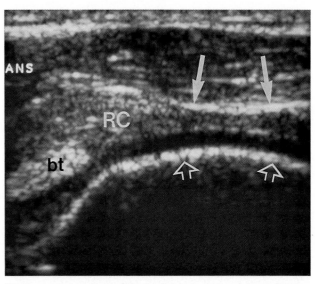

Figure 48–3 Illustration of difference in appearance between fluid-filled and nonfluid-filled rotator cuff tear. **A:** Short axis view of the rotator cuff (RC) and the intraarticular portion of the biceps tendon (bt) demonstrates a small fluid-filled full-thickness tear (t). **B:** Similar image obtained with slight transducer pressure (so that fluid is compressed out of the tear) demonstrates closer apposition of the peribursal fat (**arrows**) and the humeral head and overlying articular cartilage (**open arrows**). This changes the contour of the peribursal fat from convex to concave.

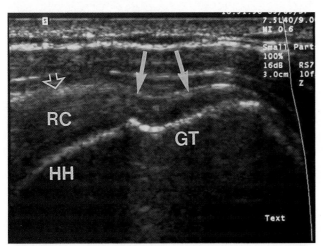

Figure 48–4 Full-thickness rotator cuff tears seen as a contour abnormality. Long axis view of the rotator cuff (RC) demonstrates normal convex contour of the peribursal fat (**open arrow**) overlying the humeral head (HH). An abnormal concave contour of the peribursal fat (**arrows**) is seen overlying the greater tuberosity (GT). This concavity defines the location of the tear.

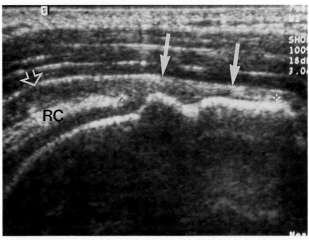

Figure 48–5 Full-thickness rotator cuff tears seen as a contour abnormality. Long axis view of the rotator cuff (RC) demonstrates normal convex contour of the peribursal fat (**open arrow**) in the region where the cuff is intact. Straightening of the contour of the peribursal fat (**arrows**) is seen in a region where the rotator cuff is torn.

In addition to the rotator cuff, the other major tendon that should be evaluated in patients with shoulder pain is the long head of the biceps.[23] As with the rotator cuff, the normal appearance of the biceps tendon is well described.[24] **Fig. 48–9** illustrates this normal appearance. Abnormalities of the biceps tendon can both simulate rotator cuff disease and often coexist with rotator cuff lesions. Rupture of the biceps tendon will usually be appreciated as no detectable tendon within the biceps groove or in the joint above the groove (**Fig. 48–10**). If the tendon retracts distally, there will be shortening of the biceps muscle, and a palpable mass will usually be present in the arm. This is readily apparent on physical exam and also on ultrasound (**Fig. 48–10**). If the tendon scars in or at the entrance to the groove (autotenodesis), it will not retract and it will not be detectable on physical exam. In the latter case, inability to detect the intraarticular tendon on sonography will be the only way to make the diagnosis.

Another abnormality of the biceps tendon that is detectable on sonography is dislocation.[25] With dislocation or subluxation, the biceps tendon migrates medially out of the tendon groove (**Fig. 48–11**). It can be positioned anterior to the lesser tuberosity or anterior to,

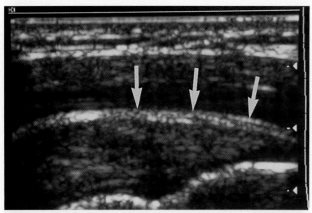

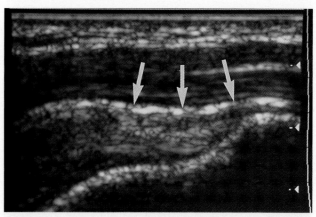

Figure 48–6 Use of compression to help identify a full-thickness rotator cuff tear. Reprinted with permission from **Sonography of the Shoulder** by WD Middleton, SA Teefey, and K Yamaguchi. **Sem Musculoskel Rad** 1998;2:211—221. **A:** Long axis view of the insertion of the supraspinatus demonstrates normal convex con-

tour of the peribursal fat (**arrows**). **B:** Similar view obtained with transducer compression now demonstrates concavity of the peribursal fat (**arrows**), indicating an underlying small, nonretracted, but full-thickness rotator cuff tear.

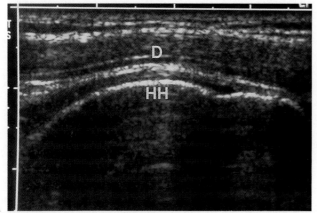

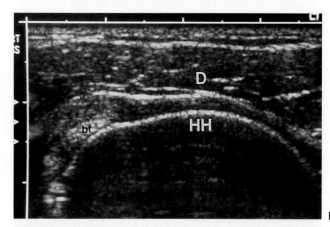

Figure 48–7 Massive rotator cuff tear with nonvisualization of the cuff. Reprinted with permission from **Sonography of the Shoulder** by WD Middleton, SA Teefey, and K Yamaguchi. **Sem Musculoskel Rad** 1998;2:211—221. **A:** Long axis view of the shoulder demonstrates deltoid muscle (D) in close apposition to the

humeral head (HH). No normal rotator cuff is seen overlying the humeral head. **B:** Short axis view of the same patient demonstrates similar finding with respect to the deltoid muscle (D) and humeral head (HH). Again, no normal rotator cuff is visualized. The intraarticular portion of the biceps tendon (bt) is seen anteriorly.

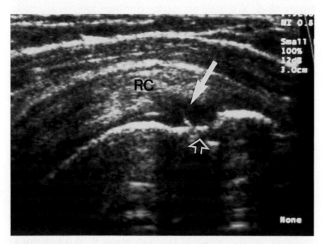

Figure 48–8 Partial-thickness rotator cuff tear. Longitudinal view of the rotator cuff (RC) demonstrates a mixed hypo- and hyperechoic defect (**arrow**) along the deep surface of the insertion to the greater tuberosity. Bony pitting and irregularity (**open arrow**) is seen at the greater tuberosity.

within, or deep to the subscapularis tendon. Dislocation of the biceps tendon medial to the lesser tuberosity almost always is accompanied by a subscapularis tear, although the tear may not be associated with tendon retraction. The supraspinatus tendon contributes to the anchoring mechanism of the biceps tendon and is also frequently torn in cases of biceps tendon dislocation.

In addition to rotator cuff disease, other intrinsic shoulder problems that are common sources of pain include glenohumeral instability, degenerative arthritis, adhesive capsulitis, and fractures. Sonography is not indicated in the initial workup of any of these problems. Glenohumeral instability is generally evaluated with MR arthrography as the labrum, capsule, and glenohumeral ligaments can be seen with this technique. Degenerative arthritis is evaluated with radiographs. Adhesive capsulitis generally is a clinical diagnosis that requires no imaging evaluation unless other possibilities

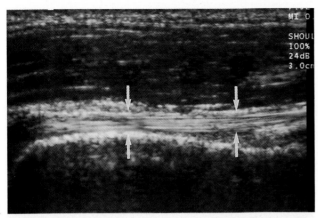

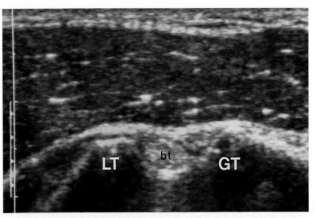

A

Figure 48–9 Normal biceps tendon. **A:** Longitudinal view of the biceps tendon (**arrows**) demonstrates the normal parallel linear reflectors within the tendon. **B:** Transverse view demonstrates the

B

ovoid echogenic biceps tendon (bt) located in the biceps tendon groove between the lesser tuberosity (LT) and the greater tuberosity (GT).

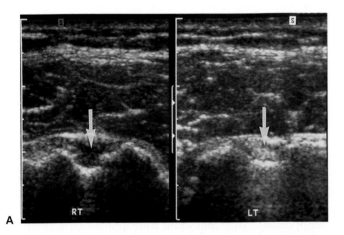

A

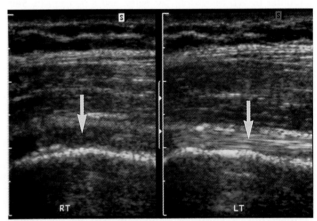

B

Figure 48–10 Biceps tendon rupture. **A:** Dual transverse images of the right (RT) and left (LT) biceps tendon grooves. A normal appearing biceps tendon is readily visible in the left biceps tendon groove (**arrow**), but no tendon is detectable in the right biceps tendon groove (**arrow**). **B:** Longitudinal view of the biceps tendon groove in the same patient demonstrates normal appearing biceps tendon on the left (**arrow**) and no detectable biceps tendon on the right (**arrow**). **C:** Longitudinal extended field of view scan of the right arm demonstrates the shortened biceps muscle (B) and the blunt retracted superior margin of the tendon (**arrow**). Refractive shadowing (s) is seen at the edge of the retracted biceps muscle. Reprinted with permission from **Sonography of the Shoulder** by WD Middleton, SA Teefey, and K Yamaguchi. **Sem Musculoskel Rad** 1998;2:211—221.

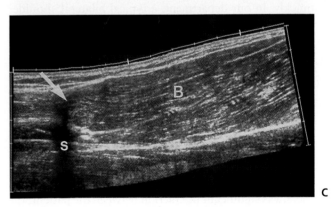

C

are being considered. Suspected fractures are evaluated with radiographs and only under unusual circumstances require other tests. One should remember, however, that radiographs are occasionally negative in the setting of an acute, minimally displaced fracture. Such patients with occult fractures may occasionally be referred for a shoulder sonogram because of persistent unexplained pain. In this situation, fractures can be detected with sonography.[26] They appear as a cortical step-off or discontinuity (**Fig. 48–12**).

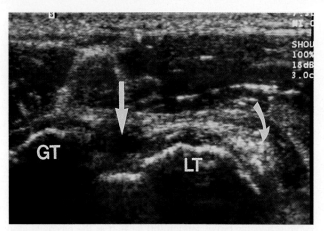

Figure 48–11 Biceps tendon dislocation. Transverse view of the right biceps tendon groove demonstrates no visible tendon within the groove (**straight arrow**). The dislocated biceps tendon (**curved arrow**) is seen located just medial to the lesser tuberosity (LT). The greater tuberosity (GT) is seen lateral to the biceps tendon groove. Reprinted with permission from **Sonography of the Shoulder** by WD Middleton, SA Teefey, and K Yamaguchi. **Sem Musculoskel Rad** 1998;2:211—221.

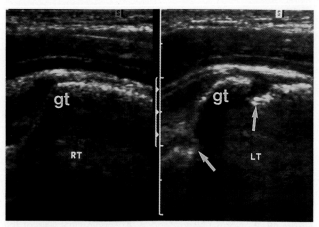

Figure 48–12 Fracture of the greater tuberosity. Dual longitudinal views of the right (RT) and left (LT) greater tuberosities (gt). The right greater tuberosity appears normal. Cortical breaks (**arrows**) are seen at the superior and inferior aspect of the left greater tuberosity.

Benefits of Ultrasound

Sonography has many benefits in the detection of rotator cuff tears. As is stressed throughout this book, the inexpensive, noninvasive nature of ultrasound is very attractive to patients and to third-party payers. Both shoulders can be examined with sonography: this is not practical with MRI or arthrography. Once the technique is mastered, a shoulder sonogram can be performed quickly. In our department, a typical bilateral shoulder ultrasound examination usually requires about 10 and 5 minutes of sonographer and radiologist time, respectively. The exam is well accepted by patients, and almost all exams can be successfully completed: rare exceptions are patients with severely limited range of motion, marked obesity, or marked bony distortion. Scheduling the exam is generally easy and results of the exam are immediately available. In addition, patients are generally satisfied at the end of a shoulder ultrasound exam. The results of one study comparing MRI and arthrography indicated that patient satisfaction was increased when there was significant interaction between the patient, the technologist, and/or the radiologist.[27] This was one of the reasons the patients in this study were more likely to find MRI unpleasant or extremely unpleasant when compared to arthrography. One could reasonably assume that ultrasound would be even better tolerated than arthrography as it is noninvasive but like arthrography, involves continuous patient interaction with a professional (technologist and/or radiologist).

Multiple studies have examined the accuracy of sonography in evaluating the rotator cuff. As with most new techniques, the initial studies that appeared in the mid 1980s showed encouraging results with sensitivity and specificity values for full-thickness rotator cuff tears of greater than 90%.[28—30] These initial reports stimulated others to attempt shoulder sonography. Although some were able to reproduce the excellent results reported in the earlier series,[31, 32] others were not.[33—35] The poor results obtained by some were likely due to a number of causes. Most important were limitations in equipment, lack of consensus about the proper criteria for diagnosing rotator cuff tears, and lack of agreement regarding optimal scan technique. In addition, the development and rapid refinement of MRI afforded another noninvasive means of imaging the rotator cuff resulting in less incentive to learn how to perform shoulder sonography. Regardless of the reasons, sonography of the shoulder did not become widely adopted and instead remained a technique that was largely confined to isolated centers where there was local expertise.

However, in the past 5 years, there have been dramatic advances in high-resolution transducer technology that have resulted in improved images. This, in turn, has made the technique easier to learn and has made the examinations faster to perform and easier to interpret. New sonographic techniques such as color Doppler, tissue harmonic imaging, and extended field of view imaging have been developed which increase the amount of information available with ultrasound. The technique of the examination has been further standardized, and the criteria for diagnosing rotator cuff tears have been refined. For all of these reasons, ultrasound has become less intimidating to most radiologists, and there is now a renewed interest in it.

This renewed interest is supported by several recent studies that indicate that sonography can detect rotator cuff tears with an accuracy equivalent to what is reported with MRI. **Table 1** shows the results of a study of 225 surgically proven cases that included 67 normal cuffs, 68 partial-thickness tears, and 90 full-thickness tears.[22] In this study, sensitivity and specificity for full-thickness tears was 93% and 99%, respectively. Sensitivity and specificity for partial-thickness tears was 94% and 97%, respectively. Another sonographic study that specifically looked at partial-thickness tears showed a sensitivity of 93%.[21] Thus, ultrasound may be better than MRI in detecting partial tears. Our own data from 100 consecutive patients with arthroscopic proof showed a sensitivity of 100% for full-thickness rotator cuff tears and a sensitivity of 67% for partial-thickness tears.

Based on these data, it is clear that in experienced hands, sonography is as effective as MRI in the detection of rotator cuff tears. It is also evident that there will be more "experienced hands" in the near future. Given this, the current American College of Radiology Appropriateness Criteria for imaging patients over 40 years of age with shoulder pain and suspected rotator cuff tears or impingement are hard to understand. On a scale of 1 to 9 with 1 being least appropriate and 9 being most appropriate, ultrasound was given a score of 1 and MRI a score of 8.[36] Even if ultrasound is assumed to be too operator dependent to be used on a widescale basis, it can be, and, in fact, is used by many radiologists both within, and especially outside, of the United States. Therefore, a score of 1 seems unjustified and is certainly not supported by the literature.

At our institution, ultrasound is used when the primary clinical question is to rule out a rotator cuff tear. In those patients with prolonged shoulder pain, differentiating an intact cuff from full-thickness rotator cuff tear disease can help the treating clinician determine the appropriate amount of time to administer nonoperative care. Additionally, when surgical procedures are necessary, there are multiple surgical options that must be considered. In order of increasing complexity they include simple arthroscopy with debridement, arthroscopy with decompression and debridement, complete arthroscopic rotator cuff repair, mini-open rotator cuff repair, and formal open rotator cuff repair. Information on the presence or absence of a full-thickness tear and the location and size of a tear, if it exists, is important in deciding which of these available treatment options would be most appropriate. Sonography can reliably provide this information at approximately one quarter of the cost of an MRI.

Table 48–1 Detection of rotator cuff tears. Results of shoulder sonography compared with surgery

	Thickness tears	
	Full	**Partial**
Sensitivity	93% (84/90)	94% (64/68)
Specificity	99% (134/135)	97% (152/157)
PPV	99% (84/85)	93% (64/69)
NPV	96% (134/140)	97% (152/156)

PPV, positive predictive value.
NPV, negative predictive value.

Summary

In summary, ultrasound can function as the primary imaging modality in patients who present with shoulder pain in whom initial clinical and radiographic evaluation suggest the diagnosis of rotator cuff disease. At our institution, the sonographic results are used to help determine if management should be conservative or surgical. When surgery is necessary, the information obtained from the ultrasound exam is used to formulate an operative approach and strategy.

References

1. Glockner SM. Shoulder pain: a diagnostic dilemma. *Am Fam Physician* 1995;51:1677—1687.
2. Iannotti JP. Evaluation of the painful shoulder. *J Hand Ther* 1994;7:77—83.
3. Frieman BG, Albert TJ, Fenlin JM Jr. Rotator cuff disease: a review of diagnosis, pathophysiology, and current trends in treatment. *Arch Phys Med Rehabil* 1994;75:604—609.
4. DePalma AF, Callery G, Bennett CA. Variational anatomy and degenerative lesions of the shoulder joint. In: American Academy of Orthopaedic Surgeons Chicago, Instructional Course Lectures 1949;6:255—281.
5. Sher JS, Uribe JW, Posada A, et al. Abnormal findings on magnetic resonance images of asymptomatic shoulders. *J Bone Joint Surg A* 1995;77:10—15.
6. Milgrom C, Schaffler M, Gilbert S, et al. Rotator cuff changes in asymptomatic adults: the effect of age, hand dominance and gender. *J Bone Joint Surg [Br]* 1995;77:296—298.
7. Lyons PM, Orwin JF. Rotator cuff tendinopathy and subacromial impingement syndrome. *Med Sci Sports Exerc* 1998;30:S12—S17.
8. Paavolainen P, Ahovuo J. Ultrasonography and arthrography in the diagnosis of tears of the rotator cuff. *J Bone Joint Surg* 1994;76(A):335—340.
9. Mink JH, Harris E, Rappaport M. Rotator cuff tears: evaluation using double-contrast shoulder arthrography. *Radiology* 1985;157:621—623.
10. Reinus WR, Shady KL, Mirowitz SA, et al. MR diagnosis of rotator cuff tears of the shoulder: value of using T2-weighted fat-saturated images. *AJR* 1995;164:1451—1455.
11. Balich SM, Sheley RC, Brown TR, et al. MR imaging of the rotator cuff tendon: interobserver agreement and analysis of interpretive errors. *Radiology* 1997;204:191—194.
12. Quinn SF, Sheley RC, Demlow TA, et al. Rotator cuff tendon tears: evaluation with fat-suppressed MR imaging with ar-

throscopic correlation in 100 patients. *Radiology* 1995;195:497—501.

13. Iannotti JP, Zlatkin MB, Esterhai JL, et al. Magnetic resonance imaging of the shoulder. *J Bone Joint Surg* 1991;73(A):17—29.

14. Hodler J, Kursunoglu-Brahme S, Snyder SJ, et al. Rotator cuff disease: assessment with MR arthrography versus standard MR imaging in 36 patients with arthroscopic confirmation. *Radiology* 1992;182:431—436.

15. Farley TE, Neumann CH, Steinbach LS, et al. Full-thickness tears of the rotator cuff of the shoulder: diagnosis with MR imaging. *AJR* 1992;158:347—351.

16. Middleton WD, Edelstein G, Reinus WR, et al. Ultrasonography of the rotator cuff: technique and normal anatomy. *J Ultrasound Med* 1984;3:549—551.

17. Middleton WD. Ultrasonography of the shoulder. *Radiol Clin North Am* 1992;30:927—940.

18. Middleton WD. Status of rotator cuff sonography. *Radiology* 1989;173:307—309.

19. Middleton WD. Sonographic detection and quantification of rotator cuff tears. *AJR* 1993;160:109—110.

20. Wohlwend JR, van Holsbeeck M, Craig J, et al. The association between irregular greater tuberosities and rotator cuff tears: a sonographic study. *AJR* 1998;171:229—233.

21. van Holsbeeck MT, Kolowich PA, Eyler WR, et al. US depiction of partial-thickness tear of the rotator cuff. *Radiology* 1995;197:443—446.

22. Wiener SN, Seitz WH, Jr. Sonography of the shoulder in patients with tears of the rotator cuff: accuracy and value for selecting surgical options. *AJR* 1993;160:103—107.

23. Ptasznik R, Hennessy O. Abnormalities of the biceps tendon of the shoulder: sonographic findings. *AJR* 1995;164:409—414.

24. Middleton WD, Reinus WR, Totty WG, et al. Ultrasonography of the biceps tendon apparatus. *Radiology* 1985;157:211—215.

25. Farin PU, Jaroma H, Harju A, et al. Medial displacement of the biceps brachii tendon: evaluation with dynamic sonography during maximal external shoulder rotation. *Radiology* 1995;195:845—848.

26. Patten RM, Mack LA, Wang KY, et al. Nondisplaced fractures of the greater tuberosity of the humerus: sonographic detection. *Radiology* 1992;182:201—204.

27. Blanchard TK, Bearcroft PW, Dixon AK, et al. Magnetic resonance imaging or arthrography of the shoulder: which do patients prefer? *Br J Radiol* 1997;70:786—790.

28. Middleton WD, Reinus WR, Totty WG, et al. Ultrasonographic evaluation of the rotator cuff and biceps tendon. *J Bone Joint Surg* 1986;68(A):440—450.

29. Mack LA, Matsen FA, Kilcoyne JF, et al. US evaluation of the rotator cuff. *Radiology* 1985;157:205—209.

30. Crass JR, Craig EV, Thompson RC, et al. Ultrasonography of the rotator cuff: surgical correlation. *J Clin Ultrasound* 1984;12:487—492.

31. Hodler J, Fretz CJ, Terrier F, et al. Rotator cuff tears: correlation of sonographic and surgical findings. *Radiology* 1988;169:791—794.

32. Soble MG, Kaye AD, Guay RC. Rotator cuff tear: clinical experience with sonographic detection. *Radiology* 1989;173:319—321.

33. Brandt TD, Cardone BW, Grant TH, et al. Rotator cuff sonography: a reassessment. *Radiology* 1989;173:323—327.

34. Miller CL, Karasick D, Kurtz AB, et al. Limited sensitivity of ultrasound for detection of rotator cuff tears. *Skel Radiol* 1989;18:179—183.

35. Vick CW, Bell SA. Rotator cuff tears: diagnosis with sonography. *AJR* 1990;154:121—123.

36. American College of Radiology Task Force on Appropriateness Criteria. Shoulder pain: suspect rotator cuff tear. In American College of Radiology Appropriateness Criteria for Imaging and Treatment Decisions, 1996, American College of Radiology, Reston VA.

49 Ultrasound Evaluation of Wrist Diseases

Doohi Lee

Introduction

The wrist is one of the most complex anatomic sites in the body. It comprises the distal radius, ulna, carpal bones, and the base of the metacarpals, held together by numerous ligaments and other supporting soft tissues structures. The multiarticulated joint derives its flexibility and strength from the arrangement of the bony structures and the interosseous ligaments. The numerous tendons that traverse the wrist also give it support and strength while transferring the force and coordinating motions from the arm and the forearm. The wrist is truly a universal joint, able to articulate in many directions while supporting the hand, to give it strength and ability for fine coordination.

The location and the function of the wrist, however, subject it to a welter of diseases and injuries. Injury to the wrist accounts for the majority of its illnesses, with the vast majority of them from falling on outstretched hand. Fracture of the distal radius occurs most commonly in the upper extremity.[1] Falls and other trauma to the wrist also result in compressive fractures of the carpal bones, dislocations, tears, and disruption of ligaments and other supporting structures. Aside from trauma, arthritis (both inflammatory and degenerative), tumors, neuropathies, and vascular diseases also involve the wrist.

The susceptibility of the wrist to a great number of diseases and the critical nature of its function make accurate diagnosis essential. It anatomy is complex, however, and we are frequently challenged in the evaluation of its internal structures and derangement. Imaging techniques including the plain X-ray, arthrography, fluoroscopy, scintigraphy, computed tomography (CT), and magnetic resonance imaging (MRI) all contribute important information in diagnosis. But each modality has its own strengths and limitations, and, frequently, a combination of techniques is necessary to adequately assess a particular condition. And recently, ultrasound is proving to be a valuable additional diagnostic modality in the evaluation and diagnosis of wrist disease.[2,3]

The wrist presents an ideal anatomic region for evaluation by high frequency ultrasound. It is readily available and inexpensive. Highly detailed anatomy can be demonstrated while patients remain comfortable without being subjected to radiation and/or prolonged immobilization. Its greatest strength as an imaging modality, however, lies in its dynamic capability in elucidating both the normal and pathological anatomy. This feature is especially applicable to the evaluation of a mobile structure such as the wrist.

Indications for Wrist Ultrasound

The clinical indications for ultrasound of the wrist are indicated in **Table 49–1**. Of these, we will discuss the common injuries to tendons, bones and joints, nerves, and masses around the wrist.

Table 49-1 Indications for wrist ultrasound

Tendons	Tears and ruptures
	Tendinitis
	Tenosynovitis
	Calcific tendinitis
Nerves	Median neuropathy
	Ulnar neuropathy
	Perineural edema
Masses	Ganglion
	Giant cell tumor
	Amyloid deposits
	Hematoma
	Accessory muscle enchroachment
	Lumbrical muscle
	Metastases
	Synovioma
Vascular	Aneurism
	Hemangioma
Bone	Fractures
	Subluxations
	Osteochondral defects
Muscles	Tears/ruptures
	Contusion
	Myositis
Other	Foreign bodies
	Loose bodies

Technique

Ultrasound examination of the wrist is technically simple. The patient is positioned either sitting facing the examiner or lying down with the affected wrist toward the examiner. A small roll of towel under the dorsal surface of the wrist places the wrist in neutral position and allows greater manipulation during the examination.

A high frequency linear array transducer is used to obtain images in transverse and longitudinal orientations. Frequency range of 7.5—13 MHz allows good penetration through the shallow wrist anatomy while providing excellent resolution. The four compartments of the wrist (volar, dorsal, radial, and ulnar) are examined beginning with the specific area of the greatest interest. For example, in a patient with carpal tunnel syndrome, the volar aspect of the wrist is examined first, concentrating on the contents of the carpal tunnel, followed by the other areas that may secondarily contribute to the disease. In a patient with suspected extensor tenosynovitis, the approach would be reversed and the examination would begin with the extensor tendons. While manipulating the transducer to accommodate the changing surface angles, images are obtained in transverse and longitudinal orientations according to the fundamentals of orthogonal imaging.

Wrist Diseases

Wrist

Acute Wrist Trauma

Typical patients with acute wrist trauma present with a history of falling on outstretched hand. Other mechanisms of acute injury include a direct blow to the wrist as well as extension from injury to either the hand or forearm. Acute trauma results in sudden local anatomic derangement, inflammation, and edema. There also are associated physical findings of swelling, pain, and diminished range of motion. These features greatly aid the ultrasound evaluation and diagnosis. Ultrasound findings vary depending on the predominant area of injury, be it bone, joint, or tendons. Edema and inflammation almost always accompany acute trauma, usually depicted as areas of heterogeneous low echogenicity of fluid, inflamed connective tissues, and debris. In most trauma cases, X-rays of the wrist are obtained and they provide important correlating information.

The types of acute injury to the wrist that can be easily evaluated with ultrasound include tendon rupture, tendinitis, tenosynovitis, and sequelae of fracture such as hematoma, ligament tears, and disruption of the triangular fibrocartilage complex (TFCC).

Chronic Trauma

Evaluation of the wrist for chronic trauma can be difficult. Formation of scars and other repair processes often hide signs of trauma such as edema, synovitis, and focal anatomic derangement. One must rely on history and physical examination more than with acute injury. The examination is generally focused to the area of ab-

normality or pain, and the examiner must be aware of often subtle accompanying pathologies of chronic disease.

Chronic diseases of the wrist that can be diagnosed with ultrasound include carpal tunnel syndrome (median nerve neuropathy), Guyon canal syndrome (ulnar nerve neuropathy), chronic tendinitis, and tenosynovitis. Sequelae of chronic arthritis and degeneration of the bony surfaces with occasional loose bodies can also be readily evaluated with ultrasound.

Tendon Diseases

There are numerous extensor and flexor tendons traversing the wrist to provide function and force transfer from the forearm to the hand. The extensor tendons are distributed in six compartments over the dorsum of the wrist while the flexor tendons cross the wrist in a tight bundle through the carpal tunnel. As they play an integral role in the function of the hand, they are vulnerable to many types of injuries including tears, tendinitis, and tenosynovitis, occurring alone or in conjunction with other injuries.

Tenosynovitis and Tendinitis

Tenosynovitis is nonspecific inflammation of the sheath covering the tendon and can occur alone or with involvement of the tendon. Tenosynovitis can result from inflammation, infection, or trauma. The hallmark of tenosynovitis is swelling of the tendon sheath, which becomes filled with fluid and debris with or without synovial proliferation.[4] On ultrasound, the tendon sheath becomes enlarged and ill defined. If the tendon is also inflamed, the normal fibrillary pattern of the tendon becomes less apparent in the longitudinal view as fluid and inflammatory materials fill the spaces between the tendon fibers. (**Fig. 49–1 A**)   In the transverse orientation, fluid and edematous tendon sheath surround the enlarged tendon. (**Fig. 49–1 B**) Anechoic fluid generally indicates inflammatory tenosynovitis, while infectious and traumatic tenosynovitis often results in heterogeneous fluid because of exudative material and debris. (**Fig. 49–1 C**)

Infectious tenosynovitis is associated with diabetes mellitus, puncture wounds, and animal bites. It is a surgical emergency, requiring immediate incision and drainage. Inflammatory tenosynovitis is associated with chronic disease, such as inflammatory arthritis [rheumatoid, gout, calcium pyrophosphate deposition disease (CPPD)], amyloidosis, and chronic hemodialysis.[5] Persistent inflammatory tenosynovitis can progress into frank infectious tenosynovitis. Other complications in the wrist include carpal tunnel syndrome, abscess formation, muscle necrosis, infectious angiopathies, and osteomyelitis.

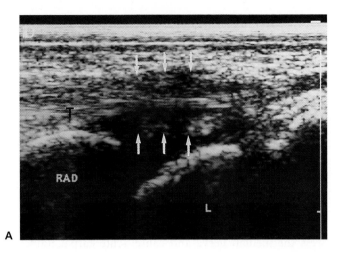

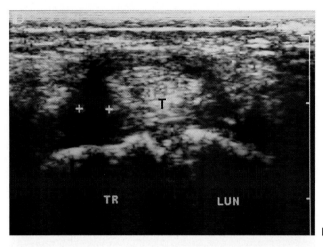

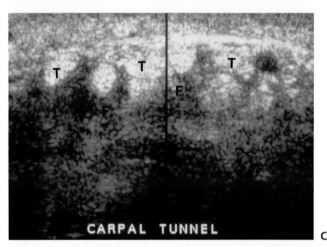

Figure 49–1 A: Extensor tendinitis and tenosynovitis. Focal tenosynovitis and tendinitis of the extensor digitorum tendons. There is focal distension and fluid collection of the tendon sheath (**arrows**). The tendons (T) are edematous and hypoechoic, indicating inflammation. (RAD, radius; L, lunate). **B:** Extensor tenosynovitis. Transverse view of the extensor tendon illustrates swelling of the tendon sheath (++) without inflammation of the tendon (T), which demonstrates normal hyperechoic architecture (TR, triquetrum; LUN, lunate). **C:** Traumatic tenosynovitis. Transverse view of the carpal tunnel demonstrates heterogenous fluid (F) filling the space between flexor tendons (T) after acute fracture of the wrist.

In traumatic tenosynovitis, the clinical and ultrasound manifestations are the result of the underlying trauma, such as a fracture of the distal radius.[6] Fracture fragments, debris, joint effusion, and other soft tissue abnormalities often accompany tenosynovitis.

Acute tenosynovitis is often associated with trauma and bacterial infection (e.g., diabetes mellitus). Fall on the wrist with fractures or tendon tears can result in accompanying tenosynovitis. Chronic tenosynovitis is associated with chronic inflammatory disease such as rheumatoid arthritis, De Quervain's syndrome, and gout. Longstanding, slow infections such as tuberculosis can also result in chronic tenosynovitis. Complex fluid and synovial proliferation is more commonly seen with chronic tenosynovitis than with acute tenosynovitis.

Tendon Tears

Tendon tears can occur either as result of acute trauma or chronic degeneration. Tears can manifest in many ways, from small, subtle partial tears to full-thickness tears with retraction of the tendon within the tendon sheath and hemorrhage.

In the evaluation of tendon injury, physical examination yields a great deal of information by correlating the mechanism of injury with the physical findings. Functional testing of flexion and extension can yield valuable information regarding the integrity of the tendons after trauma. With full-thickness tears and retraction, the tendon may form a palpable lump on examination. There will a loss of function specific to the injured tendon.

On ultrasound, tendon tears appear as either a partial or complete defect in the tendon substance, often with accompanying fluid and inflammation in the tendon sheath. (**Fig. 49–2**) The size of the tear and the extent of the tears can be readily delineated by ultrasound. In full-thickness tears with retraction, the path of the tendon can be traced by ultrasound, and the position of the torn edge can be identified. This feature is useful in planning for surgical repair. In difficult cases, flexion and extension of the digits and the wrist can aid in the diagnosis by functional evaluation of the tendon in real-time. Associated injuries to the muscles of the forearm and the myotendinous junction can also be evaluated.

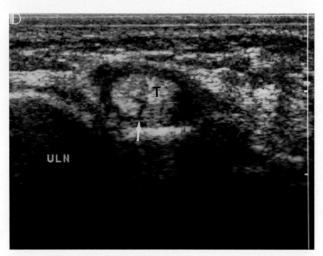

Figure 49–2 Tendon tear. Transverse view of an extensor tendon demonstrates an irregular cleft (**arrow**) at the undersurface of the tendon. The tendon sheath is distended by anechoic fluid. (ULN, ulna).

Nerve Diseases

Nerves can be affected by a variety of diseases, including tumors (primary and secondary), infection, inflammation, and trauma (acute and chronic). Within the wrist, tumors involving the nerves (median, ulnar and radial) are relatively rare. The most common disease affecting the nerves of the wrist involves the median and the ulnar nerve in the carpal tunnel syndrome and the Guyon syndrome, respectively. These are compression neuropathies, usually resulting from chronic inflammation of the median or the ulnar nerve, either from direct compression or from surrounding inflammation. Repetitive stress or overuse injuries of these nerves occur from activities and occupations that require high wrist load such as fencing, racquet sports, gymnastics, weight lifting, sewing, typing, and instrument playing.

Median Nerve

Carpal tunnel syndrome (CTS) is neuropathy of the median nerve, occurring in either acute or chronic setting. It is the fastest growing occupational disease in the United States and the world.[7] Each year, over one million workers will not be able to perform his or her duties due to this debilitating disorder. The loss of ability to perform routine daily activities and productivity in businesses is staggering. CTS most commonly affects garment workers, auto workers, seamstresses, typists, writers, and musicians. It is also associated with patients on chronic hemodialysis, and with rheumatoid arthritis and wrist trauma.

Carpal tunnel syndrome is a part of the repetitive stress syndromes that affect the wrist. It is theorized that chronic, repetitive microtrauma to the wrist starts an in-

flammatory process[8] within the carpal tunnel. This, in turn, brings about inflammatory changes of the median nerve, and carpal tunnel syndrome ensues. The changes of median nerve neuropathy are manifest by various degrees of enlargement of the median nerve, ill-definition of its margins and irregularities of the nerve contour, with and without inflammation of the surrounding tendons (**Fig. 49–3 A,B**). As the inflamed nerve enlarges in the narrow carpal tunnel, the segment that passes through the tunnel becomes compressed[9, 10] (**Fig. 49–4**) and neuropathy ensues. Carpal tunnel syndrome is usually a chronic disease, but acute form can occur in association with trauma to the bone and joints of the wrist. Edema of the injured tissues and/or hematoma can compress the median nerve and cause acute carpal tunnel syndrome.

For the purpose of diagnosing carpal tunnel syndrome, electromyography of the median nerve has been the mainstay and the "gold-standard" for the diagnosis of median nerve neuropathy. MRI has also been used to image the morphological changes of the median nerve associated with CTS.[10, 11] Aside from MRI of the wrist, radiological imaging of the median nerve has been limited.

Recent studies, however, have illustrated the efficacy of ultrasound in evaluating the median nerve in patients with CTS.[12–14] These studies demonstrated the ability of ultrasound to depict subtle changes in the median nerve and the surrounding structures in the carpal tunnel. Furthermore, high correlation between the changes in the cross-sectional area of the median nerve with CTS and abnormalities in nerve conduction studies was also reported.[14] These studies are indicating ultrasound to be the ideal modality to diagnose the changes in the median nerve associated with CTS. Considering the pain and difficulties associated with electromyography, continued development of the ultrasound technique should be a welcome relief for those suffering from this disease.

Ultrasound is capable of depicting not only the enlargement of the median nerve with CTS, but also postsurgical changes after carpal tunnel release (**Fig. 49–5**). The median nerve enlarges with return of symptoms after surgery,[14] and ultrasound provides a painless and convenient method of following the progress of disease in these patients. Additional advantages of ultrasound over electromyogram (EMG) include lower costs and faster examination time (average 12 versus 40 min).

Ulnar Nerve

Compressive neuropathy can also involve the ulnar nerve. The ulnar nerve traverses the wrist through a narrow channel called the *Guyon canal*. It is bounded posteriorly by the flexor retinaculum, medially by the ulnar head, and laterally by the pisiform. The ulnar nerve normally measures approximately 2 mm in diameter through the Guyon canal. It is hypoechoic in character in

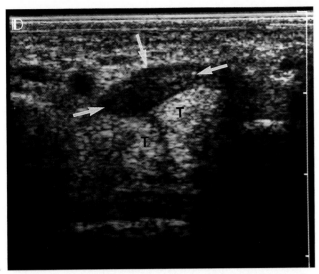

A

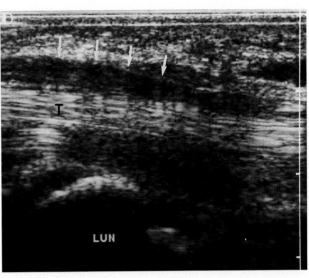

B

Figure 49–3 A: Carpal tunnel syndrome. Transverse view of a massively enlarged median nerve (**arrows**). It is markedly hypoechoic with effacement of nerve fascicles and outer margins. It presses upon the flexor tendons (T). **B:** Longitudinal view of the me-

dian nerve (**arrows**) demonstrates enlarged, hypoechoic nerve traversing over the flexor tendons (T). The nerve contour is irregular and the definition of the nerve sheath is lost due to edema. (LUN, lunate).

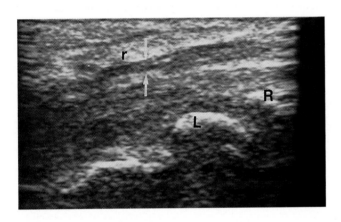

Figure 49–4 Carpal tunnel syndrome. Enlarged and inflamed median nerve is compressed by the flexor retinaculum (r) as it enters the carpal tunnel (**arrows**). (L, lunate; R, radius).

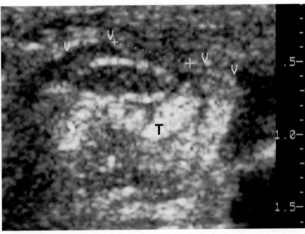

Figure 49–5 Carpal tunnel release. Transverse view of the volar wrist after carpal tunnel release demonstrates the cleft (++) in the flexor retinaculum (V). Enlarged median nerve lies over the flexor tendons (T).

relation to the surrounding fascia and other connective tissues. The ulnar artery travels lateral to the nerve and provides a useful, pulsatile landmark for identifying the ulnar nerve. Neuropathy of the ulnar nerve through this region of the wrist is also commonly referred to as the *Guyon syndrome.*

Neuropathy of the ulnar nerve can occur from a variety of causes, in many ways similar to those related to the median nerve. Compressive neuropathy most commonly results from ganglion and sequelae of

trauma, especially fractures involving the distal radioulnar joint. Repetitive stress to the wrist from various occupations and activities that require continual flexion and ulnar deviation of the wrist can also result in ulnar neuropathy. The ulnar nerve responds by focal enlargement in inflammatory conditions and focal narrowing in compressive disease (**Fig. 49–6**). Due to its small size, subtle alterations in the ulnar nerve can be technically difficult to demonstrate. Electromyogram studies of the nerve usually correlate positive ultrasound findings.

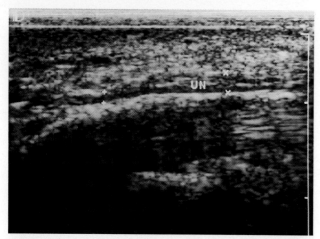

Figure 49–6 Ulnar neuropathy (Guyon canal syndrome): Longitudinal view of the ulnar nerve at the level of the wrist in a patient with ulnar neuropathy (EMG confirmed) demonstrates focal narrowing of the ulnar nerve (UN) as it passes through the Guyon canal (xx vs. ++).

Disease of the Bone and Cartilage

Triangular Fibrocartilage Complex

Damage to the triangular fibrocartilage complex (TFCC) is a common occurrence in the spectrum of wrist diseases.[15] The TFCC is a complex anatomic unit comprising triangular fibrocartilage, a meniscus homologue, an articular disc, the ulnar collateral ligament, the dorsal and volar radioulnar ligaments, and the sheath of the extensor carpi ulnaris tendon. It separates the carpal bones from the radius and ulna, serves as a major stabilizer of the radioulnar joint, and functions as a cushion for ulnar axial loads.

Injury to the TFCC is associated with collision or contact sports such as gymnastics, skiing, and mountain climbing in which rotation and dorsiflexion forces are applied to the wrist. Physical examination may reveal ulnar head instability manifested by dorsal subluxation of the ulna. Volar compression between the ulnar head and triquetrum may cause pain or crepitus. A painful clunk in the ulnar region may occur with passive supination or pronation of the wrist.

Standard imaging methods for TFCC consist of CT or MRI of the wrist.[15] Arthrography provides high specificity for tear when communication of contrast material between the radiocarpal joint and the radioulnar joint, but it can be difficult to perform and interpret. MRI has become the imaging modality of choice in the evaluation of TFCC defects. Using T2-weighted and gradient-echo sequences in the coronal plane, small tears can be detected with a high degree of accuracy.

Ultrasound application for this aspect of wrist diseases is being developed. Examination of this part of the wrist can be technically challenging. On ultrasound, the TFCC is best visualized in the coronal plane, distal to the ulnar styloid, and deep to the extensor carpi ulnaris tendon. The TFCC disc appears as a triangular structure of medium to high echogenicity between the distal ulna and the triquetrum (**Fig. 49–7 A**). In severe, chronic degeneration of TFCC, there may be complete absence of the articular disc. In other instances, tears in TFCC are demonstrated as irregular, linear hypoechoic clefts within the disc substance. (**Fig. 49–7 B**) Acute trauma and tears of the TFCC are associated with synovitis and edema.

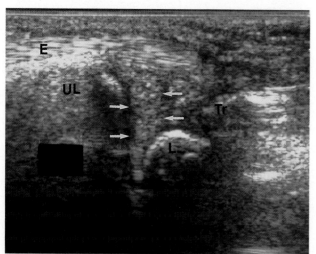

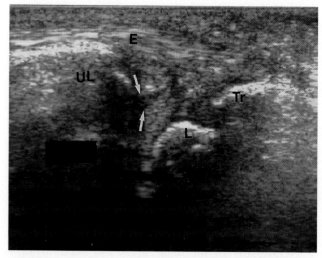

Figure 49–7 A: Triangular fibrocartilage complex (TFCC), Normal articular disc (**arrows**) of the TFCC is triangular in shape and echogenic. It is bounded by the extensor carpi ulnaris tendon (E), distal ulnar (UL), and the triquetrum (Tr). (L, lunate). **B:** TFCC tear. Focal tear of the articular disc appears as a focal hypoechoic cleft (**arrows**) in the substance of the disc. This represents chronic disease, as no edema or inflammation is present with the defect. (E, ext. carpi ulnaris; UL, ulna; L, lunate; Tr, triquetrum).

Masses in the Wrist

Ganglion

Ganglia or synovial cysts are common soft tissue tumors of the wrist.[16] They are nonsynovial cystic masses of a myxoid matrix attached to tendon sheaths, muscles, and semilunar cartilage, occasionally communicating with synovium or joint spaces. Ganglia may press on bone, producing resorption or periosteal changes. Patients present with focal wrist pain associated with a palpable firm and rubbery mass that gets larger and smaller periodically. A history of minor trauma is often given. Ganglion is often a secondary or incidental finding in the wrist examination by MRI.[17] It generally displays signal characteristics of fluid, bright on T2-weighted images and dark on T1-weighted images.

On ultrasound, ganglia appear as uniform, fluid-filled structures with posterior acoustic enhancement (**Fig. 49–8 A**). They generally lie close to or adhering to tendon sheaths or synovial lining, and may be compressible during real-time sonography. Occasionally, they demonstrate internal echoes, mimicking a solid tumor. Careful examination may reveal a tract connecting the ganglion to a nearby joint space (**Fig. 49–8 B**). Although they can occur anywhere within the wrist, the most common location is in the dorsal compartment, between the carpal bones and the extensor tendons.

Bone and Joint Diseases

Wrist disease commonly includes abnormalities of the bone and joint spaces. In acute injury, such as fracture or dislocation, there is edema, debris, and disruption of joint capsule and ligaments. Associated tendon pathologies such as tendon tears and tenosynovitis were demonstrated earlier. In the chronic setting, much of edema may subside, leaving changes of scarring, joint malalignment, or subluxations, debris, and loose bodies. Chronic capsular disruption may persist, with synovitis of the joint spaces.

Ligament Tears

Numerous interosseous ligaments stabilize the wrist. Ligament injury is common after a fall. The scapholunate ligament is one of the most common ligaments injured.[18] Tear of this ligament is typically seen on the radiograph as an increased gap between the scaphoid and the lunate bones. In subtle tears, additional imaging may be required to detect small abnormalities. As in the diagnosis of TFCC diseases, MRI has been the mainstay in imaging the carpal bones and ligament pathologies, especially in the detection of scapho-lunate ligament tears.[17]

Recently, however, ultrasound is rapidly gaining acceptance as a modality that can readily evaluate and diagnose even small ligament disruptions of the wrist, especially involving the scapho-lunate ligament, the radio-lunate ligament, and the luno-traquetral ligament. The diagnosis of these abnormalities is also aided by the dynamic capability of ultrasound. The wrist can be manipulated during scanning to elicit stresses to the joint spaces to elucidate often subtle pathology. On ultrasound, the cortical margins of the scaphoid and the lunate, for example, appear as hyperechoic arcs. The joint space between them is hypoechoic. With scapholunate ligament disruption, the thin fibers of the ligament are no longer apparent, and the joint gap becomes wide (**Fig. 49–9**).

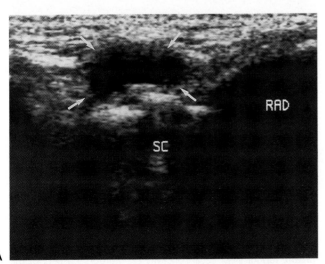

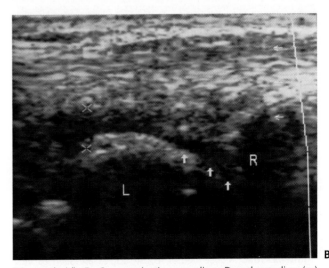

A

B

Figure 49–8 A: Ganglion. Focal cystic mass (**arrows**) with acoustic enhancement at the radio-scaphoid recess demonstrates typical appearance of a ganglion — anechoic and without a definitive wall. These can become complex and mimic a solid mass (RAD, radius; SC, scaphoid). **B:** Communicating ganglion. Dorsal ganglion (xx) demonstrates a thin tail that extends into and communicates with the radio-lunate joint (**arrows**). R, radius; L, lunate).

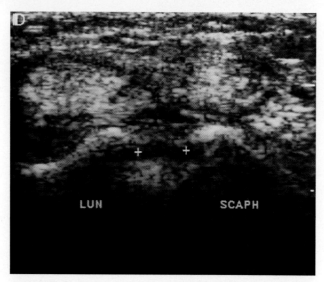

Figure 49–9 Torn scapho-lunate ligament. Wide hypoechoic gap is present between the scaphoid and the lunate (++). No residual ligament fibers are present. (LUN, lunate; SCAPH, scaphoid).

Loose Bodies

Loose bodies originate from a variety of causes, most often trauma and chronic degenerative diseases. Because of their small size, they often elude the usual diagnostic modalities including X-ray, arthrogram, and cross-sectional imaging and present a diagnostic and therapeutic challenge. Ultrasound, however, is the ideal modality for the diagnosis of loose bodies in the joints and soft tissues: Diagnosis can be made from its appearance of a well-defined, hyperechoic lesion (**Fig. 49–10 A**). They do not usually cause acoustic shadowing, but when present,

they are highly specific signs. Movement of the loose bodies can also be detected in real-time, allowing definitive diagnosis. With high-frequency transducers available today, loose bodies as small as 0.5 mm in size can be detected. Although sonographic beam does not penetrate bone, it can delineate the cortex, enabling detection of subtle cortical defects (**Fig. 49–10 B**). Examination of the bony structures around the loose body may reveal tiny defects of bone and cartilage representing the donor sites. With continuing development of ultrasound technology and interventional techniques, ultrasound-guided removal of loose bodies presents an intriguing possibility.

Conclusion

Ultrasound is a reliable and highly accurate method of evaluating common and uncommon wrist diseases. Diseases affecting the joint space, ligaments, cartilage, and bony defects, nerves and tumors can be evaluated quickly and efficiently. Due to its high-resolution capability and inherent advantage of real-time imaging, ultrasound represents the ideal modality to diagnose loose bodies within the wrist. The same features are important in the diagnosis of tendon diseases affecting the wrist.

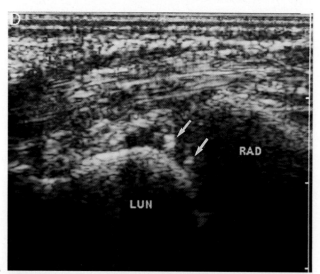

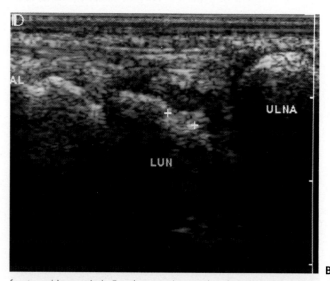

Figure 49–10 A: Loose bodies. Loose bodies are seen as very small, well-defined, hyperechoic foci (**arrows**) within the joint space. Their mobility can be demonstrated by manipulating the joint while scanning. Generally, no posterior acoustic shadow is cast due to their small size. (LUN, lunate; RAD, radius). **B:** Osteochondral fracture (donor site). Focal concavity on the dorsal aspect of the lunate represents a small osteochondral fracture and the donor site (++) for the intraarticular loose bodies detected in the volar aspect of the joint (LUN, lunate).

References

1. Palmer AK. Fractures of the distal radius. In: Green DP, ed. *Operative Hand Surgery*, 2nd ed. New York: Churchill Livingstone, 1988, p. 991—1026.
2. Flaviis LD, Musso MG. Hand and wrist. In Fornage BD, ed. *Musculoskeletal Ultrasound.* New York: Churchill Livingstone, 1995.
3. Fornage BD, Rifkin MD. Ultrasound examination of the hand and foot. *Radiol Clin North Am* 1988;26:109—129.
4. Reicher MA, Kellerhouse LE. *MRI of the Wrist and Hand.* New York: Raven Press, 1990.
5. Savage RC, Mustafa ED. Giant cell tumor of tendon sheath (localized nodular tenosynovitis). *Plastic Surg* 1947;13:205—930.
6. Linscheid RL, Dobyns JH, Beabout JW, et al. Traumatic instability of the wrist: diagnosis, classification, and pathomechanics. *J Bone Surg* 1972;54 A:1612.
7. Cummings K, Maizlisch N, Rudolph L, Dervin K, Ervin A. Occupational disease surveillance: carpal tunnel syndrome. *JAMA* 1989;262(7):886—887.
8. Makamichi K, Tachibana S. The use of ultrasonography in detection of synovitis in carpal tunnel syndrome. *J Hand Surg* 1993;18 B:176—179.
9. Lee D, van Holsbeeck M. Ultrasound of the median nerve in carpal tunnel syndrome (abstract). *RSNA* 1992.
10. Skie M, Zeiss J, Ebraheim NA, Jackson WT. Carpal tunnel changes and median nerve compression during wrist flexion and extension seen by magnetic resonance imaging. *J Hand Surg* 1990;15 A:934—939.
11. Middleton WD, Kneeland JB, Kellman GM, et al. MR imaging of the carpal tunnel: normal anatomy and preliminary findings in the carpal tunnel syndrome. *AJR* 1987;148:307—316.
12. Buchberger W, Judmaier W, Birbamer G, Lener M, Schmidauer C. Carpal tunnel syndrome: diagnosis with high-resolution sonography. *AJR* 1992;159:793—798.
13. Buchberger W, Schon G, Strasser K, Jungwirth W. High-resolution ultrasonography of the carpal tunnel. *J Ultrasound Med* 1991;10:531—537.
14. Lee D, van Holsbeeck M, Janevski Pi, Ditmars D, Darian V. Correlation of electromyogram and ultrasound of the median nerve in carpal tunnel syndrome (abstract). *RSNA* 1993.
15. Totterman SM, Miller RJ. MR imaging of the triangular fibrocartilage complex. *MRI Clin North Am* 1995;3(2):213—228.
16. Kransdorf MJ, Murphey MD. MR imaging of musculoskeletal tumors of the hand and wrist. *MRI Clin North Am* 1995;3(2):327.
17. Rettig ME, Raskin KB, Melone CP. Clinical applications of MR imaging in hand and wrist surgery. MRI Clin North Am 1995;38(2):361—368.
18. Berger RA, Blair WF, Crowinschield RD, Flatt AE. The scapholunate ligament. *J Hand Surg* 1982;1A:87–91.

50 Ultrasound of the Knee, Ankle and Foot

Ronald S. Adler

Introduction

Ultrasonography is particularly useful to evaluate soft tissue structures, especially those that contain fluid. Lesions, which are superficial in relation to the body surface, are more easily evaluated than deep-seated lesions. It is more operator dependent than the other imaging modalities and in experienced hands, can be quite effective in identifying and characterizing joint effusions and lesions of tendons, ligaments, and skeletal muscle. Imaging in "real-time" allows performance of provocative maneuvers (e.g., flexion-extension) which may enhance the appearance of a pathologic process. Simple fluid appears homogeneously dark (anechoic), while structures such as tendons appear bright (echogenic) and linearly oriented (anisotropic). Because of its noninvasive nature, availability, cost-effectiveness, and exquisite ability to image the soft tissues, ultrasound has much to offer in imaging of the musculoskeletal system.

Differential Considerations and Imaging Workup

Any clinical problem in which imaging is being considered should begin with plain radiographs. In many instances, these may obviate the need for further imaging or may better direct it. Abnormalities of bone or the articular surfaces (i.e., cartilage, interosseus ligaments, etc.) are best evaluated with magnetic resonance imaging or computed tomography. Ultrasound is best suited for a targeted exam, such as a palpable mass or suspected tendon rupture. In some instances, it may provide a useful screening to exclude several of the more common etiologies for a specific condition. An example would be evaluation of the posterior tibial tendon as a possible cause for painful flat foot.

In the knee, ultrasound is best suited to evaluate localized masses or pain, in order to determine if they correspond to a bursitis, ganglion, meniscal cyst, solid mass, or tendinitis. Trauma involving the extensor mechanism, in which injury to the quadriceps or patella tendons is clinically suspect without more extensive joint pathology, is well suited to sonographic evaluation. Finally, acute pain and swelling in the posterior aspect of the knee and leg may result from ruptured Baker's cyst, localized muscle rupture, or deep venous thrombosis, all of which are well evaluated on ultrasound.

In the ankle, inversion injuries with negative radiographs are common. Differentiating peroneal tendon injury and anterior talofibular injury may be difficult clinically; both are well evaluated with ultrasound or magnetic resonance imaging (MRI).

Evaluation of heel pain may reflect a localized bursitis, Achilles tendonitis/tear, plantar fasciitis or calcaneal stress fracture. The soft tissue processes are well evaluated both on ultrasound and MRI. The presence of an occult fracture can be readily assessed by scintigraphy or MRI.

Palpable masses about the ankle and foot most often relate to localized ganglia, synovial cysts/bursa, neuromas, and lipomas. Ultrasound can easily distinguish these and provide guidance for therapy. Magnetic resonance imaging in these cases is best reserved for surgical planning or when a more complex mass is suspected, such as a synovial sarcoma, vascular malfunction, etc. Finally, the presence of suspected foreign bodies in the setting of a negative radiographic examination is best evaluated by ultrasound. Foreign bodies such as glass or wood are easily detected and localized in three dimensions for surgical extraction.

General Principles of Musculoskeletal Ultrasound

Normal Sonographic Appearances

Tendons may have a synovial sheath surrounding them or have a relatively dense connective tissue layer adherent to them, the paratenon. This is brightly echogenic and sharply demarcates the tendon (**Fig. 50–1**). The tendon itself consists of dense connective tissue in which collagen fibrils are arranged in bundles surrounded by loose connective tissue. These bundles are further arranged in a parallel linear fashion. The resultant gray scale ultrasound image reflects this anatomic configuration by displaying marked anisotropy; the tendon is echogenic (bright) when scanned perpendicular to its long axis with a linear array transducer. Reduction of the angle by as little as between two and seven degrees produces isoechogenicity relative to muscle, and further reduction produces hypoechogenicity (dark). Due to its fibrillar nature, the tendon is not diffusely echogenic but appears as a series of echogenic parallel linear bands. These features make tendons easy to recognize ultrasonographically.[1,2]

Power Doppler — Applications to Musculoskeletal US

Power Doppler imaging is a technique that displays significantly improved sensitivity relative to conventional color Doppler imaging.[3] The technique appears exquisitely sensitive to soft tissue hyperemia associated with a number of musculoskeletal lesions (**Fig. 50–2**).

More importantly, the resolution of hyperemia appears to parallel clinical improvement even with a continued abnormal gray scale appearance.[4] We believe the detection of hyperemia may provide additional specificity in the diagnosis of inflammatory musculoskeletal lesions, as well as a means of following response to therapy.

Pathological Findings

Tendons

Tendonitis can be diffuse or nodular (**Fig. 50–3**).[1,2,5] A diffuse tendonitis is visualized sonographically as diffuse thickening and hypoechogenicity of the tendon. The appearance of hypoechoic intratendinous clefts may be seen. Measurements of various tendons have been suggested, but it must be remembered that gender, size, and training contribute to tendon thickness and the final arbiter often relies on comparison to the opposite side. The tendon may lose its normal sharp outline displaying indistinct margins. Focal tendonitis will display localized areas of thickening and hypoechogenicity. A chronic tendonitis may slowly calcify. Calcification is easily recognized sonographically when it appears as a discrete echogenic area with posterior acoustic shadowing. Al-

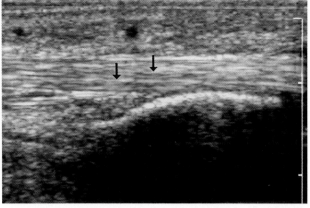

Figure 50–1 Longitudinal sonogram of normal Achilles tendon. The tendon appears bright (echogenic) and demonstrates a characteristic fibrillar pattern (**arrows**). The tendon margins are not easily separable from the paratenon, but the tendon/paratenon complex has a distinct margin with respect to the adjacent fat.

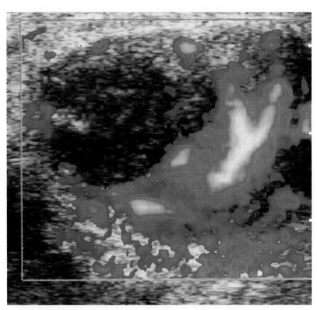

Figure 50–2 Transverse image of a muscle abscess seen as a rounded dark (hypoechoic) area. Increased blood flow (colored region) on power Doppler imaging surrounds the abscess.

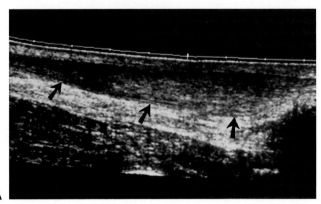

A

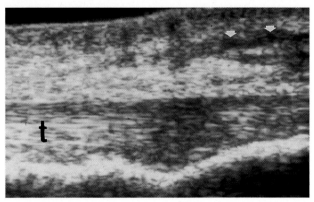

B

Figure 50–3 A: Longitudinal sonogram of the Achilles tendon (**arrows**) demonstrates it to be diffusely enlarged and hypoechoic compatible with diffuse tendinitis. **B:** Longitudinal sonogram of the patellar tendon (t) near its insertion onto the tibia shows a poorly marginated hypoechoic area corresponding to a localized tendinitis. **Short arrows** depict a crescentic hypoechoic collection corresponding to an associated superficial infrapatellar bursitis.

ternatively, posterior shadowing is not always present, and the calcification may appear as an amorphous echogenic mass.

An acute tenosynovitis is seen as a pathological quantity of fluid or thickening of the tendon sheath (**Fig. 50–4**).[6] This may be secondary to inflammation, infection, acute trauma or due to an effusion within an adjacent joint. A chronic tenosynovitis may be associated with diffuse synovial thickening and secondary inflammation of the tendon, which appears thickened and hypoechoic.[7] Increased peritendinous flow is frequently evident on power Doppler imaging, and may be striking relative to the amount of fluid or synovial thickening (**Fig. 50–5**).

Complete rupture is easily recognized in the acute phase both clinically and sonographically. The tendon retracts and the gap between the retracted ends is filled with hematoma (**Fig. 50–6**).[5] The tendon itself may appear diffusely thickened, heterogeneous, and nodular in contour. Partial rupture is similar in that there is a discontinuity in the parallel linear echoes of the tendon, with the gap filled by material of variable, but usually decreased echogenicity (**Fig. 50–7**). Because of the number of intact fibrils, there may only be minimal retraction in a partial tear. This is manifested as a contour deformity or focal thinning. Partial tears may also be manifest as splits paralleling the long axis of a tendon. This is particularly prevalent in the ankle.

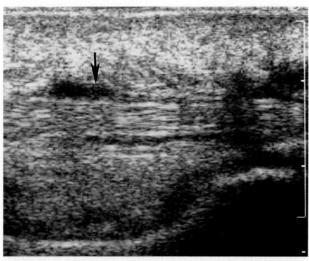

A

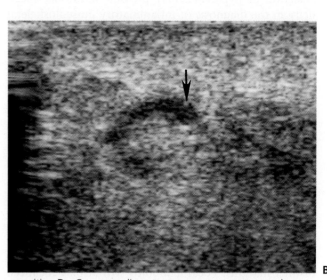

B

Figure 50–4 A: Longitudinal sonogram of the flexor hallucis longus tendon showing hypoechoic thickening (**arrow**) of the synovial sheath. The tendon appears mildly heterogeneous, but for the most part, normal. The appearances are consistent with acute teno-synovitis. **B:** Corresponding transverse sonogram produces a characteristic target appearance of acute tenosynovitis with hypoechoic halo (**arrow**) corresponding to the thickened synovial membrane.

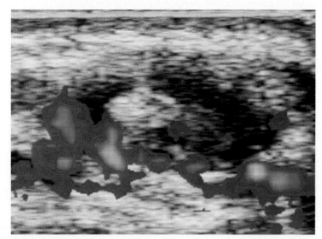

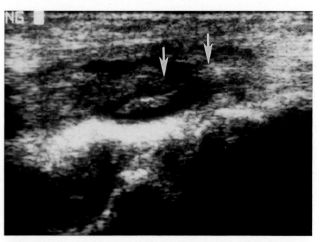

Figure 50–5 Acute tenosynovitis of the extensor hallucis longus tendon in a patient with Rieter's disease. Transverse sonogram depicts typical target appearance with peripherally increased blood flow on power Doppler imaging.

Figure 50–6 Acute rupture of peroneous longus tendon in a runner. Longitudinal sonogram shows retracted ends (**arrows**) surrounded by hypoechoic fluid, which distends the tendon sheath.

Bursitis, Synovial Cysts, Tenson Sheath Effusions

Bursae are synovial-lined structures situated about joint capsules, ligaments, and tendinous insertions that facilitate motion.[1,2] These may be deep or superficial. They may develop secondary to sites of abnormal friction and are then referred to as an *adventitial bursa*.

The synovial-lined sheath surrounding various tendons is another form of specialized bursa. Normal, nondistended bursae may be imperceptible by ultrasound or may be evident as a thin hypoechoic structure, representing a small amount of synovial fluid. The normal bursa should not exceed 2 mm in thickness. Distention of a bursa with fluid is described as bursitis, unless the bursa communicates with the joint. In this way, the distended gastrocnemius/semimembranosus bursa is not thought of as bursitis but is given the title of a Baker's cyst (**Fig. 50–8**). Such distended bursae are perhaps best thought of as synovial cysts, since they can be seen in many other locations and in association with other arthropathies.

In an acute bursitis the fluid can be anechoic or complex. This may be secondary to inflammation, infection, or acute trauma (**Fig. 50–9**). Ultrasound is ideal for evaluation of such a mass, demonstrating its cystic nature and enabling a firm diagnosis. Directed aspiration and/or injection of these under ultrasound guidance may be performed. The presence of hyperemic nodular soft tissue within the collection or in a peribursal distribution, as assessed by color or power Doppler imaging, can more readily denote an inflammatory origin.[3,8]

Joint Effusions

Joint effusions are easily detected sonographically as fluid displacing the joint capsule.[1,2,9] The presence of low-level echoes, septations, or solid material within the joint fluid may suggest infection, hemarthrosis, or other noninfective inflammatory debris, such as fibrin (**Fig. 50–10**). Fine echoes within the fluid can be seen following intraarticular corticosteroid administration. An anechoic effusion does not necessarily imply a simple synovial collection, and although its exact incidence is not well documented, infection cannot be excluded in such a case. Similarly, differentiating the various causes of a complex effusion is not usually possible based on the sonographic appearances alone. The major usefulness of ultrasound in these circumstances is the demonstration of an effusion and to provide localization for aspiration.

With a prosthesis in place, ultrasound may be the only modality to demonstrate the nature and extent of fluid, as both CT and MR are limited by artifact.[10]

Osteochondral bodies are usually suggested by their sharp margins and they will usually display posterior shadowing. Proliferation and edema of the synovium is most prominent in the pannus of rheumatoid

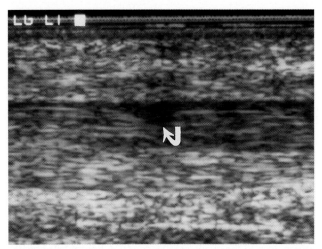

Figure 50–7 Partial tear of the Achilles tendon. Longitudinal sonogram of Achilles tendon with small discrete defect (**arrow**) along superficial margin of tendon. Hypoechoic material fills the defect and distributes along the superficial margin of the tendon. The tendon is inhomogenous in appearance.

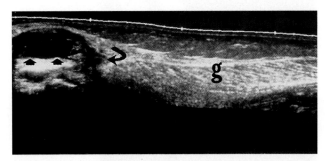

Figure 50–8 Longitudinal sonogram of a complex Baker's cyst appearing as an elliptical hypoechoic mass (**short arrow**). An ill-defined hypoechoic area at the caudal aspect of the cyst (**curved arrow**) depicts a partial rupture. The letter "g" denotes the medial head of the gastrocnemius muscle.

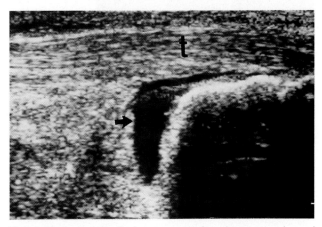

Figure 50–9 Longitudinal sonogram of a deep retrocalcaneal bursitis. Crescentic hypoechoic fluid (**arrow**) is present deep to the Achilles tendon (t) along the margin of the calcaneus.

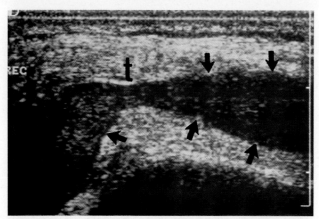

Figure 50–10 Patient with a knee hemarthrosis. Transverse sonogram over the suprapatellar pouch depicts complex hypoechoic collection deep to the quadraceps tendon (t). A horizontally oriented line denotes a plasma-hematocrit level within the fluid (**arrows**).

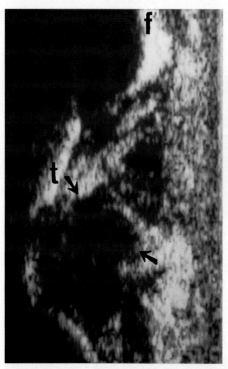

Figure 50–11 Coronal image over the lateral subtalar joint in a patient with pigmented vilonodular synovitis. The fibular (f), talus (t), and calcaneus are depicted with a nodular hypoechoic mass (**arrows**) centered at the subtalar joint and partially eroding the calcaneus.

arthritis, but a similar appearance can be seen in other inflammatory arthritides, chronic infections, pigmented villonodular synovitis, synovial osteochondromatosis and amyloid (**Fig. 50–11**). Hemophilia might also be expected to produce a similar picture. The synovium in these cases is hypoechoic and nodular in appearance.

Ganglion Cysts

These consist of well-marginated, often multiloculated pseudocysts that may form in relation to joint capsules, tendons, tendon sheaths, ligaments, and muscles.[1,2,11,12] They characteristically contain clear gelatinous material and are often hard to palpation. These are most commonly located along the dorsal surfaces of the wrist and ankle, although they can occur almost anywhere in the musculoskeletal soft tissues. These are presumably degenerative in nature and may be associated with traumatic origin. While they may be asymptomatic, it is not uncommon for these to produce direct compression of an adjacent neurovascular bundle, tendon, or synovial-lined structure. In these cases, these lesions can produce chronic intermittent pain, weakness, and diminished mobility. While surgery is considered as a definitive treatment, intracystic injection of long-acting corticosteroids is often successful.

Ultrasound has been shown to be a reliable method to ensure intracystic localization of the injected material, using real-time guidance for needle placement, as well as defining the relation of the cyst to surrounding structures.[13]

Meniscal Cysts

These constitute pseudocysts that form adjacent to a meniscal tear (**Fig. 50–12**).[14] Similar to synovial cysts, their fluid content presumably relates to a decompressive mechanism in which joint fluid escapes unidirectionally into the collection. These are often multiloculated and can occur either medially or laterally along the femorotibial joint. The presence of a cyst adjacent to meniscal fibrocartilage containing a well-defined hypoechoic defect establishes the diagnosis on ultrasound. While ultrasound can usually identify the nature of the cyst, an MRI is necessary to fully evaluate the extent of internal derangement.

Muscle

Pyomyositis appears as a complex collection within the muscle (**Fig. 50–2**).[1,2,15] The presence of punctate echogenic foci with associated "dirty" shadowing in the nondependent portions of the collection may indicate a gas-forming organism. Likewise, intramuscular hematoma may be seen as a complex collection surrounded by granulation tissue.[16] When large, these lesions display an irregular cavity with shaggy borders. The sonographic appearance is dominated by the hematoma and follows typical evolutionary changes with time. Distraction injuries differ in that the hematoma is confined usually to a single muscle, and torn fragments of muscle are more likely to be identified within the cavity, producing the "bell-clapper" sign.

Ultrasound can be useful to assess healing of these lesions. The cavity gradually decreases in size, and hypoechoic granulation tissue in the margins of the cavity advances to fill in the defect. Eventually, organization can be demonstrated with the reappearance of fibroadipose septa.

Knee

The most useful application of ultrasound in assessing the knee consists of evaluation of the extensor mechanism and soft tissue masses.[1,2] Differentiation of cystic and solid masses has been and continues to be a good use of ultrasound. Localization of the cyst enables appropriate characterization as to whether it is a bursa, ganglion, or meniscal cyst. Acute rupture of a Baker's cyst is one cause for acute pain. Cyst rupture is documented by loss of the well-defined distal cyst margin, and abnormal fluid tracking deep to the subcutaneous fat (**Fig. 50–8**). It should be recognized that ultrasound is well suited to eliminating other causes of acute posterior leg pain as well (**Fig. 50–13**).

If a fluid collection corresponds to a bursa and increased peribursal blood flow is demonstrated on Doppler imaging, then the collection is likely inflammatory in nature.[8] Ultrasound-guided aspiration can readily be performed at the time that the collection is documented. Further, secondary changes in adjacent soft tissue structures can be documented. Patients with rheumatoid arthritis, for example, often manifest secondary tendonitis and tears. Similarly, the appearance of hyperemic nodular soft tissue within a bursa is indicative of nodular synovitis.

When the fluid relates to a tendon, tendon sheath, capsular structure, etc., and bears no direct relationship to the menisci or known bursae, then the collection will likely correspond to a ganglion. The viscous nature of the material often results in these masses presenting clinically as hard, but mobile to palpation. When these are located in relation to the tibiofibular joint, they can cause common peroneal nerve compression. Superficial ganglia are usually easily documented on ultrasound. Diagnosis can be confirmed by ultrasound-guided aspiration, producing a characteristically clear gelatinous fluid, and these may then be treated at the time of diagnosis, using ultrasound-guided injection of one of the commonly utilized antiflammatory agents. Differentiation from a meniscal cyst relies on demonstration of the meniscal tear. In most cases, the adjacent tear will be detected, unless the cyst is significantly removed from the meniscal pathology. The presence of joint fluid can likewise be easily documented and aspirated.

The extensor mechanism consists of the quadriceps muscles, tendon, patella tendon, and medial and lateral

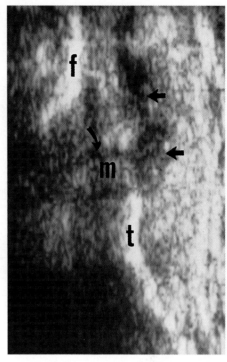

Figure 50–12 Coronal image over medial knee joint depicts a crescentic collection (**arrows**) contiguous with a horizontal hypoechoic cleft (**curved arrow**) corresponding to a tear in the medial meniscus. The femur (f) and tibia (t) are indicated and effectively determine upper and lower boundaries of the medial meniscus (m).

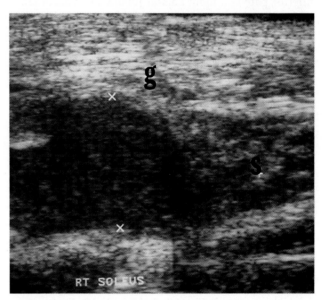

Figure 50–13 Longitudinal sonogram of posteromedial leg in a patient with acute onset of leg pain and history of systemic lupus erythematosis. Evaluation for ruptured Baker's cyst was requested. Instead, a large rupture of the soleus muscle(s) was detected filled with a complex hematoma (x). The letter "g" denotes the medial head of gastrocnemius muscle.

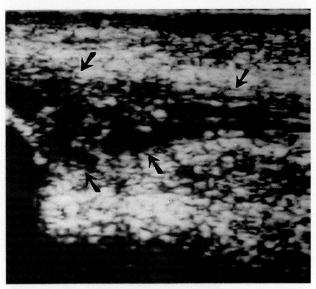

Figure 50–14   Longitudinal sonogram of focal tendinitis of the proximal patella tendon (**arrows**), also known as Jumper's Knee.

patella retinacula. These structures are well seen on ultrasound, and pathologic conditions, including tendinosis, and partial or complete tear, are readily documented. Secondary changes in the tendons and surrounding bursa can occur in individuals with osteochondrosis of the anterior tibial tubercle (Osgood Schlatter disease) or inferior patella (Sindig Larson Johansson syndrome). A common cause of knee pain results from tendinitis at the proximal insertion of the patellar tendon (Jumper's Knee, **Fig. 50–14**).

Sonographers with experience in musculoskeletal ultrasound and detailed knowledge of the knee anatomy can likewise accurately assess pathology in the surrounding tendons and collateral ligaments. Although, in situations for which the full extent of pathology is not readily appreciated clinically, or if internal derangement, bone, or cartilage pathology is suspect, magnetic resonance imaging remains the imaging study of choice.

Ankle and Foot

The superficial nature of the tendons and their synovial sheaths in the ankle make them good candidates for sonographic evaluation.[1,2,5,17] Tendinosis and tears of the Achilles tendon, posterior tibial tendon, and peroneal tendons are common abnormalities, which can easily be assessed (**Fig. 50–2 through 50–7**). Likewise the plantar fascia is often a source of heel pain. The presence of pathologic thickening, cystic degeneration, and frank tears can be documented. The real-time nature of the examination permits provocative maneuvers, which can be helpful in the assessment of tendon subluxation. Distension of the tendon sheath by fluid or synovial proliferation can be confused clinically with direct tendon pathology and the presence of synovial cysts or ganglia.

Cysts arising in the tarsal sinus can produce lateral foot pain, while those arising in the tarsal tunnel may directly compress the posterior tibial nerve, giving rise to a tarsal tunnel syndrome. Differentiation of these processes is important for appropriate therapy to proceed. Ultrasound provides a method to both document these abnormalities as well as allow guidance for therapeutic injection and/or aspiration. Likewise, in cases of tenosynovitis, needle placement into the tendon sheath before injection can be ascertained on real-time examination. Displacement of the anterior or posterior recess of the tibiotalar joint by complex material or fluid can be demonstrated. Aspiration and/or injection of the joint can be similarly performed. When there is adequate acoustic access, the presence of joint bodies can be identified. Intraarticular injection of sterile saline can often accentuate the ultrasound appearance of joint bodies or proliferative synovium.

In the forefoot, ultrasound is well suited to the diagnosis of adventitial bursae. These may form at sites of increased pressure, such as bunion deformities, plantar aspect of the foot or intermetatarsal region (**Fig. 50–15**). Again, because of its real-time nature, needle placement and therapeutic injection is well suited to sonographic guidance. Neuromas are a common source of pain along the plantar aspect of the foot, generally localized to the second or third web space. Ultrasound has been documented as an accurate means to diagnose these lesions, which often appear as hypoechoic nodules (**Fig. 50–16**).[1,17,18] These pseudotumors are usually intimately related to the plantar digital nerves, which can sometimes be seen. Ultrasound is not specific in that other soft tissue masses, such as giant cell tumor of tendon sheath or various malignant processes, may not be readily differentiated.[1] Ultrasound provides a simple screen to evaluate for cystic masses and neuromas, that form the large majority of foot and ankle masses. Ultrasound-guided biopsy of more complex masses can be performed, but often additional imaging is required to fully evaluate the extent of a soft tissue mass.

Ultrasound has been established as probably the best method to detect foreign bodies.[1,19] Objects as small as 1 to 2 mm can be detected. Many of these may not be apparent on conventional radiography, i. e., wood splinters. These typically appear as discrete echogenic foci with or without a posterior acoustic shadow. A surrounding halo of inflammatory tissue may be present or a discrete nodule, corresponding to a foreign body granuloma.

Summary

A wide variety of soft tissue and articular abnormalities of the knee, foot, and ankle can be assessed using ultrasound. It is a modality that is both cost effective and readily available. Yet it is significantly underutilized in

Figure 50–15 Longitudinal sonogram of an infected adventitial bursa seen as a complex, septated fluid collection with a surrounding hypoechoic halo (h). A curvilinear bright echo seen at the bottom of the image (**arrow**) corresponds to the plantar aspect of the metatarsal head. ▷

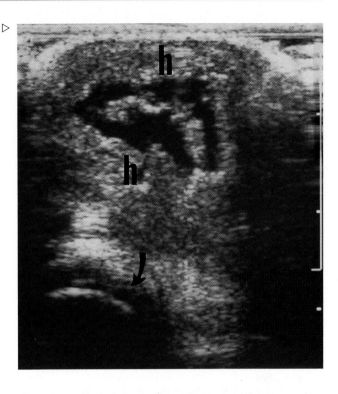

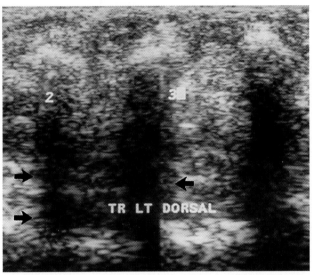

A

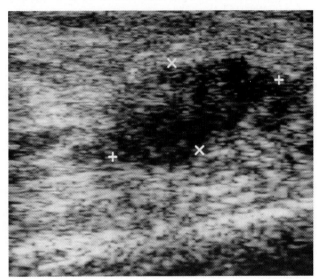

B

Figure 50–16 A: Transverse sonogram of the forefoot in a young woman with pain in the second web space. The second and third metatarsals are seen in cross-section and labeled in the image. The normal web space appears bright, while the dark area (**arrow**) situated between metatarsals 2 and 3 corresponds to the neuroma. **B:** Longitudinal sonogram obtained over the plantar aspect of the second web space depicts an elliptical hypoechoic nodule (x) corresponding to the neuroma.

the United States. The current chapter has touched on some of the more practical applications with respect to abnormalities of muscles, tendons, and synovial lined spaces of the lower extremity. In addition, the real-time nature of the examination has been emphasized in order to illustrate ultrasound's capability to assess response to provocative maneuvers and provide guidance for a variety of simple interventions.

References

1. Fornage BD. *Musculoskeletal Ultrasound*, New York: Churchill Livingstone, 1995.
2. Van Holsbeeck M, Introcaso JH. *Musculoskeletal Ultrasound*. St Louis: Mosby Year Book, 1991.
3. Newman JS, Adler RS, Bude RO, Rubin JM. Detection of soft-tissue hyperemia: value of power Doppler sonography. *AJR* 1994;163:385—389.
4. Newman JS, Laing TJ, McCarthy CJ, Adler RS. Power Doppler sonography in synovitis: assessment of therapeutic response: preliminary observations. *Radiology* 1996;198:582—584.
5. Bouffard JA, Eyler WR, Introcaso JH, van Holsbeeck M. Sonography of tendons. Ultrasound Q 1993;11(4):259—286.
6. Jeffrey RB Jr, Laing FC, Schechter WP, Markison RE, Barton RM. Acute suppurative tenosynovitis of the hand: diagnosis with US. *Radiology* 1987;162:741—742.
7. Stephenson CA, Seibert JJ, McAndrew MP, et al. Sonographic diagnosis of tenosynovitis of the posterior tibial tendon. *J Clin Ultrasound* 1990;18:114—116.
8. Breidahl WH, Newman JS, Taljanovic MS, et al. Power Doppler sonography in the assessment of musculoskeletal fluid collections. *AJR* 1996;166:1443—1446.
9. Marchal G, Van Holsbeeck M, Raes M, et al. Transient synovitis of the hip in children; role of US. *Radiology* 1987;162:825—828.
10. Van Holsbeeck M, Eyler W, Sherman L, et al. Detection of infection in loosened hip protheses: efficiency of sonography. *AJR* 1994;163:381—384.
11. DeFlaviis L, Nessi R, Delbo P, Calori G, Bakoni G. High resolution ultrasonography of wrist ganglia. *J Clin Ultrasound* 1987;15:17—22.
12. Paivansalo M, Jalovaara P. Ultrasound findings in ganglions of the wrist. *Eur J Radiol* 1991;13(3):178—180.
13. Breidahl WH, Adler RS. Ultrasound-guided injection of ganglia with corticosteroids. *Skel Radiol* 1996;25:635—638.
14. Coral A, van Holsbeeck M, Adler RS. Imaging of meniscal cyst of the knee in three cases. *Skel Radiol* 1989;18:451—455.
15. van Sonnenburg E, Wittich G, Casola G, et al. Sonography of thigh abscess: detection, diagnosis and drainage. *AJR* 1987;149:769—472.
16. Fornage B, Touche D, Segal P, et al. Ultrasonography in the evaluation of muscular trauma. *J Ultrasound Med* 1983;2(12):549—554.
17. Fornage B, Ritkin M. Ultrasound examination of the hand and foot. *Radiol Clin North Am* 1988;26(1):109—129.
18. Reed R, Peters V, Emery S, et al. Morton neuroma: sonographic evaluation. *Radiology* 1989;171:415—417.
19. Fornage B, Schernberg F. Sonographic diagnosis of foreign bodies of the distal extremities. *AJR* 1986;147(3):567—569.

Superficial Organs

51 The Palpable Neck Mass

Carl C. Reading

The palpable neck mass is a frequent diagnostic dilemma. Many pathologic processes, including congenital, inflammatory, neoplastic, and metabolic disorders, can cause palpable neck abnormalities. The radiologist who evaluates such a patient should have a working knowledge of the regional anatomy of the neck and of the disorders likely to occur in the area of the neck in which the mass is found. The diagnostic possibilities can then be reduced to a minimum, and appropriate imaging and nonimaging diagnostic examinations and procedures can be performed. When imaging studies are indicated, high-frequency sonography is often the method of choice because it demonstrates the superficial neck structures with remarkable clarity. In addition, the capability of sonography to precisely guide the percutaneous insertion of small-caliber needles into superficial pathologic processes, under continuous real-time visualization, greatly enhances the usefulness of sonography as a diagnostic, as well as, in some cases, a therapeutic procedure in the neck.

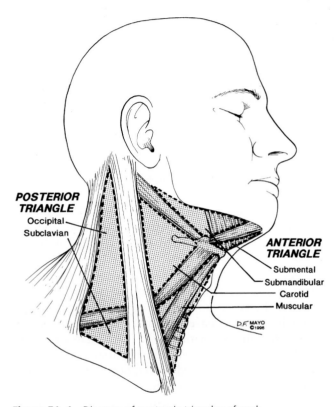

Figure 51–1 Diagram of anatomic triangles of neck.

Differential Diagnosis

Anatomy

The location of a cervical mass is described by categorizing the mass as lying within one of a number of anatomic triangles of the neck. The large sternocleidomastoid muscle, which runs obliquely across the neck, subdivides the neck into anterior and posterior triangles (**Fig. 51–1**). These two large triangles thus share a common side. Structures located anterior to the sternocleidomastoid muscle lie within the anterior triangle; structures that lie deep to and posterior to this muscle lie within the posterior triangle.

The anterior triangle is formed by the anterior edge of the sternocleidomastoid muscle, the midline of the neck from the manubrium, inferiorly, to the mandibular symphysis, superiorly, and the inferior margin of the mandible. It is subdivided into four smaller triangles: submental, submandibular, carotid, and muscular.

The submental triangle is bounded laterally by the anterior belly of the digastric muscle, inferiorly by the hyoid bone, and medially by the midline of the neck. It contains small submental lymph nodes, but otherwise contains no major structures or glands.

The submandibular triangle is bounded inferiorly by the anterior and posterior bellies of the digastric muscles and superiorly by the mandible. It contains the submandibular glands and several small submandibular lymph nodes.

The carotid triangle is bounded posteriorly by the sternocleidomastoid muscle, anteriorly by the superior belly of the omohyoid muscle, and superiorly by the posterior belly of the digastric muscle. It contains the carotid sheath which envelopes the carotid artery, internal jugular vein, the vagus nerve, and the cervical sympathetic trunk. Numerous lymph nodes in the upper internal jugular chain lie within this triangle.

The muscular triangle is formed superiorly by the superior belly of the omohyoid muscle, inferiorly by the anterior border of the sternocleidomastoid muscle, and medially by the midline of the neck. The tissues deep to the triangle contain many important structures, including the thyroid and parathyroid glands, recurrent laryngeal nerves, larynx, hypopharynx, trachea, and esophagus.

The posterior triangle of the neck is bounded anteriorly by the sternocleidomastoid muscle, posteriorly by the trapezius muscle, and inferiorly by the body of the clavicle. It is further subdivided into the occipital and subclavian triangles.

The occipital triangle is bounded inferiorly by the posterior belly of the omohyoid muscle, posteriorly by the trapezius muscle, and anteriorly by the sternocleidomastoid muscle. It contains several small occipital and accessory lymph nodes.

The subclavian triangle is bounded inferiorly by the body of the clavicle, superiorly by the posterior belly of the omohyoid muscle, and anteriorly by the sternocleidomastoid muscle. Small transverse and superficial cervical nodes are located in this triangle.

Common Neck Masses

The three most common neck masses that are evaluated by imaging examinations are thyroid nodules, parathyroid adenomas, and enlarged cervical lymph nodes. In the patient who presents with a palpable nodule in the caudal aspect of the muscular triangle, this most commonly represents a thyroid nodule. Nodular thyroid disease is a relatively common disorder. Epidemiologic studies have estimated that between 4% and 7% of the adult population in the United States have palpable thyroid nodules, with women more frequently affected than men. Thyroid cancer, however, is rare. The annual detection rate of clinically significant thyroid cancer is only 0.005%. Therefore, the overwhelming majority of thyroid nodules are benign. Most thyroid "nodules" are not true neoplasms of the thyroid but are due to cycles of hyperplasia and involution of thyroid lobules which result in fusion of localized colloid-filled follicles and are known as colloid or adenomatous nodules. In the patient with nodular thyroid disease, the clinical challenge is to distinguish the few clinically significant malignant nodules from the many benign ones and, thus, to identify those patients for whom surgical excision is indicated.

Parathyroid adenomas are usually situated within the muscular triangle of the neck, as are thyroid nodules. Primary hyperparathyroidism was once considered to be a rare endocrine disorder but now it is recognized as a common disease. The prevalence of primary hyperparathyroidism in the United States is estimated to be 100—200 per 100 000 population. Women have this disease two to three times more frequently than men and it is particularly common in postmenopausal women. The diagnosis is made biochemically by the findings of elevated serum calcium and parathyroid hormone levels.

Primary hyperparathyroidism is caused by a single parathyroid adenoma in 80—90% of cases, by multiple gland enlargement in 10—20%, and by carcinoma in less than 1% of cases.

A large number of lymph nodes lie within the neck.[1] Many of these nodes are clustered into localized groups or chains of nodes. These chains follow anatomic structures in the neck, such as the internal jugular vein, throughout the length of the neck. These chains, however, may cross throughout several of the previously described anatomic triangles of the neck and, therefore, will not be localized to a single specific triangle. For purposes of discussion, however, some general points can be made about some key anatomic and drainage patterns of lymph nodes in the neck.

In the anterior triangle of the neck, lymph nodes in the submental and submandibular triangles can become metastatically involved by primary neoplasms of the lower anterior face and upper neck such as the lower lip, anterior tongue, and submandibular gland. Lymph nodes in the muscular triangle include many of the most important nodes in the neck. For example, nodes in the mid and lower portions of the internal jugular chain, which is part of the deep portion of the lateral cervical chain, are located in this triangle. Pathologic conditions commonly involve these particular nodes because they serve as a common route of drainage for all of the major regional structures including the nasopharynx, larynx, hypopharynx, esophagus, and thyroid gland. Lymph nodes in the carotid triangle receive drainage from the nasopharynx and oral cavity and can be involved by metastases from these structures. However, care should be taken in overinterpreting enlargement of these nodes because benign reactive lymph node hyperplasia can occur frequently in this location due to inflammatory episodes that involve the neighboring teeth, gums, tonsils, and pharynx.

In the posterior cervical triangle, lymph nodes in the caudal aspect of the neck within the subclavian triangle are frequently involved by metastatic carcinoma from below the clavicle, such as the breast, lung, kidney, stomach, and lower gastrointestinal tract. Nodes in the occipital triangle receive drainage from the nasopharynx, lateral neck, and upper chest and can be involved by metastases from primary malignancies in these locations.

In addition to thyroid nodules, parathyroid adenomas, and enlarged cervical lymph nodes, other types of neck masses that may come to imaging studies include thyroglossal duct cysts, branchial cleft cysts, lymphangiomas, and carotid body tumors. The typical thyroglossal duct cyst lies in the superior aspect of the muscular triangle, at or inferior to the level of the hyoid bone.[2, 3] It is the most common clinically important congenital anomaly and accounts for 70% of congenital neck masses. Embryologically, these cysts are the result of the failure of a portion of the thyroglossal duct to involute during embryonic development which results in a tract or cyst. The cyst can occur anywhere along the course of the duct from the foramen cecum of the tongue to the pyramidal lobe of the thyroid gland. The cysts are classified as suprahyoid (20%), hyoid (15%), and infrahyoid (65%), and may occasionally occur in the suprasternal area. Usually, the cyst is less than 2 cm in size, and is midline; however, the convexity of the thyroid cartilage and hyoid bone may push the cyst to one side of midline.[4] On physical examination, the mass is smooth and well demarcated and may slide superiorly in the neck when the patient swallows or sticks out the tongue. They are usually nontender but can present with recurrent episodes of acute swelling and tenderness. Most are diagnosed by 30 years of age. Other cystic-appearing lesions, such as necrotic lymphadenopathy, sebaceous cysts, abscess, or thrombosed anterior jugular veins, may have a similar appearance to thyroglossal duct cyst. Surgical treatment is recommended because of the potential for infection and uncommon malignant transformation. Because the thyroglossal tract extends in a loop deep to the hyoid bone, removal of the hyoid bone is necessary at the time of surgery to prevent recurrence.

The vast majority (95%) of branchial cleft cysts arise from the second branchial cleft.[5–8] Embryologically, they are the result of incomplete obliteration of the second branchial apparatus or buried rest cells which enlarge and form branchial cysts later in life. If they communicate externally to the skin or internally to the foregut, they become sinuses or fistulas. Second branchial cleft cysts are usually located in the anterior triangle of the neck anterior to or along the anterior border of the sternocleidomastoid muscle. Larger cysts may extend posteriorly under the sternocleidomastoid muscle. Most are located superiorly near the angle of the mandible at the junction of the submandibular space and carotid space, but they can occur anywhere along the residual cleft tract extending from the supraclavicular region to the tonsillar fossa. Uncommon first branchial cleft cysts most commonly arise as a mass near the lower pole of the parotid gland or external auditory canal. Rare third and fourth branchial cleft cysts usually lie at the anterior margin of the lower third of the sternocleidomastoid muscle.

Most branchial cleft cysts present as painless, fluctuant, smooth lateral neck masses. They are usually found in patients who are between the ages of 10 and 40 years, most commonly in their late teens. The cysts may become painful and tender, particularly after upper respiratory tract infections. Other cervical lesions that may mimic a second branchial cleft cyst include hemangioma, lymphangioma, thymic cyst, lymphoma, dermoid, necrotic neural tumor, and necrotic metastases. In addition, some lymph node metastases from thyroid cancer can be predominately cystic and should not be misinterpreted as a benign branchial cleft cyst.[9]

Lymphangiomas are congenital lymphatic malformations that occur most commonly in the head, neck, or axilla; however, they can arise anywhere in the developing lymphatic system.[10] There are four histologic types of lymphangioma: cystic hygroma, cavernous lymphangioma, capillary (or simple) lymphangioma, and vasculolymphatic malformation. They are differentiated from one another on the basis of the size of their lymphatic spaces; otherwise, they are virtually pathologically identical. Combinations of these various forms of lymphangioma may be present within a single lesion and they may reside within vascular malformations. They probably arise from sequestrations of primitive embryonic lymph sacs and enlarge either because of inadequate drainage of the central lymphatic channels into the internal jugular veins or because of excessive secretion from the lining cells. Cystic hygroma is the most common form of lymphangioma, and it is composed of hugely dilated cystic lymphatic spaces. Seventy-four percent of these masses are located in the neck, and most of these are in the posterior compartment. Three to 10% expand into the mediastinum. They present as a painless soft, multilobular, semifirm mass. Size fluctuation is not infrequent with upper respiratory tract infections. Ninety percent are detected by age 2. Usually these tumors proliferate, sometimes rapidly and extensively during early childhood, but all will regress eventually. Surgery is indicated only to preserve the airway or for extensive tumors affecting multiple head and neck structures. Residual lesions are often removed during the teens and early 20s for cosmetic reasons.

Carotid body tumors present as a painless slowly growing mass in the carotid triangle at the carotid bifurcation. Occasionally, a bruit may be present. The tumor is difficult to separate from the carotid artery by palpation. These tumors usually present between the third and sixth decades of life. There is a familial predisposition in 20–30% of patients and multiple tumors are not uncommon.[11] Neural invasion or associated adenopathy is suggestive of malignancy. Carotid body tumors and other glomus-type tumors are found throughout the carotid sheath from the skull base to the carotid bifurcation and are named according to their location: skull base/jugular foramen — glomus jugulare; nasopharyngeal and oropharyngeal — glomus vagale; carotid bifurcation — carotid body tumor. They receive their vascular supply from the external carotid artery. The differential diagnosis of a neck mass at the carotid bifurcation includes neurogenic tumor, nodal metastases, and branchial cleft cyst. The marked hypervascularity seen in carotid body tumors by imaging techniques excludes most other diagnostic possibilities except for a rare hypervascular neurogenic tumor. Aneurysm of the carotid artery is also often considered in the clinical differential diagnosis of a carotid bifurcation mass but can readily be ruled out by imaging techniques. The treatment of choice for carotid body tumor is surgery. Radiation therapy may be considered if the risk of morbidity and mortality in a given patient is high.

In addition to the neck masses described earlier, a wide variety of other less common solid and cystic masses can occur in the neck. Solid masses include head and neck hemangiomas, most of which present soon after birth.[12] Two-thirds of the hemangiomas involve the skin alone, and the remainder are subcutaneous or mixed. Lipomas occur throughout the body and can also be found in the neck, commonly in the posterior triangle. They are distinguished by their soft consistency on physical examination, superficial location, and sonographic appearance which is similar to that of the surrounding soft tissues. Cystic masses that can occur in the neck include dermoid cysts.[13] Most of these occur in the orbit, nasal, and oral regions. Those located in the oral region are usually in the midline or slightly off midline and may extend into the sublinguinal and submental regions. The presence of fat within these lesions differentiates them from other cystic masses. Abscesses can occur in the neck, particularly in patients who are immunocompromised, or as a complication of skin infections, dental disease, trauma, endocarditis, and systemic infections such as tuberculosis. The clinical features of pain, tenderness, and swelling help to differentiate abscess from other neck masses. On imaging studies, abscesses are seen as single or multiloculated, partially fluid-filled masses which conform to adjacent facial planes. Thymic cysts, parathyroid cysts, and cervical bronchogenic cysts can also occur in the neck, but are rare.

Diagnostic Workup

Nonimaging Tests: Fine Needle Aspiration

The single most important nonimaging test that is used in the evaluation of neck masses is fine needle aspiration (FNA). Usually this procedure is performed during the workup of a thyroid nodule, but it can be used in patients with other neck masses as well.

Because it is difficult to precisely define the nature of a thyroid nodule based on its sonographic features, in our practice and in many others, FNA is the primary method of evaluating a palpable thyroid nodule. This procedure obtains thyroid follicular epithelial cells and minute tissue fragments for cytologic evaluation. It is safe, inexpensive, and provides more direct information than other available diagnostic techniques.[14—19]

Technique

FNA of the neck is most commonly performed by the clinician as an office procedure under direct palpation guidance. However, if the nodule is too poorly palpable to be biopsied in this way or if the palpation-guided biopsy is nondiagnostic, then the biopsy can be performed under ultrasound guidance. Ultrasound-guided FNA of the neck is performed with the patient in a supine position with the neck hyperextended by a pad centered under the shoulders. The radiologist sits at the head of the table to perform the procedure. Before the biopsy the skin is cleansed with a povidone-iodine solution. The transducer can also be cleansed or a separate sterile plastic sheath can be placed over the transducer. Sterile gel is used as a coupling agent. Following the procedure the transducer is soaked in a bacterocidal dialdehyde solution. Special biopsy transducers are available for needle guidance with built-in needle canals and slots or attachable guides mounted to the side of the transducer. Alternatively, a "free-hand" method of needle biopsy, utilizing standard 5.0- to 10.0-MHz linear transducers, can be performed. With this approach, the needle is inserted through the skin at an oblique angle within the plane of view of the transducer without the help of a guide. This method provides great flexibility by allowing subtle adjustments in needle position to be made during the course of the biopsy to compensate for patient movement and slight deflections of the biopsy needle.

Thyroid

The typical needle used to perform a thyroid FNA is a standard 1.5-inch, 25-gauge, noncutting, stiff, bevel-edge needle attached to a suction device such as a 10-mL disposable syringe with a self-locking plunger. This small, sharp needle easily penetrates the soft tissues of the neck and causes little deflection or displacement of highly mobile superficial structures (**Fig. 51–2**). The needle is moved gently but rapidly through the nodule with suction applied by the syringe. The aspirated material is then expelled onto a glass slide. An ideal specimen for cytologic analysis consists of one or two drops of orange-red fluid. In most cases, three to six separate needle passes, each with a new needle, is necessary to obtain an adequate specimen. If the specimen contains much blood, then a "nonaspiration" technique can be used, in which the 25-gauge needle is inserted without suction. Capillary action causes cells to move into the needle as it is moved in a back and forth excursion through the nodule, and this often yields a less bloody specimen than when suction is used.[20] If a specimen is needed for histologic examination or if the 25-gauge needle biopsy is nondiagnostic, then small-caliber (20- to 25-gauge) cutting needles, or 18-to 22-gauge biopsy guns, can be used. Cutting needles and biopsy guns generally yield very cellular specimens, but are more difficult to insert through the tough, superficial structures of the neck than are the sharper, smaller, noncutting, 25-gauge aspiration needles.

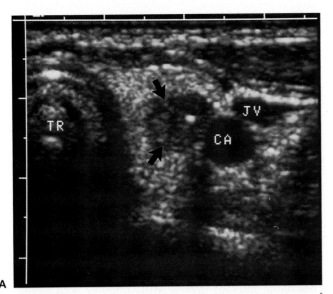

A

B

Figure 51–2 Ultrasound-guided FNA. **A:** Transverse sonogram of left neck shows 1 cm hypoechoic solid mass (**arrows**) containing a fleck of internal calcification. TR, trachea. CA, common carotid artery. JV, jugular vein. **B:** 25-gauge needle (**curved arrow**) has been inserted into nodule. Cytologic specimen showed papillary carcinoma.

Parathyroid Adenoma

In addition to the evaluation of thyroid nodules, sonographically guided percutaneous aspiration/biopsy is a very useful technique for the preoperative confirmation of a suspected parathyroid adenoma, particularly in the patient who is a candidate for reoperation.[21–23] Biopsy specimens can be analyzed for parathyroid hormone levels as well as cytology.[24] This technique has increased the specificity of sonography by permitting the reliable differentiation of parathyroid adenomas from other pathologic structures such as thyroid nodules and cervical lymph nodes. A positive biopsy reassures the reluctant reoperative patient, in addition to its value to the surgeon.

Lymph Nodes

Because of the considerable overlap in the size and appearance of the benign and malignant lymph nodes, percutaneous aspiration and biopsy of nodes suspicious for malignancy can be performed with the techniques described previously for fine-needle aspiration of thyroid nodules and parathyroid adenomas.[25–28] In one recent large multicenter study of patients with squamous cell carcinoma of the head and neck,[29] the sensitivity of US imaging and US-guided biopsy was comparable to the sensitivity of computed tomography (CT) and magnetic resonance (MR) imaging, and the specificity was higher. In one series of over 300 patients who had previous thyroidectomies for thyroid malignancy, 52 underwent sonographically guided needle biopsy of a mass in the thyroid bed or an enlarged cervical lymph node. Forty-four of the masses were nonpalpable. In 94% of the patients, the biopsy specimens were adequate for accurate interpretation as positive or negative for malignancy. Of the 29 patients with positive biopsy results, 11 had concomitant nuclear scintigraphy, but only five of the nuclear scans were positive. This study underscores the excellent sensitivity of sonography for the detection of occult metastatic cervical adenopathy in patients with previous thyroid cancer.[27] In patients with metastatic differentiated (papillary and follicular) or medullary thyroid cancer, analysis of tissue levels of thyroglobulin and calcitonin, respectively, may be useful as an adjunct to the cytopathological examination.[30]

Imaging Tests Other than Ultrasonography

Thyroid

Scintigraphy has traditionally been the most commonly used imaging method for thyroid nodule evaluation. Nodules can be classified as either hyperfunctioning ("hot") or hypofunctioning ("cold"). Cold nodules have a higher risk of malignancy than hot nodules; however, the use of this technique is decreasing in many practices in the evaluation of euthyroid patients with nodular thyroid disease since the advent of FNA. Pathologists are becoming more accurate in interpreting FNA specimens and clinicians more comfortable in making treatment decisions based on FNA results. Scintigraphy still plays an important role in the evaluation and possible treatment of patients with hyperthyroidism when blood measurements show abnormal thyroid hormone and TSH levels. CT, MR, and other imaging studies are rarely used in the evaluation of thyroid masses. However, in some patients who have a thyroid mass that extends into the mediastinum, CT or MR can be used to define the extent of the intrathoracic goiter and its relationship to adjacent vessels.

Parathyroid

A number of imaging methods are available which can be used for parathyroid adenoma localization. These modalities comprise a spectrum in terms of accuracy, degree of invasiveness, availability, and expense, and include scintigraphy, CT, MR, angiography, and venous sampling. Scintigraphy, utilizing technetium-99 m Sestamibi as the radionuclide agent, has proved to be an excellent method for parathyroid adenoma localization which has high levels of accuracy and is being used in an increasing number of medical centers, [31, 32]. It has proved to be more accurate than older nuclear medicine methods which used thallium-201 as the radionuclide agent. It is particularly useful in the reoperative setting in the localization of ectopic adenomas which may be located in the mediastinum or unusual locations in the neck. CT and MR are not used routinely in the localization of parathyroid adenomas because of the high accuracy and wide availability of ultrasound and scintigraphy. Angiography and venous sampling are relatively invasive and expensive and are reserved for very difficult cases. Their use is becoming restricted to a limited number of centers where expertise with this technique remains available.

Lymphadenopathy

In patients with cervical lymphadenopathy, contrast-enhanced CT and MR studies are very useful to define the location and extent of enlarged lymph nodes. These imaging techniques are particularly useful for adenopathy which lies deep in the neck or near the base of the skull, which are difficult areas to evaluate sonographically. In patients with metastatic differentiated thyroid cancer, scintigraphy is also useful to detect and treat functioning metastases.

Cystic Neck Masses

Cystic neck masses such as thyroglossal duct cysts and branchial cleft cysts can be evaluated with CT or MR. On CT scans, these lesions are of low attenuation and have a well-circumscribed rim. Peripheral rim enhancement usually indicates coexisting infection. On MR imaging the cysts are hypointense or slightly hyperintense to muscle on T-1 weighted images and hyperintense on T-2 weighted images. Inflammatory changes in the adjacent soft tissues are often hyperintense to fat on T-2 weighted images.[33]

Carotid Body Tumors

Other neck masses such as carotid body tumors can be evaluated with angiography, CT, or MRI which will be confirmatory of their highly vascular nature unless a significant amount of thrombosis has occurred within the lesion.[34, 35] Octreotide scintigraphy can also be used for the detection of paragangliomas.[36]

Ultrasound Imaging

Thyroid

Sonographically, thyroid nodules can be visualized with a high degree of clarity. However, no single sonographic criterion differentiates all benign thyroid nodules from malignant nodules with reliability. Thyroid nodules can be thought of as a constellation of several sonographic features, each of which may aid in predicting the benign or malignant nature of a given thyroid nodule.[37—39] However, there is considerable overlap in this sonographic spectrum of appearances of benign and malignant nodules, and caution should be used in relying on sonographic features, alone, to characterize thyroid nodules. Features that suggest a benign nature include nodules that are mostly cystic, almost always containing internal debris. Most nodules with significant cystic components are benign adenomatous nodules that have undergone degeneration or hemorrhage. When detected by older lower-resolution ultrasound equipment, the internal debris and wall thickening often could not be appreciated. However, with current generation equipment, wall irregularity, internal solid elements, and debris are visualized in virtually all nodules. Small echogenic foci with posterior reverberation, or "comet-tail," artifacts are frequently encountered in cystic nodules and are thought to represent colloid micro-crystals (**Fig. 51–3**).[40] Nodules which are hyperechoic relative to the adjacent parenchyma, and nodules which have peripheral egg-shell-type calcification — both of which are uncommonly identified are typical of benign thyroid nodules (**Fig. 51–4**). Malignant nodules, on the other hand, usually have a different appearance. Most thyroid cancer is solid and hypoechoic. However, at the same time, any given hypoechoic nodule is more likely to be benign because benign nodules have a much higher prevalence in the general population than malignant ones. Punctate, internal calcifications seen either with or without acoustic shadowing is a feature commonly found in papillary cancer and is caused by the deposition of calcium within psammona bodies within the tumor (**Fig. 51–5**). Medullary carcinoma has a similar appearance to papillary carcinoma. It is usually hypoechoic and solid and also frequently contains bright punctate echogenic foci. These are usually coarser than the calcification in papillary cancer and are thought to be due to collections of calcium and amyloid. Follicular carcinomas are usually indistinguishable from benign follicular adenomas given the cytologic and histologic similarities of their tumors, but features that suggest malignancy include irregular tumor margins and a thick irregular halo. Anaplastic cancer is rare but when seen is usually large, solid, hypoechoic, and frequently surrounds and invades adjacent muscles and vessels.

Color Doppler, spectral Doppler, and power Doppler have been applied to the evaluation of thyroid

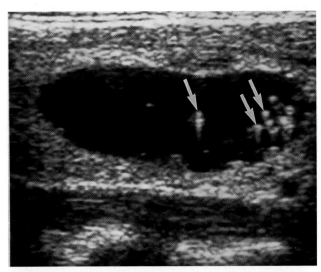

Figure 51–3   Benign thyroid nodule. Longitudinal sonogram of the right neck mass shows a 3-cm cystic nodule containing multiple echogenic foci (**arrows**) with posterior reverberation artifacts.

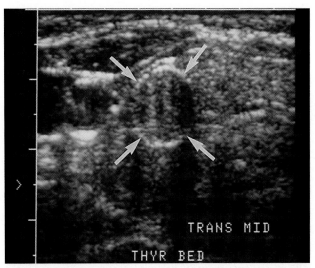

Figure 51–4   Benign thyroid nodule. Transverse sonogram of the right neck shows a 1-cm nodule with peripheral egg-shell calcification (**arrows**).

nodules.[41—45] The presence of rim vascularity may help in the initial detection of a subtle thyroid mass, but the characterization of thyroid nodules on the basis of their Doppler findings can be difficult. In general, benign hyperplastic nodules show minimal or no flow within the nodule itself and low-velocity flow about the periphery of the nodule (**Fig. 51–6**). Adenomas and carcinomas, on the other hand, show more intra- and perilesional flow than hyperplastic nodules (**Fig. 51–7**).[41] Some investigators feel that the marked hypervascularity of some carcinomas can assist in the diagnosis of these malignancies. However, other investigators have found no correlation between pathologic findings and either the presence or amount of internal flow.[44] In one study it was felt that the color Doppler flow patterns depended more on the size of the lesion than histologic type and that larger nodules, regardless of histology, had more flow than smaller nodules.[45] Additional studies will be necessary to determine what role Doppler evaluation will play in the evaluation of nodular thyroid disease.

Parathyroid

Normal parathyroid glands, which typically measure 5.0 by 3.0 by 1 mm in size, are similar in echogenicity to the adjacent thyroid and surrounding tissues and are difficult to visualize sonographically. Occasionally, normal glands are visualized in young adults. The typical parathyroid adenoma is seen sonographically as an oval, solid mass of homogeneous low echogenicity that usually measures slightly over 1 cm in length; however, the shape, echogenicity, internal architecture, and size can vary.[46]

Most parathyroid adenomas acquire a characteristic oblong, oval shape as they dissect between longitudi-

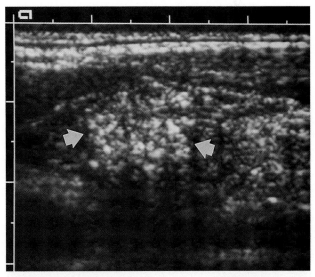

Figure 51–5   Malignant papillary carcinoma. Longitudinal sonogram of left lobe of thyroid shows 1.5-cm nodule (**arrows**) containing innumerable punctate microcalcifications.

nally oriented tissue planes in the neck. If the process is more exaggerated, they can become more elongated or tubelike. The characteristic hypoechoic echogenicity of parathyroid adenomas is due to the uniform hypercellularity of the gland, which leaves few interfaces for reflecting sound. Rare functioning parathyroid lipoadenomas can occur which contain large amounts of fat and are more echogenic than the adjacent thyroid gland. The vast majority of parathyroid adenomas are homogeneously solid. About 2% have internal cystic components due to cystic degeneration, most commonly, or true simple cysts, less commonly. Rare adenomas may

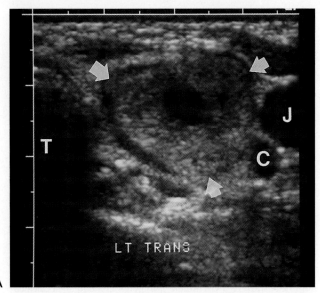

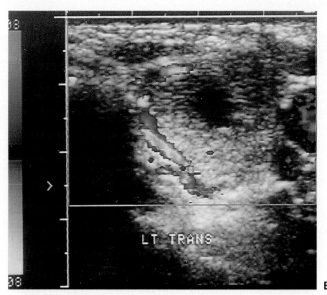

Figure 51–6 Benign adenomatous nodule. **A:** Transverse sonogram of left neck shows a 2-cm solid mass (**arrows**) containing a small internal central fluid component. J, internal jugular vein. C, common carotid artery. T, trachea. **B:** Color Doppler imaging shows minimal blood flow about the periphery of the nodule.

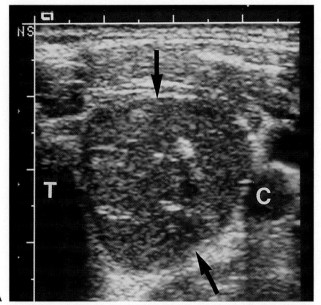

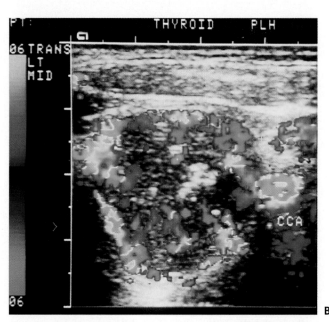

Figure 51–7 Malignant papillary carcinoma. **A:** Transverse sonogram of left neck shows a 2.5-cm solid mass (**arrows**) containing internal calcifications. T, trachea. C, common carotid artery. **B:** Color Doppler imaging shows large amounts of blood flow throughout the nodule. CCA, common carotid artery.

contain focal internal calcification. Most parathyroid adenomas are 0.8—1.5 cm long and weigh 500—1000 mg. The smallest adenomas are minimally enlarged glands that appear virtually normal during surgery but are found to be hypercellular on pathologic examination. The largest adenomas can be over 5 cm in length and weigh more than 10 g. Parathyroid carcinoma is uncommon and accounts for less than one in 200 cases of clinical hyperparathyroidism. In most cases, parathyroid carcinomas are prospectively indistinguishable sono-graphically from large benign adenomas unless there is gross evidence of invasion of adjacent structures.

Color Doppler sonography of a parathyroid adenoma may demonstrate a hypervascular pattern or a peripheral vascular arc, usually arising from the inferior thyroid artery, which can aid in the differentiation from regional lymph nodes which have hilar flow (**Fig. 51–8**).[47] Superior parathyroid adenomas are usually located adjacent to the posterior aspect of the midportion of the thyroid. The location of inferior adenomas is more vari-

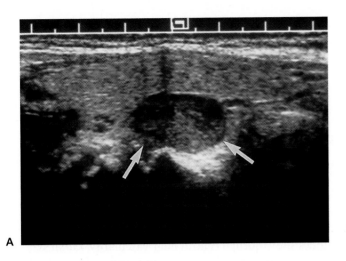

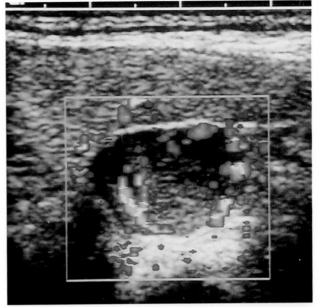

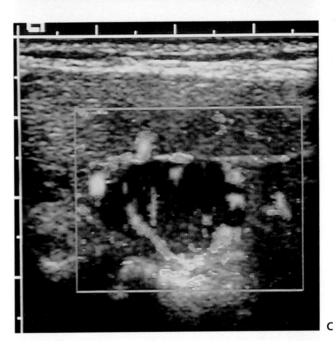

Figure 51–8 Parathyroid adenoma. **A:** Longitudinal sonogram of left neck shows a 2-cm oval, hypoechoic, solid mass (**arrows**) adjacent to the posterior aspect, midportion, left lobe of thyroid. **B:** Color Doppler imaging shows large amount of flow within and about periphery of mass. **C:** Color Doppler energy imaging shows large amount of flow within and about periphery of mass.

able, but they usually lie in close proximity to the caudal tip of the lower pole of the thyroid. Most of these inferior adenomas are adjacent to the posterior aspect or in the soft tissues 1—2 cm inferior to the thyroid. The vast majority of superior and inferior adenomas will be found in these typical locations, adjacent to the thyroid. One to 3% of adenomas are ectopic. Ectopic glands can be a cause of failure of sonographic localization and subsequent failed operations. The four most common ectopic locations are mediastinal, retrotracheal, carotid sheath, and undescended, high in the lateral neck. Ectopic adenomas are more challenging to detect than adenomas in more typical anatomic locations, but many can be visualized sonographically.

Lymph Nodes

During the course of examination of the neck normal, inflammatory, and malignant nodes will be readily identified with high-frequency sonography.[48] A number of studies have attempted to use morphologic criteria such as lymph node size, shape, and internal architecture to differentiate benign from malignant nodes.[49–51] Most normal and inflammatory cervical lymph nodes have a flattened, oblong, oval shape with their greatest dimension in the longitudinal axis. This is presumably due to compression by the adjacent longitudinally oriented tissue planes in the neck. Most normal nodes measure only a few millimeters in size. Enlarged, benign, inflammatory nodes occur with great frequency in the neck, however, and differentiation of these nodes from malignant nodes in patients with a known cervical malignancy can be difficult. The size, shape, and internal architecture of sonographically visualized nodes are important features to evaluate to help make this distinction.

In the neck, lymph node shape is probably the best method to attempt this differentiation. It has been suggested that cervical lymph nodes with a short-to-long axis ratio of greater than 0.5 show a much higher prevalence of malignancy than those with a ratio of less than 0.5.[25, 52] In other words, the more rounded the shape of a lymph node, the more likely it is to be malignant. Care must be taken, however, in translating these principles to other regions of the body. In the breast or axilla, for example, normal nodes, which are surrounded by pliable fat, can have a normal rounded configuration due to lack of surrounding constricting tissue planes that are found in the neck.

The internal architecture of cervical lymph noes can also be a useful method to distinguish benign from malignant lymph nodes. Benign nodes have a homogeneous, uniform echogenicity. Malignant nodes often have a more heterogeneous, irregular echogenicity. In patients with papillary thyroid cancer, the presence of punctate calcifications or internal fluid components within cervical lymph nodes is highly suspicious for metastatic disease (**Fig. 51–9**).[9, 53] Color Doppler sonography often shows abnormal flow patterns in malignant nodes, when compared with benign nodes. Most benign nodes show normal central hilar vascularity, radial symmetric central vascularity, and no peripheral vascularity (**Fig. 51–10**). Malignant nodes, on the other hand, may show eccentric or absent hilar vascularity, deformed or absent central vascularity, and increased peripheral vascularity (**Fig. 51–11**). However, these differences can be subtle and are unlikely to obviate the need for biopsy.[54]

Other Neck Masses

Sonographically, thyroglossal duct cysts can be fluid-filled or may contain internal debris or solid components, and the cysts may be anechoic, homogeneously hypoechoic, or heterogeneous.[55] The presence of thick walls and internal echoes does not correlate well with the presence or absence of inflammation on pathologic examination. Thyroid tissue may be present in the cyst wall. It is important to perform sonography of the thyroid bed to confirm a source of thyroid hormone sepa-

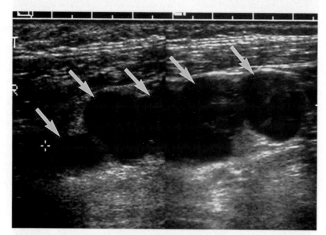

Figure 51–9 Papillary carcinoma metastatic to cervical lymph nodes. Longitudinal sonogram of the right neck shows multiple fluid-filled lymph nodes (**arrows**) consistent with metastatic papillary cancer.

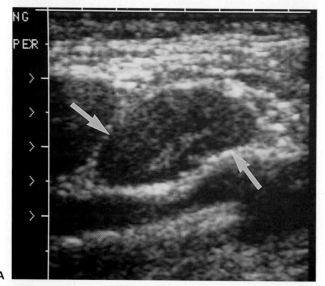

A

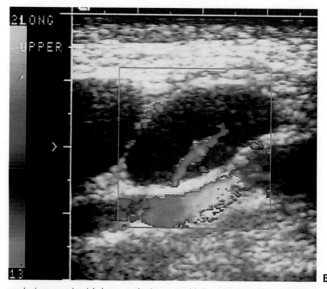

B

Figure 51–10 Benign lymph node. **A:** Longitudinal sonogram of left neck shows a 2-cm oval, homogeneous, hypoechoic lymph node (**arrows**) with hyperechoic central hilus. **B:** Color Doppler imaging shows central blood flow within hilus of node.

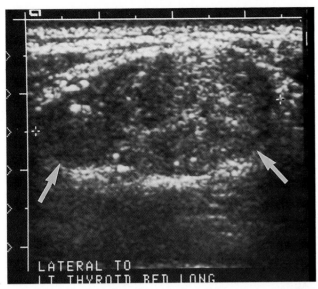

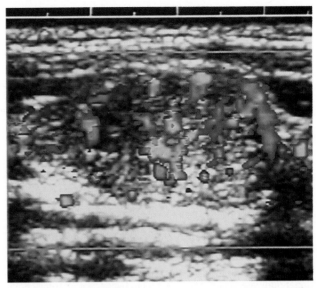

Figure 51–11 Malignant metastatic lymph node from papillary thyroid carcinoma. **A:** Longitudinal sonogram of left neck shows a 3-cm lobulated, enlarged lymph node (**arrows**) with multiple internal microcalcifications. **B:** Color Doppler imaging shows irregular, increased flow throughout the node.

rate from the thyroglossal duct cyst and thus exclude the possibility of complete ectopic thyroid in this location. Routine scintigraphy is not necessary unless the sonographic results are inconclusive.[56,57] Although rare, malignancies, the majority of which are papillary carcinoma, have been reported within thyroglossal duct cysts (**Fig. 51–12**).[58—62]

The sonographic appearance of a typical branchial cleft cyst is a cystic oval to round mass that displaces the sternocleidomastoid muscle posteriorly or posterolaterally, the carotid artery and internal jugular vein medially or posteromedially, and the submandibular gland anteriorly. Characteristically, they are of uniform, low echogenicity (**Fig. 51–13**).[63,64] Internal debris or septations may be present.

Sonographically, cystic hygromas are hypoechoic and multilocular with septa of variable thickness.[65] Solitary cystic masses are found occasionally. The cyst wall is typically very thin. The borders of the mass may be ill-defined sonographically, and it can be difficult to precisely delineate the boundaries of the mass. Other diagnostic imaging methods such as CT and MR often pro-

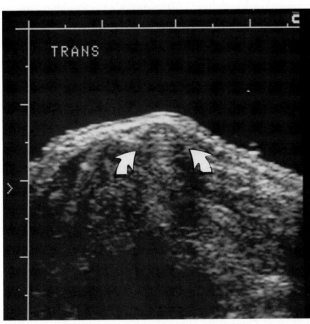

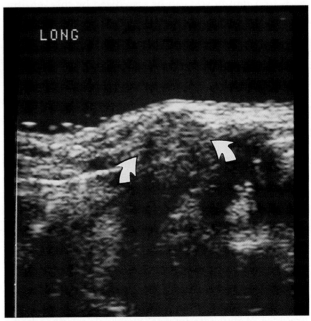

Figure 51–12 Thyroglossal duct cyst containing papillary carcinoma. **A:** Longitudinal sonogram of midline of infrahyoid neck shows a superficial 8-mm solid nodule (**arrows**). **B:** Transverse sonogram shows nodule (**arrows**) protruding superficially in midline of neck.

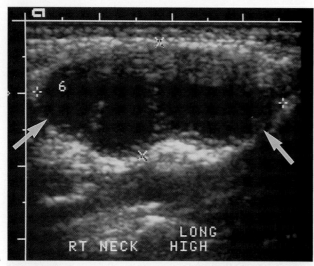

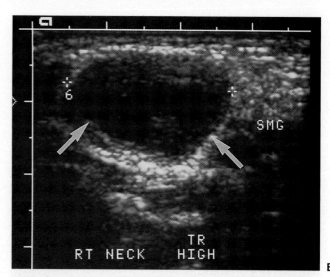

Figure 51–13 Branchial cleft cyst. **A:** Longitudinal sonogram of upper right lateral neck shows a 3.5-cm hypoechoic, partially fluid-filled mass (**arrows**) with internal septations. **B:** Transverse sono-

gram shows mass (**arrows**) adjacent to submandibular gland (SMG).

vide a better delineation of tumor extent, particularly retropharyngeal, axillary, and mediastinal extension.

Sonographically, carotid body tumors are highly vascular, and a high diastolic Doppler flow pattern in the external carotid artery is suggestive of their presence (**Fig. 51–14**).

Benefits of Ultrasound

The ability of sonography to detect small neck masses is unsurpassed by any other imaging method. Thyroid, parathyroid, and lymph node masses as small as 3- to 5-mm in size can be visualized by this sensitive technique. Because of the exquisite sensitivity of sonograpy in nodule detection, over 50% of patients with presumed solitary thyroid nodules on physical examination will have additional nodules detected sonographically.[66] Therefore, the presence of multiple nodules detected sonographically should not be presumed to have the same benign implications that it has with a less sensitive technique such as nuclear medicine. In one sonographic study of 259 thyroid nodules, 35% of 109 solitary nodules were malignant, but 26% of 150 nodules which were present in glands with multiple nodules were malignant as well.[67]

In the patient with a suspected thyroid nodule, ultrasound is most commonly used to confirm the presence of a nodule and guide FNA if the nodule is poorly palpable. Ultrasound is not commonly used to predict the histology of a nodule, but some sonographic features, as described earlier in this chapter (ultrasound Imaging-Thyroid), can suggest the nature of a thyroid nodule. The presence of punctate internal microcalcifications had a high positive predictive value for malignancy of 70% in one recent large study.[67] Punctate microcalcifications

should not be confused with the amorphous denser larger calcifications that are found in both benign and malignant lesions and which, therefore, are not specific for malignancy. The presence of a large internal cystic component is the best predictive feature of a benign thyroid nodule. The presence of punctate echogenic foci with posterior reverberation or comet-tail artifacts within the fluid has recently been reported. This feature has only been reported in benign nodules to date.[40]

The sensitivity of sonographic parathyroid adenoma localization in primary hyperparathyroidism varies, but most reports range between 70% and 85%.[38,46,68—71] Postoperatively, in patients with persistent or recurrent hyperparathyroidism, ultrasound can visualize up to 82% of abnormal parathyroid glands in the neck and 63% when all glands, including those in the mediastinum, are included.[72,73] Potential pitfalls in interpretation of these examinations include normal cervical structures, such as perithyroid veins, the esophagus, and the longus colli muscles of the neck, which can simulate parathyroid adenomas and produce false-positive results during neck sonography. Pathologic structures that are causes of false-positive results include thyroid nodules and cervical lymph nodes. The three major situations in which sonographic examinations for hyperparathyroidism give false-negative results are minimally enlarged adenomas, adenomas displaced posteriorly and obscured by a markedly enlarged thyroid goiter, and ectopic adenomas.

An outgrowth of the success of sonographically guided FNA of parathyroid adenomas is the use of sonography to guide percutaneous injections of ethanol to ablate abnormal, enlarged parathyroid glands (**Fig. 51–15**).[74—77] Currently, ethanol ablation most commonly is used postoperatively in patients with recurrent or persistent hyperparathyroidism who have a sonographically

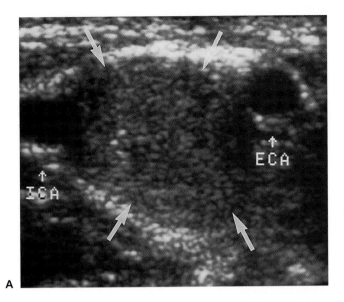

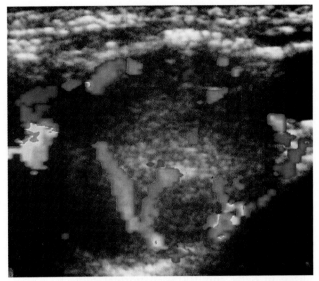

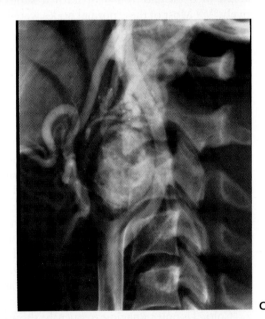

Figure 51–14 Carotid body tumor. **A:** Transverse sonogram of right neck shows a 2-cm solid mass (**arrows**) between internal carotid artery (ICA) and external carotid artery (ECA). **B:** Color Doppler imaging shows highly vascular nature of mass. **C:** Angiogram shows vascular mass situated in notch between internal and external carotid arteries.

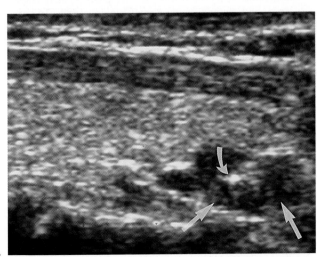

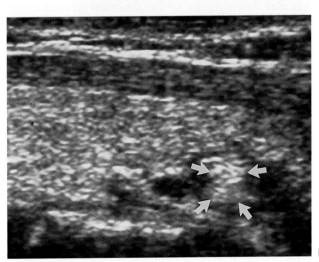

Figure 51–15 Ethanol ablation of parathyroid adenoma. **A:** Longitudinal sonogram of right neck shows 25-gauge needle (**curved arrow**) inserted into a 1.5-cm parathyroid adenoma (**straight arrows**). **B:** Injection of ethanol causes tissues surrounding the needle tip to become hyperechoic (**arrowheads**).

visualized, FNA biopsy-proven parathyroid adenoma but who are not good candidates for reoperation. This technique also is used as alternative therapy for the small number of patients with primary hyperparathyroidism who refuse surgical treatment, who are not good surgical candidates, or who present with an emergent life-threatening malignant hypercalcemia. The results of percutaneous injections of ethanol in patients with primary hyperparathyroidism have been encouraging. After long-term follow-up (mean, 39 months) of 11 patients, Karstrup et al.[74] concluded that partial or complete long-term remission of primary hyperparathyroidism could be achieved with ultrasound-guided chemical parathyroidectomy.

Cervical lymph nodes can be readily identified in normal individuals sonographically. In two large studies performed in Europe and China, lymph nodes were visualized in 67% and 100% of normal subjects, respectively.[48,78] Most of these normal nodes were identified in the submandibular, upper cervical, and posterior triangle regions. Nodes were less commonly visualized in other regions of the neck. In a separate study directed solely to the evaluation of supraclavicular lymph nodes, nodes were visualized in this location in 16% of normal subjects.[79]

Because of the high degree of accuracy and ease of performance of FNA of cervical lymph nodes, most studies that have studied the accuracy of sonography in the detection of malignant cervical adenopathy have combined the results of both ultrasound and ultrasound-guided FNA. In one large study which separated the imaging from the FNA results, ultrasound imaging alone had an accuracy of 80% in predicting malignancy in cervical lymph nodes on the basis of a minimal to maximal axial nodal diameter ratio of greater than 0.55.[80] When ultrasound-guided biopsy was added, the accuracy increased to 88%.

Color Doppler imaging frequently shows abnormal vascular flow patterns within abnormal cervical lymph nodes. One study found that 98% of malignant nodes showed an abnormal flow pattern, while only 6% of benign inflammatory disease showed an abnormal flow pattern.[81] Another similar study of flow patterns in cervical adenopathy, however, concluded that the specificity and sensitivity of power Doppler sonography cannot compare with those of FNA in the characterization of adenopathy.[82] Further studies will be necessary to determine the ultimate clinical utility of Doppler studies in the evaluation of cervical adenopathy.

Summary

The patient who presents with a palpable neck mass represents a diagnostic challenge for both the clinician and the radiologist. The differential diagnosis of a neck mass includes many pathologic processes and encompasses a large number of disease entities including congenital, inflammatory, neoplastic, and metabolic disorders. Therefore, the radiologist must follow a strategy of classifying masses by their anatomic location, which can aid in limiting the number of diagnostic possibilities. The sonographic features of the mass as well as the features of the mass by other imaging methods such as CT, MR, and scintigraphy can further narrow the diagnostic possibilities. FNA, performed either by palpation or ultrasound guidance, can obtain cytologic material which can provide a definitive diagnosis in many cases. Therefore, the combination of ultrasound and other imaging and nonimaging examinations such as FNA provides a wide variety of effective tools for the radiologist to use to evalute the palpable neck mass.

References

1. Som PM. Lymph nodes of the neck. *Radiology* 1987;165:593—600.
2. Roback SA, Telander RL. Thyroglossal duct cysts and brachial cleft anomalies. *Sem Pediatr Surg* 1994;3:142—146.
3. Som PM, Sacher M, Lanzieri CF, et al. Parenchymal cysts of the lower neck. *Radiology* 1985;157:399.
4. O'Hanlon DM, Walsh N, Corry J, et al. Aberrant thyroglossal cyst. *J Laryngol Otol* 1994;108:1105—1107.
5. Benson, MT, Dalen K, Mancuso AA, et al. Congenital anomalies of the branchial apparatus: embryology and pathologic anatomy. *RadioGraphics* 1992;12:943—960.
6. Golledge J, Ellis H. The etiology of lateral cervical (branchial) cysts: past and present theories. *J Laryngol Otol* 1994;108:653—659.
7. Choi SS, Zalzal GH. Branchial anomalies: a review of 52 cases. *Laryngoscope* 1995;105:909—913.
8. Shankar L, Josephson R, Hawke M. The branchial cleft cyst. *J Otolaryngol* 1991;20:62—64.
9. Loughran, CF. Case report: cystic lymph node metastasis from occult thyroid carcinoma: a sonographic mimic of a branchial cleft cyst. *Clin Radiol* 1991;43:213—214.
10. Zadvinskis DP, Benson MT, Kerr HH, et al. Congenital malformations of the cervicothoracic lymphatic system: embryology and pathogenesis. *RadioGraphics* 1992;12:1175—1189.
11. McCaffrey TV, Meyer FB, Michels VV, et al. Familial paragangliomas of the head and neck. *Arch Otolaryngol Head Neck Surg* 1994;120:1211—1216.
12. Filston HC. Hemangiomas, cystic hygromas, and teratomas of the head and neck. *Sem Pediatr Surg* 1994;3:147—159.
13. Miller MB, Rao VM, Tom BM. Cystic masses of the head and neck: pitfalls in CT and MR interpretation. *AJR* 1992;159:601—607.
14. Gharib H, Goellner JR. Fine-needle aspiration biopsy of the thyroid: an appraisal. *Ann Intern Med* 1993;118:282—289.
15. Goellner JR, Gharib H, Grant CS, et al: Fine needle aspiration cytology of the thyroid, 1980 to 1986. *ACTA Cytologica* 1987;31:587—590.
16. Yokozawa T, Miyauchi A, Kuma K, Sugawara M. Accurate and simple method of diagnosing thyroid nodules by the modified technique of ultrasound-guided fine needle aspiration biopsy. *Thyroid* 1995;5:141—149.
17. Woeber KA. Cost-effective evaluation of the patient with a thyroid nodule. *Surg Clin North Am* 1995;75:357—363.
18. Takashima S, Fukuda H, Kobayashi T. Thyroid nodules: clini-

cal effect of ultrasound-guided fine-needle aspiration biopsy. *J Clin Ultrasound* 1994;22:535—542.

19. Sanchez RB, van Sonnenberg E, D'Agosting HB, et al. Ultrasound-guided biopsy of nonpalpable and difficult to palpate thyroid masses. *J Amer Coll Surg* 1994;178:33—36.

20. Santos JEC, Leiman G. Nonaspiration fine needle cytology: application of a new technique to nodule thyroid disease. *ACTA Cytologica* 1988;32:353—356.

21. Bergenfelz A, Forsberg L, Hederstrom E, Ahren B. Preoperative localization of enlarged parathyroid glands with ultrasonically guided fine needle aspiration for parathyroid hormone assay. *ACTA Radiol* 1991;32:403—405.

22. Winkler B, Gooding GAW, Montgomery CK, et al. Immunoperoxidase confirmation of parathyroid origin of ultrasound-guided fine needle aspirates of the parathyroid glands. *ACTA Cytol* 1987;31:40—44.

23. Karstrup S, Glenthoj A, Hainau B, et al. Ultrasound-guided, histological, fine-needle biopsy from suspect parathyroid tumours: success-rate reliability of histologic diagnosis. *Br J Radiol* 1989;62:981—985.

24. Sacks BA, Pallotta JA, Cole A, Hurwitz J. Diagnosis of parathyroid adenomas: Efficacy of measuring parahormone levels in needle aspirates of cervical masses. *AJR* 1994;163:1223—1226.

25. van Overhagen H, Lameris JS, Berger MY, et al. Supraclavicular lymph node metastases in carcinoma of the esophagus and gastroesophageal junction: assessment with CT, US, and US-guided fine-needle aspiration biopsy. *Radiology* 1991;179:155—158.

26. Chang D, Yang PC, Yu CJ, et al. Ultrasonography and ultrasonographically guided fine-needle aspiration biopsy of impalpable cervical lymph nodes in patients with non-small cell lung cancer. *Cancer* 1992;70:1111—1114.

27. Sutton RT, Reading CC, Charboneau JW, et al. Ultrasound-guided biopsy of neck masses in postoperative management of patients with thyroid cancer. *Radiology* 1988;168:769—772.

28. Van Den Brekel MWM, Castelijins JA, Stel HV, et al. Occult metastatic neck disease: detection with ultrasound and ultrasound-guided fine needle aspiration cytology. *Radiology* 1991;180:457—461.

29. Takes RP, Knegt P, Manni JJ, et al. Regional metastasis in head and neck squamous cell carcinoma: revised value of ultrasound with ultrasound-guided fine needle aspiration biopsy. *Radiology* 1996;198:819—823.

30. Lee MJ, Ross DS, Mueller PR, et al. Fine needle biopsy of cervical lymph nodes in patients with thyroid cancer: a prospective comparison of cytopathologic and tissue marker analysis. *Radiology* 1993;187:851—854.

31. Billy HT, Rimkus DR, Hartzman S, Latimer RG. Technetium-99 m-Sestamibi single agent localization versus high-resolution ultrasonography for the preoperative localization of parathyroid glands in patients with primary hyperparathyroidism. *Am Surg* 1995;61:882—888.

32. Lee VS, Wilkinson RH, Leight GS, et al. Hyperparathyroidism in high-risk surgical patients: evaluation with double-phase technetium-99 m Sestamibi imaging. *Radiology* 1995;197:624—633.

33. Mukherji SK, Tart RP, Slattery WH. Evaluation of first branchial anomalies by CT and MR. *J Comp Assist Tomog* 1993;17:576—581.

34. Win T, Lewin JS. Imaging characteristics of carotid body tumors. *Am J Otolaryngol* 1995;16:325—328.

35. van Gils AP, van den Berg R, Falke TH, et al. MR diagnosis of paraganglioma of the head and neck: value of contrast enhancement. *AJR* 1994;162:147—153.

36. Kwekkeboom DJ, van Urk H, Pauw BK, et al. Octreotide scintigraphy for the detection of paragangliomas. *J Nuclear Med* 1993;34:873—878.

37. Solbiati L, Cioffi V, Ballarati E. Ultrasonography of the neck. *Radiol Clin North Am* 1992;30:941—954.

38. Gooding GA. Sonography of the thyroid and parathyroid. *Radiol Clin North Am* 1993;31:967—989.

39. Brkljacic B, Cuk V, Tomic-Brzac H, et al. Ultrasonic evaluation of benign and malignant nodules in echographically multinodular thyroids. *J Clin Ultrasound* 1994;22:71—76.

40. Ahuja A, Chick W, King CS, Metreweli C. Clinical significance of the comet-tail artifact in thyroid ultrasound. *J Clin Ultrasound* 1996;24:129—133.

41. Argalia G, D'Ambrosio F, Lucarelli F, et al. Doppler thyroid nodule characterization. *Radiol Med (Torino)* 1995;89:651—657.

42. Barreda R, Kaude JV, Fagein M, et al. Hypervascularity of nontoxic goiter as shown by color-coded Doppler sonography. *AJR* 1991;156:199.

43. Kerr L. High resolution thyroid ultrasound: the value of color Doppler. *Ultrasound Q* 1994;12:21—43.

44. Clark KJ, Cronan JJ, Scola FH. Color Doppler sonography: anatomic and physiologic assessment of the thyroid. *J Clin Ultrasound* 1995;23:215—223.

45. Shimamoto K, Endo T, Ishigaki T, et al. Thyroid nodules: evaluation with color Doppler ultrasonography. *J Ultrasound Med* 1993;12:673—678.

46. Reading CC, Charboneau JW, James EM, et al. High-resolution parathyroid sonography. *AJR* 1982;39:539—546.

47. Wolf RJ, Cronan JJ, Monchik JM. Color Doppler sonography: an adjunctive technique in assessment of parathyroid adenomas. *J Ultrasound Med* 1994;13:303—308.

48. Bruneton JN, Balu-Maestro C, Marcy PY, et al. Very high frequency (13 MHz) ultrasonographic examination of the normal neck. *J Ultrasound Med* 1994;13:87—90.

49. Evans, RM, Ahuja A, Metreweli C. The linear echogenic hilus in cervical lymphadenopathy — a sign of benignity or malignancy? *Clin Radiol* 1993;47:262—264.

50. Vassallo P, Wernecke K, Roos N, et al. Differentiation of benign from malignant superficial lymphadenopathy: the role of high-resolution ultrasound. *Radiology* 1992;183:215—220.

51. Rubaltelli L, Proto E, Salmaso R, et al. Sonography of abnormal lymph nodes in vitro. *AJR* 1990;155:1241—1244.

52. Thnosu N, Onoda S, Isono K. Ultrasonographic evaluation of cervical lymph node metastases in esophageal cancer with special reference to the relationship between the short to long axis ration (S/L) and the cancer content. *J Ultrasound Med* 1989;17:101—107.

53. Ahuja AT, Chow L, Chick W, et al. Metastatic cervical nodes in papillary carcinoma of the thyroid: ultrasound and histologic correlation. *Clin Radiol* 1995;50:229—231.

54. Chang D, Yuan A, Yu CJ, et al. Differentiation of benign and malignant cervical lymph nodes with color Doppler sonography. *AJR* 1994;162:965—968.

55. Wadsworth DT, Siegel MJ. Thyroglossal duct cysts: variability of sonographic findings. *AJR* 1994;163:1475—1477.

56. Pinczower E., Crockett DM, Atkinson JB, et al. Preoperative thyroid scanning in presumed thyroglossal duct cysts. *Arch Otolaryngol Head Neck Surg* 1992;118:985—988.

57. Lim-Dunham JE, Feinstein KA, Yousefzadeh DK, et al. Sonographic demonstration of a normal thyroid gland excludes ectopic thyroid in patients with thyroglossal duct cyst. *AJR* 1995;164:1489—1491.

58. Hilger AW, Thompson SD, Smallman LA, et al. Papillary carcinoma arising in a thyroglossal duct cyst: a case report and literature review. *J Laryngol Otol* 1995;109:1124—1127.

59. Deshpande A, Bobhate SK. Squamous cell carcinoma in thyroglossal duct cyst. *J Laryngol Otol* 1995;109:1001—1004.

60. Woods RH, Saunders JR Jr, Perlman S, et al. Anaplastic carcinoma arising in a thyroglossal duct tract. *Otolaryngol Head Neck Surg* 1993;109:945—949.

61. Van Vuuren PA, Balm AJ, Gregor RT, et al. Carcinoma arising in thyroglossal remnants. *Clin Otolaryngol* 1994;19:509—515.

62. Boswell WC, Zoller M, Williams JS, et al. Thyroglossal duct carcinoma. *Am Surg* 1994;60:650—655.

63. Reynolds JH, Wolinski AP. Sonographic appearance of branchial cysts. *Clin Radiol* 1993;48:109—110.

64. Baatenburg de Jong RJ, Rongen RJ, Lameris JS, et al. Evaluation of branchiogenic cysts by ultrasound. *ORL J Otorhinolaryngol Relat Spec* 1993;55:294–298.

65. Borecky N, Gudinchet F, Laurini R, et al. Imaging of cervicothoracic lymphangiomas in children. *Pediatric Radiology* 1995;25:127—130.

66. Tan GH, Charib H. Reading CC. Solitary thyroid nodule. comparison between palpation and ultrasonography. *Arch Intern Med* 1995;155:2418—2423.

67. Takashima S, Fukuda H, Nomura N, et al. Thyroid nodules: reevaluation with ultrasound. *J Clin Ultrasound* 1995;23:179—184.

68. Kohri K, Ishikawa Y, Kodama M, et al. Comparison of imaging methods for localization of parathyroid tumors. *Am J Surg* 1992;164:140—145.

69. Weinberger MS, Robbins KT. Diagnostic localization studies for primary hyperparathyroidism: a suggested algorithm. *Arch Otolaryngol Head Neck Surg* 1994;120:1187—1189.

70. Rodriquez JM, Tezelman S, Siperstein AE, et al. Localization procedures in patients with persistent or recurrent hyperparathyroidism. *Arch Surg* 1994;129:870—875.

71. Mitchell BK, Merrell RC, Kinder BK. Localization studies in patients with hyperparathyroidism. *Surg Clin North Am* 1995;75:483—498.

72. Reading CC, Charboneau JW, James EM, et al. Postoperative parathyroid high-frequency sonography: evaluation of persistent or recurrent hyperparathyroidism. *AJR* 1985;144:399–402.

73. Grant CS, van Heerden JA, Charboneau JW, James EM, Reading CC. Clinical management of persistent and/or recurrent primary hyperparathyroidism. *World J Surg* 1986 ;10:555–565.

74. Karstrup S, Hegedus L, Holm HH. Ultrasonically guided chemical parathyroidectomy in patients with primary hyperparathyroidism: a follow-up study. *Clin Endocrinol (Oxf)* 1993;38:523–530.

75. Solbiati L, Giangrande A, De Pra L, et al. Percutaneous ethanol injection of parathyroid tumors under US guidance: treatment for secondary hyperparathyroidism. *Radiology* 1985;155:607–610.

76. Karstrup S, Transbol I, Holm HH, Glenthoj A, Hegedus L. Ultrasound-guided chemical parathyroidectomy in patients with primary hyperparathyroidism: a prospective study. *Br J Radiol* 1989;62:1037–1042.

77. Kitaoka M, Fukagawa M, Ogata E, Kurokawa K. Reduction of functioning parathyroid cell mass by ethanol injection in chronic dialysis patients. *Kidney Int* 1994;46:1110–1117.

78. Ying M, Ahuja A, Brook F, Brown B, Metreweli C. Sonographic appearance and distribution of normal cervical lymph nodes in a Chinese population. *J Ultrasound Med* 1996;15:431—436.

79. Tsunoda-Shimizu H, Saida Y. Ultrasonographic visibility of supraclavicular lymph nodes in normal subjects. *J Ultrasound Med* 1997;16:481—483.

80. Takashima S, Sone S, Nomura N, et al. Nonpalpable lymph nodes of the neck: assessment with US and US-guided fine-needle aspiration biopsy. *J Clin Ultrasound* 1997;25(6):283—292.

81. Na DG, Lim HK, Byun HS, et al. Differential diagnosis of cervical lymphadenopathy: usefulness of color Doppler sonography. *AJR* 1997;168:1311—1316.

82. Giovagnorio F, Caiazzo R, Avitto A. Evaluation of vascular patterns of cervical lymph nodes with power Doppler sonography. *J Clin Ultrasound* 1997;25:71—76.

52 The Breast Nodule: Sonographic Characterization

Christopher R.B. Merritt

Mammography is currently the most sensitive method for detection of preclinical breast carcinoma. Unfortunately, its specificity is poor and many abnormalities identified by mammography require biopsy to determine whether they are benign or malignant. In North America, intraductal or invasive cancers are found in only 10—35% of referrals for biopsy based on mammographic findings.[1—3] As an adjunct to mammography, ultrasound makes a significant contribution to the evaluation and management of patients with abnormalities detected by mammographic screening. As a result of improvements in ultrasound instrumentation and the introduction of new sonographic methods, including color and power Doppler, the role of breast ultrasound has been extended well beyond the traditional tasks of differentiation of cystic and solid masses and guidance for aspiration and biopsy. Today, ultrasound, when used with mammography, aids in the differentiation of benign and malignant masses and in the selection of patients for biopsy (**Fig. 52–1**).[4] Carefully controlled studies performed under strict protocols have shown the ability of modern ultrasound instruments to add both sensitivity and specificity to mammography in the characterization of breast masses (**Fig. 52–2**). Because as many as 65—90% of women referred by mammography for breast biopsy prove to have benign disease, the use of ultrasound to identify benign lesions may markedly reduce the number of unnecessary breast biopsies. In this setting, ultrasound, being both inexpensive and noninvasive, makes a major contribution to patient care.

Attempts to use ultrasound to differentiate benign from malignant breast tissues date to the very beginning of diagnostic medical ultrasonography. Investigations in ultrasound by Wild and Reid 5 and Howry et al. in the early 1950s were underway at about the same time that mammography was beginning to be recognized as a reliable method for identification of malignant breast lesions.[5,6] During the 1960s work continued to develop instruments to overcome the peculiar challenges of imaging the breast with ultrasound, namely, those of coupling sonic energy to the breast, and problems with spatial and contrast resolution related to the thickness and acoustical inhomogeneity of breast tissue.[7] During these years the attenuation characteristics of a variety of breast lesions were observed, including cysts, fibroadenomas, and carcinomas. In the mid 1970s, following the introduction of gray scale display and real-time imaging, breast ultrasound attracted serious clinical attention, and by the early 1980s commercial systems designed specifically for breast imaging were being actively promoted to the medical community. These automated systems allowed systematic evaluation of the entire breast, usually with the patient prone with the breasts suspended in a water bath.[8] Confusion regarding the re-

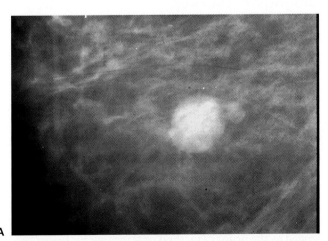

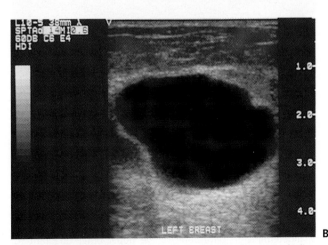

A B

Figure 52–1 Simple cyst. Mammography (**A**) reveals a circumscribed nodule with benign features, but cannot differentiate a simple cyst from a complicated cyst or solid mass. Ultrasound (**B**) of the lesion shows classical features of a benign simple cyst, including anechoic matrix, thin, smooth wall, and acoustical enhancement.

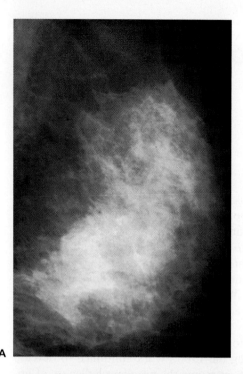

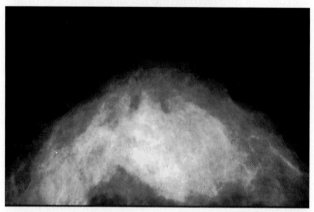

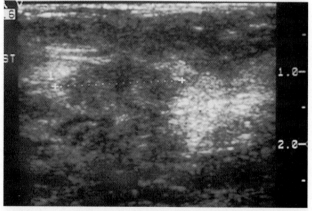

Figure 52–2 Dense breast with palpable mass. Mammograms were requested to evaluate a palpable fullness in the upper outer quadrant of the breast. The mammogram (**A, B**) shows dense breast parenchyma. In the area of the palpable abnormality only mild architectural distortion was present (Level of suspicion (LOS) = 3, indeterminate). Ultrasound of the upper outer quadrant (**C**) shows a solid mass with irregular margins and central attenuation indicating malignancy (LOS = 5, definitely malignant). Excision confirmed presence of infiltrating carcinoma.

spective roles of ultrasound and mammography and the unrealistic promotion of ultrasound as a screening modality in the early 1980s resulted in considerable uncertainty in the radiology community as to the true place, if any, of ultrasound in the evaluation of the breast. Fortunately, this uncertainty has been replaced by an appreciation of the valuable contributions of modern ultrasound to the evaluation of patients with breast disease.

Compared with earlier scanners, modern ultrasound instruments display significant improvements in image quality when used to examine the breast. Excellent contrast and spatial resolution, as well as sensitive methods to evaluate tumor neovascularity, have expanded the role of ultrasonography in the evaluation of breast nodules. In addition to allowing highly reliable characterization of masses as solid or cystic, recent studies have shown that ultrasound, when used with mammography, aids in the characterization of solid masses as benign or malignant.[9] Analysis of contour, margins, matrix, and attenuation of solid nodules permits confident identification of many benign nodules and provides the option of follow-up rather than biopsy. This leads, in turn, to reduced cost, reduced physical and emotional trauma for patients, and reduced scarring of breast tissue from biopsy.

Today, with issues regarding the safety and efficacy of mammography for screening largely resolved, the place of ultrasonography in the imaging approach to breast disease is better defined. In most breast centers ultrasonography is viewed as essential for the complete evaluation of patients with breast disease and should be available wherever mammography is provided. To obtain the full benefits of the capabilities of modern ultrasound in the evaluation of the breast a knowledge of the rationale, indications, examination techniques, and diagnostic criteria for the characterization of breast nodules is required. Each of these topics will be explored in the following pages.

Diagnostic Workup

Rationale

The imaging evaluation of women at risk for breast cancer has two important and distinct goals — screening and diagnosis.[10] The purpose of screening is to exclude an abnormality in the population at risk. The function of diagnosis is to determine the nature of an abnormality. For screening, high sensitivity is required to detect asymptomatic disease, and a reasonably high false-positive rate is acceptable. To encourage use, a screening test should also be safe, noninvasive, and of reasonable cost. Mammography fulfills these criteria and, when performed using modern dedicated equipment, is unchallenged as the primary method of screening for breast carcinoma. For diagnosis, mammography fares less well, particularly in the absence of the classical mammographic changes of malignancy. Despite its excellent sensitivity, mammography alone is not capable of resolving many common clinical problems that arise in evaluation of the breast. This limitation results from the relatively nonspecific nature of many mammographic findings, and from the decreased sensitivity of mammography in the identification of abnormalities in breasts that are extremely dense. It is in these settings that ultrasonography may provide its major contributions by adding diagnostic specificity.

Because ultrasound is based on acoustical principles, ultrasound images possess totally different (and often complementary) information from mammograms. This allows ultrasound to accurately characterize masses as solid or cystic and aids in the differentiation of some benign and malignant masses. In addition, ultrasound produces tomographic images, eliminating the problems associated with the superimposition of dense breast structures encountered with mammography. Ultrasound is not impeded by the presence of breast implants to the same extent as mammography. Finally, Doppler ultrasound permits detection and, to some extent, the characterization of the blood flow to masses. This gives ultrasound several distinct advantages over mammography in differentiation of breast abnormalities and where clarification of findings is required. Disadvantages of ultrasound include problems in imaging the fatty breast and limitations in detecting microcalcifications. Mammography, on the other hand, is superior to ultrasound in the detection and characterization of microcalcifications, particularly if no mass is present, and has a proven role in screening. The selective use of complementary methods of diagnosis including mammography, ultrasonography, as well as clinical examination, aspiration, and biopsy provides the greatest opportunity to obtain the most accurate and clinically relevant information for patient management. The advantages of such a multimodality approach are summarized in **Table 52–1**.

Properly used, breast ultrasound can contribute to efficient patient management by reducing or eliminating delays in reaching a specific diagnosis. If the ultrasound findings are suspicious for malignancy and the clinical or mammographic findings are indeterminate, the ultrasound will encourage biopsy and reduce the likelihood that a negative mammographic report will result in delay in biopsy of a lesion. Conversely, clearly benign sonographic features may eliminate the need for an unnecessary aspiration or biopsy of benign pathology. In making management decisions regarding biopsy, aspiration, and follow-up, the addition of ultrasound often allows greater confidence in either a positive or negative conclusion and provides information necessary for clinical management which is tailored to the patient.

Table 52–1   Rationale for a multimodality approach to breast evaluation

Eliminates of delay in reaching a specific diagnosis
Reduces of the likelihood that a negative mammographic report will result in delay in biopsy of a lesion
Eliminates of unnecessary aspiraton or biopsy
Encourages biopsy of a lesion on mammography that otherwise might be ignored
Provides information which is qualitatively different from mammography and is often complementary
Allows greater confidence in either a positive or negative conclusion
Provides information necessary for clinical management
Permits the evaluation to be tailored to the patient

Patient Selection and Indications

Patients selected for breast ultrasound should be those in whom ultrasound is likely to add information useful for management. Conditions in which the information provided by ultrasound is likely to have little impact on management or disease outcome should be excluded. In most cases, the management question is whether or not biopsy of an abnormality is warranted. An additional management decision is whether biopsy should be performed by aspiration, core sampling, or surgical excision. A final issue relates to defining specific areas that warrant biopsy or excision. Indications for ultrasound of the breast are summarized in **Table 52–2**.

Table 52–2   Indications for ultrasound of the breast

To characterize of breast masses in terms of level of suspicion for malignancy
Indeterminate masses found by mammography
Palpable masses not detected on mammography
To evaluate of equivocal mammographic or clinical findings
To complement mammography in patients with dense breast parenchyma
For initial evaluation of patients with dense breasts who are less than 30 years old
To provide localization for biopsy or aspiration

Ultrasound Imaging

Instrumentation and Technique

The quality of diagnostic information available for interpretation and management decision-making is highly related to the performance of the instrument used for the examination and the skill of the examiner in using the equipment to its maximum capability. Management decisions regarding breast abnormalities can only be made with confidence if images with adequate spatial, contrast, and temporal resolution are obtained.

Duplex and color Doppler require high flow sensitivity. Recently, significant improvements in ultrasound image quality have been introduced into practice. These include the use of broad bandwidth technology to improve both contrast and spatial resolution of the ultrasound image, as well as new methods to evaluate tumor neovascularity.

For breast imaging, a scanner operating at a frequency of 7.0 MHz or greater with adjustable focus and flexible image processing is required. High-resolution real-time scanners operating at these frequencies allow evaluation of masses as small as 2—4 mm within the breast and under ideal conditions are capable of showing submillimeter margin features that are important in identifying invasion (**Fig. 52–3**). Linear array and mechanical or electronically steered sector scanners may be used, although the larger near-field coverage of a linear array transducer is an advantage. Ultrasound instruments with excellent small parts imaging capability are available in most radiology departments and are ideal for breast imaging applications.

A standardized examination protocol should be used for ultrasound examination of the breast. This protocol should address patient positioning, transducer selection, and image processing including dynamic range, pre- and postprocessing, focal zone placement, standardized views, measurements, and image labeling. Positioning for the examination should elevate the shoulder and upper chest on the side being examined so that the breast being examined is flattened against the chest wall by gravity. This results in a more uniform thickness of the tissues being examined. Standard and consistently used positioning for breast ultrasound is essential for correlating the location of mammographic abnormalities with those observed with ultrasound and for serial follow-up of abnormalities.

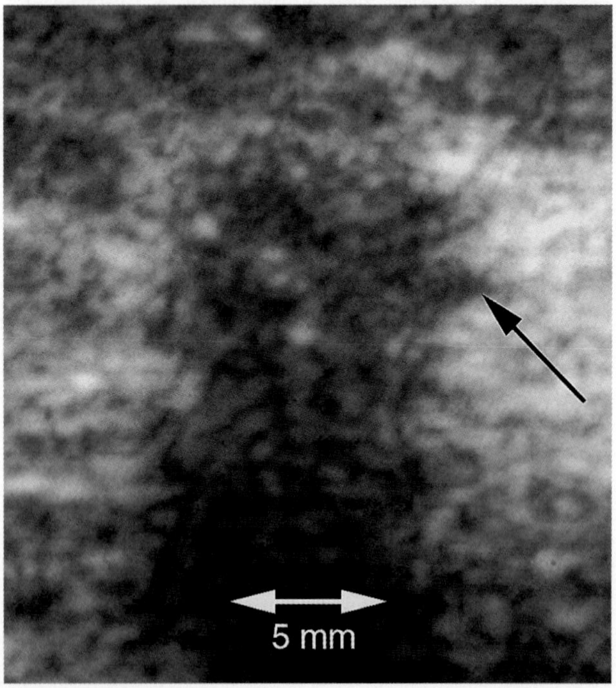

For reliable application of diagnostic criteria and comparison in follow-up studies, the transducer(s) used for breast examination should be standardized, along with instrument presets for dynamic range (a wide dynamic range of 55—65 dB is preferred) along with standard settings for preprocessing and image display postprocessing. If the instrumentation used does not have adequate near-field resolution, the use of a standoff may be required as a routine part of the imaging protocol.

The complex nature of breast tissue and its interaction with ultrasound make the adjustment of system gain and Time Gain Compensation (TGC) settings especially critical. Gain and TGC must be carefully adjusted throughout the examination to reject noise without eliminating any low-level signal that may contribute to diagnosis. When Doppler (either duplex or color) is used, standardized pulse repetition frequencies, wall filter, and display parameters must be used to permit comparison and follow-up. Likewise a consistent approach to the placement of focal zone(s), lesion measurements, and image annotation must be used.

Diagnostic Criteria

To obtain maximum benefit from ultrasound in the evaluation of breast pathology, standardized criteria based on lesion features including shape, orientation, margin definition, margin regularity, matrix echogenicity and homogeneity, and attenuation should be used and applied in a consistent fashion. In addition to lesion features, findings of architectural distortion, retraction or angulation of Cooper ligaments, and changes in the skin, subcutaneous fat, and retromammary fascia must be recorded as well. The matrix should be described as anechoic, hypoechoic, or hyperechoic relative to the surrounding breast tissue (**Fig. 52–4**). The margin should be described as well- or poorly-defined and smooth or irregular, taking particular note of subtle irregularities such as spiculation (**Fig. 52–3**), microlobulation (**Fig. 52–5**) and poor border definition (**Fig. 52–6**). Orientation of the mass to the skin surface with respect to its long axis should be described, and the degree to which the lesion attenuates or enhances sound transmission should also be noted along with whether attenuation is central or confined to the edges of the mass (**Fig. 52–7—52–8**). Diagnostic criteria for common benign and malignant breast lesions are summarized in **Table 52–3**.

Figure 52–3 High resolution ultrasound. A nonpalpable 8 mm solid breast mass with central attenuation is shown. Detail of the margin of the mass reveals tiny angular irregularities extending from the mass (arrow) in this 10 MHz image. These features indicate infiltration of fat by malignant tumor sond are characteristic of many invasive breast cancers.

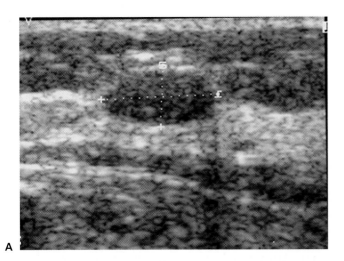

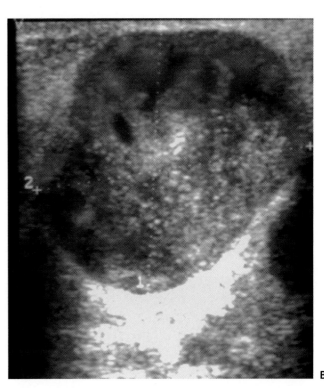

Figure 52–4 Lesion matrix. The homogenous matrix of a benign fibroadenoma (**A**) is compared with the inhomogeneous matrix of carcinoma (**B**). The cancer contains areas of hypoechoic necrosis as well as multiple microcalcifications. The presence of a homogenous matrix does not exclude malignancy as some breast cancers may be very homogeneous. On the other hand, a heterogeneous lesion should always be viewed with suspicion.

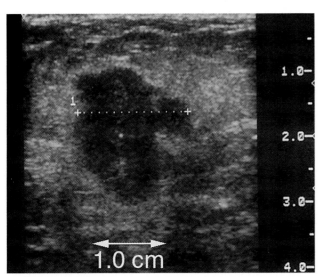

Figure 52–5 Lobulation and microlobulation. Ultrasound of a palpable abnormality shows an 18 mm mildly inhomogeneous lobulated mass without significant attenuation. In addition to its generally irregular shape, the margin contains subtle microlobulations which are indicators of malignancy (LOS = 4, probably malignant). Biopsy revealed an invasive ductal carcinoma. This mass was not seen on mammography.

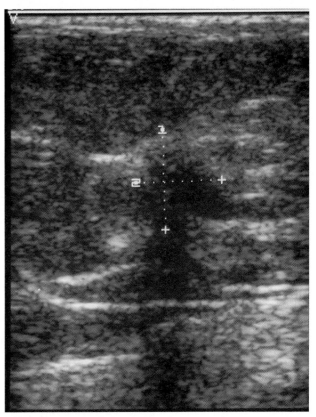

Figure 52–6 Indistinct margins. An irregular mass is shown with a hypoechoic matrix and central attenuation. The mass is not clearly delineated and the margins are indistinct. Any solid mass with indistinct margins is suspicious for malignancy (LOS = 4, probably malignant). Biopsy revealed an invasive ductal carcinoma.

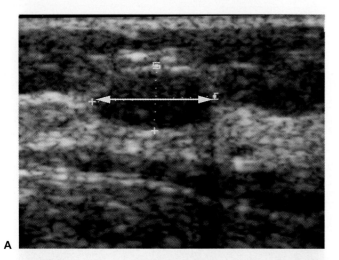

A

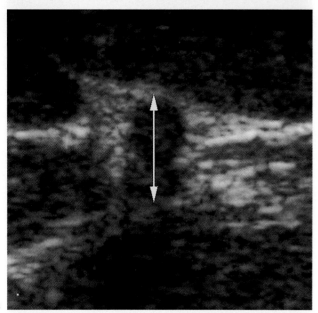

B

Figure 52–7   Lesion Orientation. Parallel orientation of the long axis of a benign fibroadenoma to the surface is shown in (**A**). The mass has a homogenous matrix, smooth regular margins, and insignificant central attenuation. A parallel orientation is more typical of benign than malignant lesions and, in association with the margin, matrix, and attenuating characteristics indicates a benign etiology (LOS = 2, probably benign) consistent with fibroadenoma. This diagnosis was confirmed by biopsy. Contrast this to **Figure 52-7 B** in which the lesion is oriented with its long axis perpendicular to the surface. Subtle margin irregularities are present along with minimal central attenuation, indicating malignancy (LOS = 4, probably malignant). Biopsy confirmed invasive carcinoma.

Cysts

Cysts are among the most common breast nodules, accounting for approximately 25% of masses found on mammography.[11] Cysts may arise as a product of ductal hyperplasia or may result from accumulation of inspissated milk (galactoceles) or in association with intraductal papillomas and fat necrosis. Cysts vary in size from less than 2 mm (microcysts) to several centimeters in diameter. With high-resolution scanners, cysts as small as 2 mm in diameter may be identified. Ultrasound is highly reliable in the identification of cysts, with accuracy approaching 100% if strict criteria for diagnosis are met. These include a round or oval shape and an anechoic matrix (unless complicated by bleeding or infection). Artifacts related to excessive gain or improper placement of focal zone may create the appearance of low-level echoes within a simple cyst and must be avoided. These problems are more common with small cysts where slice thickness and side lobe artifacts may also contribute to the generation of echoes within the cyst. The walls of a cyst are clearly defined and the margins smooth and regular (**Fig. 52–1**). Acoustical enhancement should be seen deep to the cyst, although refractive edge shadows are common. Depending on the tension of fluid within the cyst, the mass may be somewhat compressible, in contrast to solid masses which are generally not compressible. Because cysts are extremely common, the use of ultrasound to identify these may reduce the need for further investigation, including aspiration or biopsy.

Benign Solid Nodules

Sonographic features of benign solid masses in the breast include smooth regular margins, acoustical enhancement, ovoid or spherical shape and parallel orientation to skin surface. Fibroadenomas are the most common benign breast neoplasms. Incidence is highest in late adolescence and early adulthood. It is believed that most growth of fibroadenomas occurs at an early stage with later quiescence and frequent persistence into the menopause. In older women calcification is common. Typical fibroadenomas consist of epithelial tissue similar to normal ducts and fibrous or myxoid stromal com-

Table 52–3   Ultrasound criteria for diagnosis of common breast lesions

Sign	Cyst	Fibroadenoma	Ductal carcinoma	Medullary carcinoma
Margin	Smooth	Smooth	Irregular	Slightly irregular
—	Thin	Thin	Poorly defined	—
—	Well defined	Well defined	Angular	—
Shape	Spherical	Ovoid	Variable	Variable
Orientation	Parallel	Parallel	Not parallel	Not parallel
Matrix	Anechoic	Hypoechoic	Mixed	Hypoechoic
Attenuation	Little	Some	Much	Some
Shadowing	Edge	Edge	Central	Varies
Enhancement	Much	Sometimes	No	Minimal
Distortion	No	No	Yes	No

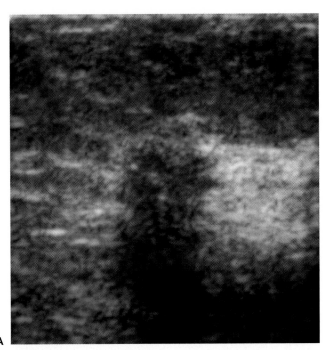

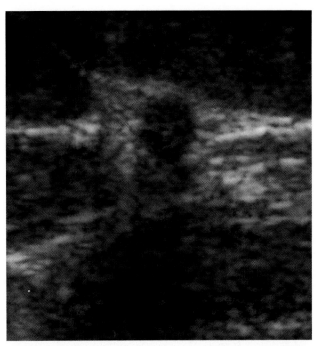

A

B

Figure 52–8   Attenuation. Small carcinomas producing central attenuation are shown. Central acoustical shadowing and poor definition of the deep margin is common with malignant nodules. The 8 mm cancer shown in (**A**) also has an irregular margin indicating invasion (LOS = 5, malignant). Biopsy confirmed an invasive car- cinoma. In (**B**) the malignant features are more subtle. In addition to central attenuation, the lesion shows nonparallel orientation of its long axis to the surface and microlobulation (LOS = 4, probably malignant). A diagnosis of invasive ductal carcinoma was confirmed by excisional biopsy.

ponents. The masses are usually spherical or ovoid in shape and are encapsulated with smooth margins. The matrix is usually homogenous with low-amplitude echoes unless calcification has occurred (**Fig. 52–9**). Depending on the attenuation characteristics of the matrix and surrounding tissues, there may be slight acoustical enhancement or slight shadowing deep to the mass. Refractive edge shadows are a common feature. Cystosarcoma phylloides or giant fibroadenomas have sonographic features that may resemble fibroadenomas. Cystic areas within the mass may be present. Cystosarcoma phylloides is uncommon and may be found at any age. The masses may grow rapidly, causing increase in breast size.

Fibrocystic Condition

With ultrasound, highly echogenic areas of fibrous reaction containing small cysts or dilated ducts are shown. In some cystic masses low-level echoes may be present. These are most often associated with galactocele, but may occur when there is bleeding or infection involving a simple cyst. Intraductal papillomas may cause duct obstruction, giving rise to cystic lesions. With ultrasound the characteristic features include a cystic mass containing an intracystic mass (intracystic papilloma). Bleeding may result in the appearance of low-level echoes or debris within the cyst.

Malignant Nodules

The most characteristic feature of a malignant breast nodule is that of irregular margins with spiculation or microlobulation (**Fig. 52–3, 52–5**). These features indicate invasion and are similar to characteristic mammographic signs of malignancy. In contrast to most benign lesions in which the long axis lies parallel to the skin surface, malignant lesions are more likely to be oriented with their long axis perpendicular to the surface (**Fig. 52–7**). Typically ductal cancers have inhomogenous internal echoes and moderate to marked central attenuation (**Fig. 52–8**). The attenuation of breast cancers is thought to be related to the amount of fibrous reaction accompanying the tumor. Thus scirrhous cancers tend to be more attenuating than those that have relatively little fibrous reaction. Although shadowing is common with carcinoma, it is not specific and may be seen with scarring as well as large calcifications accompanying some benign nodules. In contrast to scirrhous carcinoma, medullary carcinomas often show only mild attenuation, and in some cases may exhibit slight acoustical enhancement. These tumors tend to have margins that are less clearly defined than with fibroadenomas, which have similar transmission properties. Cystic carcinomas are uncommon, although it is estimated that 1—2% of breast carcinomas will appear cystic. The finding of a cyst with irregular borders or wall irregularities, internal debris, or an adjacent nodule or mass warrants suspi-

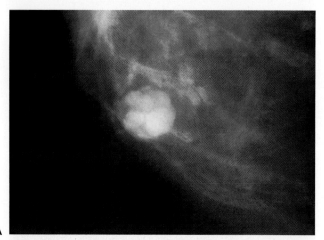

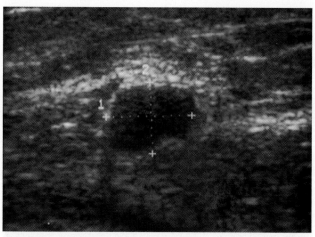

Figure 52–9 Fibroadenoma. Mammography (**A**) reveals a circumscribed lobulated mass (LOS = 2, probably benign). Ultrasound (**B**) shows typical features of a fibroadenoma with a smooth well-defined margin, homogenous matrix, parallel orientation and refractive edge shadowing. (LOS = 2, probably benign).

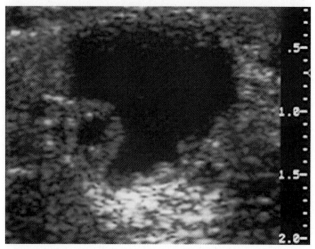

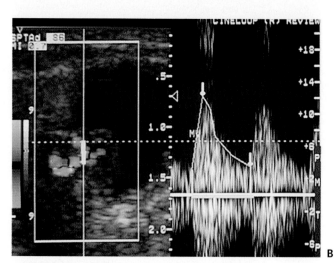

Figure 52–10 Cystic cancer. Real time ultrasound (**A**) reveals a cystic mass with acoustical enhancement. The wall is poorly defined and is slightly irregular, with a prominent mural nodule. Doppler (**B**) provides further evidence of malignancy, showing the mural nodule to be highly vascular.

cion, and the diagnosis of a simple cyst should be avoided (**Fig. 52–10**). Ultrasound can assist in differentiation of benign and malignant solid masses, and sonographic demonstration of the typical features of carcinoma have a high positive predictive value.

Recent studies have shown benefit in using a scoring system based on lesion features and odds ratios of benign or malignant etiology to characterize masses in terms of levels of suspicion (LOS).[12] Using this approach, masses may be categorized as benign (LOS = 1), probably benign (LOS = 2), indeterminate (LOS = 3), probably malignant (LOS = 4), and definitely malignant (LOS = 5). This classification, coupled with the mammographic level of suspicion, aids in reaching confident decisions regarding biopsy or follow-up (**Fig. 52–11— 52–12**).

The Role of Doppler in the Evaluation of Breast Lesions

In tumors, growth of new capillaries occurs as a result of tumor angiogenesis factors. The importance of angiogenesis in tumor development has been appreciated for many years. Doppler methods permit the evaluation of tumor vascularity. Doppler characteristics of tumor neovascularity include high-flow velocity and low vascular impedance due to arteriovenous shunting. Doppler ultrasound has been used to evaluate breast cancers for over 15 years with varying success.[13–15] Following early observations using continuous wave (CW) Doppler, there have been numerous reports of the association of characteristic Doppler findings associated with benign and malignant breast masses. These include Dop-

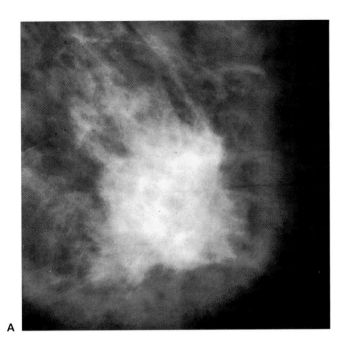

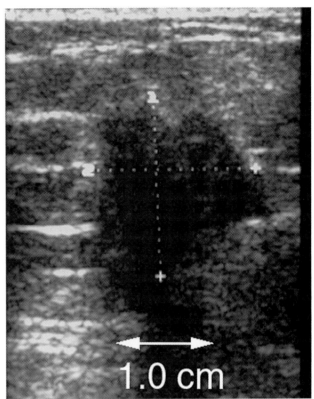

Figure 52–11 Mammographic and sonographic correlation. The mammogram (**A**) reveals dense breast tissue with an area of architectural distortion which was regarded as indeterminate (LOS = 3, indeterminate). Ultrasound of the area (**B**) shows an irregular mass with lobulated and ill defined margins, central attenuation, nonparallel orientation, and inhomogeneous matrix, resulting in a LOS = 5, definitely malignant. Biopsy confirmed the presence of an infiltrating cancer.

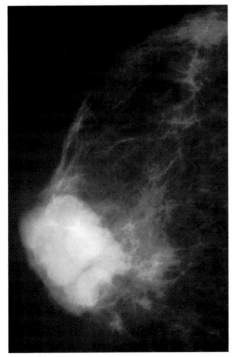

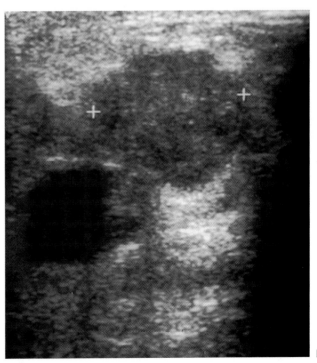

Figure 52–12 Cyst and cancer. Mammographic and clinical findings (**A**) were felt to represent cystic disease. Aspiration confirmed presence of cysts suggesting a benign process (LOS = 2, probably begin). After cyst aspiration, some residual fullness was present, prompting sonography. The ultrasound (**B**) shows a solid mass adjacent to a cyst. The mass has a homogenous matrix, enhancement and parallel orientation, but the margins are irregular and poorly defined, resulting in a LOS = 5, malignant. Biopsy was positive for an invasive cancer.

pler waveforms associated with arteriovenous shunting and low-impedance vasculature, as well as color Doppler patterns of increased flow in and around tumors. Doppler analysis contributes to improved specificity in breast lesion evaluation (**Fig. 52–10**). At the present time, ultrasound imaging is the mainstay of breast ultrasound, and the role of Doppler evaluation is still evolving.

Benefits of Ultrasound

The most important indication for breast ultrasound is the presence of a mass within the breast. This includes both lesions seen on mammography as well as palpable masses not shown with mammography. In some settings as many as 8—10% of all patients referred for mammography have masses that may benefit from ultrasound evaluation. The role of ultrasound is first to characterize the mass as solid or cystic, a determination which mammography cannot achieve (**Fig. 52–1**). Because many masses found with mammography will be cysts, ultrasonography can provide a specific diagnosis avoiding an equivocal mammographic report. The positive predictive value for ultrasound in the identification of cysts approaches 100%, provided strict adherence to the classical sonographic characteristics of a cyst are observed. If the mass is not cystic, its sonographic features, along with the mammographic findings, may be used to generate a level of suspicion for malignancy and determine whether follow-up or biopsy is necessary.

When a patient has a palpable mass which is not visible on mammography due to dense breast tissue, ultrasound is of particular value (**Fig. 52–2**). Rather than issuing a negative mammographic report, the radiologist can report the nature of the mass as solid or cystic, along with a differential diagnosis if the lesion is solid or complex. Ultrasound may thus prevent the unfortunate failure to biopsy a significant palpable lesion because the mammographic report is "negative". When ultrasound is used with mammography in the diagnostic evaluation of a breast nodule, all important information necessary for management can be reported to the referring clinician.

A second indication for ultrasound mammography is a patient with equivocal mammographic or clinical findings. With ultrasound, cysts as small as 2 mm in size can be identified in a dense glandular background, permitting recognition of localized areas of fibrocystic change producing clinical or mammographic abnormalities. In lactating women, and in women with extremely dense breasts or implants, whole breast ultrasound may improve the confidence in interpretation by allowing a more thorough inspection of the breast parenchyma than is possible using mammography. Finally, in young women, less than 30 years of age, the density of breast parenchyma usually renders mammography unsatis-

factory. In these patients, ultrasound, which performs well in the dense breast, may provide more information than mammography and is often preferred as the initial imaging method. Most masses will be detected by ultrasound; however, microcalcifications may go undetected if a mass is not present. In the very dense breast, mammography and ultrasonography are truly complementary. Masses are occasionally felt or imaged with mammography and not seen on ultrasound, or the converse may occur. In a series of breast cancers studied with dedicated ultrasound and mammography, 14 of 186 cancers were seen with ultrasound but not mammography, due to superimposition of tissue, dense parenchyma, or a lesion lying close to the chest wall.[16] The main limitation of ultrasound is encountered in the fatty breast, where differentiation of small hypoechoic masses from hypoechoic fat lobules is difficult. Fortunately, mammography generally provides excellent information in this environment.

Another important application of ultrasound in breast diagnosis is in the localization of breast lesions for biopsy or aspiration.[17] Successful localization of nonpalpable abnormalities requires accurate three-dimensional information related to the location of the abnormality. Ultrasound permits accurate three-dimensional location of the abnormality if the lesion is visible. If lesions are not evident with sonography, then conventional mammographic methods using compression grid techniques may be used if the lesion is visible in more than one view or stereotactic devices may be employed. If a lesion is visible with ultrasound it usually can be localized more conveniently with ultrasound than with other methods. Real-time ultrasound guidance is rapid and highly effective, permitting high accuracy and less discomfort than stereotactic radiographic methods.

Conclusions

Ultrasound of the breast using modern high-resolution scanners is essential for complete breast evaluation. In many cases, ultrasound permits breast nodules identified by mammography or clinical examination to be classified as benign or malignant, aiding effective management. Although ultrasound is not necessary in the majority of patients receiving mammography, it is indispensable in resolving common clinical problems likely to be encountered on a daily basis. As a supplemental examination to characterize nodules and aid in the inspection of the dense breast, ultrasound allows the radiologist to add specificity to his interpretation and thereby provide the referring clinician with more relevant information than might be available from the mammogram alone, thus aiding promoting cost-effective patient management.

References

1. Rosenberg AL, Schwartz GF, Feig SA, Patchefsky AS. Clinically occult breast lesions: localization and significance. *Radiology* 1987;162:167—170.

2. Bassett LW, Liu TH, Giuliano AE, Gold RH. The prevalence of carcinoma in palpable vs impalpable, mammographically detected lesions. *AJR* 1991;157:21—24.

3. Gisvold JJ, Martin JK Jr. Prebiopsy localization of nonpalpable breast lesions. *AJR* 1984;143:477—481.

4. Stavros AT, Thickman D, Rapp CL, et al. Solid breast nodules: use of sonography to distinguish between benign and malignant lesions. *Radiology* 1995;196:123—134.

5. Wild JJ, Reid JM. Further pilot echographic studies on the histologic structure of tumors of the living intact human breast. *Am J Pathol* 1952;28:839—861.

6. Howry DH, Scott DA, Bliss WR. The ultrasonic visualization of carcinoma of the breast and other soft tissue structures. *Cancer* 1954;7:354—358.

7. Fry WJ, Leichner GH, Okuyama D, et al. Ultrasound visualization system employing new scanning and presentation methods. *J Acoust Soc Am* 1968;44:1325—1338.

8. Kelly-Fry E. Influences on the development of ultrasound pulse-echo breast instrumentation in the United States. In: *Ultrasound Mammography*. Harper P, ed. Baltimore: University Park Press; 1985, p. 1—20.

9. Taylor KJW. Can complementary US reduce the number of biopsies of benign breast masses (abst). *Radiology* 1993;1898(P) (suppl):179.

10. Moskowitz M. Screening is not diagnosis. *Radiology* 1979;133:265—268.

11. Hilton SV, Leopold GR, Olson LK, Willson SA. Real-time breast sonography: application in 300 consecutive patients. *AJR* 1986;147:479—486.

12. Mendelson EB, Tobin CE, Merritt CB, et al. Marginal analysis of breast masses with high resolution-US (abst). *Radiology* 1994;193(P) (suppl):177.

13. Wells PNT, Halliwell M, Skidmore R, et al. Tumour detection by ultrasonic doppler blood-flow signals. *Ultrasonics* 1977;15:231—236.

14. Minasian H, Bamber JC. A preliminary assessment of an ultrasonic Doppler method for the study of blood flow in human breast cancer. *Ultrasound Med Biol* 1982;8:357—364.

15. Burns PN, Halliwell M, Wells PNT, et al. Ultrasonic Doppler studies of the breast. *Ultrasound Med Biol* 1982;8:127—143.

16. Dempsey PJ. The value of ultrasound examination in diagnosing breast disease. *Curr Opin Radiol* 1989;1:188—192.

17. Stavros AT, Thickman D, Rapp CL, et al. Solid breast nodules: use of sonography to distinguish between benign and malignant lesions. *Radiology* 1995;196:123—134.

Interventional

53 Biopsy or Drainage of a Mass: The Role of Sonography

Gerald D. Dodd, III

The clinical request for a biopsy or drainage of a mass should always be made as part of a consultation between the requesting physician and the radiologist who will perform the procedure on the patient. This consultation should include a review of the patient's pertinent clinical history, the objectives of the requested procedure, a review of pertinent imaging studies, an assessment of whether the procedure is indicated and technically feasible, the determination of the disposition of tissue or fluid to be obtained, and an assessment of the patient's willingness and ability to tolerate the procedure. After the decision to perform the procedure has been made, the radiologist must choose a method of guidance.

Guidance Techniques

Three primary modalities can be used to guide percutaneous interventional procedures: fluoroscopy, computed tomography (CT), and sonography. In a few situations, the pathologic condition or the patient's anatomy may dictate a particular method of guidance. In most instances, however, sonographic guidance has proved to be quicker and easier than the other methods. In Asia and many parts of Europe, sonography is the dominant method used to guide the performance of most nonvascular and interventional procedures. At several academic and private hospitals in the United States, sonography is used to guide 95% of all biopsies and drainages of abdominal, pelvic, pleural and mediastinal masses. The advantages of sonography include real-time guidance, multidirectional imaging, identification and avoidance of major vessels, portability, excellent anatomic resolution, and reduced cost. The cost savings of sonography result from the lower capital expenses and operating costs of sonographic equipment and the potential use of CT scanners for diagnostic purposes, rather than for intervention.

Methods

The two primary methods of performing sonography-guided intervention are the free-hand technique and the attached-guide technique. Advocates of the free-hand technique claim that it allows greater freedom in the choice of needle placement and better needle visibility. Advocates of guides claim that they provide greater accuracy for deep biopsies, quicker needle localization, diminished teaching time, and improved coordination in procedures performed with nonradiologists. Because few companies manufacture needle guides for high-frequency probes, most near-field biopsies are performed by using the free-hand technique. However, it is my belief that use of an attachable guide makes a biopsy or drainage of a mass more than 5 cm deep easier and quicker.

The success of sonographic guidance depends highly on optimization of the sonographic equipment. Important parameters that should be controlled are the type of probe, the gray scale, the field of view, and the focus. All of these variables have a direct effect on the visualization of the pathologic condition and the needle. For near-field biopsies, the best results are usually obtained with 7- to 10-MHz linear probes. Most abdominal biopsies are best performed with 3.5- or 2.5-MHz sector probes. The field of view should be chosen to maximize visualization of the pathologic condition and the needle. As a general rule, the field of view should be adjusted so that the needle traverses at least one-third of the image. Under no circumstances should a large field of view be used when performing a biopsy of a small near-field lesion. The probes should be focused at the level at which the needle is expected to enter the lesion. Visualization of the needle can be improved by needle motion (use of an in-and-out motion with approximately a 1-cm excursion) and a slight rocking motion of the probe. This rocking motion can bring a needle that has deviated slightly out of the ultrasound (US) plane back into the field of view.

With the attached-guide technique, the speed and success of the procedure can be improved by using two sets of hands: One person holds the probe and directs it, and the second person places the needle or catheter. Although the use of two people requires precise communication, it can produce less traumatic and more accurate results. In academic centers, the second person is usually a resident or fellow. In private practice, the most logical choice for the second person would be a sonographer. The most crucial task in the two-person technique is holding the probe, which is usually performed by the attending radiologist. The delivery of the anesthetic and placement of the needle are easier tasks and are usually done by the second person.

Technique

Percutaneously guided intervention may seem difficult and dangerous; however, in most instances, it is relatively simple and safe. Its success requires adherence to a few basic principles:

1. Check for and correct coagulopathy in all patients with a prothrombin time greater than 15 s, a partial thromboplastin time greater than 45 s, or fewer than 50 000/mm³ platelets.
2. Defer the procedure if the patient has taken aspirin during the prior week.
3. Use abundant amounts of local anesthetic for procedures performed with needles larger than 22 gauge.
4. Do not use a local anesthetic for simple 22-gauge aspirations.
5. Confirm the location of all needle or catheter tips before obtaining a biopsy specimen or deploying drainage catheters.
6. Avoid crossing major vessels.
7. Do not aspirate potentially sterile fluid collections through the bowel.
8. Use a subcostal approach when possible.

The following discussion provides examples of the standard approaches used to perform a biopsy or to drain masses.

Percutaneous Biopsy

When performing percutaneous biopsies, I use only a 20-gauge end cutting needle and an 18-gauge core biopsy gun. After the patient has been prepared for the procedure, the probe is covered with a sterile sheath, and a biopsy guide is attached. The pathologic condition is located, and the path of the biopsy chosen. When possible, a subcostal approach is used to prevent the potential complications (pneumothorax, contaminated pleural space, and lacerated intercostal artery) of an intercostal approach. If the procedure is a biopsy of a liver tumor, then every attempt is made to perform the biopsy through a mantle of normal liver parenchyma. This precaution reduces the risk of bleeding, as normal liver tissue is less likely to bleed than a tumor. Additionally, the risk of bleeding can be reduced further by choosing a biopsy path through the least vascular portion of the tumor. Anesthetic is administered through the biopsy guide with a 10-cm-long 22-gauge spinal needle. Conceptually, an attempt is made to create a cylinder of anesthesia from the skin to the mass or organ from which the biopsy specimen is to be obtained. A traditional skin

wheal is not raised. No skin nick is made. When the 20-gauge biopsy needle is used, the needle is placed into the lesion, and the stylet removed. The specimen is obtained by moving the needle back and forth across the lesion without aspiration. When using the 18-gauge gun, the tip of the needle is advanced to a location approximately 5 mm from the margin of the lesion and then fired across the transition zone. Care is taken to ensure that there is adequate room for needle excursion.

Percutaneous Catheter Drainage

Catheters are placed using either the trocar or Seldinger technique. With either technique, copious amounts of anesthetic are administered both through the guide and as a skin wheal. A skin nick is made and blunt dissection is performed. Because it is difficult to pass a catheter through the thoracic or abdominal fascia, adequate dissection is often the key to successful catheter placement. The trocar technique is best reserved for large "cannot-miss" fluid collections. This conviction is based on the poor sono-visibility of most catheters, which makes confirmation of location difficult, and on the marked risk associated with making multiple passes with a large-diameter trocar catheter. The Seldinger technique is used to place catheters in fluid collections that are small or hard to reach. The advantage of this technique is that it uses small diameter, echogenic access needles. Small access needles can be placed and repositioned with a greater margin of safety than trocar drainage catheters. After satisfactory access has been obtained, a drainage catheter is exchanged over a wire. The use of locking loop catheters markedly decreases the frequency of accidental catheter removal. I do not use any of the commercially available fasteners to secure a catheter to a patient; I prefer to suture the catheter in place. Physician's orders for the care of indwelling catheters should include in-and-out flushing of the catheter with 10 mL of sterile saline solution every 8 h and monitoring the input and output of the catheter.

Paracentesis and Thoracentesis

Diagnostic aspirations of localized fluid collections, pleural effusions, and ascites are performed without anesthetic. A single 22-gauge needle is placed in one pass into the fluid collection. If no fluid is obtained with this puncture, however, lidocaine is administered along the needle track as the initial needle is withdrawn. When a 22-gauge aspiration fails (that is, when the needle is in area of interest but no fluid has been obtained), an 18-gauge needle is used for aspiration. If the 18-gauge needle fails to obtain fluid, the procedure may be canceled or continued with a drainage catheter.

General Applications

The general techniques described above can be used to evaluate a wide spectrum of pathologic conditions. Obvious applications include random biopsies of the liver or kidneys, biopsies of hepatic or renal masses (**Fig. 53–1**), and aspiration or drainage of fluid collections of the solid organs or the peritoneal cavity of the abdomen (**Fig. 53–2 through 53–3**).[1,2] Less obvious applications, such as the guidance of percutaneous transhepatic cholangiography, nephrostomy (**Fig. 53–4**), and cholecystostomy (**Fig 53–5**), are more easily performed with sonography than with fluoroscopy.[3] Why puncture a patient five to 20 times under fluoroscopic guidance, hoping for a chance encounter of the needle with a bile duct or the urinary collecting system? Why irradiate both the patient and the medical personnel needlessly? With sonography, the desired anatomy can be directly visualized and often punctured only once.

Sonography is underused for the biopsies or the aspiration of pulmonary or mediastinal masses. Most pulmonary masses that abut the pleura can be visualized and a biopsy performed with sonography (**Fig. 53–6**). Likewise, mediastinal masses that can be visualized by sonography are easily and safely sampled using sonographic guidance (**Fig. 53–7**).[4] In these instances, the two-dimensional resolution and real-time imaging capability of sonography provide a much greater safety margin than CT or fluoroscopy.

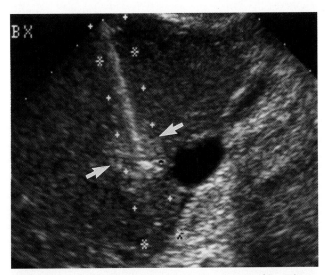

Figure 53–1 Liver mass biopsy. Transverse US scan of liver shows 1-cm hyperechoic nodule (**arrows**) with an echogenic needle traversing most of its diameter.

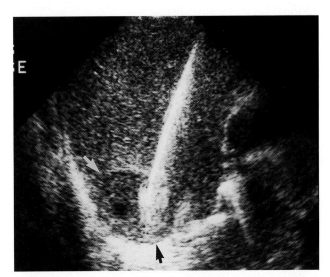

Figure 53–2 Hepatic abcess drainage. Transverse US scan shows 4-cm abscess (**arrows**) in posterior right lobe of liver. Note presence of the needle and wire.

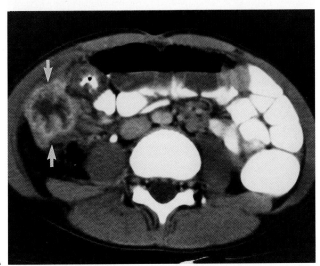

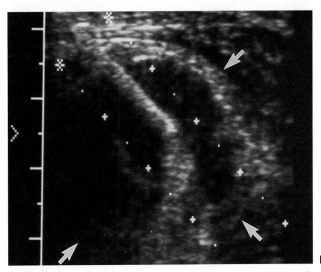

A   B

Figure 53–3 Periappendiceal abscess drainage. (**A**) CT image of the lower abdomen shows 3-cm heterogeneous periappendiceal abscess (**arrows**). (**B**) Transverse US scan of right lower quadrant obtained from the same patient shows spherical abscess (**arrows**), with needle within cavity.

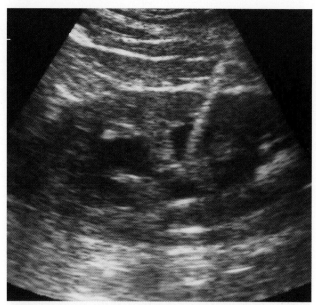

Figure 53–4 Nephrostomy. Posterior oblique US scan through right kidney shows marked hydronephrosis. Needle is puncturing one of the middle calices.

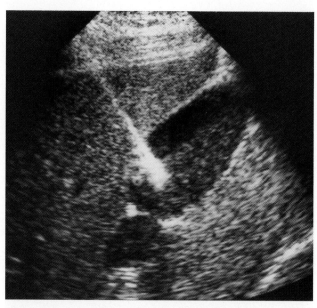

Figure 53–5 Percutaneous cholecystostomy. Sagittal US scan of right upper quadrant shows needle traversing anterior aspect of liver to enter the gallbladder lumen.

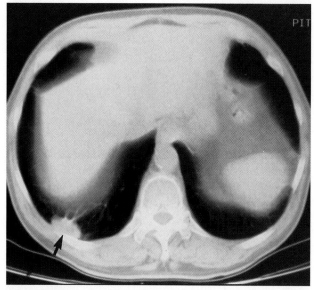

A

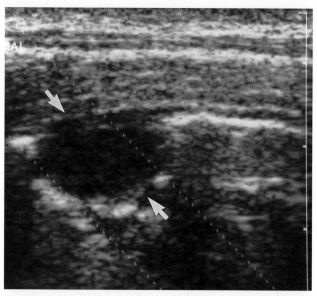

B

Figure 53–6 Biopsy of lung. (**A**) CT image of lower thorax shows 2 x 3 cm lung mass (**arrow**) abutting the pleura in the right lower lobe. (**B**) Corresponding oblique intercostal US scan clearly shows lung mass (**arrows**). A biopsy was performed under sonographic guidance. Its results showed the mass to be a metastatic tumor.

After general confidence in the use of sonographic guidance has been achieved, the technique can be applied more aggressively to perform procedures traditionally believed to be outside the realm of sonography. The biopsy of small retroperitoneal lymph nodes is a good example. My colleagues and I have found that biopsies of most retroperitoneal lymph nodes can be successfully performed by using sonographic guidance. This success is independent of the patient's size. We have successfully performed biopsies of numerous 1-cm paraaortic lymph nodes in markedly obese patients and have rarely needed to switch to CT guidance because we were unable to see the node (**Fig. 53–8**).[5] Another aggressive but ultimately simple procedure is the biopsy or drainage of a pelvic mass with a transvaginal or transrectal approach (**Fig. 53–9**).[6] Both procedures are easy to perform and

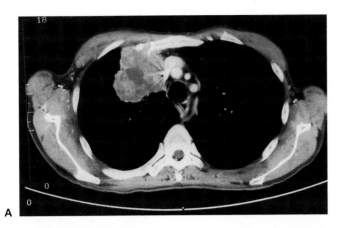

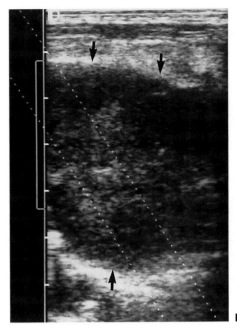

Figure 53–7 Lung mass invading mediastinum. (**A**) Axial CT image of upper thorax shows large heterogeneous anterior mass that abuts the pleura and projects laterally beyond the lateral sternal margin. (**B**) Corresponding intercostal parasternal US scan clearly shows mass (**arrows**). A biopsy was performed under sonographic guidance.

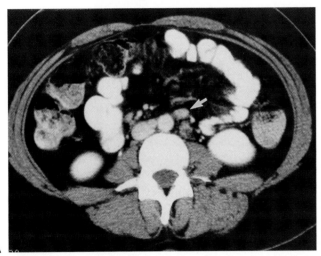

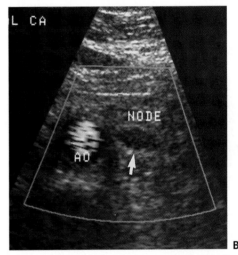

Figure 53–8 Biopsy of retroperitoneal lymph node. (**A**) Axial CT image of lower abdomen shows 1-cm periaortic lymph node (**arrow**). (**B**) Corresponding transverse US scan through lower ab- domen shows a hypoechoic node (**arrow**) adjacent to the aorta (AO).

well tolerated by patients. Finally, sonography is an excellent guidance technique for percutaneous treatment of hepatic masses by chemical or thermal ablation (**Fig. 53–10**).[7] In this application, sonography is used to direct the needle or probe into the lesion and also to monitor the degree of ablation during the procedure.

Summary

The request for a biopsy or drainage of a mass should always be approached with the patient's best interest in mind. If a procedure is indicated, the guidance technique of choice should be the one with which the radiologist is most comfortable. However, radiologists who are capable of using all guidance techniques will be best equipped to handle any situation. In particular, the radiologist who is skilled in the use of sonography as a guidance technique will have a distinct advantage over those who are not.

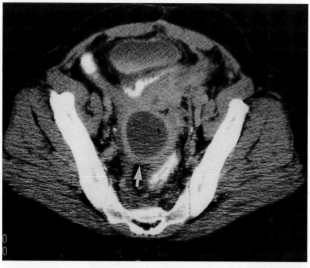
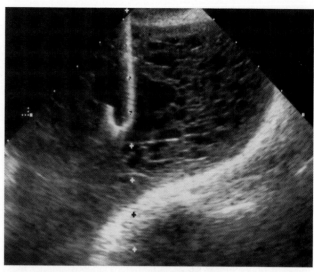

Figure 53–9 Transvaginal drainage of pelvic abscess. (**A**) Axial CT image of pelvis demonstrates 4-cm pelvic abscess (**arrow**), just anterior to rectum. (**B**) Corresponding transvaginal US scan shows J wire in complex cavity of the abscess.

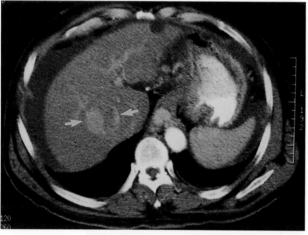
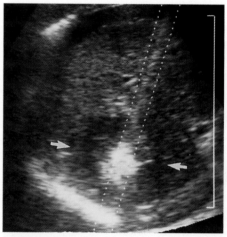

Figure 53–10 Ethanol ablation of hepatocellular carcinoma. (**A**) Axial CT image shows hypervascular 3-cm hepatocellular carcinoma (**arrows**) in posterior right lobe of liver. (**B**) Corresponding oblique US scan of liver shows hyperechoic region that represents injected alcohol within larger hypoechoic hepatocellular carcinoma (**arrows**).

References

1. Reading CC, Charboneau JW, James EM, Hurt MR. Sonographically guided percutaneous biopsy of small (3 cm or less) masses. *AJR* 1988;151:189—192.
2. vanSonnenberg E, D'Agostino HB, Casola G, et al. Percutaneous abscess drainage: current concepts. *Radiology* 1991;181:617—626.
3. McGahan JP, Lindfors KK. Percutaneous cholecystostomy: An alternative to surgical cholecystostomy for acute cholecystitis. *Radiology* 1989;173:481—485.
4. Yu C-J, Yang P-C, Chang D-B, et al. Evaluation of ultrasonically guided biopsies of mediastinal masses. *Chest* 1991;100:399–405.
5. Nagano T, Nakai Y, Taniguchi F, et al. Diagnosis of paraaortic and pelvic lymph node metastasis of gynecologic malignant tumors by ultrasound-guided percutaneous fine-needle aspiration biopsy. *Cancer* 1991;68:2571–2574.
6. Bret PM, Guibaud L, Atri M, Gillett P, et al. Transvaginal US-guided aspiration of ovarian cysts and solid pelvic masses. *Radiology* 1992;185:377–380.
7. Livraghi T, Giorgio A, Marin G, et al. Hepatocellular carcinoma and cirrhosis in 746 patients: long-term results of percutaneous ethanol injection. *Radiology* 1995;197:101—108.

54 Intraoperative Ultrasound

Robert A. Kane

Intraoperative ultrasound (IOUS) is a dynamic and highly interactive imaging study and is one of the most rapidly developing areas within ultrasonography. Unfortunately, many radiologists have been reluctant to spend a significant portion of time out of the department during the workday to perform and interpret IOUS studies, fearing that they will lose 1 or 2 h of work time while waiting in the operating suite until the surgeon is ready for the scans to be performed. However, the information obtained during IOUS is often crucial for accurate diagnostic assessment and planning of surgical approaches to resection of the disease processes. Studies have shown that the impact of IOUS imaging on surgical decision making justifies the time and effort involved, both from an efficacious as well as a cost benefit standpoint.[1] Our opinion, as well as that of many others with experience in this field, is that the benefits gained by IOUS imaging definitely justify the time spent by the radiologists performing the procedure.

We have evolved several means to improve the radiologists efficiency when performing IOUS scans, and utilization of these strategies typically allows a radiologist to perform the IOUS and return to the radiology department in approximately 30 min. The most effective strategies are as follows:

1. IOUS studies are booked in advance with the ultrasound section whenever possible, which allows more planning and manipulation of the work schedule within the ultrasound section, and anticipation of the approximate time for performing the study.
2. Prepositioning the IOUS scanner in the operating suite in advance of the examination may save a few minutes waiting time for elevators.
3. The radiologist who will perform the examination may choose to work in surgical scrubs, thereby eliminating the need to change into scrubs when the call from the operating room arrives.
4. Mutual cooperation and respect between the surgeons and radiologists has resulted in an agreement that the surgeons will call for the IOUS scan 10—15 min before they are actually ready for scanning, and the radiologists and technologists guarantee their readiness to perform the scan within 10—15 min of the telephone call. This arrangement is usually successful in avoiding any unnecessary waiting either by the surgical team or the radiologic team, and thus maximizes efficiency.

In our institution the radiologist scrubs in on the case and is gowned and gloved and performs the actual scanning. A typical intraoperative study can be completed within 5—10 min assuming that the sonologist is experienced. Scanning performed by the surgeon with the radiologist observing at the bedside or by remote teleradiography is less optimal compared to the radiologist actually performing the scan himself or herself. Scanning provides important hand-to-eye information, and the scanning technique of most surgeons cannot compare to that of a skilled and experienced sonologist. Even though IOUS scanning has removed many of the noise-generating barriers to excellent image quality, nonetheless proper scanning technique, understanding of image artifacts, and recognition of subtle findings such as small isoechoic tumor nodules are best achieved by someone with extensive experience in ultrasonography.

If possible, it is optimal to sterilize the IOUS probes before the operation. We have had excellent success using gas sterilization with ethylene oxide for many of our intraoperative probes. However, many manufacturers are reluctant to allow gas sterilization, fearing that the transducers will be damaged by the high temperatures of aeration which are required by ethylene oxide gas sterilization, although we have not experienced any problems. Some operating suites will allow prolonged immersion in Cidex (glutaraldehyde; Johnson & Johnson, Arlington, Texas) as an adequate method of probe sterilization, but other institutions do not consider this sufficiently sterile for open intraoperative use. Therefore, sterile probe covers are available and provide a third and most frequently used alternative. The use of probe covers may add 1 or 2 min to the time of the procedure as the cover is being applied, and there is some risk of compromise of sterile technique should the probe cover rip, which can occur occasionally. Therefore, when we are using equipment with sterile probe covers, we soak the probes in glutaraldehyde for at least 30 min before the procedure in case there is a break in sterile technique. It is preferable to use specifically designed transducer sheathes that fit snugly over the transducer head, as loose fitting covers may cause imaging artifacts due to trapped gas or folds in the sheath. Standard endoscopic sheathes can be used to cover the entire transducer cord.

IOUS has many uses, and the applications are extensive and growing. In neurosurgery, IOUS is used effectively in both surgery on the brain and spinal cord, and in intraabdominal surgery the uses are principally in the liver, biliary tract, and pancreas. Intraoperative assessment of vascular surgical disease and IOUS imaging postendarterectomy or reconstructive procedures is now on the increase. Other newly developing areas of use include intraoperative localization of breast tumors, applications in the genitourinary system such as evaluation of small renal cell carcinomas, as well as in gynecologic surgery, and finally to provide guidance for interventional procedures such as prostate cryosurgery and tumor ablations in the liver. One of the most exciting and rapidly developing new areas is that of laparoscopic ultrasound (LUS) imaging, which is being applied to assessment of diseases of the liver, pancreas, and biliary tract within the abdomen and has also been used to help detect lung tumors during thoracoscopic resections. Another new and exciting application is the use of catheter-mounted, high-frequency ultrasound transducers for endoluminal intraoperative use in the bile ducts and ureters, for gynecologic procedures and for vascular intraluminal assessment. Given the limitations of space, we will concentrate this discussion on selected neurosurgical and intraabdominal applications.

Neurosurgical Applications

Brain

IOUS scans of the brain can be obtained either through a burr hole, using specially designed small burr hole probes or endoluminal probes, such as are used for prostate or transvaginal scanning. More commonly, IOUS scans are obtained through an open craniotomy flap. Excellent images can be obtained transdurally as well as directly on the brain surface after incision of the dura. The optimal frequency for brain imaging ranges from 5 to 7.5 MHz in frequency, and the best probe configuration is the endfire sector type probes, either mechanical or electronic convex array or phased array probes. The dura or brain surface is moistened with a small amount of sterile saline solution which provides acoustic coupling for the transducer. Meticulous scanning technique is essential, with particular care to avoid applying significant pressure on the brain. A very light contact with the moistened dura or brain surface is sufficient for adequate acoustic coupling.

The principal use of IOUS is to accurately locate and localize masses within the brain substance that cannot be visualized directly by the neurosurgeon, and of course the brain cannot be palpated. Even masses a few millimeters deep to the cortical surface are difficult or impossible to detect visually. The vast majority of primary and metastatic brain tumors are markedly hyperechoic in comparison to the surrounding normal brain structures.[2] The sulcal convolutions on the brain surface are somewhat echogenic, but most of the brain substance is of relatively low and homogeneous echogenicity. Consequently, most tumors stand out dramatically as hyperechoic lesions against a relatively hypoechoic background (**Fig. 54–1**). The reactive edema associated with brain tumors can decrease even further the echogenicity of brain substance and increase the conspicuity of focal masses.[3] Meningiomas are the most highly echogenic primary brain tumors, and usually have a relatively smooth contour and sharp margination. Calcifications within meningiomas occur frequently and result in a further increase in echogenicity. Glioblastomas are also markedly hyperechoic and often are well marginated, but may have less well-defined margins when they are aggressive and invasive.[4] Cystic degeneration may occur in glioblastomas as well as in cystic astrocytomas (**Fig. 54–2**), and the septations, cyst cavities, and areas of solid tumor and mural nodularity are well depicted by IOUS.[5,6] The complex nature of these cystic neoplasms is more completely portrayed with IOUS than with other imaging modalities including CT and even MRI. Complete definition of the various spaces and cystic compartments may be important to guide surgical decompression of cystic tumors by aspiration.

Most brain metastases are also hyperechoic and well circumscribed (**Fig. 54–3**), with an appearance similar to

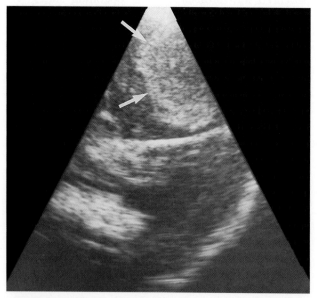

Figure 54–1 Hyperechoic glioma. US scan shows glioma (**arrows**) in occipital lobe.

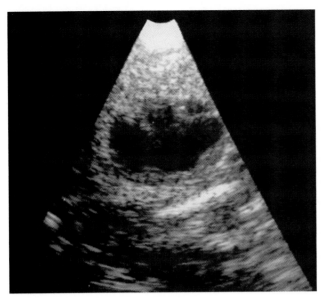

Figure 54–2 Predominately cystic astrocytoma. US scan clearly shows mural nodularity and septation.

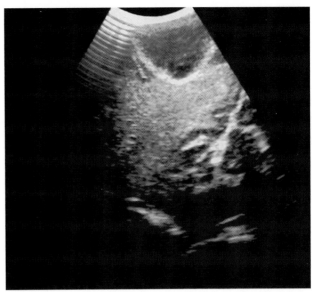

Figure 54–3 Poorly differentiated brain metastasis from primary lung carcinoma. US scan shows echogenic rim, but central portion is hypoechoic due to liquefaction necrosis. Note gyral and sulcal detail, which is obliterated by brain edema surrounding tumor nodule.

meningiomas and gliomas.[7] Liquefaction necrosis, which may occur spontaneously or as the result of therapy, may diminish the echogenicity of tumors centrally (**Fig. 54–3**). Low-grade astrocytomas can present a much more difficult imaging problem, as they tend to be less echogenic and also to have very poorly defined infiltrative margins, insinuating into the adjacent brain substance in a very ill-defined manner.[8,9] In addition, chronic edema associated with low-grade astrocytomas may actually increase brain echogenicity adjacent to the tumor, thus making tumor margins even more ill-defined.[10]

In addition to defining the tumor site and assessing margins, IOUS is helpful to the neurosurgeon in selecting an approach to resection of the tumor that will hopefully minimize damage to surrounding functional brain tissue. Following resection, IOUS can be utilized to evaluate completeness of surgical resection by rescanning after filling the surgical cavity with sterile saline and seeking any residual tumor nodules.

IOUS imaging is also very helpful in guiding biopsy procedures, again with the goal of minimizing trauma to adjacent brain tissues.[11] Specially designed probes can be used through a modified burr hole to allow precise needle placement with minimal patient trauma.[12] Biopsies can be performed with electronic real-time biopsy guides, or free hand under direct real-time visualization.[13] High-resolution endfire endoluminal probes have been quite useful to perform accurate real-time biopsies through small craniotomy sites utilizing electronic biopsy guidance (**Fig. 54–4**). Utilization of color flow imaging may help to choose a path for the biopsy needle

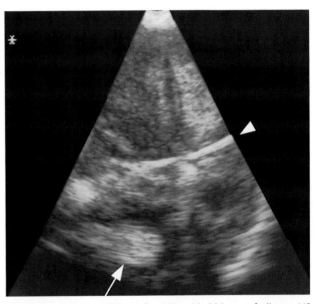

Figure 54–4 Linear defect after US-guided biopsy of glioma. US scan shows excellent penetration of the brain at 5 MHz with visualization of deep choroid plexus (**arrow**) on far side of tentorium (**arrowhead**).

that will minimize disruption of major blood vessels between the cortical surface and the tumor site.

Real-time guidance can also be successfully used for tumor ablative techniques, placement of ventricular shunt catheters, and drainage of intracranial fluid collections and abscesses (**Fig. 54–5**).[14] Following ultrasound-guided needle biopsies, we routinely rescan the patient for several minutes after the biopsy to assess for any bleeding within the lesion. Acute bleeding may appear as

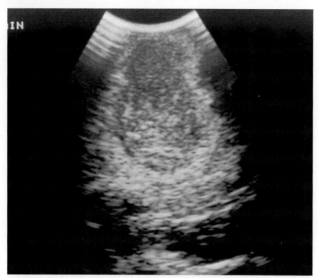

Figure 54–5 Frontal lobe abscess. US scan shows echogenic rim and centrally located, moderately echogenic purulent material. US-guided aspiration and evacuation of abscess was performed.

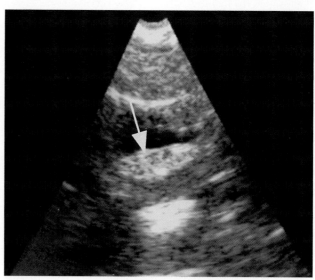

Figure 54–6 Astrocytoma. US scan shows fluid-blood level (**arrow**) within cystic cavity of astrocytoma after needle biopsy.

a small highly echogenic foci within the mass or in the surrounding brain parenchyma. Occasionally, fluid—fluid levels may be seen, particularly when there is bleeding into a mass with cystic degeneration (**Fig. 54–6**). Scanning for several minutes time is usually sufficient to ensure that any bleeding has stabilized.

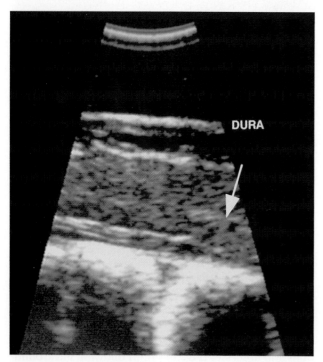

Figure 54–7 Lower thoracic cord. Sagittal US scan shows the central spinal canal (**arrow**) as a paired echogenic linear structure. The dura is well seen through the sonic window provided by sterile saline solution, which fills the surgical site.

Gray scale, Doppler, and color flow imaging have been used in neurosurgical approaches to aneurysms and arteriovenous malformations (AVMs).[15] Assessment of blood flow is important during clipping or resection of aneurysms. Many AVMs are poorly visualized on gray scale IOUS imaging, but the use of color flow imaging has been very helpful in defining their location and boundaries.

Spine

The uses of IOUS imaging in the evaluation of spinal cord abnormalities are similar to those for brain imaging. Endfire probes are essential and the optimal frequency would be in the 7- to 10-MHz range, although 5-MHz probes can be successfully utilized. Electronic curved array or linear array probes are preferable as they allow concomitant utilization of color flow imaging, but mechanical endfire probes can be also utilized. The surgical laminenectomy site is filled with sterile degassed saline to provide an acoustic coupling medium. The probe is then placed into the pool of degassed saline solution and images are usually obtained without direct contact with the spinal cord.

Both axial and sagittal planes are utilized. The spinal cord itself has a relatively low to moderate echogenicity and is quite homogeneous in texture.[16] The central spinal canal or indentation of the cord at the site of the central canal can be visualized as an echogenic single or paired set of lines relatively centrally within the spinal cord, which is otherwise featureless (**Fig. 54–7**). The central spinal canal is an important normal landmark that is frequently disrupted by pathologic conditions within the cord. The arachnoid membrane is difficult to visualize, but the dura is well seen both dorsally and ventrally, and a small amount of fluid is usually present between the dura and the arachnoid. The dentate ligaments are well visualized in axial views (**Fig. 54–8**). They arise from the dorsal and lateral margins of the sac and extend laterally to the adjacent spinal canal. Nerve roots are inconsistently imaged in the cervical and thoracic spine, but are well seen at the conus medullaris and distally in the region of the cauda equina. Nerve roots appear to be hypoechoic or anechoic, but are readily visualized within the spinal fluid by highly reflective dorsal and ventral margins, appearing as two parallel echogenic lines. Pulsations can be imaged in real-time from the anterior spinal artery which is deep to the cord. Color flow imaging and power Doppler imaging will show the vascularity in a more complete fashion.

Assessment of the location and extent of masses is one of the principal uses of spinal IOUS. Lesion location can be assessed as intramedullary or extramedullary, and intradural and extradural components can be evaluated.[17] This capability can be particularly useful in depicting tumors such as neurofibromas which may have both intradural and extradural components. The spinal cord cannot be retracted extensively, and IOUS imaging can provide important information as to the full extent of such tumors.[18] Many intramedullary tumors of the cord including ependymomas, dermoids and many metastases are hyperechoic. Astrocytomas, however, are frequently isoechoic with extremely ill-defined margins, and consequently are very poorly visualized. These lesions may be recognized by effacement of the landmark echoes from the central spinal canal, as well as by fusiform swelling of the cord. Other nonneoplastic inflammatory and posttraumatic conditions can also cause swelling of the cord and may not be readily distinguishable from astrocytomas.[19] Astrocytomas may show cystic degeneration, which can also be seen in ependymomas and hemangioblastomas (**Fig. 54–9**). These tumors can form fairly large cystic cavities and simulate syringomyelia. However, the presence of solid masses, mural nodules or irregularly thickened septations help to distinguish cystic tumors from a benign syrinx.[20,21]

Extramedullary tumors include meningiomas (**Fig. 54–10**), neurofibromas, lipomas, and dermoids, as well as malignant tumors, which are most often metastatic. Other conditions can also produce an extramedullary mass effect, including protruding discs, bony lesions (spurs and fracture fragments), hematomas, abscesses, and arachnoid cyst. Most of the neoplastic lesions appear as moderately echogenic masses with displacement or compression of the adjacent spinal cord and displacement of other structures including nerve roots. Bony spurs and fragments are highly echogenic and may be associated with acoustic shadow. Herniated disc fragments are moderately echogenic but substantially less so than bony spurs.[22] Hematomas may

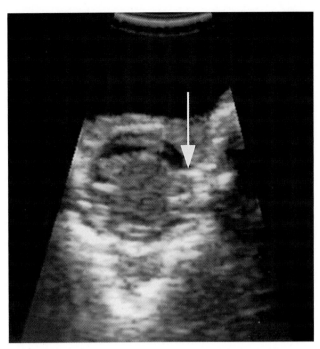

Figure 54–8 US scan shows spinal cord and dentate ligament (**arrow**).

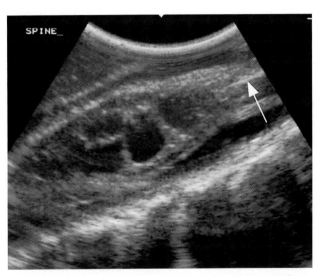

Figure 54–9 Hemangioblastoma of cervical cord. US scan shows multiple cystic components and interruption of central spinal canal (**arrow**), which indicates the presence of an intramedullary mass.

have a variable appearance, depending on their age and degree of liquefaction, while most abscesses and cysts have predominantly fluid components and increased transmission of sound through the fluid.

IOUS is very useful in evaluating the extent of surgical resections,[23] as well as in guiding biopsies, particularly biopsies of tumors with extensive cystic or necrotic components. IOUS and color flow imaging can be useful in identifying the more viable solid components of the tumor, thereby avoiding the necrotic components and diminishing the number of biopsies required to establish a diagnosis. Drainage of epidural abscesses and hema-

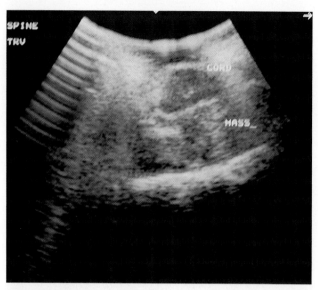

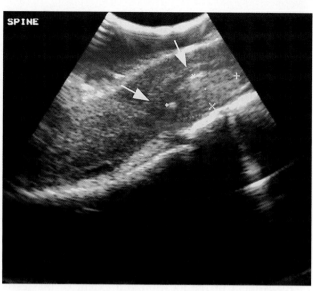

Figure 54–10 Meningioma of cervical cord. **A:** Axial US scan shows solid isoechoic ventral mass deforming the cord. **B:** Sagittal US image shows the mass (calipers). Note preservation of central spinal canal (**arrows**), which is consistent with extramedullary tumor.

tomas can also be aided by ultrasound guidance, as well as the drainage of cystic tumor cavities and the cavities of syringomyelia, both by real-time guidance of needle placement into the various component cavities as well as evaluation of the completeness of evacuation of cyst fluid. Finally, placement of intracystic shunt catheters within a syrinx can also be facilitated by IOUS guidance.

Abdominal Applications

Gallbladder and Bile Ducts

Intraoperative imaging of the gallbladder and extra hepatic bile ducts is best performed using an endfire probe with a center frequency of 7 or 7.5 MHz. Either linear array or sector formats are acceptable. Imaging at 5 MHz is probably also acceptable but may require a standoff mechanism, such as filling the abdominal cavity with sterile saline or using a water-filled glove, in order to avoid near field artifacts which may detract from imaging these structures. Scanning is performed directly in contact with the common bile duct or gallbladder, and scanning can be performed in any anatomical plane desired. If a complete study requires imaging of the intrahepatic bile ducts, then the endfire probe may be satisfactory for the central ducts, but a complete evaluation of the peripheral ducts may require a side fire liver-type probe.

IOUS of the gallbladder is not frequently required as preoperative ultrasound studies are usually more than adequate. Routine screening for gallstones is performed on patients with morbid obesity who are undergoing gastric bypass or stapling procedures, because these

patients frequently develop acute cholecystitis after substantial weight loss. Therefore, if stones are present, then the gallbladder is usually removed at the time of gastric surgery. These patients may be difficult if not impossible to image adequately because of their body habitus, and therefore, if the preoperative study is unsatisfactory, IOUS imaging of the gallbladder can be rapidly performed and may be capable of demonstrating stones which were not visualized preoperatively (**Fig. 54–11**).[24]

IOUS may be useful in assessing gallbladder masses discovered incidentally at surgery (**Fig. 54–12**) or to assess the extent of a known gallbladder carcinoma, particularly regarding potential invasion into the adjacent liver bed, which would require a more aggressive surgical resection.[25] If the tumor is resectable, but also invading the liver, most surgeons would advocate a wedge resection of liver parenchyma in order to obtain a tumor free margin. At the time of IOUS, a careful search for more distant hepatic metastases or lymph node metastases should be performed in order to avoid unnecessary radical surgery in patients with advanced metastatic disease.

IOUS of the bile ducts has been regarded as a competitive or possibly superior modality to radiographic intraoperative cholangiography by several surgical groups.[26, 27] There is also a substantial amount of interest in the use of laparoscopic ultrasound imaging for bile duct assessment in patients with potential choledocholithiasis undergoing laparoscopic cholecystectomy. The common bile duct, common hepatic duct, and intrahepatic bile ducts can be well visualized both with open and laparoscopic IOUS (**Fig. 54–13**).[28, 29] Therefore, IOUS or LUS can be quite effective in demonstrating bile duct stones, and because laparoscopic cholangiography is somewhat arduous and difficult to perform, LUS may provide a superior alternative, although no directly comparative studies have been performed. In our own institution, however, when choledocholithiasis is suspected clinically, endoscopic retrograde cholangiopancreatography is performed preoperatively both for diagnosis and, when positive, for therapeutic intervention via endoscopic sphincterotomy and stone extraction. If this approach is undertaken, the need for any form of intraoperative bile duct evaluation is substantially diminished.

Benign strictures and malignant obstructions in the biliary tract can be well evaluated by IOUS imaging to define the precise site and extent of the obstruction and help plan the type of biliary bypass procedure to be performed. The sclerosing form of cholangiocarcinoma can be difficult to fully assess even with IOUS imaging, as the tumor is an infiltrative and intensely sclerosing type lesion with poorly identified margins. Other forms of cholangiocarcinoma, particularly the papillary types, can be well defined by IOUS imaging (**Fig. 54–14**). In patients with central Klatzkin type cholangiocarcinomas, we have occasionally been asked to scan the liver to identify large dilated intrahepatic ducts which might prove suitable for a peripheral hepaticojejunostomy, when a central decompression is mechanically impossible. This has been successfully accomplished in particular in the left lobe along the ligamentum teres, where large ducts draining segments 2 and 3 can at times be identified. More frequently now, however, patients with this large central type tumor are drained externally by percutaneous or endoscopic techniques.

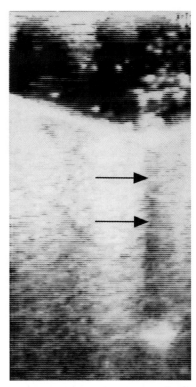

Figure 54–11 Gallbladder stones. Intraoperative US scan of gallbladder shows numerous tiny submillimeter stones not seen on preoperative studies. **Arrows** indicate acoustic shadowing from the conglomeration of these tiny stones.

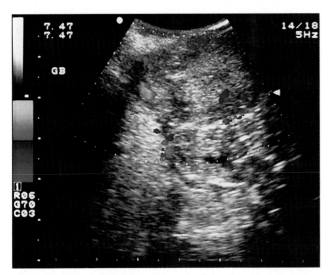

Figure 54–12 Gallbladder carcinoma. Color flow Doppler image shows vascularity within the gallbladder tumor and the contiguous hepatic parenchyma suggesting local invasion.

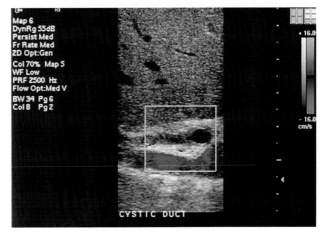

Figure 54–13 Transverse view of common duct. Color flow Doppler image allows distinction of the biliary ducts from adjacent portal vein (red) and hepatic artery (blue). This image shows the entry of the cystic duct into the common duct.

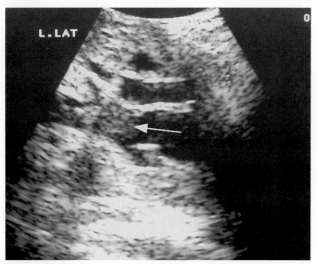

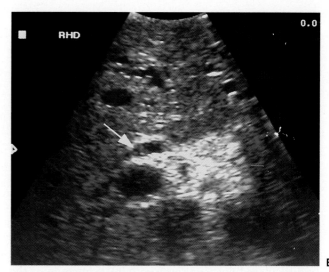

Figure 54–14   Klatzkin-type cholangiocarcinoma. **A:** US scan shows dilatation of left hepatic duct, with tumor invasion (**arrow**). **B:** US scan shows dilatation of peripheral ducts in left medial seg- ment, but right hepatic duct (**arrow**) has normal caliber and is free of tumor. This finding allowed a left hepatectomy and right hepaticojejunostomy to be performed.

Liver

Intraoperative ultrasound of the liver is most frequently performed on patients who are undergoing possible surgical resection of liver cancer, either primary or metastatic. This examination is best performed using a side fire probe with center frequency of 5 MHz, which allows full penetration of the liver from front to back, even in the right lobe where 12 cm of tissue can be adequately imaged. While higher center frequencies of 7 or 7.5 MHz are excellent for biliary and pancreatic imaging, only approximately 6 cm of liver can be effectively imaged at this higher frequency, and therefore a complete examination of the liver would be significantly lengthened in time and made more difficult, as scans along the under surface of the liver are less satisfactory due to the irregular contours and possible adhesions. A side fire linear array or convex array configuration is also important in order to fit the probe in between the liver and the diaphragm or the liver and the lateral ribcage, where there is very little space. By cradling the side fire probe in the fingers, all portions of the liver can be adequately reached and scanned even without full mobilization of the liver. Scanning is optimal in the transverse plane beginning at the dome of the left edge of the liver and proceeding from cephalad to caudad. The next field should slightly overlap the original field while moving from left to right across the liver. With this overlapping field of view, the entire liver can be adequately assessed in 5—10 min.[30]

The principal advantages of intraoperative ultrasound imaging of the liver are as follows:

1. IOUS offers the most complete detection of primary and metastatic tumors in the liver, with approximately 25—30% more lesions detected compared to conventional preoperative imaging and 10—15% more lesions compared to CT arterial portography.

2. Real-time definition of lobar and segmental liver anatomy as well as normal and aberrant vascular supply and drainage.
3. Assessment of the feasibility of resection, planning of the most appropriate type of resection and identification of deep tumor margins in patients undergoing non segmental wedge type resections.
4. Real-time guidance for tumor biopsy procedures and aspiration of fluid collections.
5. Real-time guidance for ablative techniques such as cryosurgery or alcohol ablation.

The spatial resolution of IOUS imaging in the liver is unsurpassed, allowing for imaging of cysts as small as 1—3 mm and solid lesions as small as 3—5 mm (**Fig. 54–15**). The vast majority of lesions detected by IOUS but not by preoperative imaging studies or palpation are 1 cm or less in diameter, which in part reflects the spatial resolution limits of preoperative studies.[31,32] CT arterial portography can definitely increase the sensitivity for detection of liver lesions to the range of 85—90%,[33] but this results in somewhat less specificity, particularly when attempting to detect lesions well under 1 cm in size. False-positive results for CT arterial portography are encountered with some frequency due to perfusion abnormalities (**Fig. 54–16**) and small hepatic cysts (**Fig. 54–17**).[34,35]

In our institution and others, patients who may be candidates for resection of liver tumors initially undergo laparoscopy, in order to attempt to identify patients with diffusely metastatic disease outside the liver, which would render the patient inoperable. Laparoscopic ultrasound of the liver can be combined with this approach to identify the maximum number of detectable liver lesions, as additional tumors detected by LUS but not on preoperative imaging may also render a patient

Figure 54–15 Nonpalpable colorectal liver metastases seen only with intraoperative US imaging. Scans show (**A**) 1.2-cm isoechoic lesion visible only because of hypoechoic rim (**arrows**) and (**B**) additional 0.4-cm metastasis in same patient.

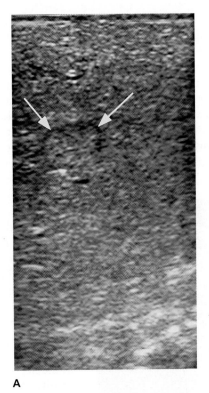

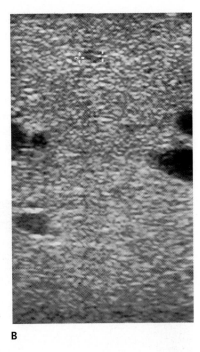

B

A

Figure 54–16 Diffuse fatty infiltration of liver. US scan shows diffuse fatty infiltration with sparing (**arrows**) at porta hepatis. This sparing caused false-positive results on CT arterial portography.

Figure 54–17 Hepatic cyst. US scan shows enhanced 5-mm cyst (**arrowheads**), which caused a false-positive CT reading.

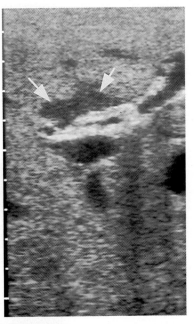

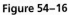

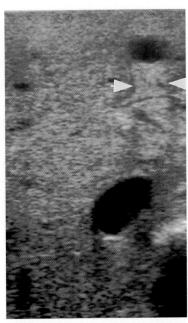

Figure 54–16   **Figure 54–17**

inoperable due to multiplicity of lesions or involvement of multiple lobes of the liver. LUS has the same capacity for detecting small liver lesions as open IOUS and is even more important in this situation, because the surgeon is unable to palpate the liver, and only a minority of small liver tumors can be directly visualized with the laparoscope.[36,37] LUS is technically more challenging and much more time consuming than open IOUS imaging of the liver, and may have slightly less sensitivity for lesion detection, as has been suggested in preliminary studies. However, with further evolution of the technique and improvement in the equipment for laparoscopic ultrasound imaging, the small differences in sensitivity may diminish.

State-of-the-art IOUS equipment allows the use of color flow or power Doppler imaging to assess the vascularity of liver tumors (**Fig. 54–18**). In addition, careful assessment of the vascular supply of the liver can have a major impact on surgical approach (**Fig. 54–19**). The presence of an accessory inferior right hepatic vein which drains into the inferior vena cava distal to the hepatic venous confluence may allow performance of a more extensive left trisegmentectomy. Similarly, an accessory or replaced left hepatic artery arising from the

left gastric artery (**Fig. 54–20**), or a right hepatic artery arising from the superior mesenteric artery may influence the type of resection performed.[38] The demonstration of major vessels surrounding masses or cystic lesions may influence the direct surgical approach to excision, drainage or unroofing of a cyst (**Fig. 54–21**).

Lymphadenopathy can be readily assessed both in the porta hepatis as well as in the peripancreatic and celiac nodal groups. Demonstration of enlarged nodes in these areas may be important (**Fig. 54–22**) in determing resectability of a liver lesion, because metastatic lymphadenopathy would generally render the patient inoperable for cure. Confirmation of lymph node metastases can be obtained directly by ultrasound-guided lymph node biopsies. IOUS is not effective in demonstrating serosal implants or seeding of the mesentery by tumor, but this type of metastatic disease is often well detected by palpation or direct visual inspection or inspection via the laparoscope.

From patients with primary hepatocellular carcinoma, venous invasion is a frequent occurrence and is well detected both in the portal venous system as well as in the hepatic venous system.[39] Hepatic venous invasion can be life-threatening at time of surgery if the clot extends into the inferior vena cava or into the right atrium. Careful assessment of the full extent of venous invasion is therefore essential. Occasionally, during assessment of a patient with liver tumor of unknown origin, the site of the primary tumor may be visualized. In particular, the pancreas should be closely assessed as a possible source of an unknown primary adenocarcinoma.

Most interventional IOUS guided procedures, including biopsies, aspirations, and drainages, can be success-

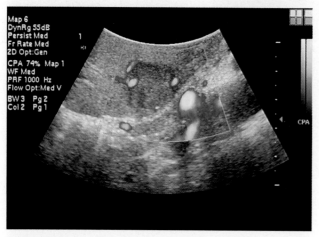

Figure 54–18 Colorectal metastasis. Power Doppler image demonstrates a hypovascular tumor with vessels being displaced around the periphery of the tumor nodule.

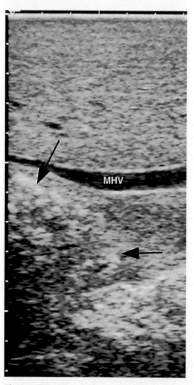

Figure 54–19 Colon metastasis. US scan shows large, partially calcified colon metastasis (**arrows**) abutting and deforming middle hepatic vein (MHV). Extended right hepatic lobectomy was required to achieve adequate surgical margins.

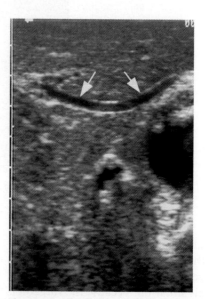

Figure 54–20 Replaced left hepatic artery. US scan shows point at which replaced left hepatic artery (**arrows**) enters the liver, along the ligamentum venosum.

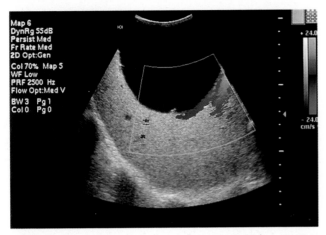

Figure 54–21 Hepatic cyst. Color flow imaging demonstrates displacement of hepatic vasculature deep to the large hepatic cyst, distant from the area of planned surgical unroofing.

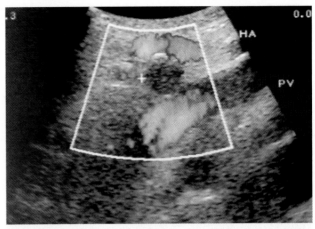

Figure 54–22 Metastatic lymphadenopathy. Laparoscopic US scan shows periportal metastatic lymphadenopathy between hepatic artery (HA) and portal vein (PV).

fully performed with free-hand real-time ultrasound guidance. Tumor ablation techniques, such as cryosurgery and ethanol injection (**Fig. 54–23**) are successfully performed and monitored under real-time IOUS guidance. At present however, guidance for procedures under laparoscopic ultrasound control is much more difficult. There are no commercially available systems equipped with electronic biopsy guidance systems similar to those used extensively and successfully in the diagnostic ultrasound laboratory. Consequently LUS-guided interventional procedures are much more difficult, whether they involve biopsies, drainages, or tumor abla-

tions. Free-hand biopsies can be performed with LUS guidance (**Fig. 54–24**), by using specially designed long needles that puncture through the abdominal wall and enter the liver adjacent to the LUS probe, with the angle and depth of penetration controlled with real-time guidance. The degree of difficulty in performing these procedures is substantially greater than with open IOUS imaging, however, particularly for small deep-seated lesions. It is hoped that eventually electronic biopsy guidance systems will be developed by the manufacturers for use with LUS probes.

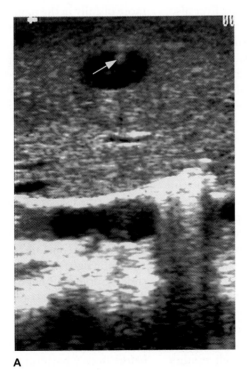
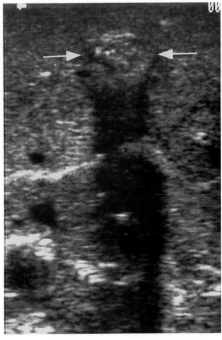

Figure 54–23 Hepatocellular carcinoma. **A:** US scan shows needle tip (**arrow**) penetrating small tumor nodule. **B:** On US scan, nodule (**arrows**) is echogenic, with acoustic shadowing, after ethanol injection for tumor ablation.

A

B

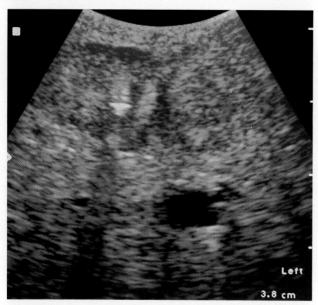

Figure 54–24 Hepatocellular carcinoma. During free-hand laparoscopic US-guided biopsy. US scan shows needle tip as an echogenic line within tumor nodule.

Pancreas

Intraoperative ultrasound imaging of the pancreas requires an endfire probe, either linear or sector format, with a center frequency ranging from 5 to 7.5 MHz. The side fire configuration which serves well for liver imaging is unsuited for imaging the pancreas because this configuration will not allow satisfactory contact with the pancreas, particularly in large deep abdominal cavities. The sector format is favored as it shows a wider area of anatomy in each image section. When IOUS is used to evaluate neoplastic lesions in the pancreas, the liver also should be scanned for evidence of metastatic disease which is commonly seen both in ductal adenocarcinoma as well as islet cell tumors of the pancreas.

Virtually all islet cell tumors of the pancreas produce hormones that can be detected by pathologic studies using special stains or electron microscopy, but only a subset of these tumors produce clinical symptomatology. Patients with symptomatic islet cell tumors often have extremely small-sized tumors that are difficult to image by preoperative techniques. Many competitive and complementary strategies have evolved including the use of spiral CT, MRI with Gadolinium, super-selective angiographic techniques and portal venous sampling as well as endoscopic ultrasound imaging. While each technique has its advocates, none are wholly satisfactory with sensitivities ranging from 70% to 85%. IOUS imaging is the single most effective technique for detection of functioning islet cell tumors,[40] and at times can detect even nonpalpable lesions as small as 3—5 mm. Most islet cell tumors are homogeneus and therefore hypoechoic, and are thus well detected against the background of hyperechoic pancreatic parenchyma. Most islet cell tumors

have smooth well-marginated borders, whether benign or malignant, as these tumors seldom are locally aggressive, even when malignant.

The pancreas can be scanned from the head and uncinate process to the tail in a matter of minutes, either before or after mobilization techniques have been performed. It may be useful to fill the abdominal cavity with degassed saline solution to serve as an acoustic window, although excellent images can often be obtained with direct contact imaging or even by scanning through compressed bowel and mesentery. Occasionally, the lateral segment of the liver may provide an acoustic window to the pancreatic body and tail. As with the liver and biliary tract, a systematic imaging study with overlapping fields is essential to evaluate the entire pancreas.

Insulinomas are usually solitary (**Fig. 54–25**) and benign,[41] but all islet cell tumors have malignant potential. Gastrinomas have a much higher rate of malignancy, and often are multiple rather than solitary. Gastrinomas are also frequently extrapancreatic in location,[42] lying in the so-called "gastrinoma triangle," between the common duct, head of pancreas, and second and third portions of the duodenum. In patients with the multiple endocrine neoplasia syndrome (MEN-1), the insulinomas may also be multiple.[43] In fact, these tumors often arise in the wall of the duodenum or in extra pancreatic tissues and adjacent lymph nodes (**Fig. 54–26**). Malignant islet cell tumors frequently involve local lymph nodes in the pancreatic, portal, and celiac beds. Liver metastases are also frequent and may be widespread and very small, exhibiting either a decreased or increased echogenecity. Glucagonomas and somatostatinomas are frequently somewhat larger than the other functional islet cell tumors and are frequently located more distally in the pancreas, are usually solitary and are also most often malignant. The so-called nonfunctional islet cell tumors (those that do not produce clinical symptomatology) often present as very large pancreatic masses, which usually exhibit locally benign behavior even when malignant and metastatic. Therefore, these tumors are usually well margined with passive displacement of surrounding vessels and infrequent vascular or neural invasion (**Fig. 54–27**).

IOUS imaging is seldom required for detection of ductal adenocarcinoma of the pancreas, because this lesion is usually readily palpable, although identification of tumor by palpation can be difficult when there is extensive surrounding pancreatitis, and in this setting IOUS imaging may be of help. Intraoperative and especially laparoscopic ultrasound imaging can be useful to assess for signs of unresectability in small pancreatic adenocarcinomas. Preoperative imaging studies, especially high-quality contrast-enhanced spiral CT arteriography can be very accurate in predicting unresectability, but these techniques are still evolving and are not yet widely available. In many settings, laparoscopy is performed before open laparotomy and resection,[44] in order to visu-

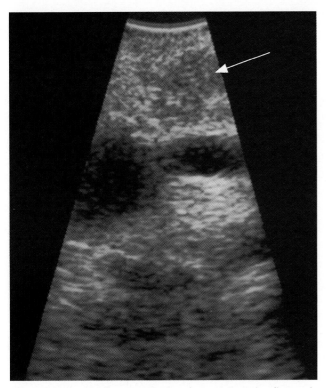

Figure 54–25 Insulinoma. US scan shows 1.2-cm insulinoma in neck of pancreas (**arrow**), just anterior to splenic-portal vein confluence.

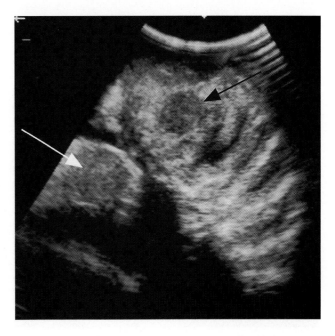

Figure 54–26 Gastrinoma. US scan shows 0.7-cm gastrinoma arising in wall of duodenum (**black arrow**), with adjacent 1.2-cm metastasis (**white arrow**) in lymph node.

ally assess for metastatic disease in the mesentery and peritoneal surfaces as well as on the surface of the liver. LUS can be utilized in conjunction with this approach to assess local resectability of pancreatic tumors (**Fig. 54–28**) by assessing the integrity of the pancreatic vasculature, particularly the superior mesenteric vein, splenic vein, as well as the SMA and celiac artery. Direct vascular invasion of the SMV/portal vein confluence or the celiac artery or SMA would render the patient inoperable. As with other type tumors, assessment of metastatic disease to local lymph nodes and to the liver can also be performed. A combination of the visual laparoscopic and LUS techniques can help to minimize the number of patients subjected to open laparotomy, only to prove ultimately unresectable.[45]

IOUS can also be used in assessing cystic neoplasms of the pancreas. Serous microcystic adenomas of the pancreas, which are almost always benign, can be well assessed by IOUS imaging (**Fig. 54–29**). The cyst cavities should be thin walled, as well as the septations, and most of the cysts are under 1—2 cm in size, many as small a few millimeters in diameter. Conversely, the presence of thick irregular septi, mural nodules, or solid components are most consistent with a mucinous cystadenoma or cystadenocarcinoma (**Fig. 54–30**) both of which require surgical resection because malignancy cannot be excluded by imaging criteria, and even the benign cystadenoma is considered premalignant.

Occasionally, IOUS imaging can be useful in patients with pancreatitis who are undergoing surgery for biliary

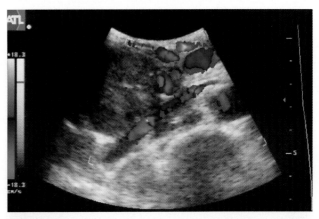

Figure 54–27 Nonfunctioning pancreatic islet cell tumor. Color flow Doppler imaging demonstrates passive displacement of pancreatic vasculature around the large 5-cm hypoechoic mass, without evidence of vascular invasion. These tumors tend to be locally non aggressive, even when malignant.

bypass or pancreatic drainage procedures (**Fig. 54–31**). The extent of pseudocysts and pancreatic ductal abnormalities can be well demonstrated as well as the potential communications between the pancreatic duct and the pseudocyst cavities.[46] If the pancreatic duct is obstructed, drainage of the pseudocysts may prove inadequate and drainage of the pancreatic duct itself may be required for adequate therapy. The use of color flow imaging and power Doppler can be important in evaluating focal peripancreatic fluid collections in order to assess

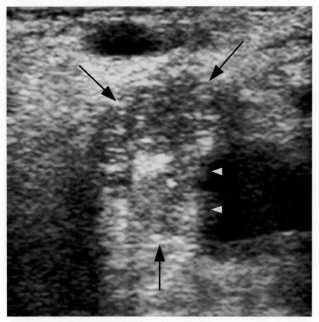

Figure 54–28 Pancreatic ductal adenocarcinoma. US scan shows mass (**black arrows**), which has invaded the lateral wall of superior mesenteric vein (**arrowheads**). This invasion makes the tumor unresectable.

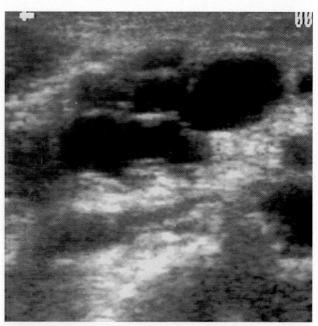

Figure 54–29 Microcystic pancreatic adenoma. US scan shows multiple thin-walled cysts, all well under 2 cm in size, with no septal thickening or nodularity.

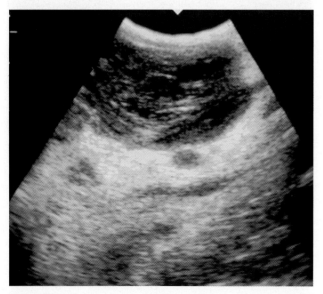

Figure 54–30 Mucinous cystadenocarcinoma of pancreas. US scan shows large 3-cm cystic mass with thickened irregular septations and adjacent small solid nodule.

for possible pseudoaneurysms. IOUS guidance can also be employed for biopsy of pancreatic masses, drainage of fluid collections, and diagnostic punctures of the pancreatic duct.

Conclusion

Intraoperative ultrasound is an important and rapidly expanding field. The demand from surgeons for access to this highly effective modality is growing continuously. The rapidly developing capacity of laparoscopic surgery is adding further to increased demand for ultrasound imaging via laparoscopic approaches.

The techniques and applications presented in this chapter will hopefully increase the interest of radiologists in performing and interpreting IOUS and LUS studies, as well as assist them in a more efficient use of their time when performing these studies. Intraoperative ultrasound studies have a profound impact on patient care and strongly influence surgical decision making. The necessity for high-quality IOUS scans is unquestionable, and in my opinion, the best quality scans will be obtained when the radiologist scrubs in and both performs and interprets the study using the scanning skills and observational ability that can only be acquired by years of experience with ultrasound imaging studies.

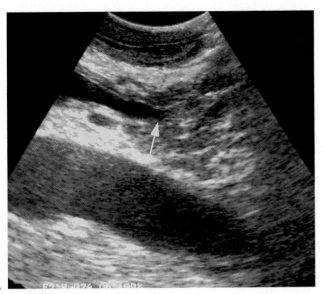
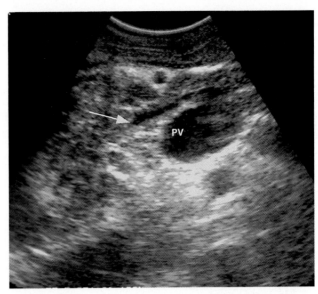

Figure 54–31 Calcific pancreatitis. **A:** Sagittal US scan demonstrates stricture of common bile duct (**arrow**) at entrance of enlarged head of pancreas. **B:** Transverse US scan shows obstruction of pancreatic duct (**arrow**). Pancreatitis rather than neoplasm was suggested by the lack of a hypoechoic mass and by diffuse enlargement with calcification. This diagnosis was confirmed by multiple biopsies. A biliary bypass was performed, and pancreatic resection was avoided. PV, portal vein.

References

1. Kane RA, Hughes LA, Cua EJ, et al. The impact of intraoperative ultrasonography on surgery for liver neoplasms. *J Ultrasound Med* 1994;13:1—6.

2. Knake JE, Chandler WF, McGillicuddy JE, et al. Intraoperative sonography for brain tumor localization and ventricular shunt placement. *AJR* 1982;139:733—738.

3. Enzmann DR, Wheat R, Marshall WH, et al. Tumors of the central nervous system studied by computed tomography and ultrasound. *Radiology* 1985;154:393—399.

4. Rubin JM, Dohrmann GJ. Intraoperative neurosurgical ultrasound in the localization and characterization of intracranial masses. *Radiology* 1983;148:519—524.

5. Latchaw RE, Gold LHA, Moore JS Jr, et al. The nonspecificity of absorption coefficients in the differentiation of solid tumors and cystic lesions. *Radiology* 1977;125:141—144.

6. Kjos BO, Brant-Zawadzki M, Kucharczyk W, et al. Cystic intracranial lesions: magnetic resonance imaging. *Radiology* 1985;155:363—369.

7. Lange SC, Howe JF, Shuman WP, et al. Intraoperative ultrasound detection of metastatic tumors in the central cortex. *Neurosurgery* 1982;11:219—222.

8. Knake JE, Chandler WJ, Gabrielson TO, et al. Intraoperative sonographic delineation of low-grade brain neoplasms defined poorly by computed tomography. *Radiology* 1984;151:735—739.

9. Hatfield MK, Rubin JM, Gebarski SS, et al. Intraoperative sonography in low-grade gliomas. *J Ultrasound Med* 1989;8:131—134.

10. Smith SJ, Vogelzang RL, Marzano MI, et al. Brain edema: ultrasound examination. *Radiology* 1985;155:379—382.

11. Tsutsumi Y, Andoh Y, Inoue N. Ultrasound-guided biopsy for deep-seated brain tumors. *J Neurosurg* 1982;57:164—167.

12. Berger MS. Ultrasound guided stereotactic biopsy using the Diasonics neuro-biopsy device for deep-seated intracranial lesions. Presented at the Annual Meeting of the American Association of Neurological Surgeons, Atlanta, GA, April 11—15, 1985.

13. Sutcliffe JC, Battersby RD. Intraoperative ultrasound-guided biopsy of intracranial lesions: comparison with freehand biopsy. *Br J Neurosurg* 1991;5:163—168.

14. Shanley DJ, Eline MJ. Intracerebral hematoma localization and removal using intraoperative ultrasound. *Milit Med* 1992;157:622—624.

15. Black KL, Rubin JM, Chandler WF, et al. Intraoperative color flow Doppler imaging of AVM's and aneurysm. *J Neurosurg* 1988;68:635–639.

16. Rubin JM, Dohrmann GJ. Intraoperative ultrasonography of the spine. *Radiology* 1983;146:173—175.

17. Platt JF, Rubin JM, Chandler WF, et al. Intraoperative spinal sonography in the evaluation of intramedullary tumors. *J Ultrasound Med* 1988;7:317—325.

18. Quencer RM, Montalvo BM, Green BA, et al. Intraoperative spinal sonography of soft-tissue masses of the spinal cord and spinal canal. *AJR* 1984;143:1307—1315.

19. Post MJD, Quencer RM, Montalvo MB, et al. Spinal infection: evaluation with magnetic resonance imaging and intraoperative ultrasound. *Radiology* 1988;169:765—771.

20. Hutchins WW, Vogelzang RL, Neiman HL, et al. Differentiation of tumor from syringohydromyelia: intraoperative neurosonography of the spinal cord. *Radiology* 1984;151:171—174.

21. Quencer RM, Montalvo BM, Naidich TP, et al. Intraoperative sonography and spinal dysraphism and syringohydromyelia. *AJR* 1987;148:1005—1013.

22. Montalvo BM, Quencer RM, Brown MD, et al. Lumbar disk herniation and canal stenosis: value of intraoperative sonography in diagnosis and surgical management. *AJR* 1990;154:821—830.

23. Lunardi P, Acqui M, Ferrante L, Fortuna A. The role of intraoperative ultrasound imaging in the surgical removal of intramedullary cavernous angiomas. *Neurosurgery* 1994;34:520—523.

24. Herbst CA, Mittlestaedt CA, Staab EV, et al. Intraoperative ultrasonography evaluation of the gallbladder in morbidly obese patients. *Ann Surg* 1984;200:691—692.

25. Machi J, Sigel B, Zaren HA, Kurohiji T, Yamashita Y. Opera-

tive ultrasonography during hepatobiliary and pancreatic surgery. *World J Surg* 1993;17:640—645.

26. Sigel B, Coelho JCU, Nyhus LM, et al. Comparison of cholangiography and ultrasonography in the operative screening of the common bile duct. *World J Surg* 1982;6:440—444.

27. Sigel B, Machi J, Beitler JG, et al. Comparative accuracy of operative ultrasonography and cholangiography in detecting common duct calculi. *Surgery* 1983;94:715—720.

28. Yamashita Y, Kurohiji T, Hayashi J, et al. Intraoperative ultrasonography during laparoscopic cholecystectomy. *Surg Laparoscopy Endoscopy* 1993;3:167—171.

29. Stiegmann GV, McIntyre R, Yamamoto M, et al. Laparoscopy-guided intracorporeal ultrasound accurately delineates hepatobiliary anatomy. *Surg Endoscopy* 1993;7:325—330.

30. Kane RA. Intraoperative ultrasound. In: Wilson SR, Charboneau JW, Leopold GR, eds. *Ultrasound: A Categorical Course Syllabus*. San Francisco, CA: American Roentgen Ray Society, 1993;241—250.

31. Clarke MP, Kane RA,. Steele DG, et al. Prospective comparison of preoperative imaging and intraoperative ultrasonography in the detection of liver tumors. *Surgery* 1989;106:849—855.

32. Kane RA, Longmaid HE, Costello P, Finn JP, Roizental M. Noninvasive imaging in patients with hepatic masses: a prospective comparison of ultrasound, CT and MR imaging (abstr). *AJR* 1993;160(suppl): 133.

33. Soyer P, Levesque M, Elias D, Zeitoun G, Roche A. Detection of liver metastases from colorectal cancer: comparison of intraoperative US and CT during arterial portography. *Radiology* 1992;1983:541—544.

34. Matsui O, Takahashi S, Kadoya M, et al. Pseudolesion in segment IV of the liver at CT during arterial portography: correlation with aberrant gastric venous drainage. *Radiology* 1994;193:31—35.

35. Nelson RC, Thompson GH, Chezmar JL, Harned RK, Fernandez MP. CT during arterial portography; diagnostic pitfalls. *RadioGraphics* 1992;12:705—718.

36. Kane RA, Roizental M, Kruskal JB, et al. Preliminary investigation of liver and biliary imaging with a dedicated laparoscopic US system (abstr). *Radiology* 1994;193(P):287.

37. John TG, Greig JD, Crosbie JL, Miles WF, Garden OJ. Superior staging of liver tumors with laparoscopy and laparoscopic ultrasound (comments). *Ann Surg* 1994;220:709—711.

38. Kruskal JB, Kane RA. Intraoperative ultrasonography of the liver. *Crit Rev Diagn Imaging* 1995;36:175—226.

39. Kruskal JB, Kane RA. Correlative imaging of malignant liver tumors. *Semin Ultrasound CT MR* 1992;13:336—354.

40. Gorman B, Charboneau JW, James EM, et al. Benign pancreatic insulinoma: preoperative sonographic localization. *AJR* 1986;147:929—934.

41. Charboneau JW, Gorman B, Reading CC, et al. Intraoperative ultrasonography of pancreatic endocrine tumors. In: Rifkin MD, ed. *Intraoperative and Endoscopic Ultrasonography*. New York, NY: Churchill Livingstone, 1987;123—134.

42. Sugg SL, Norton JA, Fraker DL, et al. A prospective study of intraoperative methods to diagnose and resect duodenal gastrinomas. *Ann Surg* 1993;218:138—144.

43. Akerstrom G, Johansson H, Grama D. Surgical treatment of endocrine pancreatic lesions in MEN-1 (review). *Acta Oncol* 1991;30:541—545.

44. John TG, Greig JD, Carter DC, Garden OJ. Carcinoma of the pancreatic head and periampullary region: tumor staging with laparoscopy and laparoscopic ultrasonography. *Ann Surg* 1995;221:156—164.

45. Hann LE, Conlon KC, Bach AM, Doughtery EC, Brennan MF. Laparoscopic gray-scale spectral Doppler ultrasound: applications in management of pancreatic carcinoma (abstr). *J Ultrasound Med* 1996;15:63.

46. Sigel B, Machi J, Ramos JR, et al. The role of ultrasound imaging during pancreatic surgery. *Ann Surg* 1984;200:486—493.

Index

Note: Page numbers in italics indicate figures or tables